Withdrawn from stock

UCC Library

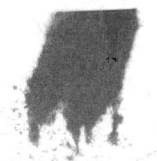

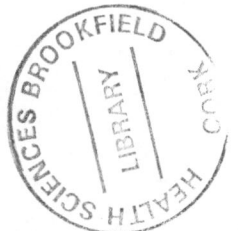

HS 618

KU-733-256

Pediatric Clinical Practice Guidelines & Policies

•••

A Compendium of Evidence-based Research for Pediatric Practice

Fourth Edition

American Academy of Pediatrics
141 Northwest Point Blvd
Elk Grove Village, IL 60007

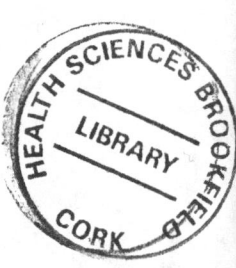

Fourth Edition—2004
Third Edition—2003
Second Edition—2002
First Edition—2001

Library of Congress Control Number: 2003112919

ISBN: 1-58110-132-5

MA0270

The recommendations in this publication do not indicate an exclusive course of treatment or serve as a standard of medical care. Variations, taking into account individual circumstances, may be appropriate.

Copyright © 2004 by the American Academy of Pediatrics. All rights reserved. No part of this publication may be reproduced, stored in a retrieval system, or transmitted, in any form or by any means, electronic, mechanical, photocopying, recording, or otherwise, without prior written permission from the publisher. Printed in the United States of America.

INTRODUCTION TO
PEDIATRIC CLINICAL PRACTICE GUIDELINES & POLICIES: A COMPENDIUM OF EVIDENCE-BASED RESEARCH FOR PEDIATRIC PRACTICE

Clinical practice guidelines have long provided physicians with a scientific-based decision-making tool for managing common pediatric conditions. Policy statements issued and endorsed by the American Academy of Pediatrics (AAP) are developed to provide physicians with a quick reference guide to the Academy's position on child health care issues. We have combined these 2 authoritative resources into one comprehensive manual/CD-ROM resource to provide easy access to important clinical and policy information.

This manual contains
- Clinical practice guidelines
- Technical report summaries
- Policy statements issued through December 2003, including abstracts where applicable

The CD-ROM, which is located on the inside back cover of this manual, builds on the content of the book and includes
- Clinical practice guidelines
- Technical reports
- Full text of the policy statements listed in this manual

We welcome your feedback on *Pediatric Clinical Practice Guidelines & Policies: A Compendium of Evidence-based Research for Pediatric Practice,* 4th edition.

Additional information regarding AAP policy can be found in a variety of professional publications such as
Guidelines for Perinatal Care, 5th Edition
Pediatric Environmental Health, 2nd Edition
Pediatric Nutrition Handbook, 5th Edition
Red Book®, 26th Edition

Parenting information consistent with AAP policy is available in a variety of consumer publications such as
ADHD: A Complete and Authoritative Guide
Caring for Your Baby and Young Child: Birth to Age 5
Caring for Your School-Age Child: Ages 5 to 12
Caring for Your Teenager
Guide to Toilet Training
New Mother's Guide to Breastfeeding

For more information on these titles and similar products, or for ordering information, please call 888/227-1770 or visit our online bookstore at www.aap.org/bookstore.

VISION STATEMENT OF THE AMERICAN ACADEMY OF PEDIATRICS

Core Values

We believe in the inherent worth of all children. They are our most enduring and vulnerable legacy. Children deserve optimum health and require the highest quality health care. Pediatricians (primary care pediatricians, pediatric medical subspecialists, and pediatric surgical specialists) are the best qualified of all health professionals to provide child health care. A dynamic organization is necessary to advance these values. The American Academy of Pediatrics is that organization.

Vision

The American Academy of Pediatrics exists to prepare its members with the tools, skills, and knowledge to be the best qualified health professionals: 1) to advocate for infants, children, adolescents, and young adults and provide for their care; 2) to collaborate with others to ensure child health; and 3) to ensure that decision-making affecting the health and well-being of children and their families is based upon the needs of those children and families. The American Academy of Pediatrics also exists to support members' professional satisfaction and personal growth. By providing these services, the American Academy of Pediatrics will be the most valuable professional organization to which those eligible for membership can belong.

Mission

The mission of the American Academy of Pediatrics is to attain optimal physical, mental, and social health and well-being for all infants, children, adolescents, and young adults. To this purpose, the Academy and its members dedicate their efforts and resources. The American Academy of Pediatrics will accomplish this mission by addressing the needs of children, their families, and their communities, and by supporting Academy members through advocacy, education, research, service, and improving the systems through which they deliver pediatric care.

Table of Contents

POLICY STATEMENTS BY COMMITTEE

Clinical Practice Guidelines

FOREWORD

In response to the growing trend toward the practice of evidence-based medicine, the American Academy of Pediatrics (AAP) Committee on Quality Improvement developed an organizational process and methodology for developing clinical practice guidelines. These guidelines provide physicians with a scientific-based decision-making tool for managing common pediatric conditions.

The evidence-based approach to developing clinical practice guidelines requires carefully defining the problem and identifying interventions and health outcomes. An extensive literature review and data analysis provide the basis for guideline recommendations. The practice guidelines also are subjected to a thorough peer-review process prior to publication and subsequent dissemination, implementation, and evaluation. Clinical practice guidelines are periodically reviewed to ensure that they are based on the most current data available.

American Academy of Pediatrics guidelines are designed to provide physicians with an analytic framework for evaluating and treating common childhood conditions and are not intended as an exclusive course of treatment or as standards of care. When using AAP practice guidelines, clinicians should continue to consider other sources of information as well as variations in individual circumstances. The AAP recognizes the incompleteness of data and acknowledges the use of expert consensus in cases where data do not exist. Thus, AAP practice guidelines allow for flexibility and adaptability at the local level and should not replace sound clinical judgment.

This text contains practice guidelines and technical report summaries developed and published by the AAP. Full technical reports are available on the CD-ROM included with this book. The full technical reports contain summaries of the data reviewed, results of data analyses, complete evidence tables, and bibliographies of articles included in the review. This collection of AAP policy also includes evidence-based practice guidelines from other organizations that the AAP has endorsed. Practice guidelines will continually be added to the compendium as they are released or updated. We encourage you to look forward to these future guidelines.

If you have any questions about current or future practice guidelines, please contact the AAP Department of Practice and Research at 800/433-9016, ext 7917. To order copies of the patient education brochures that accompany each guideline, please call the AAP at 888/227-1770.

Charles J. Homer, MD
Chairperson, Steering Committee on Quality Improvement and Management

Practical Guide for the Diagnosis and Management of Asthma

• •

*The following guideline for diagnosis and management of asthma,
developed by the National Heart, Lung, and Blood Institute,
has been endorsed by the American Academy of Pediatrics.*

Additional resource for asthma management:

Guide for Managing Asthma in Children

*This guide is intended to help pediatricians, primary care physicians, and other clinicians/
health care professionals diagnose and manage patients with allergic diseases. It was
developed by a Pediatric Asthma Committee, a multidisciplinary and multi-organizational
group of US asthma and health care experts. An AAP representative served on this committee.
This guide can be downloaded from the American Academy of Allergy, Asthma, and Immunology
(AAAAI) Web site at www.aaaai.org/media/pressreleases/1999/10/991022.html or by mail for
a fee by calling 414/272-6071.*

PRACTICAL GUIDE FOR THE DIAGNOSIS AND MANAGEMENT OF ASTHMA

Based on the *Expert Panel Report 2:*

Guidelines for the Diagnosis and Management of Asthma

Second Expert Panel on the Management of Asthma

*Shirley Murphy, M.D., *Chair*
University of New Mexico

Eugene R. Bleecker, M.D.
University of Maryland

*Homer Boushey, M.D.
University of California at San Francisco

*A. Sonia Buist, M.D.
Oregon Health Sciences University

*William Busse, M.D.
University of Wisconsin

Noreen M. Clark, Ph.D.
University of Michigan

Howard Eigen, M.D.
Riley Hospital for Children

Jean G. Ford, M.D.
Columbia University

*Susan Janson, D.N.Sc., R.N.
University of California, San Francisco

*H. William Kelly, Pharm.D.
University of New Mexico

Robert F. Lemanske, Jr., M.D.
University of Wisconsin

Carolyn C. Lopez, M.D.
Rush Medical College

Fernando Martinez, M.D.
University of Arizona

*Harold S. Nelson, M.D.
National Jewish Medical and Research Center

Richard Nowak, M.D., M.B.A.
Henry Ford Hospital

Thomas A.E. Platts-Mills, M.D., Ph.D.
University of Virginia

Gail G. Shapiro, M.D.
University of Washington

Stuart Stoloff, M.D.
Private Family Practice and University of Nevada

Kevin Weiss, M.D., M.P.H.
Rush Primary Care Institute

Federal Liaison Representatives
Clive Brown, M.B.B.S., M.P.H.
Centers for Disease Control and Prevention

Peter J. Gergen, M.D.
(formerly with the National Institute of Allergy and
    Infectious Diseases)
Agency for Health Care Policy and Research

Edward L. Petsonk, M.D.
National Institute for Occupational Safety and Health

National Heart, Lung, and Blood Institute Staff
Ted Buxton, M.P.H.
Robinson Fulwood, M.S.P.H.
Michele Hindi-Alexander, Ph.D.
Suzanne S. Hurd, Ph.D.
Virginia S. Taggart, M.P.H.

R.O.W. Sciences, Inc., Support Staff
Ruth Clark
Daria Donaldson
Lisa Marcellino
Donna Selig
Keith Stanger
Eileen Zeller, M.P.H.

* Executive Committee Member

National Asthma Education and Prevention Program
Coordinating Committee Organizations

Allergy and Asthma Network/Mothers of Asthmatics, Inc.

American Academy of Allergy, Asthma, and Immunology

American Academy of Family Physicians

American Academy of Pediatrics

American Academy of Physician Assistants

American Association for Respiratory Care

American Association of Occupational Health Nurses

American College of Allergy, Asthma, and Immunology

American College of Chest Physicians

American College of Emergency Physicians

American Lung Association

American Medical Association

American Nurses Association, Inc.

American Pharmaceutical Association

American Public Health Association

American School Health Association

American Society of Health-System Pharmacists

American Thoracic Society

Association of State and Territorial Directors of Health Promotion and Public Health Education

Asthma and Allergy Foundation of America

Centers for Disease Control and Prevention

National Association of School Nurses

National Black Nurses Association, Inc.

National Center for Environmental Health

National Center for Health Statistics

NHLBI Ad Hoc Committee on Minority Populations

National Heart, Lung, and Blood Institute

National Institute for Occupational Safety and Health

National Institute of Allergy and Infectious Diseases

National Institute of Environmental Health Sciences

National Medical Association

Society for Public Health Education

U.S. Environmental Protection Agency

U.S. Food and Drug Administration

U.S. Public Health Service

INTRODUCTION

PRACTICAL AND EFFECTIVE ASTHMA CARE

This *Practical Guide for the Diagnosis and Management of Asthma* describes how primary care clinicians can improve the asthma care they provide within the time constraints of their current clinical practice. More than 130 primary care professionals reviewed this guide to help assure that it is relevant and practical for primary care practitioners.

The recommendations in the Practical Guide are summarized from the National Asthma Education and Prevention Program, *Expert Panel Report 2: Guidelines for the Diagnosis and Management of Asthma* (EPR-2).[1] See page 13 for a summary of some major recommendations from EPR-2.

ASTHMA CARE IN THE UNITED STATES CAN BE IMPROVED

Undertreatment and inappropriate therapy are major contributors to asthma morbidity and mortality in the United States. A few examples of data that support this assertion are presented below.

- Hospitalizations due to asthma are preventable or avoidable when patients receive appropriate primary care.[2]
  - Asthma is the third leading cause of preventable hospitalizations in the United States.[2]
  - There are about 470,000 hospitalizations and more than 5,000 deaths a year from asthma.
- Studies from two metropolitan areas of children with asthma who used the emergency department[3] and adults hospitalized with asthma[4] found that:
  - Less than half of these patients were receiving anti-inflammatory therapy as recommended in the EPR-2.[1]
  - Only 28 percent of the adult patients hospitalized for asthma had written action plans that told how to manage their asthma and control an exacerbation.[4]

The Practical Guide will help clinicians improve the asthma care they provide and reduce the hospitalizations and emergency department visits needed by their patients.

AIRWAY INFLAMMATION PLAYS A CENTRAL ROLE IN ASTHMA AND ITS MANAGEMENT

The management of asthma needs to be responsive to the characteristics that define asthma. The relationships between these characteristics are illustrated in figure 1.

- **Asthma is a chronic inflammatory disorder of the airways.** Many cells and cellular elements play a role, in particular, mast cells, eosinophils, T-lymphocytes, macrophages, neutrophils, and epithelial cells.

- **Environmental and other factors "cause" or provoke the airway inflammation in people with asthma.** Examples of these factors include inhaled allergens to which the patient is sensitive, some irritants, and viruses. This inflammation is always present to some degree, regardless of the level of asthma severity.

- **Airway inflammation causes recurrent episodes** in asthma patients of wheezing, breathlessness, chest tightness, and coughing, particularly at night and in the early morning.

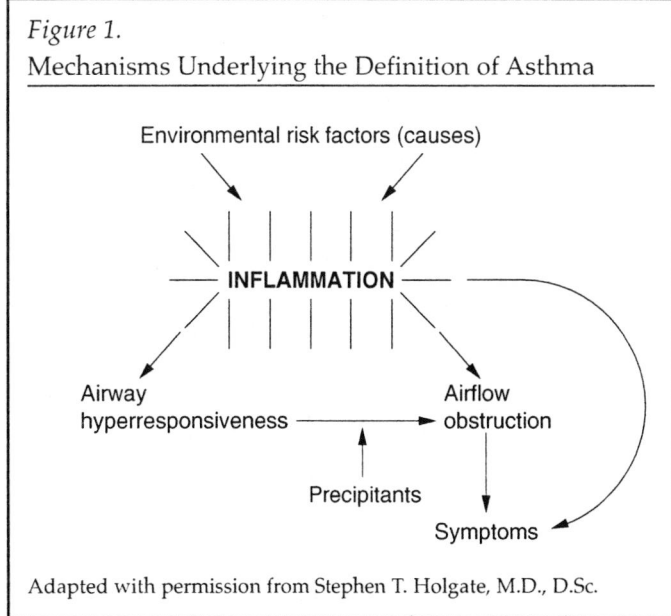

Figure 1.

Mechanisms Underlying the Definition of Asthma

Adapted with permission from Stephen T. Holgate, M.D., D.Sc.

- These episodes of asthma symptoms are usually associated with wide-spread but **variable airflow obstruction that is often reversible** either spontaneously or with treatment. Airflow obstruction is caused by a variety of changes in the airway, including bronchoconstriction, airway edema, chronic mucus plug formation, and airway remodeling.

- **Inflammation causes an associated increase in the existing airway hyperresponsiveness** to a variety of stimuli, such as allergens, irritants, cold air, and viruses. These stimuli or **precipitants result in airflow obstruction** and asthma symptoms in the patient with asthma.

ASTHMA CHANGES OVER TIME, REQUIRING ACTIVE MANAGEMENT

The condition of a patient's asthma will change depending on the environment, patient activities, management practices, and other factors (see figure 2). Thus, even when patients have their asthma under control, monitoring and treatment are needed to maintain control.

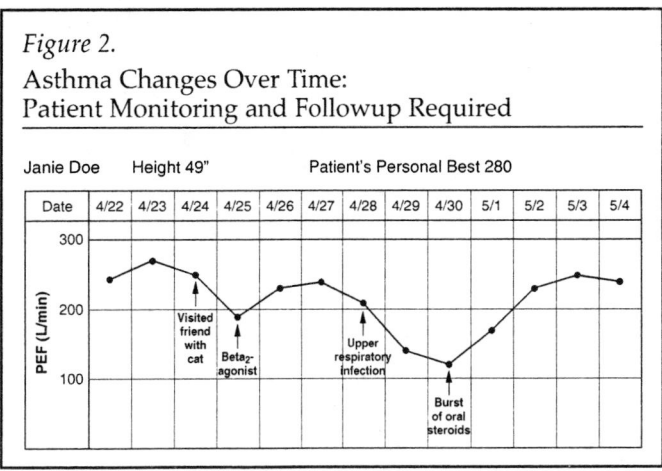

Figure 2.

Asthma Changes Over Time:
Patient Monitoring and Followup Required

FOUR KEY COMPONENTS FOR
LONG-TERM CONTROL OF ASTHMA

The four components of asthma therapy respond to the basic nature of asthma described previously. The four components are listed below and will be described in this guide.

Assessment and monitoring

Pharmacologic therapy

Control of factors contributing to asthma severity

Patient education for a partnership

REFERENCES

In EPR-2, the Expert Panel cites the scientific literature to support its recommendations or clearly indicates they are "based on the opinion of the Expert Panel." The Panel submitted multiple drafts of EPR-2 for review by more than 140 outside reviewers, including members of the NAEPP Coordinating Committee. This Practical Guide summarizes the recommendations in EPR-2, provides practical information to aid the implementation of those recommendations, and cites selected references from EPR-2. For complete documentation of the recommendations, refer to EPR-2. Copies of the full report can be accessed through the Internet (http://www.nhlbi.nih.gov/nhlbi/lung/asthma/prof/asthgdln.htm) or purchased from the NHLBI Information Center, P.O. Box 30105, Bethesda, MD 20824-0105 (phone 301-251-1222; fax 301-251-1223).

This guide presents basic recommendations for the diagnosis and management of asthma that will help clinicians and patients make appropriate decisions about asthma care. Of course, the clinician and patient need to develop an individual treatment plan that is tailored to the specific needs of the patient. This report is not an official regulatory document of any Government agency.

Major Recommendations From the *Expert Panel Report 2: Guidelines for the Diagnosis and Management of Asthma*[1]

Diagnose asthma and initiate partnership with patient.

- **Diagnose** asthma by establishing:
  - A history of recurrent symptoms,
  - Reversible airflow obstruction using spirometry, and
  - The exclusion of alternative diagnoses.
- **Establish patient-clinician partnership.**
  - Address patient's concerns.
  - Agree upon the goals of asthma therapy.
  - Agree upon a written action plan for patient self-management.

Reduce inflammation, symptoms, and exacerbations.

- **Prescribe anti-inflammatory medications to patients with mild, moderate, or severe persistent asthma** (i.e., inhaled steroids, cromolyn, or nedocromil).
- **Reduce exposures to precipitants of asthma symptoms.**
  - Assess patient's exposure and sensitivity to individual precipitants (e.g., allergens, irritants).
  - Provide written and verbal instructions on how to avoid or reduce factors that make the patient's asthma worse.

Monitor and manage asthma over time.

- **Train all patients to monitor their asthma.**
  - All patients should monitor symptoms.
  - Patients with moderate-to-severe persistent asthma should also monitor their peak flow.
- **See patients at least every 1 to 6 months**
  - Assess attainment of goals of asthma therapy and patient's concerns,
  - Adjust treatment, if needed,
  - Review the action plan with patient, and
  - Check patient's inhaler and peak flow technique.

Treat asthma episodes promptly.

- Prompt use of short-acting inhaled beta$_2$-agonists and, if episode is moderate to severe, a 3- to 10-day course of oral steroids.
- Prompt communication and followup with clinician.

1. INITIAL ASSESSMENT AND DIAGNOSIS OF ASTHMA

Diagnosis of Asthma in Adults and Children Over 5 Years of Age

Recurrent episodes of coughing or wheezing are almost always due to asthma in both children and adults. Cough can be the sole symptom.

Findings that increase the probability of asthma include:

Medical history:

- Episodic wheeze, chest tightness, shortness of breath, or cough.
- Symptoms worsen in presence of aeroallergens, irritants, or exercise.
- Symptoms occur or worsen at night, awakening the patient.
- Patient has allergic rhinitis or atopic dermatitis.
- Close relatives have asthma, allergy, sinusitis, or rhinitis.

Physical examination of the upper respiratory tract, chest, and skin:

- Hyperexpansion of the thorax
- Sounds of wheezing during normal breathing or a prolonged phase of forced exhalation
- Increased nasal secretions, mucosal swelling, sinusitis, rhinitis, or nasal polyps
- Atopic dermatitis/eczema or other signs of allergic skin problems

Diagnosis in Infants and Children Younger Than 5 Years of Age

Because children with asthma are often mislabeled as having bronchiolitis, bronchitis, or pneumonia, many do not receive adequate therapy.

- The diagnostic steps listed previously are the same for this age group except that spirometry is not possible. A trial of asthma medications may aid in the eventual diagnosis.
- **Diagnosis is not needed to *begin* to treat wheezing associated with an upper respiratory viral infection, which is the most common precipitant of wheezing in this age group.** Patients should be monitored carefully.
- There are two general patterns of illness in infants and children who have wheezing with acute viral upper respiratory infections: a remission of symptoms in the preschool years and persistence of asthma throughout childhood. The factors associated with continuing asthma are allergies, a family history of asthma, and perinatal exposure to aeroallergens and passive smoke.

Patient Education After Diagnosis

Identify the concerns the patient has about being diagnosed with asthma by asking: "What worries you most about having asthma? What concerns do you have about your asthma?"

Address the patient's concerns and make at least these key points (see patient handout, "What Everyone Should Know About Asthma Control"):

- **Asthma can be managed and the patient can live a normal life.**

▶ Assessment and monitoring

Pharmacologic therapy

Control of factors contributing to asthma severity

▶ Patient education for a partnership

To establish an asthma diagnosis, determine the following:

1. **History or presence of episodic symptoms of airflow obstruction** (i.e., wheeze, shortness of breath, tightness in the chest, or cough). Asthma symptoms vary throughout the day; absence of symptoms at the time of the examination does not exclude the diagnosis of asthma.

2. **Airflow obstruction is at least partially reversible.** Use spirometry to:
   Establish airflow obstruction: FEV_1 <80 percent predicted; FEV_1/FVC^* <65 percent or below the lower limit of normal. (If obstruction is absent, see Additional Tests, page 16.)
   Establish reversibility: FEV_1 increases ≥12 percent and at least 200 mL after using a short-acting inhaled beta$_2$-agonist (e.g., albuterol, terbutaline).
   NOTE: Older adults may need to take oral steroids for 2 to 3 weeks and then take the spirometry test to measure the degree of reversibility achieved. Chronic bronchitis and emphysema may coexist with asthma in adults. The degree of reversibility indicates the degree to which asthma therapy may be beneficial.

3. **Alternative diagnoses are excluded** (e.g., vocal cord dysfunction, vascular rings, foreign bodies, or other pulmonary diseases). See page 16 for additional tests that may be needed.

In general, FEV_1 predicted norms or reference values used for children should also be used for adolescents.

---

*FEV_1, forced expiratory volume in 1 second
FVC, forced vital capacity

- **Asthma can be controlled when the patient works together with the medical staff.** The patient plays a big role in monitoring asthma, taking medications, and avoiding things that can cause asthma episodes.

- **Asthma is a chronic lung disease characterized by inflammation of the airways.** There may be periods when there are no symptoms, but the airways are swollen and sensitive to some degree all of the time. Long-term anti-inflammatory medications are important to control airway inflammation.

- **Many things in the home, school, work, or elsewhere can cause asthma attacks** (e.g., secondhand tobacco smoke, allergens, irritants). An asthma attack (also called episodes, flareups, or exacerbations) occurs when airways narrow, making it harder to breathe.

- **Asthma requires long-term care and monitoring.** Asthma cannot be cured, but it can be controlled. Asthma can get better or worse over time and requires treatment changes.

Patient education should begin at the time of diagnosis and continue at every visit.

Additional Tests for Adults and Children

Additional tests may be needed when asthma is suspected but spirometry is normal, when coexisting conditions are suspected, or for other reasons. These tests can aid diagnosis or confirm suspected contributors to asthma morbidity (e.g., allergens and irritants).

Reasons for Additional Tests	The Tests
• Patient has symptoms but spirometry is normal or near normal	• Assess diurnal variation of peak flow over 1 to 2 weeks. • Refer to a specialist for bronchoprovocation with methacholine, histamine, or exercise; negative test may help rule out asthma.
• Suspect infection, large airway lesions, heart disease, or obstruction by foreign object	• Chest x-ray
• Suspect coexisting chronic obstructive pulmonary disease, restrictive defect, or central airway obstruction	• Additional pulmonary function studies • Diffusing capacity test
• Suspect other factors contribute to asthma (These are not diagnostic tests for asthma.)	• Allergy tests—skin or in vitro • Nasal examination • Gastroesophageal reflux assessment

Assessment of Asthma Severity

See figure 3 to estimate the severity of chronic asthma in patients of all age groups. These levels of severity correspond to the "steps" of pharmacologic therapy discussed later.

General Guidelines for Referral to an Asthma Specialist

Based on the opinion of the Expert Panel, referral for consultation or care to a specialist in asthma care is recommended if assistance is needed for:

- **Diagnosis and assessment** (e.g., differential diagnosis is problematic, other conditions aggravate asthma, or confirmation is needed on the contribution of occupational or environmental exposures)

- **Specialized treatment and education** (e.g., considering patient for immunotherapy or providing additional education for allergen avoidance)

- **Other cases:**

  — Patient is not meeting the goals of asthma therapy (defined in next section) after 3 to 6 months. An earlier referral or consultation is appropriate if the physician concludes that the patient is unresponsive to therapy.

  — Life-threatening asthma exacerbation occurred.

  — Patient requires step 4 care (see figure 4 on page 17) or has used more than two bursts of oral steroids in 1 year. (Referral may be considered for patients requiring step 3 care.)

  — Patient is younger than age 3 and requires step 3 or 4 care. Referral should be considered for patients under age 3 who require step 2 care (see figure 5 on page 18).

An asthma specialist is usually a fellowship-trained allergist or pulmonologist or, occasionally, a physician with expertise in asthma management developed through additional training and experience.

Patients with significant psychiatric, psychosocial, or family problems that interfere with their asthma therapy should be referred to an appropriate mental health professional for counseling or treatment.

Figure 3.

Classification of Asthma Severity: Clinical Features Before Treatment

	Days With Symptoms	Nights With Symptoms	PEF or FEV$_1$*	PEF Variablity
Step 4 Severe Persistent	Continual	Frequent	≤60%	>30%
Step 3 Moderate Persistent	Daily	≥5/month	>60%- <80%	>30%
Step 2 Mild Persistent	3-6/week	3-4/month	≥80%	20-30%
Step 1 Mild Intermittent	≤2/week	≤2/month	≥80%	<20%

* Percent predicted values for forced expiratory volume in 1 second (FEV$_1$) and percent of personal best for peak expiratory flow (PEF) (relevant for children 6 years old or older who can use these devices).

NOTES:
- Patients should be assigned to the most severe step in which *any* feature occurs. Clinical features for individual patients may overlap across steps.
- An individual's classification may change over time.
- Patients at any level of severity of chronic asthma can have mild, moderate, or severe exacerbations of asthma. Some patients with intermittent asthma experience severe and life-threatening exacerbations separated by long periods of normal lung function and no symptoms.
- Patients with two or more asthma exacerbations per week (i.e., progressively worsening symptoms that may last hours or days) tend to have moderate-to-severe persistent asthma.

Figure 4.

Stepwise Approach for Managing Asthma in Adults and Children Over 5 Years Old: Treatment

Long-Term Control

Preferred treatments are in bold print.

Step 4
Severe
Persistent

Daily medications:
- **Anti-inflammatory: inhaled steroid (high dose)*** AND
- Long-acting bronchodilator: either **long-acting inhaled beta$_2$-agonist** (adult: 2 puffs q 12 hours; child: 1–2 puffs q 12 hours), sustained-release theophylline, or long-acting beta$_2$-agonist tablets AND
- Steroid tablets or syrup long term; make repeated attempts to reduce systemic steroid and maintain control with high-dose inhaled steroid.

Step 3
Moderate
Persistent

Daily medication:
- Either
  —**Anti-inflammatory: inhaled steroid (medium dose)***
  OR
  —**Inhaled steroid (low-to-medium dose)*** and add a long-acting bronchodilator, especially for nighttime symptoms: either **long-acting inhaled beta$_2$-agonist** (adult: 2 puffs q 12 hours; child: 1-2 puffs q 12 hours), sustained-release theophylline, or long-acting beta$_2$-agonist tablets.
- If needed
  —Anti-inflammatory: **inhaled steroids (medium-to-high dose)***
  AND
  —Long-acting bronchodilator, especially for nighttime symptoms; either **long-acting inhaled beta$_2$-agonist**, sustained-release theophylline, or long-acting beta$_2$-agonist tablets.

Step 2
Mild
Persistent

Daily medication:
- **Anti-inflammatory: either inhaled steroid (low dose)*** or **cromolyn** (adult: 2–4 puffs tid-qid; child: 1–2 puffs tid-qid) or **nedocromil** (adult: 2–4 puffs bid-qid; child: 1–2 puffs bid-qid) (children usually begin with a trial of cromolyn or nedocromil).
- Sustained-release theophylline to serum concentration of 5–15 mcg/mL is an alternative, but not preferred, therapy. Zafirlukast or zileuton may also be considered for those ≥12 years old, although their position in therapy is not fully established.

Step 1
Mild
Intermittent

- No daily medication needed.

Quick-Relief

All Patients

Short-acting bronchodilator: **inhaled beta$_2$-agonist** (2–4 puffs) as needed for symptoms. Intensity of treatment will depend on severity of exacerbation.

*See Estimated Comparative Daily Dosages for Inhaled Steroids on page 41.

NOTES:
- *The stepwise approach presents general guidelines to assist clinical decisionmaking. Asthma is highly variable; clinicians should tailor medication plans to the needs of individual patients.*
- **Gain control** as quickly as possible. Either start with aggressive therapy (e.g., *add* a course of oral steroids or a higher dose of inhaled steroids to the therapy that corresponds to the patient's initial step of severity); or start at the step that corresponds to the patient's initial severity and step up treatment, if necessary.
- **Step down:** Review treatment every 1 to 6 months. Gradually decrease treatment to the least medication necessary to maintain control.
- **Step up:** If control is not maintained, consider step up. Inadequate control is indicated by increased use of short-acting beta$_2$-agonists and in: step 1 when patient uses a short-acting beta$_2$-agonist more than two times a week; steps 2 and 3 when patient uses short-acting beta$_2$-agonist on a daily basis or more than three to four times in 1 day. But before stepping up: Review patient inhaler technique, compliance, and environmental control (avoidance of allergens or other precipitant factors).
- A course of oral steroids may be needed at any time and at any step.
- Patients with exercise-induced bronchospasm should take two to four puffs of an inhaled beta$_2$-agonist 5 to 60 minutes before exercise.
- Referral to an asthma specialist for consultation or comanagement is *recommended* if there is difficulty maintaining control or if the patient requires step 4 care. Referral may be *considered* for step 3 care.
- For a list of brand names, see glossary.

Figure 5.

Stepwise Approach for Managing Infants and Young Children (5 Years of Age and Younger) With Acute or Chronic Asthma Symptoms

Long-Term Control

Step 4 **Severe** **Persistent**	• Daily anti-inflammatory medication — High-dose inhaled steroid* with spacer and face mask — If needed, add oral steroids (2 mg/kg/day); reduce to lowest daily or alternate-day dose that stabilizes symptoms
Step 3 **Moderate** **Persistent**	• Daily anti-inflammatory medication. Either: — Medium-dose inhaled steroid* with spacer and face mask Once control is established, consider: — Lower medium-dose inhaled steroid* with spacer and face mask and nedocromil (1–2 puffs bid-qid) OR — Lower medium-dose inhaled steroid* with spacer and face mask and theophylline (10 mg/kg/day up to 16 mg/kg/day for children ≥1 year of age, to a serum concentration of 5–15 mcg/mL)**
Step 2 **Mild** **Persistent**	• Daily anti-inflammatory medication. — Infants and young children usually begin with a trial of cromolyn (nebulizer is preferred—1 ampule tid-qid; or MDI—1–2 puffs tid-qid) or nedocromil (MDI only—1–2 puffs bid-qid) OR — Low-dose inhaled steroid* with spacer and face mask
Step 1 **Mild** **Intermittent**	• No daily medication needed.

Quick-Relief

All Patients	Bronchodilator as needed for symptoms: Short-acting inhaled beta$_2$-agonist by nebulizer (0.05 mg/kg in 2–3 cc of saline) or inhaler with face mask and spacer (2–4 puffs; for exacerbations, repeat q 20 minutes for up to 1 hour) or oral beta$_2$-agonist. **With viral respiratory infection,** use short-acting inhaled beta$_2$-agonist q 4 to 6 hours up to 24 hours (longer with physician consult) but, in general, if repeated more than once every 6 weeks, consider moving to next step up. Consider oral steroids if the exacerbation is moderate to severe or at the onset of the infection if the patient has a history of severe exacerbations.

* See Estimated Comparative Dosages for Inhaled Steroids on page 41
** For children <1 year of age: usual max mg/kg/day = 0.2 (age in weeks) + 5.

NOTES:
• *The stepwise approach presents general guidelines to assist clinical decisionmaking. Asthma is highly variable; clinicians should tailor medication plans to the needs of individual patients.*
• **Gain control** as quickly as possible. Either start with aggressive therapy (e.g., *add* a course of oral steroids or a higher dose of inhaled steroids to the therapy that corresponds to the patient's initial step of severity); or start at the step that corresponds to the patient's initial severity and step up treatment, if necessary.
• **Step down.** Review treatment every 1 to 6 months. If control is sustained for at least 3 months, a gradual stepwise reduction in treatment may be possible.
• **Step up.** If control is not achieved, consider step up. Inadequate control is indicated by increased use of short-acting beta$_2$-agonists and in: step 1 when patient uses a short-acting beta$_2$-agonist more than two times a week; steps 2 and 3 when patient uses short-acting beta$_2$-agonist on a daily basis OR more than three to four times a day. But before stepping up: review patient inhaler technique, compliance, and environmental control (avoidance of allergens or other precipitant factors).
• A course of oral steroids (prednisolone) may be needed at any time and step.
• Referral to an asthma specialist for consultation or comanagement is *recommended* for patients requiring step 3 or 4 care. Referral may be *considered* for step 2 care.
• For a list of brand names, see glossary.

2. PHARMACOLOGIC THERAPY: MANAGING ASTHMA LONG TERM

Establish the Goals of Asthma Therapy With the Patient

The goals of asthma therapy provide the criteria that the clinician and patient will use to evaluate the patient's response to therapy. The goals will provide the focus for all subsequent interactions with the patient.

First, determine the patient's personal goals of therapy by asking a few questions, such as: "What would you like to be able to do that you can't do now or can't do well because of your asthma?" "What would you like to accomplish with your asthma treatment?"

Then, share the general goals of asthma therapy with the patient and the family.

Finally, agree on the goals you and the patient will set as the foundation for the patient's treatment plan.

The Asthma Medications: Long-Term Control and Quick Relief

- **Long-term-control asthma medications are taken daily to achieve and maintain control of persistent asthma** (for dosage information, see pages 39–40). The most effective long-term-control medications for asthma are those that reduce inflammation. Inhaled steroids are the most potent inhaled anti-inflammatory medication currently available (see next page).

  Inhaled steroids are generally well tolerated and safe at recommended doses. To reduce the potential for adverse effects, **patients taking inhaled steroids should:**
  — Use a spacer/holding chamber.
  — Rinse and spit following inhalation.
  — Use the lowest possible dose to maintain control. Consider adding a long-acting inhaled beta$_2$-agonist to a low-to-medium dose of inhaled steroid rather than using a higher dose of inhaled steroid.[17,18]

- **Quick-relief medications are used to provide prompt treatment of acute airflow obstruction and its accompanying symptoms** such as cough, chest tightness, shortness of breath, and wheezing. These medications include short-acting inhaled beta$_2$-agonists and oral steroids. Anticholinergics are included in special circumstances.

STEPWISE APPROACH TO MANAGING ASTHMA IN ADULTS AND IN CHILDREN OVER 5 YEARS OF AGE

All patients need to have a short-acting inhaled beta$_2$-agonist to take as needed for symptoms. Patients with mild, moderate, or severe persistent asthma require daily long-term-control medication to control their asthma.

See figure 4 for the recommended pharmacologic therapy at each level of asthma severity and pages 39–40 for dosage information. Also, see the glossary for the brand names of the medications mentioned in this guide.

Gaining Control of Asthma

The physician's judgment of an individual patient's needs and circumstances will determine at what step to initiate therapy. There are two appropriate approaches to gaining control of asthma:

Assessment and monitoring
Pharmacologic therapy
Control of factors contributing to asthma severity
Patient education for a partnership

General Goals of Asthma Therapy

- **Prevent chronic asthma symptoms and asthma exacerbations during the day and night.** (Indicators: No sleep disruption by asthma. No missed school or work due to asthma. No or minimal need for emergency department visits or hospitalizations.)
- **Maintain normal activity levels**—including exercise and other physical activities.
- **Have normal or near-normal lung function.**
- **Be satisfied with the asthma care received.**
- **Have no or minimal side effects** while receiving optimal medications.

- Start treatment at the step appropriate to the severity of the patient's asthma at the time of evaluation. If control is not achieved, gradually step up therapy until control is achieved and maintained.

OR

- At the onset, give therapy at a higher level to achieve rapid control and then step down to the minimum therapy needed to maintain control. A higher level of therapy can be accomplished by either adding a course of oral steroids to inhaled steroids, cromolyn, or nedocromil or using a higher dose of inhaled steroids.
- In the opinion of the Expert Panel, the **preferred approach is to start with more intensive therapy** in order to more rapidly suppress airway inflammation and thus gain prompt control.

If control is not achieved with initial therapy (e.g., within 1 month), the step selected, the therapy in the step, and possibly the diagnosis should be reevaluated.

Maintaining Control

Increases or decreases in medications may be needed as asthma severity and control vary over time. The Expert Panel's opinion is that **followup visits every 1 to 6 months are essential for monitoring asthma.** In addition, patients should be instructed to monitor their symptoms (and peak flow if used) and adjust therapy as described in the action plan (see Patient Handouts).

Step Down Therapy

Gradually reduce or "step down" long-term-control medications after several weeks or months of controlling persistent asthma (i.e., the goals of asthma therapy are achieved). In general, the last medication added to the medical regimen should be the first medication reduced.

Inhaled steroids may be reduced about 25 percent every 2 to 3 months until the lowest dose required to maintain control is reached. For patients with persistent asthma, anti-inflammatory medications should be continued.

Inhaled Steroids: The Most Effective Long-Term-Control Medication for Asthma

The daily use of inhaled steroids results in the following:[5,6,10-16]

- Asthma symptoms will diminish. Improvement will continue gradually (see study 1).
- Occurrence of severe exacerbations is greatly reduced.
- Use of quick-relief medication decreases (see study 2).
- Lung function improves significantly, as measured by peak flow, FEV_1, and airway hyperresponsiveness.

Problems due to asthma may return if patients stop taking inhaled steroids.

Frequency of dosing

Once-daily dosing with inhaled steroids for patients with mild asthma and twice-a-day dosing for many other patients, even with high doses of some preparations, have been effective.[7-9]

Study 1.

Daily Inhaled Steroids Control Moderate Persistent Asthma in Children 7 to 16 Years Old: Reduced Symptomatic Days*

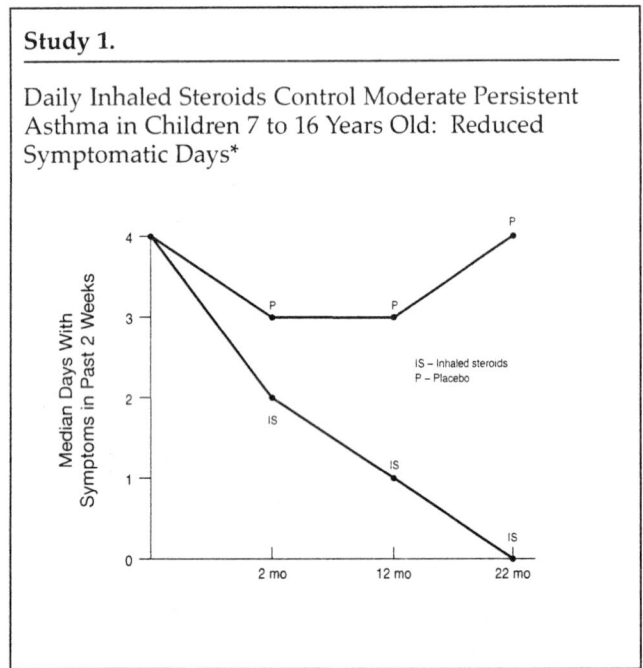

IS – Inhaled steroids
P – Placebo

Study 2.

Inhaled Steroids Control Asthma in Adults: Significant Reduction in Need for Quick-Relief Medicine*

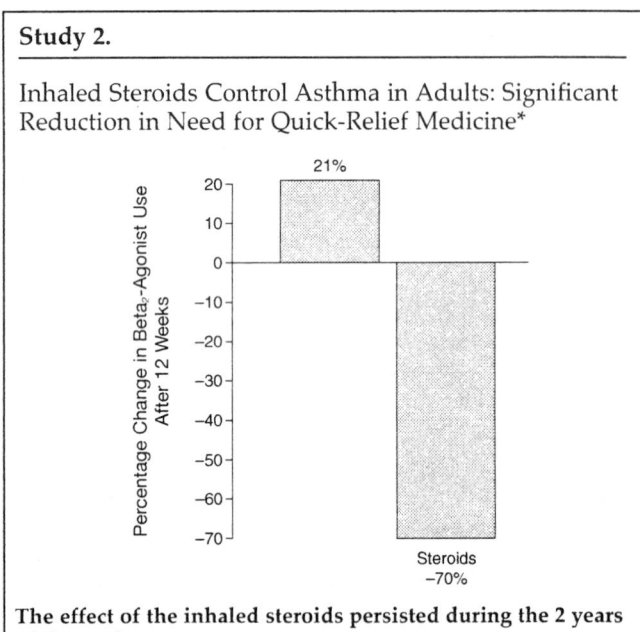

The effect of the inhaled steroids persisted during the 2 years of the study.

*Other endpoints—FEV_1, peak flow, airway hyperresponsiveness, and symptoms—significantly improved relative to the placebo group over 22 months of the children's study (N=116)[5] and over 2 years in the adult study (N=103).[6]

For patients who are taking oral steroids daily on a long-term basis, referral for consultation or care by an asthma specialist is recommended. Patients should be closely monitored for adverse side effects. **Continuous attempts should be made to reduce daily use of oral steroids when asthma is controlled:**

- Maintain patients on the lowest possible dose of oral steroids (single dose daily or on alternate days).
- Use high doses of inhaled steroids to eliminate or reduce the need for oral steroids.

Step Up Therapy

The presence of one or more indicators of poor asthma control (see figure 6) **may suggest a need to increase or "step up" therapy.** Before increasing therapy, alternative reasons for poorly controlled asthma should be considered (see figure 7). Referral to a specialist for comanagement or consultation may be appropriate.

The addition of a 3- to 10-day course of oral steroids may be needed to reestablish control during a period of gradual deterioration or a moderate-to-severe exacerbation (see Managing Asthma Exacerbations, page 32). If symptoms do not recur after the course of steroids (and peak flow remains normal), the patient should continue in the same step. However, if the steroid course controls symptoms for less than 1 to 2 weeks, or if courses of steroids are repeated frequently, the patient should move to the next higher step in therapy.

SPECIAL CONSIDERATIONS FOR INFANTS, CHILDREN, AND ADOLESCENTS

Infants and Preschool Children

Treatment of acute or chronic wheezing or cough should follow the stepwise approach presented in figure 5. In general, physicians should do the following when infants and young children consistently require treatment for symptoms more than two times per week:

- Prescribe daily inhaled anti-inflammatory medication (inhaled steroids, cromolyn, or nedocromil) as long-term-control asthma therapy. A trial of cromolyn or nedocromil is often given to patients with mild persistent asthma.

- Monitor the response to therapy carefully (e.g., frequency of symptoms over 2 to 4 weeks).
- If benefits are sustained for at least 3 months, a step down in therapy should be attempted.
- If clear benefit is not observed, treatment should be stopped. Alternative therapies or diagnoses should be considered.
- Consider oral steroids if an exacerbation caused by a viral respiratory infection is moderate to severe. If the patient has a history of severe exacerbations, consider steroids at the onset of the viral infection.

Medication delivery devices should be selected according to the child's ability to use them. Be aware that the dose received can vary considerably among delivery devices:

- **Children aged 2 or less**—nebulizer therapy is preferred for administering cromolyn or high doses of short-acting inhaled beta$_2$-agonists. A metered-dose inhaler (MDI) with a spacer/holding chamber that has a face mask may be used to take inhaled steroids.
- **Children 3 to 5 years of age**—MDI plus spacer/holding chamber may be used by many children of this age. If the desired therapeutic effects are not achieved, a nebulizer or an MDI plus spacer/holding chamber with a face mask may be required.

Spacers/holding chambers are devices that hold the aerosol medication so the patient can inhale it easily. This reduces the problem of coordinating the actuation of the MDI with the inhalation. Spacers/holding chambers come in many different shapes. These devices are not simply tubes that put space between the patient's mouth and the MDI. Examples of spacers/holding chambers are illustrated in the box on page 22.

Parents or caregivers need to be instructed in the proper use of appropriately sized face masks, spacers with face masks, and holding chamber devices. Acceptable use of the delivery device should be demonstrated in the office before the patient leaves. The ability of children to use the devices may vary widely.

Figure 6.

Indicators of Poor Asthma Control—Consider Increasing Long-Term Medications*

- **Awakened at night with symptoms**
- **An urgent care visit**
- **Patient has increased need for short-acting inhaled beta$_2$-agonists** (excludes use for upper respiratory viral infections and exercise-induced bronchospasm) OR
  - At step 1: Used short-acting inhaled beta$_2$-agonists more than two times in a week
  - At steps 2–3: Used short-acting inhaled beta$_2$-agonists more than three to four times a day OR used this medication on a daily basis for a week or less
  - Patient used more than one canister of short-acting inhaled beta$_2$-agonist in one month

* This may mean a temporary increase in anti-inflammatory medication to regain control or a "step up" in long-term therapy. This will depend on the frequency of the above events, reasons for poor control (see figure 7), and the clinician's judgment.

Figure 7.

Assess Reasons for Poor Asthma Control Before Increasing Medications—ICE

• **I**nhaler technique	Check patient's technique.
• **C**ompliance	Ask when and how much medication the patient is taking.
• **E**nvironment	Ask patient if something in his or her environment has changed.

Also consider:

• **Alternative diagnosis**	Assess patient for presence of concomitant upper respiratory disease or alternative diagnosis.

SCHOOL-AGE CHILDREN AND ADOLESCENTS

The pharmacologic management of school-age children and adolescents follows the same basic principles as those for adults, but with special consideration of growth, school, and social development.

- **Cromolyn or nedocromil is often tried first in children with mild or moderate persistent asthma.** This is because these medications are often effective anti-inflammatory therapies and have no known long-term systemic effects.

- **For children with severe persistent asthma, and for many with moderate persistent asthma, inhaled steroids are necessary for long-term-control therapy.** Cromolyn and nedocromil do not provide adequate control for these patients. See stepwise approach to pharmacotherapy (figure 4 on page 17) for treatment recommendations.

Inhaled Steroids and Growth

The potential but small risk of adverse effects on linear growth from the use of inhaled steroids is well balanced by their efficacy. Poor asthma control itself can result in retarded linear growth. Most studies do not demonstrate a negative effect on growth with dosages of 400 to 800 mcg a day of beclomethasone,[21-23] although a few short-term studies have.[24,25] Adverse effects on linear growth appear to be dose dependent. High doses of inhaled steroids have greater potential for growth suppression, but less potential than the alternative of oral steroids. Some caution (e.g., monitoring growth, stepping down therapy when possible) is suggested while this issue is studied further.

Action Plan for Schools

The clinician should prepare a written action plan for the student's school that explains when medications may be needed to treat episodes and to prevent exercise-induced bronchospasm. Recommendations to limit exposures to offending allergens or irritants and a written request for the child to carry quick-relief medications at school could be helpful. When possible, schedule daily medications so they do not need to be taken at school. (See patient hand-out, "School Self-Management Plan.")

MANAGING ASTHMA IN OLDER ADULTS

- Make adjustments or avoid asthma medications that can aggravate other conditions:
  - **Inhaled steroids.** Give supplements of calcium (1,000 to 1,500 mg per day), vitamin D (400 units a day), and, where appropriate, estrogen replacement therapy, especially for women using high doses of inhaled steroids.
  - **Oral steroids** may provoke confusion, agitation, and changes in glucose metabolism.
  - **Theophylline and epinephrine** may exacerbate underlying heart conditions. Also, the risk of theophylline overdose may be higher because of reduced theophylline clearance in older patients.

- Inform patients about potential adverse effects on their asthma from medications used for other conditions, for example:

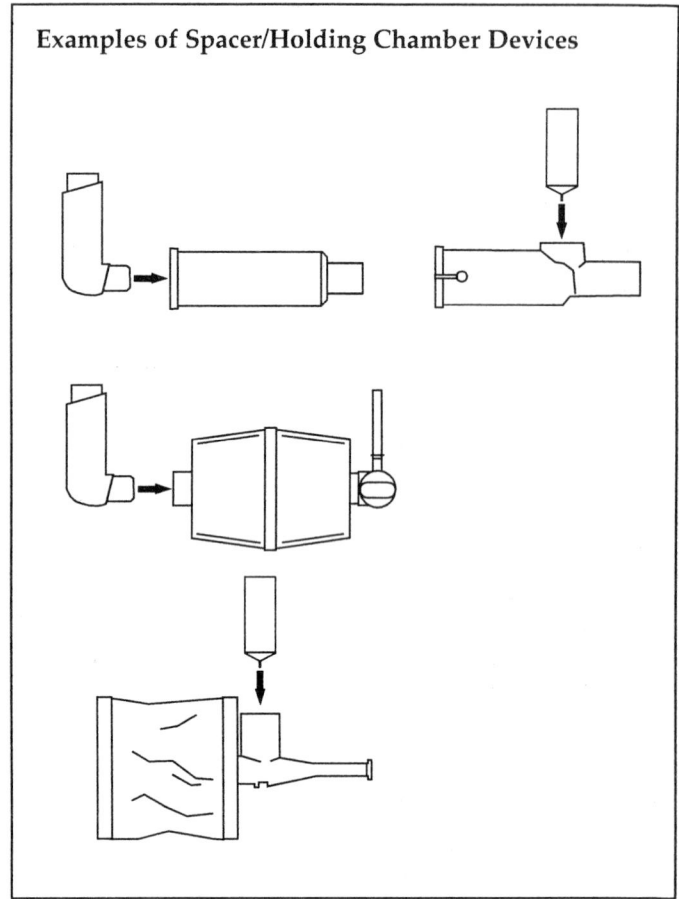

Examples of Spacer/Holding Chamber Devices

  - **Aspirin and other oral nonsteroidal anti-inflammatory medications** (arthritis, pain relief)
  - **Nonselective beta-blockers** (high blood pressure)
  - **Beta-blockers in some eye drops** (glaucoma)

- Chronic bronchitis and emphysema may coexist with asthma. A 2- to 3-week trial with oral steroids can help determine the presence of reversibility of airway obstruction and indicate the extent of potential benefit from asthma therapy.

MANAGING SPECIAL SITUATIONS

Managing Exercise-Induced Bronchospasm

Exercise-induced bronchospasm generally begins during exercise and reaches its peak 5 to 10 minutes after stopping. The symptoms often spontaneously resolve in another 20 to 30 minutes.

A diagnosis of exercise-induced bronchospasm is suggested by a history of cough, shortness of breath, chest pain or tightness, wheezing, or endurance problems during and after vigorous activity. The diagnosis can be confirmed by an objective measure of the problem (i.e., a 15 percent decrease in peak flow or FEV_1 between measurements taken before and after vigorous activity at 5-minute intervals for 20 to 30 minutes.)

For the vast majority of patients, exercise-induced bronchospasm should not limit either participation or success in vigorous activities. The following are the **recommended control measures:**

- **Two to four puffs of short-acting beta$_2$-agonist 5 to 60 minutes before exercise,** preferably as close to the start of exercise as possible. The effects of this pretreatment should last approximately 2 to 3 hours. A long-acting inhaled beta$_2$-agonist taken at least 30 minutes before exercise will last 10 to 12 hours.[26] Cromolyn or nedocromil can also be used before exercise with a duration of effect of 1 to 2 hours.[27–29]

- **A 6- to 10-minute warmup period before exercise** may benefit patients who can tolerate continuous exercise with minimal symptoms. The warmup may preclude a need for repeated medications.

- **Increase in long-term-control medications, if appropriate.** If symptoms occur with usual activities or exercise, a step up in long-term-control therapy may be warranted. Long-term control of asthma with anti-inflammatory medication (i.e., inhaled steroid, cromolyn, or nedocromil) can reduce the frequency and severity of exercise-induced bronchospasm.[30]

Teachers and coaches need to be notified that a child has exercise-induced bronchospasm. They should be told that the child is able to participate in activities but may need inhaled medication before activity. Athletes should disclose the medications they use and adhere to standards set by the U.S. Olympic Committee.[31] A complete, easy-to-use list of prohibited and approved medications can be obtained from the U.S. Olympic Committee's Drug Control Hotline (1-800-233-0393).

Managing Seasonal Asthma Symptoms

- **During the allergy season:** Use the stepwise approach to the long-term management of asthma to control symptoms.

- **Before the season:** If symptoms during a season are predictable, start daily anti-inflammatory therapy (inhaled steroids, cromolyn, or nedocromil) just before the anticipated onset of symptoms and continue this throughout the season.

Managing Asthma in Patients Undergoing Surgery

- Evaluate the patient's asthma over the past 6 months.
- Improve lung function to predicted values before surgery, possibly with a short course of oral steroids.
- Give patients who have received oral steroids for longer than 2 weeks during the past 6 months 100 mg of hydrocortisone every 8 hours intravenously during the surgical period. Reduce the dose rapidly within 24 hours following surgery.

Managing Asthma in Pregnant Women

Management of asthma in pregnant women is essential and is achieved with basically the same treatment as for nonpregnant women. Poorly controlled asthma during pregnancy can result in reduced oxygen supply to the fetus, increased perinatal mortality, increased prematurity, and low birth weight.[32] There is little to suggest an increased risk to the fetus for most drugs used to treat asthma.

Drugs or drug classes with potential risk to the fetus include brompheniramine, epinephrine, and alpha-adrenergic compounds (other than pseudoephedrine),[33-35] decongestants (other than pseudoephedrine), antibiotics (tetracycline, sulfonamides, and ciprofloxacine), live virus vaccines, immunotherapy (initiation or increase in doses), and iodides.

3. CONTROL OF FACTORS CONTRIBUTING TO ASTHMA SEVERITY

Avoiding or controlling factors that contribute to asthma severity will reduce symptoms and the need for medications. (See figure 8.)

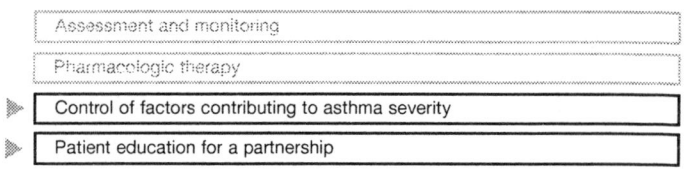

PATIENT ASSESSMENT AND EDUCATION

Have each patient complete the "Patient Self-Assessment Form for Environmental and Other Factors That Can Make Asthma Worse" to assess exposures and identify factors that may contribute to asthma severity.

Educate patients in how to reduce their exposures to these factors (see patient handout, "How To Control Things That Make Your Asthma Worse," and box on page 26). Confirm suspected occupational exposures by having the patient record over 2 to 3 weeks symptoms, exposures, bronchodilator use, and peak flow at and away from work.

INHALED ALLERGENS AND PERSISTENT ASTHMA

To reduce the effects of specific allergens on a patient with persistent asthma (see figure 9):

• **Identify the specific allergens to which patient is exposed** (use "Patient Self-Assessment Form for Environmental and Other Factors That Can Make Asthma Worse").
• **Determine and confirm sensitivity to the allergens** (skin or in vitro tests, medical history).
• **Obtain agreement with the patient to initiate one or two simple control measures** (see patient handout, "How To

Control Things That Make Your Asthma Worse," and box on page 26).
• **Follow up with patient, adding control measures after first ones are implemented.**

Let the patient know that the benefits of many control measures will take some time to be felt. For dust-mite control it can take less than a month, whereas the benefits from removing an animal from the home may take 6 months or longer to become apparent. This is how long it may take before all the dander is out of the environment.

Allergy Testing

Skin or in vitro (e.g., RAST) tests are *alternative* methods to assess the sensitivity to the year-round allergens to which patients with persistent asthma are exposed (i.e., animal, house-dust mite, cockroach, or indoor mold allergens). Allergy testing is the only reliable way to determine sensitivity to year-round indoor allergens[40,41] and is important for justifying the expense and effort involved in implementing environmental controls. Allergy tests also reinforce for the patients the need to take environmental

---

Figure 8.

Allergen Control Significantly Improves Even Mild Asthma: An Illustrative Study with House-Dust Mites

Many studies support the effectiveness of allergen control in improving asthma and reducing the need for medication.[36-39] The controlled study of 20 children with mild asthma and house-dust mite allergy illustrates the effect control measures can have.[39]

• Major components of treatment used in the study:
  — Encased pillows, mattresses, and box springs in allergen-impermeable covers.
  — Washed blankets and mattress pads every 2 weeks in hot water.
  — Removed toys, upholstered furniture, and carpets from bedroom.
• After 1 month, the treatment group had:
  — Symptom days and days needing medicine significantly reduced to a minimal number
  — Airway hyperresponsiveness reduced significantly relative to the control group.

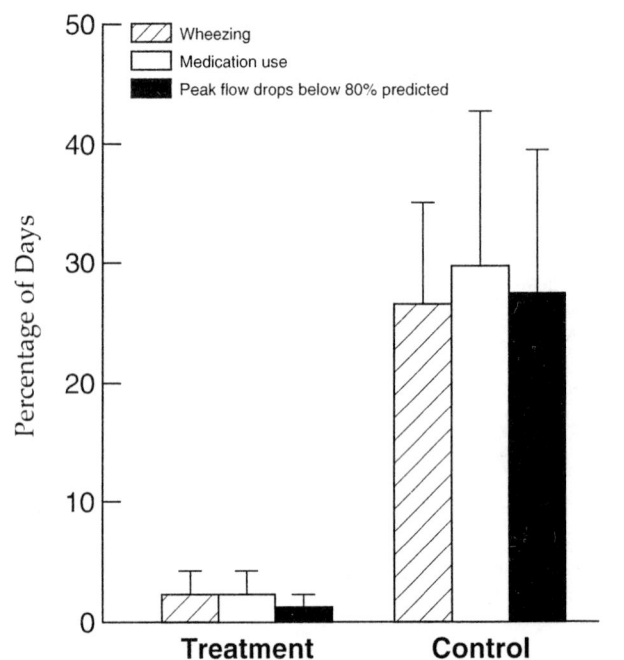

Percentage of days (± standard error) in which wheezing was noticed, medication was used, or peak flow dropped below 80% predicted.[39]
Reproduced with permission.

Figure 9.

Determining the Need for Allergen Control in Patients With Persistent Asthma

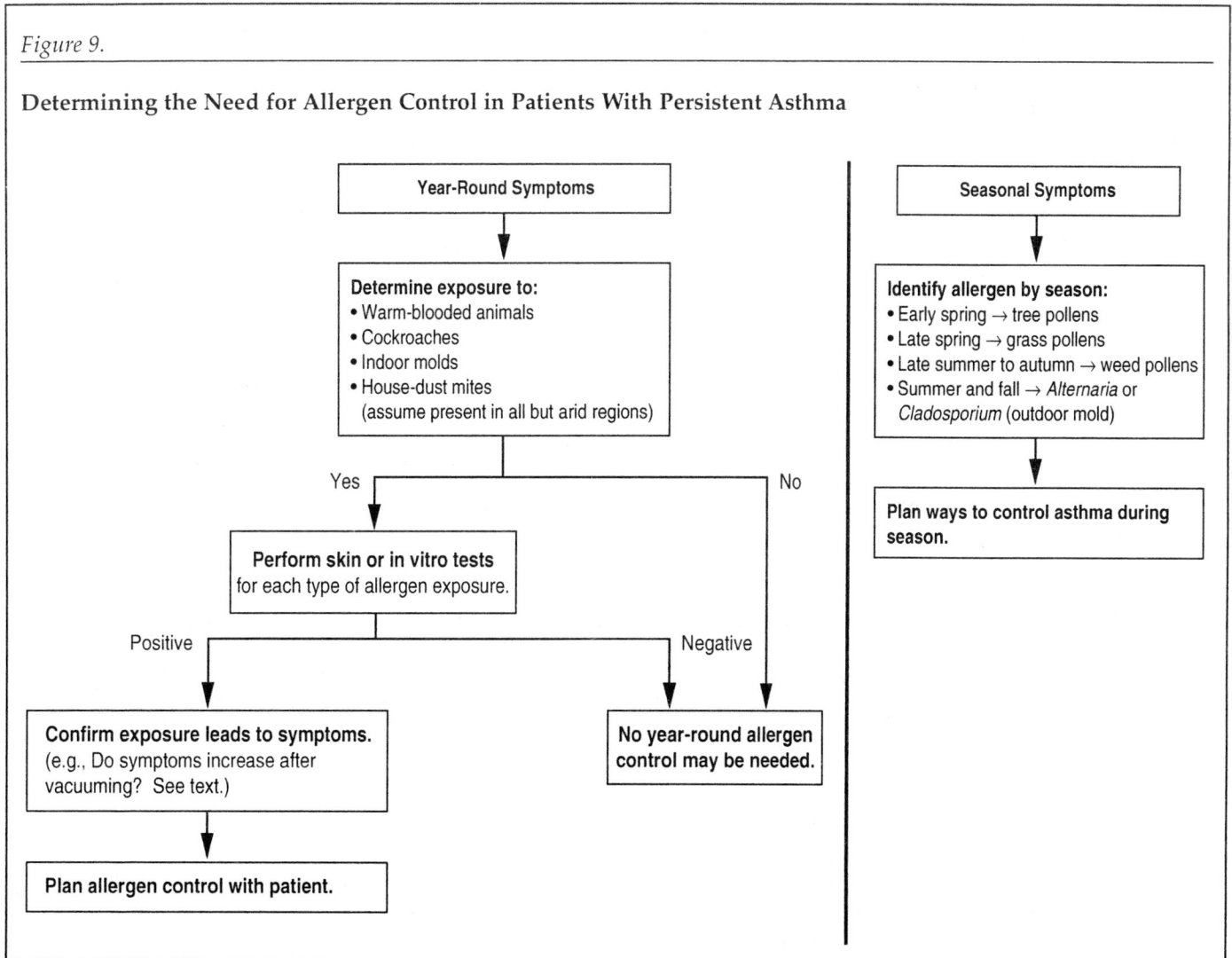

control measures. Whether skin or in vitro tests are used will probably depend on whether the physician is knowledgeable about skin testing technique.

Order tests only for those substances to which you have determined the patient is exposed (i.e., do not order a panel of tests). **When allergy tests are positive, ask patients about the onset of symptoms when they are in contact with the allergen.** Positive answers to these questions confirm the likelihood that the allergy is contributing to asthma symptoms. However, lack of a positive response to these questions does not exclude the possibility that the allergen may be contributing to the patient's symptoms.

- **For animals and dust mites:** "Do nasal, eye, or chest symptoms occur in a room where carpets are being or have just been vacuumed?"
- **For indoor mold:** "Do nasal, eye, or chest symptoms appear when in damp or moldy rooms, such as basements?"

Immunotherapy

In the opinion of the Expert Panel and based on the evidence,[42-46] allergen immunotherapy may be considered for asthma patients when (1) there is clear evidence of a relationship between symptoms and exposure to an unavoidable allergen to which the patient is sensitive, (2) symptoms occur all year or during a major portion of the year, and (3) there is difficulty controlling symptoms with pharmacologic management because multiple medications are required or medications are ineffective or not accepted by the patient. The course of allergen immunotherapy is typically of 3 to 5 years' duration. If use of allergen immunotherapy is elected, it should be administered only in a medical office where facilities and trained personnel are available to treat any life-threatening reaction that can, but rarely does, occur.[47,48] In the Expert Panel's opinion, referral to an allergist should be made when patients are being considered for immunotherapy.

Control Measures for Factors Contributing to Asthma Severity

Factors Contributing to Asthma Severity	Control Measures: Instructions to Patients
Allergens	See patient handout, "How To Control Things That Make Your Asthma Worse."
Tobacco smoke	Strongly advise patient and others living in the home to *stop smoking*. Discuss ways to reduce exposure to other sources of tobacco smoke, such as from day care providers and the workplace.
Rhinitis	Intranasal steroids. Antihistamine/decongestant combinations may also be used.
Sinusitis	Medical measures to promote drainage. Antibiotic therapy is appropriate when complicating acute bacterial infection is present.
Gastroesophageal reflux	No eating within 3 hours of bedtime, head of bed elevated 6 to 8 inches, and appropriate medications (e.g., H_2-antagonist).
Sulfite sensitivity	No eating of shrimp, dried fruit, processed potatoes. No drinking of beer or wine.
Medication interactions	No beta-blockers (including ophthalmological preparations). Aspirin and other nonsteroidal anti-inflammatory medications. Inform adult patients with severe persistent asthma, nasal polyps, or a history of aspirin sensitivity about the risk of severe and even fatal episodes from using these drugs. Usually safe alternatives are acetaminophen or salsalate.
Occupational exposures	Discuss with asthma patients the importance of avoidance, ventilation, respiratory protection, and a tobacco smoke-free environment. If occupationally induced asthma, recommend complete cessation of exposure to initiating agent. Obtain permission from patient before contacting management or onsite health professionals about workplace exposure.
Viral respiratory infections	Annual influenza vaccinations should be given to patients with persistent asthma.

4. PERIODIC ASSESSMENT AND MONITORING

Periodic clinical assessments every 1 to 6 months and patient self-monitoring are essential for asthma care because:

- Asthma symptoms and severity change, requiring changes in therapy.
- Patients' exposure to precipitants of asthma will change.
- Patients' memories and self-management practices fade with time. Reinforcement, review, and reminders are needed.

The frequency of patient visits depends on the severity of the asthma and the patient's ability to control and monitor symptoms. The first followup visit usually needs to be sooner than 1 month.

WORKING WITHIN THE TIME CONSTRAINTS OF THE TYPICAL OFFICE VISIT

Each physician develops his or her own way of accomplishing the periodic assessment and patient education (see box below for an example). Here are ways some primary care physicians have been able to perform the recommended periodic assessment and patient education within the time constraints of routine office visits:

- **Give patients an assessment questionnaire to complete in the waiting room.** The answers to these questions determine the issues to be addressed during that visit. See "Patient Self-Assessment Form for Followup Visits" on page 55 for such an assessment questionnaire. This helps set priorities to be addressed.

- **Have patients come back to the office more often, especially at the beginning.** Break the assessment and education the patient needs into segments and perform these over a number of visits. For example, after the diagnosis of asthma, a patient could be given the "Patient Self-Assessment Form for Environmental and Other Factors That Can Make Asthma Worse" to be completed at home. A visit in a week or so could be set to review the form and your recommendations to the patient. Similarly, initial education on the use of a peak flow meter and action plan might be scheduled for a separate visit. An example of how the necessary patient education can be divided and conducted across

| Assessment and monitoring |
| Pharmacologic therapy |
| Control of factors contributing to asthma severity |
| Patient education for a partnership |

visits is outlined in figure 10 on page 30. Review this and make adjustments, as needed, for your own practice.

- **Use nurses or office staff to do some of the tasks,** like checking MDI technique.

- Some managed care organizations have a home case manager to do followup assessments and education.

PATIENT SELF-MONITORING

All patients should be taught to recognize symptoms and what to do when symptoms occur (see patient handout, "Asthma Action Plan"). Review the information in the Asthma Action Plan often, optimally at each office visit.

Long-term daily peak flow monitoring is recommended for those with moderate or severe persistent asthma or patients with a history of severe exacerbations. If long-term daily peak flow monitoring is not used by these patients, short-term monitoring (2 to 3 weeks) can be used to evaluate the severity of exacerbations to guide treatment decisions, evaluate response to changes in long-term treatment, and identify environmental or occupational exposures.

Educate patients on how to use the peak flow meter to help monitor and manage their asthma (see patient handout, "How To Use Your Peak Flow Meter," for details). Ask patients to demonstrate the use of their peak flow meter at every visit and use the reading as part of the clinical assessment. This will take less than a minute and should become a routine component of the clinic visit.

Specific recommendations regarding peak flow monitoring include:

- Use the patient's own personal best peak flow (see patient handout, "How To Use Your Peak Flow Meter") as the standard against which peak flow measurements should be compared.

- Use the same peak flow meter and, when needed, replace with same brand.

Spirometry and Peak Flow Measurement at Office Visits

The Expert Panel recommends that spirometry tests be done (1) at the initial assessment, (2) after treatment has stabilized symptoms and peak flow (to document a baseline of "normal" airway function), and (3) at least every 1 to 2 years when asthma is stable, more often when asthma is unstable, or at other times the clinician believes it is needed.

How I Organized My Visits To Accomplish the Periodic Assessment and Patient Education

- My staff gives asthma patients a self-assessment form to complete in the waiting room.
- My nurse evaluates the patients' inhaler technique and checks their peak flow before they see me.
- I am then able to direct my care to the patients' and families' concerns, problems in achieving the goals of therapy, medication issues, and other concerns I may identify with open-ended questions.

I feel my office has been very successful with this organized approach to the asthma office visit. It obviously required energy to organize the system and practice on the part of myself and my staff to make it work. But the routine periodic assessment and patient education needed for good asthma care are doable in the typical office visit.

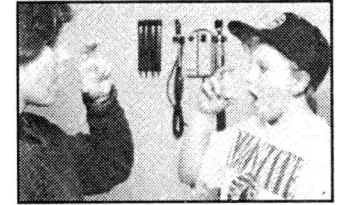

Stuart Stoloff, MD
Private Family Practice
Carson City, Nevada

- Measure peak flow first thing in the morning before medications.
- A drop in peak flow below 80 percent of personal best indicates a need for added medications.
- A drop in peak flow below 50 percent of personal best indicates a severe exacerbation.

CLINICIAN ASSESSMENT

At each visit, (1) identify patient's concerns about asthma and expectations for the visit, (2) assess achievement of the patient's goals and the general goals of asthma therapy, (3) review medications usage, and (4) teach and reinforce patient's self-management activities (the latter is addressed in the next chapter on "Education for a Partnership in Asthma Care"). These four activities can be achieved within the time constraints of routine medical visits, particularly when the patient completes the "Patient Self-Assessment Form for Followup Visits" in the waiting room.

Identify Patient Concerns and Expectations of the Visit

Review the self-assessment questionnaire and address the patient's concerns during the visit.

Assess Achievement of the Goals of Asthma Therapy

If the patient is not meeting the following goals of asthma therapy, assess the reasons (see figure 7 on page 21) and consider increasing the patient's medications.

Prevent chronic asthma symptoms and asthma exacerbations during the day and night.

- Perform physical examination (respiratory tract).
- Review patient's symptom history at each visit:
  — Daytime symptoms in the past 2 weeks
  — Nighttime symptoms in the past 2 weeks
  — Symptoms while exercising
  — Cause(s) of the symptoms
  — What the patient did to control the symptoms

- Use of quick-relief medications:
  — Number of times short-acting inhaled beta$_2$-agonists are used per week
  — Number of short-acting inhaled beta$_2$-agonist inhalers used in past month
- Emergency or hospital care.
- Missed any work or school due to asthma.

Maintain normal activity levels — including exercise and other physical activities.

- Reduction in usual activities or exercise.
- Disruption of caregivers' or parents' routine by their child's asthma.

Have normal or near-normal lung function.

- Objective measure of lung function—either spirometry or peak flow at each visit (see box on page 27).
- Number of times peak flow went below 80 percent personal best in past 2 weeks, if peak flow monitoring is performed.

Be satisfied with the asthma care received and the level of control—ask patient about this.

Have no or minimal side effects—shakiness, nervousness, bad taste, sore throat, cough, upset stomach—while receiving optimal medications.

REVIEW MEDICATIONS USAGE AND SKILLS

- Ask patients to review for you what medications they are taking, when they take them, and how often.
- Identify any problems patients have had taking medications as prescribed (e.g., missed doses). Note: Patients should bring all of their medications to each office visit.
- Ask patients to demonstrate their use of a placebo inhaler at each followup visit. Assess their performance using the checklist in the patient handout (see patient handout, "How To Use Your Metered-Dose Inhaler the Right Way"). Ask patients to demonstrate use of their peak flow meter, if used.

5. EDUCATION FOR A PARTNERSHIP IN ASTHMA CARE

The goal of all patient education is to help patients take the actions needed to control their asthma.

These actions are listed below and are described more fully in the patient handouts. See figure 10 on page 30 for an example of how to address these issues during routine office visits.

- Taking daily medications for long-term control as prescribed
- Using delivery devices effectively—metered-dose inhalers, spacers, nebulizers
- Identifying and controlling factors that make asthma worse
- Monitoring peak flow and/or symptoms
- Following the written action plan when symptoms or episodes occur

HOW TO INCREASE THE LIKELIHOOD OF COMPLIANCE

Patients cannot be expected to perform a task they never agreed to do or one that is only mentioned once to them. Thus, two essential clinician activities for successful patient education are:

1. **Asking the patient for a verbal, sometimes written, agreement** to take specific action(s). You will need to explain the recommended action(s) and the benefits the patient can expect from doing them.

2. **Following up** and reinforcing the patient for the actions during subsequent visits or phone calls.

Other ways to increase compliance are:

- **Develop an Asthma Action Plan with the patient** (see patient handout). Involve adolescents and school-age children in developing their plan, as appropriate. Minimize the number of medications and daily doses to the fewest clinically possible. Give parents additional copies of the plan to give to day care providers and schools.

- **Fit the daily medication regimen into the patient's and family's routine.** Explain the difference between long-term-control and quick-relief medicines and how to use them. Ask patients (and parents) when would be the easiest times for them to take their daily medicines.

- **Identify and address obstacles and concerns. Ask patients about problems they think they might have doing the recommended action(s).** Ask questions that start with "what" or "how" to identify the obstacles (e.g., "What are things that might make it hard for you to take the action each day?"). Discuss ways to address the problems or provide alternative actions.

- **Ask for agreement/plans to act.** Ask patients to summarize what recommended action(s) they plan to take, especially at the end of each visit.

- **Encourage or enlist family involvement.**

- **Follow up. At each visit, review the performance of the agreed-upon actions.** Praise appropriate actions and discuss how to improve other actions. Share evidence of the patient's improvement in lung function and symptoms. Remain encouraging when patients do not take the agreed-upon actions.

- **Assess the influence of the patient's cultural beliefs and practices that might affect asthma care.** Ask open-ended questions (e.g., "What will your friends and family think when you tell them you have asthma? What advice might they give to you?") If harmless or potentially beneficial folk remedies are mentioned by the patients, consider incorporating them into the treatment plan.

Assessment and monitoring
Pharmacologic therapy
Control of factors contributing to asthma severity
▶ **Patient education for a partnership**

TEACH USE OF INHALER AND PEAK FLOW METER

Most patients use their inhalers incorrectly, and this skill deteriorates over time. Patients' poor technique results in less medication getting to the airways. The initial inhaler training can be done in minutes with the simple skills-training method described below. Note that different inhalers may require different inhalation techniques. The necessary reviews at each visit are quick and easy and can be done by other staff members in the office.

Effective skills-training steps for teaching inhaler techniques are as follows:

1. **Tell** the patient the steps and give written instructions. (For written instructions, see patient handouts.)

2. **Demonstrate** how to use the inhaler following each of these steps.

3. Ask the patient to **demonstrate** how to use the inhaler. Let the patient refer to the handout on the first training. Subsequently, use the handout as a checklist to assess the patient's technique.

4. **Tell** patients what they did right and what they need to improve. Have them demonstrate their technique again, if needed. Focus the patient on improving one or two key steps (e.g., timing of actuation and inhalation) if the patient made multiple errors.

At each subsequent visit, perform the last two steps: patient demonstration and telling what they did right and what they need to improve. Train patients to use their peak flow meter using the same four skills-training steps above and the patient handout, "How To Use Your Peak Flow Meter."

TIPS FOR REPLACING METERED-DOSE INHALERS

The *only* reliable way to determine whether a metered-dose inhaler is empty is to count the number of puffs used and subtract that number from the total number of sprays in the canister. Unfortunately, many patients believe they know when their inhalers are empty by floating the canister, spraying into the air, or tasting the medicine.

Clinicians and pharmacists can help patients determine the life of their long-term-control canisters by referring to the chart in figure 11 ("How Often To Change Long-Term-Control Canisters") or by dividing the number of sprays per canister (written on the canister and listed in the dosage chart on pages 39–40) by the number of puffs prescribed per day. Determine the corresponding calendar date. Make an appointment before that date or make refills available after that date.

Figure 10.

Example of Delivery of Asthma Education by Clinicians During Patient Care Visits

Recommendations for Initial Visit

Assessment Questions Focus on: • Concerns • Goals of Therapy • Quality of Life • Expectations	Teach information in simple language	Teach and demonstrate skills

"What worries you most about your asthma?"
 	
"What do you want to accomplish at this visit?"
 	
"What do you want to be able to do that you can't do now because of your asthma?"
 	
"What do you expect from treatment?"
 	
"What medicines have you tried?"
 	
"What other questions do you have for me today?"
	What is asthma? A chronic lung disease. The airways are very sensitive. They become inflamed and narrow; breathing becomes difficult.
	
	Two types of medicines are needed:
	• Long-term control: medications that prevent symptoms, often by reducing inflammation
	• Quick relief: short-acting bronchodilator relaxes muscles around airways
	
	Bring all medications to every appointment.
	
	When to seek medical advice. Provide appropriate telephone number.
		Inhaler (see patient handout) and spacer/holding chamber use. Check performance.
		
		Self-monitoring skills tied to action plan:
		• Recognize intensity and frequency of asthma symptoms
		• Review the signs of deterioration and the need to reevaluate therapy:
		  — Waking at night with asthma
		  — Increased medication use
		  — Decreased activity tolerance
		
		Use of an action plan (see patient handout)

Recommendations for First Followup Visit (2 to 4 weeks or sooner as needed)

Ask relevant questions from previous visit and also ask: "What medications are you taking?" "How and when are you taking them?" "What problems have you had using your medications?" "Please show me how you use your inhaled medications."	Use of two types of medications. Remind patient to bring all medications and the peak flow meter to every appointment for review. Self-evaluation of progress in asthma control using symptoms and peak flow as a guide.	Use of an action plan. Review and adjust as needed. Peak flow monitoring (see patient handout) and daily diary recording. Correct inhaler and spacer/holding chamber technique.

Recommendations for Second Followup Visit

Ask relevant questions from previous visits and also ask: "Have you noticed anything in your home, work, or school that makes your asthma worse?" "Describe for me how you know when to call your doctor or go to the hospital for asthma care." "What questions do you have about the action plan?" "Can we make it easier?" "Are your medications causing you any problems?"	Relevant environmental control/avoidance strategies (see patient handout). • How to identify and control home, work, or school exposures that can cause or worsen asthma • How to avoid cigarette smoke (active and passive) Review all medications and review and interpret peak flow and symptom scores from daily diary	Inhaler/spacer/holding chamber technique. Peak flow monitoring technique. Review use of action plan. Confirm that patient knows what to do if asthma gets worse.

Recommendations for All Subsequent Visits

Ask relevant questions from previous visits and also ask: "How have you tried to control things that make your asthma worse?" "Please show me how you use your inhaled medication."	Review and reinforce all: • Educational messages • Environmental control strategies at home, work, or school • Medications Review and interpret peak flow and symptom scores from daily diary.	Inhaler/spacer/holding chamber technique. Peak flow monitoring technique. Review use of action plan. Confirm that patient knows what to do if asthma gets worse. Periodically review and adjust written action plan.

Figure 11.

How Often To Change Long-Term-Control Canisters

# Sprays	2 Sprays/ Day	4 Sprays/ Day	6 Sprays/ Day	8 Sprays/ Day	9 Sprays/ Day	12 Sprays/ Day	16 Sprays/ Day
60	30 days	15 days	n/a	n/a	n/a	n/a	n/a
100	n/a	25 days	16 days	12 days	n/a	n/a	n/a
104	n/a	26 days	17 days	13 days	n/a	n/a	n/a
112	n/a	28 days	18 days	14 days	n/a	n/a	n/a
120	60 days	30 days	20 days	15 days	n/a	n/a	n/a
200	n/a	50 days	33 days	25 days	22 days	16 days	12 days
240	n/a	60 days	40 days	30 days	26 days	20 days	15 days

* If the medication is taken as prescribed, the canister should be discarded as indicated above. Otherwise, the remaining puffs may not contain sufficient medication.

6. **MANAGING ASTHMA EXACERBATIONS AT HOME, IN THE EMERGENCY DEPARTMENT, AND IN THE HOSPITAL**

HOME MANAGEMENT: PROMPT TREATMENT IS KEY

Educating patients to recognize and treat exacerbations early is the best strategy.

Education and preparation of patients to manage their exacerbations* are essential and should include:

- A written action plan and clear instructions on how to follow it. (See patient handout, "Asthma Action Plan," and figure 12).

- Instructions on how to recognize signs of worsening asthma and signs that indicate the need to call the doctor or seek emergency care.

- Prompt use of short-acting beta$_2$-agonists (two puffs every 20 minutes for 1 hour) and, for moderate-to-severe exacerbations, the addition of oral steroids. Increased therapy should be maintained for several days to stabilize symptoms and peak flow.

- Monitoring the response to the medications.

- Followup with patients to assess overall asthma control, the need to increase long-term-control medications, and the need to remove or withdraw from allergens or irritants that precipitated the exacerbation.

*Asthma exacerbations are episodes of progressively worsening shortness of breath, cough, wheezing, chest tightness, or some combination of these symptoms.

Assessment and monitoring
▷ Pharmacologic therapy
Control of factors contributing to asthma severity
▷ Patient education for a partnership

Patients at high risk of asthma-related death (see box below) **require special attention** — intensive education, monitoring, and care. They should be counseled to seek medical care early during an exacerbation and instructed about when and how to call for an ambulance. Patients with moderate-to-severe persistent asthma or a history of severe exacerbations should have the medication (e.g., steroid tablets or liquid) and equipment (e.g., peak flow meter, compressor-driven nebulizer for young children) for assessing and treating exacerbations at home.

PREHOSPITAL EMERGENCY MEDICINE/ AMBULANCE MANAGEMENT

It is recommended that emergency workers administer short-acting inhaled beta$_2$-agonists and supplemental oxygen to patients who have signs or symptoms of asthma.[53] Subcutaneous epinephrine or terbutaline are NOT recommended but can be used if inhaled medication is not available (see dosage information on page 42).

EMERGENCY DEPARTMENT AND HOSPITAL MANAGEMENT OF EXACERBATIONS

Treat Without Delay
Assess patient's peak flow or FEV$_1$ and administer medication(s) upon patient's arrival without delay. After ther-

Risk Factors for Death From Asthma

History of Severe Exacerbations

- Past history of sudden severe exacerbations
- Prior intubation for asthma
- Prior admission for asthma to an intensive care unit

Asthma Hospitalizations and Emergency Visits

- ≥ 2 hospitalizations in the past year
- ≥ 3 emergency care visits in the past year
- Hospitalization or emergency visit in past month

Beta$_2$-Agonist and Oral Steroid Usage

- Use of >2 canisters per month of short-acting inhaled beta$_2$-agonist
- Current use of oral steroids or recent withdrawal from oral steroids

Complicating Health Problems

- Comorbidity (e.g., cardiovascular diseases or COPD)
- Serious psychiatric disease, including depression, or psychosocial problems
- Illicit drug use

Other Factors

- Poor perception of airflow obstruction or its severity
- Sensitivity to *Alternaria* (an outdoor mold)
- Low socioeconomic status and urban residence

Sources: See references 19, 49–52.

Figure 12.

Management of Asthma Exacerbations: Home Treatment
Give patients the Asthma Action Plan (page 47), which corresponds to this figure.

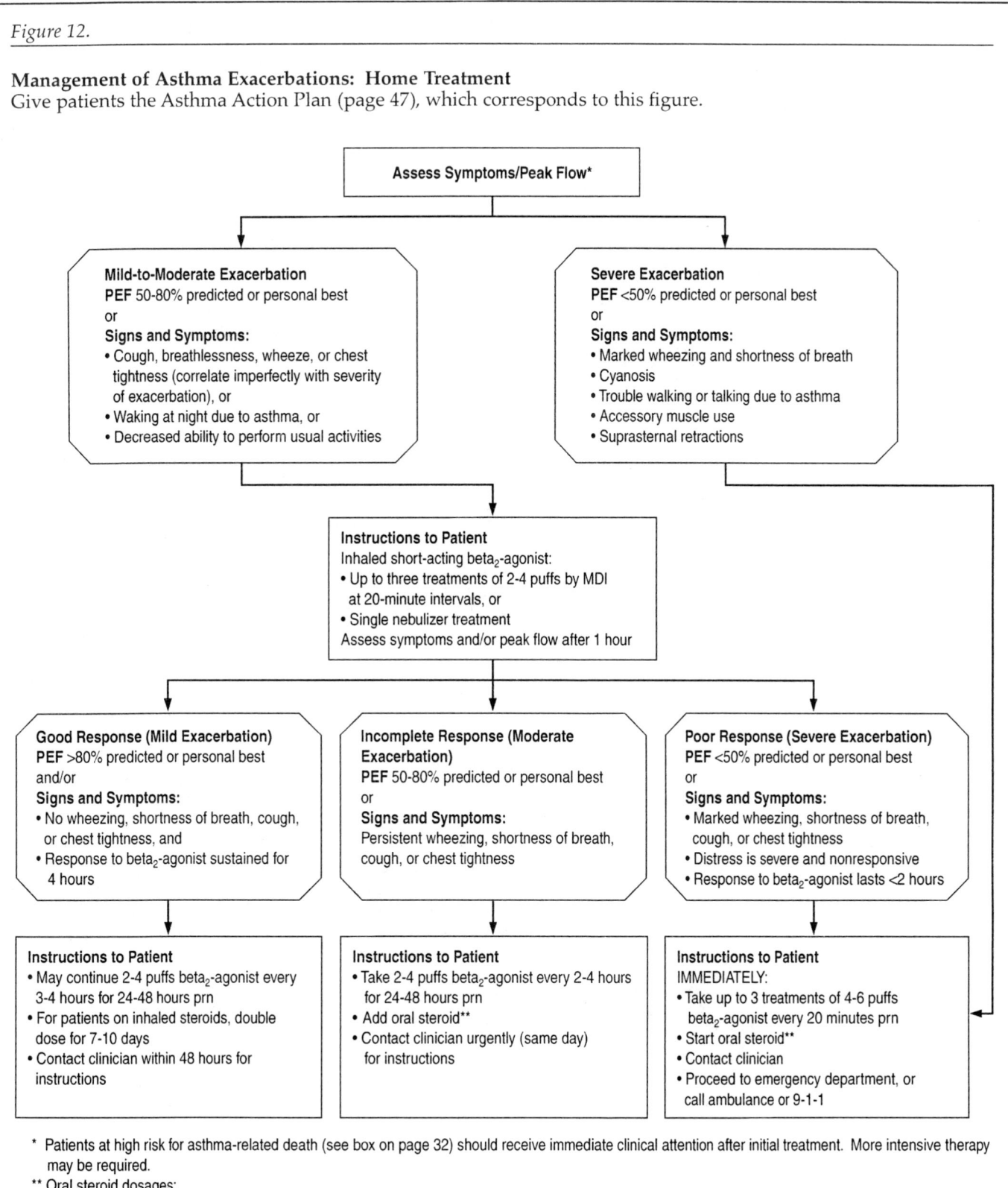

Assess Symptoms/Peak Flow*

Mild-to-Moderate Exacerbation
PEF 50-80% predicted or personal best
or
Signs and Symptoms:
• Cough, breathlessness, wheeze, or chest tightness (correlate imperfectly with severity of exacerbation), or
• Waking at night due to asthma, or
• Decreased ability to perform usual activities

Severe Exacerbation
PEF <50% predicted or personal best
or
Signs and Symptoms:
• Marked wheezing and shortness of breath
• Cyanosis
• Trouble walking or talking due to asthma
• Accessory muscle use
• Suprasternal retractions

Instructions to Patient
Inhaled short-acting beta$_2$-agonist:
• Up to three treatments of 2-4 puffs by MDI at 20-minute intervals, or
• Single nebulizer treatment
Assess symptoms and/or peak flow after 1 hour

Good Response (Mild Exacerbation)
PEF >80% predicted or personal best
and/or
Signs and Symptoms:
• No wheezing, shortness of breath, cough, or chest tightness, and
• Response to beta$_2$-agonist sustained for 4 hours

Incomplete Response (Moderate Exacerbation)
PEF 50-80% predicted or personal best
or
Signs and Symptoms:
Persistent wheezing, shortness of breath, cough, or chest tightness

Poor Response (Severe Exacerbation)
PEF <50% predicted or personal best
or
Signs and Symptoms:
• Marked wheezing, shortness of breath, cough, or chest tightness
• Distress is severe and nonresponsive
• Response to beta$_2$-agonist lasts <2 hours

Instructions to Patient
• May continue 2-4 puffs beta$_2$-agonist every 3-4 hours for 24-48 hours prn
• For patients on inhaled steroids, double dose for 7-10 days
• Contact clinician within 48 hours for instructions

Instructions to Patient
• Take 2-4 puffs beta$_2$-agonist every 2-4 hours for 24-48 hours prn
• Add oral steroid**
• Contact clinician urgently (same day) for instructions

Instructions to Patient
IMMEDIATELY:
• Take up to 3 treatments of 4-6 puffs beta$_2$-agonist every 20 minutes prn
• Start oral steroid**
• Contact clinician
• Proceed to emergency department, or call ambulance or 9-1-1

* Patients at high risk for asthma-related death (see box on page 32) should receive immediate clinical attention after initial treatment. More intensive therapy may be required.

** Oral steroid dosages:
  Adult: 40-60 mg, single or 2 divided doses for 3-10 days.
  Child: 1-2 mg/kg/day, maximum 60 mg/day, for 3-10 days

apy is initiated, obtain a brief, focused history and physical examination pertinent to the exacerbation. Perform a more detailed history, physical, and lab studies only after therapy has started.

The goals for treating asthma exacerbations are rapid reversal of airflow obstruction, reduction in the likelihood of recurrence, and correction of significant hypoxemia. To achieve these goals, the management of asthma exacerbations in the emergency department and hospital (see figure 13 and dosage chart on page 42) includes:

*   **Oxygen for most patients** to maintain $SaO_2 \geq 90$ percent (>95 percent in pregnant women, infants, and patients with coexistent heart disease). Monitor oxygen saturation until a significant clinical improvement has occurred.

*   **Short-acting inhaled beta$_2$-agonists every 20 to 30 minutes for three treatments for all patients** (see box on page 42). The onset of action is about 5 minutes. Subsequent therapy depends on response (see figure 13). Subcutaneous beta$_2$-agonists provide no proven advantage over inhaled medication.

*   **Oral steroids should be given to most patients** — those with moderate-to-severe exacerbations, patients who fail to respond promptly and completely to an inhaled beta$_2$-agonist, and patients admitted into the hospital. Oral steroids speed recovery and reduce the likelihood of recurrence. Onset of action is greater than 4 hours.[57-59] Often, a 3- to 10-day course of oral steroids at discharge is useful.

NOTE: Anticholinergics added to albuterol may be considered. Adding high doses of ipratropium bromide (0.5 mg in adults, 0.25 mg in children) to albuterol in a nebulizer has been shown to cause additional bronchodilation in some but not all studies,[54-56] particularly in patients with severe airflow obstruction.

— For patients who take oral steroids long term, give supplemental doses, even if the exacerbation is mild.

— In infants and children, give oral steroids early in the course of an asthma exacerbation.

— Oral administration of prednisone is usually preferred to intravenous methylprednisolone because it is less invasive and the effects are equivalent.[60,61]

Repeat Assessment

The Expert Panel recommends repeat assessments of patients with severe exacerbations after the first dose and the third dose (about 60 to 90 minutes after initiating treatment) of short-acting inhaled beta$_2$-agonists. Evaluate the patient's subjective response, physical findings, and

---

Effectiveness of MDI Plus Spacer/Holding Chamber vs. Nebulizer

Equivalent bronchodilation can be achieved by a beta$_2$-agonist given by MDI with a spacer/holding chamber under the supervision of trained personnel or by nebulizer therapy.[62-64] Continuous administration with a nebulizer may be more effective in children and severely obstructed adults[65-68] and patients who have difficulty with an MDI plus spacer/holding chamber.

---

lung function. Consider arterial blood gas measurement for evaluating arterial carbon dioxide (PCO_2) in patients with suspected hypoventilation, severe distress, or with FEV_1 or peak flow ≤ 30 percent of predicted after treatment.

SPECIAL CONSIDERATIONS FOR INFANTS

Infants require special attention due to their greater risk for respiratory failure.

*   Use oral steroids early in the episode.

*   Monitor oxygen saturation by pulse oximetry. SaO_2 should be >95 percent at sea level.

*   Assess infants for signs of serious distress, including use of accessory muscles, paradoxical breathing, cyanosis, a respiratory rate >60, or oxygen saturation <91 percent.

*   Assess response to therapy. A lack of response to beta$_2$-agonist therapy noted by physical exam or oxygen saturation is an indication for hospitalization.

THERAPIES NOT RECOMMENDED FOR TREATING EXACERBATIONS

Theophylline/aminophylline is NOT recommended therapy in the emergency department because it appears to provide no additional benefit to short-acting inhaled beta$_2$-agonists and may produce adverse effects.[69-73] In hospitalized patients, intravenous methylxanthines are not beneficial in children with severe asthma[74-76] and their addition remains controversial for adults.[77,78]

Chest physical therapy and mucolytics are not recommended. Anxiolytic and hypnotic drugs are contraindicated. Antibiotics are NOT recommended for asthma treatment but may be needed for comorbid conditions (e.g., patients with fever and purulent sputum or with evidence of bacterial pneumonia). Aggressive hydration is NOT recommended for older children and adults. Assess fluid status and make appropriate corrections for infants and young children to reduce their risk of dehydration.

HOSPITAL ASTHMA CARE

In general, the principles of care in the hospital are similar to those for care in the emergency department and involve treatment with aerosolized bronchodilators, systemic steroids, oxygen, and frequent assessments (see figure 13). Clinical assessment of respiratory distress and fatigue and objective measurement of airflow (peak flow or FEV_1) and oxygen saturation with pulse oximetry should be performed. Most patients respond well to therapy; however, a small minority will show signs of worsening ventilation.

Signs of impending respiratory failure include declining mental clarity, worsening fatigue, and a PCO_2 of ≥ 42 mm Hg. Respiratory failure tends to progress rapidly and is hard to reverse. The decision to intubate is based on clinical judgment; however, intubation is best done semi-electively, before the crisis of respiratory arrest. Therefore, the Expert Panel recommends that intubation should not be delayed once it is deemed necessary. Intubation should be performed by physicians with extensive experience in intubation and airway management. Consultation or comanagement by a physician expert in ventilator management is appropriate.

Figure 13.

Management of Asthma Exacerbations: Emergency Department and Hospital-Based Care

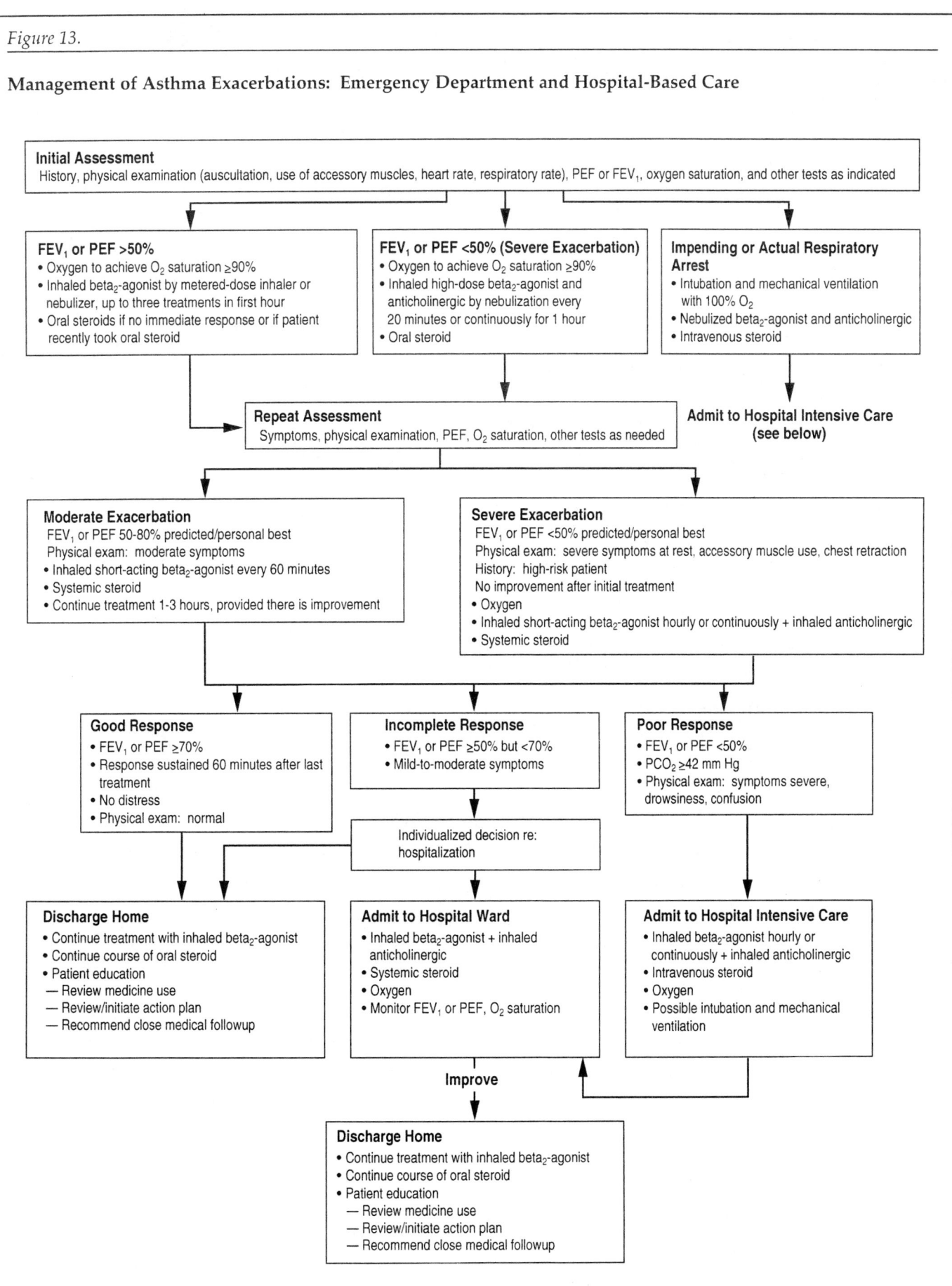

PATIENT DISCHARGE FROM THE EMERGENCY DEPARTMENT OR HOSPITAL

Patients can be discharged from the emergency department and hospital when peak flow or FEV$_1$ is ≥70 percent of predicted or personal best and symptoms are minimal. Patients should be assessed for discharge on an individual basis if they have a peak flow or FEV$_1$ of ≥50 but <70 percent of predicted or personal best and mild symptoms. Take into consideration the risk factors for asthma-related death (see box on page 32). Hospitalized patients should have their medications changed to an oral or inhaled regimen and then be observed for 24 hours before discharge.

BEFORE DISCHARGE, PROVIDE PATIENTS WITH THE FOLLOWING:

- **Sufficient short-acting inhaled beta$_2$-agonist and oral steroids** to complete the course of therapy or to continue therapy until the followup appointment. Patients given oral steroids should continue taking them for 3 to 10 days. **Patients may be asked to start taking or to increase inhaled steroids** in an attempt to improve the patient's long-term-control regimen.

- **Written and verbal instructions** on when to increase medications or return for care should asthma worsen. The plan provided in the emergency department can be quite simple. Before discharge from the hospital, patients should receive a more complete written action plan (see patient handout, page 47) on when to take their medicines.

- **Training on how to monitor peak flow** should be *provided* in the hospital and *considered* for patients in the emergency department. Also, consider issuing peak flow meters. Patients in both settings should receive instruction on monitoring their symptoms.

- **Training on necessary environmental control measures and inhaler technique, whenever possible.**

- **Referral for a followup medical appointment.** Tell patients from the emergency department to go to a followup appointment within 3 to 5 days or set up an appointment for them. When possible, phone or fax a notice to the patient's physician that the patient came to the emergency department. For both emergency department and hospital patients, emphasize the need for continual, regular care in an outpatient setting. If patients do not have a physician, refer them or arrange a followup visit with a primary care physician, a clinic, or an asthma specialist.

REFERENCES

1. National Heart, Lung, and Blood Institute, National Asthma Education and Prevention Program. *Expert Panel Report 2: Guidelines for the Diagnosis and Management of Asthma.* National Institutes of Health pub no 97-4051. Bethesda, MD, 1997.

2. Pappas G, Hadden WC, Kozak LJ, Fisher GF. Potentially avoidable hospitalizations: inequalities in rates between US socioeconomic groups. *Am J Public Health* 1997;87:811-16.

3. Friday GA Jr, Khine H, Lin MS, Caliguiri LA. Profile of children requiring emergency treatment for asthma. *Ann Allergy Asthma Immunol* 1997; 78:221-224.

4. Hartert TV, Windom HH, Peebles RS Jr, Freidhoff LR, Togias A. Inadequate outpatient medical therapy for patients with asthma admitted to two urban hospitals. *Am J Med* 1996;100:386-394.

5. van Essen-Zandvliet EE, Hughes MD, Waalkens HJ, Duiverman EJ, Pocock SJ, Kerrebijn KF. Effects of 22 months of treatment with inhaled steroids and/or beta$_2$-agonists on lung function, airway responsiveness, and symptoms in children with asthma. *Am Rev Respir Dis* 1992;146:547-54.

6. Haahtela T, Jarvinen M, Kava T, et al. Comparison of a beta$_2$-agonist, terbutaline, with an inhaled corticosteroid, budesonide, in newly detected asthma. *N Engl J Med* 1991;325:388-92.

7. Jones AH, Langdon CG, Lee PS, et al. Pulmicort Turbuhaler once daily as initial prophylactic therapy for asthma. *Respir Med* 1994;88:293-9.

8. Pincus DJ, Szefler SJ, Ackerson LM, Martin RJ. Chronotherapy of asthma with inhaled steroids: the effect of dosage timing on drug efficacy. *J Allergy Clin Immunol* 1995;95:1172-8.

9. Noonan M, Chervinsky P, Busse WW, et al. Fluticasone propionate reduces oral prednisone use while it improves asthma control and quality of life. *Am J Respir Crit Care Med* 1995;152:1467-73.

10. Haahtela T, Jarvinen M, Kava T, et al. Effects of reducing or discontinuing inhaled budesonide in patients with mild asthma. *N Engl J Med* 1994; 331:700-5.

11. Waalkens HJ, Van Essen-Zandvliet EE, Hughes MD, et al. Cessation of long-term treatment with inhaled corticosteroid (budesonide) in children with asthma results in deterioration. *Am Rev Respir Dis* 1993;148:1252-7.

12. Dahl R, Lundback E, Malo JL, et al. A dose-ranging study of fluticasone propionate in adult patients with moderate asthma. *Chest* 1993;104:1352-8.

13. Fabbri L, Burge PS, Croonenborgh L, et al. on behalf of an International Study Group. Comparison of fluticasone propionate with beclomethasone dipropionate in moderate to severe asthma treated for one year. *Thorax* 1993;48:817-23.

14. Gustafsson P, Tsanakas J, Gold M, Primhak R, Radford M, Gillies E. Comparison of the efficacy and safety of inhaled fluticasone 200 mcg/day with inhaled beclomethasone dipropionate 400 mcg/day in mild and moderate asthma. *Arch Dis Child* 1993;69:206-11.

15. Jeffery PK, Godfrey RW, Adelroth E, Nelson F, Rogers A, Johansson SA. Effects of treatment on airway inflammation and thickening of basement membrane reticular collagen in asthma. *Am Rev Respir Dis* 1992;145:890-9.

16. Rafferty P, Tucker LG, Frame MH, Fergusson RJ, Biggs BA, Crompton GK. Comparison of budesonide and beclomethasone dipropionate in patients with severe chronic asthma: assessment of relative prednisolone-sparing effects. *Br J Dis Chest* 1985;79:244-50.

17. Greening AP, Wind P, Northfield M, Shaw G. Added salmeterol versus higher-dose steroid in asthma patients with symptoms on existing inhaled steroid. *Lancet* 1994;344:219-24.

18. Woolcock A, Lundback B, Ringdal N, Jacques LA. Comparison of addition of salmeterol to inhaled steroids with doubling of the dose of inhaled steroid. *Am J Respir Crit Care Med* 1996;153:1481-8.

19. Suissa S, Ernst P, Bolvin JF, et al. A cohort analysis of excess mortality in asthma and the use of inhaled beta$_2$-agonists. *Am J Respir Crit Care Med* 1994;149(3 Pt 1):604-10.

20. Drazen JM, Israel E, Boushey HA, et al. Comparison of regularly scheduled with as-needed use of albuterol in mild asthma. *N Engl J Med* 1996;335:841-7.

21. Wolthers OD. Long-, intermediate- and short-term growth studies in asthmatic children treated with inhaled glucosteroids. *Eur Respir J* 1996;9:821-7.

22. Kamada AK, Szefler SJ, Martin RJ, et al. and the Asthma Clinical Research Network. Issues in the use of inhaled glucocorticoids. *Am J Respir Crit Care Med* 1996;153:1739-48.

23. Barnes PJ, Pedersen S. Efficacy and safety of inhaled steroids in asthma. *Am Rev Respir Dis* 1993;148:S1-S26.

24. Tinkelman DG, Reed CE, Nelson HS, Offord KP. Aerosol beclomethasone dipropionate compared with theophylline as primary treatment of chronic, mild to moderately severe asthma in children. *Pediatrics* 1993;92:64-77.

25. Doull IJM, Freezer NJ, Holgate ST. Growth of pre-pubertal children with mild asthma treated with inhaled beclomethasone dipropionate. *Am J Respir Crit Care Med* 1995;151:1715-9.

26. Kemp JP, Dockhorn RJ, Busse WW, Bleecker ER, Van As A. Prolonged effect of inhaled salmeterol against exercise-induced bronchospasm. *Am J Respir Crit Care Med* 1994;150:1612-5.

27. Albazzaz MK, Neale MG, Patel KR. Dose-response study of nebulized nedocromil sodium in exercise induced asthma. *Thorax* 1989;44:816-9.

28. de Benedictis FM, Tuteri G, Pazzelli P, Bertotto A, Bruni L, Vaccaro R. Cromolyn versus nedocromil: duration of action in exercise-induced asthma in children. *J Allergy Clin Immunol* 1995;96:510-4.

29. Woolley M, Anderson SD, Quigley BM. Duration of terbutaline sulfate and cromolyn sodium alone and in combination on exercise-induced asthma. *Chest* 1990;97:39-45.

30. Vathenen AS, Knox AJ, Wisniewski A, Tattersfield AE. Effect of inhaled budesonide on bronchial reactivity to histamine, exercise, and eucapnic dry air hyperventilation in patients with asthma. *Thorax* 1991;46:811-6.

31. Nastasi KJ, Heinly TL, Blaiss MS. Exercise-induced asthma and the athlete. *J Asthma* 1995;32:249-57.

32. Nelson HS, Weber RW. Endocrine aspects of allergic diseases. In: Bierman CW, Pearlman DS, eds. *Allergic Diseases From Infancy to Adulthood.* Philadelphia: WB Saunders, 1988. ch. 15.

33. Schatz M, Zeiger RS, Harden KM, et al. The safety of inhaled beta-agonist bronchodilators during pregnancy. *J Allergy Clin Immunol* 1988;82:686-95.

34. *Federal Register.* 21 CFR Parts 201, 202. 1979;44(124):37434-37467.

35. Briggs GG, Freeman RK, Yaffe SJ. *Drugs in Pregnancy and Lactation: A Reference Guide to Fetal and Neonatal Risk,* 2nd ed. Baltimore, MD: Williams & Wilkins, 1986.

36. Peroni DG, Boner AL, Vallone G, Antolini I, Warner JO. Effective allergen avoidance at high altitude reduces allergen-induced bronchial hyperresponsiveness. *Am J Respir Crit Care Med* 1994;149(6):1442-6.

37. Piacentini GL, Martinati L, Fornari A, et al. Antigen avoidance in a mountain environment: influence on basophil releasability in children with allergic asthma. *J Allergy Clin Immunol* 1993;92(5):644-50.

38. Simon HU, Grotzer M, Nikolaizik WH, Blaser K, Schoni MH. High altitude climate therapy reduces peripheral blood T lymphocyte activation, eosinophilia, and bronchial obstruction in children with house-dust mite allergic asthma. *Pediatr Pulmonol* 1994;17(5):304-11.

39. Murray AB, Ferguson AC. Dust-free bedrooms in the treatment of asthmatic children with house dust or house dust mite allergy: a controlled trial. *Pediatrics* 1983;71:418-22.

40. Murray AB, Milner RA. The accuracy of features in the clinical history for predicting atopic sensitization to airborne allergens in children. *J Allergy Clinical Immunol* 1995;96:588-96.

41. Adinoff AD, Rosloniec DM, McCall LL, Nelson HS. Immediate skin test reactivity to Food and Drug Administration-approved standardized extracts. *J Allergy Clin Immunol* 1990;86:766-74.

42. Abramson MJ, Puy RM, Weiner JM. Is allergen immunotherapy effective in asthma? A meta-analysis of randomized controlled trials. *Am J Respir Crit Care Med* 1995;151:969-74.

43. Reid MJ, Moss RB, Hsu YP, Kwasnicki JM, Commerford TM, Nelson BL. Seasonal asthma in northern California: allergic causes and efficacy of immunotherapy. *J Allergy Clin Immunol* 1986;78:590-600.

44. Malling HJ, Dreborg S, Weeke B. Diagnosis and immunotherapy of mould allergy. V. Clinical efficacy and side effects of immunotherapy with *Cladosporium herbarum. Allergy* 1986;41:507-19.

45. Creticos PS, Reed CE, Norman PS, et al. Ragweed immunotherapy in adult asthma. *N Engl J Med* 1996;334(8):501-6.

46. Horst M, Hejjaoui A, Horst V, Michel FB, Bousquet J. Double-blind, placebo-controlled rush immunotherapy with a standardized *Alternaria* extract. *J Allergy Clin Immunol* 1990;85:460-72.

47. American Academy of Allergy and Immunology Board of Directors. Guidelines to minimize the risk from systemic reactions caused by immunotherapy with allergenic extracts. *J Allergy Clin Immunol* 1994;93:811-2.

48. Frew AJ. Injection immunotherapy. British Society for Allergy and Clinical Immunology Working Party. *BMJ* 1993; 307:919-23.

49. Kallenbach JM, Frankel AH, Lapinsky SE, et al. Determinants of near fatality in acute severe asthma. *Am J Med* 1993;95:265-72.

50. Rodrigo C, Rodrigo G. Assessment of the patient with acute asthma in the emergency department. A factor analytic study. *Chest* 1993;104:1325-8.

51. Greenberger PA, Miller TP, Lifschultz B. Circumstances surrounding deaths from asthma in Cook County (Chicago) Illinois. *Allergy Proc* 1993;14:321-6.

52. O'Hollaren MT, Yunginger JW, Offord KP, et al. Exposure to an aeroallergen as a possible precipitating factor in respiratory arrest in young patients with asthma. *N Engl J Med* 1991;324:359-63.

53. Fergusson RJ, Stewart CM, Wathen CG, Moffat R, Crompton GK. Effectiveness of nebulised salbutamol administered in ambulances to patients with acute severe asthma. *Thorax* 1995;50:81-2.

54. Schuh S, Johnson DW, Callahan S, Canny G, Levison H. Efficacy of frequent nebulized ipratropium bromide added to frequent high-dose albuterol therapy in severe childhood asthma. *J Pediatr* 1995;126:639-45.

55. Kelly HW, Murphy S. Corticosteroids for acute, severe asthma. *DICP* 1991;25:72-9.

56. Karpel JP, Schacter EN, Fanta C, et al. A comparison of ipratropium and albuterol vs. albuterol alone for the treatment of acute asthma. *Chest* 1996;110:611-6.

57. Rowe BH, Keller JL, Oxman AD. Effectiveness of steroid therapy in acute exacerbations of asthma: a meta-analysis. *Am J Emerg Med* 1992;10:301-10.

58. Scarfone RJ, Fuchs SM, Nager AL, Shane SA. Controlled trial of oral prednisone in the emergency department treatment of children with acute asthma. *Pediatrics* 1993;2:513-8.

59. Connett GJ, Warde C, Wooler E, Lenney W. Prednisolone and salbutamol in the hospital treatment of acute asthma. *Arch Dis Child* 1994;70:170-3.

60. Harrison BD, Stokes TC, Hart GJ, Vaughan DA, Ali NJ, Robinson AA. Need for intravenous hydrocortisone in addition to oral prednisolone in patients admitted to hospital with severe asthma without ventilatory failure. *Lancet* 1986;1(8474):181-4.

61. Ratto D, Alfaro C, Sipsey J, Glovsky MM, Sharma OP. Are intravenous corticosteroids required in status asthmaticus? *JAMA* 1988;260:527-9.

62. Idris AH, McDermott MF, Raucci JC, Morrabel A, McGorray S, Hendeles L. Emergency department treatment of severe asthma. Metered-dose inhaler plus holding chamber is equivalent in effectiveness to nebulizer. *Chest* 1993;103: 665-72.

63. Colacone A, Afilalo M, Wolkove N, Kreisman H. A comparison of albuterol administered by metered dose inhaler (and holding chamber) or wet nebulizer in acute asthma. *Chest* 1993;104:835-41.

64. Kerem E, Levison H, Schuh S, et al. Efficacy of albuterol administered by nebulizer versus spacer device in children with acute asthma. *J Pediatr* 1993;123:313-7.

65. Lin RY, Sauter D, Newman T, Sirleaf J, Walters J, Tavakol M. Continuous versus intermittent albuterol nebulization in the treatment of acute asthma. *Ann Emerg Med* 1993;22:1847-53.

66. Rudnitsky GS, Eberlein RS, Schoffstall JM, Mazur JE, Spivey WH. Comparison of intermittent and continuously nebulized albuterol for treatment of asthma in an urban emergency department. *Ann Emerg Med* 1993;22:1842-6.

67. Papo MC, Frank J, Thompson AE. A prospective, randomized study of continuous versus intermittent nebulized albuterol for severe status asthmaticus in children. *Crit Care Med* 1993;21:1479-86.

68. Kelly HW, Murphy S. Beta-adrenergic agonists for acute, severe asthma. *Ann Pharmacother* 1992;26:81-91.

69. Fanta CH, Rossing TH, McFadden ER Jr. Treatment of acute asthma: is combination therapy with sympathomimetics and methylxanthines indicated? *Am J Med* 1986;80:5-10.

70. Rossing TH, Fanta CH, Goldstein DH, Snapper JR, McFadden ER Jr. Emergency therapy of asthma: comparison of the acute effects of parenteral and inhaled sympathomimetics and infused aminophylline. *Am Rev Respir Dis* 1980;122:365-71.

71. Murphy DG, McDermott MF, Rydman RJ, Sloan EP, Zalenski RJ. Aminophylline in the treatment of acute asthma when beta$_2$-adrenergics and steroids are provided. *Arch Intern Med* 1993;153:1784-88.

72. Rodrigo C, Rodrigo G. Treatment of acute asthma. Lack of therapeutic benefit and increase of the toxicity from aminophylline given in addition to high doses of salbutamol delivered by metered-dose inhaler with a spacer. *Chest* 1994;106:1071-6.

73. Coleridge J, Cameron P, Epstein J, Teichtahl H. Intravenous aminophylline confers no benefit in acute asthma treated with intravenous steroids and inhaled bronchodilators. *Aust N Z J Med* 1993;23:348-54.

74. Strauss RE, Wertheim DL, Bonagura VR, Valacer DJ. Aminophylline therapy does not improve outcome and increases adverse effects in children hospitalized with acute asthmatic exacerbations. *Pediatrics* 1994;93:205-10.

75. Carter E, Cruz M, Chesrown S, Shieh G, Reilly K, Hendeles L. Efficacy of intravenously administered theophylline in children hospitalized with severe asthma. *J Pediatr* 1993;122:470-6.

76. DiGiulio GA, Kercsmar CM, Krug SE, Alpert SE, Marx CM. Hospital treatment of asthma: lack of benefit from theophylline given in addition to nebulized albuterol and intravenously administered corticosteroid. *J Pediatr* 1993;122:464-9.

77. Huang D, O'Brien RG, Harman E, et al. Does aminophylline benefit adults admitted to the hospital for an acute exacerbation of asthma? *Ann Intern Med* 1993;119:1155-60.

78. Self TH, Abou-Shala N, Burns R, et al. Inhaled albuterol and oral prednisone therapy in hospitalized adult asthmatics. Does aminophylline add any benefit? *Chest* 1990;98:1317-21.

APPENDICES

Usual Dosages for Long-Term-Control Medications*

Medication	Dosage Form	Adult Dose	Child Dose	Comments
Inhaled Steroids (see Estimated Comparative Daily Dosages for Inhaled Steroids, page 41)				• Most effective anti-inflammatory currently available.
Oral Steroids				
Methylprednisolone	2, 4, 8, 16, 32 mg tablets	• 7.5–60 mg daily in a single dose or qod as needed for control	• 0.25–2 mg/kg daily in single dose or qod as needed for control	• For long-term treatment of severe persistent asthma, administer single dose in a.m. either daily or on alternate days (which may lessen adrenal suppression). One study suggests improved efficacy and no increase in adrenal suppression when administered at 3:00 p.m.
Prednisolone	5 mg tabs, 5 mg/5 cc, 15 mg/5 cc	• Short-course "burst": 40–60 mg per day as single or 2 divided doses for 3–10 days	• Short course "burst": 1–2 mg/kg/day, maximum 60 mg/day, for 3–10 days	• Short courses or "bursts" are effective for establishing control when initiating therapy or during a period of gradual deterioration.
Prednisone	1, 2.5, 5, 10, 20, 25 mg tabs; 5 mg/cc, 5 mg/5 cc			• The burst should be continued until patient achieves 80% of peak flow personal best or symptoms resolve. This usually requires 3–10 days but may require longer. There is no evidence that tapering the dose following improvement prevents relapse.
Cromolyn and Nedocromil				
Cromolyn	MDI 1 mg/puff (200 sprays/canister) Nebulizer solution 20 mg/ampule	2–4 puffs tid-qid 1 ampule tid-qid	1–2 puffs tid-qid 1 ampule tid-qid	• An initial trial in children with mild-to-moderate persistent asthma is often given due to strong safety profile. • Can usually see therapeutic effect of cromolyn within 2 weeks; takes 4 to 6 weeks to determine maximum effect. • Dose of cromolyn by MDI may be inadequate, so nebulizer may be preferred.
Nedocromil	MDI 1.75 mg/puff (104 sprays/canister)	2–4 puffs bid-qid	1–2 puffs bid-qid	
Long-Acting Bronchodilators				
Salmeterol	*Inhaled* MDI 21 mcg/puff, 60 or 120 puffs (120 sprays/canister) DPI 50 mcg/blister	2 puffs q 12 hours 1 blister q 12 hours	1–2 puffs q 12 hours 1 blister q 12 hours	• Should not be used in place of anti-inflammatory therapy. • Use with inhaled steroids in step 3. • May use one dose nightly for symptoms. • Duration of bronchodilation is 12 hours. • **Should not be used for symptom relief or for exacerbations.**
Sustained-release albuterol	*Tablet* 4 mg tablet	4 mg q 12 hours	0.3–0.6 mg/kg/day, not to exceed 8 mg/day	

Usual Dosages for Long-Term-Control Medications* *continued*

Medication	Dosage Form	Adult Dose	Child Dose	Comments
Theophylline	Liquids Sustained-release tablets and capsules	Starting dose 10 mg/kg/day up to 300 mg max; usual max 800 mg/day	Starting dose 10 mg/kg/day; usual max: • ≥1 year of age: 16 mg/kg/day • <1 year: 0.2 (age in weeks) + 5 = mg/kg/day	• Adjuvant to inhaled steroids for nocturnal symptoms. • Alternative, but not preferred, long-term therapy at step 2. • Adjust dosage to achieve peak serum concentration of 5-15 mcg/mL at steady-state (at least 48 hours on same dosage). • Due to wide interpatient variability in theophylline metabolic clearance, **routine serum theophylline level monitoring is important.**
Leukotriene Modifiers				
Zafirlukast	20 mg tablet	40 mg daily (1 tablet bid)		• May be considered at step 2 for patients ≥12 years of age, although their position in therapy is not fully established. • For zafirlukast, administration with meals decreases bioavailability; take at least 1 hour before or 2 hours after meals. • For patients taking zafirlukast and warfarin, closely monitor prothrombin and adjust warfarin dosage. • For zileuton, monitor hepatic enzymes (ALT).
Zileuton	300 mg tablet 600 mg tablet	2,400 mg daily (two 300-mg tablets or one 600-mg tablet, qid)		

NOTE: All chlorofluorocarbon (CFC)-propelled inhalers are being phased out. The new non-CFC products should have similar effectiveness and safety levels as the original product.

* For a list of brand names, see glossary, page 43.

Estimated Comparative Daily Dosages for Inhaled Steroids

Adults

Inhaled Steroid	Low Dose	Medium Dose	High Dose
Beclomethasone dipropionate	168–504 mcg	504–840 mcg	>840 mcg
42 mcg/puff	**4–12 puffs—42 mcg**	**12–20 puffs—42 mcg**	**>20 puffs—42 mcg**
84 mcg/puff	**2–6 puffs—84 mcg**	**6–10 puffs—84 mcg**	**>10 puffs—84 mcg**
Budesonide DPI	200–400 mcg	400–600 mcg	>600 mcg
200 mcg/dose	**1–2 inhalations**	**2–3 inhalations**	**>3 inhalations**
Flunisolide	500–1,000 mcg	1,000–2,000 mcg	>2,000 mcg
250 mcg/puff	**2–4 puffs**	**4–8 puffs**	**>8 puffs**
Fluticasone	88–264 mcg	264–660 mcg	>660 mcg
MDI:			
44, 110, 220 mcg/puff	**2–6 puffs—44 mcg or 2 puffs—110 mcg**	**2–6 puffs—110 mcg**	**>6 puffs—110 mcg or >3 puffs—220 mcg**
DPI:			
50, 100, 250 mcg/dose	**2–6 inhalations—50 mcg**	**3–6 inhalations—100 mcg**	**>6 inhalations—100 mcg or >2 inhalations—250 mcg**
Triamcinolone acetonide	400–1,000 mcg	1,000–2,000 mcg	>2,000 mcg
100 mcg/puff	**4–10 puffs**	**10–20 puffs**	**>20 puffs**

Children ≤12 years

Inhaled Steroid	Low Dose	Medium Dose	High Dose
Beclomethasone dipropionate	84–336 mcg	336–672 mcg	>672 mcg
42 mcg/puff	**2–8 puffs—42 mcg**	**8–16 puffs—42 mcg**	**>16 puffs—42 mcg**
84 mcg/puff	**1–4 puffs—84 mcg**	**4–8 puffs—84 mcg**	**>8 puffs—84 mcg**
Budesonide DPI	100–200 mcg	200–400 mcg	>400 mcg
200 mcg/dose		**1–2 inhalations—200 mcg**	**>2 inhalations—200 mcg**
Flunisolide	500–750 mcg	1,000–1,250 mcg	>1,250 mcg
250 mcg/puff	**2–3 puffs**	**4–5 puffs**	**>5 puffs**
Fluticasone	88–176 mcg	176–440 mcg	>440 mcg
MDI:			
44, 110, 220 mcg/puff	**2–3 puffs—44 mcg**	**4–10 puffs—44 mcg or 2–4 puffs—110 mcg**	**>4 puffs—110 mcg or >2 puffs—220 mcg**
DPI:			
50, 100, 250 mcg/dose	**2–4 inhalations—50 mcg**	**2–4 inhalations—100 mcg**	**>4 inhalations—100 mcg or >2 inhalations—250 mcg**
Triamcinolone acetonide	400–800 mcg	800–1,200 mcg	>1,200 mcg
100 mcg/puff	**4–8 puffs**	**8–12 puffs**	**>12 puffs**

- *Clinician judgment of patient response is essential to appropriate dosing.* Once asthma is controlled, medication doses should be carefully titrated to the minimum dose required to maintain control, thus reducing the potential for adverse effect.
- Data from *in vitro* and clinical trials suggest that different inhaled corticosteroid preparations are not equivalent on a per puff or microgram basis. However, few data directly compare the preparations. *The Expert Panel developed recommended dose ranges for different preparations based on available data.*
- Inhaled corticosteroid safety data suggest dose ranges for children equivalent to beclomethasone dipropionate 200–400 mcg/day (low dose), 400–800 mcg/day (medium dose), and >800 mcg/day (high dose).

Dosages of Drugs for Asthma Exacerbations in Emergency Medical Care or Hospital*

Medication	Dosages		Comments
	Adults	Children	
Inhaled short-acting beta₂-agonists			
Albuterol Nebulizer solution (5 mg/mL)	2.5–5 mg every 20 min for 3 doses, then 2.5–10 mg every 1–4 hours as needed, or 10–15 mg/hour continuously.	0.15 mg/kg (minimum dose 2.5 mg) every 20 min for 3 doses, then 0.15–0.3 mg/kg up to 10 mg every 1–4 hours as needed, or 0.5 mg/kg/hour by continuous nebulization.	Only selective beta₂-agonists are recommended. For optimal delivery, dilute aerosols to minimum of 4 mL at gas flow of 6–8 L/min.
Metered-dose inhaler (90 mcg/puff)	4–8 puffs every 20 min up to 4 hours, then every 1–4 hours as needed.	4–8 puffs every 20 min for 3 doses, then every 1–4 hours as needed.	As effective as nebulized therapy if patient is able to coordinate inhalation maneuver. Use spacer/holding chamber.
Bitolterol and pirbuterol			Have not been studied in severe asthma exacerbations.
Systemic (injected) beta₂-agonists			
Epinephrine 1:1000 (1 mg/mL)	0.3–0.5 mg every 20 min for 3 doses SQ.	0.01 mg/kg up to 0.3–0.5 mg every 20 min for 3 doses SQ.	No proven advantage of systemic therapy over aerosol.
Terbutaline (1 mg/mL)	0.25 mg every 20 min for 3 doses SQ.	0.01 mg/kg every 20 min for 3 doses then every 2–6 hours as needed SQ.	No proven advantage of systemic therapy over aerosol.
Anticholinergics			
Ipratropium bromide Nebulizer solution (0.25 mg/mL)	0.5 mg every 30 min for 3 doses then every 2–4 hours as needed.	0.25 mg every 20 min for 3 doses, then every 2 to 4 hours.	May mix in same nebulizer with albuterol. Should not be used as first-line therapy; should be added to beta₂-agonist therapy. Dose delivered from MDI is low and has not been studied in asthma exacerbations.
Metered-dose inhaler (18 mcg/puff)	4–8 puffs as needed.	4–8 puffs as needed.	
Steroids			
Prednisone Methylprednisolone Prednisolone	120–180 mg/day in 3 or 4 divided doses for 48 hours, then 60–80 mg/day until PEF reaches 70% of predicted or personal best.	1 mg/kg every 6 hours for 48 hours then 1–2 mg/kg/day (maximum = 60 mg/day) in 2 divided doses until PEF 70% of predicted or personal best.	Adult "burst" at discharge: 40–60 mg in single or 2 divided doses for 3–10 days. Child "burst" at discharge: 1–2 mg/kg/day, maximum 60 mg/day for 3–10 days.

* For a list of brand names, see glossary page 43.

Glossary*

Asthma Long-Term-Control Medications

Generic name	Brand name
Corticosteroids: Inhaled	
beclomethasone	Beclovent®
	Vanceril®, Vanceril®—Double Strength
budesonide	Pulmicort Turbuhaler®
flunisolide	AeroBid®, AeroBid-M®
fluticasone	Flovent®
triamcinolone	Azmacort®
Cromolyn and Nedocromil: Inhaled	
cromolyn sodium	Intal®
nedocromil sodium	Tilade®
Leukotriene Modifiers: Oral	
zafirlukast	Accolate®
zileuton	Zyflo®
Long-Acting Beta₂-Agonists	
salmeterol (inhaled)	Serevent®
albuterol (extended release)	Volmax®
	Proventil Repetabs®
Theophylline: Oral	
	Aerolate® III
	Aerolate® JR
	Aerolate® SR
	Choledyl® SA
	Elixophyllin®
	Quibron®-T
	Quibron®-T/SR
	Slo-bid®
	Slo-Phyllin®
	Theo-24®
	Theochron®
	Theo-Dur®
	Theolair®
	Theolair®-SR
	T-Phyl®
	Uni-Dur®
	Uniphyl®

Asthma Quick-Relief Medications

Generic name	Brand name
Short-Acting Beta₂-Agonists: Inhaled	
albuterol	Airet®
	Proventil®
	Proventil HFA®
	Ventolin®
	Ventolin® Rotacaps
bitolterol	Tornalate®
pirbuterol	Maxair®
terbutaline	Brethaire®
	Brethine® (tablet only)
	Bricanyl® (tablet only)

** This list does not include metaproterenol, which is not recommended for relief of acute bronchospasm due to its potential for excessive cardiac stimulation, especially in high doses.

Generic name	Brand name
Anticholinergics: Inhaled	
ipratropium bromide	Atrovent®
Corticosteroids: Oral	
methylprednisolone	Medrol®
prednisone	Prednisone
	Deltasone®
	Orasone®
	Liquid Pred®
	Prednisone Intensol®
prednisolone	Prelone®
	Pediapred®

* This glossary is a complete list of brand names associated with the appropriate generic names of asthma medications, as listed in the United States Pharmacopeial Convention, Inc., *Approved Drug Products and Legal Requirements*, Volume III, 17th edition, 1997, and the USP DI *Drug Information for Health Care Professionals*, Volume I, 17th edition, 1997. This list does not constitute an endorsement of these products by the National Heart, Lung, and Blood Institute.

What Everyone Should Know About Asthma Control

You will learn to take care of your asthma over time. For now, you will be off to a good start if you know just five key things. These five things should guide your efforts to take care of your asthma.

Asthma can be managed so that you can live a normal life.

Your asthma should not keep you from doing what you want. It should not keep you from going to work or school. If it does, talk to your doctor about your treatment.

Asthma is a disease that makes the airways in your lungs inflamed.

This means your airways are swollen and sensitive. The swelling is there all of the time, even when you feel just fine. The swelling can be controlled with medicine and by staying away from things that bother your airways.

Many things in your home, school, work, and other places can cause asthma attacks.

An asthma attack occurs when your airways narrow, making it harder to breathe. Asthma attacks are sometimes called flareups, exacerbations, or episodes.

Things in the air that you are allergic to (like pollen) can cause an asthma attack. So can things that bother your airways like tobacco smoke. You can learn to stay away from the things that cause you to have asthma attacks.

Asthma needs to be watched and cared for over a very long time.

Asthma cannot be cured, but it can be treated. You can become free of symptoms all or most of the time. But your asthma does NOT go away when your symptoms go away. You will need to keep taking care of your asthma.

Also, over the years your asthma may change. Your asthma could get worse so you need more medicine. That's why you need to keep in touch with your doctor.

Asthma can be controlled when you manage your asthma and work with your doctor.

You play a big role in taking care of your asthma with your doctor's help. Your job is to:

- Take your medicines as your doctor suggests,
- Watch for signs that your asthma is getting worse and act quickly to stop the attack,
- Stay away from things that can bother your asthma,
- Ask your doctor about any concerns you have about your asthma, and
- See your doctor at least every 6 months.

When you do these things, you will gain—and keep—control of your asthma.

How To Control Things That Make Your Asthma Worse

You can help prevent asthma attacks by staying away from things that make your asthma worse. This guide suggests many ways to help you do this.

You need to find out what makes your asthma worse. Some things that make asthma worse for some people are not a problem for others. You do not need to do all of the things listed in this guide.

Look at the things listed in dark print below. Put a check next to the ones that you know make your asthma worse. Ask your doctor to help you find out what else makes your asthma worse. Then, decide with your doctor what steps you will take. Start with the things in your bedroom that bother your asthma. Try something simple first.

☐ **TOBACCO SMOKE**

- ☐ If you smoke, ask your doctor for ways to help you quit. Ask family members to quit smoking, too.
- ☐ Do not allow smoking in your home or around you.
- ☐ Be sure no one smokes at a child's day care center.

☐ **DUST MITES**

Many people with asthma are allergic to dust mites. Dust mites are like tiny "bugs" you cannot see that live in cloth or carpet.

Things that will help the most:

- ☐ Encase your mattress in a special dust-proof cover.*
- ☐ Encase your pillow in a special dust-proof cover* or wash the pillow each week in hot water. Water must be hotter than 130°F to kill the mites.
- ☐ Wash the sheets and blankets on your bed each week in hot water.

Other things that can help:

- ☐ Reduce indoor humidity to less than 50 percent. Dehumidifiers or central air conditioners can do this.
- ☐ Try not to sleep or lie on cloth-covered cushions or furniture.
- ☐ Remove carpets from your bedroom and those laid on concrete, if you can.
- ☐ Keep stuffed toys out of the bed or wash the toys weekly in hot water.

☐ **ANIMAL DANDER**

Some people are allergic to the flakes of skin or dried saliva from animals with fur or feathers.

The best thing to do:

- ☐ Keep furred or feathered pets out of your home.

If you can't keep the pet outdoors, then:

- ☐ Keep the pet out of your bedroom and keep the bedroom door closed.
- ☐ Cover the air vents in your bedroom with heavy material to filter the air.*
- ☐ Remove carpets and furniture covered with cloth from your home. If that is not possible, keep the pet out of the rooms where these are.

☐ **COCKROACH**

Many people with asthma are allergic to the dried droppings and remains of cockroaches.

- ☐ Keep all food out of your bedroom.
- ☐ Keep food and garbage in closed containers (never leave food out).
- ☐ Use poison baits, powders, gels, or paste (for example, boric acid). You can also use traps.
- ☐ If a spray is used to kill roaches, stay out of the room until the odor goes away.

☐ **VACUUM CLEANING**

- ☐ Try to get someone else to vacuum for you once or twice a week, if you can. Stay out of rooms while they are being vacuumed and for a short while afterward.
- ☐ If you vacuum, use a dust mask (from a hardware store), a double-layered or microfilter vacuum cleaner bag,* or a vacuum cleaner with a HEPA filter.*

☐ **INDOOR MOLD**

- ☐ Fix leaky faucets, pipes, or other sources of water.
- ☐ Clean moldy surfaces with a cleaner that has bleach in it.

☐ **POLLEN AND OUTDOOR MOLD**

What to do during your allergy season (when pollen or mold spore counts are high):

- ☐ Try to keep your windows closed.
- ☐ Stay indoors with windows closed during the midday and afternoon, if you can. Pollen and some mold spore counts are highest at that time.
- ☐ Ask your doctor whether you need to take or increase anti-inflammatory medicine before your allergy season starts.

☐ **SMOKE, STRONG ODORS, AND SPRAYS**

- ☐ If possible, do not use a wood-burning stove, kerosene heater, or fireplace.
- ☐ Try to stay away from strong odors and sprays, such as perfume, talcum powder, hair spray, and paints.

☐ **EXERCISE, SPORTS, WORK, OR PLAY**

- ☐ You should be able to be active without symptoms. See your doctor if you have asthma symptoms when you are active—like when you exercise, do sports, play, or work hard.
- ☐ Ask your doctor about taking medicine before you exercise to prevent symptoms.
- ☐ Warm up for about 6 to 10 minutes before you exercise.
- ☐ Try not to work or play hard outside when the air pollution or pollen levels (if you are allergic to the pollen) are high.

☐ **OTHER THINGS THAT CAN MAKE ASTHMA WORSE**

- ☐ **Flu:** Get a flu shot.
- ☐ **Sulfites in foods:** Do not drink beer or wine or eat shrimp, dried fruit, or processed potatoes if they cause asthma symptoms.
- ☐ **Cold air:** Cover your nose and mouth with a scarf on cold or windy days.
- ☐ **Other medicines:** Tell your doctor about all the medicines you may take. Include cold medicines, aspirin, and even eye drops.

---

*To find out where to get products mentioned in this guide, call:

Asthma and Allergy Foundation of America
(800-727-8462)

Allergy and Asthma Network/Mothers of
Asthmatics, Inc. (800-878-4403)

American Academy of Allergy, Asthma, and Immunology
(800-822-2762)

National Jewish Medical and Research Center
(Lung Line) (800-222-5864)

HOW TO USE YOUR METERED-DOSE INHALER THE RIGHT WAY

Using an inhaler seems simple, but most patients do not use it the right way. When you use your inhaler the wrong way, less medicine gets to your lungs. (Your doctor may give you other types of inhalers.)

For the next 2 weeks, read these steps aloud as you do them or ask someone to read them to you. Ask your doctor or nurse to check how well you are using your inhaler.

Use your inhaler in one of the three ways pictured below (A or B are best, but C can be used if you have trouble with A and B).

Steps for Using Your Inhaler

Getting ready
1. Take off the cap and shake the inhaler.
2. Breathe out all the way.
3. Hold your inhaler the way your doctor said (A, B, or C below).

Breathe in slowly
4. As you start breathing in **slowly** through your mouth, press down on the inhaler **one** time. (If you use a holding chamber, first press down on the inhaler. Within 5 seconds, begin to breathe in slowly.)
5. Keep breathing in **slowly**, as deeply as you can.

Hold your breath
6. Hold your breath as you count to 10 slowly, if you can.
7. For inhaled quick-relief medicine (beta$_2$-agonists), wait about 1 minute between puffs. There is no need to wait between puffs for other medicines.

A. Hold inhaler 1 to 2 inches in front of your mouth (about the width of two fingers).

B. Use a spacer/holding chamber. These come in many shapes and can be useful to any patient.

C. Put the inhaler in your mouth. Do not use for steroids.

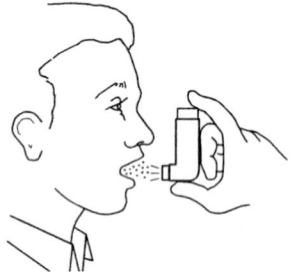

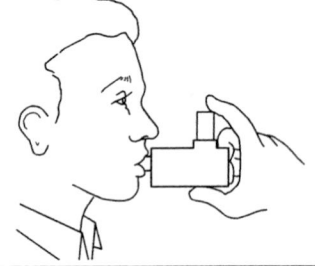

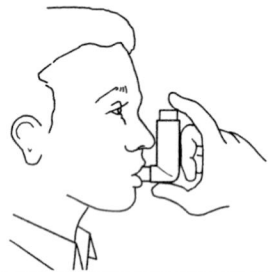

Clean Your Inhaler as Needed

Look at the hole where the medicine sprays out from your inhaler. If you see "powder" in or around the hole, clean the inhaler. Remove the metal canister from the L-shaped plastic mouthpiece. Rinse only the mouthpiece and cap in warm water. Let them dry overnight. In the morning, put the canister back inside. Put the cap on.

Know When To Replace Your Inhaler

For medicines you take each day (an example):
Say your new canister has 200 puffs (number of puffs is listed on canister) and you are told to take 8 puffs per day.

$$8 \text{ puffs per day} \overline{)200 \text{ puffs in}\atop \text{canister}}^{\displaystyle 25 \text{ days}}$$

So this canister will last 25 days.

If you started using this inhaler on May 1, replace it on or before May 25.

You can write the date on your canister.

For quick-relief medicine take as needed and count each puff.

Do not put your canister in water to see if it is empty. This does not work.

ASTHMA ACTION PLAN FOR _____

Doctor's Phone Number _____ Doctor's Name _____ Date _____

Hospital / Emergency Room Phone Number _____

GREEN ZONE: Doing Well

- No cough, wheeze, chest tightness, or shortness of breath during the day or night
- Can do usual activities

And, if a peak flow meter is used,
Peak flow: more than _____
(80% or more of my best peak flow)

My best peak flow is: _____

Take These Long-Term-Control Medicines Each Day (include an anti-inflammatory)

Medicine	How much to take	When to take it

| Before exercise | ☐ | ☐ 2 or ☐ 4 puffs | 5 to 60 minutes before exercise |

YELLOW ZONE: Asthma Is Getting Worse

- Cough, wheeze, chest tightness, or shortness of breath, or
- Waking at night due to asthma, or
- Can do some, but not all, usual activities

-Or-

Peak flow: _____ to _____
(50% - 80% of my best peak flow)

FIRST → Add: **Quick-Relief Medicine – and keep taking your GREEN ZONE medicine**

_____ ☐ 2 or ☐ 4 puffs, every 20 minutes for up to 1 hour
(short-acting beta₂-agonist) ☐ Nebulizer, once

SECOND → If your symptoms (and peak flow, if used) *return to GREEN ZONE* after 1 hour of above treatment:
- ☐ Take the quick-relief medicine every 4 hours for 1 to 2 days.
- ☐ Double the dose of your inhaled steroid for _____ (7-10) days.

-Or-

If your symptoms (and peak flow, if used) *do not return to GREEN ZONE* after 1 hour of above treatment:

- ☐ Take: _____ ☐ 2 or ☐ 4 puffs or ☐ Nebulizer
  (short-acting beta₂-agonist)
- ☐ Add: _____ _____ mg. per day For _____ (3-10) days
  (oral steroid)
- ☐ Call the doctor ☐ before/ ☐ within _____ hours after taking the oral steroid.

RED ZONE: Medical Alert!

- Very short of breath, or
- Quick-relief medicines have not helped, or
- Cannot do usual activities, or
- Symptoms are same or get worse after 24 hours in Yellow Zone

-Or-

Peak flow: less than _____
(50% of my best peak flow)

Take this medicine:

☐ _____ ☐ 4 or ☐ 6 puffs or ☐ Nebulizer
(short-acting beta₂-agonist)

☐ _____ _____ mg.
(oral steroid)

Then call your doctor *NOW*. Go to the hospital or call for an ambulance if:
- You are still in the red zone after 15 minutes AND
- You have not reached your doctor.

DANGER SIGNS

- Trouble walking and talking due to shortness of breath
- Lips or fingernails are blue

→ Take ☐ 4 or ☐ 6 puffs of your quick-relief medicine *AND*
■ Go to the hospital or call for an ambulance (_____) *NOW!*

School Self-Management Plan

Asthma and Allergy
Foundation of America
1125 15th St., N.W., Suite 502
Washington, DC 20005

STUDENT ASTHMA ACTION CARD

Endorsed by

National Asthma
Education Program

ID Photo

Name: _____ Grade: _____ Age: _____

Teacher: _____ Room: _____

Parent/Guardian Name: _____ Ph: (H) _____

Address: _____ Ph: (W) _____

Parent/Guardian Name: _____ Ph: (H) _____

Address: _____ Ph: (W) _____

Emergency Phone Contact #1 _____
                            Name   Relationship   Phone

Emergency Phone Contact #2 _____
                            Name   Relationship   Phone

Physician Student Sees for Asthma: _____ Ph: _____

Other Physician: _____ Ph: _____

DAILY ASTHMA MANAGEMENT PLAN

- **Identify the things which start an asthma episode (Check each that applies to the student.)**

  ☐ Exercise   ☐ Strong odors or fumes   ☐ Other _____

  ☐ Respiratory infections   ☐ Chalk dust   _____

  ☐ Change in temperature   ☐ Carpets in the room

  ☐ Animals   ☐ Pollens

  ☐ Food _____   ☐ Molds

  Comments _____

- **Control of School Environment**

  (List any environmental control measures, pre-medications, and/or dietary restrictions that the student needs to prevent an asthma episode.)

  _____

  _____

  _____

- **Peak Flow Monitoring**

  Personal Best Peak Flow number: _____

  Monitoring Times: _____   _____   _____

- **Daily Medication Plan**

	Name	Amount	When to Use
1.	_____	_____	_____
2.	_____	_____	_____
3.	_____	_____	_____
4.	_____	_____	_____

School Self-Management Plan (continued)

EMERGENCY PLAN

Emergency action is necessary when the student has symptoms such as _____, _____,

_____, _____ or has a peak flow reading of _____.

- **Steps to take during an asthma episode:**

  1. Give medications as listed below.

  2. Have student return to classroom if _____

  _____

  3. Contact parent if _____

  4. Seek emergency medical care if the student has any of the following:

     ✔ No improvement 15-20 minutes after initial treatment
        with medication and a relative cannot be reached.

     ✔ Peak flow of _____

     ✔ Hard time breathing with:

        • Chest and neck pulled in with breathing

        • Child is hunched over

        • Child is struggling to breathe

     ✔ Trouble walking or talking

     ✔ Stops playing and can't start activity again

     ✔ Lips or fingernails are gray or blue

  } *IF THIS HAPPENS, GET EMERGENCY HELP NOW!*

- **Emergency Asthma Medications**

	Name	Amount	When to Use
1.	_____	_____	_____
2.	_____	_____	_____
3.	_____	_____	_____
4.	_____	_____	_____

COMMENTS / SPECIAL INSTRUCTIONS

_____

_____

_____

FOR INHALED MEDICATIONS

☐ I have instructed _____ in the proper way to use his/her medications. It is my professional opinion that _____ should be allowed to carry and use that medication by him/herself.

☐ It is my professional opinion that _____ should not carry his/her inhaled medication by him/herself.

_____   _____
Physician Signature   Date

_____   _____
Parent Signature   Date

How To Use Your Peak Flow Meter

A peak flow meter helps you check how well your asthma is controlled. Peak flow meters are most helpful for people with moderate or severe asthma.

This guide will tell you (1) how to find your personal best peak flow number, (2) how to use your personal best number to set your peak flow zones, (3) how to take your peak flow, and (4) when to take your peak flow to check your asthma each day.

Starting Out: Find Your Personal Best Peak Flow Number

To find your personal best peak flow number, take your peak flow each day for 2 to 3 weeks. Your asthma should be under good control during this time. Take your peak flow as close to the times listed below as you can. (These times for taking your peak flow are only for finding your personal best peak flow. To check your asthma each day, you will take your peak flow in the morning. This is discussed below.)

- Between noon and 2:00 p.m. each day.
- Each time you take your quick-relief medicine to relieve symptoms. (Measure your peak flow <u>after</u> you take your medicine.)
- Any other time your doctor suggests.

Write down the number you get for each peak flow reading. The highest peak flow number you had during the 2 to 3 weeks is your personal best. Your personal best can change over time. Ask your doctor when to check for a new personal best.

Your Peak Flow Zones

Your peak flow zones are based on your personal best peak flow number. The zones will help you check your asthma and take the right actions to keep it controlled. The colors used with each zone come from the traffic light.

 Green Zone (80 to 100 percent of your personal best) signals **good control.** Take your usual daily long-term-control medicines, if you take any. Keep taking these medicines even when you are in the yellow or red zones.

 Yellow Zone (50 to 79 percent of your personal best) signals **caution: your asthma is getting worse.** Add quick-relief medicines. You might need to increase other asthma medicines as directed by your doctor.

 Red Zone (below 50 percent of your personal best) signals **medical alert**! Add or increase quick-relief medicines and call your doctor **now**.

Ask your doctor to write an action plan for you that tells you:

- The peak flow numbers for <u>your</u> green, yellow, and red zones. Mark the zones on your peak flow meter with colored tape or a marker.
- The medicines you should take while in each peak flow zone.

How To Take Your Peak Flow

1. Move the marker to the bottom of the numbered scale.
2. Stand up or sit up straight.
3. Take a deep breath. Fill your lungs all the way.
4. Hold your breath while you place the mouthpiece in your mouth, between your teeth. Close your lips around it. Do **not** put your tongue inside the hole.
5. Blow out as hard and fast as you can. Your peak flow meter will measure how fast you can blow out air.
6. Write down the number you get. But if you cough or make a mistake, do not write down the number. Do it over again.
7. Repeat steps 1 through 6 two more times. Write down the highest of the three numbers. This is your peak flow number.
8. Check to see which peak flow <u>zone</u> your peak flow number is in. Do the actions your doctor told you to do while in that zone.

Your doctor may ask you to write down your peak flow numbers each day. You can do this on a calendar or other paper. This will help you and your doctor see how your asthma is doing over time.

Checking Your Asthma: When To Use Your Peak Flow Meter

- **Every morning** when you wake up, *before* you take medicine. Make this part of your daily routine.

- **When you are having asthma symptoms or an attack.** And after taking medicine for the attack. This can tell you how bad your asthma attack is and whether your medicine is working.

- Any other time your doctor suggests.

  If you use more than one peak flow meter (such as at home and at school), be sure that both meters are the same brand.

Bring to Each of Your Doctor's Visits:

- Your peak flow meter.
- Your peak flow numbers if you have written them down each day.

Also, ask your doctor or nurse to check how you use your peak flow meter—just to be sure you are doing it right.

Patient Self-Assessment Form for Environmental and Other Factors That Can Make Asthma Worse

PATIENT NAME: _____ DATE: _____

Do you cough, wheeze, have chest tightness, or feel short of breath year-round? (If no, go to next question)	No _____	Yes _____
If yes:		
• Are there **pets** or animals in your home, school, or day care?	No _____	Yes _____
• Is there moisture or **dampness** in any room of your home?	No _____	Yes _____
• Have you seen **mold** or smelled musty odors any place in your home?	No _____	Yes _____
• Have you seen **cockroaches** in your home?	No _____	Yes _____
• Do you use a **humidifier** or swamp cooler in your home?	No _____	Yes _____
Does your coughing, wheezing, chest tightness, or shortness of breath get worse at certain times of the year? (If no, go to next question)	No _____	Yes _____
If yes:		
Do your symptoms get worse in the:		
• Early spring? (Trees)	No _____	Yes _____
• Late spring? (Grasses)	No _____	Yes _____
• Late summer to autumn? (Weeds)	No _____	Yes _____
• Summer and fall? (*Alternaria, Cladosporium*)	No _____	Yes _____
Do you **smoke**?	No _____	Yes _____
Does anyone smoke at home, work, or day care?	No _____	Yes _____
Is a **wood-burning stove or fireplace** used in your home?	No _____	Yes _____
Are **kerosene, oil, or gas stoves or heaters** used without vents in your home?	No _____	Yes _____
Are you exposed to **fumes or odors** from cleaning agents, sprays, or other chemicals?	No _____	Yes _____
Do you cough or wheeze during the week, but not on weekends when away from **work or school**?	No _____	Yes _____
Do your eyes and nose get irritated soon after you get to work or school?	No _____	Yes _____
Do your coworkers or classmates have symptoms like yours?	No _____	Yes _____
Are isocyanates, plant or animal products, smoke, gases, or fumes used where you work?	No _____	Yes _____
Is it cold, hot, dusty, or humid where you work?	No _____	Yes _____
Do you have a **stuffy nose** or postnasal drip, either at certain times of the year or year-round?	No _____	Yes _____
Do you sneeze often or have itchy, watery eyes?	No _____	Yes _____
Do you have **heartburn**?	No _____	Yes _____
Does food sometimes come up into your throat?	No _____	Yes _____
Have you had coughing, wheezing, or shortness of breath at night in the past 4 weeks?	No _____	Yes _____
Does your infant vomit then cough or have wheezy cough at night?	No _____	Yes _____
Are these symptoms worse after feeding?	No _____	Yes _____

Patient Self-Assessment Form for Environmental and Other Factors That Can Make Asthma Worse, *continued*

Have you had wheezing, coughing, or shortness of breath **after eating** shrimp, dried fruit, or canned or processed potatoes?	No _____	Yes _____
After drinking beer or wine?	No _____	Yes _____
Are you taking any prescription medicines or over-the-counter **medicines**?	No _____	Yes _____
If yes, which ones?	No _____	Yes _____
_____		
Do you use eye drops?	No _____	Yes _____
Do you use any medicines that contain beta-blockers (e.g., blood pressure medicine)?	No _____	Yes _____
Do you ever take aspirin or other nonsteroidal anti-inflammatory drugs (like ibuprofen)?	No _____	Yes _____
Have you ever had coughing, wheezing, chest tightness, or shortness of breath after taking any medication?	No _____	Yes _____
Do you cough, wheeze, have chest tightness, or feel short of breath during or after **exercising**?	No _____	Yes _____

Patient Self-Assessment Form for Followup Visits

PATIENT NAME: _____　DATE: _____

Please answer the questions below in the space provided on the right.

Since your last visit:

1. Has your asthma been any worse?　　　　　　　　　　　　　　　No _____　Yes _____

2. Have there been any changes in your home, work, or school environment (such as a new pet, someone smoking)?　　　　　　　No _____　Yes _____

3. Have you had any times when your symptoms were a lot worse than usual?　　　　　　　　　　　　　　　　　　　　　No _____　Yes _____

4. Has your asthma caused you to miss work or school or reduce or change your activities?　　　　　　　　　　　　　　No _____　Yes _____

5. Have you missed any regular doses of your medicines for any reason?　No _____　Yes _____

6. Have your medications caused you any problems? (shakiness, nervousness, bad taste, sore throat, cough, upset stomach)　　No _____　Yes _____

7. Have you had any emergency room visits or hospital stays for asthma?　No _____　Yes _____

8. Has the cost of your asthma treatment kept you from getting the medicine or care you need for your asthma?　　　　　　No _____　Yes _____

In the past 2 weeks,

9. Have you had a cough, wheezing, shortness of breath or chest tightness during:

   • the day　　　　　　　　　　　　　　　　　　　　　　No _____　Yes _____

   • night　　　　　　　　　　　　　　　　　　　　　　　No _____　Yes _____

   • exercise or play?　　　　　　　　　　　　　　　　　　No _____　Yes _____

10. (If you use a peak flow meter) Did your peak flow go below 80 percent of your personal best?　　　　　　　　　　　　No _____　Yes _____

11. How many days have you used your inhaled quick-relief medicine?　Number of days _____

12. Have you been satisfied with the way your asthma has been?　　No _____　Yes _____

13. What are some concerns or questions you would like us to address at this visit?

_____

_____

_____

_____

For staff use.

☐ Peak Flow Technique

☐ MDI Technique

☐ Reviewed Action Plan:　　☐ Daily meds　　☐ Emergency meds

Diagnosis and Evaluation of the Child With Attention-Deficit/Hyperactivity Disorder

- *Clinical Practice Guideline*
- *Technical Report Summary*

AMERICAN ACADEMY OF PEDIATRICS

Committee on Quality Improvement, Subcommittee on Attention-Deficit/Hyperactivity Disorder

Clinical Practice Guideline: Diagnosis and Evaluation of the Child With Attention-Deficit/Hyperactivity Disorder

ABSTRACT. This clinical practice guideline provides recommendations for the assessment and diagnosis of school-aged children with attention-deficit/hyperactivity disorder (ADHD). This guideline, the first of 2 sets of guidelines to provide recommendations on this condition, is intended for use by primary care clinicians working in primary care settings. The second set of guidelines will address the issue of treatment of children with ADHD.

The Committee on Quality Improvement of the American Academy of Pediatrics selected a committee composed of pediatricians and other experts in the fields of neurology, psychology, child psychiatry, development, and education, as well as experts from epidemiology and pediatric practice. In addition, this panel consists of experts in education and family practice. The panel worked with Technical Resources International, Washington, DC, under the auspices of the Agency for Healthcare Research and Quality, to develop the evidence base of literature on this topic. The resulting evidence report was used to formulate recommendations for evaluation of the child with ADHD. Major issues contained within the guideline address child and family assessment; school assessment, including the use of various rating scales; and conditions seen frequently among children with ADHD. Information is also included on the use of current diagnostic coding strategies. The deliberations of the committee were informed by a systematic review of evidence about prevalence, coexisting conditions, and diagnostic tests. Committee decisions were made by consensus where definitive evidence was not available. The committee report underwent review by sections of the American Academy of Pediatrics and external organizations before approval by the Board of Directors.

The guideline contains the following recommendations for diagnosis of ADHD: 1) in a child 6 to 12 years old who presents with inattention, hyperactivity, impulsivity, academic underachievement, or behavior problems, primary care clinicians should initiate an evaluation for ADHD; 2) the diagnosis of ADHD requires that a child meet *Diagnostic and Statistical Manual of Mental Disorders, Fourth Edition* criteria; 3) the assessment of ADHD requires evidence directly obtained from parents or caregivers regarding the core symptoms of ADHD in various settings, the age of onset, duration of symptoms, and degree of functional impairment; 4) the assessment of ADHD requires evidence directly obtained from the classroom teacher (or other school professional) regarding the core symptoms of ADHD, duration of symptoms, degree of functional impairment, and associated conditions; 5) evaluation of the child with ADHD should include assessment for associated (coexisting) conditions; and 6) other diagnostic tests are not routinely indicated to establish the diagnosis of ADHD but may be used for the assessment of other coexisting conditions (eg, learning disabilities and mental retardation).

This clinical practice guideline is not intended as a sole source of guidance in the evaluation of children with ADHD. Rather, it is designed to assist primary care clinicians by providing a framework for diagnostic decisionmaking. It is not intended to replace clinical judgment or to establish a protocol for all children with this condition and may not provide the only appropriate approach to this problem.

ABBREVIATIONS. ADHD, attention-deficit/hyperactivity disorder; DSM-IV, *Diagnostic and Statistical Manual of Mental Disorders, Fourth Edition*; AAP, American Academy of Pediatrics; DSM-PC, *Diagnostic and Statistical Manual for Primary Care.*

Attention-deficit/hyperactivity disorder (ADHD) is the most common neurobehavioral disorder of childhood. ADHD is also among the most prevalent chronic health conditions affecting school-aged children. The core symptoms of ADHD include inattention, hyperactivity, and impulsivity.[1,2] Children with ADHD may experience significant functional problems, such as school difficulties, academic underachievement,[3] troublesome interpersonal relationships with family members[4,5] and peers, and low self-esteem. Individuals with ADHD present in childhood and may continue to show symptoms as they enter adolescence[6] and adult life.[7] Pediatricians and other primary care clinicians frequently are asked by parents and teachers to evaluate a child for ADHD. Early recognition, assessment, and management of this condition can redirect the educational and psychosocial development of most children with ADHD.[8,9]

Recorded prevalence rates for ADHD vary substantially, partly because of changing diagnostic criteria over time,[10–13] and partly because of variations in ascertainment in different settings and the frequent use of referred samples to estimate rates. Practitioners of all types (primary care, subspecialty, psychiatry, and nonphysician mental health providers) vary greatly in the degree to which they use *Diagnostic and Statistical Manual of Mental Health Disorders, Fourth Edition* (DSM-IV) criteria to diagnose ADHD. Reported rates also vary substantially in different geographic areas and across countries.[14]

With increasing epidemiologic and clinical research, diagnostic criteria have been revised on mul-

The recommendations in this statement do not indicate an exclusive course of treatment or serve as a standard of medical care. Variations, taking into account individual circumstances, may be appropriate.
PEDIATRICS (ISSN 0031 4005). Copyright © 2000 by the American Academy of Pediatrics.

tiple occasions over the past 20 years.[10–13] A recent review of prevalence rates in school-aged community samples (rather than referred samples) indicates rates varying from 4% to 12%, with estimated prevalence based on combining these studies of ~8% to 10%. In the general population,[15–23,24] 9.2% (5.8%–13.6%) of males and 2.9% (1.9%–4.5%) of females are found to have behaviors consistent with ADHD. With the *DSM-IV* criteria (compared with earlier versions), more females have been diagnosed with the predominantly inattentive type.[25,26] Prevalence rates also vary significantly depending on whether they reflect school samples 6.9% (5.5%–8.5%) versus community samples 10.3% (8.2%–12.7%).

Public interest in ADHD has increased along with debate in the media concerning the diagnostic process and treatment strategies.[27] Concern has been expressed about the over-diagnosis of ADHD by pointing to the several-fold increase in prescriptions for stimulant medication among children during the past decade.[28] In addition, there are significant regional variations in the amount of stimulants prescribed by physicians.[29] Practice surveys among primary care pediatricians and family physicians reveal wide variations in practice patterns about diagnostic criteria and methods.[30]

ADHD commonly occurs in association with oppositional defiant disorder, conduct disorder, depression, anxiety disorder,[16] and with many developmental disorders, such as speech and language delays and learning disabilities.

This diagnostic guideline is intended for use by primary care clinicians to evaluate children between 6 and 12 years of age for ADHD, consistent with best available empirical studies. Special attention is given to assessing school performance and behavior, family functioning, and adaptation. In light of the high prevalence of ADHD in pediatric practice, the guideline should assist primary care clinicians in these assessments. The diagnosis usually requires several steps. Clinicians will generally need to carry out the evaluation in more than 1 visit, often indeed 2 to 3 visits. The guideline is not intended for children with mental retardation, pervasive developmental disorder, moderate to severe sensory deficits such as visual and hearing impairment, chronic disorders associated with medications that may affect behavior, and those who have experienced child abuse and sexual abuse. These children too may have ADHD, and this guideline may help clinicians in considering this diagnosis; nonetheless, this guideline primarily reviews evidence relating to the diagnosis of ADHD in relatively uncomplicated cases in primary care settings.

METHODOLOGY

To initiate the development of a practice guideline for the diagnosis and evaluation of children with ADHD directed toward primary care physicians, the American Academy of Pediatrics (AAP) worked with several colleague organizations to organize a working panel representing a wide range of primary care and subspecialty groups. The committee, chaired by 2 general pediatricians (1 with substantial additional experience and training in developmental and behavioral pediatrics), included representatives from the American Academy of Family Physicians, the American Academy of Child and Adolescent Psychiatry, the Child Neurology Society, and the Society for Pediatric Psychology, as well as developmental and behavioral pediatricians and epidemiologists.

This group met over a period of 2 years, during which it reviewed basic literature on current practices in the diagnosis of ADHD and developed a series of questions to direct an evidence-based review of the prevalence of ADHD in community and primary care practice settings, the rates of coexisting conditions, and the utility of several diagnostic methods and devices. The AAP committee collaborated with the Agency for Healthcare Research and Quality in its support of an evidence-based review of several of these key items in the diagnosis of ADHD. David Atkins, MD, provided liaison from the Agency for Healthcare Research and Quality, and Technical Resources International conducted the evidence review.

The Technical Resources International report focused on 4 specific areas for the literature review: the prevalence of ADHD among children 6 to 12 years of age in the general population and the coexisting conditions that may occur with ADHD; the prevalence of ADHD among children in primary care settings and the coexisting conditions that may occur; the accuracy of various screening methods for diagnosis; and the prevalence of abnormal findings on commonly used medical screening tests. The literature search was conducted using Medline and PsycINFO databases, references from review articles, rating scale manuals, and articles identified by the subcommittee. Only articles published in English between 1980 and 1997 were included. The study population was limited to children 6 to 12 years of age, and only studies using general, unselected populations in communities, schools, or the primary clinical setting were used. Data on screening tests were taken from studies conducted in any setting. Articles accepted for analysis were abstracted twice by trained personnel and a clinical specialist. Both abstracts for each article were compared and differences between them resolved. A multiple logistic regression model with random effects was used to analyze simultaneously for age, gender, diagnostic tool, and setting using EGRET software. Results were presented in evidence tables and published in the final evidence report.[24]

The draft practice guideline underwent extensive peer review by committees and sections within the AAP, by numerous outside organizations, and by other individuals identified by the subcommittee. Liaisons to the subcommittee also were invited to distribute the draft to entities within their organizations. The resulting comments were compiled and reviewed by the subcommittee co-chairpersons, and relevant changes were incorporated into the draft based on recommendations from peer reviewers.

The recommendations contained in the practice guideline are based on the best available data (Fig 1).

Where data were lacking, a combination of evidence and expert consensus was used. Strong recommendations were based on high-quality scientific evidence, or, in the absence of high-quality data, strong expert consensus. Fair and weak recommendations were based on lesser quality or limited data and expert consensus. Clinical options were identified as interventions because the subcommittee could not find compelling evidence for or against. These clinical options are interventions that a reasonable health care provider might or might not wish to implement in his or her practice.

RECOMMENDATION 1: In a child 6 to 12 years old who presents with inattention, hyperactivity, impulsivity, academic underachievement, or behavior problems, primary care clinicians should initiate an evaluation for ADHD (strength of evidence: good; strength of recommendation: strong).

The major justification for this recommendation is the high prevalence of ADHD in school-aged populations. School-aged children with a variety of developmental and behavioral concerns present to primary care clinicians.[31] Primary care pediatricians and family physicians recognize behavior problems that may impact academic achievement in 18% of school-aged children seen in their offices and clinics. Hyperactivity or inattention is diagnosed in 9% of children.[32]

Presentations of ADHD in clinical practice vary. In many cases, concerns derive from parents, teachers, other professionals, or nonparental caregivers. Common presentations include referral from school for academic underachievement and failure, disruptive classroom behavior, inattentiveness, problems with social relationships, parental concerns regarding similar phenomena, poor self-esteem, or problems with establishing or maintaining social relationships. Children with core ADHD symptoms of hyperactivity and impulsivity are identified by teachers, because they often disrupt the classroom. Even mild distractibility and motor symptoms, such as fidgetiness, will be apparent to most teachers. In contrast, children with the inattentive subtype of ADHD, where hyperactive and impulsive symptoms are absent or minimal, may not come to the attention of teachers. These children may present with school underachievement.

Symptoms may not be apparent in a structured clinical setting that is free from the demands and distraction of the home and school.[33] Thus, if parents do not bring concerns to the primary clinician, then early detection of ADHD in primary care may not occur. Clinical practices during routine health supervision may assist in early recognition of ADHD.[34,35] Options include direct history from parents and children. The following general questions may be useful at all visits for school-aged children to heighten attention about ADHD and as an initial screening for school performance.

1. How is your child doing in school?
2. Are there any problems with learning that you or the teacher has seen?
3. Is your child happy in school?
4. Are you concerned with any behavioral problems in school, at home, or when your child is playing with friends?
5. Is your child having problems completing classwork or homework?

Alternatively, a previsit questionnaire may be sent to parents or given while the family is waiting in the reception area.[36] When making an appointment for a health supervision visit for a school-aged child, 1 or 2 of these questions may be asked routinely to sensitize parents to the concerns of their child's clinician. For example, "Your child's clinician is interested in how your child is doing in school. You might check with her teacher and discuss any concerns with your child's physician." Wall posters, pamphlets, and books in the waiting area that focus on educational achievements and school-aged behaviors send a message that this is an office or clinic that considers these issues important to a child's development.[37]

RECOMMENDATION 2: The diagnosis of ADHD requires that a child meet DSM-IV criteria (strength of evidence: good; strength of recommendation: strong).

Establishing a diagnosis of ADHD requires a strategy that minimizes over-identification and under-identification. Pediatricians and other primary care health professionals should apply *DSM-IV* criteria in the context of their clinical assessment of a child. The use of specific criteria will help to ensure a more accurate diagnosis and decrease variation in how the diagnosis is made. The *DSM-IV* criteria, developed through several iterations by the American Psychiatric Association, are based on clinical experience and an expanding research foundation.[13] These criteria have more support in the literature than other available diagnostic criteria. The *DSM-IV* specification of behavior items, required numbers of items, and levels of impairment reflect the current consensus among clinicians, particularly psychiatry. The consensus includes increasing research evidence, particularly in the distinctions that the *DSM-IV* makes for the dimensions of attention and hyperactivity-impulsivity.[38]

The *DSM-IV* criteria define 3 subtypes of ADHD (see Table 1 for specific inattention and hyperactive-impulsive items).

- ADHD primarily of the inattentive type (ADHD/I, meeting at least 6 of 9 inattention behaviors)
- ADHD primarily of the hyperactive-impulsive type (ADHD/HI, meeting at least 6 of 9 hyperactive-impulsive behaviors)
- ADHD combined type (ADHD/C, meeting at least 6 of 9 behaviors in both the inattention and hyperactive-impulsive lists)

Children who meet diagnostic criteria for the behavioral symptoms of ADHD but who demonstrate no functional impairment do not meet the diagnostic criteria for ADHD.[13] The symptoms of ADHD should be present in 2 or more settings (eg, at home and in school), and the behaviors must adversely affect

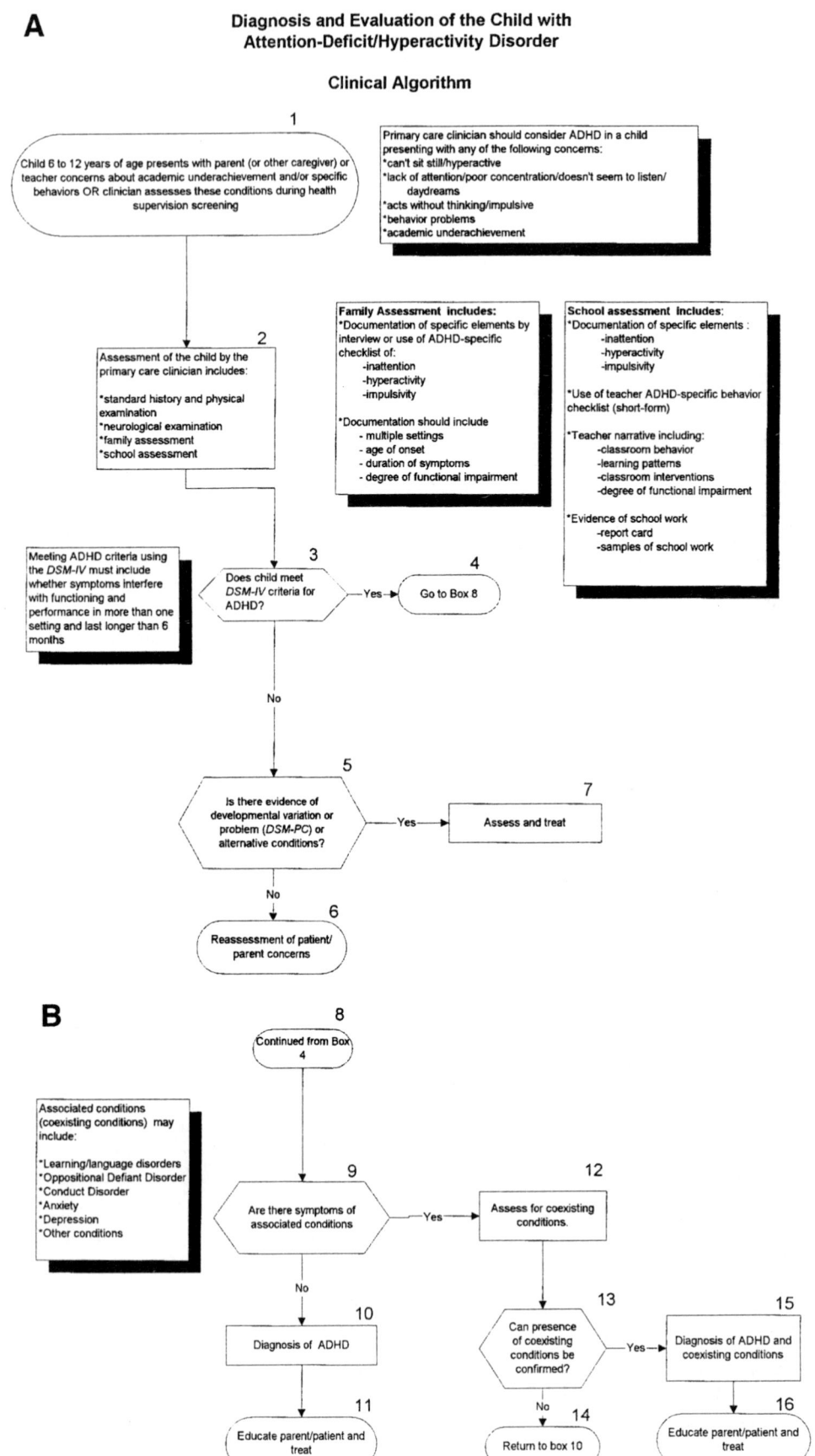

Fig 1. Clinical algorithm.

TABLE 1. Diagnostic Criteria for ADHD

A. Either 1 or 2
  1) Six (or more) of the following symptoms of **inattention** have persisted for at least 6 months to a degree that is maladaptive and inconsistent with developmental level:

Inattention
  a) Often fails to give close attention to details or makes careless mistakes in schoolwork, work, or other activities
  b) Often has difficulty sustaining attention in tasks or play activities
  c) Often does not seem to listen when spoken to directly
  d) Often does not follow through on instructions and fails to finish schoolwork, chores, or duties in the workplace (not due to oppositional behavior or failure to understand instructions)
  e) Often has difficulty organizing tasks and activities
  f) Often avoids, dislikes, or is reluctant to engage in tasks that require sustained mental effort (such as schoolwork or homework)
  g) Often loses things necessary for tasks or activities (eg, toys, school assignments, pencils, books, or tools)
  h) Is often easily distracted by extraneous stimuli
  i) Is often forgetful in daily activities
  2) Six (or more) of the following symptoms of **hyperactivity-impulsivity** have persisted for at least 6 months to a degree that is maladaptive and inconsistent with developmental level:

Hyperactivity
  a) Often fidgets with hands or feet or squirms in seat
  b) Often leaves seat in classroom or in other situations in which remaining seated is expected
  c) Often runs about or climbs excessively in situations in which it is inappropriate (in adolescents or adults, may be limited to subjective feelings of restlessness)
  d) Often has difficulty playing or engaging in leisure activities quietly
  e) Is often "on the go" or often acts as if "driven by a motor"
  f) Often talks excessively

Impulsivity
  g) Often blurts out answers before questions have been completed
  h) Often has difficulty awaiting turn
  i) Often interrupts or intrudes on others (eg, butts into conversations or games)
B. Some hyperactive-impulsive or inattentive symptoms that caused impairment were present before 7 years of age.
C. Some impairment from the symptoms is present in 2 or more settings (eg, at school [or work] or at home).
D. There must be clear evidence of clinically significant impairment in social, academic, or occupational functioning.
E. The symptoms do not occur exclusively during the course of a pervasive developmental disorder, schizophrenia, or other psychotic disorder and are not better accounted for by another mental disorder (eg, mood disorder, anxiety disorder, dissociative disorder, or personality disorder).
Code based on type:
314.01 Attention-Deficit/Hyperactivity Disorder, Combined Type: if both criteria A1 and A2 are met for the past 6 months
314.00 Attention-Deficit/Hyperactivity Disorder, Predominantly Inattentive Type: if criterion A1 is met but criterion A2 is not met for the past 6 months
314.01 Attention-Deficit/Hyperactivity Disorder, Predominantly Hyperactive, Impulsive Type: if criterion A2 is met but criterion A1 is not met for the past 6 months
314.9 Attention-Deficit/Hyperactivity Disorder Not Otherwise Specified

Reprinted with permission from the *Diagnostic and Statistical Manual of Mental Disorders, 4th Ed. (DSM-IV)*. Copyright 1994. American Psychiatric Association.

functioning in school or in a social situation. Reliable and clinically valid measures of dysfunction applicable to the primary care setting have been difficult to develop. The diagnosis comes from a synthesis of information obtained from parents; school reports; mental health care professionals, if they have been involved; and an interview/examination of the child. Current *DSM-IV* criteria require evidence of symptoms before 7 years of age. In some cases, the symptoms of ADHD may not be recognized by parents or teachers until the child is older than 7 years of age, when school tasks become more challenging. Age of onset and duration of symptoms may be obtained from parents in the course of a comprehensive history.

Teachers, parents, and child health professionals typically encounter children with behaviors relating to activity, impulsivity, and attention who may not fully meet *DSM-IV* criteria. The *Diagnostic and Statistical Manual for Primary Care (DSM-PC), Child and Adolescent Version*,[39] provides a guide to the more common behaviors seen in pediatrics. The manual describes common variations in behavior, as well as more problematic behaviors, at levels less than those

specified in the *DSM-IV* (and with less impairment). The behavioral descriptions of the *DSM-PC* have not yet been tested in community studies to determine the prevalence or severity of developmental variations and moderate problems in the areas of inattention and hyperactivity or impulsivity. They do, however, provide guidance to clinicians in the evaluation of children with these symptoms and help to direct clinicians to many elements of treatment for children with problems with attention, hyperactivity, or impulsivity (Tables 2 and 3). The *DSM-PC* also considers environmental influences on a child's behavior and provides information on differential diagnosis with a developmental perspective.

Given the lack of methods to confirm the diagnosis of ADHD through other means, it is important to recognize the limitations of the *DSM-IV* definition. Most of the development and testing of the *DSM-IV* has occurred through studies of children seen in psychiatric settings. Much less is known about its use in other populations, such as those seen in general pediatric or family practice settings. Despite the agreement of many professionals working in this field, the *DSM-IV* criteria remain a consensus with-

TABLE 2.   *DSM-PC: Developmental Variation: Impulsive/Hyperactive Behaviors*

Developmental Variation	Common Developmental Presentations
V65.49 Hyperactive/impulsive variation Young children in infancy and in the preschool years are normally very active and impulsive and may need constant supervision to avoid injury. Their constant activity may be stressful to adults who do not have the energy or patience to tolerate the behavior. During school years and adolescence, activity may be high in play situations and impulsive behaviors may normally occur, especially in peer pressure situations. High levels of hyperactive/impulsive behavior do not indicate a problem or disorder if the behavior does not impair function.	*Early childhood* The child runs in circles, doesn't stop to rest, may bang into objects or people, and asks questions constantly. *Middle childhood* The child plays active games for long periods. The child may occasionally do things impulsively, particularly when excited. *Adolescence* The adolescent engages in active social activities (eg, dancing) for long periods, may engage in risky behaviors with peers.

	Special Information
	Activity should be thought of not only in terms of actual movement, but also in terms of variations in responding to touch, pressure, sound, light, and other sensations. Also, for the infant and young child, activity and attention are related to the interactions between the child and caregiver, eg, when sharing attention and playing together. Activity and impulsivity often normally increase when the child is tired or hungry and decrease when sources of fatigue or hunger are addressed. Activity normally may increase in new situations or when the child may be anxious. Familiarity then reduces activity. Both activity and impulsivity must be judged in the context of the caregiver's expectations and the level of stress experienced by the caregiver. When expectations are unreasonable, the stress level is high, and/or the parent has an emotional disorder (especially depression), the adult may exaggerate the child's level of activity/impulsivity. Activity level is a variable of temperature. The activity level of some children is on the high end of normal from birth and continues to be high throughout their development.

Taken from: American Academy of Pediatrics. *The Classification of Child and Adolescent Mental Diagnoses in Primary Care. Diagnostic and Statistical Manual for Primary Care (DSM-PC), Child and Adolescent Version.* Elk Grove Village, IL: American Academy of Pediatrics; 1996

out clear empirical data supporting the number of items required for the diagnosis. Current criteria do not take into account gender differences or developmental variations in behavior. Furthermore, the behavioral characteristics specified in the *DSM-IV*, despite efforts to standardize them, remain subjective and may be interpreted differently by different observers. Continuing research will likely clarify the validity of the *DSM-IV* criteria (and subsequent modifications) in the diagnosis. These complexities in the diagnosis mean that clinicians using *DSM-IV* criteria must apply them in the context of their clinical judgment.

No instruments used in primary care practice reliably assess the nature or degree of functional impairment of children with ADHD. With information obtained from the parent and school, the clinician can make a clinical judgment about the effect of the core and associated symptoms of ADHD on aca-

demic achievement, classroom performance, family and social relationships, independent functioning, self-esteem, leisure activities, and self-care (such as bathing, toileting, dressing, and eating).

The following 2 recommendations establish the presence of core behavior symptoms in multiple settings.

RECOMMENDATION 3: The assessment of ADHD requires evidence directly obtained from parents or caregivers regarding the core symptoms of ADHD in various settings, the age of onset, duration of symptoms, and degree of functional impairment (strength of evidence: good; strength of recommendation: strong).

Behavior symptoms may be obtained from parents or guardians using 1 or more methods, including open-ended questions (eg, "What are your concerns about your child's behavior in school?"), focused

TABLE 3. *DSM-PC: Developmental Variation: Inattentive Behaviors*

Developmental Variation	Common Developmental Presentations
V65.49 Inattention variation A young child will have a short attention span that will increase as the child matures. The inattention should be appropriate for the child's level of development and not cause any impairment.	*Early childhood* The preschooler has difficulty attending, except briefly, to a storybook or a quiet task such as coloring or drawing. *Middle childhood* The child may not persist very long with a task the child does not want to do such as read an assigned book, homework, or a task that requires concentration such as cleaning something. *Adolescence* The adolescent is easily distracted from tasks he or she does not desire to perform.

	Special Information
	Infants and preschoolers usually have very short attention spans and normally do not persist with activities for long, so that diagnosing this problem in younger children may be difficult. Some parents may have a low tolerance for developmentally appropriate inattention. Although watching television cartoons for long periods of time appears to reflect a long attention span, it does not reflect longer attention spans because most television segments require short (2- to 3-minute) attention spans and they are very stimulating. Normally, attention span varies greatly depending upon the child's or adolescent's interest and skill in the activity, so much so that a short attention span for a particular task may reflect the child's skill or interest in that task.

Taken from: American Academy of Pediatrics. *The Classification of Child and Adolescent Mental Diagnoses in Primary Care. Diagnostic and Statistical Manual for Primary Care (DSM-PC), Child and Adolescent Version.* Elk Grove Village, IL: American Academy of Pediatrics; 1996

questions about specific behaviors, semi-structured interview schedules, questionnaires, and rating scales. Clinicians who obtain information from open-ended or focused questions must obtain and record the relevant behaviors of inattention, hyperactivity, and impulsivity from the *DSM-IV*. The use of global clinical impressions or general descriptions within the domains of attention and activity is insufficient to diagnose ADHD. As data are gathered about the child's behavior, an opportunity becomes available to evaluate the family environment and parenting style. In this way, behavioral symptoms may be evaluated in the context of the environment that may have important characteristics for a particular child.

Specific questionnaires and rating scales have been developed to review and quantify the behavioral characteristics of ADHD (Table 4). The ADHD-specific questionnaires and rating scales have been shown to have an odds ratio greater than 3.0 (equivalent to sensitivity and specificity greater than 94%) in studies differentiating children with ADHD from normal, age-matched, community controls.[24] Thus, ADHD-specific rating scales accurately distinguish between children with and without the diagnosis of ADHD. Almost all studies of these scales and checklists have taken place under ideal conditions, ie, comparing children in referral sites with apparently

healthy children. These instruments may function less well in primary care clinicians' offices than indicated in the tables. In addition, questions on which these rating scales are based are subjective and subject to bias. Thus, their results may convey a false sense of validity and must be interpreted in the context of the overall evaluation of the child. Whether these scales provide additional benefit beyond careful clinical assessment informed by *DSM-IV* criteria is not known. *RECOMMENDATION 3A: Use of these scales is a clinical option when evaluating children for ADHD (strength of evidence: strong; strength of recommendation: strong).*

Global, nonspecific questionnaires and rating scales that assess a variety of behavioral conditions, in contrast with the ADHD-specific measures, generally have an odds ratio <2.0 (equivalent to sensitivity and specificity <86%) in studies differentiating children referred to psychiatric practices from children who were not referred to psychiatric practices (Table 5). Thus, these broadband scales do not distinguish well between children with and without ADHD. *RECOMMENDATION 3B: Use of broadband scales is not recommended in the diagnosis of children for ADHD, although they may be useful for other purposes (strength of evidence: strong; strength of recommendation: strong).*

TABLE 4.   Total ADHD-Specific Checklists: Ability to Detect ADHD vs Normal Controls

Study	Behavior Rating Scale	Age	Gender	Effect Size	95% Confidence Limits
Conners (1997)	CPRS-R:L-ADHD Index (Conners Parent Rating Scale—1997 Revised Version: Long Form, ADHD Index Scale)	6–17	MF	3.1	2.5, 3.7
Conners (1997)	CTRS-R:L-ADHD Index (Conners Teacher Rating Scale—1997 Revised Version: Long Form, ADHD Index Scale)	6–17	MF	3.3	2.8, 3.8
Conners (1997)	CPRS-R:L-*DSM-IV* Symptoms (Conners Parent Rating Scale—1997 Revised Version: Long Form, *DSM-IV* Symptoms Scale)	6–17	MF	3.4	2.8, 4.0
Conners (1997)	CTRS-R:L-*DSM-IV* Symptoms (Conners Teacher Rating Scale—1997 Revised Version: Long Form, *DSM-IV* Symptoms Scale)	6–17	MF	3.7	3.2, 4.2
Breen (1989)	SSQ-O-I Barkley's School Situations Questionnaire-Original Version, Number of Problem Settings Scale	6–11	F	1.3	0.5, 2.2
Breen (1989)	SSQ-O-II Barkley's School Situations Questionnaire-Original Version, Mean Severity Scale	6–11	F	2.0	1.0, 2.9
Combined				2.9	2.2, 3.5

Taken from: Green M, Wong M, Atkins D, et al. *Diagnosis of Attention Deficit/Hyperactivity Disorder. Technical Review 3.* Rockville, MD: US Department of Health and Human Services, Agency for Health Care Policy and Research; 1999. AHCPR publication 99-0050

TABLE 5.   Total Scales of Broadband Checklists: Ability to Detect Referred vs Nonreferred

Study	Behavior Rating Scale	Age	Gender	Effect Size	95% Confidence Limits
Achenbach (1991b)	CBCL/4-18-R, Total Problem Scale (Child Behavior Checklist for Ages 4–18, Parent Form)	4–11	M	1.4	1.3, 1.5
Achenbach (1991b)	Same as above	4–11	F	1.3	1.2, 1.4
Achenbach (1991c)	CBCL/TRF-R, Total Problem Scale (Child Behavior Checklist, Teacher Form)	5–11	M	1.2	1.0, 1.4
Achenbach (1991c)	Same as above	5–11	F	1.1	1.0, 1.3
Naglieri, LeBuffe, Pfeiffer (1994)	DSMD-Total Scale (Devereaux Scales of Mental Disorders)	5–12	MF	1.0	0.8, 1.3
Conners (1997)	CPRS-R:L-Global Problem Index (1997 Revision of Conners Parent Rating Scale, Long Version)	—	MF	2.3	1.9, 2.6
Conners (1997)	CTRS-R:L-Global Problem Index (1997 Revision of Conners Teacher Rating Scale, Long Version)	—	MF	2.0	1.7, 2.3
Combined				1.5	1.2, 1.8

Taken from: Green M, Wong M, Atkins D, et al. *Diagnosis of Attention Deficit/Hyperactivity Disorder. Technical Review 3.* Rockville, MD: US Department of Health and Human Services, Agency for Health Care Policy and Research; 1999. AHCPR publication 99-0050.

More research is needed on the use of the ADHD-specific and global rating scales in pediatric practices for the purposes of differentiating children with ADHD from other children with different behavior or school problems.

RECOMMENDATION 4: The assessment of ADHD requires evidence directly obtained from the classroom teacher (or other school professional) regarding the core symptoms of ADHD, the duration of symptoms, the degree of functional impairment, and coexisting conditions. A physician should review any reports from a school-based multidisciplinary evaluation where they exist, which will include assessments from the teacher or other school-based professional (strength of evidence: good; strength of recommendation: strong).

The evaluation of ADHD must establish whether core behavior symptoms of inattention, hyperactiv-ity, and impulsivity are present in >1 setting to meet *DSM-IV* criteria for the condition. Children 6 to 12 years of age generally are students in an elementary school setting, where they spend a substantial proportion of waking hours. Therefore, a description of their behavioral characteristics in the school setting is highly important to the evaluation. With permission from the legal guardian, the clinician should review a report from the child's school. The classroom teacher typically has more information about the child's behavior than do other professionals at the school and, when possible, should provide the report. Alternatively, a school counselor or principal often is helpful in coordinating the teacher's reporting and may be able to provide the required information.

Behavior symptoms may be obtained using 1 or more methods such as verbal narratives, written narratives, questionnaires, or rating scales. Clinicians who obtain information from narratives or interviews must obtain and record the relevant behaviors of inattention, hyperactivity, and impulsivity from the *DSM-IV*. The use of global clinical impressions or general descriptions within the domains of attention and activity is insufficient to diagnose ADHD.

The ADHD-specific questionnaires and rating scales also are available for teachers (Table 4). Teacher ADHD-specific questionnaires and rating scales have been shown to have an odds ratio >3.0 (equivalent to sensitivity and specificity greater than 94%) in studies differentiating children with ADHD from normal peers in the community.[24] Thus, teacher ADHD-specific rating scales accurately distinguish between children with and without the diagnosis of ADHD. Whether these scales provide additional benefit beyond narratives or descriptive interviews informed by *DSM-IV* criteria is not known. *RECOMMENDATION 4A: Use of these scales is a clinical option when diagnosing children for ADHD (strength of evidence: strong; strength of recommendation: strong).*

Teacher global questionnaires and rating scales that assess a variety of behavioral conditions, in contrast with the ADHD-specific measures, generally have an odds ratio <2.0 (equivalent to sensitivity and specificity <86%) in studies differentiating children referred to psychiatric practices from children who were not referred to psychiatric practices (Table 5). Thus, these broadband scales do not distinguish between children with and without ADHD. *RECOMMENDATION 4B: Use of teacher global questionnaires and rating scales is not recommended in the diagnosing of children for ADHD, although they may be useful for other purposes (strength of evidence: strong; strength of recommendation: strong).*

If a child 6 to 12 years of age routinely spends considerable time in other structured environments such as after-school care centers, additional information about core symptoms can be sought from professionals in those settings, contingent on parental permission. The ADHD-specific questionnaires may be used to evaluate the child's behavior in these settings. For children who are educated in their homes by parents, evidence of the presence of core behavior symptoms in settings other than the home should be obtained as an essential part of the evaluation.

Frequently there are significant discrepancies between parent and teacher ratings.[40] These discrepancies may be in either direction; symptoms may be reported by teachers and not parents or vice versa. These discrepancies may be attributable to differences between the home and school in terms of expectations, levels of structure, behavioral management strategies, and/or environmental circumstances. The finding of a discrepancy between the parents and teachers does not preclude the diagnosis of ADHD. A helpful clinical approach for understanding the sources of the discrepancies and whether the child meets *DSM-IV* criteria is to obtain additional information from other informants, such as former teachers, religious leaders, or coaches.

RECOMMENDATION 5: Evaluation of the child with ADHD should include assessment for coexisting conditions (strength of evidence: strong; strength of recommendation: strong).

A variety of other psychological and developmental disorders frequently coexist in children who are being evaluated for ADHD. As many as one third of children with ADHD have 1 or more coexisting conditions (Table 6). Although the primary care clinician may not always be in a position to make a precise diagnosis of coexisting conditions, consideration and examination for such a coexisting condition should be an integral part of the evaluation. A review of all coexisting conditions (such as motor disabilities, problems with parent-child interaction, or family violence) is not possible within the scope of this review. More common psychological disorders include conduct and oppositional defiant disorder, mood disorders, anxiety disorders, and learning disabilities. The pediatrician should also consider ADHD as a coexisting condition when considering these other conditions. Evidence for most of these coexisting disorders may be readily detected by the primary care clinician. For example, frequent sadness and preference for isolated activities may alert the physician to the presence of depressive symptoms, whereas a family history of anxiety disorders coupled with a patient history characterized by frequent fears and difficulties with separation from caregivers may be suggestive of symptoms associated with an anxiety disorder. Several screening tests are available that can detect areas of concern for many of the mental health disorders that coexist with ADHD. Although these scales have not been tested for use in primary care settings and are not diagnostic tests for either ADHD or associated mental health conditions, some clinicians may find them useful to establish high risk for coexisting psychological conditions. Similarly, poor school performance may indicate a learning disability. Testing may be required to determine whether a discrepancy exists between the child's learning potential (intelligence quotient) and his actual academic progress (achievement test scores), indicating the presence of a learning disability. Most studies of rates of coexisting conditions have come from referral populations. The following data generally reflect the relatively small number of studies from community or primary care settings.

TABLE 6. Summary of Prevalence of Selected Coexisting Conditions in Children With ADHD

Comorbid Disorder	Estimated Prevalence (%)	Confidence Limits for Estimated Prevalence (%)
Oppositional defiant disorder	35.2	27.2, 43.8
Conduct disorder	25.7	12.8, 41.3
Anxiety disorder	25.8	17.6, 35.3
Depressive disorder	18.2	11.1, 26.6

Taken from: Green M, Wong M, Atkins D, et al. *Diagnosis of Attention Deficit/Hyperactivity Disorder. Technical Review* 3. Rockville, MD: US Dept of Health and Human Services. Agency for Health Care Policy and Research; 1999. AHCPR publication 99-0050

Conduct Disorder and Oppositional Defiant Disorder

Oppositional defiant or conduct disorders coexist with ADHD in ~35% of children.[24] The diagnostic features of conduct disorder include "a repetitive and persistent pattern of behavior in which the basic rights of others or major age-appropriate social norms or rules are violated."[13] Oppositional defiant disorder (a less severe condition) includes persistent symptoms of "negativistic, defiant, disobedient, and hostile behaviors toward authority figures."[13] Frequently, children and adolescents with persisting oppositional defiant disorder later develop symptoms of sufficient severity to qualify for a diagnosis of conduct disorder. Longitudinal follow-up for children with conduct disorders that coexist with ADHD indicates that these children fare more poorly in adulthood relative to their peers diagnosed with ADHD alone.[41] For example, 1 study has reported the highest rates of police contacts and self-reported delinquency in children with ADHD and coexisting conduct disorder (30.8%) relative to their peers diagnosed with ADHD alone (3.4%) or conduct disorder alone (20.7%). Preliminary studies suggest that these coexisting conditions are more frequent in children with the predominantly hyperactive-impulsive and combined subtypes.[25,26]

Mood Disorders/Depression

The coexistence of ADHD and mood disorders (eg, major depressive disorder and dysthymia) is ~18%.[39] Frequently, the family history of children with ADHD includes other family members with a history of major depressive disorder.[42] In addition, children who have coexisting ADHD and mood disorders also may have a poorer outcome during adolescence relative to their peers who do not have this pattern of co-occurrence.[43] For example, adolescents with coexisting mood disorders and ADHD are at increased risk for suicide attempts.[44] Preliminary studies suggest that these coexisting conditions are more frequent in children with the predominantly inattentive and combined subtypes.[25,26]

Anxiety

The coexisting association between ADHD and anxiety disorders has been estimated to be ~25%.[24] In addition, the risk for anxiety disorders among relatives of children and adolescents diagnosed with ADHD is higher than for typically developing children, although some research suggests that ADHD and anxiety disorders transmit independently from families.[45] In either case, it is important to obtain a careful family history. Preliminary studies suggest that these coexisting conditions are more frequent in children with the predominantly inattentive and combined subtypes.[25,26]

Learning Disabilities

Only 1 published study examined the coexistence of ADHD and learning disabilities in children evaluated in general pediatric settings using *DSM-IV* criteria for the diagnosis of ADHD.[46] The prevalence of learning disabilities as a coexisting condition can-not be determined in the same manner as other psychological disorders because studies have employed dimensional (looking at the condition on a spectrum) rather than categorical diagnoses. Rates of learning disabilities that coexist with ADHD in settings other than primary care have been reported to range from 12% to 60%.[24]

To date, no definitive data describe the differences among groups of children with different learning disabilities coexisting with ADHD in the areas of sociodemographic characteristics, behavioral and emotional functioning, and response to various interventions. Nonetheless, the subgroup of children with learning disabilities, compared with their ADHD peers who do not have a learning disability, is most in need of special education services. Preliminary studies suggest that these coexisting conditions are more frequent in children with the predominantly inattentive and combined subtypes.[25,26]

RECOMMENDATION 6: Other diagnostic tests are not routinely indicated to establish the diagnosis of ADHD (strength of evidence: strong; strength of recommendation: strong).

Other diagnostic tests contribute little to establishing the diagnosis of ADHD. A few older studies have indicated associations between blood lead levels and child behavior symptoms, although most studies have not.[47–49] Although lead encephalopathy in younger children may predispose to later behavior and developmental problems, very few of these children will have elevated lead levels at school age. Thus, regular screening of children for high lead levels does not aid in the diagnosis of ADHD.

Studies have shown no significant associations between abnormal thyroid hormone levels and the presence of ADHD.[50–52] Children with the rare disorder of generalized resistance to thyroid hormone have higher rates of ADHD than other populations, but these children demonstrate other characteristics of that condition. This association does not argue for routine screening of thyroid function as part of the effort to diagnose ADHD.

Brain imaging studies and electroencephalography do not show reliable differences between children with ADHD and controls. Although some studies have demonstrated variation in brain morphology comparing children with and without ADHD, these findings do not discriminate reliably between children with and without this condition. In other words, although group means may differ significantly, the overlap in findings among children with and without ADHD creates high rates of false-positives and false-negatives.[53–55] Similarly, some studies have indicated higher rates of certain electroencephalogram abnormalities among children with ADHD,[56–58] but again the overlap between children with and without ADHD and the lack of consistent findings among multiple reports indicate that current literature do not support the routine use of electroencephalograms in the diagnosis of ADHD.

Continuous performance tests have been designed to obtain samples of a child's behavior (generally measuring vigilance or distractibility), which may correlate with behaviors associated with ADHD. Several such tests have been developed and tested, but all of these have low odds ratios (all <1.2, equivalent to a sensitivity and specificity <70%) in studies differentiating children with ADHD from normal comparison controls.[24,45,59,60] Therefore, current data do not support the use of any available continuous performance tests in the diagnosis of ADHD.

AREAS FOR FUTURE RESEARCH

The research issues pertaining to the diagnosis of ADHD relate to the diagnostic criteria themselves as well as the methods used to establish the diagnosis. The *DSM-IV* has helped to define behavioral criteria for ADHD more specifically. Although research has established the dimensional concepts of inattention and hyperactivity-impulsivity, further research is required to validate these subtypes. Because most of the existing research has been conducted with referred convenience samples, primarily in psychiatric settings, further research is required to determine whether the findings of previous research are generalizable to the type of children currently diagnosed and treated by primary care clinicians. Although the current *DSM-IV* criteria are appropriate for the age range included in this guideline, there is, as yet, inadequate information about its applicability to individuals younger or older than the age range for this guideline. Further research should clarify the developmental course of ADHD symptomatology. An additional difficulty for primary care is that existing evidence indicates that the behaviors used in making a *DSM-IV* diagnosis of ADHD fall on a spectrum. Currently, decisions about the inappropriateness of the behaviors in children depend on subjective judgments of observers/reporters. There are no data to offer precise estimates of when diagnostic behaviors become inappropriate. This is particularly problematic to primary care clinicians, who care for a number of patients who fit into borderline or gray areas. The inadequacy of research on this aspect is central to the issue of which children should be diagnosed with ADHD and treated with stimulant medication. Further research using normative or community-based samples to develop more valid and precise diagnostic criteria is essential.

The diagnostic process is also an area requiring further research. Because no pathognomonic findings currently establish the diagnosis, further research should examine the utility of existing methods, with the goal of developing a more definitive process. Specific examples include the need for additional information about the reliability and validity of teacher and parent rating scales and the reliability and validity of different interviewing methods. Further, given the prominence of impairment in the current diagnostic requirements, it is imperative to develop and assess better measurements of impairment that can be applied practically in the primary care setting. The research into diagnostic methods also should include those methods helpful in identifying clinically relevant coexisting conditions.

Lastly, research is required to identify more clearly the current practices of primary care physicians beyond using self-report. Such research is critical in determining the practicality of guideline recommendations as a method to determine changes in practice and to determine whether changes have an actual impact on the treatment and outcome of children with the diagnosis of ADHD.

CONCLUSION

This guideline offers recommendations for the diagnosis and evaluation of school-aged children with ADHD in primary care practice. The guideline emphasizes: 1) the use of explicit criteria for the diagnosis using *DSM-IV* criteria; 2) the importance of obtaining information regarding the child's symptoms in more than 1 setting and especially from schools; and 3) the search for coexisting conditions that may make the diagnosis more difficult or complicate treatment planning. The guideline further provides current evidence regarding various diagnostic tests for ADHD. It should help primary care providers in their assessment of a common child health problem.

COMMITTEE ON QUALITY IMPROVEMENT, 1999–2000
Charles J. Homer, MD, MPH, Chairperson
Richard D. Baltz, MD
Gerald B. Hickson, MD
Paul V. Miles, MD
Thomas B. Newman, MD, MPH
Joan E. Shook, MD
William M. Zurhellen, MD

LIAISON REPRESENTATIVES
Betty A. Lowe, MD, National Association of
    Children's Hospitals and Related Institutions
Ellen Schwalenstocker, MBA, National Association of
    Children's Hospitals and Related Institutions
Michael J. Goldberg, MD, Council on Sections
Richard Shiffman, MD, Section on Computers and
    Other Technologies
Jan Ellen Berger, MD, Committee on Medical Liability
F. Lane France, MD, Committee on Practice and
    Ambulatory Medicine

SUBCOMMITTEE ON ATTENTION-DEFICIT/
    HYPERACTIVITY DISORDER
James M. Perrin, MD, Co-chairperson
Martin T. Stein, MD, Co-chairperson
Robert W. Amler, MD
Thomas A. Blondis, MD
Heidi M. Feldman, MD, PhD
Bruce P. Meyer, MD
Bennett A. Shaywitz, MD
Mark L. Wolraich, MD

CONSULTANTS
Anthony DeSpirito, MD
Charles J. Homer, MD, MPH

LIAISON REPRESENTATIVES
Karen Pierce, MD, American Academy of Child and
    Adolescent Psychiatry
Theodore G. Ganiats, MD, American Academy of
    Family Physicians
Brian Grabert, MD, Child Neurology Society
Ronald T. Brown, PhD, Society for Pediatric
    Psychology

ACKNOWLEDGMENTS

The Practice Guideline, "Diagnosis and Evaluation of the Child With Attention-Deficit/Hyperactivity Disorder," was reviewed by appropriate committees and sections of the AAP, including the Chapter Review Group, a focus group of office-based pediatricians representing each AAP District: Gene R. Adams, MD; Robert M. Corwin, MD; Diane Fuquay, MD; Barbara M. Harley, MD; Thomas J. Herr, MD, Chair Person; Kenneth E. Mathews, MD; Robert D. Mines, MD; Lawrence C. Pakula, MD; Howard B. Weinblatt, MD; and Delosa A. Young, MD. The Practice Guideline was also reviewed by relevant outside medical organizations as part of the peer review process as well as by several patient advocacy organizations.

REFERENCES

1. Reiff MI, Banez GA, Culbert TP. Children who have attentional disorders: diagnosis and evaluation. *Pediatr Rev.* 1993;14:455–465
2. Barkley RA. *Attention Deficit Hyperactivity Disorder: A Handbook for Diagnosis and Treatment.* 2nd ed. New York, NY: Guilford Press; 1996
3. Zentall SS. Research on the educational implications of attention deficit hyperactivity disorder. *Exceptional Child.* 1993;60:143–153
4. Schachar R, Taylor E, Wieselberg MB, Ghorley G, Rutter M. Changes in family functioning and relationships in children who respond to methylphenidate. *J Am Acad Child Adolesc Psychiatry.* 1987;26:728–732
5. Almond BW Jr, Tanner JL, Goffman HF. *The Family Is the Patient: Using Family Interviews in Children's Medical Care.* 2nd ed. Baltimore, MD: Williams & Wilkins; 1999:307–313
6. Biederman J, Faraone SV, Milberger S, et al. Predictors of persistence and remissions of ADHD into adolescence: results from a four-year prospective follow-up study. *J Am Acad Child Adolesc Psychiatry.* 1996; 35:343–351
7. Biederman J, Faraone SV, Spencer T, et al. Patterns of psychiatric comorbidity, cognition, and psychosocial functioning in adults with attention deficit hyperactivity disorder. *Am J Psychiatry.* 1993;150: 1792–1798
8. Baumgaertel A, Copeland L, Wolraich ML. Attention deficit-hyperactivity disorder. In: *Disorders of Development and Learning: A Practical Guide to Assessment and Management.* 2nd ed. St Louis, MO: Mosby Yearbook, Inc; 1996:424–456
9. Cantwell DP. Attention deficit disorder: a review of the past 10 years. *J Am Acad Child Adolesc Psychiatry.* 1996;35:978–987
10. American Psychiatric Association. *Diagnostic and Statistical Manual for Mental Disorders.* 2nd ed. Washington, DC: American Psychiatric Association; 1967
11. American Psychiatric Association. *Diagnostic and Statistical Manual for Mental Disorders.* 3rd ed. Washington, DC: American Psychiatric Association; 1980
12. American Psychiatric Association. *Diagnostic and Statistical Manual for Mental Disorders-Revised.* 3rd ed. Washington, DC: American Psychiatric Association; 1987
13. American Psychiatric Association. *Diagnostic and Statistical Manual for Mental Disorders.* 4th ed. Washington, DC: American Psychiatric Association; 1994
14. Drug Enforcement Agency. Washington, DC (personal communication)
15. August GJ, Garfinkel BD. Behavioral and cognitive subtypes of ADHD. *J Am Acad Child Adolesc Psychiatry.* 1989;28:739–748
16. August GJ, Realmuto GM, MacDonald AW III, Nugent SM, Crosby R. Prevalence of ADHD and comorbid disorders among elementary school children screened for disruptive behavior. *J Abnorm Child Psychol.* 1996; 24:571–595
17. Bird H, Canino G, Rubio-Stipec M, et al. Estimates of the prevalence of childhood maladjustment in a community survey in Puerto Rico. *Arch Gen Psychiatry.* 1988;45:1120–1126
18. Cohen P, Cohen J, Kasen S, Velez CN. An epidemiological study of disorders in late childhood and adolescence I: age and gender-specific prevalence. *J Child Psychol Psychiatry.* 1993;34:851–867
19. King C, Young RD. Attentional deficits with and without hyperactivity: teacher and peer perceptions. *J Abnorm Child Psychol.* 1982;10:483–495
20. Kuperman S, Johnson B, Arndt S, Lingren S, Wolraich M. Quantitative EEG differences in a nonclinical sample of children with ADHD and undifferentiated ADD. *J Am Acad Child Adolesc Psychiatry.* 1996;35: 1009–1017
21. Newcorn J, Halperin JM, Schwartz S, et al. Parent and teacher ratings of attention-deficit hyperactivity disorder symptoms: implications for case identification. *J Dev Behav Pediatr.* 1994;15:86–91
22. Shaffer D, Fisher P, Dulcan MK, et al. The NIMH Diagnostic Interview Schedule for Children Version 2.3 (DISC-2.3): description, acceptability,

prevalence rates, and performance in the MECA study. Methods for the Epidemiology of Child and Adolescent Mental Disorders Study. *J Am Acad Child Adolesc Psychiatry.* 1996;35:865–877
23. Shekim WO, Kashani J, Beck N, et al. The prevalence of attention deficit disorders in a rural midwestern community sample of nine-year-old children. *J Am Acad Child Adolesc Psychiatry.* 1985;24:765–770
24. Green M, Wong M, Atkins D, et al. *Diagnosis of Attention Deficit/Hyperactivity Disorder: Technical Review 3.* Rockville, MD: US Department of Health and Human Services, Agency for Health Care Policy and Research; 1999. Agency for Health Care Policy and Research publication 99-0050
25. Wolraich ML, Hannah JN, Pinnock TY, Baumgaertel A, Brown J. Comparison of diagnostic criteria for attention deficit/hyperactivity disorder in a county-wide sample. *J Am Acad Child Adolesc Psychiatry.* 1996; 35:319–324
26. Wolraich M, Hannah JN, Baumgaertel A, Pinnock TY, Feurer I. Examination of *DSM-IV* criteria for attention deficit/hyperactivity disorder in a county-wide sample. *J Dev Behav Pediatr.* 1998;19:162–168
27. Gibbs N. Latest on Ritalin. *Time.* 1998;152:86–96
28. Safer DJ, Zito JM, Fine EM. Increased methylphenidate usage for attention deficit disorder in the 1990s. *Pediatrics.* 1996;98:1084–1088
29. Rappley MD, Gardiner JC, Jetton JR, Houang RT. The use of methylphenidate in Michigan. *Arch Pediatr Adolesc Med.* 1995;149:675–679
30. Wolraich ML, Lindgren S, Stromquist A, et al. Stimulant medication use by primary care physicians in the treatment of attention deficit hyperactivity disorder. *Pediatrics.* 1990;86:95–101
31. Mulhern S, Dworkin PH, Bernstein B. Do parental encounters predict a diagnosis of attention deficit hyperactivity disorder? *J Dev Behav Pediatr.* 1994;15:348–352
32. Wasserman R, Kelleher KJ, Bocian A, et al. Identification of attentional and hyperactivity problems in primary care: a report from Pediatric Research in Office Settings and the Ambulatory Sentinel Practice Network. *Pediatrics.* 1999;103(3). URL: http://www.pediatrics.org/cgi/content/full/103/3/e38
33. Sleator EK, Ullmann RK. Can the physician diagnose hyperactivity in the office? *Pediatrics.* 1981;67:13–17
34. American Academy of Pediatrics. *Guidelines for Health Supervision III.* 3rd ed. Elk Grove Village, IL: American Academy of Pediatrics; 1997
35. Green M, ed. National Center for Education in Maternal and Child Health. *Bright Futures: Guidelines for Health Supervision of Infants, Children, and Adolescents.* Arlington, VA: National Center for Education in Maternal and Child Health; 1994
36. Stein MT. Preparing families for the toddler and preschool years. *Contemp Pediatr.* 1998;15:88
37. Dixon S, Stein M. *Encounters With Children: Pediatric Behavior and Development.* 3rd ed. St Louis, MO: Mosby; 1999
38. McBurnett K, Pfiffner LJ, Willcutt E, et al. Experimental cross-validation of *DSM-IV* types of attention-deficit/hyperactivity disorder. *J Am Acad Child Adolesc Psychiatry.* 1999;38:17–24
39. American Academy of Pediatrics. *The Classification of Child and Adolescent Mental Diagnoses in Primary Care: Diagnostic and Statistical Manual for Primary Care (DSM-PC) Child and Adolescent Version.* Elk Grove Village, IL: American Academy of Pediatrics; 1996
40. Lahey BB, McBurnett K, Piacentini JC, et al. Agreement of parent and teacher rating scales with comprehensive clinical assessments of attention deficit disorder with hyperactivity. *J Psychopathol Behav Assess.* 1987;9:429–439
41. Ingrams S, Hechtman L, Morganstern G. Outcome issues in ADHD: adolescent and adult long term outcome. In: *Mental Retardation and Developmental Disabilities.* In press
42. Biederman J, Milberger S, Farone SV, Guite J, Warburton R. Associations between childhood asthma and ADHD: issues of psychiatric comorbidity and familiarity. *J Am Acad Child Adolesc Psychiatry.* 1994;33: 842–848
43. Biederman J, Newcorn PJ, Sprich S. Comorbidity of attention deficit hyperactivity disorder with conduct, depressive, anxiety, and other disorders. *Am J Psychiatry.* 1991;148:564–577
44. Brent DA, Perper JA, Goldstein CE, Kolko DJ, Zelenak JP. Risk factors for adolescent suicide: a comparison of adolescent suicide victims with suicidal inpatients. *Arch Gen Psychiatry.* 1988;45:581–588
45. Faraone SV, Biederman J, Mennin D, Gershon J, Tsuang MT. A prospective four-year follow-up study of children at risk for ADHD: psychiatric, neuropsychological, and psychosocial outcome. *J Am Acad Child Adolesc Psychiatry.* 1996;35:1449–1459
46. August GJ, Garfinkel BD. Behavioral and cognitive subtypes of ADHD. *J Am Acad Child Adolesc Psychiatry.* 1989;28:739–748
47. Kahn CA, Kelly PC, Walker WO Jr. Lead screening in children with

attention deficit hyperactivity disorder and developmental delay. *Clin Pediatr (Phila)*. 1995;34:498–501

48. Tuthill RW. Hair lead levels related to children's classroom attention-deficit behavior. *Arch Environ Health*. 1996;51:214–220
49. Gittelman R, Eskenazi B. Lead and hyperactivity revisited: an investigation of non-disadvantaged children. *Arch Gen Psychiatry*. 1983;40:827–833
50. Elia J, Gulotta C, Rose SR, Marin G, Rapoport JL. Thyroid function and attention-deficit hyperactivity disorder. *J Am Acad Child Adolesc Psychiatry*. 1994;33:169–172
51. Spencer T, Biederman J, Wilens T, Guite J, Harding M. ADHD and thyroid abnormalities: a research note. *J Child Psychol Psychiatry*. 1995;36:879–885
52. Weiss RE, Stein MA, Trommer B, Refetoff S. Attention-deficit hyperactivity disorder and thyroid function. *J Pediatr*. 1993;123:539–545
53. Shaywitz BA, Shaywitz SE, Byrne T, Cohen DJ, Rothman S. Attention deficit disorder: quantitative analysis of CT. *Neurology*. 1983;33:1500–1503
54. Castellanos FX, Giedd JN, Marsh WL, et al. Quantitative brain magnetic

resonance imaging in attention-deficit hyperactivity disorder. *Arch Gen Psychiatry*. 1996;53:607–616
55. Lyoo IK, Noam GG, Lee CK, et al. The corpus callosum and lateral ventricles in children with attention-deficit hyperactivity disorder: a brain magnetic resonance imaging study. *Biol Psychiatry*. 1996;40:1060–1063
56. Matsuura M, Okubo Y, Toru M, et al. A cross-national EEG study of children with emotional and behavioral problems: a WHO collaborative study in the Western Pacific Region. *Biol Psychiatry*. 1993;34:59–65
57. Lahat E, Avital E, Barr J, et al. BAEP studies in children with attention deficit disorder. *Dev Med Child Neurol*. 1995;37:119–123
58. Kuperman S, Johnson B, Arndt S, et al. Quantitative EEG differences in a nonclinical sample of children with ADHD and undifferentiated ADD. *J Am Acad Child Adolesc Psychiatry*. 1996;35:1009–1017
59. Seidel WT, Joschko M. Assessment of attention in children. *Clin Neuropsychology*. 1991;5:53–66
60. Dykman RA, Ackerman PT. Attention deficit disorder and specific reading disability: separate but often overlapping disorders. *J Learn Disabil*. 1991;24:96–103

Technical Report Summary:
Diagnosis of Attention-Deficit/
Hyperactivity Disorder

Author:
Agency for Health Care Policy and Research

SUMMARY

The Agency for Health Care Policy and Research (AHCPR) is developing scientific information for other agencies and organizations on which to base clinical guidelines, performance measures, and other quality improvement tools, under the Agency's Evidence-Based Practice Initiative, which was launched in the fall of 1996. This technical review summarizes current scientific evidence on the prevalence of attention-deficit/hyperactivity disorder and on the value of various evaluation methods.

OVERVIEW

Attention-deficit/hyperactivity disorder (ADHD) is one of the most common childhood-onset psychiatric disorders. It is distinguished by symptoms of inattention, hyperactivity, and impulsivity. ADHD may be accompanied by learning disabilities, depression, anxiety, conduct disorder, and oppositional defiant disorder. The etiology of ADHD is unknown, and the disorder may have several different causes. Investigators have studied, for example, the relation of ADHD to elevated lead levels, abnormal thyroid function, morphologic brain differences, and electroencephalograph (EEG) patterns.

With current public awareness of ADHD, pediatricians and health care providers are reporting increases in referral rates of children with suspected ADHD. Numerous rating scales and medical tests for evaluation and diagnosis of ADHD are available, with mixed expert opinion on their usefulness.

The Agency for Health Care Policy and Research (AHCPR) sponsored the development of this technical review to summarize current scientific evidence from the literature on the prevalence of ADHD and on the value of various evaluation methods. The following questions provided a framework for the analysis:

1. What percentage of the U.S. general population ages 6 to 12 years has ADHD? Of those with ADHD, what percentage has one or more of the following comorbidities: learning disabilities, depression, anxiety, conduct disorder, and oppositional defiant disorder?
2. What percentage of children ages 6 to 12 years presenting at pediatricians' or family physicians' offices in the United States meets diagnostic criteria for ADHD? Of those with ADHD, what percentage has one or more of the following comorbidities: learning disabilities, depression, anxiety, conduct disorder, and oppositional defiant disorder?
3. What is the accuracy (i.e., sensitivity, specificity, positive predictive value) and reliability (i.e., inter/intra-rater agreement) of behavioral rating screening tests for ADHD compared with a reference standard?
4. What is the prevalence of abnormal findings on selected medical screening tests commonly recommended as standard components of an evaluation of a child with suspected ADHD?

Diagnostic screening tests, as analyzed under questions 3 and 4, were of two types: behavioral rating scales and medical screening tests. The behavior rating scales selected for consideration consisted of both ADHD-specific scales and "broad-band" scales designed to screen for various symptoms (including ADHD symptoms). The medical screening tests considered included commonly recommended tests that are standard components of an evaluation of a child with suspected ADHD: electroencephalography, lead concentration level testing, thyroid hormone level testing, hearing and vision screening, imaging tests, neurological screening, and continuous performance tests (CPTs).

REPORTING THE EVIDENCE

The evidence on ADHD prevalence and diagnosis reported here was gathered from 87 published articles and 10 behavioral scale manuals. Studies must have been peer reviewed and published in the English language between 1980 and 1997. These 97 sources were identified during searches of the databases MEDLINE and PsycINFO and from reference lists in review articles, research study articles, and a draft guideline on ADHD obtained from the American Academy of Child and Adolescent Psychiatry (currently in development), recent journal publications, citations suggested by members of the American Academy of Pediatricians, and a database of bibliographies on studies that used or evaluated the Child Behavior Checklists (CBCL). Abstracts of more than 4,000 identified citations were reviewed, from which 507 articles and 10 manuals were retrieved and subjected to further consideration. The published studies had to be soundly designed and conform to specified inclusion and exclusion criteria to qualify for consideration.

METHODOLOGY

Data from the 97 accepted articles/manuals were abstracted, tabulated systematically, and subjected to statistical analysis. A multiple logistic regression model with random effects was used to analyze simultaneously for the effect of age, gender, diagnostic tool, and setting. This model accommodates the fact that each study estimated ADHD rates under slightly different conditions. The analysis was done using the EGRET software.

FINDINGS

The significant findings derived from the analysis are summarized below.

Prevalence of ADHD in General Population

- Gender, diagnostic tool (DSM-III or DSM-III-R), and setting (community or school setting) are significant contributors to the ADHD rate, but age (5 to 9 years versus 10 to 12 years) is not a significant factor.
- ADHD prevalence is much higher when academic and behavioral functioning impairment criteria are not considered (16.1 percent without impairment criteria versus 6.8 percent with). Boys have higher rates of ADHD than do girls.

Prevalence of Comorbid ADHD in General Population

- One-third of children diagnosed with ADHD also qualify for a diagnosis of oppositional defiant disorder (ODD).
- One-fourth of children diagnosed with ADHD also qualify for a diagnosis of conduct disorder (CD).
- Less than one-fifth of children with ADHD also have a depressive disorder.
- More than one-fourth of children with ADHD qualify for a diagnosis of anxiety disorder.
- Almost one-third of children with ADHD also have more than one comorbid condition.

- Overall, the prevalence rates of comorbid ADHD are high. Estimates of the prevalence rates of various comorbid conditions in children with ADHD range from 12.36 percent (learning disorders) to 35.15 percent (conduct disorder).

Prevalence of ADHD in Pediatric Clinic Setting

- Results on prevalence of ADHD in a pediatric clinic setting are varied. A 1997 study finds prevalence conforms to that of the general population; a 1988 study shows much smaller prevalence.

Prevalence of Comorbid ADHD in Pediatric Clinic Setting

- Results on prevalence of comorbid ADHD in a pediatric clinic setting are varied. A 1997 study finds a high prevalence, similar to that in the general population; a 1988 study gives much lower rates.

Behavior Rating Scales, ADHD Specific

- The Conners Rating Scales, 1997 Revision, contain two highly effective indices for discriminating between ADHD children and normal controls. The Barkley School Situations Questionnaire is less effective. These results are based on studies conducted under ideal conditions; actual performance of the scales in physicians' offices is expected to be poorer.
- Hyperactivity subscales that effectively discriminate between ADHD children and normal controls include DSM-III-R SNAP and Conners Abbreviated Teacher Questionnaire (CATQ, HI). The ACTeRS scale performed poorly. These results are based on studies conducted under ideal conditions; actual performance of the scales in physicians' offices is expected to be poorer.
- An inattention subscale that effectively discriminates between ADHD children and normal controls is the DSM-III-R SNAP checklist. The ACTeRS scale performed poorly. These results are based on studies conducted under ideal conditions; actual performance of the scales in physicians' offices is expected to be poorer.
- An impulsivity subscale that effectively discriminates between ADHD children and normal controls is the DSM-III-R SNAP checklist.

Broad-Band Behavioral Rating Scales

- None of the broad-band scales analyzed—the CPCL/4-18-R Total Problem Scale, DSMD Total Problem Scale, CPRS-R:L Global Problem Index, and CTRS-R:L Global Problem Index—effectively discriminate between referred and nonreferred children. Thus, they are not useful as tools to detect clinical-level problems in children presenting at a pediatrician's office.
- Externalizing, internalizing, and adaptive functioning scales did not effectively detect referred versus nonreferred children.

Medical Screening Tests

- Analysis of six studies on the relation between elevated lead levels and ADHD showed that lead levels are not useful as a general diagnostic tool for ADHD. This is strengthened by the fact that ADHD prevalence appears to be increasing even as lead levels in the population appear to be decreasing.

- Analysis of four studies showed no relation between abnormal thyroid function and ADHD. Thus, the evidence does not support the use of tests of thyroid function to screen for ADHD.
- Analysis of seven imaging studies of the brain (computed tomography [CT], computerized axial tomography [CAT], and magnetic resonance imaging [MRI]) that were performed to detect morphologic differences in brain structures of children with ADHD yielded sparse and diverse evidence. Thus, none of the imaging procedures analyzed are considered useful as a screening or diagnostic tool for ADHD.
- Eight studies of electroencephalogram (EEG) patterns and ADHD found no serious EEG abnormalities in ADHD children, although many studies found significant differences in brain wave activity between ADHD children and normal controls. The heterogeneity of results across studies indicates that the EEG should not be routinely used as a screening tool for ADHD.
- Evidence from studies of neurological screening tests did not yield any clues to the etiology of ADHD. Thus, these tests are not deemed effective for screening ADHD.
- Continuous performance tests measure impulsivity, inattention, and vigilance. Statistical analysis of studies using these tests indicated that CPTs would not serve as useful screening tools for ADHD.

FUTURE RESEARCH

- There is a need for continued work to gather data on prevalence of ADHD using the following factors, which are lacking in much of the work already done: DSM-IV, use of both genders as subjects, rates of ADHD—Primarily Inattentive Type, and wider-scale studies across regions of the country or across countries using the same criteria.
- Comparison studies are needed to assess the ability of broad-band behavior checklists to discriminate between clinical and nonclinical samples (the studies available at this time have only presented results of the ability of these tests to discriminate between referred and nonreferred samples). Clinically severe problems are present in both of these groups, as are subclinical problems.
- Continued work is needed in the area of magnetic resonance imaging and PET, when possible, to continue to explore structural and functional differences in the brains of children diagnosed with ADHD and each of the types of ADHD.

AVAILABILITY OF THE FULL REPORT

The full technical review from which this summary was taken was prepared by Technical Resources International, Inc., located in Rockville, Maryland. It was developed for AHCPR under contract No. 290-94-2024, and is expected to be available in 2001.

When the technical review is available, printed copies may be obtained free of charge from the AHCPR Publications Clearinghouse by calling 1-800-358-9295. Requestors should ask for Technical Review No. 3, *Diagnosis of Attention-Deficit/Hyperactivity Disorder* (AHCPR Publication No. 99-0050). Internet users will be able to access the review online at: http://www.ahrq.gov/clinic/epcix.htm.

For more information on AHCPR's Evidence-Based Practice Initiative or the development of this report, contact the Center for Practice and Technology Assessment, Agency for Health Care Policy and Research, 6000 Executive Boulevard, Suite 310, Rockville, MD 20852; phone (301) 594-4015; fax (301) 594-4027.

AHCPR Publication No. 99-0049
Current as of October 1999

Treatment of the School-Aged Child With Attention-Deficit/Hyperactivity Disorder

• *Clinical Practice Guideline*

AMERICAN ACADEMY OF PEDIATRICS

Subcommittee on Attention-Deficit/Hyperactivity Disorder

Committee on Quality Improvement

Clinical Practice Guideline: Treatment of the School-Aged Child With Attention-Deficit/Hyperactivity Disorder

ABSTRACT. This clinical practice guideline provides evidence-based recommendations for the treatment of children diagnosed with attention-deficit/hyperactivity disorder (ADHD). This guideline, the second in a set of policies on this condition, is intended for use by clinicians working in primary care settings. The initiation of treatment requires the accurate establishment of a diagnosis of ADHD; the American Academy of Pediatrics (AAP) clinical practice guideline on diagnosis of children with ADHD[1] provides direction in appropriately diagnosing this disorder.

The AAP Committee on Quality Improvement selected a subcommittee composed of primary care and developmental-behavioral pediatricians and other experts in the fields of neurology, psychology, child psychiatry, education, family practice, and epidemiology. The subcommittee partnered with the Agency for Healthcare Research and Quality and the Evidence-based Practice Center at McMaster University, Ontario, Canada, to develop the evidence base of literature on this topic.[2] The resulting systematic review, along with other major studies in this area, was used to formulate recommendations for treatment of children with ADHD. The subcommittee also reviewed the multimodal treatment study of children with ADHD[3] and the Canadian Coordinating Office for Health Technology Assessment report (CCOHTA).[4] Subcommittee decisions were made by consensus where definitive evidence was not available. The subcommittee report underwent extensive review by sections and committees of the AAP as well as by numerous external organizations before approval from the AAP Board of Directors.

The guideline contains the following recommendations for the treatment of a child diagnosed with ADHD:

- Primary care clinicians should establish a treatment program that recognizes ADHD as a chronic condition.
- The treating clinician, parents, and child, in collaboration with school personnel, should specify appropriate target outcomes to guide management.
- The clinician should recommend stimulant medication and/or behavior therapy as appropriate to improve target outcomes in children with ADHD.
- When the selected management for a child with ADHD has not met target outcomes, clinicians should evaluate the original diagnosis, use of all appropriate treatments, adherence to the treatment plan, and presence of coexisting conditions.
- The clinician should periodically provide a systematic follow-up for the child with ADHD. Monitoring should be directed to target outcomes and adverse effects, with information gathered from parents, teachers, and the child.

This guideline is intended for use by primary care clinicians for the management of children between 6 and 12 years of age with ADHD. In light of the high prevalence of ADHD in pediatric practice, the guideline should assist primary care clinicians in treatment. Although many of the recommendations here also may apply to children with coexisting conditions, this guideline primarily addresses children with ADHD but without major coexisting conditions. The guideline is not intended for use in the treatment of children with mental retardation, pervasive developmental disorder, moderate to severe sensory deficits such as visual and hearing impairment, chronic disorders associated with medications that may affect behavior, and those who have experienced child abuse and sexual abuse. This guideline is not intended as a sole source of guidance for the treatment of children with ADHD. Rather, it is designed to assist the primary care clinician by providing a framework for decision-making. It is not intended to replace clinical judgment or to establish a protocol for all children with this condition, and may not provide the only appropriate approach to this problem.

ABBREVIATIONS. AAP, American Academy of Pediatrics; ADHD, attention-deficit/hyperactivity disorder; *DSM-IV, Diagnostic and Statistical Manual of Mental Disorders, Fourth Edition*; MTA, multimodal treatment study of children with ADHD; CCOHTA, Canadian Coordinating Office for Health Technology Assessment.

The American Academy of Pediatrics (AAP) recognizes the importance of accurate diagnosis and management of children with attention-deficit/hyperactivity disorder (ADHD). The AAP developed a practice guideline for the diagnosis of ADHD among children from 6 to 12 years of age who are evaluated by primary care clinicians.[1] The significant components of the diagnostic guideline include 1) the use of explicit criteria for the diagnosis using the *Diagnostic and Statistical Manual of Mental Health Disorders, Fourth Edition (DSM-IV)* criteria[5]; 2) the importance of obtaining information about the child's symptoms in more than 1 setting (especially from schools); and 3) the search for coexisting conditions that may make the diagnosis more difficult or complicate treatment planning.

This guideline is based on an extensive review of the medical, psychological, and educational literature. The objectives of the literature review were to determine the long- and short-term effectiveness and

The recommendations in this statement do not indicate an exclusive course of treatment or serve as a standard of medical care. Variations, taking into account individual circumstances, may be appropriate.
PEDIATRICS (ISSN 0031 4005). Copyright © 2001 by the American Academy of Pediatrics.

safety of pharmacological and nonpharmacological interventions for ADHD in children from 6 to 12 years of age, and to compare single treatment methods (eg, medications alone) with combined management strategies. Two systematic, evidence-based reviews were used extensively in the development of this guideline.[2,4] In addition, other resources were used to gather more information.[6,7]

Primary care clinicians cannot work alone in the treatment of school-aged children with ADHD. Ongoing communication with parents, teachers, and other school-based professionals is necessary to monitor the progress and effectiveness of specific interventions. Parents are key partners in the management plan as sources of information and as the child's primary caregiver. Integration of services with psychologists, child psychiatrists, neurologists, educational specialists, developmental-behavioral pediatricians, and other mental health professionals may be appropriate for children with ADHD who have coexisting conditions and may continue to have problems in functioning despite treatment. Attention to the child's social development in community settings other than school requires clinical knowledge of a variety of activities and services in the community.

METHODOLOGY

The AAP collaborated with several organizations to develop a working subcommittee representing a wide range of primary care and subspecialty groups. The subcommittee, chaired by 2 general pediatricians, included representatives from the American Academy of Family Physicians, the American Academy of Child and Adolescent Psychiatry, the Child Neurology Society, the Society for Pediatric Psychology, the Society for Developmental and Behavioral Pediatrics, and the Society for Developmental Pediatrics.

This subcommittee met over a period of 3 years, during which it reviewed basic literature on current practices in the treatment of children with ADHD. The subcommittee developed a series of research questions to direct an extensive evidence-based review, in partnership with the Agency for Healthcare Research and Quality.

In 1997, the McMaster University Evidence-based Practice Center received the contract for reviewing the literature related to treatment of children with ADHD. The McMaster report[2] focused on the evidence from comparative studies on the effectiveness and safety of pharmacological and nonpharmacological interventions for ADHD in children and adults and whether combined interventions are more effective than individual interventions. This resulted in several questions in the following 7 areas: 1) studies with drug-to-drug comparisons of pharmacological interventions; 2) placebo-controlled studies evaluating the effect of tricyclic antidepressants; 3) studies comparing pharmacological and nonpharmacological interventions; 4) studies evaluating the effect of long-term therapies; 5) studies evaluating therapies for ADHD in adults (ie, those older than 18 years of age); 6) studies evaluating therapies given in

combination; and 7) studies evaluating adverse effects of pharmacological interventions.

Several systematic reviews and meta-analyses have examined placebo-controlled trials of stimulant medication and have established the short-term efficacy of these agents for core symptoms. Placebo-controlled trials of stimulant medication were reviewed in the McMaster report only if they met the criteria for inclusion in any of the other 6 areas. The report also focused on head-to-head comparisons of pharmacological interventions and of pharmacological and nonpharmacological interventions because these were identified as of prime interest to clinicians.

The McMaster report of the literature on treatment of ADHD followed current standards for analyzing research evidence.[2] Studies in this report were selected for evaluation if they were randomized, controlled trials that focused on the treatment of ADHD in humans and if they were published in peer-reviewed journals. Nonrandomized, controlled trials were included only if they provided data on adverse effects that were collected for more than 16 weeks. Studies of multiple conditions that included separate analyses for patients with ADHD were also included. The literature search was conducted using MEDLINE (from 1966), CINAHL (from 1982), HEALTHStar (from 1975), PsycINFO (from 1984), and EMBASE (from 1984). The Cochrane Library (issue 4, 1997) was also used in reviewing the literature. A total of 2405 citations were identified by the search strategies, and 92 reports, describing 78 different studies, were identified for further analysis.

In addition to the McMaster report, other sources of data were used to support clinical practice guideline recommendations. Although the McMaster report included results of the multimodal treatment study of children with ADHD (MTA),[3,7] the subcommittee also carefully evaluated the results of this large study separately.[8–16] The subcommittee used data from the Canadian Coordinating Office for Health Technology Assessment (CCOHTA) study.[4] The CCOHTA review addressed the following 3 major issues related to treatment of children with ADHD: 1) a clinical evaluation of the use of methylphenidate for ADHD; 2) the efficacy of stimulant medications and other therapies; and 3) an economic evaluation of the pharmacological and behavioral therapies for ADHD. Many studies of behavioral interventions for ADHD use crossover techniques, where effects were determined on the same children when they did and did not receive treatment.[6,17] The McMaster report excluded these crossover trials.[2]

The draft clinical practice guideline underwent extensive peer review by committees and sections within the AAP, numerous outside organizations, and other individuals identified by the subcommittee. Liaisons to the subcommittee were also invited to distribute the draft to entities within their organizations. Comments were compiled and reviewed by the subcommittee cochairpersons, and relevant changes were incorporated into the guideline.

The recommendations contained in this guideline (see Fig 1) are based on the best available data. For

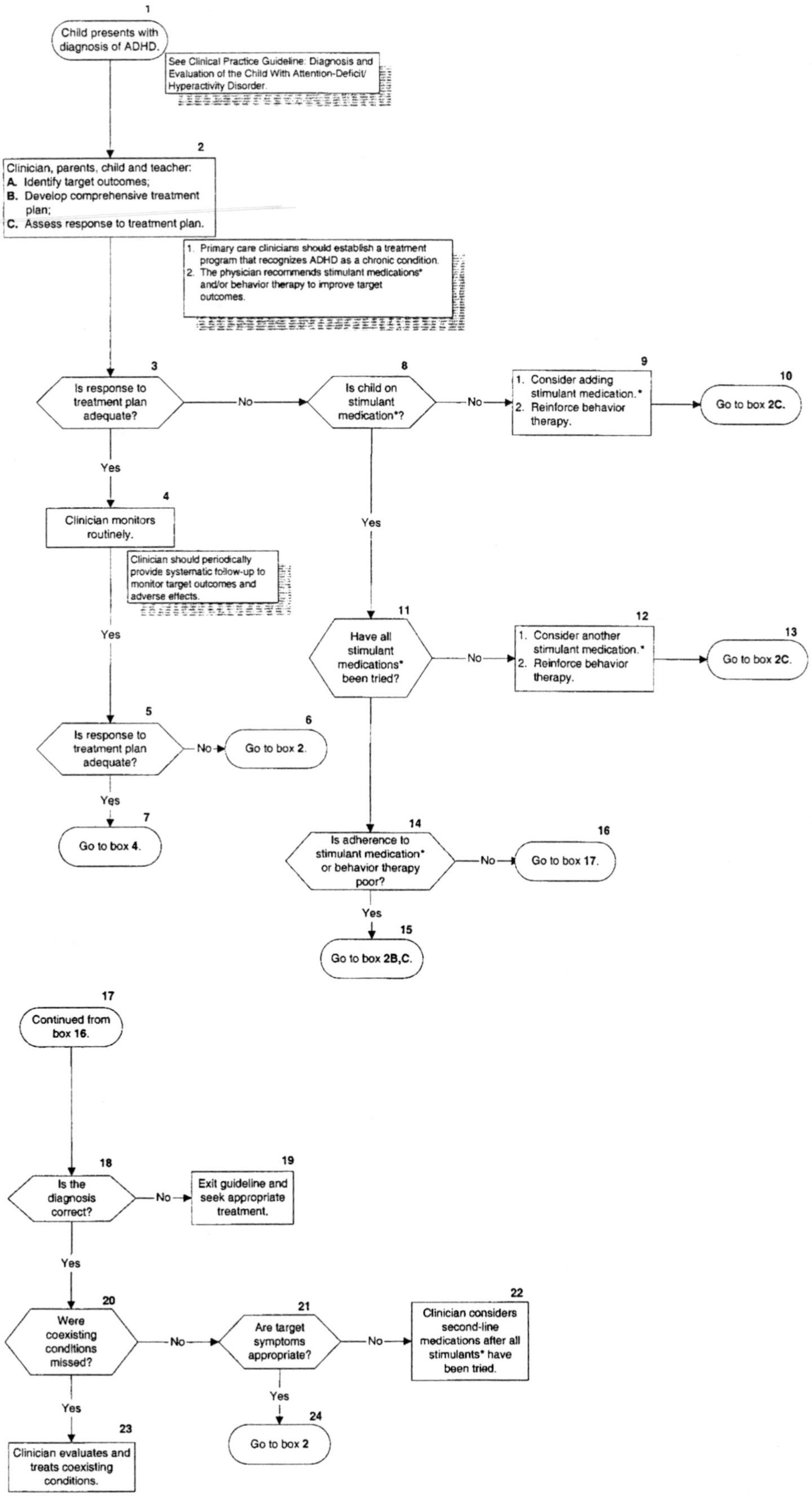

1
Child presents with diagnosis of ADHD.

See Clinical Practice Guideline: Diagnosis and Evaluation of the Child With Attention-Deficit/Hyperactivity Disorder.

2
Clinician, parents, child and teacher:
A. Identify target outcomes;
B. Develop comprehensive treatment plan;
C. Assess response to treatment plan.

1. Primary care clinicians should establish a treatment program that recognizes ADHD as a chronic condition.
2. The physician recommends stimulant medications* and/or behavior therapy to improve target outcomes.

3
Is response to treatment plan adequate? —No→

8
Is child on stimulant medication*? —No→

9
1. Consider adding stimulant medication.*
2. Reinforce behavior therapy. →

10
Go to box **2C**.

4
Clinician monitors routinely.

Clinician should periodically provide systematic follow-up to monitor target outcomes and adverse effects.

11
Have all stimulant medications* been tried? —No→

12
1. Consider another stimulant medication.*
2. Reinforce behavior therapy. →

13
Go to box **2C**.

5
Is response to treatment plan adequate? —No→

6
Go to box **2**.

7
Go to box **4**.

14
Is adherence to stimulant medication* or behavior therapy poor? —No→

16
Go to box **17**.

15
Go to box **2B,C**.

17
Continued from box **16**.

18
Is the diagnosis correct? —No→

19
Exit guideline and seek appropriate treatment.

20
Were coexisting conditions missed? —No→

21
Are target symptoms appropriate? —No→

22
Clinician considers second-line medications after all stimulants* have been tried.

23
Clinician evaluates and treats coexisting conditions.

24
Go to box **2**.

*Excluding Pemoline

Fig 1. Algorithm for the treatment of the school-aged child with Attention-Deficit/Hyperactivity Disorder.

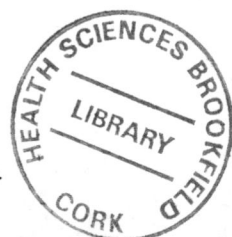
HEALTH SCIENCES BROOKFIELD LIBRARY CORK

each recommendation, the subcommittee graded the *quality of evidence* on which the recommendation was based and the *strength* of the recommendation. Grades of evidence were grouped into 3 categories—good, fair, or poor. Recommendations were made at 3 levels. Strong recommendations were based on high-quality scientific evidence or, in the absence of high-quality data, strong expert consensus. Fair and weak recommendations were based on lesser quality or limited data and expert consensus. Clinical options are identified as interventions for which the subcommittee could not find compelling evidence for or against. Clinical options are defined as interventions that a reasonable health care provider might or might not wish to implement in his or her practice.

RECOMMENDATION 1: Primary care clinicians should establish a management program that recognizes ADHD as a chronic condition (strength of evidence: good; strength of recommendation: strong).

Attention-deficit/hyperactivity disorder is one of the more common chronic conditions of childhood. Studies using parent reports indicate persistence of ADHD of 60% to 80% into adolescence.[18-20] Given the high prevalence of ADHD among school-aged children (4% to 12%),[1] primary care clinicians will encounter children with ADHD in their practices regularly and should have a strategy for diagnosis and long-term management of this condition. The primary care of children with ADHD includes attention to the main principles of care for children with any chronic condition, such as

- Providing information about the condition
- Updating and monitoring family knowledge and understanding on a periodic basis
- Counseling about family response to the condition
- Developmentally appropriate education of the child about ADHD, with updates as the child grows
- Availability to answer family questions
- Ensuring coordination of health and other services
- Helping families set specific goals in areas related to the child's condition and its effects on daily activities
- Linking families with other families with children who have similar chronic conditions as needed and available[21-26]

As with other chronic conditions, treatment of ADHD requires the development of child-specific treatment plans that describe methods and goals of treatment and means of monitoring care over time, including specific plans for follow-up (See Recommendation 5.)

Primary care clinicians should educate parents and children about the ways in which ADHD can affect learning, behavior, self-esteem, social skills, and family function. This initial phase of patient education is critical to demystifying the diagnosis and providing parents and children with knowledge about the condition. Education enables parents to work with clinicians, educators, and, in some cases, mental health

professionals to develop an effective treatment plan. A therapeutic alliance among clinicians, parents, and the child is enhanced when attention is directed toward cultural values that affect the child's health and health care. The long-term care of a child with ADHD requires an ongoing partnership among clinicians, parents, teachers, and the child. Other school personnel—nurses, psychologists, and counselors—can also help with developing and monitoring plans.

Studies of children and adults with several chronic conditions indicate better adherence to treatment plans, improved health and disease status measures, and higher levels of satisfaction in the context of a comprehensive treatment plan with specific goals, follow-up activities, and monitoring.[27-28] Thus, careful attention to the key elements of chronic care can lead to improved outcomes for children and families.

Activities specific to the care of children with ADHD include providing current information on the etiology of ADHD, its treatment, long-term outcomes, and effects on daily life and family activities. Thorough family understanding of the problem is essential before discussing treatment options and side effects. What distinguishes this condition from most other chronic conditions managed by primary care clinicians is the important role that the education system plays in the treatment and monitoring of children with ADHD.

Like other chronic conditions, new research on ADHD will change the information available to parents and clinicians over time and fill many gaps in diagnosing and understanding the etiology, treatment, long-term effects, and complications related to ADHD. Families should have access to this information. In addition, national, grassroots, parent-run associations provide support and/or education to caregivers and families of individuals with ADHD (eg, Children and Adults with Attention-Deficit/Hyperactivity Disorder [CHADD]). The clinician should be aware of community resources that provide these services and know how to make referrals. Primary care providers may offer this information directly or collaborate with other providers, especially subspecialists and mental health providers, to ensure families' access to needed information.

RECOMMENDATION 2: The treating clinician, parents, and the child, in collaboration with school personnel, should specify appropriate target outcomes to guide management (strength of evidence: good; strength of recommendation: strong).

The core symptoms of ADHD (ie, inattention, impulsivity, hyperactivity) can result in multiple areas of dysfunction relating to a child's performance in the home, school, or community. The primary goal of treatment should be to maximize function. Desired results include

- improvements in relationships with parents, siblings, teachers, and peers
- decreased disruptive behaviors
- improved academic performance, particularly in volume of work, efficiency, completion, and accuracy

- increased independence in self-care or homework
- improved self-esteem
- enhanced safety in the community, such as in crossing streets or riding bicycles. Target outcomes should follow from the key symptoms the child manifests and the specific impairments these symptoms cause.

The process of developing target outcomes requires input from parents, children, and teachers, as well as other school personnel where available and appropriate.[29] They should agree on at least 3 to 6 key targets and desired changes as prerequisites to constructing the treatment plan. The goals should be realistic, attainable, and measurable. The methods of treatment and of monitoring change will vary as a function of the target outcomes.

RECOMMENDATION 3: The clinician should recommend stimulant medication (strength of evidence: good) and/or behavior therapy (strength of evidence: fair), as appropriate, to improve target outcomes in children with ADHD (strength of recommendation: strong).

The clinician should develop a comprehensive management plan focused on the target outcomes. For most children, stimulant medication is highly effective in the management of the core symptoms of ADHD. For many children, behavioral interventions are valuable as primary treatment or as an adjunct in the management of ADHD, based on the nature of coexisting conditions, specific target outcomes, and family circumstances.

Stimulant Medication

Many studies have documented the efficacy of stimulants in reducing the core symptoms of ADHD. In many cases, stimulant medication also improves the child's ability to follow rules and decreases emotional overreactivity, thereby leading to improved relationships with peers and parents. Three formal meta-analyses[30–32] and 1 review of reviews[33] support the short-term efficacy of stimulant medications in reducing core symptoms of ADHD as well as improving function in a number of domains. The most powerful effects[4] are found on measures of observable social and classroom behaviors and on core symptoms of attention, hyperactivity, and impulsivity.* The effects on intelligence and achievement tests are more modest. Most studies of stimulants have been short-term, demonstrating efficacy over several days or weeks. The MTA study extends the demonstrated efficacy to 14 months.[3] In that study, 579 children 7 to 9.9 years of age with ADHD were randomized to 4 treatment groups: medication management alone, medication and behavior management, behavior management alone, and a standard community care group. The medication management groups followed specific protocols and algorithms in

distinction to routine community practice based on clinicians' best judgments. School-aged children with ADHD showed a marked reduction in core ADHD symptoms over a 14-month period when they were treated with medication management alone or a combination of medication and behavior management. Eighty-five percent of the children treated with medication received a stimulant medication.[3] Despite the efficacy of stimulant medications in improving behaviors, many children who receive them do not demonstrate fully normal behavior (eg, only 38% of medically managed children in the MTA study received scores in the normal range at 1-year follow-up). Although the MTA study demonstrated that efficacy of stimulants lasts at least to 14 months, the longer term effects of stimulants remain unclear, attributable in part to methodologic difficulties in other studies.[35]

Stimulant medications currently available include short-, intermediate-, and long-acting methylphenidate, and short-, intermediate-, and long-acting dextroamphetamine. The latter 2 formulations are mixed amphetamine salts (75% dextroamphetamine and 25% levoamphetamine). Pemoline, a long-acting stimulant, is rarely used now because of its rare but potentially fatal hepatotoxicity.[36] Primary care clinicians should not use it routinely, and this guideline does not include it as a first- or second-line treatment for ADHD. Table 1 indicates available medications and their doses. The McMaster report reviewed 22 studies and showed no differences comparing methylphenidate with dextroamphetamine or among different forms of these stimulants.[2] Each stimulant improved core symptoms equally. Individual children, however, may respond to one of the stimulants but not to another. Recommended stimulants require no serologic, hematologic, or electrocardiogram monitoring. Current evidence supports the use of only 2 other medications for ADHD, tricyclic antidepressants[2] and bupropion.[37] Nine studies carefully evaluated tricyclic antidepressants (6 evaluated desipramine, 3 evaluated imipramine); all indicated positive effects on ADHD symptoms.[2] Four trials comparing tricyclic antidepressants with methylphenidate indicated either no differences in response or slightly better results with stimulant use.[2] The use of nonstimulant medications falls outside this practice guideline, although clinicians should select tricyclic antidepressants after the failure of 2 or 3 stimulants and only if they are familiar with their use. Desipramine use has been associated, in rare cases, with sudden death.[38] Clonidine, one of the antihypertensive drugs occasionally used in the treatment of ADHD, also falls outside the scope of this guideline. Limited studies of clonidine indicate that it is better than placebo in the treatment of core symptoms (although with effect sizes lower than those for stimulants). Its use has been documented mainly in children with ADHD and coexisting conditions, especially sleep disturbances.[39,40]

Detailed instructions for determining the dose and schedule of stimulant medications are beyond the scope of this guideline. However, a few basic principles guide the available clinical options.

---

*The effect size for classroom and social behavior in the CCOHTA meta-analysis averaged 0.81; for core symptoms, 0.78; and for intelligence and achievement, 0.34. The first two of these would be considered a large change, the third, a minor to moderate change.[34]

TABLE 1.   Medications Used in the Treatment of Attention-Deficit/Hyperactivity Disorder

Generic Class (Brand Name)	Daily Dosage Schedule	Duration	Prescribing Schedule
Stimulants (First-Line Treatment)			
Methylphenidate			

Short-acting
    (Ritalin, Metadate, Methylin)
	Twice a day (BID) to 3
	  times a day (TID)
		3–5 hr	5–20 mg BID to TID

Intermediate-acting
    (Ritalin SR, Metadate ER, Methylin ER)
	Once a day (QD) to
	  BID
		3–8 hr	20–40 mg QD or 40 mg in the
			  morning and 20 early afternoon

Extended Release (Concerta, Metadate CD, Ritalin LA*)	QD	8–12 hr	18–72 mg QD
Amphetamine			
Short-acting (Dexedrine, Dextrostat)	BID to TID	4–6 hr	5–15 mg BID or 5–10 mg TID
Intermediate-acting (Adderall, Dexedrine spansule)	QD to BID	6–8 hr	5–30 mg QD or 5–15 mg BID
Extended Release (Adderall-XR*)	QD		10–30 mg QD
Antidepressants (Second-Line Treatment)			
Tricyclics (TCAs) Imipramine, Desipramine	BID to TID		2–5 mg/kg/day†
Bupropion			
(Wellbutrin)	QD to TID		50–100 mg TID
(Wellbutrin SR)	BID		100–150 mg BID

* Not FDA approved at time of publication.
† Prescribing and monitoring information in *Physicians' Desk Reference*.

Unlike most other medications, stimulant dosages usually are not weight dependent. Clinicians should begin with a low dose of medication and titrate upward because of the marked individual variability in the dose-response relationship. The first dose that a child's symptoms respond to may not be the best dose to improve function. Clinicians should continue to use higher doses to achieve better responses.[3] This strategy may require reducing the dose when a higher dose produces side effects or no further improvement. The best dose of medication for a given child is the one that leads to optimal effects with minimal side effects. The dosing schedules vary depending on target outcomes, although no consistent controlled studies compare different dosing schedules. For example, if there is a need for relief of symptoms only during school, a 5-day schedule may be sufficient. By contrast, a need for relief of symptoms at home and school suggests a 7-day schedule.

Stimulants are generally considered safe medications, with few contraindications to their use. Side effects occur early in treatment and tend to be mild and short-lived.[35] The most common side effects are decreased appetite, stomachache or headache, delayed sleep onset, jitteriness, or social withdrawal. Most of these symptoms can be successfully managed through adjustments in the dosage or schedule of medication. Approximately 15% to 30% of children experience motor tics, most of which are transient, while on stimulant medications. In addition, approximately half of children with Tourette syndrome have ADHD. The effects of medication on tics are unpredictable. The presence of tics before or during medical management of ADHD is not an absolute contraindication to the use of stimulant medications.[41,42] A review of 7 studies comparing stimulants with placebo or with other medications indicated no increase in tics in children treated with stimulants.[2]

According to the *Physicians' Desk Reference*[43] and medication package insert, methylphenidate is contraindicated in children with seizure disorders, a history of seizure disorder, or abnormal electroencephalograms. Studies of the use of methylphenidate have not, however, demonstrated an increase in seizure frequency or severity when it is added to appropriate anticonvulsant medications.[44–46]

Children who receive too high a dose or who are overly sensitive may become overfocused on the medication or appear dull or overly restricted. Many times this side effect can be addressed by lowering the dose. Rarely, with high doses, some children experience psychotic reactions, mood disturbances, or hallucinations.

No consistent reports of behavioral rebound, motor tics, or dose-related growth delays have been found in controlled studies,[47] although they are reported clinically.[33] Appetite suppression and weight loss are common side effects of stimulant medication, with no apparent difference between methylphenidate and dextroamphetamine. Concern for growth delay has been raised, but a prospective follow-up study into adult life[48] has found no significant impairment of height attained. Studies of stimulant use have found little or no decrease in expected height, with any decrease in growth early in treatment compensated for later on.[49–54] Many clinicians recommend drug holidays during summers, although no controlled trials exist to indicate whether holidays have gains or risks, especially related to weight gain.

3A: For children on stimulants, if one stimulant does not work at the highest feasible dose, the clinician should recommend another.

At least 80%[3] of children will respond to one of the stimulants if they are tried in a systematic way. Children who fail to show positive effects or who experience intolerable side effects on one stimulant medication should be tried on another of the recommended stimulant medications. The reasons for this recommendation include the following:

- The finding that most children who fail to respond to one medication will have a positive response to an alternative stimulant
- The safety and efficacy of stimulants in the treatment of ADHD compared with nonstimulant medications
- The numerous crossover trials that indicate the efficacy of different stimulants in the same child[2,4]
- The idiosyncratic responses to medication[55]

Children who fail 2 stimulant medications can be tried on a third type or formulation of stimulant medication for the same reason. (As indicated in Recommendation 4, lack of response to treatment also should lead clinicians to assess the accuracy of the diagnosis and the possibility of undiagnosed coexisting conditions.)

Behavior Therapy

Behavior therapy represents a broad set of specific interventions that have a common goal of modifying the physical and social environment to alter or change behavior. Along with behavior therapy, most clinicians, parents, and schools address a variety of changes in the child's home and school environment, including more structure, closer attention, and limitations of distractions. Such environmental modifications have not undergone careful efficacy assessment, but most treatment plans include them.

Behavior therapy usually is implemented by training parents and teachers in specific techniques of improving behavior. Behavior therapy then involves providing rewards for demonstrating the desired behavior (eg, positive reinforcement) or consequences for failure to meet the goals (eg, punishment). Repetitive application of the rewards and consequences gradually shapes behavior. Although behavior therapy shares a set of principles, it includes different techniques with many of the strategies often combined into a comprehensive program.

Behavior therapy should be differentiated from psychological interventions directed to the child and designed to change the child's emotional status (eg, play therapy) or thought patterns (eg, cognitive therapy or cognitive-behavior therapy). Although these psychological interventions have great intuitive appeal, they have little documented efficacy in the treatment of children with ADHD,[56] and gains achieved in the treatment setting usually do not transfer into the classroom or home. By contrast, parent training in behavior therapy and classroom behavior interventions have successfully changed the behavior of children with ADHD.[6]

Parent training typically begins with 8 to 12 weekly group sessions with a trained therapist. The focus is on the child's behavior problems and difficulties in family relationships. A typical program aims to improve the parents' or caregivers' understanding of the child's behavior and teaching them skills to deal with the behavioral difficulties posed by ADHD. Programs offer specific techniques for giving commands, reinforcing adaptive and positive social behavior, and decreasing or eliminating inappropriate behavior. Programs plan for maintenance and relapse prevention. Parent training improves the child's functioning and decreases disruptive behavior but (as with stimulant medications) does not necessarily bring the behavior of a child with ADHD into the normal range on parent rating scales.[56,57]

Classroom management also focuses on the child's behavior and may be integrated into classroom routines for all students or targeted for a selected child in the classroom. Classroom management often begins with increasing the structure of activities. Systematic rewards and consequences, including point systems or use of token economy (see Table 2), are included to increase appropriate behavior and eliminate inappropriate behavior. A periodic (often daily) report card can record the child's progress or performance with regard to goals and communicate the child's progress to the parents, who then provide reinforcers or consequences based on that day's performance. Classroom behavior management also may improve a child's functioning but may not bring the child's behavior into the normal range on teacher behavior rating scales.[57] Table 2 outlines specific behavior therapies that have been demonstrated as effective for ADHD.[17]

Evidence for the effectiveness of behavior therapy in children with ADHD comes from a variety of studies. The diversity of interventions and outcome

TABLE 2. Effective Behavioral Techniques for Children With Attention-Deficit/Hyperactivity Disorder

Technique	Description	Example
Positive reinforcement	Providing rewards or privileges contingent on the child's performance.	Child completes an assignment and is permitted to play on the computer.
Time-out	Removing access to positive reinforcement contingent on performance of unwanted or problem behavior.	Child hits sibling impulsively and is required to sit for 5 minutes in the corner of the room.
Response cost	Withdrawing rewards or privileges contingent on the performance of unwanted or problem behavior.	Child loses free time privileges for not completing homework.
Token economy	Combining positive reinforcement and response cost. The child earns rewards and privileges contingent on performing desired behaviors and loses the rewards and privileges based on undesirable behavior.	Child earns stars for completing assignments and loses stars for getting out of seat. The child cashes in the sum of stars at the end of the week for a prize.

measures makes meta-analysis of the effects of behavior therapy alone or in association with medications very difficult. Double-blind, randomized, placebo-controlled trials are difficult to perform, in part because of the difficulty of keeping examiners and participants unaware of whether the child is receiving treatment or placebo. Thus, the usual evidence-based medicine searches turn up few studies for review.[2] Alternative experimental methods, such as rigorous single-subject designs, are used frequently in the psychological literature. Studies that compare the behavior of children during periods on and off behavior therapy demonstrate the effectiveness of behavior therapy[17]; however, behavior therapy has been demonstrated to be effective only while it is implemented and maintained.

A number of individual studies indicate positive effects of behavior therapy in addition to medications. Almost all studies comparing behavior therapy with stimulants alone indicate a much stronger effect from stimulants than from behavior therapy. When comparing behavior therapy to stimulant medications, efficacy of their combined treatment could not be demonstrated to be greater than medication alone for the core symptoms of ADHD.[2] The MTA study[3] found that the combined treatment (medication management with behavior therapy), compared with medication alone, offered improved scores on academic measures, measures of conduct, and some specific ADHD symptoms (although not on global ADHD symptom scales). Although these trends were consistent, few reached statistical significance. In addition, parents and teachers of children receiving combined therapy were significantly more satisfied with the treatment plan.[13,14,58–60]

A wide range of clinicians, including psychologists, school personnel, community mental health therapists, or the primary care clinician, can implement behavior therapy directly or train others to implement behavior therapy. Many clinicians prefer to refer to community resources for behavior therapy because behavior therapy with parents is time-consuming and often does not lend itself to the structure and schedule of the primary care office. Schools may provide behavior therapy with teachers in the context of a Rehabilitation Act (Section 504) plan or an individual education plan. Where ADHD has a significant impact on a child's educational abilities, Section 504 requires schools to make classroom adaptations to help children with ADHD function in that setting. Adaptations may include preferential seating, decreased assignment and homework load, and behavior therapy implemented by the teacher.

RECOMMENDATION 4: When the selected management for a child with ADHD has not met target outcomes, clinicians should evaluate the original diagnosis, use of all appropriate treatments, adherence to the treatment plan, and presence of coexisting conditions (strength of evidence: weak; strength of recommendation: strong).

Most school-aged children with ADHD respond to a therapeutic regimen that includes stimulant medications and/or behavioral/environmental interventions. As noted in 3A, when one stimulant medication appears ineffective (despite appropriate titration), clinicians should carry out a trial of a second stimulant medication. Continuing lack of response to treatment may reflect 1) unrealistic target symptoms; 2) lack of information about the child's behavior; 3) an incorrect diagnosis; 4) a coexisting condition affecting the treatment of the ADHD; 5) lack of adherence to the treatment regimen; or 6) a treatment failure. As discussed previously, treatment of ADHD, while decreasing a child's level of impairment, may not fully eliminate the core symptoms of inattention, hyperactivity, and impulsivity. Similarly, children with ADHD may continue to have difficulties with peer relationships despite adequate treatment, and treatment for ADHD frequently shows no association with improvements in academic achievement as measured by standardized instruments.

Evaluation of treatment outcomes requires a careful collection of information from multiple sources, including parents, teachers, other adults in the child's environment (eg, coaches), and the child. If the target symptoms are realistic and the lack of effectiveness is clear, the primary care clinician should reassess the accuracy of the diagnosis of ADHD. This reassessment should include review of the data initially obtained to make the diagnosis, as described in the AAP clinical practice guideline for the diagnosis of children with ADHD.[1] Reassessment usually will require gathering new information from the child, school, and family about the core symptoms of ADHD and their impact on the child's functioning. Clinicians should reconsider other conditions that can mimic ADHD.

As indicated in the diagnostic clinical practice guideline,[1] other conditions commonly accompany ADHD in children, especially oppositional/conduct disorders, anxiety, depression, and learning disorders. These conditions often complicate the treatment of ADHD; clinicians should determine if children who do not respond to treatment have these conditions, either by direct determination in their offices or by referral to appropriate subspecialists (eg, developmental-behavioral pediatricians, child psychiatrists, psychologists, or other mental health clinicians) or the school system (eg, school psychologists for learning disabilities) for further evaluation. These coexisting conditions may not have been fully evaluated initially because of the severity of the ADHD, or the child may have developed another condition with time. Standard psycho-educational testing may clarify the role of learning and language disorders, although other disorders require different assessments.

Treatment plans for ADHD typically require children, families, and schools to enter into a long-term plan that includes a complex medication schedule along with environmental and behavioral interventions. Environmental and behavioral interventions will require ongoing efforts by parents, teachers, and the child. A common cause of nonresponse to treatment is lack of adherence to the treatment plan.

Ongoing monitoring of a child's progress should assess the implementation of the plan and determine key problems with, and barriers to, implementation. The clinician should assess adherence to medication and behavior therapy. Lack of adherence is not the equivalent of treatment failure; clinicians should help families find solutions to adherence problems before considering a plan as a failure.

The following can be considered true treatment failure: 1) lack of response to 2 or 3 stimulant medications at maximum dose without side effects or at any dose with intolerable side effects; 2) inability of behavioral therapy or combination therapy to control the child's behaviors; and 3) the interference of a coexisting condition. In each of these situations, referral to mental health specialists who are knowledgeable about behavioral interventions in children is the next step unless the primary care clinician has expertise and experience in managing these situations.

RECOMMENDATION 5: The clinician should periodically provide a systematic follow-up for the child with ADHD. Monitoring should be directed to target outcomes and adverse effects by obtaining specific information from parents, teachers, and the child (strength of evidence: fair; strength of recommendation: strong).

Clinicians should establish a plan for periodic monitoring of the effects of treatment. Research on adherence to medical regimens in chronic diseases highlights the importance of identifying patient and family concerns and goals and jointly designing a management plan in a way that addresses these concerns and promotes these goals.[61] Plans should include obtaining information about target behaviors, educational output, and medication side effects periodically through office visits, written reports, and phone calls. Monitoring data should include the date of refills, the medication type, dosage, frequency, quantity, and responses to treatment (both medication and behavior therapy). Data can be recorded in a flow sheet, ideally, or in a progress note within each patient's chart. The plan also should include a system for communication among parent, child, and clinician between visits as well as a method for periodic contact with the teacher or other school personnel before a follow-up visit. The monitoring plan should consider normal developmental changes in behavior over time, educational expectations that increase with each grade, and the dynamic nature of a child's home and school environment, because changes in any of these factors may alter target behaviors. All participants should share the plan agenda. Clinicians should provide information and support at frequent intervals in a way that enables the child and family to make informed decisions that promote the child's long-term health and well-being.

Information about target symptoms will continue to come from the parents, child, and teacher. Office interviews, telephone conversations, teacher narratives, and periodic behavior report cards and checklists are among the methods used to obtain needed information. As with the diagnosis of ADHD, clinicians should have active and direct communication with schools. The MTA study indicates the benefit of teacher information over parent-derived information when titrating the medication to maximum benefit.[3,62] Adherence to medication and the behavior therapy program should be reviewed at each encounter.

The frequency of monitoring depends on the degree of dysfunction, complications, and adherence. No controlled trials clearly document the appropriate frequency of follow-up visits. In the MTA trial, children in the medical management groups had better outcomes and more frequent follow-up than those in the standard community category, but whether the frequency of follow-up was a determining factor in outcomes cannot be determined from currently published materials.[3] Once the child is stable, an office visit every 3 to 6 months allows for assessment of learning and behavior. These visits also allow assessment of potential side effects of stimulants, such as decreased appetite and alteration of weight, height, and growth velocity. Periodic requests for medication refills offer an additional opportunity for communication with the family. At the refill request, the family can be asked about the child's functioning in school and interpersonal relationships, as well as updates on communication from the school. If any of the follow-up evaluations reveal a decrease in the targeted outcomes, the clinician must first establish that the family is adhering to the treatment plan.

AREAS FOR FUTURE RESEARCH

Tailoring Treatments to Children and Outcomes

At the present time, the clinician's initial choice of a specific treatment program—the exact stimulant medication and the precise form of behavior therapy—is an area of uncertainty. Research to date has not shown clear advantages of one stimulant medication over others. The process of prescribing an effective and comprehensive plan based on the characteristics of the child and family and tailored in terms of type, intensity, and frequency would help clinicians to improve treatment plans. What is required is information relating specific sociodemographic characteristics (eg, age or sex) or clinical characteristics (eg, subtype of ADHD) to optimal responses to stimulant medication or type of behavior therapy. Moreover, relating treatments to specific behaviors or components of ADHD rather than the whole symptom complex would allow the clinician to better tailor the treatment plan.

Many children with ADHD have coexisting conditions, including anxiety, depression, oppositional defiant disorder, conduct disorder, and learning disabilities. The literature provides minimal information about how to treat these coexisting conditions in conjunction with ADHD and how the conditions affect the effectiveness and safety of treatments. Research on how ADHD and coexisting conditions interact to affect treatment and outcomes will help determine if children require multiple concurrent treatments. Such studies can identify sensible, effective, and comprehensive treatment plans for children with these conditions.

Expanded Treatment Options

A major research challenge pertaining to the treatment of ADHD is the development and evaluation of new treatments for this condition. The 2 current treatments (stimulant medication and behavior therapy) reduce the symptoms and functional consequences of ADHD, but only for as long as they are administered. Treatments with more lasting or even curative effects are needed. A significant number of children do not respond to stimulant medications or have severe side effects. Some families cannot implement behavioral programs. Expanding the available medical and behavioral treatment regimens with additional safe and effective options would be useful for such a prevalent chronic condition where not all children respond to current treatments or adhere to them. Studying common-sense approaches, such as decreasing environmental distraction, should be done. There is also the need for well-designed rigorous studies of currently promoted but less well-established therapies such as occupational therapy, biofeedback, herbs, vitamins, and food supplements. These interventions are not supported by evidence-based studies at the present time.

Long-term Outcomes

Most studies about ADHD and its treatment have been short-term. The long-term outcome of children with ADHD with or without coexisting conditions has not been well studied. Furthermore, there is minimal information about the role of stimulant medication and/or behavior therapy in the natural history of the disorder. Future research should correct these deficits. For this chronic condition, efficacy and safety studies must be extended from weeks or months to years. Long-term outcome studies must be prospective in design and consider changes over time in core symptoms of ADHD, coexisting conditions, and functional outcomes such as occupational successes and long-term relationships.

Service Delivery

Another major research area should address the optimal services and procedures for successful management of ADHD in the real world (ie, in clinical practice and classrooms). Much of the popular controversy over the inappropriate use of stimulant medication relates to how clinicians actually prescribe them. Future research needs to study how medications are actually prescribed and what factors affect physician practice patterns. Research that includes monitoring the outcomes of training will lead to the ability to develop better methods to assist clinicians in using effective treatment practices. Specifically, basic information such as who are the most appropriate clinicians to manage ADHD; the best schedule for follow-up; and the most valid, reliable, sensitive, and cost-effective ways to monitor treatment is essential. Such research must go beyond physician self-reporting and into scrutinizing and evaluating actual practices in clinics and offices. The

most effective and efficient methods for affecting change in clinician practices need to be determined. This determination must be broad, taking into account clinician, practice, family, community, and policy issues that affect treatment. Research also should evaluate the role of school- and community-based professionals, as well as primary care clinicians, in delivering treatment services. Little is known about how short- or long-term effectiveness varies as a function of the school and community-based professional involvement. Further, the studies of service delivery need to include a public health and service system approach. They should consider child and family outcomes and cost-effectiveness of care. Linking outcomes to service parameters is an important step in encouraging practice or system change.

Epidemiology and Etiology

The great growth in the diagnosis of ADHD has led to major new work in the study of treatments. As indicated previously, these efforts should continue and expand. Less investigation has addressed the etiology of ADHD (ie, its biological and socioenvironmental causes) and the opportunities arising from that understanding for prevention. For example, would different social and behavioral arrangements in young families affect the onset of ADHD symptoms? Would early intervention in some way decrease rates of ADHD? A clear need exists for active work in understanding the etiology and prevention of ADHD.

CONCLUSION

This clinical practice guideline offers recommendations for the treatment of school-aged children with ADHD in primary care practice. The guideline emphasizes 1) consideration of ADHD as a chronic condition; 2) explicit negotiations about target symptoms; 3) use of stimulant medication and behavior therapy; and 4) close monitoring of treatment outcomes and failures. The guideline further provides suggestions for pediatric office-based management of ADHD. It should help primary care clinicians in their treatment of a common child health problem.

SUBCOMMITTEE ON
 ATTENTION-DEFICIT/HYPERACTIVITY DISORDER
James M. Perrin, MD, Cochairperson
Martin T. Stein, MD, Cochairperson
Robert W. Amler, MD
Thomas A. Blondis, MD
Heidi M. Feldman, MD, PhD
Bruce P. Meyer, MD
Bennett A. Shaywitz, MD
Mark L. Wolraich, MD

CONSULTANTS
Anthony DeSpirito, MD
Charles J. Homer, MD, MPH
Esther Wender, MD

LIAISON REPRESENTATIVES
Ronald T. Brown, PhD
 Society for Pediatric Psychology

Theodore G. Ganiats, MD
   American Academy of Family Physicians
Brian Grabert, MD
   Child Neurology Society
Karen Pierce, MD
   American Academy of Child and Adolescent
   Psychiatry

STAFF
Carla T. Herrerias, BS, MPH

COMMITTEE ON QUALITY IMPROVEMENT
Charles J. Homer, MD, MPH, Chairperson
Richard D. Baltz, MD
Gerald B. Hickson, MD
Paul V. Miles, MD
Thomas B. Newman, MD, MPH
Joan E. Shook, MD
William M. Zurhellen, MD

LIAISON REPRESENTATIVES
Betty A. Lowe, MD
   National Association of Children's Hospitals
   and Related Institutions
Ellen Schwalenstocker, MBA
   National Association of Children's Hospitals
   and Related Institutions
Michael J. Goldberg, MD
   Council on Sections
Richard Shiffman, MD
   Section on Computers and Other
   Technologies
Jan Ellen Berger, MD
   Committee on Medical Liability
F. Lane France, MD
   Committee on Practice and Ambulatory
   Medicine

ACKNOWLEDGMENTS

The subcommittee wishes to acknowledge the numerous people and groups that made development of this clinical practice guideline possible. The subcommittee would like to thank the Agency for Healthcare Research and Quality and the McMaster University Evidence-based Practice Center for its work in developing the evidence report, and William E. Pelham, Jr, PhD, and Peter Jensen, MD, for their continuous input and insight into the evidence about treatment of ADHD.

REFERENCES

1. American Academy of Pediatrics, Committee on Quality Improvement and Subcommittee on Attention-Deficit/Hyperactivity Disorder. Diagnosis and evaluation of the child with attention-deficit/hyperactivity disorder. *Pediatrics.* 2000;105:1158–1170

2. Jadad AR, Boyle M, Cunningham C, et al. *Treatment of Attention Deficit/ Hyperactivity Disorder. Evidence Report/Technology Assessment No. 11.* Rockville, MD: Agency for Healthcare Research and Quality; 1999. AHRQ Publ. No. 00-E005

3. Jensen P, Arnold L, Richters J, et al. 14-month randomized clinical trial of treatment strategies for attention deficit hyperactivity disorder. *Arch Gen Psychiatry.* 1999;56:1073–1086

4. Miller A, Lee S, Raina P, et al. *A Review of Therapies for Attention-Deficit/ Hyperactivity Disorder.* Ottawa, Ontario: Canadian Coordinating Office for Health Technology Assessment (CCOHTA); 1998

5. American Psychiatric Association. *Diagnostic and Statistical Manual of Mental Disorders.* 4th ed. Washington, DC: American Psychiatric Association; 1994

6. Pelham WE Jr, Wheeler T, Chronis A. Empirically supported psychosocial treatments for attention deficit hyperactivity disorder. *J Clin Child Psychol.* 1998;27:190–205

7. MTA Cooperative Group. Moderators and mediators of treatment response for children with attention-deficit/hyperactivity disorder: the multimodal treatment study of children with ADHD. *Arch Gen Psychiatry.* 1999;56:1088–1096

8. Epstein JN, Conners CK, Erhardt D, et al. Familial aggregation of ADHD characteristics. *J Abnorm Child Psychol.* 2000;28:585–594

9. Hinshaw SP, Owens EB, Wells KC, et al. Family processes and treatment outcomes in the MTA: negative/ineffective parenting practices in relation to multimodal treatment. *J Abnorm Child Psychol.* 2000;28: 555–568

10. Hoza B, Owens JS, Pelham WE Jr, et al. Cognitions as predictors of child treatment response in attention-deficit/hyperactivity disorder. *J Abnorm Child Psychol.* 2000;28:569–583

11. March JS, Swanson JM, Arnold LE, et al. Anxiety as a predictor and outcome variable in the multimodal treatment study of children with ADHD. *J Abnorm Child Psychol.* 2000;28:527–541

12. Pelham WE Jr, Gnagy EM, Greiner AR, et al. Behavioral vs behavioral and pharmacological treatment in ADHD children attending a summer treatment program. *J Abnorm Child Psychol.* 2000;28:507–525

13. Conners CK, Epstein JN, March JS, et al. Multimodal treatment of ADHD (MTA): an alternative outcome analysis. *J Am Acad Child Adolesc Psychiatry.* 2000;40:159–167

14. Wells KC, Epstein JN, Hinshaw SP, et al. Parenting and family stress treatment outcomes in attention deficit hyperactivity disorder (ADHD): an empirical analysis in the MTA study. *J Abnorm Child Psychol.* 2000; 28:543–553

15. Wells KC, Pelham WE Jr, Kotkin RA, et al. Psychosocial treatment strategies in the MTA study. Rationale, methods, and critical issues in design and implementation. *J Abnorm Child Psychol.* 2000;28:483–505

16. Hinshaw SP, March JS, Abikoff H, et al. Comprehensive assessment of childhood attention-deficit hyperactivity disorder in the context of a multisite, multimodal clinical trial. *J Attention Disorders.* 1997;1:217–234

17. Pelham WE Jr, Fabiano G. Behavior modification. *Child Adolesc Psychiatr Clin North Am.* 2001;9:671–688

18. Barkley RA, Fischer M, Edelbrock CS, Smallish L. The adolescent outcome of hyperactive children diagnosed by research criteria: I: an 8-year prospective follow-up study. *J Am Acad Child Adolesc Psychiatry.* 1990; 29:546–557

19. Biederman J, Faraone S, Milberger S, et al. A prospective 4-year follow-up study of attention-deficit hyperactivity and related disorders. *Arch Gen Psychiatry.* 1996;53:437–446

20. Mannuzza S, Klein R, Bessler A, Malloy P, LaPudula M. Adult psychiatric status of hyperactive boys grown up. *Am J Psychiatry.* 1998;155: 493–498

21. American Academy of Pediatrics, Committee on Children With Disabilities. Pediatric services for infants and children with special health care needs. *Pediatrics.* 1993;92:163–165

22. American Academy of Pediatrics, Committee on Children With Disabilities. General principles in the care of children and adolescents with genetic disorders and other chronic health conditions. *Pediatrics.* 1997; 99:643–644

23. American Academy of Pediatrics, Committee on Children With Disabilities. Care coordination: integrating health and related systems of care for children with special health care needs. *Pediatrics.* 1999;104:978–981

24. American Academy of Pediatrics, Committee on Psychosocial Aspects of Child and Family Health and Committee on Children With Disabilities. Psychosocial risks of chronic health conditions in children and adolescents. *Pediatrics.* 1993;92:876–878

25. Perrin JM. Children with chronic illness. In: Behrman RE, ed. *Nelson Textbook of Pediatrics.* 16th ed. Philadelphia, PA: WB Saunders Co; 2000:123–125

26. Perrin JM, Shayne MW, Bloom SR. *Home and Community Care for Chronically Ill Children.* New York, NY: Oxford University Press; 1993

27. Fireman P, Friday GA, Gira C, Vierthaler WA, Michaels L. Teaching self-management skills to asthmatic children and parents in an ambulatory care setting. *Pediatrics.* 1981;68:341–348

28. Jessop DJ, Stein REK. Providing comprehensive health care to children with chronic illness. *Pediatrics.* 1994;93:602–607

29. Nader PR, ed. *School Health: Policy and Practice.* 5th ed. Elk Grove Village, IL: American Academy of Pediatrics; 1993

30. Kavale K. The efficacy of stimulant drug treatment for hyperactivity: a meta-analysis. *J Learn Disabil.* 1982;15:280–289

31. Ottenbacher KJ. Drug treatment of hyperactivity in children. *Dev Med Child Neurol.* 1983;25:358–366

32. Thurber S. Medication and hyperactivity. A meta-analysis. *J Gen Psychol.* 1983;108:79–86

33. Swanson JM, McBurnett K, Wigal T, et al. Effect of stimulant medication on children with attention-deficit disorder—a review of reviews. *Except Child.* 1993;60:154–162

34. Cohen J. *Statistical Power Analysis for the Behavioural Sciences.* New York, NY: Academic Press; 1977

35. Ingram S, Hechtman L, Morgenstern G. Outcomes issues in ADHD: adolescent and adult long-term outcomes. *Ment Retard Dev Disabil Res Rev.* 1999;5:243–250

36. Sheveli M, Schreiber R. Pemoline-associated hepatic failure: a critical analysis of the literature. *Pediatr Neurol.* 1997;16:14–16

37. Connors CK, Casat CD, Guaitieri CT, et al. Bupropion hydrochloride in attention deficit disorder with hyperactivity. *J Am Acad Child Adolesc Psychiatry.* 1996;35:1314–1321

38. Biederman J, Thisted RA, Greenhill LL, Ryan ND. Estimation of the association between desipramine and the risk for sudden death in 5- to 14-year-old children. *J Clin Psychiatry.* 1995;56:87–93

39. Connor DF, Fletcher KE, Swanson JM. A meta-analysis of clonidine for symptoms of attention-deficit hyperactivity disorder. *J Am Acad Child Adolesc Psychiatry.* 1999;38:1551–1559

40. Prince JB, Wilens TE, Biederman J Spencer TJ, Wozniak JR. Clonidine for sleep disturbances associated with attention-deficit hyperactivity disorder: a systematic chart review of 62 cases. *J Am Acad Child Adolesc Psychiatry.* 1996;35:499–605

41. Gadow KD, Sverci J, Sprafkin J, Nolan EE, Grossman S. Long-term methylphenidate therapy in children with co-morbid attention-deficit hyperactivity disorder and chronic multiple tic disorder. *Arch Gen Psychiatry.* 1999;56:330–336

42. Castellanos FX, Giedd JN, Elia J, et al. Controlled stimulant treatment of ADHD and comorbid Tourette's syndrome: effects of stimulant and dose. *J Am Acad Child Adolesc Psychiatry.* 1997;36:589–596

43. PDR Electronic Library. Available at: www.pdrel.com. Accessed March 14, 2001

44. Gross-Tsur V, Manor O, van der Meere J, Joseph A, Shalev RS. Epilepsy and attention deficit hyperactivity disorder: is methylphenidate safe and effective? *J Pediatr.* 1997;130:670–674

45. Wroblewski BA, Leary JM, Phelan AM, Whyte J, Manning K. Methylphenidate and seizure frequency in brain injured patients with seizure disorders. *J Clin Psychiatry.* 1992;53:86–89

46. Feldman H, Crumrine P, Handen BL, Alvin R, Teodori J. Methylphenidate in children with seizures and attention-deficit disorder. *Am J Dis Child.* 1989;143:1081–1086

47. Greenhill LL, Halperin JM, Abikoff H. Stimulant medications. *J Am Acad Child Adolesc Psychiatry.* 1999;38:503–528

48. Mannuzza S, Klein RG, Bonagura N, Malloy P, Giampino TL, Addali KA. Hyperactive boys almost grow up V: replication of psychiatric status. *Arch Gen Psychiatry.* 1991;48:77–83

49. Gross MD. Growth of hyperkinetic children taking methylphenidate, dextroamphetamine or imipramine/desipramine. *Pediatrics.* 1976;58:423–431

50. Satterfield JH, Cantwell DP, Schell A, Blaschke T. Growth of hyperactive children treated with methylphenidate. *Arch Gen Psychiatry.* 1979;36:212–217

51. Kent JD, Blader JC, Koplewicz HS, Abikoff H, Foley CA. Effects of late-afternoon methylphenidate administration on behavior and sleep in attention-deficit hyperactivity disorder. *Pediatrics.* 1995;96:320–325

52. Efron D, Jarman F, Barker M. Side effects of methylphenidate and dextroamphetamine in children with attention deficit hyperactivity disorder: a double-blind, crossover trial. *Pediatrics.* 1997;100:662–666

53. Schertz M, Adesman A, Alfieri N, Bienkowski RS. Predictors of weight loss in children with attention deficit hyperactivity disorder treated with stimulant medication. *Pediatrics.* 1996;98:763–769

54. Rappaport JL, Zahn TP, Ludlow C, Mikkelsen EJ. Dextroamphetamine: cognitive and behavioral effects in normal prepubertal boys. *Science.* 1978;199:560–563

55. Arnold LE. Methylphenidate versus amphetamine: a comparative review. In: Greenhill LL, Osman BB, eds. *Ritalin: Theory and Practice.* 2nd ed. Larchmont, NY: Mary Ann Liebert, Inc; 2000:127–140

56. Barkley RA. *Handbook of Attention Deficit Hyperactivity Disorder.* 2nd ed. New York, NY: Guildford; 1998

57. Pelham WE Jr, Hinshaw S. *Handbook of Clinical Behavior Therapy.* Turner S, ed. New York, NY: Wiley; 1992

58. Swanson JM, Kraemer HC, Hinshaw SP, et al. Clinical relevance of the primary findings of the MTA: success rates based on severity of symptoms at the end of treatment. *J Am Acad Child Adolesc Psychiatry.* 2001;40:168–179

59. Jensen PS, Hinshaw SP, Kraemer HC, et al. ADHD comorbidity findings from the MTA study: comparing comorbid subgroups. *J Am Acad Child Adolesc Psychiatry.* 2001;40:147–158

60. Pelham WE Jr, MTA Cooperative Group. Presented at: Association for the Advancement of Behavioral Therapy. November 2000; New Orleans, LA

61. Clark N, Gong M. Management of chronic disease by practitioners and patients: are we teaching the wrong things? *BMJ.* 2000;320:572–575

62. Greenhill LL, Swanson JM, Vitiello B, et al. Determining the best dose of methylphenidate under controlled conditions: lessons from the MTA titration. *J Am Acad Child Adolesc Psychiatry.* 2001;40:180–198

Screening and Diagnosis of Autism

• •

The following guideline for screening and diagnosis of autism, developed by the Quality Standards Subcommittee of the American Academy of Neurology and the Child Neurology Society, has been endorsed by the American Academy of Pediatrics.

Special Article

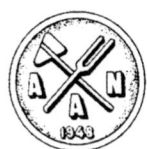

Practice parameter: Screening and diagnosis of autism

Report of the Quality Standards Subcommittee of the American Academy of Neurology and the Child Neurology Society

P.A. Filipek, MD; P.J. Accardo, MD; S. Ashwal, MD; G.T. Baranek, PhD, OTR/L; E.H. Cook, Jr., MD;
G. Dawson, PhD; B. Gordon, MD, PhD; J.S. Gravel, PhD; C.P. Johnson, MEd, MD; R.J. Kallen, MD;
S.E. Levy, MD; N.J. Minshew, MD; S. Ozonoff, PhD; B.M. Prizant, PhD, CCC-SLP; I. Rapin, MD;
S.J. Rogers, PhD; W.L. Stone, PhD; S.W. Teplin, MD; R.F. Tuchman, MD; and F.R. Volkmar, MD

Article abstract—Autism is a common disorder of childhood, affecting 1 in 500 children. Yet, it often remains unrecognized and undiagnosed until or after late preschool age because appropriate tools for routine developmental screening and screening specifically for autism have not been available. Early identification of children with autism and intensive, early intervention during the toddler and preschool years improves outcome for most young children with autism. This practice parameter reviews the available empirical evidence and gives specific recommendations for the identification of children with autism. This approach requires a dual process: 1) routine developmental surveillance and screening specifically for autism to be performed on all children to first identify those at risk for any type of atypical development, and to identify those specifically at risk for autism; and 2) to diagnose and evaluate autism, to differentiate autism from other developmental disorders.

NEUROLOGY 2000;55:468–479

This statement has been endorsed by the American Academy of Audiology, the American Occupational Therapy Association, the American Speech–Language–Hearing Association, the Autism National Committee, Cure Autism Now, the National Alliance for Autism Research, and the Society for Developmental Pediatrics.

From the Departments of Pediatrics and Neurology (Dr. Filipek), University of California, Irvine, College of Medicine; Department of Pediatrics (Dr. Accardo), New York Medical College, Valhalla; Department of Pediatrics (Dr. Ashwal), Loma Linda University School of Medicine, California; Departments of Allied Health Sciences (Dr. Baranek) and Pediatrics (Dr. Teplin), University of North Carolina at Chapel Hill; Departments of Psychiatry (Dr. Cook) and Pediatrics (Drs. Cook and Kallen), University of Chicago, Illinois; Department of Psychology (Dr. Dawson), University of Washington, Seattle; Department of Neurology and Cognitive Science (Dr. Gordon), The Johns Hopkins Medical Institutions, Baltimore, Maryland; Departments of Otolaryngology (Dr. Gravel), Neurology and Pediatrics (Dr. Rapin), Albert Einstein College of Medicine, Yeshiva University, Bronx, New York; Department of Pediatrics (Dr. Johnson), University of Texas Health Science Center, San Antonio; Department of Pediatrics (Dr. Levy), University of Pennsylvania School of Medicine, Philadelphia; Department of Psychiatry and Neurology (Dr. Minshew), University of Pittsburgh School of Medicine, Pennsylvania; Departments of Psychology and Psychiatry (Dr. Ozonoff), University of Utah, Salt Lake City; Center for Study of Human Development (Dr. Prizant), Brown University, Providence, Rhode Island; Department of Psychiatry (Dr. Rogers), University of Colorado Health Sciences Center, Denver; Department of Pediatrics (Dr. Stone), Vanderbilt University Medical Center, Nashville, Tennessee; Department of Neurology (Dr. Tuchman), University of Miami School of Medicine, Florida; and Department of Child Psychiatry and the Child Study Center (Dr. Volkmar), Yale University School of Medicine, New Haven, Connecticut.

Supported by the National Institute of Child Health and Human Development; the National Institute of Deafness and Communication Disorders; the National Institute of Mental Health; the National Institute of Neurologic Disorders and Stroke; the NIH Office of Behavioral and Social Sciences Research; the Maternal and Child Health Bureau, Health Resources; and Services Administration, Department of Health and Human Resources. Supported in part by HD28202/ HD27802/ HD35458 (P.A.F.), HD35482 (E.H.C. and F.R.V.), HD34565 (G.D.), HD36080 (J.S.G.), HD35469 (N.J.M.), HD35468 (S.J.R.) and HD03008 (F.R.V.) from the National Institute of Child Health and Human Development; DC00223 (J.S.G.) from the National Institute of Deafness and Communication Disorders; MH01389/ MH52223 (E.H.C.), MH47117 (G.D.), and MH50620 (W.L.S.) from the National Institute of Mental Health; NS35896 (P.A.F.), NS33355 (N.J.M.), NS20489 (I.R.), from the National Institute of Neurologic Disorders and Stroke, and by the NIH Office of Behavioral and Social Sciences Research, National Institutes of Health, Bethesda, MD. Supported by MCJ-369029 (P.J.A.) from the Maternal and Child Health Bureau, Health Resources and Services Administration, Department of Health and Human Resources. The Panel also gratefully acknowledges the unrestricted educational grants provided for this endeavor by the AAN Foundation, Janssen Pharmaceutica, the SK Corporation, Abbott Laboratories, Novartis, and Athena Neurosciences, Inc.

The authors and coauthors have read and agree with the content of this publication and acknowledge their compliance with the "Disclosure" requirements of *Neurology*. There is no pertinent financial interest of any author (i.e., ownership, equity position, stock options, patent-licensing arrangements), consulting fees, or honoraria associated with this publication or its products.

Approved by the AAN Quality Standards Subcommittee on April 1, 2000. Approved by the AAN Practice Committee on May 3, 2000. Approved by the AAN Board of Directors on June 9, 2000.

Address correspondence and reprint requests to QSS, American Academy of Neurology, 1080 Montreal Avenue, St. Paul, MN 55116; phone: 1-800-879-1960.

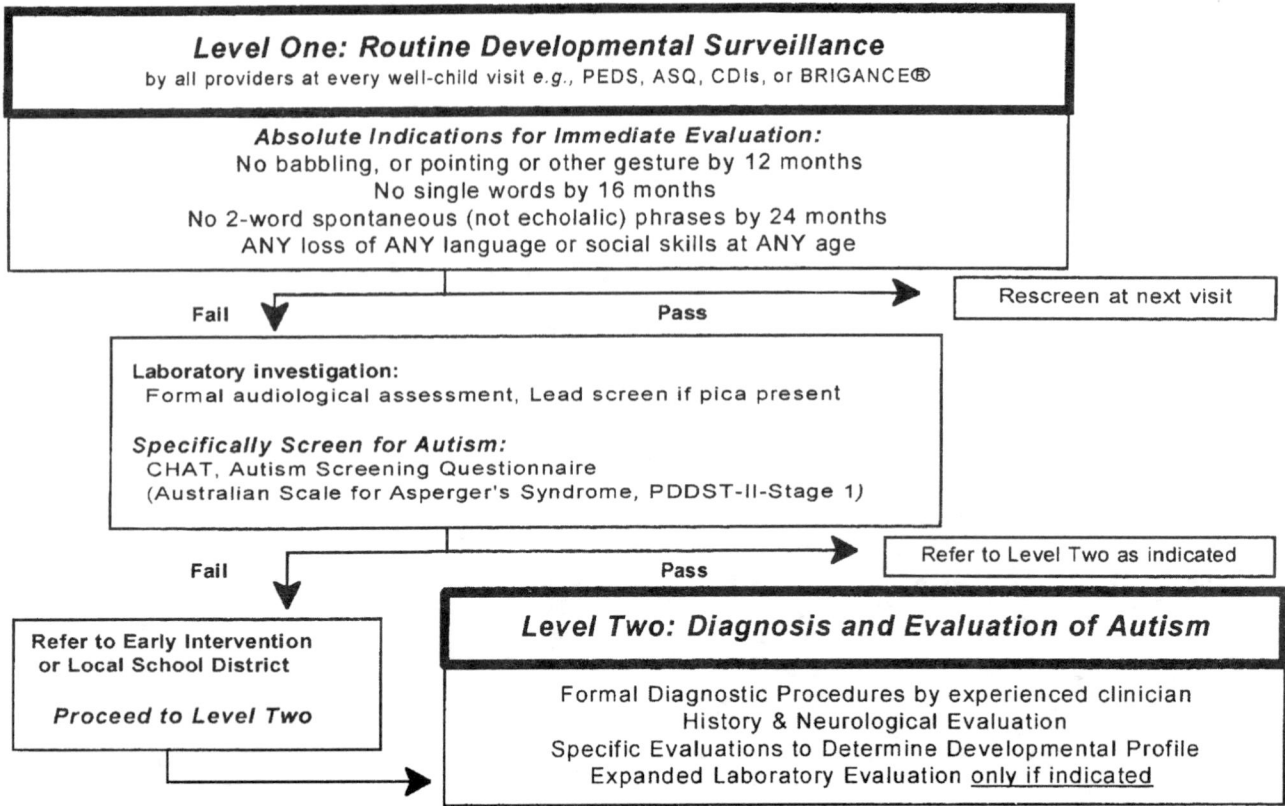

Figure. Practice parameter algorithm.

Autism, autistic spectrum, and pervasive developmental disorders encompass a wide continuum of associated cognitive and neurobehavioral disorders, including the core-defining features of impaired socialization, impaired verbal and nonverbal communication, and restricted and repetitive patterns of behavior (table).[1] Between 60,000 and 115,000 children under 15 years of age in the United States meet diagnostic criteria for autism based on recent prevalence estimates of 10 to 20 cases per 10,000 people. In 1,300 families recently surveyed, the average age at diagnosis of autism was about 6 years, despite the fact that most parents felt something was wrong by 18 months of age and usually sought medical assistance by age 2 years.[2] Fewer than 10% of the children were diagnosed at initial presentation; another 10% were either told to return if their worries persisted, or that their child "would grow out of it." The rest were referred to another professional (at a mean age of 40 months), of which only 40% were given a formal diagnosis, 25% were told "not to worry," and 25% were referred to a third or fourth professional. Almost 20% reported that they either had to exert considerable pressure to obtain the referrals or pay privately. Over 30% of parents referred to subsequent professionals reported that no help was offered (e.g., with education, therapy, or referrals to parent support groups), and only about 10% reported that a professional explained their child's problems. Almost

half of the families reported that the school system and other parents were the major source of assistance over time, rather than the medical health care community.

The diagnosis of autism often is not made until 2 to 3 years after symptoms are recognized, primarily because of concerns about labeling or incorrectly diagnosing the child. Identifying children with autism and initiating intensive, early intervention during the preschool years results in improved outcomes for most young children with autism.[3-7] Early diagnosis of autism and early intervention facilitates earlier educational planning, provisions for family supports and education, management of family stress and anguish, and delivery of appropriate medical care and treatment.[3-7]

Clinically identifying children with autism requires two levels of investigation, each addressing a distinct component of patient management (figure).[1] The first level, *Routine Developmental Surveillance and Screening Specifically for Autism*, should be performed on all children and involves first identifying those at risk for any type of atypical development, followed by identifying those specifically at risk for autism. Mental retardation or other medical or neurodevelopmental conditions require separate evaluations and are not within the scope of this document.

The second level, *Diagnosis and Evaluation of Autism*, involves a more in-depth investigation of already identified children and differentiates autism from other developmental disorders. In-depth diagnosis and

Table Diagnostic Criteria for 299.00 Autistic Disorder

A. A total of six (or more) items from (1), (2), and (3), with two from (1), and at least one each from (2) and (3):

1. Qualitative impairment in social interaction, manifest by at least two of the following:

   - Marked impairment in the use of multiple nonverbal behaviors, such as eye-to-eye gaze, facial expression, body postures, and gestures, to regulate social interaction

   - Failure to develop peer relationships appropriate to developmental level

   - Lack of spontaneous seeking to share enjoyment, interests, or achievements with other people (e.g., by lack of showing, bringing, or pointing out objects of interest)

   - Lack of social or emotional reciprocity

2. Qualitative impairment in communication, as manifest by at least one of the following:

   - Delay in, or total lack of, the development of spoken language (not accompanied by an attempt to compensate through alternative modes of communication such as gesture or mime)

   - In individuals with adequate speech, marked impairment in the ability to initiate or sustain a conversation with others

   - Stereotyped and repetitive use of language, or idiosyncratic language

   - Lack of varied, spontaneous make-believe, or social imitative play appropriate to developmental level

3. Restrictive repetitive and stereotypic patterns of behavior, interests, and activities, as manifested by at least one of the following:

   - Encompassing preoccupation with one or more stereotyped and restricted patterns of interest that is abnormal either in intensity or focus

   - Apparently inflexible adherence to specific nonfunctional routines or rituals

   - Stereotyped and repetitive motor mannerisms (e.g., hand or finger flapping or twisting, or complex whole-body movements)

   - Persistent preoccupation with parts of objects.

B. Delays or abnormal functioning in at least one of the following areas, with onset prior to age 3 years:

1. Social interaction

2. Language as used in social communication

3. Symbolic or imaginative play

C. The disturbance is not better accounted for by Rett's disorder or childhood disintegrative disorder.

The other pervasive developmental disorders include Asperger's disorder, Rett syndrome, childhood disintegrative disorder, pervasive developmental disorder—not otherwise specified (PDD-NOS), or atypical autism.

Reprinted with permission from the *Diagnostic and Statistical Manual of Mental Disorders, 4th edition.* Washington, DC: American Psychiatric Association, 1994:70–71.

Detailed information on other PDD diagnoses can be found in the comprehensive background paper.[1]

evaluation are important in determining optimal interventional strategies based on the child's profile of strengths and weaknesses. For these two areas of in-

vestigation, specific clinical questions were defined (see Appendix 2), clinical evidence was summarized, and diagnostic recommendations were developed.

Evidence and recommendations are presented in three sections. The first two sections, *Level One: Routine Developmental Surveillance and Screening Specifically for Autism,* and *Level Two: Diagnosis and Evaluation of Autism,* first present the empiric data for each question and are followed by recommendations linked to the specific evidence. Each is followed by a section on *Recommendations for Research.* The third section, *Consensus-Based General Principles of Management,* presents additional recommendations based on broad consensus. Additional information about autism, including behavioral aspects associated with the core defining deficits, methodology, and clinical evidence are described in the background paper.[1] Specific information about the recommended developmental screening and diagnostic tools can be found at *http://www.aan.com* under *AAN Resources: Practice Statements: Official AAN Practice Statements: Autism, Screening and diagnosis of.*

Description of the process. Experts in the surveillance/screening and diagnosis of autism were selected by 11 professional organizations (see Appendix 1) and convened in June 1998 and January 1999. They reviewed and evaluated the quality of the evidence from the published literature, developed a consensus of evidence-based management recommendations, and published a comprehensive background paper on the surveillance, screening, and diagnosis of autism.[1] Evidence reviewed for this parameter was identified through literature searches using MEDLINE and PsychINFO. Relevant articles were included from all languages using the following search terms: autistic; OR autism; OR pervasive, and NOT treatment. This search produced over 4,000 citations, from which 2,750 studies met the following inclusion criteria: clinical papers published since 1990; review papers and meta-analyses developed for DSM-IV; and the overview of the *National Institutes of Health State of the Science Conference on Autism in 1995.* Relevant book chapters and books were also included, as identified by the expert panel.

The strength of the evidence for each relevant article and book chapter was ranked using the defined criteria shown in Appendix 3. Recommendations were thereby derived based on the strength of the evidence and stratified (**Standard, Guideline,** or **Practice Option**) as defined in Appendix 3.

Level one: routine developmental surveillance and screening specifically for autism. *Analysis of the evidence.* When and how often should developmental surveillance/screening be performed? Approximately 25% of children in any primary care practice show developmental issues. However, fewer than 30% of primary care providers conduct standardized screening tests at well-child appointments.[8-10] The American Academy of Pediatrics (AAP) stresses the importance of a flexible, continual developmental surveillance process at each well-child visit, and recommends eliciting and valuing parental concerns, probing regarding age-appropriate skills in each developmental domain, and observing each child.[11]

What are the appropriate developmental screening questionnaires that provide sensitive and specific information? Developmental screening tools have been formulated based on screening of large populations of children with standardized test items. Sensitive and specific developmental screening instruments include: the Ages and Stages Questionnaire, the BRIGANCE Screens, the Child Development Inventories, and the Parents' Evaluations of Developmental Status.[1]

The Denver-II (DDST-II, formerly the Denver Developmental Screening Test-Revised) has been the traditional tool used for developmental screening, but research has found that it is insensitive and lacks specificity. The Revised Denver Pre-Screening Developmental Questionnaire (R-DPDQ) was designed to identify a subset of children who needed further screening. However, studies have shown that it detected only 30% of children with language impairments and 50% of children with mental retardation.[12-15]

How are conventional developmental milestones defined? Conventional developmental language milestones are based on normative data from numerous standardized language instruments for infants.[16-19] Lack of acquisition of the following milestones within known accepted and established ranges is considered abnormal: no babbling by 12 months; no gesturing (e.g., pointing, waving bye-bye) by 12 months; no single words by 16 months; no 2-word spontaneous (not just echolalic) phrases by 24 months; and any loss of any language or social skills at any age. Failure to meet these milestones is associated with a high probability of a developmental disability.

Do parents provide reliable information regarding their child's development? Several studies encompassing 737 children showed that parental concerns about speech and language development, behavior, or other developmental issues were highly sensitive (i.e., 75% to 83%) and specific (79% to 81%) in detecting global developmental deficits.[20-22] However, the absence of such concerns had modest specificity in detecting normal development (47%).[20] An additional study that combined parental concern with a standardized parental report found this to be effective for early behavioral and developmental screening in the primary care setting.[23]

Can autism be reliably diagnosed before 36 months of age? Because there are no biological markers for autism, screening must focus on behavior. Recent studies comparing 109 autistic and 33 typically developing children demonstrated that problems with eye contact, orienting to one's name, joint attention, pretend play, imitation, nonverbal communication, and language development are measurable by 18 months of age.[24-27] These symptoms are stable in children from toddler age through preschool

age. Retrospective analysis of home videotapes have also identified behaviors that distinguish infants with autism from other developmental disabilities as early as 8 months of age.[28-30]

Current screening methods may not identify children with milder variants of autism, those without mental retardation or language delay, such as verbal individuals with high-functioning autism and Asperger's disorder, or older children, adolescents, and young adults.

Is there an increased risk of having another child with autism (recurrence)? The incidence of autism in the general population is 0.2%, but the risk of having a second (or additional) autistic child increases almost 50-fold to approximately 10 to 20%.[31-34]

What tools are available with appropriate psychometric properties to specifically screen for autism? Appropriately sensitive and specific autism screening tools for infants and toddlers have only recently been developed, and this continues to be the current focus of many research centers. The Checklist for Autism in Toddlers (CHAT) for 18-month-old infants, and the Autism Screening Questionnaire for children 4 years of age and older, have been validated on large populations of children. However, it should be noted that the CHAT is less sensitive to milder symptoms of autism, as children later diagnosed with PDD-NOS, Asperger's, or atypical autism did not routinely fail the CHAT at 18 months.[27,35]

The Pervasive Developmental Disorders Screening Test–II (PDDST-II) for infants from birth to 3 years of age, the Modified Checklist for Autism in Toddlers (M-CHAT) for infants at 2 years of age, and the Australian Scale for Asperger's Syndrome for older verbal children, are currently under development or validation phases.[1]

What screening laboratory investigations are available for developmental delay, with or without suspicion of autism? *Formal audiologic evaluation.* The Committee on Infant Hearing of the American Speech–Language–Hearing Association developed guidelines for the audiologic assessment of children from birth through 36 months of age.[36] They recommended that all children with developmental delays, particularly those with delays in social and language development, have a formal audiologic hearing evaluation. Three studies have documented that conductive, sensorineural, or mixed hearing loss can co-occur with autism, and that some children with autism may be incorrectly thought to have peripheral hearing loss.[37,38] In addition, transient conductive hearing loss associated with otitis media with effusion can also occur in children with autism.

Audiologic assessment of such children requires modifications of traditional test techniques and environments (e.g., operant test procedures).[39,40] Electrophysiologic procedures are useful for estimating hearing sensitivity and for examining middle ear, cochlear, and VIIIth nerve or auditory brainstem pathway integrity.[41,42] Evoked otoacoustic emissions are useful for examining cochlear (sensory) function, and is a frequency-specific, as well as a time- and cost-efficient procedure.[43] Frequency-specific auditory brainstem response (ABR) is the single most useful electrophysiologic procedure for use in estimating hearing thresholds, and has been demonstrated to be highly correlated with behavioral hearing thresholds in children who hear normally and in children who have sensorineural hearing loss.[42]

Lead screening. Children with developmental delays who spend an extended period in the oral–motor stage of play (where everything "goes into their mouths") are at increased risk for lead toxicity, especially in certain environments. The prevalence of pica in this group can result in high rates of substantial or recurrent exposure to lead. The National Center for Environmental Health of the Centers for Disease Control and Prevention recommends that children with developmental delays, even without frank pica, should be screened for lead poisoning.[44] Blood lead levels in children with autism are elevated.[1] In one study, the mean blood lead level in 18 autistic children was higher than in 16 nonautistic "psychotic" children or in 10 normal siblings; 44% of the autistic and psychotic children had lead levels significantly above the mean compared with control subjects.[45] In a more recent study, 17 autistic children treated for lead poisoning were compared with 30 children without autism. The autistic children were older at diagnosis, had higher lead levels, and most were reexposed despite close monitoring of their environment.[46]

Level one evidence-based recommendations.
Clinical practice recommendations.

1. Developmental surveillance should be performed at all well-child visits from infancy through school-age, and at any age thereafter if concerns are raised about social acceptance, learning, or behavior (**Guideline**).
2. Recommended developmental screening tools include the Ages and Stages Questionnaire, the BRIGANCE Screens, the Child Development Inventories, and the Parents' Evaluations of Developmental Status (**Guideline**).
3. Because of the lack of sensitivity and specificity, the Denver-II (DDST-II) and the Revised Denver Pre-Screening Developmental Questionnaire (R-DPDQ) are not recommended for appropriate primary-care developmental surveillance (**Guideline**).
4. Further developmental evaluation is required whenever a child fails to meet any of the following milestones (**Guideline**): babbling by 12 months; gesturing (e.g., pointing, waving bye-bye) by 12 months; single words by 16 months; two-word spontaneous (not just echolalic) phrases by 24 months; loss of any language or social skills at any age.
5. Siblings of children with autism should be carefully monitored for acquisition of social, communi-

cation, and play skills, and the occurrence of maladaptive behaviors. Screening should be performed not only for autism-related symptoms but also for language delays, learning difficulties, social problems, and anxiety or depressive symptoms (**Guideline**).
6. Screening specifically for autism should be performed on all children failing routine developmental surveillance procedures using one of the validated instruments—the CHAT or the Autism Screening Questionnaire (**Guideline**).
7. Laboratory investigations recommended for any child with developmental delay and/or autism include audiologic assessment and lead screening (**Guideline**). Early referral for a formal audiologic assessment should include behavioral audiometric measures, assessment of middle ear function, and electrophysiologic procedures using experienced pediatric audiologists with current audiologic testing methods and technologies (**Guideline**). Lead screening should be performed in any child with developmental delay and pica. Additional periodic screening should be considered if the pica persists (**Guideline**).

Recommendations for research.

1. Develop and validate appropriate autism screening tools with adequate sensitivity and specificity in children younger than 1 year of age that could be used by a wide range of practitioners.
2. Current methods of screening for autism may not identify: 1) children with milder variants of the disorder; 2) children without mental retardation or language delay, such as verbal individuals with high functioning autism and Asperger's disorder; or 3) older children, adolescents, and young adults. Additional tools are needed to help identify and evaluate these groups of patients.
3. Studies are needed to provide insight into the emergence of early auditory behaviors that are considered atypical and may be prevalent in children with autism. Studies are also needed on the audiologic characteristics of individuals with autism to help assess peripheral hearing sensitivity and suprathreshold responses.

Level two: diagnosis and evaluation of autism.
Analysis of the evidence. Who should diagnose autism? Although educators, parents, and other health care professionals identify signs and symptoms characteristic of autism, a clinician experienced in the diagnosis and treatment of autism is usually necessary for accurate and appropriate diagnosis.[25,47,48] Clinicians must rely on their clinical judgment, aided by guides to diagnosis, such as DSM-IV and the *Tenth Edition of the International Classification of Diseases* (ICD-10), as well as by the results of various assessment instruments, rating scales, and checklists. These instruments and criteria should be used by practitioners not as experienced in the diagnosis of autism.

What are the medical and neurologic concerns in evaluating children with autism? *Familial prevalence.* Family studies have shown that there is a 50-fold to 100-fold increase in the rate of autism in first-degree relatives of autistic children. Within these families, there are also elevated rates of social difficulties; higher incidences of cognitive, communication, learning and executive function deficits; increased stereotyped behaviors; and anxiety, affective, language, and pragmatic disorders.[33,49-55] Monozygotic twin pair studies have also shown a high concordance rate (60%) for DSM-IV Autistic Disorder, 71% for the broader autistic spectrum phenotype, and 92% for an even broader phenotype of social and communication deficits with stereotyped behaviors that nonetheless were clearly differentiated from normal. In contrast, no concordance for autism was noted in dizygotic twin pairs and only 10% were concordant for some form of cognitive, social or language deficit.[56,57]

Large head circumference without frank neuropathology. Children with autism have a larger head circumference; only a small proportion have frank macrocephaly.[33,57-61] Large head size may not necessarily be present at birth, but may appear in early to mid-childhood, perhaps indicating an increased rate of brain growth. Neuroimaging studies in autism also found larger brain volumes without associated neuropathology.[62,63]

Association with tuberous sclerosis complex (TSC) and less often with Fragile X (FraX) syndrome. Seventeen to over 60% of mentally retarded individuals with TSC are also autistic, and these patients commonly have epilepsy.[64-67] In contrast, the number of autistic individuals with TSC has been estimated to be between 0.4% and 3%.[66] This rate increases to 8% to 14% if epilepsy is also present.[66]

Clinical studies report that 3% to 25% of patients with FraX have autism.[68-70] However, no evidence of FraX in autistic individuals was found using cytogenetic (not DNA analysis) techniques;[71] with molecular genetic analyses, only a few autistic individuals were shown to have FraX.[72]

What are the specific deficits of the autistic child's developmental profile? *Speech, language, and verbal and nonverbal communication.* Verbal and nonverbal communication deficits seen in autism are far more complex than simple speech delay, but overlap with developmental language disorders or specific language impairments. Expressive language function ranges from complete mutism (as often seen in children 2 to 3 years of age) to verbal fluency, though verbal abilities are often accompanied by many errors in word meaning (semantics) or language and communicative deficits in social contexts (social-pragmatics).[73-75]

Cognitive deficits. Many autistic individuals demonstrate a particular pattern on intellectual tests that is characteristic of autism, i.e., performance IQ (PIQ) higher than verbal IQ (VIQ), and specific intersubtest scatter, with Block Design typically the highest and Comprehension usually the lowest. However, the PIQ–VIQ split is severity dependent. When Full Scale IQ (FSIQ) and VIQ are both above 70, 80% of autistic individuals will have no significant VIQ–PIQ disparity, and the remainder are evenly divided between those with PIQ > VIQ and those with PIQ < VIQ.[76]

The DSM-IV defines the diagnosis of mental retardation as the combination of subaverage intellectual functioning (IQ < 70) and concurrent deficits in adaptive functioning. Autistic individuals have poorer adaptive function than would be predicted by IQ alone.[77]

Sensorimotor deficits. Impairments of gross and fine motor function are reported as being common in autistic individuals, and are recognized as hypotonia, limb apraxia, or motor stereotypies. Motor deficits are more severe in individuals with lower IQ scores.[78] Hand or finger mannerisms, body rocking, or unusual posturing are reported in 37% to 95% of individuals, and often manifest during the preschool years.[24,58,78] Sensory processing abilities are aberrant in 42% to 88% of autistic individuals and include preoccupation with sensory features of objects, over- or underresponsiveness to environmental stimuli, or paradoxical responses to sensory stimuli.[79]

Neuropsychological, behavioral, and academic impairments. Specific neuropsychological impairments can be identified, even in young children with autism, that correlate with the severity of autistic symptoms.[80] Performance on tasks that rely on rote, mechanical, or perceptual processes are typically spared; deficient performance exists on tasks requiring higher-order conceptual processes, reasoning, interpretation, integration, or abstraction. Dissociations between simple and complex processing are reported in the areas of language, memory, executive function, motor function, reading, mathematics, and perspective-taking.[80-83] There is no reported evidence that confirms or excludes a diagnosis of autism based on these cognitive patterns alone.

When and what laboratory investigations are indicated for the diagnosis of autism? *Genetic testing.* A chromosomal abnormality reported in possibly more than 1% of autistic individuals involves the proximal long arm of chromosome 15 (15q11-q13), which is a greater frequency than other currently identifiable chromosomal disorders.[84-86] Those with the 15q abnormalities typically have moderate to profound mental retardation. The duplication is usually maternally inherited, either pseudodicentric 15 (inverted duplication 15) or other atypical marker chromosomes, with one or two extra copies of the area roughly corresponding to the typical Angelman syndrome (AS)/Prader Willi Syndrome (PWS) deletion region of approximately four million base pairs. Conversely, AS is usually due to a deletion of maternally inherited 15q11-q13 material and has been found in patients with autism and profound mental retardation.[85,87]

Metabolic testing. Inborn errors in amino acid, carbohydrate, purine, peptide, and mitochondrial metabolism, as well as toxicologic studies have been studied, but the percentage of children with autism who have a metabolic disorder is probably less (and some experts agree that it is considerably less) than 5%.[88,89]

Electrophysiologic testing. The prevalence of epilepsy in autistic children has been estimated at 7[90] to 14%,[91] whereas the cumulative prevalence by adulthood is estimated at 20% to 35%.[90,91] Seizure onset peaks in early childhood and again in adolescence. Mental retardation, with or without motor abnormalities and family history of epilepsy, was a significant risk factor for the development of seizures in autistic individuals.[92-95]

It is unclear whether there is a relationship between autism and an early regressive course (before 36 months), childhood disintegrative disorder ([CDD] after 36 months), Landau–Kleffner syndrome, and electrical status epilepticus during slow wave sleep (ESES). Autism with regression and CDD have both been associated with seizures or epileptiform sleep-deprived EEG (with adequate sampling of slow wave sleep).[96-98] A higher incidence of epileptiform EEG abnormalities in autistic children with a history of regression has been reported when compared to autistic children with clinical epilepsy.[97] Seizures or epileptiform discharges were more prevalent in children with regression who demonstrated cognitive deficits. Regression in cognition and language in adolescence associated with seizure onset has also been observed, but little is known about its cause or prevalence. There may be a causal relationship between a subgroup of children with autistic regression and EEG-defined "benign focal epilepsies."[99] There is insufficient evidence to suggest a role for event-related potentials or magnetoencephalography in the evaluation of autism.

Neuroimaging. CT studies, ordered as standard assessments of children diagnosed with autism during the 1970s and 1980s, reported a wide range of brain imaging abnormalities and suggested that there was an underlying structural disorder in patients with autism. This view changed when Damasio et al.[100] demonstrated that such abnormalities were incidental to coexisting anatomic disorders unrelated to autism. A very low prevalence of focal lesions or other structural abnormalities was found; their inconsistent localization marked them as coincidental. Prevalence of lesions on MRI in children with autism is similar to normal control subjects.[101] CT and MRI studies of autistic subjects screened to exclude those with disorders other than autism confirmed the absence of significant structural brain abnormalities.[63]

Functional imaging modalities such as functional MRI (fMRI), single-photon emission CT (SPECT), or positron-emission tomography (PET) are currently only research tools in the evaluation of autism. There is no evidence to support a role for functional neuroimaging studies in the clinical diagnosis of autism at the present time.[1]

Other tests. There is insufficient evidence to support the use of other tests such as hair analysis for

trace elements, celiac antibodies, allergy testing (particularly food allergies for gluten, casein, candida, and other molds), immunologic or neurochemical abnormalities, micronutrients such as vitamin levels, intestinal permeability studies, stool analysis, urinary peptides, mitochondrial disorders (including lactate and pyruvate), thyroid function tests, or erythrocyte glutathione peroxidase studies.[1]

Level two: evidence-based recommendations. *Clinical practice recommendations.*

1. Genetic testing in children with autism, specifically high resolution chromosome studies (karyotype) and DNA analysis for FraX, should be performed in the presence of mental retardation (or if mental retardation cannot be excluded), if there is a family history of FraX or undiagnosed mental retardation, or if dysmorphic features are present (**Standard**). However, there is little likelihood of positive karyotype or FraX testing in the presence of high-functioning autism.

2. Selective metabolic testing (**Standard**) should be initiated by the presence of suggestive clinical and physical findings such as the following: if lethargy, cyclic vomiting, or early seizures are evident; the presence of dysmorphic or coarse features; evidence of mental retardation or if mental retardation cannot be ruled out; or if occurrence or adequacy of newborn screening for a birth is questionable.

3. There is inadequate evidence at the present time to recommend an EEG study in all individuals with autism. Indications for an adequate sleep-deprived EEG with appropriate sampling of slow wave sleep include (**Guideline**) clinical seizures or suspicion of subclinical seizures, and a history of regression (clinically significant loss of social and communicative function) at any age, but especially in toddlers and preschoolers.

4. Recording of event-related potentials and magnetoencephalography are research tools at the present time, without evidence of routine clinical utility (**Guideline**).

5. There is no clinical evidence to support the role of routine clinical neuroimaging in the diagnostic evaluation of autism, even in the presence of megalencephaly (**Guideline**).

6. There is inadequate supporting evidence for hair analysis, celiac antibodies, allergy testing (particularly food allergies for gluten, casein, candida, and other molds), immunologic or neurochemical abnormalities, micronutrients such as vitamin levels, intestinal permeability studies, stool analysis, urinary peptides, mitochondrial disorders (including lactate and pyruvate), thyroid function tests, or erythrocyte glutathione peroxidase studies (**Guideline**).

Recommendations for research.

1. Studies are needed to further identify the usefulness of electrophysiologic techniques to clarify the

role of epilepsy in autism, especially in children with a history of regression.

2. Additional studies to examine potential genetic and/or environmental factors and their relationship to the etiology of autism are needed.

3. Continuing efforts might focus on identifying contributing genes to determine whether the behavioral syndromes (which constitute the basis of DSM-IV and ICD-10) have actual biological validity.

4. Evaluation of environmental factors (e.g., nonspecific infections or other immunologically mediated events) that might contribute to triggering the expression of autistic symptoms or regression requires additional study.

Consensus-based general principles of management. The following recommendations are based on consensus agreement by the participating organizations involved in the development of this parameter.[1]

Surveillance and screening. In the United States, states must follow federal Public Law 105-17: the Individuals with Disabilities Education Act Amendments of 1997–IDEA'97, which mandates immediate referral for a free appropriate public education for eligible children with disabilities from the age of 36 months, and early intervention services for infants and toddlers with disabilities from birth through 35 months of age.

Diagnosis. The diagnosis of autism should include the use of a diagnostic instrument with at least moderate sensitivity and good specificity for autism. Sufficient time should be planned for standardized parent interviews regarding current concerns and behavioral history related to autism, and direct, structured observation of social and communicative behavior and play. Recommended instruments include[1]:

Diagnostic parental interviews

The Gilliam Autism Rating Scale

The Parent Interview for Autism

The Pervasive Developmental Disorders Screening Test–Stage 3

The Autism Diagnostic Interview–Revised

Diagnostic observation instruments

The Childhood Autism Rating Scale

The Screening Tool for Autism in Two-Year-Olds

The Autism Diagnostic Observation Schedule-Generic

Medical and neurologic evaluation. Perinatal and developmental history should include milestones; regression in early childhood or later in life; encephalopathic events; attentional deficits; seizure disorder (absence or generalized); depression or mania; and behaviors such as irritability, self-injury, sleep and eating disturbances, and pica. The physical and neurologic examination should include: longitudinal measurements of head circumference and examination for unusual features (facial, limb, stature, etc.) suggesting the need for genetic evaluation;

neurocutaneous abnormalities (requiring an ultraviolet [Wood's] lamp examination); gait; tone; reflexes; cranial nerves; and determination of mental status, including verbal and nonverbal language and play.

Evaluation and monitoring of autism. The immediate and long-term evaluation and monitoring of autistic individuals requires a comprehensive multidisciplinary approach, and can include one or more of the following professionals: psychologists, neurologists, speech–language pathologists and audiologists, pediatricians, child psychiatrists, occupational therapists, and physical therapists, as well as educators and special educators. Individuals with mild autism should also receive adequate assessments and appropriate diagnoses.

Reevaluation within 1 year of initial diagnosis and continued monitoring is an expected aspect of clinical practice because relatively small changes in the developmental level affect the impact of autism in the preschool years. In general, there is no need to repeat extensive diagnostic testing; however, follow-up visits can be helpful to address behavioral, environmental, and other developmental concerns.

Speech, language, and communication evaluation. A comprehensive speech–language–communication evaluation should be performed on all children who fail language developmental screening procedures by a speech–language pathologist with training and expertise in evaluating children with developmental disabilities. Comprehensive assessments of both preverbal and verbal individuals should account for age, cognitive level, and socioemotional abilities, and should include assessment of receptive language and communication, expressive language and communication, voice and speech production, and in verbal individuals, a collection and analysis of spontaneous language samples to supplement scores on formal language tests.

Cognitive and adaptive behavior evaluations. Cognitive evaluations should be performed in all children with autism by a psychologist or other trained professional. Cognitive instruments should be appropriate for the mental and chronologic age, provide a full range (in the lower direction) of standard scores and current norms independent of social ability, include independent measures of verbal and nonverbal abilities, and provide an overall index of ability. A measure of adaptive functioning should be collected for any child evaluated for an associated cognitive handicap. Consensus-based recommendations for using specific instruments include the Vineland Adaptive Behavior Scales and the Scales of Independent Behavior–Revised.[1]

Sensorimotor and occupational therapy evaluations. Evaluation of sensorimotor skills by a qualified experienced professional (occupational therapist or physical therapist) should be considered, including assessment of gross and fine motor skills, praxis, sensory processing abilities, unusual or stereotyped mannerisms, and the impact of these components on the autistic person's life. An occupational therapy evaluation is indicated when deficits exist in functional skills or occupational performance in the areas of play or leisure, self-maintenance through activities of daily living, or productive school and work tasks. Although not routinely warranted as part of all evaluations of children with autism, the Sensory Integration and Praxis Tests may be used on an individual basis to detect specific patterns of sensory integrative dysfunction.

Neuropsychological, behavioral, and academic assessments. These assessments should be performed as needed, in addition to the cognitive assessment, to include social skills and relationships, educational functioning, problematic behaviors, learning style, motivation and reinforcement, sensory functioning, and self-regulation. Assessment of family resources should be performed by appropriate psychologists or other qualified health care professionals and should include assessment of parents' level of understanding of their child's condition, family (parent and sibling) strengths, talents, stressors and adaptation, resources and supports, as well as offer appropriate counseling and education.

Disclaimer. The Quality Standards Subcommittee (QSS) of the American Academy of Neurology (AAN) seeks to develop scientifically sound, clinically relevant practice parameters for the practice of neurology. Practice parameters are strategies for patient management that assist physicians in clinical decision making. A practice parameter is one or more specific recommendations based on analysis of evidence of a specific clinical problem. These might include diagnosis, symptoms, treatment, or procedure evaluation. This evidence-based review addresses the major management issues health care providers face in surveying, screening, and diagnosing children with autism. The clinical evidence is reviewed, management recommendations provided, and areas of continued research identified. This statement is provided as an educational service of the American Academy of Neurology. It is based on an assessment of current scientific and clinical information. It is not intended to include all possible proper methods of care for choosing to use a specific procedure. Neither is it intended to exclude any reasonable alternative methodologies. The AAN recognizes that specific patient care decisions are the prerogative of the patient and the physician caring for the patient, based on all of the circumstances involved.

Acknowledgment

The authors thank the following people who contributed to this endeavor by their participation in the NIH State of the Science in Autism: Screening and Diagnosis Working Conference, June 15 to 17, 1998: George Anderson, PhD, Anthony Bailey, MD, W. Ted Brown, MD, Susan E. Bryson, PhD, Rebecca Landa, PhD, Jeffrey Lewine, PhD, Catherine Lord, PhD, William McIlvane, PhD, Joseph Piven, MD, Ricki Robinson, MD, Bryna Siegel, PhD, Vijendra K. Singh, PhD, Frank Symons, PhD, and Max Wiznitzer, MD. The current authors, participants and NIH Liaisons also participated in this working conference. The Panel acknowledges with gratitude the valuable consultations of Frances P. Glascoe, PhD, and Donald J. Siegel, PhD, and the assistance of Cheryl Jess, Jody Sallah, and Starr Pearlman, PhD, in this endeavor. Special gratitude is extended for the additional assistance of Michael L. Goldstein, MD, and Roy Elterman, MD.

Appendix 1

Participating Organizations and Authors

Pauline A. Filipek, MD—Chair (Child Neurology Society, American Academy of Neurology and American Academy of Pediatrics); Judith S. Gravel, PhD (American Academy of Audiology); Edwin H. Cook, Jr., MD, and Fred R. Volkmar, MD (American Academy of Child and Adolescent Psychiatry); Isabelle Rapin, MD, and Barry Gordon, MD, PhD (American Academy of Neurology); Stuart W. Teplin, MD, Ronald J. Kallen, MD, and Chris Plauche Johnson, MEd, MD (American Academy of Pediatrics); Grace T. Baranek, PhD, OTR/L (American Occupational Therapy Association); Sally J. Rogers, PhD, Sally Ozonoff, PhD, and Wendy L. Stone, PhD (American Psychological Association); Geraldine Dawson, PhD (American Psychological Society); Barry M. Prizant, PhD, CCC-SLP (American Speech–Language–Hearing Association); Nancy J. Minshew, MD, and Roberto F. Tuchman, MD (Child Neurology Society); Susan E. Levy, MD (Society for Developmental and Behavioral Pediatrics); Pasquale J. Accardo, MD (Society for Developmental Pediatrics); and Stephen Ashwal, MD (Child Neurology Society, American Academy of Neurology Quality Standards Subcommittee).

Representatives were named from the following associations: Barbara Cutler, EdD, and Susan Goodman, JD (Autism National Committee); Cheryl Trepagnier, PhD (Autism Society of America); Daniel H. Geschwind, MD, PhD (Cure Autism Now); and Charles T. Gordon, MD (National Alliance for Autism Research). The National Institutes of Health also named liaisons to serve on this committee, including Marie Bristol–Power, PhD (National Institute of Child Health and Human Development); Judith Cooper, PhD (National Institute of Deafness and Communication Disorders); Judith Rumsey, PhD (National Institute of Mental Health); and Giovanna Spinella, MD (National Institute of Neurological Disorders and Stroke).

Appendix 2

Clinical questions addressed for surveillance, screening and diagnosing children with autism

Routine developmental surveillance and screening for autism

1. When and how often should developmental surveillance/screening be performed?
2. What are the appropriate developmental screening questionnaires that provide sensitive and specific information?
3. How are conventional developmental milestones defined?
4. Do parents provide reliable information regarding their child's development?
5. Can autism can be reliably diagnosed before 36 months of age?
6. Is there an increased risk of having another child with autism (recurrence)?
7. What screening laboratory investigations are available for developmental delay, with or without suspicion of autism?
8. What tools are available with appropriate psychometric properties to specifically screen for autism?

Diagnosis and evaluation of autism

1. Who should diagnose autism?
2. What are the medical and neurologic concerns in evaluating children with autism?
3. What are the specific deficits of the autistic child's developmental profile?
4. When and what laboratory investigations are indicated for the diagnosis of autism?

Appendix 3

Definitions for strength of the evidence

Class I. Must have all of a through d. a) Prospective study of a well-defined cohort which includes a description of the nature of the population, the inclusion/exclusion criteria, demographic characteristics such as age and sex, and seizure type. b) The sample size must be adequate with enough statistical power to justify a conclusion or for identification of subgroups for whom testing does or does not yield significant information. c) The interpretation of evaluations performed must be done blinded to outcome. d) There must be a satisfactory description of the technology used for evaluations (e.g., EEG, MRI).

Class II. Must have a or b. a) Retrospective study of a well-defined cohort which otherwise meets criteria for class 1a, b and 1d. b) Prospective or retrospective study which lacks any of the following: adequate sample size, adequate methodology, a description of inclusion/exclusion criteria, and information such as age, sex and characteristics of the seizure.

Class III. Must have a or b. a) A small cohort or case report. b) Relevant expert opinion, consensus, or survey.

A cost-benefit analysis or a meta-analysis may be class I, II, or III, depending on the strength of the data upon which the analysis is based.

Definitions for strength of the recommendations

Standard. A principle for patient management that reflects a high degree of clinical certainty (usually requires one or more Class I studies that directly address the clinical question, or overwhelming Class II evidence when circumstances preclude randomized clinical trials).

Guideline. A recommendation for patient management that reflects moderate clinical certainty (usually requires one or more Class II studies or a strong consensus of Class III evidence).

Practice option. Strategy for patient management for which clinical utility is uncertain (inconclusive or conflicting evidence or opinion).

Appendix 4

American Academy of Neurology Quality Standards Subcommittee Members: Gary Franklin, MD, MPH—Co-Chair; Catherine A. Zahn, MD—Co-Chair; Milton Alter, MD, PhD; Stephen Ashwal, MD (facilitator); John Calverley, MD; Richard Dubinsky, MD; Jacqueline French, MD; Michael Glantz, MD; Michael K. Greenberg, MD; Gary Gronseth, MD; Deborah Hirtz, MD; Robert G. Miller, MD; James Stevens, MD; William Weiner, MD; and Wendy Edlund, AAN Manager, Clinical Practice Guidelines.

References

1. Filipek PA, Accardo PJ, Baranek GT, et al. The screening and diagnosis of autistic spectrum disorders. J Autism Dev Disord 1999;29:437–482.
2. Howlin P, Moore A. Diagnosis of autism. A survey of over 1200 patients in the UK. Autism 1997;1:135–162. (Class II).
3. Rogers SJ. Empirically supported comprehensive treatments for young children with autism. J Clin Child Psychol 1998;27: 168–179. (Class III).
4. Lovaas OI. Behavioral treatment and normal educational and intellectual functioning in young autistic children. J Consult Clin Psychol 1987;55:3–9. (Class II).
5. McEachin JJ, Smith T, Lovaas OI. Long-term outcome for children with autism who received early intensive behavioral treatment. Am J Ment Retard 1993;97:359–372. (Class II).
6. Ozonoff S, Cathcart K. Effectiveness of a home program intervention for young children with autism. J Autism Dev Disord 1998;28:25–32. (Class II).
7. Sheinkopf SJ, Siegel B. Home-based behavioral treatment of young children with autism. J Autism Dev Disord 1998;28: 15–23. (Class III).
8. Majnemer A, Rosenblatt B. Reliability of parental recall of developmental milestones. Pediatr Neurol 1994;10:304–308. (Class II).
9. Dworkin PH. British and American recommendations for developmental monitoring: the role of surveillance. Pediatrics 1989;84:1000–1010. (Class III).
10. Glascoe FP, Dworkin PH. Obstacles to effective developmental surveillance: errors in clinical reasoning. J Dev Behav Pediatr 1993;14:344–349. (Class III).
11. American Academy of Pediatrics Committee on Children with Disabilities. Screening infants and young children for developmental disabilities. Pediatrics 1994;93:863–5. (Class III).
12. Glascoe FP, Byrne KE, Ashford LG, Johnson KL, Chang B, Strickland B. Accuracy of the Denver-II in developmental screening. Pediatrics 1992;89:1221–1225. (Class I).
13. Greer S, Bauchner H, Zuckerman B. The Denver Developmental Screening Test: how good is its predictive validity? Dev Med Child Neurol 1989;31:774–781. (Class II).
14. Diamond KE. Predicting school problems from preschool developmental screening: A four-year followup of the Revised Denver Developmental Screening test and the role of parent report. J Div Early Child 1987;11:247–253. (Class I).
15. Sciarillo WG, Brown MM, Robinson NM, Bennett FC, Sells CJ. Effectiveness of the Denver Developmental Screening Test with biologically vulnerable infants. J Dev Behav Pediatr 1986;7:77–83. (Class I).
16. Fenson L, Dale P, Reznick S, et al. MacArthur communicative development inventories. San Diego, CA: Singular Publishing, 1993.
17. Hedrick DL, Prather EM, Tobin AR. Sequenced inventory of communication development–revised edition. Seattle, WA: University of Washington Press, 1984.
18. Ireton H, Glascoe FP. Assessing children's development using parents' reports. The Child Development Inventory. Clin Pediatr 1995;34:248–255. (Class I).
19. Bricker D, Squires J. The ages & stages questionnaires, second edition. Baltimore, MD: Paul H. Brookes Publishing Company, 1999.
20. Glascoe FP. It's not what it seems. The relationship between parents' concerns and children with global delays. Clin Pediatr 1994;33:292–296. (Class I).
21. Glascoe FP, Sandler H. Value of parents' estimates of children's developmental ages. J Pediatr 1995;127:831–835. (Class I).
22. Glascoe FP. Parents' concerns about children's development: prescreening technique or screening test? Pediatrics 1997;99: 522–528. (Class I).
23. Glascoe FP, Dworkin PH. The role of parents in the detection of developmental and behavioral problems. Pediatrics 1995; 95:829–836. (Class III).
24. Lord C. Follow-up of two-year-olds referred for possible autism. J Child Psychol Psychiatry 1995;36:1365–1382. (Class II).
25. Stone WL, Lee EB, Ashford L, Brissie J, Hepburn SL, Coonrod EE, Weiss BH. Can autism be diagnosed accurately in children under three years? J Child Psychol Psychiatry 1999; 40:219–226. (Class II).
26. Charman T, Swettenham J, Baron–Cohen S, Cox A, Baird G, Drew A. Infants with autism: An investigation of empathy, pretend play, joint attention, and imitation. Dev Psychol 1997;33:781–789. (Class II).
27. Cox A, Klein K, Charman T, et al. The early diagnosis of autism spectrum disorders: use of the autism diagnostic interview– revised at 20 months and 42 months of age. J Child Psychol Psychiatry 1999;40:705–718. (Class II).
28. Mars AE, Mauk JE, Dowrick P. Symptoms of pervasive developmental disorders as observed in prediagnostic home videos of infants and toddlers. J Pediatr 1998;132:500–504. (Class II).
29. Werner E, Dawson G, Osterling J, Dinno J. Recognition of autism spectrum disorders before 1 year of age. A retrospective study based on home videotapes. J Autism Dev Disord 2000;30:157–162. (Class II).
30. Baranek GT. Autism during infancy: A retrospective video analysis of sensory-motor and social behaviors at 9-12 months of age. J Autism Dev Disord 1999;29:213–224. (Class II).
31. Szatmari P, Jones MB, Tuff L, Bartolucci G, Fisman S, Mahoney W. Lack of cognitive impairment in first-degree relatives of children with pervasive developmental disorders. J Am Acad Child Adolesc Psychiatry 1993;32:1264–1273. (Class II).
32. Jorde LB, Mason-Brothers A, Waldmann R, et al. The UCLA–University of Utah epidemiologic survey of autism: genealogical analysis of familial aggregation. Am J Med Genet 1990;36:85–88. (Class I).
33. Bolton P, Macdonald H, Pickles A, et al. A case-control family history study of autism. J Child Psychol Psychiatry 1994; 35:877–900. (Class I).
34. Piven J, Gayle J, Chase GA, Fink B, Landa R, Wzorek MM, Folstein SE. A family history study of neuropsychiatric disorders in the adult siblings of autistic individuals. J Am Acad Child Adolesc Psychiatry 1990;29:177–183. (Class II).

35. Charman T, Swettenham J, Baron–Cohen S, Cox A, Baird G, Drew A. An experimental investigation of social-cognitive abilities in infants with autism: Clinical implications. Infant Mental Health Journal 1998;19:260–275.

36. American Speech–Language–Hearing Association. Guidelines for the audiologic assessment of children from birth through 36 months of age. Committee on Infant Hearing. American Speech–Language–Hearing Association (ASHA) 1991;33(suppl 5):37–43. (Class III).

37. Jure R, Rapin I, Tuchman RF. Hearing-impaired autistic children. Dev Med Child Neurol 1991;33:1062–1072. (Class II).

38. Klin A. Auditory brainstem responses in autism: brainstem dysfunction or peripheral hearing loss? J Autism Dev Disord 1993;23:15–35. (Class II).

39. Gravel JS, Kurtzberg D, Stapells D, Vaughan H, Wallace I. Case studies. Seminars in hearing 1989;10:272–287. (Class III).

40. Verpoorten RA, Emmen JG. A tactile–auditory conditioning procedure for the hearing assessment of persons with autism and mental retardation. Scand Audiol Suppl 1995;41:49–50. (Class II).

41. Gorga MP, Kaminski JR, Beauchaine KL, Jesteadt W, Neely ST. Auditory brainstem responses from children three months to three years of age. J Speech Hear Res 1989;32:281–288. (Class II).

42. Stapells DR, Gravel JS, Martin BA. Thresholds for auditory brain stem responses to tones in notched noise from infants and young children with normal hearing or sensorineural hearing loss. Ear Hear 1995;16:361–371. (Class I).

43. Grewe TS, Danhauer JL, Danhauer KJ, Thornton AR. Clinical use of otoacoustic emissions in children with autism. International J Pediatr Otorhinolaryngol 1994;30:123–132. (Class III).

44. Centers for Disease Control and Prevention. Screening young children for lead poisoning: Guidance for state and local public health officials. Atlanta, GA: Centers for Disease Control and Prevention–National Center for Environmental Health, November 1997. (Class III).

45. Cohen DJ, Johnson WT, Caparulo BK. Pica and elevated blood lead level in autistic and atypical children. Am J Dis Child 1976;130:47–48. (Class II).

46. Shannon M, Graef JW. Lead intoxication in children with pervasive developmental disorders. J Toxicol Clin Toxicol 1997;34:177–182. (Class II).

47. Volkmar FR, Klin A, Siegel B, Szatmari P, Lord C, Campbell M, Freeman BJ, Cicchetti DV, Rutter M, Kline W, et al. Field trial for autistic disorder in DSM-IV. Am J Psychiatry 1994;151:1361–1367. (Class I).

48. Lord C, Storoschuk S, Rutter M, Pickles A. Using the ADI–R to diagnose autism in preschool children. Infant Mental Hlth J 1993;14:234–252. (Class I).

49. Piven J, Wzorek M, Landa R, Lainhart J, Bolton P, Chase GA, Folstein S. Personality characteristics of the parents of autistic individuals. Psychol Med 1994;24:783–795. (Class I).

50. DeLong R. Children with autistic spectrum disorder and a family history of affective disorder. Dev Med Child Neurol 1994;36:674–687. (Class II).

51. DeLong R, Nohria C. Psychiatric family history and neurological disease in autistic spectrum disorders. Dev Med Child Neurol 1994;36:441–448. (Class II).

52. Piven J, Palmer P, Landa R, Santangelo S, Jacobi D, Childress D. Personality and language characteristics in parents from multiple-incidence autism families. Am J Med Genet 1997;74:398–411. (Class I).

53. Hughes C, Leboyer M, Bouvard M. Executive function in parents of children with autism. Psychol Med 1997;27:209–220. (Class II).

54. Piven J, Palmer P, Jacobi D, Childress D, Arndt S. Broader autism phenotype: evidence from a family history study of multiple-incidence autism families. Am J Psychiatry 1997;154:185–190. (Class I).

55. Fombonne E, Bolton P, Prior J, Jordan H, Rutter M. A family study of autism: Cognitive patterns and levels in parents and siblings. J Child Psychol Psychiatry 1997;38:667–683. (Class I).

56. Le Couteur A, Bailey A, Goode S, Pickles A, Robertson S, Gottesman I, Rutter M. A broader phenotype of autism: the clinical spectrum in twins. J Child Psychol Psychiatry 1996;37:785–801. (Class I).

57. Bailey A, Le Couteur A, Gottesman I, Bolton P, Simonoff E, Yuzda E, Rutter M. Autism as a strongly genetic disorder: evidence from a British twin study. Psychol Med 1995;25:63–77. (Class I).

58. Rapin I. Neurological examination. In: Rapin I, ed. Preschool children with inadequate communication: developmental language disorder, autism, low IQ. London, UK: MacKeith Press, 1996:98–122. (Class I).

59. Lainhart JE, Piven J, Wzorek M, Landa R, Santangelo SL, Coon H, Folstein SE. Macrocephaly in children and adults with autism. J Am Acad Child Adolesc Psychiatry 1997;36:282–290. (Class II).

60. Davidovitch M, Patterson B, Gartside P. Head circumference measurements in children with autism. J Child Neurol 1996;11:389–393. (Class II).

61. Woodhouse W, Bailey A, Rutter M, Bolton P, Baird G, Le Couteur A. Head circumference in autism and other pervasive developmental disorders. J Child Psychol Psychiatry 1996;37:665–671. (Class II).

62. Piven J, Arndt S, Bailey J, Andreasen N. Regional brain enlargement in autism: a magnetic resonance imaging study. J Am Acad Child Adolesc Psychiatry 1996;35:530–536. (Class II).

63. Filipek PA. Neuroimaging in the developmental disorders: The state of the science. J Child Psychol Psychiatry 1999;40:113–128. (Class II).

64. Gillberg IC, Gillberg C, Ahlsen G. Autistic behaviour and attention deficits in tuberous sclerosis: a population-based study. Dev Med Child Neurol 1994;36:50–56. (Class II).

65. Hunt A, Shepherd C. A prevalence study of autism in tuberous sclerosis. J Autism Dev Disord 1993;23:323–339. (Class II).

66. Smalley SL, Tanguay PE, Smith M, Gutierrez G. Autism and tuberous sclerosis. J Autism Dev Disord 1992;22:339–355. (Class II).

67. Curatolo P, Cusmai R, Cortesi F, Chiron C, Jambeque I, Dulac O. Neuropsychiatric aspects of tuberous sclerosis. New York Academy of Sciences and the National Tuberous Sclerosis Association Conference: Tuberous sclerosis and allied disorders (1990, Bethesda, Maryland). Ann NY Acad Sci 1991;615:8–16. (Class III).

68. Piven J, Gayle J, Landa R, Wzorek M, Folstein S. The prevalence of fragile X in a sample of autistic individuals diagnosed using a standardized interview. J Am Acad Child Adolesc Psychiatry 1991;30:825–830. (Class II).

69. Bolton P, Rutter M. Genetic influences in autism. Int Rev Psychiatr 1990;2:67–80. (Class II).

70. Bailey A, Bolton P, Butler L, et al. Prevalence of the fragile X anomaly amongst autistic twins and singletons. J Child Psychol Psychiatry 1993;34:673–688. (Class I).

71. Hashimoto O, Shimizu Y, Kawasaki Y. Brief report: low frequency of the fragile X syndrome among Japanese autistic subjects. J Autism Dev Disord 1993;23:201–209. (Class III).

72. Klauck SM, Munstermann E, Bieber–Martig B, et al. Molecular genetic analysis of the FMR-1 gene in a large collection of autistic patients. Hum Genet 1997;100:224–229. (Class I).

73. Wetherby AM, Prizant BM, Hutchinson T. Communicative, social-affective, and symbolic profiles of young children with autism and pervasive developmental disorder. Am J Speech-Language Pathol 1998;7:79–91. (Class III).

74. Stone WL, Ousley OY, Yoder PJ, Hogan KL, Hepburn SL. Nonverbal communication in two-and three-year-old children with autism. J Autism Dev Disord 1997;27:677–696. (Class II).

75. Rapin I. Preschool Children with Inadequate Communication: developmental language disorder, autism, low IQ. London, UK: MacKeith Press, 1996. (Class I).

76. Siegel DJ, Minshew NJ, Goldstein G. Wechsler IQ profiles in diagnosis of high-functioning autism. J Autism Dev Disord 1996;26:389–406. (Class II).

77. Volkmar FR, Carter A, Sparrow SS, Cicchetti DV. Quantifying social development in autism. J Am Acad Child Adolesc Psychiatry 1993;32:627–632. (Class II).

78. Rogers SJ, Bennetto L, McEvoy R, Pennington BF. Imitation and pantomime in high-functioning adolescents with autism

spectrum disorders. Child Dev 1996;67:2060–2073. (Class II).

79. Kientz MA, Dunn W. A comparison of the performance of children with and without autism on the Sensory Profile. Am J Occup Ther 1997;51:530–537. (Class II).

80. Dawson G, Meltzoff AN, Osterling J, Rinaldi J. Neuropsychological correlates of early symptoms of autism. Child Dev 1998;69:1276–1285. (Class II).

81. Minshew NJ, Goldstein G, Taylor HG, Siegel DJ. Academic achievement in high functioning autistic individuals. J Clin Exp Neuropsychol 1994;16:261–270. (Class I).

82. Ozonoff S, Pennington BF, Rogers SJ. Executive function deficits in high-functioning autistic individuals: relationship to theory of mind. J Child Psychol Psychiatry 1991;32:1081–1105. (Class II).

83. Minshew NJ, Goldstein G, Siegel DJ. Neuropsychologic functioning in autism: profile of a complex information processing disorder. J Int Neuropsychol Soc 1997;3:303–316. (Class II).

84. Cook EH Jr, Lindgren V, Leventhal BL, et al. Autism or atypical autism in maternally but not paternally derived proximal 15q duplication. Am J Hum Genet 1997;60:928–934.

85. Schroer RJ, Phelan MC, Michaelis RC, et al. Autism and maternally derived aberrations of chromosome 15q. Am J Med Genet 1998;76:327–336. (Class II).

86. Weidmer-Mikhail E, Sheldon S, Ghaziuddin M. Chromosomes in autism and related pervasive developmental disorders: a cytogenetic study. J Intellect Disabil Res 1998;42:8–12. (Class II).

87. Steffenburg S, Gillberg CL, Steffenburg U, Kyllerman M. Autism in Angelman syndrome: a population-based study. Pediatr Neurol 1996;14:131–136. (Class II).

88. Dykens EM, Volkmar FR. Medical conditions associated with autism. In: Cohen DJ, Volkmar FR, eds. Handbook of autism and pervasive developmental disorders, second edition. New York, NY: John Wiley & Sons, 1997:388–410. (Class III).

89. Rutter M, Bailey A, Simonoff E, Pickles A. Genetic influences and autism. In: Cohen DJ, Volkmar FR, eds. Handbook of autism and pervasive developmental disorders, second edition. New York, NY: John Wiley & Sons, 1997:370–387. (Class III).

90. Rapin I. Historical data. In: Rapin I, ed. Preschool children with inadequate communication: developmental language disorder, autism, low IQ. London, UK: MacKeith Press, 1996:58–97. (Class I).

91. Tuchman RF, Rapin I, Shinnar S. Autistic and dysphasic children. II. Epilepsy. Pediatrics 1991;88:1219–1225. (Class II).

92. Gillberg C, Steffenburg S. Outcome and prognostic factors in infantile autism and similar conditions: a population-based study of 46 cases followed through puberty. J Autism Dev Disord 1987;17:273–287. (Class II).

93. Rossi PG, Parmeggiani A, Bach V, Santucci M, Visconti P. EEG features and epilepsy in patients with autism. Brain Dev 1995;17:169–174. (Class II).

94. Volkmar FR, Nelson DS. Seizure disorders in autism. J Am Acad Child Adolesc Psychiatry 1990;29:127–129. (Class II).

95. Wong V. Epilepsy in children with autistic spectrum disorder. J Child Neurol 1993;8:316–322. (Class II).

96. Rapin I. Autism. N Engl J Med 1997;337:97–104. (Class III).

97. Tuchman RF, Rapin I. Regression in pervasive developmental disorders: seizures and epileptiform electroencephalogram correlates. Pediatrics 1997;99:560–566. (Class II).

98. Tuchman RF. Regression in pervasive developmental disorders: Is there a relationship with Landau-Kleffner Syndrome? Ann Neurol 1995;38:526. Abstract. (Class II).

99. Nass R, Gross A, Devinsky O. Autism and autistic epileptiform regression with occipital spikes. Dev Med Child Neurol 1998;40:453–458. (Class III).

100. Damasio H, Maurer R, Damasio AR, Chui H. Computerized tomographic scan findings in patients with autistic behavior. Arch Neurol 1980;37:504–510. (Class II).

101. Filipek PA, Richelme C, Kennedy DN, Rademacher J, Pitcher DA, Zidel SY, Caviness VS. Morphometric analysis of the brain in developmental language disorders and autism. Ann Neurol 1992;32:475. Abstract. (Class II).

Constipation in Infants and Children: Evaluation and Treatment

· ·

The following guideline for evaluation and treatment of constipation, developed by the North American Society for Pediatric Gastroenterology and Nutrition, has been endorsed by the American Academy of Pediatrics.

CONSTIPATION IN INFANTS AND CHILDREN: EVALUATION AND TREATMENT

A medical position statement of the
North American Society for Pediatric Gastroenterology and Nutrition

Running Title: Algorithm for Evaluation and Treatment of Constipation

Susan S. Baker[1], Gregory S. Liptak[2], Richard B. Colletti[3], Joseph M. Croffie[4]
Carlo DiLorenzo[5], Walton Ector[1], and Samuel Nurko[6]

[1]Department of Pediatrics, Medical University of South Carolina, [2] Department of Pediatrics University of Rochester, [3]Department of Pediatrics, University of Vermont College of Medicine, [4]Department of Pediatrics, J Whitcomb Riley Hospital for Children, [5]Department of Pediatrics, Children's Hospital of Pittsburgh, University of Pittsburgh, [6]Department of Pediatrics, Harvard Medical School.

ABSTRACT

Background Constipation, defined as a delay or difficulty in defecation, present for two or more weeks, is a common pediatric problem encountered by both primary and specialty medical providers.

Methods The Constipation Subcommittee of the Clinical Guidelines Committee of the North American Society for Pediatric Gastroenterology and Nutrition has formulated clinical practice guidelines for the management of pediatric constipation. The Constipation Subcommittee, consisting of two primary care pediatricians, a clinical epidemiologist and pediatric gastroenterologists, based its recommendations on an integration of a comprehensive and systematic review of the medical literature combined with expert opinion. Consensus was achieved through Nominal Group Technique, a structured quantitative method.

Results The Subcommittee developed two algorithms to assist with medical management, one for older infants and children and the second for infants less than one year of age. The guidelines provide recommendations for management by the primary care provider, including evaluation, initial treatment, follow-up management and indications for consultation by a specialist. The Constipation Subcommittee also provided recommendations for management by the pediatric gastroenterologist.

Conclusion This report, which has been endorsed by the Executive Council of the North American Society for Pediatric Gastroenterology and Nutrition, has been prepared as a general guideline to assist providers of medical care in the evaluation and treatment of constipation in children. It is not intended as a substitute for clinical judgment or as a protocol for the management of all patients with this problem.

Key Words: Constipation, Encopresis, Infants, Children, Algorithm, Evidence based, Impaction, Guideline

BACKGROUND

A normal pattern of stool evacuation is felt to be a sign of health in children of all ages. Especially during the first months of life, parents pay close attention to the frequency and the characteristics of their children's defecation. Any deviation from what is felt to be normal for children by any family member may trigger a call to the nurse or a visit to the pediatrician. Thus, it is not surprising that approximately 3% of general pediatric outpatient visits and 25% of pediatric gastroenterology consultations are related to a complaint of defecation disorder (1). Chronic constipation is a source of anxiety for parents who worry that a serious disease may be causing the symptom. Yet only a small minority of children have an organic etiology for constipation. Beyond the neonatal period, the most common cause of constipation is functional constipation, which has also been called idiopathic constipation, functional fecal retention, and withholding constipation.

In most cases the parents are worried that the child's stools are too large, too hard, painful or too infrequent. The normal frequency of bowel movements at different ages has been defined (Table 1). Infants have a mean of 4 stools per day during the first week of life. This frequency gradually declines to a mean average of 1.7 stools per day at 2 years of age and 1.2 stools per day at 4 years of age (2,3). Some normal breastfed babies do not have stools for several days or longer (4). After 4 years, the frequency of bowel movements remains unchanged.

In most children constipation is functional, that is, without objective evidence of a pathological condition. Functional constipation most commonly is due to painful bowel movements with resultant voluntary withholding of feces by a child who wishes to avoid an unpleasant defecation. Many events can lead to painful defecation such as toilet training, changes in routine or diet, stressful events, intercurrent illness, unavailability of toilets, or postponing defecation because the child is too busy. They can lead to prolonged fecal stasis in the colon, with reabsorption of fluids and an increase in the size and consistency of the stools.

The passage of large hard stools that painfully stretch the anus may frighten the child, resulting in a fearful determination to avoid all defecation. Such children respond to the urge to defecate by contracting their anal sphincter and gluteal muscles, attempting to withhold stool (5). They rise on their toes and rock back and forth while stiffening their buttocks and legs, or wriggle, fidget or assume unusual postures, often performed while hiding in a corner. This dance-like behavior is frequently misconstrued by parents who believe that the child is straining in an attempt to defecate. Eventually, the rectum habituates to the stimulus of the enlarging fecal mass and the urge to defecate subsides. With time such retentive behavior becomes an automatic reaction. As the rectal wall stretches fecal soiling may occur, angering the parents and frightening the child (6). After several days without a bowel movement, irritability, abdominal distension, cramps and decreased oral intake may result.

Although constipation is a common pediatric problem, no evidence-based guidelines for its evaluation and treatment currently exist. Therefore, the Constipation Subcommittee of the Clinical Guidelines Committee was formed by the North American Society for Pediatric Gastroenterology and Nutrition (NASPGN) to develop a clinical practice guideline.

METHODS

The Constipation Subcommittee, which consists of two primary care pediatricians, a clinical epidemiologist and five pediatric gastroenterologists, addressed the problem of constipation in infants and children without a previously established medical condition. Neonates less than 72 hours old and premature infants less than 37 weeks gestation were excluded from consideration. This clinical practice guideline is designed to assist primary care pediatricians, family practitioners, nurse practitioners, physician assistants, pediatric gastroenterologists and pediatric surgeons in the management of children with constipation in both inpatient and outpatient settings. Constipation was defined as a delay or difficulty in defecation, present for two or more weeks, sufficient to cause significant distress to the patient. The desirable outcome of optimal management was defined as a normal stooling pattern, with interventions that have few or no adverse effects, and with resultant resumption of functional health.

In order to develop evidence-based guidelines, articles on constipation published in English were found using Medline (7). A search for articles published between January 1966 and November 1997, revealed 3,839 documents on constipation. The Cochrane Center has designed a search strategy for Medline to identify randomized controlled trials. This strategy includes controlled vocabulary and free-text terms such as randomized controlled trial, clinical trial, and placebo (8). When this search strategy was run with the term constipation, 1,047 articles were identified, 809 of which were in English, and 254 of which included children.

After letters, editorials, and review articles were eliminated, 139 articles remained. Forty-four of these dealt with special populations, such as children with meningomyelocele or Hirschsprung disease, and were discarded. Ninety-five articles remained and were reviewed in depth. A second search strategy was performed to identify articles on constipation that related to treatment, including drug therapy (75 articles), surgery (64 articles), and "therapy" (144 articles). This added 148 new articles, whose abstracts were reviewed. If the abstracts indicated the article might be relevant, the article was reviewed in depth. Seven additional articles were identified from the bibliographies of the articles already catalogued. A total of 160 articles were reviewed for these guidelines.

Articles were evaluated using written criteria developed by Sackett and colleagues (9,10). These criteria had been used in previous reviews (11,12). Five articles were chosen at random and reviewed by a colleague in the Department of Pediatrics at the University of Rochester who had been trained in epidemiology. Concordance using the criteria was 92%. Using the methods of the Canadian Preventive Services Task Force (13), the quality of evidence of each of the recommendations made by the Constipation Subcommittee was determined and is summarized in Table 2. The Subcommittee based its recommendations on integration of the literature review combined with expert opinion when evidence was insufficient. Consensus was achieved through Nominal Group Technique, a structured, quantitative method (14).

The guidelines were critiqued by numerous primary care physicians in community and academic practices including members of several committees of the American Academy of Pediatrics. In addition, the guidelines were distributed to the membership of the North American

Society for Pediatric Gastroenterology and Nutrition for review and comment and finally were officially endorsed by the Society's Executive Council.

Two algorithms were developed (Figures 1 and 2). The initial discussion is based on the algorithm for children one year and older. The second algorithm is for children less than one year of age. This paper discusses the first algorithm in detail and the second algorithm is discussed only where it diverges from the first.

MEDICAL HISTORY

Based on clinical experience, a thorough history is recommended as part of a complete evaluation of a child with constipation (Table 3). There are no well-designed studies that determine which aspects of a history are pertinent. Important information includes the time after birth of the first bowel movement, what the family or child means by the term constipation (15), the length of time the condition has been present, the frequency of bowel movements, the consistency and size of the stools, whether defecation is painful, whether blood has been present on the stool or toilet paper, and if the child experiences abdominal pain. Fecal soiling may be mistaken for diarrhea by some parents. A history of stool-withholding behavior reduces the likelihood that there is an organic disorder. Medications are an important potential cause of constipation (Table 4).

Fever, abdominal distention, anorexia, nausea, vomiting, weight loss or poor weight gain could be signs of an organic disorder (Table 4). Bloody diarrhea in an infant with a history of constipation could be an indication of enterocolitis complicating Hirschsprung disease.

A psychosocial history assesses the family structure, the number of people living in the child's home and their relationship to the child, the interactions the child has with peers and the possibility of abuse. If the child is in school it is important to learn whether or not the child uses the school bathrooms and if not why. The caregiver's assessment of the child's temperament may be useful in planning a reward system for toileting behavior.

PHYSICAL EXAMINATION

Based on clinical experience, a thorough physical examination is recommended as part of a complete evaluation of a child with constipation (Table 5). No well-designed studies have determined the aspects of the physical examination that are most important. External examination of the perineum and perianal area is essential. At least one digital examination of the anorectum is recommended. The anorectal examination assesses perianal sensation, anal tone, the size of the rectum and the presence of an anal wink. It also determines the amount and consistency of stool, and its location within the rectum. It is recommended that a test for occult blood in the stool be performed in all infants with constipation, as well as in any child who also has abdominal pain, failure to thrive, intermittent diarrhea or a family history of colon cancer or colonic polyps. Detection of a physical abnormality could lead to the identification of an organic disorder (Table 6).

A thorough history and physical examination is generally sufficient to allow the practitioner to establish whether the child requires further evaluation (Figure 1, box 4) or has functional constipation (Figure 1, box 5).

MANAGEMENT OF CHILDREN WITH FUNCTIONAL CONSTIPATION

The general approach to the child with functional constipation includes the following steps: determine whether fecal impaction is present (Figure 1, box 6), treat the impaction if present (Figure 1, box 7), initiate treatment with oral medication, provide parental education and close follow-up, and adjust medications as necessary (Figure 1, box 10).

Education

The education of the family and the demystification of constipation, including an explanation of the pathogenesis of constipation, are the first steps in treatment. If fecal soiling is present, an important goal is to remove negative attributions for both the child and the parent. It is especially important for parents to understand that soiling from overflow incontinence is not a willful and defiant maneuver. Parents are encouraged to maintain a consistent, positive and supportive attitude for all aspects of treatment. It may be necessary to repeat the education and demystification processes several times during treatment (16).

Disimpaction

A fecal impaction is defined as a hard mass in the lower abdomen identified on physical examination, a dilated rectum filled with a large amount of stool on rectal examination or excessive stool in the colon on abdominal radiography (17). Disimpaction is necessary prior to starting maintenance therapy. Disimpaction may be carried out with either oral or rectal medication (Figure 1, box 7). In uncontrolled clinical trials disimpaction by the oral route, the rectal route or a combination of the two has been shown to be effective (Table 7) (18). There are no randomized studies that compare the effectiveness of one to the other. The oral approach is not invasive and gives a sense of power to the child but adherence to the treatment regimen may be a problem. The rectal approach is faster but is invasive. The choice of treatment is best determined after discussing the options with the family and child.

Disimpaction with oral medication has been shown to be effective when high doses of mineral oil, polyethylene glycol electrolyte solutions or both are used (18-20). Although there are no controlled trials demonstrating the effectiveness of high dose magnesium hydroxide, magnesium citrate, lactulose, sorbitol, senna or bisacodyl for initial disimpaction, these laxatives have been used successfully in that role (21,22). It is recommended that mineral oil, oral electrolyte solutions, or the above-mentioned laxatives be used alone or in combination for initial disimpaction when the oral route is selected.

Rectal disimpaction may be carried out with phosphate soda enemas, saline enemas, or mineral oil enemas followed by a phosphate enema (23,24). These enemas are widely used and are effective. The use of soapsuds, tap water and magnesium enemas is not recommended because of their potential toxicity. Rectal disimpaction has also been effectively carried out with glycerin suppositories in infants (25) and bisacodyl suppositories in older children.

The Subcommittee discussed the use of digital disimpaction in chronic constipation in the primary care setting. However, there was insufficient literature on the subject and the Subcommittee could not reach consensus on whether to discourage or recommend its use.

Maintenance Therapy

Once the impaction has been removed, the treatment focuses on the prevention of the re-occurrence . For the child presenting without impaction (Figure 1, box 9) or after successful disimpaction, maintenance therapy is begun. This treatment consists of dietary interventions, behavioral modification and laxatives to assure that bowel movements occur at normal intervals with a good evacuation.

Dietary changes are commonly advised, particularly increased intake of fluids and absorbable and nonabsorbable carbohydrate, as a method to soften stools. Carbohydrates and especially sorbitol, found in some juices, such as prune, pear and apple juice, can cause increased frequency and water content of stools (26-27). No randomized controlled studies were found that demonstrated a proven effect on stools of increasing intakes of fluids, nonabsorbable carbohydrates or dietary fiber in children (28). A balanced diet that includes whole grains, fruits and vegetables is recommended as part of the treatment for constipation in children. Forceful implementation is undesirable.

Behavioral Modification

An important component of treatment includes behavior modification and regular toileting (29,30). Unhurried time on the toilet after meals is recommended. As part of the treatment of constipation, with or without overflow incontinence, it is often helpful to have children and their caregivers keep diaries of stool frequency. This can be combined with a reward system. For example, a child can use a calendar with stickers to record each stool that is passed in the toilet. The calendar can then be brought to visits with the health care provider and serves as both a diary and a point for positive reinforcement. In cases where motivational or behavior problems are interfering with successful treatment referral to a mental health care provider for behavior modification or other intervention may be helpful.

The successful treatment of constipation, especially with overflow incontinence, requires a family that is well organized, can complete time-consuming interventions, and is sufficiently patient to endure gradual improvements and relapses. Close follow-up by telephone and with office visits is recommended. Some families may need counseling support to help them effectively deal with this problem.

Medication

It is often necessary to use medication to help constipated children achieve regular bowel movements (Table 7). A prospective, randomized trial showed that the addition of medications to behavior management in children with constipation is beneficial (31). Children who received medications achieved remission significantly sooner than children who did not. The use of laxatives was most advantageous for children until they were able to maintain regular toileting.

When medication is necessary in the daily treatment of constipation, mineral oil (a lubricant) or magnesium hydroxide, lactulose or sorbitol (osmotic laxatives), or a combination of the two, is recommended. At this stage in the treatment of constipation, the chronic use of stimulant laxatives is not recommended. Extensive experience with long term use of mineral oil (32), magnesium hydroxide (33) and lactulose or sorbitol (33) has been reported. Long term studies show that these therapies are effective and safe (33,34). The doses and potential adverse effects of these medications are found in Table 7. Since mineral oil, magnesium hydroxide, lactulose or sorbitol seem to be equally efficacious, the choice among these is based on safety, cost, the child's preference, ease of administration and the practitioner's experience (Figure 1, box 14).

A stimulant laxative may be necessary intermittently, for short periods of time, to avoid recurrence of an impaction (Figure 1, box 15) (35). In this situation the use of stimulant laxatives is sometimes termed rescue therapy.

Maintenance therapy may be necessary for many months. Only when the child has been having regular bowel movements without difficulty is weaning considered. Primary care providers and families need to be aware that relapses are common and difficulty with bowel movements may continue into adolescence. Long term follow-up studies have demonstrated that a significant number of children continue to require therapy to maintain regular bowel movements (36,37).

CONSULTATION WITH A SPECIALIST

Consultation with a pediatric gastrointestinal specialist becomes necessary when the child fails therapy, when there is concern that an organic disease exists, or when management is complex (Figure 1, box 20). A consultant can re-evaluate the non-responding child, exclude an underlying organic process, perform specialized tests and offer counseling. The pediatric gastroenterologist (Figure 1, boxes 21-23) can review previous therapies, consider using different or additional medications or higher doses of the current medications, and reassess previous management before performing additional studies (Figure 1, box 23).

A careful review by the primary care practitioner of the differential diagnosis (Table 4) of the organic causes of constipation may be helpful at this time in order to determine which laboratory tests are indicated before referring to a specialist. It is recommended that the primary care physician consider whether or not the children who require evaluation by a specialist need to have blood tests to identify evidence of hypothyroidism, hypercalcemia, celiac disease and lead toxicity (Figure 1, box 16). By having these tests ordered by the primary care provider just prior to referral to a pediatric gastroenterologist, patients who are found to have a medical problem that requires evaluation by a different subspecialist can be referred directly to the appropriate sub specialist. For example, a child with hypothyroidism can be referred directly to a pediatric endocrinologist.

Abdominal Radiograph and Transit Time

An abdominal radiograph is not indicated to establish the presence of a fecal impaction if the rectal exam reveals the presence of large amounts of stool. A retrospective study in encopretic children showed that moderate to large amounts of stool found on rectal examination had a high sensitivity and positive predictive value (greater than 80%) for predicting fecal retention determined by abdominal radiograph, even using the radiologists' subjective interpretation (38). However, the specificity and negative predictive value were 50% or less. When the systematic scoring system developed by Barr (17) was used for the presence of fecal retention on radiograph, the sensitivity of moderate to large amounts of stool on rectal examination improved to 92%, and the positive predictive value was 94%. However, the specificity was still only 71% and the negative predictive value was only 62% (39).

This suggests that, when there is doubt about whether the patient is constipated, a plain abdominal radiograph is reliable in determining the presence of fecal retention in the child who is obese or refuses a rectal exam, or in whom there are other psychological factors (sexual abuse) that make the rectal examination too traumatic. It may also be helpful in the child with a good history for constipation who does not have large amounts of stool on rectal examination (Figure 1, box 23). In a recent study the value of the Barr Score was compared to the colonic transit time. The Barr Score was shown to be poorly reproducible, with low inter-observer and intra-observer reliability, and there was no correlation with measurements of transit time (39).

Some patients have a history of infrequent bowel movements, but have no objective findings of constipation. The history obtained from the parents and child may not be entirely accurate (40). In these patients an evaluation of colonic transit time with radio-opaque markers may be helpful (Figure 1, box 25) (41). The quantification of transit time shows whether constipation is present and provides an objective evaluation of bowel movement frequency. If the transit time is normal, the child does not have constipation. If the transit time is normal and there is no soiling, the child needs no further evaluation (Figure 1, box 30). For children who have soiling without evidence of constipation the best results have been achieved with behavioral modification, but in some instances psychological evaluation and treatment may be necessary (Figure 1, box 29). If the transit study is abnormal or a fecal impaction is present, further evaluation will be needed (Figure 1, box 26). When a child with objective evidence of constipation is refractory to treatment, it is important to consider Hirschsprung disease (Figure 1, box 28).

Hirschsprung Disease

Hirschsprung disease is the most common cause of lower intestinal obstruction in neonates and is a rare cause of intractable constipation in toddlers and school-age children (42-44). It is characterized by a lack of ganglion cells in the myenteric and submucous plexuses of the distal colon, resulting in sustained contraction of the aganglionic segment. The aganglionic segment begins at the internal anal sphincter, extending orad in a contiguous fashion. In 75% of cases the disease is limited to the rectosigmoid area. The bowel proximal to the aganglionic zone becomes dilated due to the distal obstruction.

The incidence of Hirschsprung disease is approximately 1 in 5,000 live births. The most common associated abnormality is trisomy 21. More than 90% of normal neonates and less than 10% of children with Hirschsprung disease pass meconium in the first 24 hours of life (45,46). Thus, a delayed passage of meconium by a full term infant raises the suspicion of Hirschsprung disease. Hirschsprung disease can present with bilious vomiting, abdominal distension and refusal to feed, symptoms suggestive of intestinal obstruction. Subjects with short segment Hirschsprung disease may go undiagnosed until childhood. They have ribbon-like stools, a distended abdomen and often fail to thrive. In rare cases constipation is the only symptom. Fecal soiling is even more rare and occurs only when the aganglionic segment is extremely short.

Enterocolitis, the most feared complication of Hirschsprung disease, may be its initial manifestation. Enterocolitis presents with the sudden onset of fever, abdominal distension and explosive and, at times, bloody diarrhea (47,48). Occurring most often during the second and third months of life, it is associated with a mortality of 20%. The incidence of enterocolitis can be greatly reduced by a timely diagnosis of Hirschsprung disease.

The mean age at diagnosis decreased from 18.8 months in the 1960's to 2.6 months in the 1980's due to physician vigilance, anorectal manometry and early biopsy. However, 8-20% of children with Hirschsprung disease remain unrecognized after the age of 3 years (49,50). Physical examination reveals a distended abdomen and a contracted anal sphincter and rectum in the majority of children. The rectum is devoid of stool except in cases of short segment aganglionosis. As the finger is withdrawn, there may be an explosive discharge of foul smelling liquid stools, with decompression of the proximal normal bowel. In the older child presenting with constipation, a careful history and a thorough physical examination are sufficient to differentiate Hirschsprung disease from functional constipation in most cases.

Once Hirschsprung disease is suspected (Figure 1, box 28), it is recommended that the patient be evaluated at a medical center with a pediatric gastroenterologist and a pediatric surgeons where diagnostic studies can be performed. Delay in diagnosis increases the risk of enterocolitis. Rectal biopsy with histopathologic examination and rectal manometry are the only tests that can reliably exclude Hirschsprung disease. Rectal biopsies demonstrating the absence of ganglion cells in the submucosal plexus are diagnostic of Hirschsprung disease (51). The biopsies, obtained approximately 3 cm above the anal verge, must be deep enough to include adequate submucosa. Confirmation is obtained when special staining shows hypertrophied nerves.

However, in total colonic aganglionosis there is both an absence of ganglion cells and an absence of hypertrophied nerves. Occasionally suction biopsies are not diagnostic and a full thickness biopsy is required.

Anorectal manometry (Figure 1, box 31) evaluates the response of the internal anal sphincter to inflation of a balloon in the internal anal sphincter (52). When the rectal balloon is inflated, there is normally a reflex relaxation of the internal anal sphincter. In Hirschsprung disease this rectoanal inhibitory reflex is absent; there is no relaxation, or there may even be paradoxical contraction, of the internal anal sphincter. In a cooperative child, anorectal manometry represents a sensitive and specific diagnostic test for Hirschsprung disease. It is particularly useful when the aganglionic segment is short and radiologic or pathologic studies are equivocal. If sphincter relaxation is normal, Hirschsprung disease can be reliably excluded. In the presence of a dilated rectum, it is necessary to inflate the balloon with large volumes to elicit a normal sphincter relaxation. In the child with retentive behaviors, there may be artifacts due to voluntary contraction of the external anal sphincter and the gluteal muscles. Sedation, which does not interfere with the rectoanal inhibitory reflex, may be used in newborns and uncooperative children. If manometry is abnormal diagnosis needs to be confirmed with a biopsy.

Although a barium enema is often performed as the initial screening test to rule out Hirschsprung disease, it is usually unnecessary beyond infancy (53). When stool is present in the rectum to the level of the anus, the barium enema provides no more useful information than can be obtained with a plain radiograph. However, after the diagnosis of Hirschsprung disease has been made, the barium enema may be useful to identify the location of the transition zone, provided that laxatives or enemas have not been administered prior to the study to clean out the colon. The barium enema may not show a transition zone in cases of total colonic Hirschsprung disease, or may be indistinguishable from cases of functional consitpation when ultra-short segment Hirschsprung disease is present.

Other Medications and Testing

If a child with constipation fails to achieve resolution with the treatments outlined above, and Hirschsprung disease has been excluded, other therapies may be considered (Figure 1, box 34). Clearly, treatment may be necessary for an extended period of time, for months or years. Stimulant laxatives can be added for short periods of time. There is extensive experience with senna, bisacodyl and phenolphthalein (54,55). However, phenolphthalein is no longer available in the United States due to concerns about its carcinogenic potential.

The effectiveness of cisapride for the treatment of constipation is controversial. In some open label studies and placebo controlled trials it appears to be effective, but in another placebo controlled study cisapride had no effect (23,56-59). Polyethylene glycol electrolyte solutions have been used to achieve bowel clean out (20-61), and recently it has been suggested that the chronic administration of lower doses may be useful for long term therapy.

Biofeedback therapy has been evaluated in multiple open label studies where it was found to be efficacious (62). Some recent controlled studies, however, failed to demonstrate its long-term efficacy. Biofeedback may be beneficial for the treatment of a small subgroup of patients with intractable constipation (63-65). At times intensive psychotherapy may be needed. Rarely inpatient hospitalization with behavioral therapy may be required.

Many conditions can cause constipation (Table 4). For children who remain constipated despite conscientious adherence to the treatment outlined above, other tests may be indicated (Figure 1, box 38). Magnetic resonance imaging (MRI) of the lumbosacral spine can demonstrate intra-spinal problems, such as a tethered cord, tumors, or sacral agenesis. Other diagnostic tests such as anorectal manometry, rectal biopsy, colonic manometry, barium enema, and a psychological evaluation can at times also prove helpful. Colonic manometry, by providing objective evidence of colonic function, can exclude the presence of an underlying neuropathy or myopathy (66). Barium enema can be useful to exclude the presence of anatomic abnormalities, or of a transition zone. Full thickness rectal biopsy can be useful to detect neuronal intestinal dysplasia or other myenteric abnormalities, including Hirschsprung disease. Metabolic tests, such as a serum calcium level, thyrocalcitonin concentration or thyroid function tests, can detect metabolic causes of constipation (67).

ALGORITHM FOR INFANTS LESS THAN 1 YEAR OF AGE

The evaluation of infants differs in some aspects from that of older children. Even in infancy most constipation is functional. However, when treatment fails, or there is delayed passage of meconium (Figure 2, box 4), or red flags are present (Figure 2, box, 8), particular consideration of Hirschsprung disease and other disorders is necessary. Hirschsprung disease is described in detail above. In a constipated infant with delayed passage of meconium, if Hirschsprung disease has been excluded, it is recommended that a sweat test be performed to rule out cystic fibrosis (Figure 2, box 6). Constipation can be the presenting manifestation of cystic fibrosis, even in the absence of failure to thrive and pulmonary symptoms.

Special consideration should also be given to breast fed infants in the first year of life. Greater variability in stool frequency occurs among breast fed infants than in formula fed infants (4, 68,69). Unless a suspicion of Hirschsprung disease is present, management of a breast fed infant requires only reassurance and close follow-up if the infant is growing normally, nurses well and has no signs or symptoms of obstruction or enterocolitis,

The treatment of constipation in infancy is similar to that of older children, with important exceptions. Increased intake of fluids, particularly juices containing sorbitol, such as prune, pear and apple, is recommended within the context of a healthy diet. Barley malt extract, corn syrup, lactulose or sorbitol can be used as a stool softeners. Light and dark corn syrups are not considered to be potential sources of *C botulinum* spores (70). Mineral oil and stimulant laxatives are not recommended. Because gastroesophageal reflux and incoordination of swallowing is more common in infants, there is a greater risk of aspiration of mineral oil, which can induce a severe lipoid pneumonia (71-73). Glycerin suppositories can be useful, and enemas are to be avoided.

References

1. Molnar D, Taitz LS, Urwin OM, Wales JK. Anorectal manometry results in defecation disorders. Arch Dis Child 1983;58:257-61.

2. Nyhan WE. Stool frequency of normal infants in the first weeks of life. Pediatrics 1952;10:414-25.

3. Weaver LT, Steiner H. The bowel habits of young children. Arch Dis Child 1983;59:649-52.

4. Hyams JS, Treem WR, Etienne NL, Weinerman H, MacGilpin D, Hine P, Choy K, Burke G. Effect of infant formula on stool characteristics of young infants. Pediatrics 1995;95:50-54.

5. Partin JC, Hamill SK, Fischel JE, Partin JS. Painful defecation and fecal soiling in children. Pediatrics 1992;89:1007-9.

6. Hyman PE, Fleisher D. Functional fecal retention. Practical Gastroenterology 1992;31:29-37.

7. Medline (online database) Bethesda, MD: National Library of Medicine, 1989. Updated weekly. Available from National Library of Medicine; BRS Information Technologies, McLean, VA: DIALOG Information Services, Inc., Palo Alto, CA

8. Mulrow CD, Oxman AD (eds). Formulating the problem. Cochrane Collaboration Handbook (updated September, 1997); Section 4. In: The Cochrane Library (database on disk and CDROM). Cochrane Collaboration. Oxform: Update Software; 1997, issue 4; Appendix 5c.2; http://www.medlib.com/cochranehandbook/.

9. Sackett DL, Haynes B, Tugwell P. Clinical Epidemiology: A Basic Science for Clinical Medicine, 2nd ed. Boston; Little, Brown, 1991.

10. Evidence-Based Medicine Informatics Project. Evidence Based Medicine; Users' Guides to the Medical Literature. Http://hiru.mcmaster.ca/ebm/userguid/, revised, May, 1997.

11. Liptak GS. Tethered spinal cord: an analysis of clinical research. European J Pediatr Surg 1992;2 (Suppl1):12-17.

12. Liptak GS. Tethered spinal cord: update of an analysis of published articles. European J Pediatr Surg 1995;5:21-23.

13. Canadian Task Force on the Periodic Health Examination. The periodic health examination. Canadian Medical Assoc J 1979;121:1193-1254.

14. McMurray AR. Three decision-making aids. Brainstorming, nominal group, and delphi technique. J Nursing Staff Development 1994;10:62-65.

15. Potts MJ, Sesney J. Infant constipation: maternal knowledge and beliefs. Clin Pediatr 1992;31:143-148.

16. Rappaport LA, Levine MD. The prevention of constipation and encopresis: a developmental model and approach. Pediatr Clin North Am 1986;33:859-869.

17. Barr RG, Levine MD, Wilkinson RH, Mulvihill D. Chronic and occult stool retention. A clinical tool for its evaluation in school-aged children. Clin Pediatr 1979;18:674-686.

18. Tolia V, Lin CH, Elitsur Y. A prospective randomized study with mineral oil and oral lavage solution for treatment of faecal impaction in children. Alimentary Pharmacology and Therapeutics 1993;7:523-29.

19. Gleghorn EE, Heyman MB, Rudolph CD. No-enema therapy for idiopathic constipation and encopresis. Clinical Pediatrics 1991;30:667-672

20. Ingebo KB, Heyman MB. Polyethylene glycol-electrolyte solution for intestinal clearance in children with refractory encopresis. A safe and effective therapeutic program. Am J Dis Child 1988;142:340-42.

21. Sutphen JL, Borowitz SM, Hutchison RL, Cox DJ. Long-term follow-up of medically treated childhood constipation. Clinical Pediatrics 1995;34:576-580.

22. Loening-Baucke V. Modulation of abnormal defecation dynamics by biofeedback treatment in chronically constipated children with encopresis. J Pediatr 1990;116:214-222.

23. Nurko SS, Garcia-Aranda JA, Guerrero VY, Woroma LB. Treatment of intractable constipation in children: experience with cisapride. J Pediatr Gastroenterol Nutr 1996;22:38-44.

24. Cox DJ, Sutphen J, Borowitz S, Dickens MN, Singles J, Whitehead WE. Simple electromyographic biofeedback treatment for chronic pediatric constipation/encopresis: preliminary report. Biofeedback & Self Regulation. 1994;19:41-50.

25. Weisman LE, Merenstein GB, Digirol M, Collins J, Frank G, Hudgins C. The effect of early meconium evacuation on early-onset hyperbilirubinemia. Am J Dis Child 1983;137:666-68.

26. Kneepkens CMF. What happens to fructose in the gut? Scand J Gastroenterol 1989;24(suppl 171):1-8.

27. Gryboski JD. Diarrhea from dietetic candy. N Eng J Med 1966;266:818

28. Olness K, Tobin JS, Hanck AB, Goffin H. Chronic constipation in children: can it be managed by diet alone: Dexpanthenol (Ro 01-4709) in the treatment of constipation. Postgraduate Medicine 1982;72:149-154.

29. Lowery SP, Srour JW, Whitehead WE, Schuster NM. Habit training as treatment of encopresis secondary to chronic constipation. J Pediatr Gastro Nutr 1985;4:397-401.

30. Howe AC, Walker CE, Behavioral management of toilet training, enuresis and encopresis. Pediatr Clin North Am 1992;39:413-32.

31. Nolan T, Debelle G, Oberklaid F, Coffey C.. Randomized trial of laxatives in treatment of childhood encopresis. Lancet 1991;338:523-27.

32. McClung HJ, Boyne LJ, Linsheid T, Heitlinger LA, Murray RD, Fyda J, Li Bu. Is combination therapy for encopresis nutritionally safe: Pediatrics 1993; 91:591-4.

33. Loening-Baucke V. Chronic constipation in children. Gastroenterology 1993;105:1557-1564.

34. Clark JH, Russell GJ, Fitzgerald JF, Nagamori KE. Serum β-carotene, retinol, and α-tocopherol levels during mineral oil therapy for constipation. Am J Dis Child 1987;141:1210-12.

35. Nurko SS. Constipation. In: Walker-Smith J, Hamilton D, Walker AW, eds. Practical Pediatric Gastroenterology, Second edition. Hamilton, Ontario: BC Decker, 1996;95-106.

36. Staiano A Andreotti MR, Greco L, Basile P, Auricchio S. Long term follow up of children with chronic idiopathic constipation. Dig Dis Sci 1994;39:561-564.

37. Loening-Baucke V. Constipation in children. Current Opinion in Pediatrics. 1994;6:556-561.

38. Rockney, RM, McQuade WH, Days AL. The plain abdominal roentgenogram in the management of encopresis. Arch Pediatr Adolesc Med 1995;149:623-627.

39. Benninga, MA, Buller HA, Staalman CR, Gubler FM, Bossuyt PM, van der Plas RN, Taminiau JA. Defecation disorders in children, colonic transit vs the Barr score. European J Pediatr 1995;154:277-284.

40. Van der Plas RN, Benninga MA, Redekop WK, Taminiau JA, Buller HA. How accurate is the recall of bowel habits in children with defaecation disorders? European J Pediatr 1997;156:178-81.

41. Papadopoulou A, Clayden GS, Booth IW. The clinical value of solid marker transit studies in childhood constipation and soiling. European Journal of Pediatr 1994;153:560-64.

42. Keinhaus S, Boley SJ, Sheran M, Sieber WK. Hirschsprung's disease: a survey of the members of the surgical section of the American Academy of Pediatrics. J Pediatr Surg 1979; 14: 588-600.

43. Russell MB, Russell CA, Niebuhr E. An epidemiological study of Hirschsprung's disease and additional anomalies. Acta Paediatr 1994;83:68-71.

44. Reding R, de Ville de Goyet J, Gosseye S, Clapuyt P, Sokal E, Buts JP, Gibbs P, Otte JB. Hirschsprung's disease: a 20 year experience. J Pediatr Surg 1997;32:1221-25.

45. Sherry SN, Kramer I. The time of passage of the first stool and first urine in the newborn infant. J Pediatr 1955;46:158-9.

46. Clark DA. Times of first void and first stool in 500 newborns. Pediatrics 1977;60:457-9.

47. Marty TL, Matlak ME, Hendrickson M, Black RE, Johnson DG. Unexpected death from enterocolitis after surgery for Hirschsprung's disease. Pediatrics 1995:96;118-121.

48. Elhalaby EA, Teitelbaum DH, Coran AG, Heidelberger KP. Enterocolitis associated with Hirschsprung's disease: a clinical histopathological correlative study. J Pediatr Surg 1995;30:1023-26.

49. Klein MD, Phillippart AL. Hirschsprung's disease: three decades experience at a single institution. J Pediatr Surg 1993;28:1291-4.

50. Swenson O, Sherman JO, Fisher JH. Diagnosis of congenital megacolon: an analysis of 501 patients. J Pediatr Surg 1973;8:587-594.

51. Aldridge RT, Campbell PE. Ganglion cells distribution in the normal rectum and anal canal. A basis for diagnosis of Hirschsprung's disease by anorectal biopsy. J Pediatr Surg 1968; 3: 475-489.

52. Rosemberg AJ, Vela AR. A new simplified technique for pediatric anorectal manometry. Pediatrics 1983; 71: 240-245.

53. Taxman TL, Yulish BS, Rothstein FC. How useful is the barium enema in the diagnosis of infantile Hirschsprung's disease? Am J Dis Child 1986; 140: 881-884.

54. Berg I, Forsythe I, Holt P, Watts J. A controlled trial of 'Senokot' in faecal soiling treated by behavioral methods. J Child Psychol Psychiatry 1983;24:543-49.

55. Loening-Baucke VA, Younoszai MK. Effect of treatment on rectal and sigmoid motility in Chronically constipated children. Pediatrics 1984;73:199-205.

56. Murray RD, Li UK, McClung HJ, Heitlinger L, Rehm D. Cisapride for intractable constipation in children: observation from an open trial. J Pediatr Gastroenterol Nutr 1990;11:503-508.

57. Odeka EB, Sagher F, Miller V, Doig C. Use of cisapride in treatment of constipation in children. J Pediatr Gastroenterol Nutr 1997;25:199-203.

58. Staiano A, Cucchiara S, Andreotti MR, Minella R, Manzi G. Effect of cisapride on chronic idiopathic constipation in children. Dig Dis Sci 1991;1991: 733-36.

59. Halabi IM. Cisapride in management of chronic pediatric constipation. J Pediatr Gastroenter Nutr 1999;28:199-202.

60. Andorsky RI, Goldner F. Colonic lavage solution (polyethylene glycol electrolyte lavage solution) as a treatment for chronic constipation: a double-blind, placebo controlled study. Am J Gastroenterol 1990;85:261-65.

61. Corazziari E, Badiali D, Habib FI, Reboa GU, Mazzacca G, Sabbatini F. Small volume isosmotic polyethylene glycol electrolyte balanced solution (PMF-100) in treatment of chronic nonorganic constipation. Dig Dis Sci 1996;41: 1636-1642.

62. Loening-Baucke V. Biofeedback therapy for chronic constipation and encopresis in childhood: long term outcome. Pediatrics 1995;96:105-110.

63. Loening-Baucke V. Biofeedback training in children with constipation: a critical review. Dig Dis Sci 1996;41:65-71.

64. Van der Plas RN, Benninga MA , Redekop WK, Taminiau JA, Buller HA. Randomized trial of biofeedback training for encopresis. Arch Dis Child 1996;75:367-74.

65. Van der Plas RN, Benninga MA, Buller HA, Bossuyt PM, Akkermans LM, Redekop WK, Taminiau JA. Biofeedback training in treatment of childhood constipation: a randomized controlled study. Lancet 1996;348:776-80.

66. DiLorenzo C, Flores AF, Reddy SN, Hyman PE. Use of colonic manometry differentiates causes of intractable constipation in children. J Pediatr 1992;120:690-05.

67. De Krijer RR, Brooks A, Van Der Harst E, Hofstra RW, Bruining HA, Molenaar JC, Meijers C. Constipation as the presenting symptom in de novo multiple endocrine neoplasia type 2B. Pediatrics 1998;102:405-7.

68. Fontana M Bianchi C, Cataldo F, Conti Nibali S, Cucchiora S, Gobio Casali L, Iacono G, Sanfilippo M, Tone G. Bowel frequency in healthy children. Acta Paediatr Scand 1989;78:682-84.

69. Sievers E, Oldigs H-D, Schultz-Lell, G, Schaub J. Faecal excretion in infants. Eur J Pediatr 1993;152:452-54.

70. Committee on Infectious Diseases, American Academy of Pediatrics. Red Book , American Academy of Pediatrics, Elk Grove Village, 1997, p175.

71. Fan LL, Graham LM. Radiological cases of the month. Lipoid pneumonia from mineral oil aspiration. Archives of Pediatr and Adolescent Medicine 1994;148:205-06.

72. Rabah R, Evans RW, Yunis EJ. Mineral oil embolization and lipid pneumonia in an infant treated for Hirschspring's disease. Pediatr Path 1987;7:447-55.

73. Wolfson BJ, Allen JL, Panitch HB, Karmazin N. Lipid aspiration pneumonia due to gastroesophageal reflux. A complication of nasogastric lipid feedings. Pediatr Rad 1989;19:545-47.

74. Fisher M, Eckhard C (eds). Guide to clinical preventive services: an assessment of the effectiveness of 169 interventions. Report of the U.S. Preventive Services Task Force. Baltimore: Williams and Wilkins;1989:387-8.

75. Bar-Maor JA, Eitan A. Determination of the normal position of the anus (with reference to idiopathic constipation). J Pediatr Gastroenterol Nutr 1987;6:559-61.

76. Iacono G, Cavataio F, Montalto G, Florena A, Tumminello M, Soresi M, Notarbartolo A, Carroccio A. Intolerance of cow's milk and chronic constipation in children. New Eng J Med 1998;339:1100-4.

77. Shulman RJ, Boyle JT, Colletti RB, Friedman R, Heyman MB, Kearns G, Kirschner BS, Levy J, Mitchell AA, Van Hare G. Use of cisapride in children. J Pediatr Gastroenterol Nutr 1999;28:529-33.

Table 1. Normal Frequency of Bowel Movements*

AGE	Bowel Movements per Week**	Bowel Movements per day***
0 to 3 months old		
Breast milk	5 to 40	2.9
Formula	5 to 28	2.0
6 to 12 months old	5 to 28	1.8
1 to 3 years old	4 to 21	1.4
> 3 years old	3 to 14	1.0

*   Acta Paediatr Scand 1989;78:682-4
**   Approximately mean ± 2 SD
*** Mean

Table 2. Summary of Recommendations and the Quality of the Evidence

Recommendations	Quality of Evidence*

General Recommendations

Recommendation	Quality
A thorough history and physical examination are an important part of the complete evaluation of the infant or child with constipation	III
Performing a thorough history and physical examination is sufficient to diagnose functional constipation in most cases	III
A stool test for occult blood is recommended in all constipated infants and in those children who also have abdominal pain, failure to thrive, diarrhea or a family history of colonic cancer or polyps	III
In selected patients, an abdominal radiograph, when interpreted correctly, can be useful to diagnose fecal impaction	II-2
Rectal biopsy with histopathologic examination and rectal manometry are the only tests that can reliably exclude Hirschsprung disease	II-1
In selected patients, measurement of transit time using radio-opaque markers can determine whether constipation is present	II-2

Recommendations for Infants

Recommendation	Quality
In infants, rectal disimpaction can be carried out with glycerin suppositories. Enemas are to be avoided	II-3
In infants, juices that contain sorbitol, such as prune, pear and apple juice, can decrease constipation	II-3
Barley malt extract, corn syrup, lactulose or sorbitol (osmotic laxatives) can be used as stool softeners	III
Mineral oil and stimulant laxatives are not recommended for infants	III

Recommendations for Children

Recommendation	Quality
In children, disimpaction may be carried out with either oral or rectal medication, including enemas	II-3
In children, a balanced diet, containing whole grains, fruits and vegetables, is recommended as part of the treatment for constipation	III
The use of medications in combination with behavioral management can decrease the time to remission in children with functional constipation	I
Mineral oil (a lubricant) and magnesium hydroxide, lactulose and sorbitol (osmotic laxatives) are safe and effective medications	I
Rescue therapy with short-term administration of stimulant laxatives can be useful in selected patients	II-3
Senna and bisacodyl (stimulant laxatives) can be useful in selected patients who are more difficult to manage	II-1
Cisapride has been shown in some but not all controlled studies to be an effective laxative, and can be useful in selected patients	I
Polyethylene glycol electrolyte solution, given chronically in low dosage, may be an effective treatment for constipation that is difficult to manage	III

Biofeedback therapy can be effective short-term treatment of intractable constipation	II-2

*Categories of the Quality of Evidence (74)

I   Evidence obtained from at least one properly designed randomized controlled study.

II-1   Evidence obtained from well-designed cohort or case-controlled trials without randomization.

II-2   Evidence obtained from well-designed cohort or case-control analytic studies, preferably from more than one center or research group.

II-3   Evidence obtained from multiple time series with or without the intervention. Dramatic results in uncontrolled experiments (such as the results of the introduction of penicillin treatment in the 1940's) could also be regarded as this type of evidence.

III   Opinions of respected authorities, based on clinical experience, descriptive studies, or reports of expert committees.

Table 3. History in Pediatric Patients with Constipation

Age
Sex
Chief Complaint
Constipation History
      Frequency and consistency of stools
      Pain or bleeding with passing stools
      Abdominal pain
      Waxing and waning of symptoms
      Age of onset
      Toilet training
      Fecal soiling
      Withholding behavior
      Change in appetite
      Nausea/vomiting
      Weight loss
      Peri-anal fissures, dermatitis, abscess or fistula
      Current treatment
            Current diet (24 hour recall history)
            Current Medications (for all medical problems)
                  Oral, enema, suppository, herbal
      Previous treatment
            Diet
            Medications
                  Oral, enema, suppository, herbal
            What has helped in the past
            Behavioral treatment
            Results of studies performed in the past
            Estimate of parent/patient adherence

Family history
      Significant illnesses
      Gastrointestinal (constipation, Hirschsprung Disease)
      Other
            Thyroid, parathyroid, cystic fibrosis, celiac disease

Past Medical History
      Gestational age
      Time of passage of meconium
      Condition at birth
      Acute injury or disease
      Hospitalizations
      Immunizations
      Allergies
      Surgeries
      Delayed growth/development
      Sensitivity to cold

Table 4. Differential Diagnosis of Constipation

Nonorganic
    Developmental
        Cognitive handicaps
        Attention-deficit disorders
    Situational
        Coercive toilet training
        Toilet phobia
        School bathroom avoidance
        Excessive parental interventions
        Sexual abuse
        Other
    Depression
    Constitutional
        Colonic inertia
        Genetic predisposition
    Reduced stool volume and dryness
        Low fiber in diet
        Dehydration
        Underfeeding/malnutrition

Organic
    Anatomic malformations
        Imperforate anus
        Anal stenosis
        Anterior displaced anus (75)
        Pelvic mass (sacral teratoma)
    Metabolic and Gastrointestinal
        Hypothyroidism
        Hypercalcemia
        Hypokalemia
        Cystic fibrosis
        Diabetes mellitus
        Multiple endocrine neoplasia type 2B
        Gluten enteropathy
    Neuropathic conditions
        Spinal cord abnormalities
        Spinal cord trauma
        Neurofibromatosis
        Static encephalopathy
        Tethered cord
    Intestinal nerve or muscle disorders
        Hirschsprung disease
        Intestinal neuronal dysplasia
        Visceral myopathies
        Visceral neuropathies
    Abnormal abdominal musculature

Table 4. Differential Diagnosis of Constipation

Nonorganic
- Developmental
  - Cognitive handicaps
  - Attention-deficit disorders
- Situational
  - Coercive toilet training
  - Toilet phobia
  - School bathroom avoidance
  - Excessive parental interventions
  - Sexual abuse
  - Other
- Depression
- Constitutional
  - Colonic inertia
  - Genetic predisposition
- Reduced stool volume and dryness
  - Low fiber in diet
  - Dehydration
  - Underfeeding/malnutrition

Organic
- Anatomic malformations
  - Imperforate anus
  - Anal stenosis
  - Anterior displaced anus (75)
  - Pelvic mass (sacral teratoma)
- Metabolic and Gastrointestinal
  - Hypothyroidism
  - Hypercalcemia
  - Hypokalemia
  - Cystic fibrosis
  - Diabetes mellitus
  - Multiple endocrine neoplasia type 2B
  - Gluten enteropathy
- Neuropathic conditions
  - Spinal cord abnormalities
  - Spinal cord trauma
  - Neurofibromatosis
  - Static encephalopathy
  - Tethered cord
- Intestinal nerve or muscle disorders
  - Hirschsprung disease
  - Intestinal neuronal dysplasia
  - Visceral myopathies
  - Visceral neuropathies
- Abnormal abdominal musculature

        Prune belly
        Gastroschisis
        Down syndrome
Connective tissue disorders
        Scleroderma
        Systemic lupus erythematosus
        Ehlers-Danlos Syndrome

Drugs

        Opiates
        Phenobarbital
        Sucralfate
        Antacids
        Antihypertensives
        Anticholinergics
        Antidepressants
        Sympathomimetics

Other

        Heavy-metal ingestion (lead)
        Vitamin D intoxication
        Botulism
        Cows milk protein intolerance (76)

Table 5. Physical Examination of Children with Constipation

General appearance
Vital Signs
      Temperature
      Pulse
      Respiratory rate
      Blood pressure
Growth Parameters
Head, ears, eyes nose, throat
Neck
Cardiovascular
Lungs/chest
Abdomen
      Distention
      Liver/spleen palpable
      Fecal mass
Anal inspection:
      Position
      Stool present around anus/on clothes
      Perianal erythema
      Skin tags
      Anal fissures
Rectal examination
      Anal wink
      Anal tone
      Fecal mass
      Presence of stool
      Consistency of stool
      Other masses
      Explosive stool on withdrawal of finger
      Occult blood in stool
Back and spine examination
      Dimple
      Tuft of hair
Neurological examination:
      Tone
      Strength
      Cremasteric reflex
      Deep tendon reflexes

Table 6.   Physical Findings Distinguishing Organic Constipation From Functional Constipation

Failure to thrive
Abdominal distention
Lack of lumbo-sacral curve
Pilonidal dimple covered by a tuft of hair
Midline pigmentary abnormalities of the lower spine
Sacral agenesis
Flat buttocks
Anteriorly displaced anus
Patulous anus
Tight empty rectum in presence of palpable abdominal fecal mass
Gush of liquid stool and air from rectum on withdrawal of finger
Occult blood in stool
Absent anal wink
Absent cremasteric reflex
Decreased lower extremity tone and/or strength
Absence or delay in relaxation phase of lower extremity deep tendon reflexes

Table 7. Medications for use in treatment of constipation

Laxatives		Dosage	Side Effects	Notes
Osmotic	Lactulose*	1-3 mL/kg/day in divided doses Available as 70% solution	Flatulence, abdominal cramps Hypernatremia has been reported when used in high dosage for hepatic encephalopathy. Case reports of 'nontoxic megacolon' in elderly	Synthetic disaccharide. Well tolerated long term.
	Sorbitol*	1-3 mL/kg/day in divided doses Available as 70% solution	Same as Lactulose	Less expensive than Lactulose
	Barley malt extract*	2-10 mL/240 mL of milk or juice	U	npleasant odor. Suitable for infants drinking from a bottle
	Magnesium hydroxide*	1-3 mL/kg/day of 400 mg/5 mL Available as liquid, 400 mg/5 mL, 800 mg/5 mL and tablets	Infants are susceptible to magnesium poisoning. Overdose can lead to hypermagnesemia, hypophosphatemia and secondary hypocalcemia	Acts as an osmotic laxative Releases cholecystokinin, which stimulates gastrointestinal secretion and motility. Use with caution in renal impairment
	Magnesium citrate*	< 6 years – 1-3 mL/kg/day as QD 6-12 years – 100-150 mL/day >12 years – 150-300 ml/day Single or divided doses Available as liquid, 16.17% magnesium	Infants are susceptible to magnesium poisoning. Overdose can lead to hypermagnesemia, hypophosphatemia and secondary hypocalcemia	

Category	Agent	Dose	Adverse Effects	Comments
Osmotic Enema	Phosphate enemas	<2 year old: to be avoided ≥ 2 years old: 6 mL/kg up to 135 mL	Risk of mechanical trauma to rectal wall. Abdominal distention, vomiting. May cause severe and lethal episodes of hyperphosphatemia hypocalcemia, with tetany.	Some of the anion is absorbed, but if kidney is normal, no toxic accumulation occurs. Most side effects occur in children with renal failure or Hirschsprung disease.
Lavage	Polyethylene glycol-electrolyte solution	For disimpaction: 25 mL/kg/hr (to 1000 mL/hr) by nasogastric tube until clear Or 20 mL/kg/hr for 4 hr/day For maintenance: (older children): 5-10 mL/kg/day	Difficult to take. Nausea, bloating, abdominal cramps. Vomiting and anal irritation. Aspiration pneumonia Pulmonary edema Mallory Weiss tear Safety of long-term maintenance not well established	Information mostly obtained from use for total colonic irrigation. May require hospitalization and nasogastric tube.
Lubricant	Mineral oil*	< 1 year old: not recommended Disimpaction: 15-30 mL/year of age, up to 240 mL daily Maintenance: 1-3 mL/kg/day	Lipoid pneumonia if aspirated. Theoretical interference with absorption of fat soluble substances, but there is no evidence in the literature. Foreign body reaction in intestinal mucosa.	Softens stool and decreases water absorption More palatable if given cold Anal leakage indicates dose too high or need for clean-out
Prokinetic	Cisapride	0.2 mg/kg/dose, TID or QID. Available as suspension, 1 mg/mL and 5, 10 and 20 mg tablets	Headaches Abdominal pain Diarrhea Urinary frequency Cardiac arrhythmias	Can cause cardiac arrhythmia when given with medications that interact with cytochrome P450 3A4 (77).

Stimulants				Increased intestinal motility
			Abdominal pain. Cathartic colon (possibility of permanent gut, nerve, or muscle damage)	
	Senna	2-6 years old: 2.5-7.5 mL/day 6-12 years old: 5-15 mL/day Available as Senokot® syrup, 8.8 mg of sennosides/5 mL. Also available as granules and tablets.	Idiosyncratic hepatitis Melanosis Coli Hypertrophic osteoarthropathy Analgesic nephropathy	Melanosis Coli improves 4-12 months after stopping medications
	Bisacodyl	≥ 2 years old: 0.5-1 suppository 1-3 tablets per dose Available in 5 mg tablets and 10 mg suppositories	Abdominal pain Diarrhea and hypokalemia Abnormal rectal mucosa, and rarely proctitis Case reports of urolithiasis	
	Glycerin suppositories		No side effects	

*Adjust dose to induce a daily bowel movement for 1-2 months

Figure 1.   An algorithm for the management of constipation in children one year of age and older.   T4 = thyroxine; TSH = thyroid stimulating hormone; Ca = calcium; Pb = lead; Rx = therapy; PEG = polyethylene glycol electrolyte; psych = psychological management; MRI = Magnetic resonance imaging.

Figure 2.   An algorithm for the management of constipation in infants less than one year of age.   T4 = thyroxine; TSH = thyroid stimulating hormone; Ca = calcium; Pb = lead; Rx = therapy; PEG =polyethylene glycol electrolyte; psych = psychological management; MRI =Magnetic resonance imaging.

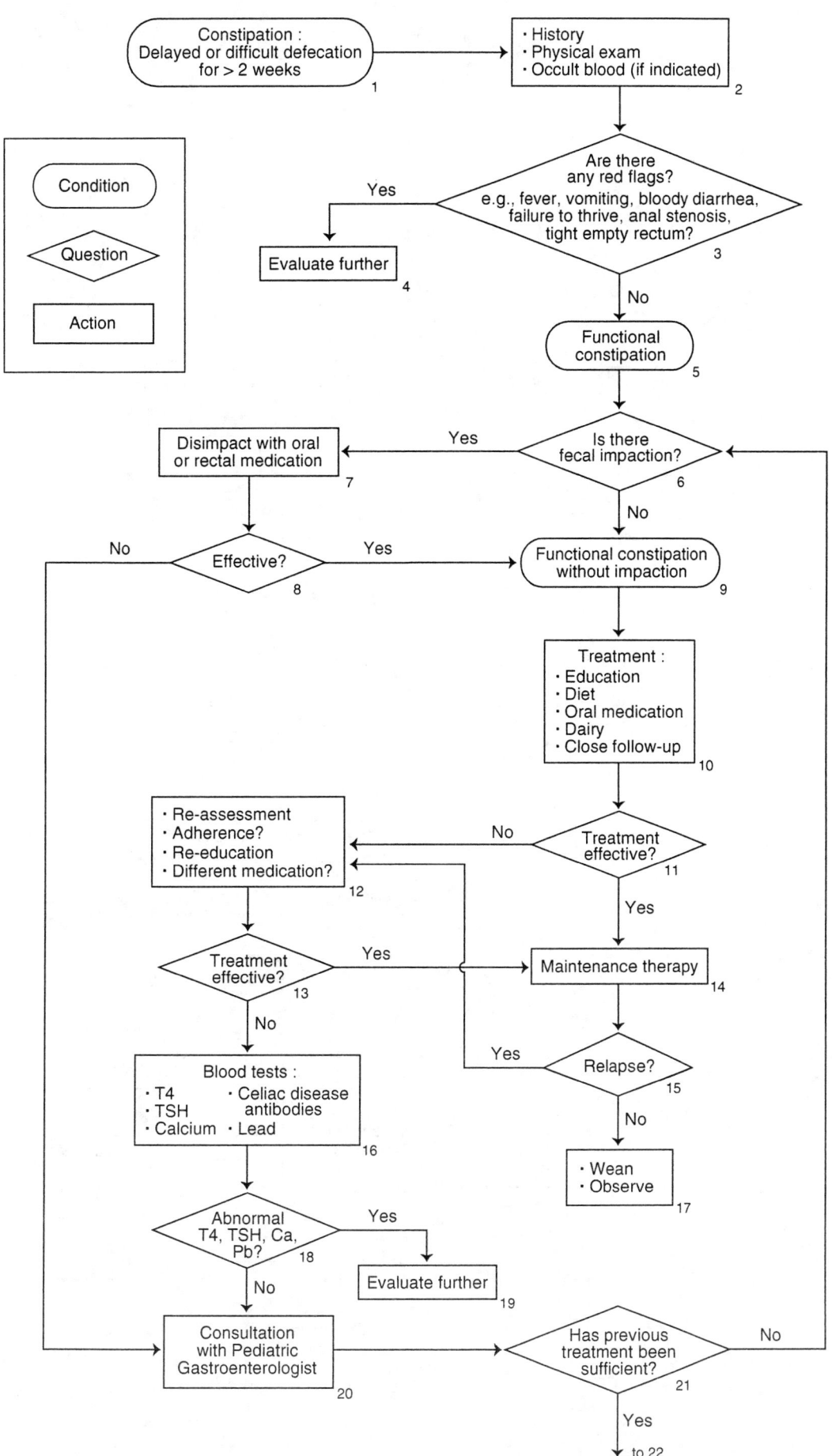

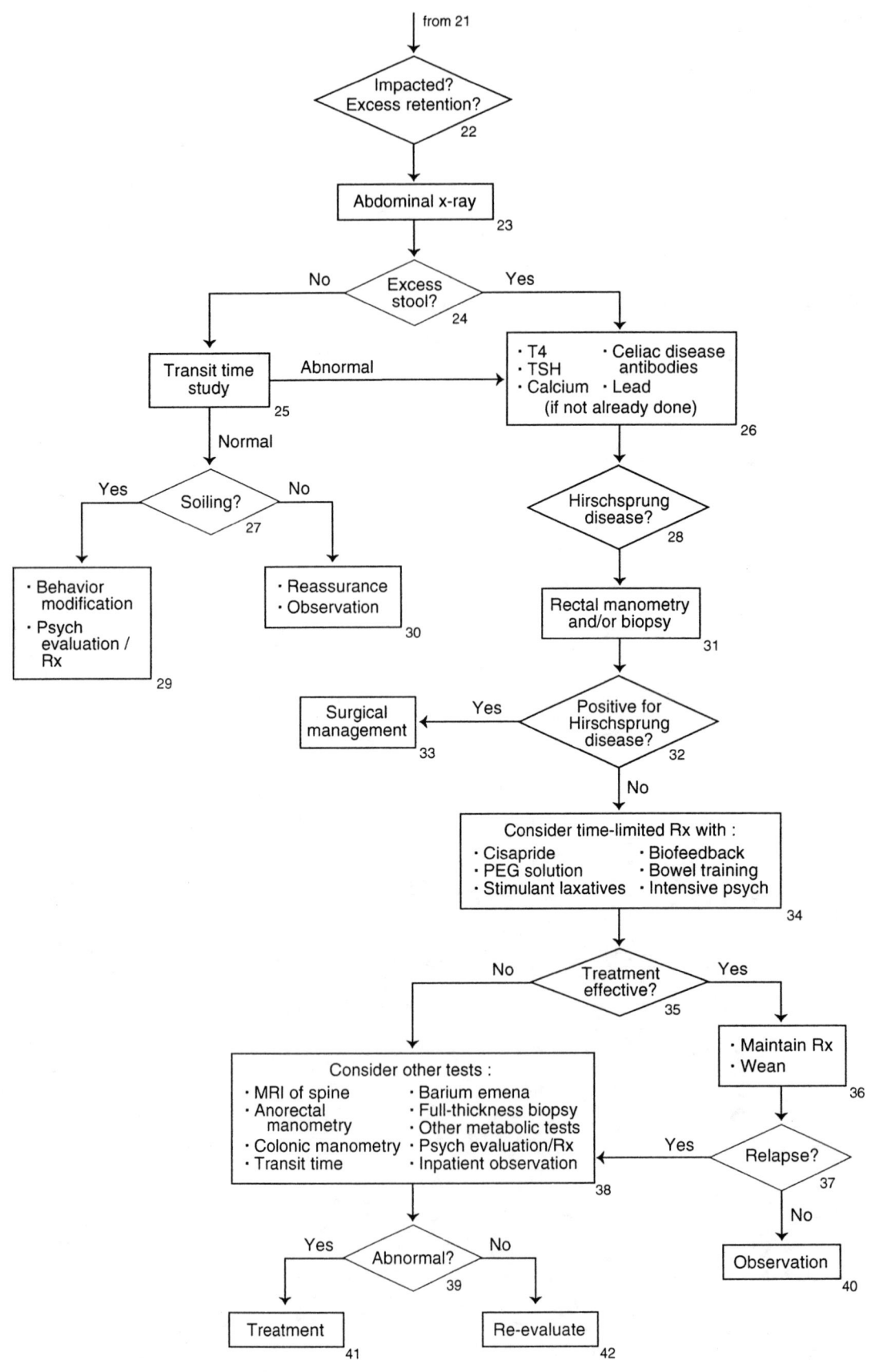

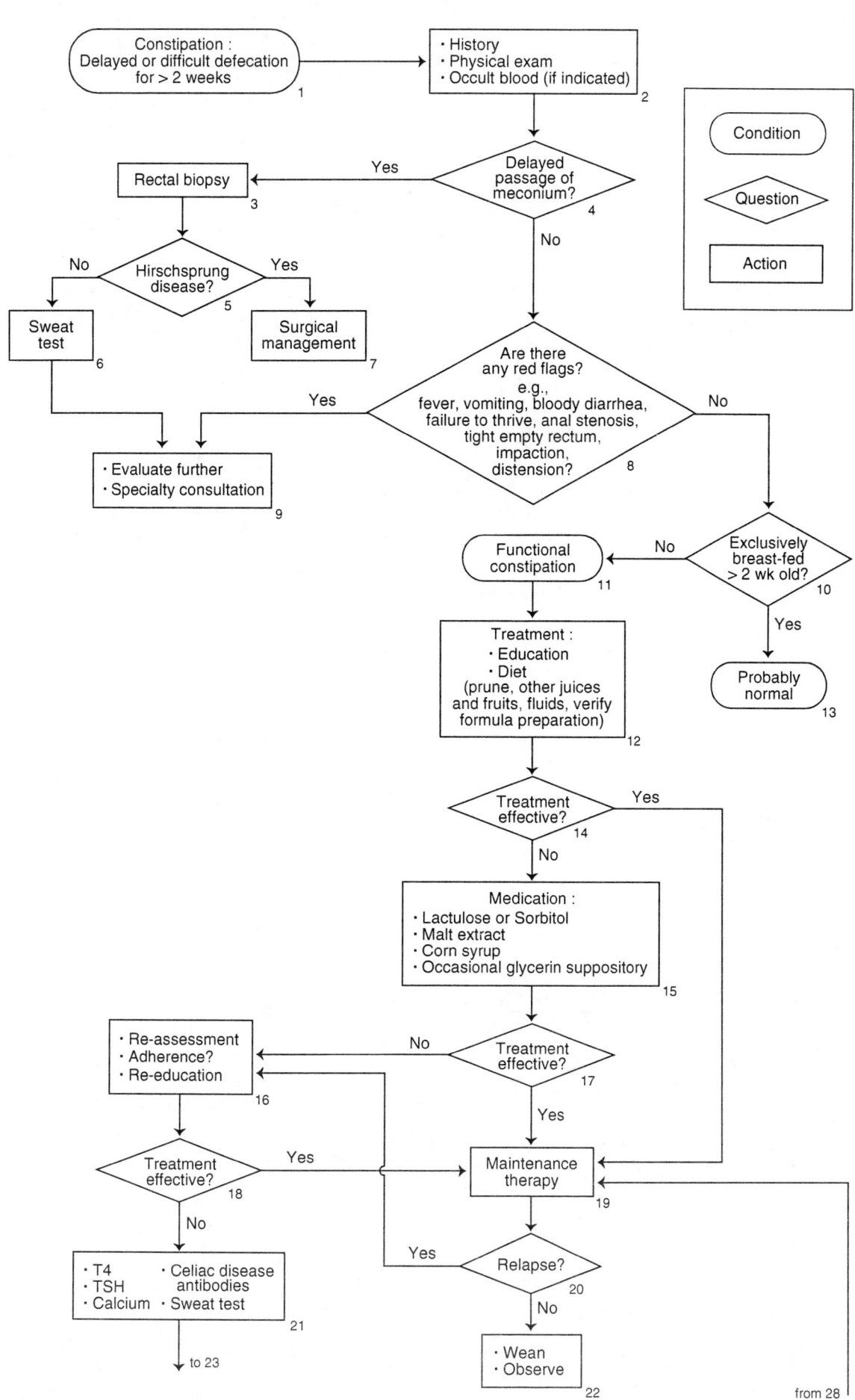

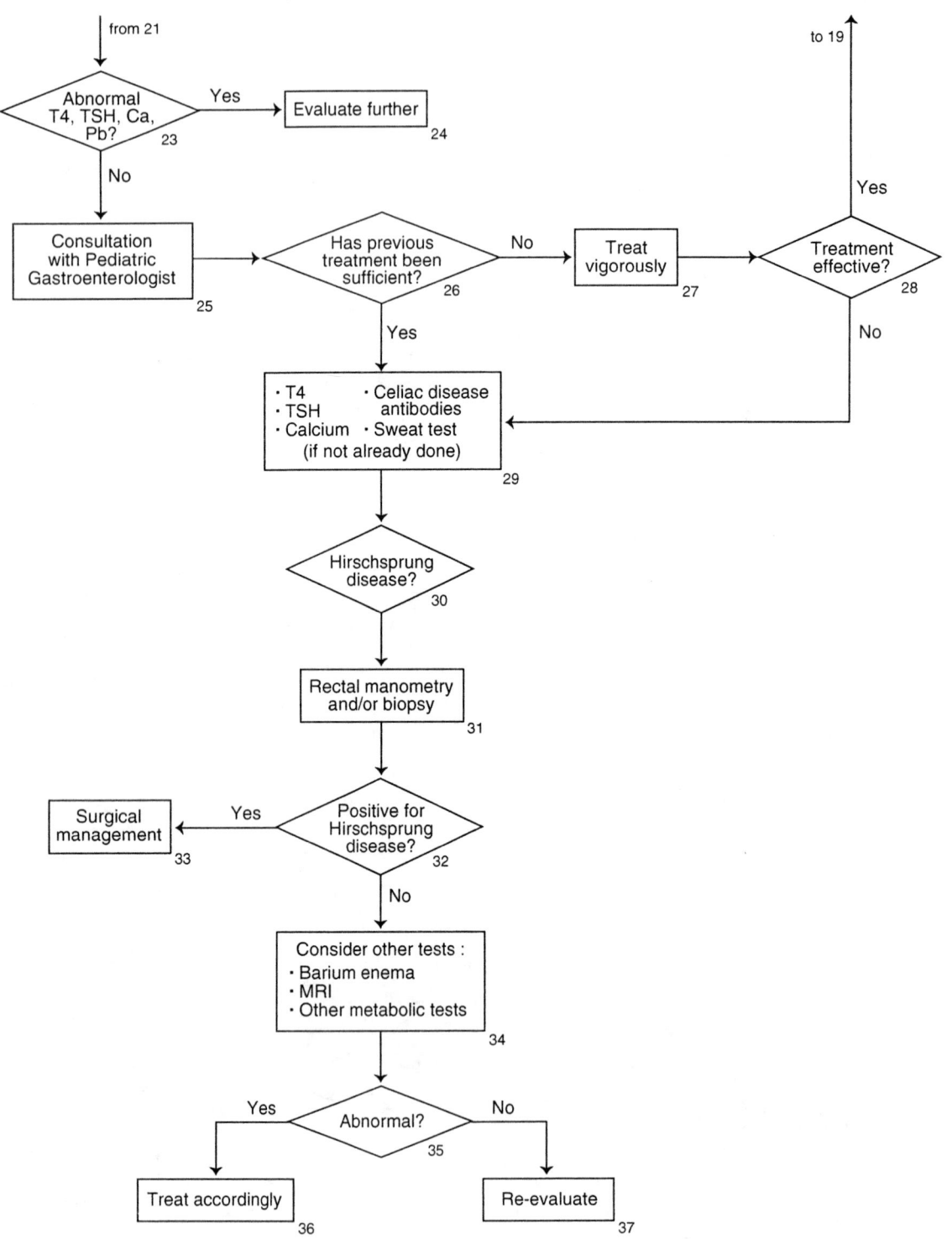

Helping the Student with Diabetes Succeed:
A Guide for School Personnel

. . . .

The following guideline for helping the student with diabetes, developed by a joint program of the National Institutes of Health and the Centers for Disease Control and Prevention, has been endorsed by the American Academy of Pediatrics.

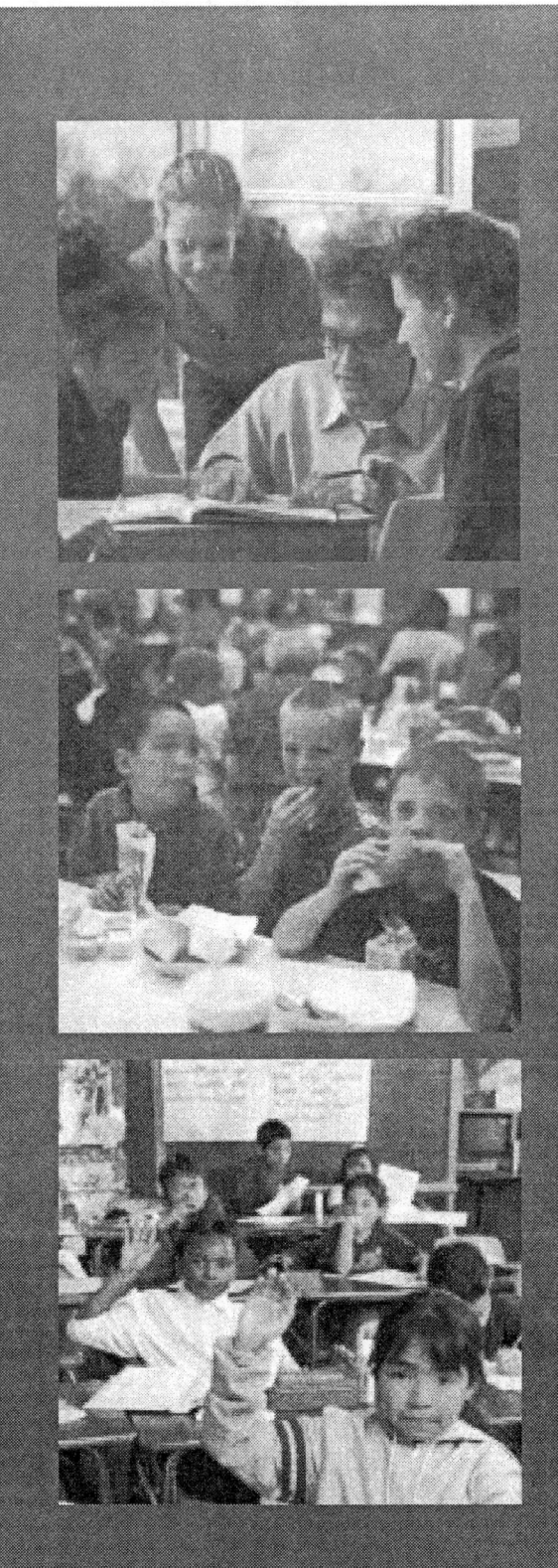

● ● ● ● ● ● ● ● ● ● ● ● ● ● ● ●

Helping the Student with Diabetes Succeed

A Guide for School Personnel

● ● ● ● ● ● ● ● ● ● ● ● ● ● ● ●

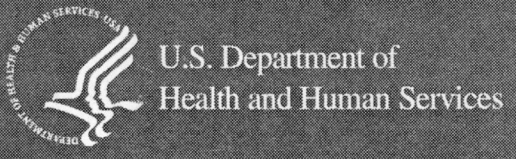

U.S. Department of
Health and Human Services

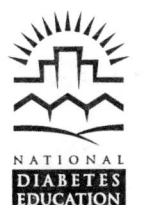

NATIONAL
DIABETES
EDUCATION
PROGRAM

A Joint Program of the
National Institutes of Health and
the Centers for Disease Control
and Prevention

This guide was produced by the National Diabetes Education Program (NDEP), a federally sponsored partnership of the National Institutes of Health, the Centers for Disease Control and Prevention, and more than 200 partner organizations. The following organizations support its use by school personnel:

American Academy of Pediatrics

American Association for Health Education

American Association of Diabetes Educators

American Diabetes Association

American Dietetic Association

American Medical Association

Barbara Davis Center for Childhood Diabetes

Centers for Disease Control and Prevention

Indian Health Service

Juvenile Diabetes Research Foundation International

Lawson Wilkins Pediatric Endocrine Society

National Association of Elementary School Principals

National Association of School Nurses

National Association of Secondary School Principals

National Association of State Boards of Education

National Diabetes Education Program

National Education Association Health Information Network

National Institute of Diabetes and Digestive and Kidney Diseases,
      National Institutes of Health

U.S. Department of Education

Acknowledgments

Many National Diabetes Education Program partners contributed to the development of this guide. A core writing and review team helped research, write, and refine drafts of the manuscript and enlisted the involvement of school personnel and parents in reviewing the guide. Their dedication and assistance were invaluable (their names appear below).

Guides developed by state departments of health and education in New York, Rhode Island, Vermont, Virginia, and Washington to address the issue of diabetes in schools and materials from the National Association of State Boards of Education provided additional background information and direction for developing this document.

American Academy of Pediatrics
Janet Silverstein, M.D.

American Association of Diabetes Educators
Jean Betschart Roemer, C.P.N.P., C.D.E.

American Diabetes Association
Shereen Arent, J.D.
Crystal Jackson
Francine Kaufman, M.D.
Regan Minners

American Dietetic Association
Alison Evert, R.D., C.D.E.

Hager Sharp Inc.
Rachel Greenberg, M.A.

National Association of School Nurses
Nichole Bobo, M.S.N., R.N., A.N.P.

National Diabetes Education Program
Joanne Gallivan, M.S., R.D.
Jane Kelly, M.D.

National Institute of Diabetes and Digestive and Kidney Diseases
Barbara Linder, M.D., Ph.D.

University of Illinois, College of Medicine, Department of Pediatrics
Rodney Lorenz, M.D.

U.S. Department of Education
Eileen Hanrahan, J.D.
Anne Hoogstraten, J.D.
Bobbi Stettner-Eaton, Ph.D.

Foreword

Major research advances have been made in diabetes management and control during the past decade. Several landmark research studies have proved conclusively that aggressive treatment to lower blood glucose (sugar) levels can help prevent or delay diabetes-related complications affecting the eyes, kidneys, nerves, and cardiovascular system. In addition, advances in medical research and technology have produced an array of treatment and management tools that have made it easier for people with diabetes to check their blood glucose levels and to control them.

For young people with diabetes, these advances mean a brighter and healthier future. Blood glucose levels that are well managed have the potential to help young people not only to stave off the long-term complications of diabetes but also to feel better and to be happier and more productive at school and at play. Accordingly, students with diabetes need a supportive environment to help them take care of their diabetes throughout the school day and at school-sponsored activities.

The National Diabetes Education Program (NDEP) developed this guide to educate and inform school personnel about diabetes, how it is managed, and how each member of the school staff can help meet the needs of students with the disease. School principals, administrators, nurses, teachers, coaches, bus drivers, health care, and lunchroom staff all play a role in making the school experience safe and sound for students with diabetes.

The NDEP convened an expert panel comprised of health care professionals, federal agency staff, and representatives from key diabetes, pediatric medicine, and educational organizations to develop this comprehensive guide and to help disseminate it throughout the country.

We hope that schools will take advantage of the important information contained in this guide, share it with school staff, parents, and students, and use it to ensure that all students with diabetes are educated in a medically safe environment and have the same access to educational opportunities as their peers.

Sincerely,

James R. Gavin III, M.D., Ph.D.
Chair, National Diabetes Education Program
May 2003

Introduction

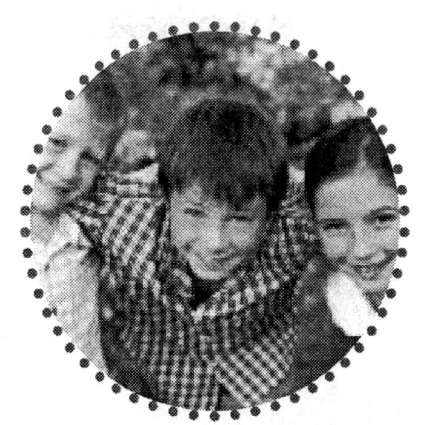

More than 17 million Americans have diabetes. In your work with children and youth in the school setting, it is likely that you already have, or will have, a student with diabetes in your care. Diabetes is one of the most common chronic diseases in school-aged children, affecting about 151,000 young people in the United States, or about 1 in every 400 to 500 young people under 20 years of age. Each year, more than 13,000 youths are diagnosed with type 1 diabetes. In addition, health care providers are finding more and more children and teens with type 2 diabetes, even though the disease is usually diagnosed in adults over age 40.

Diabetes is a serious chronic disease that impairs the body's ability to use food for energy. It is the sixth-leading cause of death by disease in the United States. Long-term complications include heart disease, stroke, blindness, kidney disease, and amputation of the foot or leg. Although there is no cure, the disease can be managed and complications delayed or prevented.

Diabetes must be managed 24 hours a day, 7 days a week. For students with type 1 diabetes, and for some with type 2 diabetes, that means careful monitoring of their blood glucose (sugar) levels throughout the school day and administering multiple doses of insulin therapy—now prescribed for most young people with diabetes. As a result, the school health team, which includes the school nurse, teachers, office personnel, and other school staff members, plays an important role in helping students manage their diabetes.

- Effective diabetes management is crucial
- for the immediate safety of students with diabetes
- for the long-term health of students with diabetes
- to ensure that students with diabetes are ready to learn and to participate fully in school activities and
- to minimize the possibility that diabetes-related emergencies will disrupt classroom activities.

> *The school nurse, teachers, office personnel, and other school staff members play an important role in helping students manage their diabetes.*

⭐ ⭐ ⭐

The purpose of this guide is to educate school personnel about diabetes and to share a set of practices that enable schools to ensure a safe learning environment for students with diabetes.

The purpose of this guide is to educate school personnel about diabetes and to share a set of practices that enable schools to ensure a safe learning environment for students with diabetes, particularly the student who uses insulin to control the disease (all students with type 1 and some with type 2 diabetes). **The team approach to school-based diabetes management presented in this guide builds on what schools already are doing for children with other chronic diseases.** Current practices and use of existing resources have been adapted for the student with diabetes.

The practices shared in this guide are not necessarily required by the federal laws enforced by the U.S. Department of Education for each student with diabetes. This guide can be used, however, in determining how to address the needs of students with diabetes. The individual situation of any particular student with diabetes will affect what is legally required for that particular student. Additionally, the guide does not address state and local laws, as the requirements of these laws may vary from state to state and school district to school district. This guide should be used in conjunction with federal as well as state and local laws.

At its core, effective school-based diabetes management requires two things:

- **All school staff members who have responsibility for a student with diabetes should receive training that provides a basic understanding of the disease** and the student's needs, how to identify medical emergencies, and which school staff members to contact with questions in case of an emergency.

- **A small group of school staff members should receive training from a qualified health care professional such as a physician or a nurse in student-specific routine and emergency care** so that a staff member is always available for younger or less-experienced students who require assistance with their diabetes management (e.g., administering insulin, checking their blood glucose, or choosing an appropriate snack) and for all students with diabetes in case of an emergency. This group may be comprised of the school nurse and other school staff who are not health care professionals. The non-medical personnel are called "trained diabetes personnel" in this guide. Other terminology may be used in your school.

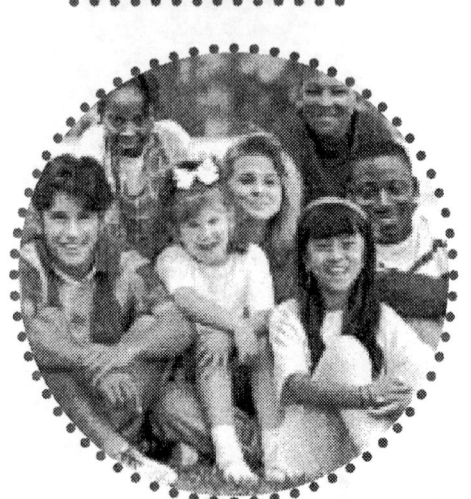

Organized in four sections, the guide includes background information and tools for school personnel to help students manage diabetes effectively.

SECTION 1, Diabetes Primer for School Personnel, provides overview information about diabetes, describes how the disease is managed, and reviews the components for planning and implementing effective diabetes management in school. **The Primer should be copied and distributed to all school personnel who may be responsible for the safety of students with diabetes.** School nurses are the likely leaders in distributing this information and providing the background and education that other school personnel will need. This leadership may vary, however, from one school system to another because of state laws, staffing levels, and other considerations.

SECTION 2, Actions for School Personnel, Parents, and Students, lays out the roles and responsibilities of individual school personnel, parents, and students. **The pages in this section should be copied and distributed to school staff members, parents, and students with diabetes** so that they understand their respective roles in diabetes management.

SECTION 3, Tools for Effective Diabetes Management, contains two important tools for helping schools implement effective diabetes management, a sample Diabetes Medical Management Plan and a sample Quick Reference Emergency Plan for a student with diabetes. **The Quick Reference Emergency Plan should be distributed to all personnel who have responsibility for the student with diabetes** during the school day and during school-sponsored activities.

SECTION 4, School Responsibilities Under Law, was developed by the U.S. Department of Education. This section provides an overview of federal laws that address schools' responsibilities to students with diabetes, including confidentiality requirements. In applying the laws, schools must consider each student on an individualized basis; what is appropriate for one student may not be appropriate for another student.

This guide may be reproduced without permission and shared with all school personnel, parents, and students.

The **APPENDICES** contain additional resources and information for diabetes management in the school setting. The **Resources** section lists government, professional, and voluntary organizations that can be contacted for more information about diabetes and youth. The **Glossary** provides additional explanations of the medical and technical terms used in this guide. The **American Diabetes Association's position statement** on "Care for Children with Diabetes in the School and Day Care Setting" lays out the diabetes medical community's recommendations that are the basis for this guide.

School personnel are encouraged to **visit the National Diabetes Education Program's website, www.ndep.nih.gov**, to download a comprehensive online resource directory on Diabetes in Children and Adolescents.

• •

www.ndep.nih.gov

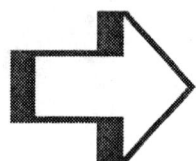 **To obtain additional copies of this guide and other diabetes information, please call the National Diabetes Education Program at 1-800-438-5383 or visit the program's website at www.ndep.nih.gov to download copies.**

• •

Section 1 | DIABETES PRIMER

Copy and distribute this section to all school personnel who may be responsible for the safety of students with diabetes.

Section 1 DIABETES PRIMER

FOR School Personnel

> ★ ★ ★
>
> Taking care of diabetes is important. If not treated, diabetes can lead to serious health problems.

WHAT IS DIABETES?

Diabetes is a chronic disease in which the body does not make or properly use insulin, a hormone needed to convert sugar, starches, and other food into energy. People with diabetes have increased blood glucose (sugar) levels because they lack insulin, have insufficient insulin, or are resistant to insulin's effects. High levels of glucose build up in the blood and spill into the urine; as a result, the body loses its main source of fuel.

When insulin is no longer made, it must be obtained from another source—insulin shots or an insulin pump. When the body does not use insulin properly, oral medications may be taken instead of, or in addition to, insulin shots. Neither insulin nor other medications, however, are cures for diabetes: they only help control the disease.

Taking care of diabetes is important. If not treated, diabetes can lead to serious health problems. The disease can affect the blood vessels, eyes, kidneys, nerves, gums, and teeth, and it is the leading cause of adult blindness, lower limb amputations, and kidney failure. People with diabetes also have a higher risk of heart disease and stroke. Some of these problems can occur in teens and young adults who develop diabetes during childhood. The good news is that research shows that these problems can be greatly reduced or delayed by keeping blood glucose levels near normal.

WHAT ARE THE TYPES OF DIABETES?

There are two main types of diabetes: type 1 and type 2 are described below. A third type—gestational diabetes—occurs only during pregnancy and ends after delivery. Women who have had gestational diabetes, however, are more likely to develop type 2 diabetes later in life.

Type 1 Diabetes

Type 1 diabetes is a disease of the immune system, the body's system for fighting infection. In people with type 1 diabetes, the immune system attacks the beta cells (the insulin-producing cells of the pancreas) and destroys them. Because the pancreas can no longer produce insulin, people with type 1 diabetes need to take insulin daily to live. Type 1 diabetes can occur at any age, but it occurs most often in children and young adults.

✚ **Symptoms.** The symptoms of type 1 diabetes usually develop over a short period of time. They include increased thirst and urination, constant hunger, weight loss, and blurred vision. Affected children also may feel very tired all the time. If not diagnosed and treated with insulin, the child with type 1 diabetes can lapse into a life-threatening condition known as diabetic ketoacidosis (KEY-toe-asi-DOE-sis), or DKA.

✚ **Risk factors.** Although scientists have made much progress in predicting who is at risk for type 1 diabetes, they do not yet know what triggers the immune system's attack on beta cells. They believe that type 1 diabetes is due to a combination of genetic and environmental factors. Researchers are working to identify these factors and to stop the autoimmune process that leads to type 1 diabetes.

Type 1 Diabetes

INFO

Symptoms:

✔ Increased thirst and urination

✔ Constant hunger

✔ Weight loss

✔ Blurred vision

✔ Fatigue

Risk Factors:

✔ Genetics

✔ Environment

Type 2 Diabetes INFO

Symptoms:

✔ Fatigue

✔ Increased thirst and urination

✔ Nausea

✔ Rapid weight loss

✔ Blurred vision

✔ Frequent infections

✔ Slow healing of wounds or sores

Risk Factors:

✔ Being overweight

✔ Having a family member who has type 2 diabetes

✔ Being African American, Hispanic/Latino American, American Indian, Asian American or Pacific Islander American

Type 2 Diabetes

The first step in the development of type 2 diabetes is often a problem with the body's response to insulin, or insulin resistance. For reasons scientists do not completely understand, the body cannot use its insulin very well. This means that the body needs increasing amounts of insulin to control blood glucose. The pancreas tries to make more insulin, but after several years, insulin production may drop off.

Type 2 diabetes used to be found mainly in overweight adults ages 40 or older. Now, as more children and adolescents in the United States become overweight and inactive, type 2 diabetes occurs more often in young people. To control their diabetes, children with type 2 diabetes may need to take oral medication, insulin, or both.

✚ **Symptoms.** Type 2 diabetes develops slowly in some children, but quickly in others. Symptoms may be similar to those of type 1 diabetes. A child or teen can feel very tired, thirsty, or nauseated and have to urinate often. Other symptoms include rapid weight loss, blurred vision, frequent infections, yeast infections, and slow healing of wounds or sores. High blood pressure may be a sign of insulin resistance. In addition, physical signs of insulin resistance, such as acanthosis nigricans (A-can-tho-sis NIG-reh-cans), may appear; here the skin around the neck or in the armpits or groin appears dark, thick, and velvety.

On the other hand, some children or adolescents with type 2 diabetes show no symptoms at all when they are diagnosed. For that reason, it is important for parents and caregivers to talk to their health care providers about screening children or teens at high risk for diabetes.

✚ **Risk factors.** Being overweight and having a family member who has type 2 diabetes are the key risk factors for type 2 diabetes. In addition, type 2 diabetes is more common in certain racial or ethnic groups, such as African Americans, Hispanic/Latino Americans, American Indians, and some Asian Americans and Pacific Islander Americans. For children and teens at risk, health care providers can encourage, support, and educate the entire family to make lifestyle changes that may delay—or prevent—the onset of type 2 diabetes. Such changes may include reaching a healthy weight and then maintaining it and engaging in regular physical activity.

WHAT IS EFFECTIVE DIABETES MANAGEMENT?

The goal of effective diabetes management is to control blood glucose levels by keeping them within a target range that is determined for each child. Optimal blood glucose control helps to promote normal growth and development and allows for optimal learning. Effective diabetes management is needed to prevent the immediate dangers of blood glucose levels that are too high or too low. As noted earlier, research has shown that maintaining blood glucose levels within the target range can prevent or delay the long-term complications of diabetes, such as heart attack, stroke, blindness, kidney failure, nerve disease, and amputations of the foot or leg.

The key to optimal blood glucose control is to carefully balance food, exercise, and insulin or medication. As a general rule, food makes blood glucose levels go up, and exercise and insulin make blood glucose levels go down. Several other factors, such as growth and puberty, mental stress, illness, or injury also can affect blood glucose levels.

☆ ☆ ☆

> *The key to optimal blood glucose control is to carefully balance food, exercise, and insulin or medication.*

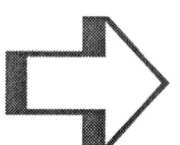 With all of these factors coming into play, maintaining good blood glucose control is a constant juggling act—24 hours a day, 7 days a week.

Students with diabetes must check (or test) their blood glucose levels throughout the day by using a blood glucose meter. The meter gives a reading of the level of glucose in the blood at the time it is being checked. If blood glucose levels are too low (hypoglycemia) or too high (hyperglycemia), students can then take corrective action, such as eating, modifying their activity level, or administering insulin. **Low blood glucose levels, which can be life-threatening, present the greatest immediate danger to people with diabetes** (see hypoglycemia, pages 166–168).

Many students will be able to handle all or almost all of their diabetes care by themselves. Others, because of age, developmental level, or inexperience, will need help from school staff.

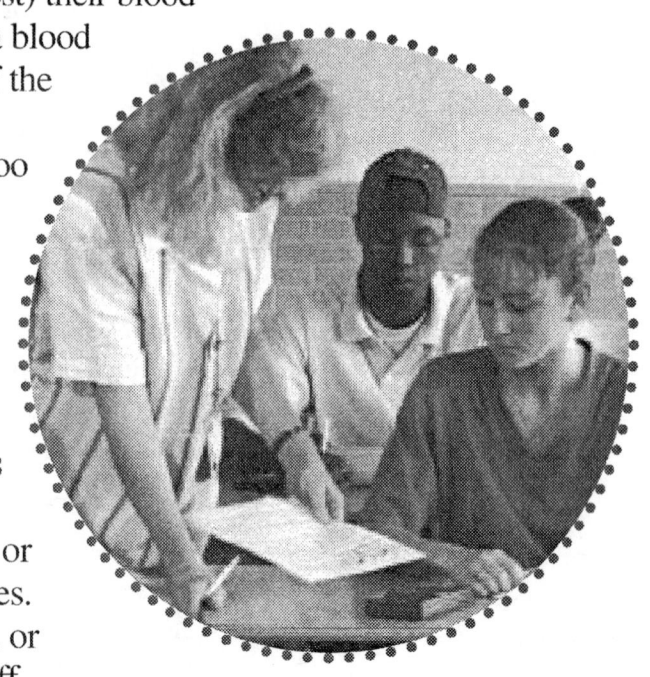

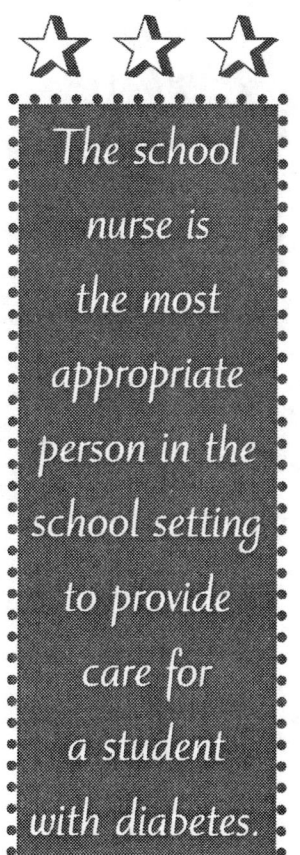

The school nurse is the most appropriate person in the school setting to provide care for a student with diabetes.

The school nurse is the most appropriate person in the school setting to provide care for a student with diabetes. Many schools, however, do not have a full-time nurse, and sometimes a single nurse must cover a large number of schools. Moreover, even when a nurse is assigned to a school full time, this staff member may not always be available during the school day, during extracurricular activities, or on field trips. Yet, because diabetes management is needed 24 hours a day, 7 days a week—and diabetes emergencies can happen at any time—school personnel should be prepared to provide diabetes care at school and at all school-sponsored activities in which a student with diabetes participates. In this case, the school nurse or another qualified health professional should be involved with training of appropriate staff and providing professional supervision and consultation regarding routine and emergency care of the student.

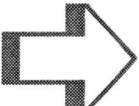 All students with diabetes will need help with emergency medical care.

Effective school-based diabetes management requires two things:

1. All school staff members who have responsibility for students with diabetes should receive training that provides a basic understanding of the disease and the students' needs, how to identify medical emergencies, and whom to contact in case of an emergency.

2. A few school staff members should receive training from a qualified health care professional in student-specific routine and emergency diabetes care tasks so that at least one staff member is always available for younger, less experienced students and for any student with diabetes in case of an emergency.

The diabetes medical community has found that nonmedical personnel (called "trained diabetes personnel" in this guide) can be trained and supervised to safely provide and assist with diabetes care tasks in the school setting, including blood glucose monitoring, insulin and glucagon administration, and urine ketone testing. These nonmedical school staff members should be trained and monitored by the school nurse or a qualified health professional. Assignment of diabetes care tasks must take into account state laws that may be relevant in determining what tasks may be performed by nonmedical personnel.

HOW CAN A SCHOOL PLAN AND IMPLEMENT EFFECTIVE DIABETES MANAGEMENT?

Collaboration, cooperation, and planning are key elements in developing and implementing successful diabetes management at school. As is true for children with other chronic diseases, students with diabetes are more likely to succeed in school when students, parents, school nurses, principals, teachers, other school personnel, and the student's health care providers (or personal health care team) work together to ensure effective diabetes management. Your school probably has similar plans and systems in place for children with other health considerations.

To work collaboratively, a school health team should be assembled that includes people who are knowledgeable about diabetes, the school environment, and federal and state education and nursing laws. Team members could include the student, parents/guardian, the school nurse and other health personnel, administrators, the principal, the student's teacher(s) and guidance counselor, and other relevant staff.

The school health team works together to implement the Diabetes Medical Management Plan (see pages 200–203) developed by the student's personal health care team and family. The team decides who needs to receive appropriate medical information about the child, who will be the trained diabetes personnel and who will monitor them, and what tasks will be delegated. In addition, the school health team should be part of the group that develops and implements the student's Section 504 Plan, Individualized Education Program (IEP), or other education plan that addresses the student's developmental and educational needs so that diabetes can be managed safely and effectively in school.

Three federal laws address the school's responsibilities to help students with diabetes:

- Section 504 of the Rehabilitation Act of 1973 (Section 504)

- Americans with Disabilities Act of 1990 (ADA)

- Individuals with Disabilities Education Act (IDEA)

These federal laws provide a framework for planning and implementing effective diabetes management in the school setting. School administrators and nursing personnel also should determine whether there are applicable state and local

School Health
TEAM

- ✔ Student with diabetes
- ✔ Parents/guardian
- ✔ School nurse
- ✔ Other school health personnel
-   Principal
- ✔ Office staff
- ✔ Student's teacher(s)
- ✔ Guidance counselor
- ✔ Other relevant staff

laws that should be factored into helping the student with diabetes (see pages 163–164 and Section 4 for additional information on these federal laws).

Written plans outlining each student's diabetes management help students, their families, school staff, and the student's health care providers know what is expected of them. These expectations should be laid out in writing in the following documents:

■ *Diabetes Medical Management Plan*, developed by the student's personal health care team and family, contains the prescribed diabetes health care regimen, tailored for each student.

■ *Quick Reference Emergency Plan*, based on the information provided in the student's Diabetes Medical Management Plan, describes how to recognize hypoglycemia and hyperglycemia and what to do as soon as signs or symptoms of these conditions are observed.

■ *Education plans, such as the Section 504 Plan or Individualized Education Program (IEP)*, explain what accommodations, education aids, and services are needed for each student with diabetes.

■ *Other documents may be generated when a school nurse is involved*, such as a nursing care plan and instructions to staff (see page 36).

> ★ ☆ ☆
>
> The Diabetes Medical Management Plan describes the diabetes regimen developed by the student's personal health care team and family.

Diabetes Medical Management Plan

The Diabetes Medical Management Plan describes the diabetes care regimen developed by the student's personal health care team and family and should be signed by the student's physician or other member of the health care team (see Section 3 for a sample plan). Although this guide uses the term "Diabetes Medical Management Plan," school districts may use other terms for this document. While this plan is not required by Section 504, the ADA, or the IDEA, the information in it can be useful in addressing the requirements of these federal laws.

Information in the Diabetes Medical Management Plan may include the following:

■ Date of diagnosis

■ Current health status

- Emergency contact information

- Student's willingness and ability to perform self-management tasks at school

- List of diabetes equipment and supplies

- Specific medical orders
  - ❏ Blood glucose monitoring
  - ❏ Insulin, glucagon, and other medications to be given at school
  - ❏ Meal and snack plan
  - ❏ Exercise requirements
  - ❏ Additional monitoring

- Typical signs, symptoms, and prescribed treatment for hypoglycemia

- Typical signs, symptoms, and prescribed treatment for hyperglycemia

The Diabetes Medical Management Plan should be reviewed and updated each school year or upon a change in the student's prescribed regimen, level of self-management, school circumstances (e.g., a change in schedule), or at the request of the student or parents/guardian. Information from this plan is used by the school nurse to develop the student's nursing care plan and may be incorporated into the 504, IEP, or other education plan.

Quick Reference Emergency Plan

The Quick Reference Emergency Plan is based on the information provided in the student's Diabetes Medical Management Plan; the school nurse will usually coordinate its development. The plan summarizes how to recognize and treat hypoglycemia and hyperglycemia and should be distributed to all personnel who have responsibility for students with diabetes (see Section 3 for a sample plan). Although this guide uses "Quick Reference Emergency Plan," school districts might use other names.

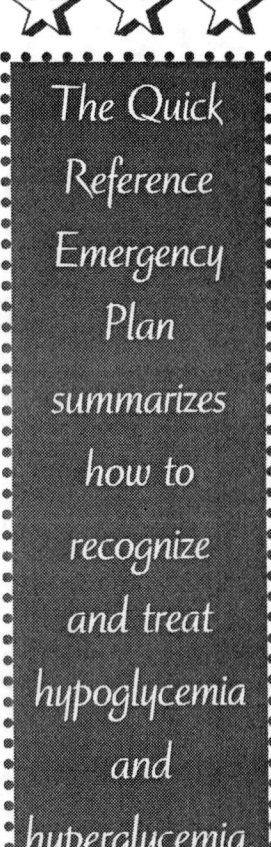

The Quick Reference Emergency Plan summarizes how to recognize and treat hypoglycemia and hyperglycemia.

Education Plans

The school health team, including the student and parents/guardian, must agree on how the Diabetes Medical Management Plan will be implemented and what medical accommodations, educational aids, and services may be needed for the student. This information might be included in a Section 504 Plan, an IEP, or other education plan.

A "504 Plan" is the commonly used term for a plan of services developed under Section 504 of the Rehabilitation Act. An IEP is required for students who receive special education and related services under the Individuals with Disabilities Education Act (IDEA). The information in the Diabetes Medical Management Plan can be used in developing either a Section 504 Plan or an IEP, but should not be a substitute for these plans.

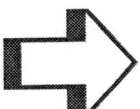 **The 504 Plan, IEP, or other education plan lays out what medical accommodations, educational aids, and services the student may need.**

Each student with diabetes has different needs, but the education-related plans developed for such students are likely to address the following common elements:

- Where and when blood glucose monitoring and treatment will take place

- Identity of trained diabetes personnel who are trained to conduct blood glucose checking, insulin and glucagon administration, and treatment of hypoglycemia and hyperglycemia

- Location of the student's diabetes management supplies

- Free access to the restroom and water fountain

- Nutritional needs, including provisions for meals and snacks

- Full participation in all school-sponsored activities and field trips, with coverage provided by trained diabetes personnel

- Alternative times for academic exams if the student is experiencing hypoglycemia or hyperglycemia

- Permission for absences, without penalty, for doctors' appointments and diabetes-related illness

- Maintenance of confidentiality and the student's right to privacy

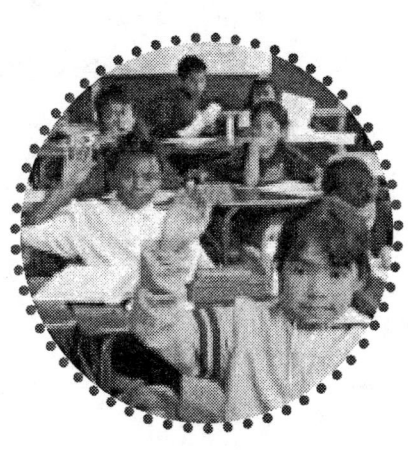

It is strongly recommended that this information be agreed upon before each school year begins (or upon diagnosis of diabetes) and that it be written down and signed by a representative of the school and the parents/guardian. This assures that school staff members, parents, and students know their responsibilities. Parents must be notified in a timely manner of any proposed changes in the provision of services and be included in related discussions.

This approach to planning and implementing effective diabetes management in school can promote a better understanding of schools' responsibilities and can prepare staff members to act in the best interest of students with diabetes.

WHAT ARE THE ELEMENTS OF EFFECTIVE DIABETES MANAGEMENT IN SCHOOL?

Diabetes management means monitoring or checking blood glucose levels throughout the day, following an individualized meal plan, getting regular physical activity, and administering insulin and/or medications to help keep blood glucose levels in the target range and to help prevent the onset of hypoglycemia or hyperglycemia. Additional elements of diabetes management in school include planning for events outside the usual school day, planning for appropriate disposal of materials that come in contact with blood, and dealing with the emotional and social aspects of living with diabetes.

Monitoring Blood Glucose

One of the most important parts of diabetes management is regular monitoring or checking of blood glucose levels. Monitoring involves pricking the skin with a lancet at the fingertip, forearm, or other test site to obtain a drop of blood and placing the drop on a special test strip that is inserted in a glucose meter. The meter gives the current blood glucose level.

Physicians generally recommend that students check their blood glucose during the school day, usually before eating snacks or lunch, before physical activity, or when there are symptoms of hypoglycemia or hyperglycemia. In young children, symptoms may be subtle; blood glucose should be checked whenever symptoms are suspected. Many students can check their own

---

Elements of Effective DIABETES MANAGEMENT

- ✔ Monitoring blood glucose
- ✔ Understanding hypoglycemia
- ✔ Understanding hyperglycemia
- ✔ Following an individualized meal plan
- ✔ Getting regular physical activity
- ✔ Administering insulin
- ✔ Planning for special events
- ✔ Planning for disasters and emergencies
- ✔ Dealing with emotional and social issues

blood glucose level; others will need supervision; and others will need to have this task performed by a school nurse or trained diabetes personnel.

It is extremely important for students to be able to check their blood glucose levels and respond to levels that are too high or too low as quickly as possible. Accordingly, if recommended by the student's physician, **it is medically preferable to permit students to check their blood glucose level and respond to the results in the classroom, at any other campus location, or at any school activity.** Taking immediate action is important so that the symptoms don't get worse and the student doesn't miss time in the classroom.

Blood glucose monitoring does not present a danger to other students or staff members when there is a plan for proper disposal of lancets and other materials that come into contact with blood. The family and the school should agree on the plan, which should be consistent with standard Universal Precautions and local waste-disposal laws. Disposal may be in a container kept at school or in the student's personal container, a heavy-duty plastic or metal container with a tight-fitting lid. Check with the student's personal health care team about health and safety requirements in your area.

Students Usually Check Their BLOOD GLUCOSE

✔ Before eating snacks or meals

✔ Before physical activity

✔ When they have symptoms of high or low blood glucose

Advantages of Checking Blood Glucose Levels Any Time and Any Place

■ The student can achieve better blood glucose control to prevent long-term complications of high blood glucose and acute complications of high and low blood glucose.

■ It is safer for students because less time is lost between recognizing symptoms, confirming low blood glucose, and obtaining treatment with a fast-acting sugar source followed by a snack or meal.

■ The student gains independence in diabetes management when the blood glucose meter is easily accessible and checks can be conducted as needed.

■ The student experiences less stigma as blood glucose monitoring loses its mystery when handled as a regular occurrence.

■ The student spends less time out of class.

Understanding Hypoglycemia (Low Blood Glucose)

HYPOglycemia means LOW blood glucose.

Hypoglycemia, also called "low blood glucose" or "low blood sugar," is one of the most frequent complications of diabetes and can happen very suddenly. Hypoglycemia occurs when a student's blood glucose level falls too low, usually as a result of administering too much insulin, skipping or delaying meals or snacks, not eating enough food as prescribed in the meal plan, exercising too long or too intensely, or a combination of two or more of these factors. It is more likely to occur before lunch, at the end of the school day, or during or after physical education classes.

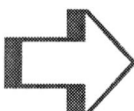 **Hypoglycemia, which often cannot be prevented, is the greatest immediate danger to students with diabetes.**

Hypoglycemia usually can be treated easily and effectively. If it is not treated promptly, however, hypoglycemia can lead to unconsciousness and convulsions and can be life threatening. Early recognition of its symptoms and prompt treatment, in accordance with the student's Diabetes Medical Management Plan, are necessary for preventing severe symptoms that may place the student in danger. This information, contained in the Quick Reference Emergency Plan, should be provided to all school personnel who have responsibility for the student with diabetes (see sample plan on page 204).

Hypoglycemia is not always completely preventable, and not all students, especially young children, will recognize its symptoms with every episode. Therefore, school personnel should be familiar with the symptoms and treatment so that an urgent problem can be handled appropriately.

Hypoglycemia can impair thinking abilities and sometimes can be mistaken for misbehavior. If a student has a sudden change in behavior, becomes lethargic, combative, or unconscious, or is having a seizure or convulsion, presume that the student has hypoglycemia. Treat the situation as a hypoglycemic emergency and check the student's blood glucose level immediately. If a blood glucose meter

Hypoglycemia occurs when a student's blood glucose level falls too low, usually as a result of

■ Administering too much insulin

■ Skipping or delaying meals or snacks

■ Not eating enough food as prescribed in the meal plan

■ Exercising longer and more intensely

■ Or a combination of these factors

is not available in the immediate area, or if the blood glucose level is otherwise unknown, treat the student for hypoglycemia.

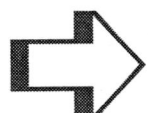 **The student should never be left alone or sent anywhere alone when experiencing hypoglycemia.**

As soon as symptoms of hypoglycemia are observed, give the student a quick-acting sugar product equivalent to 15 grams of carbohydrate, as specified in the Quick Reference Emergency Plan. This may include: 3 or 4 glucose tablets, 3 teaspoons (or three-fourths of a tube) of glucose gel, 4 ounces of juice, or 6 ounces (half a can) of non-diet soda. Recheck the student's blood glucose level 10 to 15 minutes after treatment. Repeat treatment if the blood glucose level still falls below the student's target range.

Symptoms of hypoglycemia, which are different for each student and may vary from episode to episode, can include:

Mild/Moderate Symptoms

■ shaky	■ sleepy	■ changed personality
■ sweaty	■ dizzy	■ inability to
■ hungry	■ confused	concentrate
■ pale	■ disoriented	■ weak
■ headache	■ uncoordinated	■ lethargic
■ blurry vision	■ irritable or nervous	■ changed behavior

Severe Symptoms

■ inability to swallow	■ having a seizure or convulsions	■ unconscious

---

Severe hypoglycemia is rare at school and generally can be prevented with prompt treatment when the early signs of low blood glucose are recognized. When hypoglycemia is severe, the school nurse or trained diabetes personnel must respond immediately. Symptoms may include inability to swallow, unconsciousness, unresponsiveness, seizure activity, convulsions, or jerking movements. At this point, never attempt to give the student food or a drink or to put anything in the mouth because it could cause choking.

If students become unconscious or experience convulsions or seizures, position them on their side to prevent choking. Immediately contact the school nurse or trained diabetes personnel, who will administer an injection of glucagon (see next page), if

---

How to Treat Hypoglycemia

Mild/Moderate Symptoms:

As soon as symptoms are observed, give the student a quick-acting sugar product, such as:

■ 3 or 4 glucose tablets

■ 3 teaspoons of glucose gel

■ 4 ounces of juice

■ 6 ounces of non-diet soda

Severe Symptoms:

■ Position the student on his/her side

■ Contact the school nurse or trained diabetes personnel

■ Administer glucagon, as prescribed

■ Call 911

■ Call student's parents

indicated in the student's Diabetes Medical Management Plan. While the glucagon is being administered, another school staff member should call for emergency medical assistance and then notify the parents/guardian. If glucagon is not authorized, staff should call 911 immediately.

Glucagon is a hormone that raises blood glucose levels by causing the release of glycogen (a form of stored carbohydrate) from the liver. It is administered when the student's blood glucose level gets so low that the student passes out, experiences seizures, or cannot swallow. Although it may cause nausea and vomiting when the student regains consciousness, glucagon can be a life-saving treatment that cannot harm a student.

The student's parents/guardian should supply the school with a glucagon emergency kit. This kit usually contains a bottle (vial) of glucagon in powder form and a pre-filled syringe with special liquid; the two are mixed just before a glucagon injection is given. Glucagon may be stored at room temperature. The school nurse and trained diabetes personnel must have ready access to the glucagon emergency kit at all times.

Understanding Hyperglycemia (High Blood Glucose)

HYPERglycemia means HIGH blood glucose.

Hyperglycemia, also called "high blood glucose," is a serious manifestation of diabetes that may be caused by too little insulin, illness, infection, injury, stress or emotional upset, ingestion of food that has not been covered by the appropriate amount of insulin, or decreased exercise or activity. High blood glucose symptoms include increased thirst, frequent urination, nausea, blurry vision, and fatigue. Over a long period of time, even moderately high blood glucose levels can lead to serious complications, such as heart disease, blindness, kidney failure, and amputations. In the short term, hyperglycemia can impair cognitive abilities and adversely affect academic performance.

Hyperglycemia does not usually result in acute problems. If, however, the student fails to take insulin, if a pump malfunctions and delivers less insulin, or if either physical or emotional stress

Hyperglycemia INFO

Symptoms:
- Increased thirst
- Frequent urination
- Nausea
- Blurry vision
- Fatigue

causes the insulin not to work effectively, there will be a breakdown of fat, causing ketones to form (see below).

At first, ketones will be cleared by the kidneys into the urine, but if there are more than the kidneys can handle, they will build up in the blood and may result in diabetic ketoacidosis (DKA). This complication will cause a fruity breath odor, nausea, vomiting, stomach pain, and, if untreated, deep breathing and increasing sleepiness. Students who use insulin pumps can go into DKA within hours if their pumps stop delivering insulin appropriately.

DKA can be prevented if the student's urine is checked for ketones during times of illness, especially if vomiting occurs, or whenever the blood glucose level exceeds the target range provided in the Diabetes Medical Management Plan. The test involves dipping a special strip into the urine and comparing the resulting color to a color chart.

Treatment of hyperglycemia may involve drinking extra water or diet drinks or administering supplemental insulin in accordance with the Diabetes Medical Management Plan.

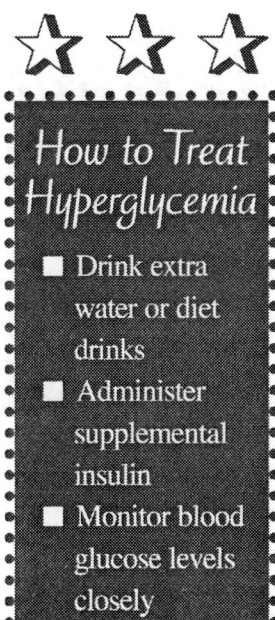

How to Treat Hyperglycemia

- Drink extra water or diet drinks
- Administer supplemental insulin
- Monitor blood glucose levels closely

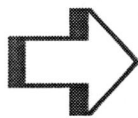 **Free and unrestricted access to liquids and the restroom must be provided, as high blood glucose levels increase urination and may lead to dehydration if the student cannot replace the fluids.**

The student's blood glucose level should be monitored closely until it returns to the target range, as outlined in the Diabetes Medical Management Plan. If treatment does not lower blood glucose levels and clear the ketones, if vomiting occurs, or if the student is lethargic or experiences breathing difficulties, call the parents/guardian or call for medical assistance if they cannot be reached. Treatment guidelines for ketones and when to call parents should be listed in the student's Diabetes Medical Management Plan. Information about the symptoms and treatment of hyperglycemia, contained in the Quick Reference Emergency Plan, should be provided to all school personnel who have responsibility for the student with diabetes (see sample plan on page 205).

Administering Insulin

Students with type 1 diabetes, and some students with type 2 diabetes, require insulin to be given at regular times each day. Some students may need additional or corrective dosages of insulin to treat hyperglycemia or to cover a rise in blood glucose levels. The Diabetes Medical Management Plan specifies the dosage, delivery system, and schedule for insulin administration, which will differ for each student. The nursing care plan, 504, IEP, or other education plan, which are based on the Diabetes Medical Management Plan, specify who will administer prescribed insulin and under what circumstances.

Today, new types of insulin and new delivery systems help keep blood glucose levels within the target range. These options may require closer monitoring and possibly more assistance for the student with diabetes.

Insulin has three characteristics:

Onset is the length of time before insulin reaches the blood-stream and begins lowering blood glucose.

Peak time is the time during which insulin is at its maximum strength in terms of lowering blood glucose.

Duration is the number of hours insulin continues to lower blood glucose levels.

There are several types of insulin that are used in combination to treat people with diabetes. These different types of insulin have been manufactured either to have immediate (rapid-acting or short-acting insulin), intermediate, or long (basal insulin) onset of action and duration of action in the body. A coordinated combination of insulins is used to allow for adequate treatment of diabetes at meals, snacks, during periods of physical activity, and through the night.

Opened vials of insulin may be left at room temperature for 30 days after opening, but will keep for 3 months if refrigerated. Unopened vials should be stored in the refrigerator and are good until the expiration date.

The **three most common ways to administer insulin** are with a syringe, an insulin pen, or an insulin pump.

Insulin syringes available today make it easier to draw up the proper dosage, and shorter, smaller needles make injections easier and relatively painless.

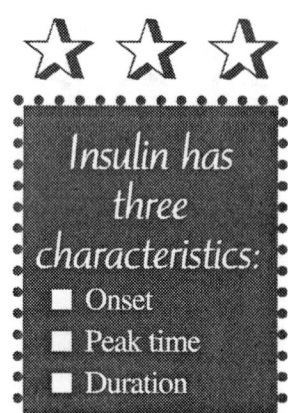

Insulin has three characteristics:
- Onset
- Peak time
- Duration

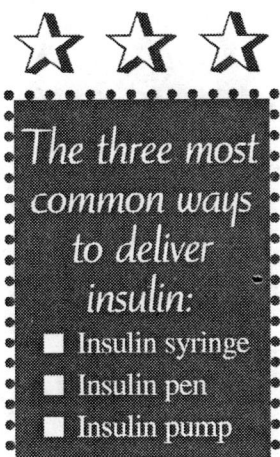

The three most common ways to deliver insulin:
- Insulin syringe
- Insulin pen
- Insulin pump

An insulin pen looks like a fountain pen. The pen holds a cartridge of insulin, and a needle is screwed onto its tip just before use. Insulin pens are convenient and most appropriate when children need a single type of insulin.

An insulin pump is a computerized device that looks like a pager and is usually worn on the student's waistband or belt. The pump is programmed to deliver small, steady doses of insulin throughout the day; additional doses are given to cover food or high blood glucose levels. The pump holds a reservoir of insulin that is attached to a system of tubing called an infusion set. Most infusion sets are started with a guide needle, then the plastic cannula (a tiny, flexible plastic tube) is left in place, taped with dressing, and the needle is removed. The cannula is usually changed every 2 or 3 days or when blood glucose levels remain above target range. More students are opting for insulin pump therapy as a means to keep blood glucose levels in better control.

Some students who need insulin during the school day are able to administer it on their own; others will need supervision; and others will need someone to administer the insulin for them. The school nurse and/or trained diabetes personnel should provide this help in accordance with the Diabetes Medical Management Plan and the nursing care plan. School personnel who are responsible for the student's care should be knowledgeable about the use and operation of that student's insulin delivery system. Information about insulin administration should appear in the student's Diabetes Medical Management Plan, nursing care plan, and education plan (504, IEP, or other education plan).

In the event a school nurse is not available to administer insulin, a nurse or another qualified health care professional should teach, monitor, and supervise trained diabetes personnel to administer insulin. Further, when the school nurse is not available to administer insulin and insulin is administered by other trained diabetes personnel, additional safety precautions may be taken, such as verification of the dose by two trained diabetes personnel before administration.

Following an Individualized Meal Plan

The nutritional needs of a student with diabetes do not differ from the needs of a student without diabetes. Both should eat a variety of foods to maintain normal growth and development. The major difference is that the timing, amount, and content of the food that the student with diabetes eats are carefully matched to the action of the insulin.

The student's meal plan is designed to balance nutritional needs with the insulin regimen and physical activity level. **There are usually no forbidden foods for people with diabetes.** The family and personal health care team create an individualized meal plan based upon carbohydrate counting or an exchange system.

Carbohydrate counting involves calculating the number of grams of carbohydrate or choices of carbohydrate the student eats. This information, which can be obtained from nutrition information on food labels, is used to determine the amount of insulin the student needs to control blood glucose for any given meal or snack.

The **exchange system** groups foods in six different lists, each with a set nutritional value. A meal plan is prepared that recommends several exchanges or servings from each food group for each meal and snack. The exchange list ensures that the meal plan is consistent in portion size and nutrient content while offering a wide variety of foods from each group. Students using this approach consume a prescribed number of exchanges at meal and snack times.

The exchange lists include the following food groups:

- Bread/starch ■ Fruit ■ Milk ■ Vegetables
- Meat/protein foods ■ Fats

With some insulin regimens, it is important to maintain consistency in the timing and content of meals and snacks. The student should eat lunch at the same time each day. Snacks are often necessary for a child with diabetes and must be eaten to balance the peak times of insulin action. **A missed or delayed snack could result in hypoglycemia.** The student also must have immediate access to a quick-acting form of glucose, such as juice, glucose

> *The student's meal plan is designed to balance the student's nutritional needs with his or her insulin routine and physical activity level.*

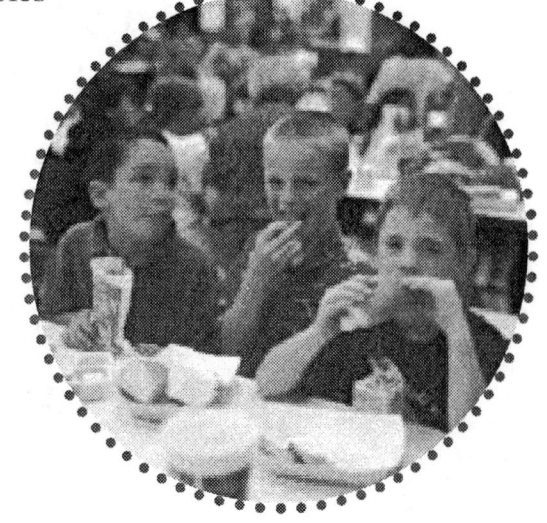

tablets or gel, or regular soda to treat hypoglycemia. The student's nursing care plan or education plan (504, IEP, or other education plan) should show the timing of meals and snacks and an alternative plan for unusual or unforeseen circumstances.

Getting Regular Physical Activity

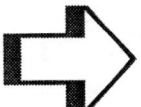

Exercise and physical activity are critical parts of diabetes management. Everyone can benefit from regular exercise, but it is even more important for a student with diabetes. In addition to maintaining cardiovascular fitness and controlling weight, physical activity can help to lower blood glucose levels.

Students with diabetes should participate fully in physical education classes and team sports. To maintain blood glucose levels within their target ranges during extra physical activity, students will make adjustments in their insulin and food intake. To prevent hypoglycemia, they also may need to check their blood glucose levels more frequently while engaging in physical activity.

Students with diabetes should participate fully in physical education classes and team sports.

Physical education instructors and sports coaches must be able to recognize and assist with the treatment of hypoglycemia. A quick-acting source of glucose and the student's glucose meter should always be available, along with plenty of water.

Students using pumps may disconnect from the pump for sports activities. If they keep the pump on, they may set a temporary, reduced rate of insulin while they are playing. School personnel should provide the student with a safe location for storing the pump when the student does not wear it. The student's Diabetes Medical Management Plan, nursing care plan, 504 Plan, IEP, or other education plan should include specific instructions.

Planning for Special Events, Field Trips, and Extracurricular Activities

Meeting the needs of students with diabetes requires advance planning for special events, such as classroom parties, field trips, and school-sponsored extracurricular activities held before or after school. With proper planning for coverage by trained diabetes personnel and possible adjustments to their insulin regimen and meal plan, students with diabetes can participate fully in all school-related activities.

While there are usually no forbidden foods in a meal plan for children or teens with diabetes, school parties often include foods high in carbohydrates and fats. Providing more nutritious snacks will be healthier for all students and encourage good eating habits. The parents/guardian should decide whether the student with diabetes should be given the same food as other students or food the parents provide. Parents should be given advance notice of parties to incorporate special foods in the meal plan or to adjust the insulin regimen.

Students often view a field trip as one of the most interesting and exciting activities of the school year, and students with diabetes must be allowed to have these school-related experiences. Although it is not unusual to invite parents to chaperone field trips, parental attendance is **not** a prerequisite for participation by the student with diabetes. **Trained diabetes personnel should accompany the student with diabetes** and ensure that all the student's supplies are brought along with the student and that there are snacks and supplies to treat hypoglycemia.

The plan for coverage and care during extracurricular activities sponsored by the school that take place outside of school hours should be carefully set out in the student's 504, IEP, or other education plan. As with field trips, trained diabetes personnel must be available at these activities.

☆ ☆ ☆

With proper planning, students with diabetes can participate fully in all school-related activities.

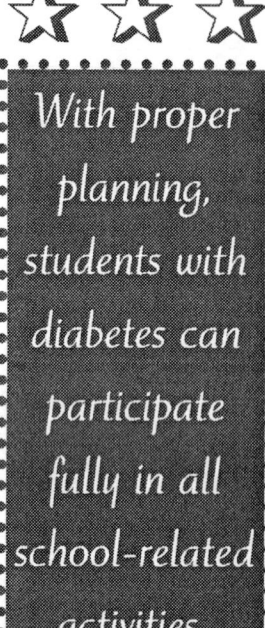

Planning for Disasters and Emergencies

To be prepared in the event of natural disasters or emergencies when students need to stay at school, the parents/guardian must provide an emergency supply kit. This kit should contain enough supplies for 72 hours, including the following items as appropriate:

- Blood glucose meter, testing strips, lancets, and batteries for the meter

- Urine ketone strips

- Insulin and supplies

- Insulin pump and supplies, including syringes

- Other medications

- Antiseptic wipes or wet wipes

- Fast-acting source of glucose

- Carbohydrate-containing snacks

- Hypoglycemia food supplies (enough for 3 episodes): quick-acting sugar and carbohydrate/protein snacks

- Glucagon emergency kit

Dealing with Emotional and Social Issues

Students with diabetes must deal not only with the usual developmental issues of growing up but also with learning to manage this complex disease. Diabetes can affect every facet of life, complicating the task of mastering normal developmental challenges.

For the most part, children do not want to be singled out or made to feel different from their peers. Diabetes care tasks, however, can set them apart and make them feel angry or resentful about their disease. Sometimes, children and teens feel pressured to please caretakers and yet cannot consistently comply with their requests. To appease concerned parents or health care providers, some children report fictitious glucose levels or do not take all their insulin.

Children react differently to having diabetes. They may be accepting, resentful, open to discussing it, or attempt to hide it. Often, the same child will experience all of these feelings over time. School personnel should be aware of the student's feelings about having diabetes and identify ways to ensure the student is treated the same as others.

Diabetes can be a focal point for conflict within families. One of the biggest tasks for children and adolescents is to become increasingly independent from their parents, but diabetes may compromise independence because parents are concerned about their children's ability to perform self-care and take responsibility for it. Parents, who are ultimately responsible for their children's well-being, may be reluctant to allow normal independence in children or teens who have not been able to take care of themselves properly. This parental concern can lead to increasing struggles with dependence, oppositional behavior, and rebellion. Some adolescent girls, for example, may rebel by not following their insulin regimen because they want to lose weight or avoid gaining weight.

Increasingly, depression is being recognized as quite common among children and teens generally, and even more so in those with diabetes. Health care providers and school personnel must be aware of emotional and behavioral issues and refer students with diabetes and their families for counseling and support as needed.

Diabetes care tasks can set children and teens apart from their peers and make them feel resentful or angry about their disease.

WHY IS DIABETES SELF-MANAGEMENT IMPORTANT?

While it is very important to provide students with assistance and supervision of their diabetes care as needed, it is equally important to enable students to take on the responsibility of learning diabetes self-management and control. The age for transfer of responsibility from caregiver to child varies from child to child and from task to task because children develop and mature at different rates. Students' ability to participate in self-care also depends upon their willingness to do so. As students are ready, they can assume more responsibility for their care.

Students' competence and capability for performing diabetes-related tasks are determined by the school health care team and the parents/guardian. **Diabetes care depends upon self-management.** Ultimately, each person with diabetes becomes responsible for all aspects of self-care, including blood glucose monitoring and insulin administration. Regardless of their level of self-management, however, all students with diabetes may require assistance when blood glucose levels are out of the target range.

WHY IS DIABETES MANAGEMENT TRAINING ESSENTIAL FOR SCHOOL PERSONNEL?

Diabetes management training teaches school nurses and staff members how to provide necessary care for students with diabetes during the school day and school-sponsored extracurricular activities. Training should occur before the beginning of the school year, when a student is diagnosed with diabetes, when a student with diabetes is enrolled in the school, or when appropriate. There also should be regular refresher sessions.

There are two levels of training appropriate for school personnel. The first level of training is for school staff members who have primary responsibility for students with diabetes (e.g., teachers and coaches), but who don't perform diabetes care tasks such as blood glucose monitoring or insulin or glucagon administration. This training should include:

■ General overview of diabetes and typical health care needs of a student with diabetes

■ Recognition of hypoglycemia and hyperglycemia

■ Identity of school nurses and/or trained diabetes personnel and how to contact them for help

The second level of training is for school personnel who will perform routine and emergency care (school nurses and trained diabetes personnel) and should include the following content based on current standards of care for children and youth with diabetes recommended by the American Diabetes Association:

■ General overview of typical health care needs of a student with diabetes and how these needs are addressed in the student's written care plans

- Explanation/overview of type 1 and type 2 diabetes

- The effect of balancing insulin, food, and exercise upon a student's blood glucose levels

- Procedures for routine care of individual students, including blood glucose monitoring, insulin administration, urine ketone testing, and recording results

- Signs and symptoms of hypoglycemia and hyperglycemia and the short- and long-term risks of these conditions

- Treatment of hypoglycemia and hyperglycemia

- Glucagon administration

- Managing nutrition and exercise in the school setting

- Tools, supplies, and equipment required for diabetes care and their storage

- Legal rights and responsibilities of schools and parents/guardian

More information on diabetes can be found in the Resource List beginning on page 213.

WHERE CAN I LEARN MORE ABOUT DIABETES?

The Resource List beginning on page 213 includes a list of the major organizations (and their websites) that offer related information, resources, and training.

Section 2 *ACTIONS*

ACTIONS

Section 2 *ACTIONS*

FOR School Personnel, Parents, and Students

• • • • • • • • • • • • • • •

The health, safety, and educational progress of a student with diabetes depend on cooperation and collaboration between the family and school staff members. Working together, they form the school health team that implements the provisions of the student's written plans and provides the necessary assistance in the school environment (see Diabetes Primer, page 155).

When available, the school nurse is the most appropriate person to plan diabetes care in the school and oversee implementation of the student's written plans. When a school nurse is not available, the diabetes medical community has found that nonmedical personnel ("trained diabetes personnel") can be trained and supervised to safely provide and assist with diabetes care tasks in the school setting, including blood glucose monitoring, insulin and glucagon administration, and urine ketone testing. Assignment of diabetes care tasks must take into account state and local laws addressing what tasks may be performed by nonmedical school personnel.

The responsibilities of each key school staff member are described in the pages that follow, along with those of the parents/guardian and the student. One person may fill more than one role. For example, a teacher or a coach also may be one of the trained diabetes personnel. The recommended actions on the following pages do not represent legal checklists of what people must do to comply with relevant federal, state, and local laws. Rather, they are steps that school personnel, parents, and students should take to ensure effective diabetes management.

The following pages should be copied and distributed to everyone involved along with the student's Quick Reference Emergency Plan (see pages 204–205). All substitute and appropriate after-school personnel should receive information relevant to their position.

Please copy and distribute to the School District Administrator.

ACTIONS for the School District Administrator

(Superintendent, 504 coordinator, or other school administrator responsible for coordinating student services)

❏ **Provide leadership** in developing district policy related to all aspects of diabetes management at school that is consistent with the standards of care* recommended for children with diabetes, including delegation of responsibilities, required staff training, medication administration policy, and blood glucose monitoring. Obtain input from local or regional experts.

❏ **Support implementation of district policy.** Support school district health professionals and other school administrators regarding: 1) development, coordination, and implementation of diabetes management training; 2) ongoing quality control and improvement of these training programs; and 3) development and implementation of a program to monitor the performance of those who receive training.

❏ **Arrange for training of school personnel.** Arrange for a health care professional, such as the school nurse or a diabetes-trained public health nurse, to provide training and ongoing monitoring for trained diabetes personnel.

❏ **Allocate sufficient resources** to manage students with diabetes.

❏ **Monitor schools** attended by students with diabetes for compliance with district policy.

❏ **Meet with members of the school health team as needed.** Address issues of concern about the provision of diabetes care by the school district, as appropriate.

❏ **Respect the student's confidentiality and right to privacy.**

❏ **Learn about diabetes** by reviewing the materials contained in this guide.

❏ **Understand and implement the federal and state laws** that may apply to students with diabetes, including Section 504 of the Rehabilitation Act of 1973, the Americans with Disabilities Act, and the Individuals with Disabilities Education Act (see Section 4).

*The American Diabetes Association (ADA) publishes "Standards of Care for Diabetes Management" annually in the journal *Diabetes Care*. These standards also appear on the association's website, www.diabetes.org. See the ADA's position statement on "Care of Children with Diabetes in the School and Day Care Setting" on pages 225–229.

Please copy and distribute to the Principal, School Administrator, or Designee.

ACTIONS for the Principal, School Administrator, or Designee

❏ **Participate in developing and implementing school policy** related to diabetes management at school and implement school district policy.

❏ **Allocate sufficient resources to manage students with diabetes.**

❏ **Develop and implement a system to inform school health services** of the pending enrollment of a student with diabetes.

❏ **Promote a supportive learning environment** for students with diabetes. Treat these students the same as other students except to respond to medical needs.

❏ **Meet annually with the school health team.** Arrange and attend a meeting of the school health team members (student, family, school nurse, 504/IEP coordinator, teacher(s), and other staff members who have primary responsibility for the student) before the school year starts, or when the child is newly diagnosed, to discuss medical accommodations and educational aids and related services the student needs.

❏ **Identify all staff members** who have responsibility for the student with diabetes.

❏ **Arrange for diabetes management training** for the school nurse, trained diabetes personnel, and other staff members with responsibility for students with diabetes. Inform staff members about how and when they should contact trained diabetes personnel. Ensure that trained diabetes personnel are available at all times when the student is on or off campus for school-sponsored activities and events.

❏ **Alert all school-related staff members** who teach or supervise a student with diabetes. Ensure that they, including the bus driver, are familiar with the accommodations and emergency procedures contained in the student's Diabetes Medical Management Plan, 504 Plan, IEP, or other education plan.

❏ **Alert all substitute personnel.** Ensure that they are aware of the needs and emergency procedures for students with diabetes.

❏ **Work with the school health team to implement the student's written plans,** including the Diabetes Medical Management Plan, and monitor compliance.

Continued on next page

ACTIONS for the Principal, School Administrator, or Designee *Continued*

❏ **Implement school policy on availability of trained staff.** The school nurse or at least one of the school's trained diabetes personnel must be available when the student with diabetes is on campus or is a participant in off-campus school-sponsored activities and events.

❏ **Respect the student's confidentiality and right to privacy.**

❏ **Help develop and implement on-campus as well as off-campus emergency protocols.**

❏ **Include diabetes awareness as part of health or cultural education.**

❏ **Support and facilitate** ongoing communication between parents/guardian of students with diabetes and school staff.

❏ **Learn about diabetes** by reviewing the materials contained in this guide.

❏ **Be able to recognize and respond to signs and symptoms of hypoglycemia and hyperglycemia** in accordance with the student's Quick Reference Emergency Plan, which includes knowing when and how to contact the school nurse or trained diabetes personnel.

❏ **Understand the federal and state laws** that may apply to students with diabetes, including Section 504 of the Rehabilitation Act of 1973, the Americans with Disabilities Act, and the Individuals with Disabilities Education Act; understand procedures for implementation (see Section 4).

Please copy and distribute to the School Nurse.

ACTIONS for the School Nurse

● ●

When a school nurse is assigned to the school (or school district), that person is the key school staff member who coordinates provision of health care services for a student with diabetes at school and at school-related activities. When notified that a student with diabetes is enrolled in the school, annually or more often as necessary, the school nurse will:

❏ **Obtain and review the student's current Diabetes Medical Management Plan** from the personal health care provider and pertinent information from the family.

❏ **Facilitate the initial school health team meeting** to discuss implementing the student's Diabetes Medical Management Plan and participate in the development and implementation of the student's 504 Plan, IEP, or other education plan. Monitor compliance with these plans and facilitate follow-up meetings of the school health team to discuss concerns, receive updates, and evaluate the need for changes to the student's plans, as appropriate.

❏ **Conduct a nursing assessment of the student and develop a nursing care plan.** Many school nurses already have systems set up to develop nursing care plans for students with chronic diseases. The plan for students with diabetes is based on assessment of the student, input from the parents/guardian and the student, and the Diabetes Medical Management Plan. For example, the nursing care plan will identify specific functional problems, establish a goal to overcome each problem, and delineate tasks or interventions to help reach the goals.

❏ **Conduct ongoing, periodic assessments of students with diabetes and update the nursing care plans.**

❏ **Coordinate development of the student's Quick Reference Emergency Plan** and provide copies to staff members who have responsibility for the student throughout the school day (e.g., teachers, coach, PE instructor, lunchroom staff, and bus driver).

❏ **Obtain materials and medical supplies necessary for diabetes care tasks** from the parents/guardian and arrange a system for notifying the student or parents/guardian when supplies need to be replenished.

❏ **Plan and implement diabetes management training** for the trained diabetes personnel and any other staff members with responsibility for the student with diabetes who require such training. Ensure that all those mentioned in the 504 Plan, IEP, or other education plan know their roles in carrying out the plan, how their roles relate to each other, and when and where to seek help.

❏ **Participate in diabetes management training** provided by health care professionals with expertise in diabetes and attend other continuing education offerings to attain and/or maintain knowledge about current standards of care for children with diabetes.

Continued on next page

ACTIONS for the School Nurse *Continued*

- ❑ **Review the information about diabetes in this guide.**

- ❑ **Distribute the Diabetes Primer in this guide to all school personnel** who have responsibility for students with diabetes.

- ❑ **Train (or oversee training of), assess competence, and monitor trained diabetes personnel** in carrying out the health care procedures defined in the Diabetes Medical Management Plan, 504 Plan, IEP, or other education plan.

- ❑ **Perform routine and emergency diabetes care tasks,** including blood glucose monitoring, urine ketone testing, insulin administration, and glucagon administration.

- ❑ **Practice universal precautions and infection control procedures** during all student encounters.

- ❑ **Maintain accurate documentation** of contacts with students and family members; communications with the student's health care provider; any direct care given, including medication administration; and the training and monitoring of trained diabetes personnel.

- ❑ **Collaborate with other co-workers** (e.g., food service) and agencies (e.g., outside nursing agencies, school bus transportation services) as necessary to provide health care services.

- ❑ **With parental permission, act as liaison between the school and the student's health care provider** regarding the student's self-management at school.

- ❑ **Communicate to parents/guardian any concerns about the student's diabetes management or health,** such as acute hypoglycemia episodes, hyperglycemia, general attitude, and emotional issues.

- ❑ **Promote and encourage independence and self-care** consistent with the student's ability, skill, maturity, and developmental level.

- ❑ **Respect the student's confidentiality and right to privacy.**

- ❑ **Act as an advocate** for students to help them meet their diabetes health care needs.

- ❑ **Provide education and act as a resource on managing diabetes** at school to the student, family, and school staff. Establish and maintain an up-to-date resource file of pamphlets, brochures, and other publications for school personnel.

- ❑ **Assist the classroom teacher** with developing a plan for substitute teachers.

- ❑ **Assist the PE instructor** with managing the student's exercise program at school.

- ❑ **Be knowledgeable about federal, state, and local laws and regulations** that pertain to managing diabetes at school (see Section 4).

Please copy and distribute to Trained Diabetes Personnel.

ACTIONS for Trained Diabetes Personnel

● ●

With proper supervision and training, and where state laws do not prohibit it, nonmedical personnel can help students manage their diabetes safely at school. This guide uses the term "trained diabetes personnel," but some schools use other names. Trained diabetes personnel may include school staff members, health aides, and licensed practical nurses. Depending on the size of the school, at least two people should be trained to perform diabetes care tasks and be trained diabetes personnel.

If a school has a nurse, the nurse takes the lead in providing diabetes care. Either the school nurse or at least one of the trained diabetes personnel should be on site throughout the school day and during school-sponsored activities that take place before or after school in which a student with diabetes participates.

❑ **Understand the student's Diabetes Medical Management Plan, 504 Plan, IEP, or other education plan.**

❑ **Understand the student's Quick Reference Emergency Plan.**

❑ **Attend the student's school health team meetings** to gain understanding of the overall goal of care.

❑ **Participate in diabetes management training.**

❑ **Learn about diabetes** by reviewing materials contained in this guide.

❑ **Perform routine and emergency diabetes care tasks,** including blood glucose monitoring, urine ketone testing, insulin administration, and glucagon administration after receiving training under the direction of the school nurse or other assigned health care professional.

❑ **Practice universal precautions and infection control procedures** in all student encounters.

❑ **Participate in planned evaluations of care.**

❑ **Document care provided** according to standards and requirements outlined by school policy.

❑ **Observe and record student health and behavior,** noting any changes over time.

❑ **Communicate directly and regularly with the school nurse or the supervising health care professional.**

❑ **Consult with appropriate members of the student's school health team** when questions arise or the student's health status changes.

Continued on next page

ACTIONS for Trained Diabetes Personnel *Continued*

❑ **Respect the student's confidentiality and right to privacy.**

❑ **Be available** on campus during regular school hours and when the student participates in school-sponsored extracurricular activities held before or after school.

❑ **Accompany the student on field trips or off-campus school-sponsored sports events** and activities, as determined by the 504 Plan, IEP, or other education plan.

❑ **Provide support and encouragement to the student.**

❑ **Help ensure that the student has a supportive learning environment** and is treated the same as students without diabetes, except to respond to medical needs.

Please copy and distribute to the Teacher.

ACTIONS for the Teacher

● ●

❏ **Participate in the school health team meeting(s).** The teacher(s) who has primary responsibility for the student participates in the school health team meeting(s) when the Diabetes Medical Management Plan, 504 Plan, IEP, or other education plans are discussed.

❏ **Work with the school health team to implement written care plans,** including the Diabetes Medical Management Plan, 504 Plan, IEP, or other education plan.

❏ **Recognize that a change in the student's behavior could be a symptom of blood glucose changes.** Be aware that a student who has low blood sugar, even mildly low, may briefly have some cognitive impairment. If changes occur, respond in accordance with the student's Quick Reference Emergency Plan.

❏ **Be prepared to recognize and respond to the signs and symptoms of hypo-glycemia and hyperglycemia** in accordance with the student's Quick Reference Emergency Plan, which speci-fies when and how to contact the school nurse or trained diabetes personnel.

❏ **Provide a supportive environment for the student** to manage diabetes effectively and safely at school, which includes eating snacks for routine diabetes management and to treat low blood glucose levels, having bathroom privileges and access to drinking water, monitoring blood glucose, and adminis-tering insulin and other medications.

❏ **Provide classroom accommodations for the student with diabetes,** as indicated in the student's 504 Plan, IEP, or other education plan.

❏ **Provide instruction to the student** if it is missed because of absence for diabetes-related care.

❏ **Provide information for substitute teachers** that communicates the day-to-day needs of the student and the Quick Reference Emergency Plan.

❏ **Notify the parents/guardian in advance of changes in school schedule,** such as class parties, field trips, and other special events.

❏ **Communicate with the school nurse, trained diabetes personnel, or parents regarding any concerns about the student.**

❏ **Attend diabetes management training,** if designated as trained diabetes personnel.

❏ **Learn about diabetes** by reviewing the materials contained in this guide.

❏ **Treat the student with diabetes the same as other students,** except to meet medical needs.

❏ **Respect the student's confidentiality and right to privacy.**

Please copy and distribute to the Coach and Physical Education Instructor.*

ACTIONS for the Coach and Physical Education Instructor

❏ Encourage exercise and participation in physical activities and sports for students with diabetes as well as for other students.

❏ Treat the student with diabetes the same as other students, except to meet medical needs.

❏ Encourage the student to have personal supplies readily accessible. Make sure blood glucose monitoring equipment is available at all activity sites.

❏ Allow the student to check blood glucose levels as outlined in the 504 Plan, IEP, or other education plan.

❏ Understand and be aware that hypoglycemia can occur during and after physical activity.

❏ Recognize that a change in the student's behavior could be a symptom of blood glucose changes.

❏ Be prepared to recognize and respond to the signs and symptoms of hypoglycemia and hyperglycemia and take initial actions in accordance with the student's Quick Reference Emergency Plan, which specifies when and how to contact the school nurse or trained diabetes personnel.

❏ To treat hypoglycemia, provide the student with immediate access to a fast-acting form of glucose, as outlined in the Quick Reference Emergency Plan.

❏ Consider taping a fast-acting form of glucose (e.g., 3 or 4 glucose tablets or hard candies) to a clipboard or include it in the First Aid pack that goes out to physical education activities, practices, and games.

❏ Learn about diabetes by reviewing materials contained in this guide.

❏ Provide input to the student's school health team as needed.

❏ Communicate with the school nurse and/or trained diabetes personnel regarding any observations or concerns about the student.

❏ Provide information for the substitute PE instructor that communicates the daily needs of the student and the Quick Reference Emergency Plan.

❏ Respect the student's confidentiality and right to privacy.

Please copy and distribute to the Food Service Manager,
Lunchroom Staff, or Lunchroom Monitor.

ACTIONS for the Food Service Manager, Lunchroom Staff, or Lunchroom Monitor

❏ Obtain a copy of the student's written meal plan from the Diabetes Medical Management Plan.

❏ Obtain a copy of the student's Quick Reference Emergency Plan and keep it in a known, yet secure, place in the lunchroom.

❏ Provide a lunch menu and lunch schedule in advance to parents along with the nutrition content of menu selections, including grams of carbohydrate and fat.

❏ Understand and be aware that hypoglycemia can occur before lunch. Supervisory lunch personnel may need to encourage the student to eat appropriate foods.

❏ Be prepared to recognize and respond to the signs and symptoms of hypoglycemia and hyperglycemia and take actions in accordance with the student's Quick Reference Emergency Plan.

❏ Recognize that a student's behavior change could be a symptom of blood glucose changes.

❏ Learn about the various kinds of diabetes meal and snack plans. Know which type of meal plan the student follows.

❏ Recognize that eating meals and snacks on time is a critical component of diabetes management. Failure to eat lunch on time could result in low blood glucose, especially if a student has missed a morning snack or has had a physically strenuous or otherwise active morning at school.

❏ Ensure that the student has timely access to food and sufficient time to finish.

❏ Know where supplies to treat hypoglycemia are kept (e.g., with the student or another place).

❏ Treat the student with diabetes the same as other students, except to respond to medical needs.

❏ Provide input to the student's school health team when requested.

❏ Communicate with the school nurse and/or trained diabetes personnel regarding any concerns about the student.

❏ Respect the student's confidentiality and right to privacy.

Please copy and distribute to the Bus Driver.

ACTIONS for the Bus Driver

❏ At the beginning of the school year, identify any students on the bus who have diabetes.

❏ Obtain a copy of the student's Quick Reference Emergency Plan and keep it on the bus in a known, yet secure, place. Leave the plan readily available for substitute drivers.

❏ Understand and be aware that although hypoglycemia normally occurs at the end of the day, it may happen at the beginning of the day if the student has not eaten breakfast.

❏ Recognize that a student's behavior change could be a symptom of blood glucose changes.

❏ Be prepared to recognize and respond to the signs and symptoms of hypoglycemia and hyperglycemia and take initial actions in accordance with the student's Quick Reference Emergency Plan, which specifies when and how to contact trained diabetes and emergency personnel.

❏ Keep supplies to treat low blood glucose on the bus and be aware of where the students with diabetes normally keep their supplies.

❏ Treat the student with diabetes the same as other students, except to respond to medical needs.

❏ Allow the student to eat snacks on the bus.

❏ Provide input to the student's school health team when requested.

❏ Communicate with the school nurse and/or trained diabetes personnel regarding any concerns about the student.

❏ Respect the student's confidentiality and right to privacy.

Please copy and distribute to the Guidance Counselor or School Psychologist.

ACTIONS for the Guidance Counselor or School Psychologist

❏ Work with school staff to promote a supportive learning environment.

❏ Ensure that the student with diabetes is treated the same as students without diabetes, except to respond to medical needs.

❏ Be aware of and be prepared to respond to the emotional needs of the student. Children react differently to having diabetes. Some are accepting and open to discussing it; others are resentful and may attempt to hide it. Often, a single child will experience both kinds of feelings. Be aware of the student's feelings about having diabetes and identify ways to ensure the student is treated the same as other students.

❏ Recognize that students with chronic illnesses such as diabetes may rebel by discontinuing all or part of their medical regimen. Adolescent girls, for example, may not follow their insulin regimen because they want to lose weight or to avoid gaining weight.

❏ Be aware that some students may not wish to share information about their diabetes with other students or school staff, particularly if it makes them feel different from others.

❏ Promote and encourage independence and self-care that are consistent with the student's ability, skill, maturity, and development.

❏ Provide input to the student's school health team when requested.

❏ Communicate with the school nurse and/or trained diabetes personnel regarding any concerns about the student.

❏ Respect the student's confidentiality and right to privacy.

Please copy and distribute to the Parents or Guardian.

ACTIONS for the Parents or Guardian

- ❑ **Inform the school principal that your child has diabetes** when the student enrolls in school or is newly diagnosed with the disease.

- ❑ **Provide accurate and current emergency contact information.**

- ❑ **Provide the signed Diabetes Medical Management Plan** to the school nurse or other member of the school health team.

- ❑ **Attend and participate in the initial and annual meetings of the school health team** (includes student, parents, school nurse, principal, 504 coordinator, teachers, and other school personnel who have responsibility for the student with diabetes) to discuss implementing the student's Diabetes Medical Management Plan, to review medical accommodations and educational aids the student may need, and to develop a 504 Plan, IEP, or other education plan.

- ❑ **Provide specific information about your child's diabetes** and performance of diabetes-related tasks at home to the school health team.

- ❑ **Permit sharing of medical information** necessary for the student's safety between the school and the student's personal health care providers.

- ❑ **Inform school staff of any changes in the student's health status.**

- ❑ **Provide all supplies and equipment necessary for implementing your child's Diabetes Medical Management Plan, 504 Plan, IEP, or other education plan,** including blood glucose monitoring equipment, supplies for insulin administration and urine ketone testing, snacks, fast-acting glucose, and a glucagon emergency kit. As appropriate, provide these supplies to school personnel. Replenish supplies as needed.

- ❑ **Provide and maintain all supplies and equipment necessary to accommodate the student's long-term needs (72 hours)** in case of an emergency.

- ❑ **Inform appropriate school staff (principal, teachers, coaches, and others) when the student plans to participate in school-sponsored activities** that take place before or after school so that health care coverage can be coordinated to ensure the health and safety of the student with diabetes.

- ❑ **Understand the federal, state, and local laws** that address the school's responsibilities to students with diabetes.

Please copy and distribute to Students with Diabetes who are able to take responsibility for their self-management.

ACTIONS for the Student with Diabetes

❏ Participate in the school meeting to discuss your Diabetes Medical Management Plan, 504 Plan, IEP, or other education plan, as appropriate.

❏ **Always wear a medical alert ID** and carry a fast-acting source of glucose.

   Tell teachers and other school staff members if you feel symptoms of low or high blood glucose, especially if you need help.

❏ **Work with school staff members if you need help** checking your blood glucose, getting insulin, or eating the right amount of food at the right time during the school day.

❏ **Take charge of your diabetes care at school** if your written school plans allow you to. This may include:

   ■ checking and writing down blood glucose levels

   ■ figuring out the right insulin doses

   ■ giving yourself insulin

   ■ throwing away needles, lancets, and other supplies you have used in the right place

   ■ eating meals and snacks as planned

   ■ treating low blood sugar

   ■ carrying diabetes equipment and supplies with you at all times

Things You Need to Know:

1. What your written school plans say to help you manage your diabetes, which person at school will help you, and what is expected of you.

2. Who to contact and what to do when you are having a low blood sugar reaction.

3. When you should check your blood glucose levels, give yourself insulin, have a snack, and eat lunch.

4. Where your diabetes supplies are stored, if you don't carry them, and who to contact when you need to use them.

Section 3 *TOOLS*

Sample Diabetes Medical Management Plan *Page 200*
Sample Quick Reference Emergency Plan *Page 204*

TOOLS

Section 3 TOOLS

FOR Effective Diabetes Management in Schools

● ● ● ● ● ● ● ● ● ● ● ● ● ● ●

This section contains examples of two important tools to help the school health team in managing the student with diabetes:

The **Sample Diabetes Medical Management Plan** is completed by the student's parents/guardian and personal health care team and can be used as the basis for developing education plans and nursing care plans for students with diabetes.

The **Sample Quick Reference Emergency Plan** addresses management of hypoglycemia and hyperglycemia emergencies. This plan should be completed for each student with diabetes and both pages should be copied and distributed to all relevant personnel, in accordance with the student's Diabetes Medical Management Plan, 504 Plan, IEP, or other education plan.

Date of Plan: _____

Diabetes Medical Management Plan

Effective Dates: _____

This plan should be completed by the student's personal health care team and parents/guardian. It should be reviewed with relevant school staff and copies should be kept in a place that is easily accessed by the school nurse, trained diabetes personnel, and other authorized personnel.

Student's Name:_____

Date of Birth:_____ Date of Diabetes Diagnosis:_____

Grade:_____ Homeroom Teacher:_____

Physical Condition: ❏ Diabetes type 1 ❏ Diabetes type 2

Contact Information

Mother/Guardian:_____

Address:_____

_____

Telephone: Home_____ Work _____ Cell _____

Father/Guardian:_____

Address:_____

_____

Telephone: Home_____ Work _____ Cell _____

Student's Doctor/Health Care Provider:

Name:_____

Address:_____

_____

Telephone:_____ Emergency Number:_____

Other Emergency Contacts:

Name:_____

Relationship:_____

Telephone: Home_____ Work _____ Cell _____

Notify parents/guardian or emergency contact in the following situations:

_____

_____

_____

Diabetes Medical Management Plan *Continued*

Blood Glucose Monitoring

Target range for blood glucose is ❏ 70-150   ❏ 70-180   ❏ Other_____

Usual times to check blood glucose _____

Times to do extra blood glucose checks (*check all that apply*)
❏ before exercise
❏ after exercise
❏ when student exhibits symptoms of hyperglycemia
❏ when student exhibits symptoms of hypoglycemia
❏ other (explain):_____

Can student perform own blood glucose checks? ❏ Yes ❏ No

Exceptions: _____

Type of blood glucose meter student uses: _____

Insulin

Usual Lunchtime Dose

Base dose of Humalog/Novolog /Regular insulin at lunch (circle type of rapid-/short-acting insulin used) is
_____ units or does flexible dosing using _____ units/ _____ grams carbohydrate.
Use of other insulin at lunch: (circle type of insulin used): intermediate/NPH/lente _____ units or
basal/Lantus/Ultralente _____ units.

Insulin Correction Doses

Parental authorization should be obtained before administering a correction dose for high blood
glucose levels. ❏ Yes ❏ No

_____ units if blood glucose is _____ to _____ mg/dl

_____ units if blood glucose is _____ to _____ mg/dl

_____ units if blood glucose is _____ to _____ mg/dl

_____ units if blood glucose is _____ to _____ mg/dl

_____ units if blood glucose is _____ to _____ mg/dl

Can student give own injections? ❏ Yes ❏ No
Can student determine correct amount of insulin? ❏ Yes ❏ No
Can student draw correct dose of insulin? ❏ Yes ❏ No

_____ Parents are authorized to adjust the insulin dosage under the following circumstances:_____

_____

For Students With Insulin Pumps

Type of pump:_____ Basal rates: _____ 12 am to _____

_____ _____ to _____

_____ _____ to _____

Type of insulin in pump:_____

Type of infusion set:_____

Insulin/carbohydrate ratio:_____Correction factor: _____

Student Pump Abilities/Skills:	*Needs Assistance*
Count carbohydrates	❏ Yes ❏ No
Bolus correct amount for carbohydrates consumed	❏ Yes ❏ No
Calculate and administer corrective bolus	❏ Yes ❏ No
Calculate and set basal profiles	❏ Yes ❏ No
Calculate and set temporary basal rate	❏ Yes ❏ No
Disconnect pump	❏ Yes ❏ No
Reconnect pump at infusion set	❏ Yes ❏ No
Prepare reservoir and tubing	❏ Yes ❏ No
Insert infusion set	❏ Yes ❏ No
Troubleshoot alarms and malfunctions	❏ Yes ❏ No

For Students Taking Oral Diabetes Medications

Type of medication:_____ Timing: _____

Other medications:_____ Timing: _____

Meals and Snacks Eaten at School

Is student independent in carbohydrate calculations and management? ❏ Yes ❏ No

Meal/Snack	*Time*	*Food content/amount*
Breakfast	_____	_____
Mid-morning snack	_____	_____
Lunch	_____	_____
Mid-afternoon snack	_____	_____
Dinner	_____	_____

Snack before exercise? ❏ Yes ❏ No

Snack after exercise? ❏ Yes ❏ No

Other times to give snacks and content/amount:_____

Preferred snack foods: _____

Foods to avoid, if any: _____

Instructions for when food is provided to the class (e.g., as part of a class party or food sampling event):
_____

_____

Exercise and Sports

A fast-acting carbohydrate such as_____ should be
available at the site of exercise or sports.

Restrictions on activity, if any:_____

Student should not exercise if blood glucose level is below_____ mg/dl or above_____ mg/dl
or if moderate to large urine ketones are present.

Diabetes Medical Management Plan *Continued*

Hypoglycemia (Low Blood Sugar)

Usual symptoms of hypoglycemia: _____

_____

Treatment of hypoglycemia: _____

_____

Glucagon should be given if the student is unconscious, having a seizure (convulsion), or unable to swallow.
Route_____, Dosage_____, site for glucagon injection: _____arm, _____thigh, _____other.

If glucagon is required, administer it promptly. Then, call 911 (or other emergency assistance) and the parents/guardian.

Hyperglycemia (High Blood Sugar)

Usual symptoms of hyperglycemia: _____

_____

Treatment of hyperglycemia: _____

_____

Urine should be checked for ketones when blood glucose levels are above _____ mg/dl.

Treatment for ketones: _____

Supplies to be Kept at School

_____Blood glucose meter, blood glucose test
        strips, batteries for meter

_____Lancet device, lancets, gloves, etc.

_____Urine ketone strips

_____Insulin vials and syringes

_____Insulin pump and supplies

_____Insulin pen, pen needles, insulin cartridges

_____Fast-acting source of glucose

_____Carbohydrate containing snack

_____Glucagon emergency kit

Signatures

This Diabetes Medical Management Plan has been approved by:

_____   _____

Student's Physician/Health Care Provider   Date

I give permission to the school nurse, trained diabetes personnel, and other designated staff members of _____ school to perform and carry out the diabetes care tasks as outlined by _____'s Diabetes Medical Management Plan. I also consent to the release of the information contained in this Diabetes Medical Management Plan to all staff members and other adults who have custodial care of my child and who may need to know this information to maintain my child's health and safety.

Acknowledged and received by:

_____   _____

Student's Parent/Guardian   Date

_____   _____

Student's Parent/Guardian   Date

Quick Reference Emergency Plan
for a Student with Diabetes
Hypoglycemia
(Low Blood Sugar)

Photo

Student's Name

Grade/Teacher   Date of Plan

Emergency Contact Information:

Mother/Guardian   **Father/Guardian**

| Home phone | Work phone | Cell | Home phone | Work phone | Cell |

School Nurse/Trained Diabetes Personnel   **Contact Number(s)**

Never send a child with suspected low blood sugar anywhere alone.

Causes of Hypoglycemia
- Too much insulin
- Missed food
- Delayed food
- Too much or too intense exercise
- Unscheduled exercise

Onset
- Sudden

Symptoms

Mild
- Hunger
- Shakiness
- Weakness
- Paleness
- Anxiety
- Irritability
- Dizziness
- Sweating
- Drowsiness
- Personality change
- Inability to concentrate
- Other: _____
  _____

Circle student's usual symptoms.

Moderate
- Headache
- Behavior change
- Poor coordination
- Blurry vision
- Weakness
- Slurred Speech
- Confusion
- Other _____
  _____

Circle student's usual symptoms.

Severe
- Loss of consciousness
- Seizure
- Inability to swallow

Circle student's usual symptoms.

Actions Needed
Notify School Nurse or Trained Diabetes Personnel. If possible, check blood sugar, per Diabetes Medical Management Plan. When in doubt, always TREAT FOR HYPOGLYCEMIA.

Mild
- Student may/may not treat self.
- Provide quick-sugar source.
  3-4 glucose tablets
  or
  4 oz. juice
  or
  6 oz. regular soda
  or
  3 teaspoons of glucose gel
- Wait 10 to 15 minutes.
- Recheck blood glucose.
- Repeat food if symptoms persist or blood glucose is less than _____.
- Follow with a snack of carbohydrate and protein (e.g., cheese and crackers).

Moderate
- Someone assists.
- Give student quick-sugar source per MILD guidelines.
- Wait 10 to 15 minutes.
- Recheck blood glucose.
- Repeat food if symptoms persist or blood glucose is less than _____.
- Follow with a snack of carbohydrate and protein (e.g., cheese and crackers).

Severe
- Don't attempt to give anything by mouth.
- Position on side, if possible.
- Contact school nurse or trained diabetes personnel.
- Administer glucagon, as prescribed.
- Call 911.
- Contact parents/guardian.
- Stay with student.

Quick Reference Emergency Plan
for a Student with Diabetes
Hyperglycemia
(High Blood Sugar)

Photo

Student's Name _____

Grade/Teacher _____   Date of Plan _____

Emergency Contact Information:

Mother/Guardian _____   **Father/Guardian** _____

Home phone   Work phone   Cell   Home phone   Work phone   Cell

School Nurse/Trained Diabetes Personnel _____   **Contact Number(s)** _____

Causes of Hyperglycemia
- Too much food   • Illness
- Too little insulin   • Infection
- Decreased activity • Stress

Onset
- Over time—several hours or days

Symptoms

Mild
- Thirst
- Frequent urination
- Fatigue/sleepiness
- Increased hunger
- Blurred vision
- Weight loss
- Stomach pains
- Flushing of skin
- Lack of concentration
- Sweet, fruity breath
- Other: _____

Circle student's usual symptoms.

Moderate
- Mild symptoms plus:
- Dry mouth
- Nausea
- Stomach cramps
- Vomiting
- Other:_____

Circle student's usual symptoms.

Severe
- Mild and moderate symptoms plus:
- Labored breathing
- Very weak
- Confused
- Unconscious

Circle student's usual symptoms.

Actions Needed
- Allow free use of the bathroom.
- Encourage student to drink water or sugar-free drinks.
- Contact the school nurse or trained diabetes personnel to check urine or administer insulin, per student's Diabetes Medical Management Plan.
- If student is nauseous, vomiting, or lethargic, _____ call the parents/guardian or _____ call for medical assistance if parent cannot be reached.

School Responsibilities Under Federal Law

The federal laws described in this section apply to a school's responsibility to help students manage diabetes, including confidentiality requirements. A particular student with diabetes could be covered under only one law or more than one law. For information on getting copies of the laws, see page 209.

Section 504 of the Rehabilitation Act of 1973 (Section 504) and Americans with Disabilities Act of 1990 (ADA)

Section 504 prohibits recipients of federal funds from discriminating against people on the basis of disability. Title II of the ADA prohibits discrimination on the basis of disability by public entities, regardless of whether the public entities receive federal funds. Public school districts that receive federal funds are covered by both Title II and Section 504 and the obligations of public schools to students with disabilities under each law are generally the same. For schools, these laws are enforced by the Office for Civil Rights (OCR) in the U.S. Department of Education.

Section 504 outlines a process for schools to use in determining whether a student has a disability and in determining what services a student with a disability needs. This evaluation process must be tailored individually, since each student is different and his or her needs will vary. Historically, students with diabetes have been covered by Section 504 and the ADA.

Under Section 504, students with disabilities must be given an equal opportunity to participate in academic, nonacademic, and extracurricular activities. The regulations also require school districts to identify all students with disabilities and to provide them with a free appropriate public education (FAPE). Under Section 504, FAPE is the provision of regular or special education and related aids and services designed to meet the individual educational needs of students with disabilities as adequately as the needs of nondisabled students are met.

However, a student does not have to receive special education services in order to receive related aids and services under Section 504. Administering insulin or glucagon, providing assistance in checking blood glucose levels, and allowing the student to eat snacks in school are a few examples of related aids and services that schools may have to provide for a particular student with diabetes. The most common practice is to include these related aids

LAWS

and services as well as any needed special education services in a written document, sometimes called a "Section 504 Plan."

Private schools that receive federal funds may not exclude an individual student with a disability if the school can, with minor adjustments, provide an appropriate education to that student. Private, nonreligious schools are covered by Title III of the ADA.

Individuals with Disabilities Education Act (IDEA)

IDEA provides federal funds to assist state educational agencies and, through them, local educational agencies in making special education and related services available to eligible children with disabilities. IDEA is administered by the Office of Special Education Programs (OSEP) in the Office of Special Education and Rehabilitative Services (OSERS) in the U.S. Department of Education.

A child with a disability must meet the criteria of one or more of 13 disability categories and need special education and related services. The IDEA category of "other health impairment" includes diabetes as one of the health conditions listed. To qualify under IDEA, the student's diabetes also must adversely affect educational performance to the point that the student requires special education and related services, as defined by state law. An example of a child with diabetes who may qualify under IDEA is a student who may have difficulty paying attention or concentrating in the learning environment because of recurring high or low blood glucose levels that adversely affect the student's educational performance.

IDEA requires school districts to find and identify children with disabilities and to provide them a free appropriate public education (FAPE). Under IDEA, FAPE means special education and related services that meet state standards and are provided in conformity with an individualized education program (IEP). The IDEA regulations specify how school personnel and parents, working together, develop and implement an IEP.

Each child's IEP must include the supplementary aids and services to be provided for, or on behalf of, the child and a statement of the program modifications or supports for school personnel that will be provided for the child to make progress and be involved in the general curriculum. Administering insulin or glucagon, providing assistance in checking blood glucose levels, and allowing the student to eat snacks in school are a few examples of related services, supplementary aids and services, or program modifications or supports that schools could provide for a particular student with diabetes who is eligible under IDEA.

Generally, if a child with diabetes needs only a related service and not special education services as defined by state law, that child is not a child with a disability under IDEA and therefore is not eligible for any services under IDEA. Such a child might still be eligible for services under Section 504.

Family Education Rights and Privacy Act (FERPA)

FERPA generally prohibits schools from disclosing personally identifiable information in a student's education record, unless the school obtains the consent of the student's parent or the eligible student (a student who is 18 years old or older or who attends an institution of postsecondary education). FERPA does allow schools to disclose this information, without obtaining consent, to school officials, including teachers, who have legitimate educational interests in the information, including the educational interests of the child. Schools that do this must include in their annual notification to parents and eligible students the criteria for determining who constitutes a school official and what constitutes a legitimate educational interest. Additionally, under FERPA, schools may not prevent the parents of students, or eligible students themselves, from inspecting and reviewing the student's education records.

How can I get copies of the federal laws?

The statutes are found in the United States Code (U.S.C.). The regulations implementing the statutes are found in the Code of Federal Regulations (CFR).

- Section 504 of the Rehabilitation Act of 1973, 29 U.S.C. 794, implementing regulations at 34 CFR Part 104. Available at www.ed.gov/ocr/disability.html.

- Title II of the Americans with Disabilities Act of 1990, 42 U.S.C. 12134 et seq., implementing regulations at 28 CFR Part 35. Available at www.ed.gov/ocr/disability.html.

- To obtain copies of the Section 504 and Title II regulations, you also may contact the Customer Service Team of the Office for Civil Rights, U.S. Department of Education, at (202) 205–5413 or toll-free at 1–800–421–3481. For TTY, call 1–877–521–2172.

- Individuals With Disabilities Education Act, 20 U.S.C. 111 et seq., implementing regulations at 34 CFR Part 300. Available at www.ed.gov/offices/OSERS/OSEP.

- For copies of the IDEA regulations, you also may contact EdPubs at 1–877–433–7827.

- Family Education Rights and Privacy Act (FERPA), 20 U.S.C.1232g, implementing regulations at 34 CFR Part 99. Available at www.ed.gov/offices/OM/fpco.

How can I get more information?

The Office for Civil Rights (OCR) and the Office of Special Education Programs (OSEP) in the U.S. Department of Education can answer questions and provide technical assistance. For more information from OCR, contact OCR's Customer Service Team at (202) 205–5413 or toll-free at 1–800–421–3481. For TTY, call 1–877–521–2172. Information is also available on the OCR website, www.ed.gov/ocr. You may also contact one of OCR's 12 Enforcement Offices around the country. Contact information is available from the OCR Customer Service Team and from the OCR website. For more information from OSEP, call (202) 205–5507 or (202) 205–5637 for TTY. More information about FERPA is available at www.ed.gov/offices/OM/fpco.

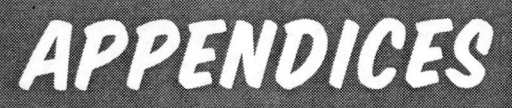

APPENDICES

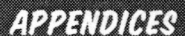

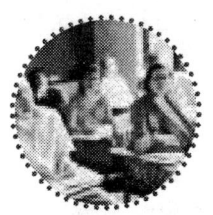

RESOURCE LIST
Help for Students with Diabetes

American Academy of Family Physicians (AAFP)

The AAFP is the national member organization of family doctors. Its website includes articles about the link between obesity and diabetes in young people and how to help children lose weight.

11400 Tomahawk Creek Parkway
Leawood, KS 66211
Phone: (913) 906–6000
www.aafp.org

American Academy of Pediatrics (AAP)

The AAP is a professional membership organization committed to the attainment of optimal physical, mental, and social health and well-being for all infants, children, adolescents, and young adults.

141 Northwest Point Boulevard
Elk Grove Village, IL 60007–1098
Phone: (847) 434–4000
www.aap.org

American Association for Health Education (AAHE)

The AAHE serves health educators and other professionals who promote the health of all people through education and other systematic strategies. Programming focuses on health promotion in schools (K-12), health care, public and community agencies, business/industry, and professional preparation. AAHE is one of six national associations within the American Alliance for Health, Physical Education, Recreation and Dance.

1900 Association Drive
Reston, VA 20191
Toll-free: 1–800–213–7193, Ext. 437
www.aahperd.org/aahe

American Association of Diabetes Educators (AADE)

The AADE is a multidisciplinary organization for health professionals who provide diabetes education and care. The AADE website provides diabetes links, including information about diabetes in children and adolescents.

100 West Monroe Street, Suite 400
Chicago, IL 60603
Toll-free: 1–800–TEAM–UP4
        (1–800–832–6874)
www.aadenet.org

American Council on Exercise (ACE)

The ACE is a nonprofit organization that promotes active, healthy lifestyles and their positive effects on the mind, body, and spirit. Its programs are directed to youths as well as adults.

4851 Paramount Drive
San Diego, CA 92123
Phone: (858) 535–8227
www.acefitness.org

American Diabetes Association (ADA)

The ADA's mission is to prevent and cure diabetes and improve the lives of people with diabetes. Founded in 1940, the association conducts programs in all 50 states and the District of Columbia, reaching hundreds of communities across the country. The ADA is a nonprofit organization that provides diabetes research, information and advocacy. The association offers a variety of programs focused on young people with diabetes.

1701 North Beauregard Street
Alexandria, VA 22311
Toll-free: 1–800–DIABETES
          (1–800–342–2383)
www.diabetes.org

For information about ADA's training curriculum for school personnel:
www.diabetes.org/schooltraining

American Dietetic Association (ADA)

The ADA is a member organization for registered dietitians and registered technicians representing special interests, including public health, sports nutrition, medical nutrition therapy, diet counseling for weight control, cholesterol reduction, and diabetes. More than 5,000 dietitians now belong to the ADA's specialty group on Diabetes Care and Education.

120 South Riverside Plaza, Suite 2000
Chicago, IL 60606–6995
Toll-free: 1–800–877–1600
Consumer referral: 1–800–366–1655
www.eatright.org

American Medical Association (AMA)

The AMA is the nation's leader in promoting professionalism in medicine and setting standards for medical education, practice, and ethics. As the largest physician membership organization in the United States, the AMA is at the forefront of every major development in medicine and is a steadfast and influential advocate for physicians and their patients. The AMA works tirelessly to promote the art and science of medicine and the betterment of public health.

American Medical Association
Science, Quality and Public Health Group
515 N. State Street
Chicago, IL 60610
Phone: (312) 464–4908

American School Health Association (ASHA)

The mission of the ASHA is to promote and improve the well-being of children and youth by supporting comprehensive school health programs. In addition to a journal, the association produces a book for school nurses and families on managing school-age children with chronic health conditions.

Route 43, P.O. Box 708
Kent, OH 44240
Phone: (330) 678–1601
www.ashaweb.org

Barbara Davis Center for Childhood Diabetes

The Barbara Davis Center for Childhood Diabetes is the largest diabetes and endocrine care program in Colorado with unique facilities and resources for clinicians, clinical researchers, and basic biomedical scientists working to help patients with type 1 diabetes. The center provides state-of-the-art clinical diabetes care to a majority of children and many adults within the Rocky Mountain Region.

4200 East Ninth Avenue
Box B -140
Denver, Colorado 80262
Phone: (303) 315–8796
www.barbaradaviscenter.org

Centers for Disease Control and Prevention (CDC)

The CDC serves as the national focus for developing and applying disease prevention and control, environmental health, and health promotion and education activities designed to improve the health of the people of the United States. CDC divisions with special relevance to diabetes in students are the Division of Diabetes Translation, the Division of Nutrition and Physical Activity, and the Division of Adolescent and School Health.

4770 Buford Highway, NE
Atlanta, GA 30341
Toll-free: 1–800-311–3435
www.cdc.gov

Division of Diabetes Translation
Toll-free: 1–877–CDC–DIAB
(1–877–232–3422)
www.cdc.gov/diabetes

Division of Nutrition and Physical Activity
www.cdc.gov/nccdphp/dnpa

Division of Adolescent and School Health
www.cdc.gov/nccdphp/dash

Disability Rights Education and Defense Fund (DREDF)

DREDF is a national law and policy center dedicated to protecting and advancing the civil rights of people with disabilities through legislation, litigation, advocacy, technical assistance, and education and training of attorneys, advocates, persons with disabilities, and parents and children with disabilities.

2212 Sixth Street
Berkeley, CA 94710
Phone: (510) 644–2555
www.dredf.org

Diabetes Exercise and Sports Association

This nonprofit service organization is dedicated to enhancing the quality of life for people with diabetes through exercise.

1647-B West Bethany Home Road
Phoenix, AZ 85015
Toll-free: 1–800–898–4322
www.diabetes-exercise.org

Educational Resources Information Center (ERIC)

The ERIC is a federally funded, nonprofit information network designed to provide ready access to education literature for teachers and parents.

1307 New York Avenue, NW, Suite 300
Washington, DC 20005–4701
Toll-free: 1–800–822–9229
www.eric.ed.gov

Indian Health Service (IHS)
IHS National Diabetes Program

The mission of the IHS is to develop, document, and sustain a public health effort to prevent and control diabetes in American Indian and Alaskan Native communities.

5300 Homestead Road, NE
Albuquerque, NM 87110
Phone: (505) 248–4182
www.ihs.gov

Joslin Diabetes Center

The Joslin Diabetes Center and its affiliates offer a full range of services for children and adults with diabetes, including programs to help youngsters with diabetes and their families to better manage the disease.

1 Joslin Place
Boston, MA 02215
Toll-free: 1–800–JOS–LIN1
        (1–800–567–5461)
www.joslin.harvard.edu

Juvenile Diabetes Research Foundation International (JDRF)

The mission of JDRF is to find a cure for diabetes and its complications through the support of research.

120 Wall Street
New York, NY 10005–4001
Toll-free: 1–800–533–CURE
        (1–800–533–2873)
www.jdrf.org

Lawson Wilkins Pediatric Endocrine Society (LWPES)

The LWPES is a membership organization that promotes the acquisition and dissemination of knowledge of endocrine and metabolic disorders from conception through adolescence. The LWPES website provides links with information about diabetes in children and adolescents.

867 Allardice Way
Stanford, CA 94305
Phone: (650) 494–3133
www.lwpes.org

National Association of Elementary School Principals (NAESP)

The NAESP promotes advocacy and support for elementary and middle level principals and other education leaders in their commitment to all children.

Linkages to Learning
1615 Duke Street
Alexandria, VA 22314
Toll-free: 1–800–38–NAESP
        (1–800–386–2377)
www.naesp.org

National Association of School Nurses (NASN)

The NASN is a nonprofit organization that represents school nurses; it offers continuing education, issues briefs, holds an annual conference, provides legislative updates and position statements, and other materials.

1416 Park Street, Suite A
Castle Rock, CO 80109
Toll-free: 1–866–NASN–SNS
        (1–866–627–6767)
www.nasn.org

For information about the National Association of School Nurses' and the Pediatric Adolescent Diabetes Research Foundation's "P.E.D.S." (Pediatric Education for Diabetes in Schools) training workshop and manual, contact NASN.

National Association of Secondary School Principals (NASSP)

The NASSP is a membership organization of middle level and high school principals, assistant principals, and aspiring school leaders from across the United States and around the world. NASSP's motto is "promoting excellence in school leadership," and the association provides members with various programs and services to guide them in administration, supervision, curriculum planning, and staff development to achieve that goal.

1904 Association Drive
Reston, VA 20191
(703) 860–0200
www.principals.org

National Association of State Boards of Education (NASBE)

The NASBE is a nonprofit association that represents state and territorial boards of education. NASBE's principal objectives include strengthening state leadership in educational policymaking, promoting excellence in the education of all students, advocating equality of access to educational opportunity, and assuring continued citizen support for public education.

277 South Washington Street, Suite 100
Alexandria, VA 22314
Phone (703) 684–4000
www.nasbe.org

National Center on Physical Activity and Disability (NCPAD)

The NCPAD provides information about current research, local programs, adapted equipment, recreation and leisure facilities, and many other aspects of physical activity for persons with disabilities, including children and adolescents with diabetes.

1640 West Roosevelt Road
Chicago, IL 60608
Toll-free: 1–800–900–8086
www.ncpad.org

National Education Association (NEA) Health Information Network

The NEA Health Information Network is the nonprofit health affiliate of the National Education Association, the nation's largest labor organization representing 2.3 million public school employees. The mission of the NEA Health Information Network is to ensure that all public school employees, students, and their communities have the health information and skills to achieve excellence in education.

1201 16th Street, NW
Suite 521
Washington, DC 20036–3290
Phone: (202) 833–4000
www.neahin.org

National Information Center for Children and Youth with Disabilities

This national information and referral clearinghouse on special education and disability-related issues provides information about local, state, or national disability groups and gives technical assistance to parents and professionals.

P.O. Box 1492
Washington, DC 20013–1492
Toll-free: 1–800–695–0285
www.nichcy.org

National Institute of Child Health and Human Development (NICHD), National Institutes of Health

The NICHD conducts and supports laboratory, clinical, and epidemiologic research on the reproductive, neurobiologic, developmental, and behavioral processes that determine and maintain the health of children, adults, families, and populations.

31 Center Drive, MSC 2425
Bethesda, MD 20892–2425
Phone: (301) 496–5133
www.nichd.nih.gov

National Institute of Diabetes and Digestive and Kidney Diseases (NIDDK), National Institutes of Health

The NIDDK conducts and supports research on many of the most serious diseases affecting public health. The Institute supports much of the clinical research on the diseases of internal medicine and related subspecialty fields as well as many basic science disciplines.

National Diabetes Education Program (NDEP)

The NDEP is a federally sponsored program of the National Institutes of Health and the Centers for Disease Control and Prevention, involving over 200 public and private partners to improve diabetes treatment and outcomes for people with diabetes, promote early diagnosis, and prevent diabetes.

1 Diabetes Way
Bethesda, MD 20892–3600
Toll-free: 1–800–438–5383
www.ndep.nih.gov

National Diabetes Information Clearinghouse (NDIC)

The NDIC is a service of the National Institute of Diabetes and Digestive and Kidney Diseases that provides information about diabetes to people with diabetes, their families, health care professionals, and the public.

1 Information Way
Bethesda, MD 20892–3560
Toll-free: 1–800–860–8747
www.niddk.nih.gov

Pediatric Endocrinology Nursing Society (PENS)

The PENS is a nonprofit professional nursing organization with the goal of advancing pediatric endocrine nursing. Its website features articles about diabetes-related topics, including insulin pump therapy, obesity in children, and development of a pediatric diabetes education program for home health nurses.

P.O. Box 2933
Gaithersburg, MD 20886–2933
Phone: Not available. All contact is through mail or email.
Email: Through website under Contact PENS.
www.pens.org

U. S. Department of Agriculture (USDA)

The USDA supports several programs of importance to students with diabetes: the Center for Nutrition Policy and Promotion, the Food and Nutrition Information Center, and the Food and Nutrition Service.

Center for Nutrition Policy and Promotion

www.usda.gov/cnpp

Food and Nutrition Information Center

www.nal.usda.gov/fnic

Food and Nutrition Service

www.fns.usda.gov/fns

U.S. Department of Education*
The mission of the Department of Education is to ensure equal access to education and to promote educational excellence throughout the nation.

400 Maryland Avenue, SW
Washington, DC 20202

Office for Civil Rights (OCR)
Toll-free: 1–800–421–3481
TTY: 1–877–521–2172
www.ed.gov/ocr

Office of Special Education Programs (OSEP)
Phone: (202) 205–5507
TTY: (202) 205–5637
www.ed.gov/offices/OSERS/OSEP

A detailed listing of organizations and programs related to children and adolescents with diabetes and related conditions may be found in

"Resource Directory: Diabetes in Children and Adolescents".

The directory is available on the NDEP website:

WWW.NDEP.NIH.GOV

---

* Resources, including websites, are mentioned in this guide as examples and are only a few of the many appropriate resource materials available. Other materials mentioned are provided as resources and examples for the reader's convenience. Listing of materials and resources in this guide should not be construed or interpreted as an endorsement by the U.S. Department of Education of any private organization or business listed herein.

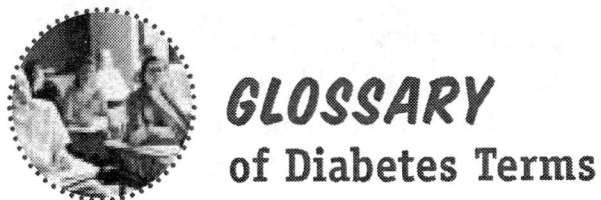

GLOSSARY
of Diabetes Terms

A

Americans with Disabilities Act. A federal law enacted in 1990 to protect people with disabilities from discrimination. Under this law, diabetes can be considered a disability.

Autoimmune disease. A disorder in which the immune system mistakenly attacks and destroys body tissue that it believes to be foreign. In type 1 diabetes, an autoimmune disease, the immune system attacks and destroys the insulin-producing beta cells.

B

Blood glucose level. The amount of glucose in the blood. The recommended blood glucose levels for most people with diabetes are from about 80 to 120 before a meal, 180 or less after a meal, and between 100 and 140 at bedtime.

Blood glucose meter. A device that measures how much glucose is in the blood. A specially coated test strip containing a fresh sample of blood (obtained by pricking the skin, usually the finger, with a lancet) is inserted in the meter, which then measures the amount of glucose in the blood.

Blood glucose monitoring. The act of checking the amount of glucose in the blood. Also called self-monitoring of blood glucose.

C

Carbohydrates. One of the three main classes of foods and a source of energy for the body. Carbohydrates are mainly sugars and starches that the body breaks down into glucose. Foods high in carbohydrates raise blood glucose levels. Carbohydrate foods include: breads, crackers, and cereals; pasta, rice, and grains; vegetables; milk and yogurt; fruit, juice, and sweetened sodas; and table sugar, honey, syrup, and molasses.

Complications of diabetes. Harmful effects that may happen when a person has diabetes. Short-term complications resulting from poorly controlled or uncontrolled diabetes include hypoglycemia (low blood glucose) and hyperglycemia (high blood glucose). Long-term complications, which may develop when a person has had diabetes for a long time, include blindness, amputation of feet or legs, kidney disease, heart disease, stroke, and nerve damage.

D

Diabetes Medical Management Plan. Describes the medical orders or diabetes regimen developed by the student's health care provider and family.

Diabetic Coma. A severe emergency in which a person is not conscious because his or her blood glucose is too low or too high. See also hyperglycemia; hypoglycemia; and diabetic ketoacidosis.

Diabetic ketoacidosis (DKA). A condition that occurs due to insufficient insulin in the body. This can be due to illness, incorrect doses of insulin, or omitting insulin injections. The acidic state that follows causes fruity smelling breath, deep and rapid breathing, stomach pain, nausea, vomiting, and sleepiness. DKA can lead to coma and death if not treated promptly.

F

Fast-acting glucose. Foods containing simple sugar that are used to raise blood glucose levels quickly during a hypoglycemic episode.

G

Glucagon. A hormone that raises the level of glucose in the blood. Glucagon, given by injection, is used to treat severe hypoglycemia.

Glucose. A simple sugar found in the blood. It is the body's main source of energy.

Glucose tablets or gel. Special products that deliver a pre-measured amount of pure glucose. They are a fast-acting form of glucose used to counteract hypoglycemia.

H

Hormone. A chemical produced by an organ that travels in the blood to affect other organs.

Hyperglycemia. A high level of glucose in the blood. High blood glucose can be due to a mismatch in insulin, food, and exercise. Symptoms include thirst, frequent urination, blurred vision, and fatigue.

Hypoglycemia. A low level of glucose in the blood. Low blood glucose is most likely to occur during or after exercise, if too much insulin is present, or not enough food is consumed. Symptoms include feeling shaky, having a headache, or being sweaty, pale, hungry, or tired.

I

Individualized Education Program (IEP). A program designed for students covered by the Individuals with Disabilities Education Act (IDEA).

Individuals with Disabilities Education Act (IDEA). A federal law that provides funds to states to support special education and related services for children with disabilities, administered by the Office of Special Education Programs in the U.S. Department of Education. To be eligible for services under IDEA, a student's diabetes must impair his or her educational performance so that he or she requires special education and related services.

Insulin. A hormone produced by the pancreas that helps the body use glucose for growth and energy. There are several types of insulin that are used in combination to treat people with diabetes. These different types of insulin have been manufactured either to have immediate (rapid-acting or short-acting insulin), intermediate, or long (basal insulin) onset of action and duration of action in the body. A coordinated combination of insulins is used to allow for adequate treatment of diabetes at meals, snacks, during periods of physical activity, and through the night.

Insulin injections. The process of putting insulin into the body with a needle and syringe or an insulin pen.

Insulin pen. A pen-like device used to put insulin into the body.

Insulin pump. A device that delivers a continuous supply of insulin. The insulin is delivered in a steady, measured dose through a system of plastic tubing (infusion set). Most infusion sets are started with a guide needle, then the plastic cannula (a tiny, flexible plastic tube) is left in place, taped with dressing, and the needle is removed.

Insulin resistance. A condition in which the body does not respond normally to the action of insulin. Many people with type 2 diabetes have insulin resistance.

K

Ketoacidosis. See Diabetic ketoacidosis.

Ketones (ketone bodies). Chemicals that the body makes when there is not enough insulin in the blood and the body must break down fat for its energy. Ketones can poison and even kill body cells. When the body does not have the help of insulin, ketones build up in the blood and "spill" over into the urine so that the body can get rid of them. Ketones that build up in the body for

a long time lead to serious illness and coma. See also: Diabetic ketoacidosis.

L

Lancet. A fine, sharp-pointed needle used by people with diabetes for pricking their skin to obtain a sample of blood for blood glucose monitoring.

M

Metabolism. The term for the way cells chemically change food so that it can be used to keep the body alive.

Medical alert identification. An identification card and necklace or bracelet indicating the student has diabetes and giving an emergency number to call.

Mg/dL. Milligrams per deciliter. This term is used in blood glucose monitoring to describe how much glucose is in a specific amount of blood.

N

Nursing Care Plan. A plan developed by the school nurse used to implement the student's diabetes medical management plan. The plan describes functional problem areas, sets goals for overcoming problems, and lists tasks/interventions to meet the goals.

P

Pallor. Abnormal paleness of the skin.

Palpitations. Abnormally rapid or violent beating of the heart.

Pancreas. The organ behind the lower part of the stomach that makes insulin.

Peak effect time. Time when insulin has its major impact on reducing blood glucose levels. See also Insulin.

Q

Quick Reference Emergency Plan. This plan provides school personnel with essential information on how to recognize and treat hypoglycemia or hyperglycemia.

S

Section 504 of the Rehabilitation Act. A federal law that prohibits recipients of federal funds from discriminating against people on the basis of disability.

Syringe. A device used to inject medications such as insulin into body tissue.

T

Target range. A selected level for blood glucose values that the person with diabetes tries to maintain. The target range is usually determined by the physician in consultation with the patient (or parents, if the patient is a child). See also blood glucose levels.

Test strips. Specially designed strips used in blood glucose meters or in urine testing.

Trained Diabetes Personnel. Nonmedical personnel who have basic diabetes knowledge and have received training in diabetes care, including the performance of blood glucose monitoring, insulin and glucagon administration, recognition and treatment of hypoglycemia and hyperglycemia, and performance of urine ketone testing.

U

Urine ketone testing. A procedure for measuring the level of ketones in the urine.

POSITION STATEMENT

Care of Children With Diabetes in the School and Day Care Setting

AMERICAN DIABETES ASSOCIATION

Diabetes is one of the most common chronic diseases of childhood, with a prevalence of ~1.7 affected individuals per 1,000 people aged <20 years (1–4). In the U.S., ~13,000 new cases are diagnosed annually in children (4–7). There are about 125,000 individuals <19 years of age with diabetes in the U.S. (8). The majority of these young people attend school and/or some type of day care and need knowledgeable staff to provide a safe school environment (9–12). Both parents and the health care team should work together to provide school systems and day care providers with the information necessary to allow children with diabetes to participate fully and safely in the school experience.

DIABETES AND THE LAW

— Federal laws that protect children with diabetes include Section 504 of the Rehabilitation Act of 1973, the Individuals with Disabilities Education Act of 1991 (originally the Education for All Handicapped Children Act of 1975), and the Americans with Disabilities Act. Under these laws, diabetes has been considered to be a disability, and it is illegal for schools and/or day care centers to discriminate against children with disabilities. In addition, any school that receives federal funding or any facility considered open to the public must reasonably accommodate the special needs of children with diabetes. Indeed, federal law requires an individualized assessment of any child with diabetes. The required accommodations should be provided within the child's usual school setting

with as little disruption to the school's and the child's routine as possible and allowing the child full participation in all school activities.

Despite these protections, children in the school and day care setting still face discrimination. For example, some day care centers may refuse admission to children with diabetes, and children in the classroom may not be provided the assistance necessary to monitor blood glucose and may be prohibited from eating needed snacks. The American Diabetes Association works to ensure the safe and fair treatment of children with diabetes in the school and day care setting (13–15).

Diabetes care in schools

Appropriate diabetes care in the school and day care setting is necessary for the child's immediate safety, long-term well being, and optimal academic performance. The Diabetes Control and Complications Trial showed a significant link between blood glucose control and the later development of diabetes complications, with improved glycemic control decreasing the risk of these complications (16,17). To achieve glycemic control, a child must monitor blood glucose frequently, follow a meal plan, and take medications. Insulin is usually taken in multiple daily injections or through an infusion pump. Crucial to achieving glycemic control is an understanding of the effects of physical activity, nutrition therapy, and insulin on blood glucose levels.

To facilitate the appropriate care of the student with diabetes, school and day care personnel must have an understanding of diabetes and must be trained in its management and in the treatment of diabetes emergencies. Knowledgeable trained personnel are essential if the student is to avoid the immediate health risks of low blood glucose and to achieve the metabolic control required to decrease risks for later development of diabetes complications. Studies have shown that the majority of school personnel have an inadequate understanding of diabetes and that parents of children with diabetes lack confidence in their teachers' ability to manage diabetes effectively (12,18,19). Consequently, diabetes education must be targeted toward day care providers, teachers, and other school personnel who interact with the child, including school administrators, school coaches, school nurses, health aides, bus drivers, secretaries, etc.

The purpose of this position statement is to provide recommendations for the management of children with diabetes in the school and day care setting.

GENERAL GUIDELINES FOR THE CARE OF THE CHILD IN THE SCHOOL AND DAY CARE SETTING

I. Diabetes Health Care Plan

An individualized Diabetes Health Care Plan should be developed by the parent/guardian, the student's diabetes care team, and the school or day care provider. Inherent in this process are delineated responsibilities assumed by all parties, including the parent/guardian, the school personnel, and the student. These responsibilities are outlined in this position statement. The Diabetes Health Care Plan should address the specific needs of the child and provide specific instructions for each of the following:

1. Blood glucose monitoring, including the frequency and circumstances requiring testing.

The recommendations in this paper are based on the evidence reviewed in the following publications: Diabetes Control and Complications Trial Research Group: The effect of intensive treatment of diabetes on the development and progression of long-term complications in insulin-dependent diabetes mellitus. *N Engl J Med* 329:977–986, 1993; and Diabetes Control and Complications Trial Research Group: The effect of intensive diabetes treatment on the development and progression of long-term complications in adolescents with insulin-dependent diabetes mellitus. *J Pediatr* 125:177–188, 1994.

The initial draft of this paper was prepared by Georgeanna Klingensmith, MD, Francine Kaufman, MD, *Desmond Schatz*, MD, and *William Clarke*, MD. The paper was peer-reviewed, modified, and approved by the Professional Practice Committee and the Executive Committee, November 1998. Most recent review/ revision, 2000.

2. Insulin administration (if necessary), including doses/injection times prescribed for specific blood glucose values and the storage of insulin.
3. Meals and snacks, including food content, amounts, and timing.
4. Symptoms and treatment of hypoglycemia (low blood glucose), including the administration of glucagon if recommended by the student's treating physician.
5. Symptoms and treatment of hyperglycemia (high blood glucose).
6. Testing for ketones and appropriate actions to take for abnormal ketone levels, if requested by the student's health care provider.

Figure 1 includes a sample Diabetes Health Care Plan. For detailed information on the symptoms and treatment of hypoglycemia and hyperglycemia, refer to the *Medical Management of Type 1 Diabetes* (20). A brief description of diabetes targeted to school and day care personnel is included in the APPENDIX; it may be helpful to include this information as an introduction to the Diabetes Health Care Plan.

II. Responsibilities of the various care providers

A. The parent/guardian should provide the school or day care provider with the following:

1. All materials and equipment necessary for diabetes care tasks, including blood glucose testing, insulin administration (if needed), and urine or blood ketone testing. The parent/guardian is responsible for the maintenance of the blood glucose testing equipment (i.e., cleaning and performing controlled testing per the manufacturer's instructions) and must provide materials necessary to ensure proper disposal of materials. A separate logbook should be kept at school with the diabetes supplies for the staff or student to record test results; blood glucose values should be transmitted to the parent/guardian for review as often as requested.
2. Supplies to treat hypoglycemia, including a source of glucose and a glucagon emergency kit, if indicated in the Diabetes Health Care Plan.
3. Information about diabetes and the performance of diabetes-related tasks.

4. Emergency phone numbers for the parent/guardian and the diabetes care team so that the school can contact these individuals with diabetes-related questions and/or during emergencies.
5. Information about the student's meal/snack schedule. The parent should work with the school to coordinate this schedule with that of the other students as closely as possible. For young children, instructions should be given for when food is provided during school parties and other activities.

B. The school or day care provider should provide the following:

1. Training to all adults who provide education/care for the student on the symptoms and treatment of hypoglycemia and hyperglycemia and other emergency procedures. An adult and back-up adult(s) trained to 1) perform fingerstick blood glucose monitoring and record the results; 2) take appropriate actions for blood glucose levels outside of the target ranges as indicated in the student's Diabetes Health Care Plan; and 3) test the urine or blood for ketones, when necessary, and respond to the results of this test.
2. Immediate accessibility to the treatment of hypoglycemia by a knowledgeable adult. The student should remain supervised until appropriate treatment has been administered, and the treatment should be available as close to where the student is as possible.
3. If indicated by the child's developmental capabilities and the Diabetes Health Care Plan, an adult and back-up adult(s) trained in insulin administration.
4. An adult and back-up adult(s) trained to administer glucagon, in accordance with the student's Diabetes Health Care Plan.
5. A location in the school to provide privacy during testing and insulin administration, if desired by the student and family, or permission for the student to check his or her blood glucose level and to take appropriate action to treat hypoglycemia in the classroom or anywhere the student is in conjunction with a school activity,

if indicated in the student's Diabetes Health Care Plan.
6. An adult and back-up adult(s) responsible for the student who will know the schedule of the student's meals and snacks and work with the parent/guardian to coordinate this schedule with that of the other students as closely as possible. This individual also will notify the parent/guardian in advance of any expected changes in the school schedule that affect the student's meal times or exercise routine. Young children should be reminded of snack times.
7. Permission for the student to see school medical personnel upon request.
8. Permission for the student to eat a snack anywhere, including the classroom or the school bus, if necessary to prevent or treat hypoglycemia.
9. Permission to miss school without consequences for required medical appointments to monitor the student's diabetes management. This should be an excused absence with a doctor's note, if required by usual school policy.
10. Permission for the student to use the restroom and have access to fluids (i.e., water) as necessary.
11. An appropriate location for insulin and/or glucagon storage, if necessary.

An adequate number of school personnel should be trained in the necessary diabetes procedures (e.g., blood glucose monitoring, insulin and glucagon administration) and in the appropriate response to high and low blood glucose levels to ensure that at least one adult is present to perform these procedures in a timely manner while the student is at school, on field trips, and during extracurricular activities or other school-sponsored events. These school personnel need not be health care professionals.

The student with diabetes should have immediate access to diabetes supplies at all times, with supervision as needed. Provisions similar to those described above must be available for field trips, extracurricular activities, other school-sponsored events, and on transportation provided by the school or day care facility to enable full participation in school activities.

It is the school's legal responsibility to provide appropriate training to school

Diabetes Care Plan for _____ (name of student) _____ School _____ Effective Dates: _____

To be completed by parents/health care team and reviewed with necessary school staff. Copies should be kept in student's classrooms and school records.

Date of Birth: _____ Grade: _____ Homeroom Teacher: _____

Contact Information:
Parent/guardian #1: _____ Address: _____
 Telephone - Home: _____ Work: _____ Cell Phone: _____
Parent/guardian #2: _____ Address: _____
 Telephone - Home: _____ Work: _____ Cell Phone: _____
Student's Doctor/Health Care Provider: _____ Telephone: _____
 Nurse Educator: _____ Telephone: _____
Other emergency contact: _____ Relationship: _____
 Telephone - Home: _____ Work: _____ Cell Phone: _____
Notify parent/guardian in the following situations: _____

Blood Glucose Monitoring
Target range for blood glucose: _____ mg/dl to _____ mg/dl   Type of blood glucose meter student uses: _____
Usual times to test blood glucose: _____
Times to do extra tests (check all that apply):   _____ Before exercise   _____ When student exhibits symptoms of hyperglycemia
                                                    _____ After exercise   _____ When student exhibits symptoms of hypoglycemia
                                                    _____ Other (explain): _____
Can student perform own blood glucose tests?   Yes   No   Exceptions: _____
School personnel trained to monitor blood glucose level and dates of training: _____

Insulin
Times, types, and dosages of insulin injections to be given during school:
Time   Type(s)   Dosage
_____   _____   _____
_____   _____   _____
_____   _____   _____
School personnel trained to assist with insulin injection and dates of
training: _____

Can student give own injections?   Yes   No
Can student determine correct amount of insulin? Yes   No
Can student draw correct dose of insulin?   Yes   No

For Students with Insulin Pumps:
Type of pump: _____
Insulin/carbohydrate ratio: _____ _____
Correction factor: _____

Is student competent regarding pump?   Yes   No
Can student effectively troubleshoot problems (e.g., ketosis,
pump malfunction)?   Yes   No
Comments: _____
_____
_____

Meals and Snacks Eaten at School (The carbohydrate content of the food is important in maintaining a stable blood glucose level.)

        Time   Food content/amount
Breakfast _____ _____
A.M. snack_____ _____
Lunch   _____ _____
P.M. snack _____ _____
Dinner   _____ _____
Snack before exercise?
  Yes   No   _____
Snack after exercise?
  Yes   No   _____

Other times to give snacks and content/amount: _____
_____
A source of glucose, such as _____,
should be readily available at all times.
Preferred snack foods: _____
Foods to avoid, if any: _____
Instructions for when food is provided to the class, e.g., as part of a class
party or food sampling: _____

Hypoglycemia (Low Blood Sugar)
Usual symptoms of hypoglycemia: _____ _____
_____
Treatment of hypoglycemia: _____
_____
School personnel trained to administer glucagon and dates of training: _____
_____
Glucagon should be given if the student is unconscious, having a seizure
(convulsion), or unable to swallow. If required, glucagon should be
administered promptly and then 911 (or other emergency assistance) and
parents should be called.

Hyperglycemia (High Blood Sugar)
Usual symptoms of hyperglycemia: _____
_____
Treatment of hyperglycemia: _____
_____
Circumstances when urine or blood ketones should be tested:
_____
_____
Treatment for ketones: _____
_____

Exercise and Sports
A snack such as _____ should be readily available at the site of exercise or sports.
Restrictions on activity, if any: _____
Student should not exercise if blood glucose is below _____ mg/dl.

Supplies and Personnel
Location of supplies: Blood glucose monitoring equipment: _____ Insulin administration supplies: _____
                       Glucagon emergency kit: _____ Ketone testing supplies: _____
                       Snack foods: _____
Personnel trained in the symptoms and treatment of low and high blood sugar and dates of training: _____
_____

Signatures
Reviewed by: __[student's health provider/ date]__ Acknowledged/received by: __[guardian/date]__ Acknowledged/received by: __[school representative/date]__

Figure 1—*Diabetes Health Care Plan.*

Position Statement

Table 1—*Resources for teachers, child care providers, parents, and health professionals*

Children with Diabetes: Information for Teachers & Child-Care Providers, Alexandria, VA, American Diabetes Association, 1999 (brochure); available online at www.diabetes.org/ ada/teacher.asp.

Your School & Your Rights: Protecting Children with Diabetes Against Discrimination in Schools and Day Care Centers, Alexandria, VA, American Diabetes Association, 2000 (brochure); available online at http://www.diabetes.org/main/type1/parents_kids/away/scrights.jsp.*

Your Child Has Type 1 Diabetes: What You Should Know, Alexandria, VA, American Diabetes Association, 1999 (brochure); available online at http://www.diabetes.org/main/community /advocacy/type1.jsp*

Treating Diabetes Emergencies: What You Need to Know, Alexandria, VA, American Diabetes Association, 1995 (video); 1-800-232-6733.

Complete Guide to Diabetes, Alexandria, VA, American Diabetes Association, 1999; 1-800-232-6733.

Raising a Child with Diabetes: A Guide for Parents, Alexandria, VA, American Diabetes Association, 2000; 1-800-232-6733.

Clarke W: Advocating for the child with diabetes. *Diabetes Spectrum* 12:230–236, 1999.

Education Discrimination Resources List, Alexandria VA, American Diabetes Association, 2000.*

Wizdom: A Kit of Wit and Wisdom for Kids with Diabetes (and their parents), Alexandria, VA, American Diabetes Association, 2000. Order information and select resources available at www.diabetes.org/wizdom.

The Care of Children with Diabetes in Child Care and School Setting (video); available from, Managed Design, Inc., P.O. Box 3067, Lawrence, KS 66046, (785) 842-9088.

Fredrickson L, Griff M: *Pumper in the School, Insulin Pump Guide for School Nurses, School Personnel and Parents. MiniMed Professional Education, Your Clinical Coach. First Edition, May 2000.* MiniMed, Inc., 1-800-440-7867.

Tappon D. Parker M, Bailey W: *Easy As ABC, What You Need to Know About Children Using Insulin Pumps in School.* Disetronic Medical Systems, Inc., 1-800-280-7801.

*These documents are available in the American Diabetes Association's Education Discrimination Packet by calling 1-800-DIABETES.

staff on diabetes-related tasks and in the treatment of diabetes emergencies. This training should be provided by health care professionals with expertise in diabetes unless the student's health care provider determines that the parent/guardian is able to provide the school personnel with sufficient oral and written information to allow the school to have a safe and appropriate environment for the child. If appropriate, members of the health care team should provide instruction and materials to the parent/guardian to facilitate the education of school staff. Educational materials from the American Diabetes Association and other sources targeted to school personnel and/or parents are available. Table 1 includes a listing of appropriate resources.

III. Expectations of the student in diabetes care

Children and youths should be able to implement their diabetes care at school with parental consent to the extent that is appropriate for the student's develop-

ment and his or her experience with diabetes. The extent of the student's ability to participate in diabetes care should be agreed upon by the school personnel, the parent/guardian, and the health care team, as necessary. The ages at which children are able to perform self-care tasks are very individual and variable, and a child's capabilities and willingness to provide self-care should be respected.

1. *Preschool and day care.* The preschool child is usually unable to perform diabetes tasks independently. By 4 years of age, children may be expected to generally cooperate in diabetes tasks.
2. *Elementary school.* The child should be expected to cooperate in all diabetes tasks at school. By age 8 years, most children are able to perform their own fingerstick blood glucose tests with supervision. By age 10, some children can administer insulin with supervision.
3. *Middle school or junior high school.* The student should be able to administer

insulin with supervision and perform self-monitoring of blood glucose under usual circumstances when not experiencing a low blood glucose level.
4. *High school.* The student should be able to perform self-monitoring of blood glucose under usual circumstances when not experiencing low blood glucose levels. In high school, adolescents should be able to administer insulin without supervision.

At all ages, individuals with diabetes may require help to perform a blood glucose test when the blood glucose is low. In addition, many individuals require a reminder to eat or drink during hypoglycemia and should not be left unsupervised until such treatment has taken place and the blood glucose value has returned to the normal range.

MONITORING BLOOD GLUCOSE IN THE CLASSROOM — It is best for a student with diabetes to obtain a blood glucose level and to respond to the results as quickly and conveniently as possible. This is important to avoid medical problems being worsened by a delay in testing/ treatment and to minimize educational problems caused by missing instruction in the classroom. Accordingly, as stated earlier, a student should be permitted to monitor his or her blood glucose level and take appropriate action to treat hypoglycemia in the classroom or anywhere the student is in conjunction with a school activity, if preferred by the student and indicated in the student's Diabetes Health Care Plan. However, some students desire privacy during testing and this preference should also be accommodated.

In summary, with proper planning and the education and training of school personnel, children and youth with diabetes can fully participate in the school experience. To this end, the family, the health care team, and the school should work together to ensure a safe learning environment.

APPENDIX: BACKGROUND INFORMATION ON DIABETES FOR SCHOOL PERSONNEL — Diabetes is a serious, chronic disease that impairs the body's ability to use food. Insulin, a hormone produced by the pancreas, helps the body convert food into energy. In people with diabetes, either the pancreas does not make insulin or the body cannot use insulin properly. Without insulin, the body's main energy source—glucose—cannot be used as fuel. Rather, glucose builds up in the blood. Over many years, high blood glucose levels can cause damage to the eyes, kidneys, nerves, heart, and blood vessels.

The majority of school-aged youth with diabetes have type 1 diabetes. People with type 1 diabetes do not produce insulin and must receive insulin through either injections or an insulin pump. Insulin taken in this manner does not cure diabetes and may cause the student's blood glucose level to become dangerously low. Type 2 diabetes, the most common form of the disease typically afflicting obese adults, has been shown to be increasing in youth (21). This may be due to the increase in obesity and decrease in physical activity in young people. Students with type 2 diabetes may be able to control their disease through diet and exercise alone or may require oral medications and/or insulin injections. All people with type 1 and type 2 diabetes must carefully balance food, medications, and activity level to keep blood glucose levels as close to normal as possible.

Low blood glucose (hypoglycemia) is the most common immediate health problem for students with diabetes. It occurs when the body gets too much insulin, too little food, a delayed meal, or more than the usual amount of exercise. Symptoms of mild to moderate hypoglycemia include tremors, sweating, light-headedness, irritability, confusion, and drowsiness. A student with this degree of hypoglycemia will need to ingest carbohydrates promptly and may require assistance. Severe hypoglycemia, which is rare, may lead to unconsciousness and convulsions and can be life-threatening if not treated promptly.

High blood glucose (hyperglycemia) occurs when the body gets too little insulin, too much food, or too little exercise; it may also be caused by stress or an illness such as a cold. The most common symptoms of hyperglycemia are thirst, frequent urination, and blurry vision. If untreated over a period of days, hyperglycemia can cause a serious condition called diabetic ketoacidosis (DKA), which is characterized by nausea, vomiting, and a high level of ketones in the blood and urine. For students using insulin infusion pumps, lack of insulin supply may lead to DKA more rapidly. DKA can be life-threatening and thus requires immediate medical attention.

References

1. LaPorte RE, Tajima N, Dorman JS, Cruick-shanks KJ, Eberhardt MS, Rabin BS, Atchison RW, Wagener DK, Becker DJ, Orchard TJ: Differences between blacks and whites in the epidemiology of insulin-dependent diabetes mellitus in Allegheny County, Pennsylvania. *Am J Epidemiol* 123:592–603, 1986
2. Libman I, Songer T, LaPorte R: How many people in the U.S. have IDDM? *Diabetes Care* 16:841–842, 1993
3. Lipman TH: The epidemiology of type 1 diabetes in children 0–14 yr of age in Philadelphia. *Diabetes Care* 16:922–925, 1993
4. Rewers M, LaPorte R, King H, Tuomilehto J: Trends in the prevalence and incidence of diabetes: insulin-dependent diabetes mellitus in childhood. *World Health Stat Q* 41:179–189, 1988
5. American Diabetes Association: *Diabetes 1996 Vital Statistics*. Alexandria, VA, American Diabetes Association, 1996, p. 13–20
6. Dokheel TM, for the Pittsburgh Diabetes Epidemiology Research Group: An epidemic of childhood diabetes in the United States? Evidence from Allegheny County, Pennsylvania. *Diabetes Care* 16:1606–1611, 1993
7. Rewers M: The changing face of epidemiology of insulin-dependent diabetes mellitus (IDDM): research designs and models of disease causation. *Ann Med* 23:419–426, 1991
8. LaPorte RE, Matsushima M, Chang Y-F: Prevalence and incidence of insulin-dependent diabetes. In *Diabetes in America*. 2nd ed. Harris MI, Cowie CC, Stern MP, Boyko EJ, Reiber GE, Bennett PH, Eds.

Washington, DC, U.S. Govt. Printing Office, 1995, p. 37–45 (NIH publ. no. 95-1468)
9. Diabetes Epidemiology Research International Group: Secular trends in incidence of childhood IDDM in 10 countries. *Diabetes* 39:858–864, 1990
10. Kostraba JN, Gay EC, Cai Y, Cruick-shanks KJ, Rewers MJ, Klingensmith GJ, Chase HP, Hamman RF: Incidence of insulin-dependent diabetes mellitus in Colorado. *Epidemiology* 3:232–238, 1992
11. Kyllo CJ, Nuttall FQ: Prevalence of diabetes mellitus in school-age children in Minnesota. *Diabetes* 27:57–60, 1978
12. Wysocki T, Meinhold P, Cox DJ, Clarke WL: Survey of diabetes professionals regarding developmental charges in diabetes self-care. *Diabetes Care* 13:65–68, 1990
13. Jesi Stuthard and ADA v. Kindercare Learning Centers, Inc., Case no. C2-96-0185 (USCD South Ohio 8/96)
14. Calvin Davis and ADA v. LaPetite Academy, Inc., Case no. CIV97-0083-PHX-SMM (USCD Arizona 1997)
15. Agreement, Loudoun County Public Schools and Office of Civil Rights, United States Department of Education (Complaints nos. 11-99-1003, 11-99-1064, 11-99-1069, 1999)
16. Diabetes Control and Complications Trial Research Group: Effect of intensive treatment of diabetes on the development and progression of long-term complications in insulin-dependent diabetes mellitus. *N Engl J Med* 329:977–986, 1993
17. Diabetes Control and Complications Trial Research Group: Effect of intensive diabetes treatment on the development and progression of long-term complications in adolescents with insulin-dependent diabetes mellitus. *J Pediatr* 125:177–188, 1994
18. Hodges L, Parker J: Concerns of parents with diabetic children. *Pediatr Nurse* 13:22–24, 1987
19. Lindsey R, Jarrett L, Hillman K: Elementary schoolteachers' understanding of diabetes. *Diabetes Educ* 13:312–314, 1987
20. Skyler JS (Ed.): *Medical Management of Type 1 Diabetes*. 3rd ed. Alexandria, VA, American Diabetes Association, 1998
21. American Diabetes Association: Type 2 diabetes in children and adolescents (Consensus Statement). *Diabetes Care* 23:381–389, 2000

Identifying and Responding to Domestic Violence: Consensus Recommendations for Child and Adolescent Health

• •

The following guideline for identifying and responding to domestic violence, developed by the Family Prevention Fund's National Health Resource Center on Domestic Violence, has been endorsed by the American Academy of Pediatrics.

IDENTIFYING AND RESPONDING TO
DOMESTIC VIOLENCE

CONSENSUS RECOMMENDATIONS
FOR CHILD AND ADOLESCENT HEALTH

Written by
BETSY MCALISTER GROVES, MSW
MARILYN AUGUSTYN, MD, AAP
DEBBIE LEE
PETER SAWIRES, MA

Produced by
THE FAMILY VIOLENCE
PREVENTION FUND
September 2002

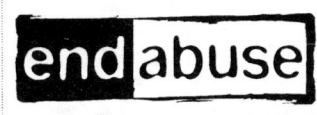

FAMILY VIOLENCE PREVENTION FUND

In partnership with
AMERICAN ACADEMY OF FAMILY PHYSICIANS
AMERICAN ACADEMY OF PEDIATRICS
AMERICAN COLLEGE OF OBSTETRICIANS AND GYNECOLOGISTS
CHILD WITNESS TO VIOLENCE PROJECT BOSTON MEDICAL CENTER
NATIONAL ASSOCIATION OF PEDIATRIC NURSE PRACTITIONERS

Funded by
OFFICE FOR
VICTIMS OF CRIME

With support from
US DEPARTMENT OF HEALTH AND HUMAN
SERVICES, ADMINISTRATION FOR CHILDREN AND
FAMILIES AND THE CONRAD N. HILTON FOUNDATION

ACKNOWLEDGEMENTS

These guidelines were guided by members of the Advisory Committee that met in Boston, MA on December 7, 2001. Their input resulted in further revisions and a final review by the Advisory Committee. The Office of Victims of Crime also reviewed it before finalization.

The Family Violence Prevention Fund (FVPF) wishes to thank the following individuals for their time and rigorous attention to the development of these guidelines. Their expertise, experience and guidance were invaluable

ADVISORY COMMITTEE

Elaine Alpert, MD, MPH
Boston University, School of Public Health
Boston, MA

Linda Chamberlain, PhD, MPH
Alaska Family Violence Prevention Project
Anchorage, AK

Sue Chandler
Center for Community Health Education, Research,
& Services
Boston, MA

Cindy Christian, MD, FAAP
Children's Hospital of Philadelphia,
Division of General Pediatrics
Philadelphia, PA

M. Denise Dowd, MD, MPH
Children's Mercy Hospital
Kansas City, MO

Rev. Dr. Bobbie Groth
Milwaukee Women's Center, Inc.
Milwaukee, WI

Joyce Haas
American Academy of Family Physicians
Leawood, KS

Leah Harrison, MSN, CPNP
National Association of Pediatric
Nurse Practitioners
Bronx, NY

Deborah L. Horan, MSW
American College of Obstetricians
and Gynecologists

Tammy Piazza Hurley
American Academy of Pediatrics
Elk Grove Village, IL

Howard S. King, MD, MPH
Newton-Wellesley Hospital
Newton, MA

Margaret M. McNamara, MD
University of California San Francisco, Department
of Pediatrics
San Francisco, CA

Robert M. Pallay, MD
American Academy of Family Physicians
Hillsborough, NJ

Anu Partap, MD, MPH
Maricopa Medical Center, Department
of Pediatric
Phoenix, AZ

Robert M. Reece, MD
American Academy of Pediatrics
West Falmouth, MA

Molly Resnik, MSW
Domestic Violence Project Safe House
Ann Arbor, MI

 Family Violence Prevention Fund

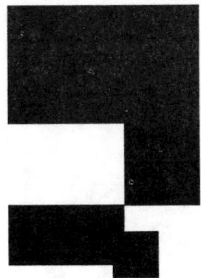

Advisory Committee

Jennifer L. Robertson
The AWAKE Project, Children's Hospital
Boston, MA

Robert D. Sege, MD, PhD
The Floating Hospital for Children,
New England Medical Center
Boston, MA

Howard R. Spivak, MD
New England Medical Center
Boston, MA

Jennifer Stallbaumer-Rouyer, LMSW, LCSW
The Children's Mercy Hospital,
Department of Emergency Medicine
Kansas City, MO

Melinda Strauss, ACSW, LICSW
Partners HealthCare System,
Inc of Newton-Wellesley Hospital
Newton, MA

Peter Stringham, MD
East Boston Neighborhood Health Center
East Boston, MA

Erin E. Tracy, MD, MPH, FACOG
Massachusetts General Hospital
Boston, MA

Therese Zink, MD, MPH
Univeristy of Cincinnati,
Department of Family Medicine
Cincinnati, OH

Barry S. Zuckerman, MD
Boston University School of Medicine/Boston
Medical Center, Department of Pediatrics
Boston, MA

SPECIAL THANKS TO:
Margaret McNamara, MD, Josephine Yeh, JD,
Robin Hassler Thompson, JD, Ariella Hyman, JD,
Nanette Falkenberg, and Sarah Stout

**AND FAMILY VIOLENCE PREVENTION
FUND (FVPF) STAFF:**
Lisa James, MA, Rebecca Whiteman,
Kiersten Stewart, Lonna Davis, Anna Marjavi,
Parry Wu, Jenn Smith, MA, Fran Navarro,
and Erika Rodriguez

ANY ADAPTATION OR REPRINTING OF THIS
PUBLICATION MUST BE ACCOMPANIED BY
THE FOLLOWING ACKNOWLEDGEMENT:

PRODUCED BY
The Family Violence Prevention Fund
383 Rhode Island Street, Suite 304
San Francisco, CA 94103-5133
(415) 252-8900 TTY (800) 595-4889
www.endabuse.org

September 2002

Graphic design by Liz Chalkley

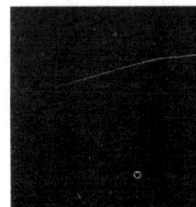

PART 1 | OVERVIEW

Over the past 15 years, there has been a growing recognition among health care professionals that domestic violence is a major health problem with devastating effects on individuals, families and communities. Health care professional associations have issued position statements or guidelines for their members that describe the impact of domestic violence on patients and suggest strategies for inquiring about domestic violence (See **Appendix I** for position statements from several professional associations). Studies show that regular screening for domestic violence in medical settings has been effective in identifying women who are victims[1,2,3] and that victims are not offended when asked about domestic violence.[4,5,6,7,8]

In 1998, the American Academy of Pediatrics (AAP) issued a position statement declaring, "The abuse of women is a pediatric issue."[9] The statement made a strong case for recognizing domestic violence in child health care settings, but did not offer specific guidelines for screening and response or discuss the policy and practice dilemmas that arise when child health providers implement screening and response protocols.

The guidelines offered here provide specific recommendations for screening and responding to domestic violence in child health settings, which provide a unique and important opportunity to screen for domestic violence and to educate parents about the impact of such violence on children. Virtually every child is seen at some point by a health provider. Thus, it is possible to screen every family that uses the health care system.

These guidelines also speak to the need for child health providers to engage in, model, and take leadership in delivering effective primary prevention of domestic violence, as well as other types of family and community violence, by highlighting violence prevention during well child and other routine visits, as a component of routine anticipatory guidance.

Part One of the Guidelines presents an overview of the impact of domestic violence on children and adolescents, and the rationale for regular and universal screening for domestic violence in child health settings. Part Two addresses dilemmas that providers may encounter in discussing domestic violence with parents of their patients and adolescents. Part Three contains the specific guidelines for screening and response. Part Four recommends elements to create a clinical environment that effectively responds to domestic violence. Several useful resources have been included in the Appendices.

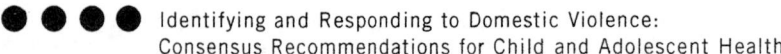

DEFINITIONS

The term **"family violence"** and sometimes **"domestic violence"** has been used to describe acts of violence between family members, including adult partners, a parent against a child, caretakers or partners against elders and between siblings. While all forms of family violence can be devastating, this monograph focuses only on domestic violence or "intimate partner violence." In this monograph, "intimate partner violence" will be used to more specifically define a range of behaviors between intimate or dating partners:

> **"Intimate partner violence"** *is a pattern of purposeful coercive behaviors that may include inflicted physical injury, psychological abuse, sexual assault, progressive social isolation, stalking, deprivation, intimidation and threats. These behaviors are perpetrated by someone who is, was or wishes to be involved in an intimate or dating relationship with an adult or adolescent victim and are aimed at establishing control of one partner over the other.*[10]

Legal definitions of domestic violence or intimate partner violence are generally more restrictive and refer specifically to threats or acts of physical or sexual violence including forced rape, stalking, harassment, certain types of psychological abuse and other crimes where civil or criminal justice remedies apply. Laws vary from state to state. Since evidence exists that non-physical intimate partner violence has many devastating physical, psychological, behavioral and developmental effects, the definition used in these Guidelines is better suited for the identification and treatment of intimate partner violence in the health care setting.

> **"Child exposure to domestic violence or intimate partner violence"** *is a term encompassing a wide range of experiences for children whose caregivers are being abused physically, sexually, or emotionally by an intimate partner. This term includes the child who actually observes his/her parents being harmed, threatened or murdered, who overhears this behavior from another part of the home or who is exposed to the short- or long-term physical or emotional aftermath of care giver's abuse without hearing or seeing a specific aggressive act. Children exposed to intimate partner violence may see their parents' bruises or other visible injuries, or bear witness to the emotional consequences of violence such as fear or intimidation without having directly witnessed violent acts.*[11]

Studies consistently show that the vast majority of victims of intimate partner violence are women. In fact, the latest United States Bureau of Justice Statistics report on intimate violence report found that 85 percent of victims are women.[12] The language in this monograph reflects this trend. However, it is important to note that some victims of intimate partner violence are men, and that violence exists in same-sex relationships as well. All victims should be responded to appropriately.

The term **"screening"** will be used to refer to direct inquiry into domestic violence victimization. It is a term that is widely used in the field referring to the initial questions that are asked regardless of whether signs or symptoms are present, or if the provider does or does not suspect abuse has occurred.

Overview

Prevalence of Intimate Partner Violence

Intimate partner violence is a health problem of enormous proportions. It is estimated that 20 percent to 30 percent of all women and 7.5 percent of men in the United States have been physically and/or sexually abused by an intimate partner at some point in their adult lives.[13,14,15] Heterosexual women are five to eight times more likely than heterosexual men to be victimized by an intimate partner.[16] From 1993 to 1998, victimization by an intimate accounted for 22 percent of the violence experienced by females and three percent of the violent crime sustained by males.[17] Females are also approximately ten times more likely to be killed by an intimate partner than males.

For adolescents, rates of experiencing some form of dating violence vary from 20 to 60 percent.[19,20,21] Women age 16 to 24 experience the highest per capita rate of intimate partner violence with 15.6 victimizations per 1,000 females age 16 to 24, as opposed to 5.8 per 1,000 females in general.[22] Teens are also at higher risk for abuse during pregnancy: 21.7 percent of pregnant teens experience abuse as opposed to 15.9 percent of pregnant adults.[23] While studies indicate that boys and girls may accept physical and sexual aggression as normal in dating and intimate partner relationships, female teens are more likely to receive more significant physical injuries and to be sexually victimized by their partners.[24] Finally, adolescent girls who have been sexually and physically hurt by dating partners are six to nine times more likely to attempt suicide or have suicidal ideation than those who reported no abuse.[25]

Far less data exist on lesbian, gay, transgender, and bisexual (LGTB) victimization, however available literature suggests similarly high rates for LGTB adolescents and adults.[26,27] Intimate partner violence occurs in every community—urban, suburban or rural; in all social classes; and in all ethnic groups. Consequently, all health care settings and professionals are affected by intimate partner violence.

The estimates of numbers of children who are exposed to intimate partner violence vary from 3.3 million to ten million children per year, depending on the specific definitions of witnessing violence, the source of interview and the age of child included in the survey.[28]

Children who are five and under are disproportionately represented in households in which there is intimate partner violence and a sizable number of these children are involved because they call for help, are identified as the cause of the dispute that led to violence, are caught in the cross fire, or are directly physically abused by the perpetrator.[29] In a study conducted in an urban outpatient pediatric clinic, 40 percent of a sample of 160 mothers had filed a restraining order against a boyfriend or husband.[30] In another study conducted in an office-based pediatric practice, 2.5 percent of mothers reported current intimate partner abuse and 14.7 percent reported abuse in past relationships.[31] In the Adverse Childhood Experiences (ACE) Study, conducted on a large sample of members

Overview

(30,000 adults) of the Kaiser Health Plan in California, 12.5 percent of respondents indicated childhood exposure to intimate partner violence and 10.8 percent indicated a history of child abuse, including physical, sexual and emotional abuse.[32] Together these studies indicate that children who witness intimate partner violence are seen with both frequency and regularity in virtually all health settings and that young children are disproportionately represented in the population of children who live with intimate partner violence.

Health Effects of Intimate Partner Violence on Adult and Teen Victims

In addition to injuries sustained by women during violent episodes, physical and psychological abuse are linked to a number of adverse physical health effects including arthritis, chronic neck or back pain, migraine and other frequent headaches, stammering, sexually transmitted infections, chronic pelvic pain, peptic ulcers, spastic colon, and frequent indigestion, diarrhea or constipation.[33] Additionally, optimal management of other chronic illnesses such as asthma, HIV/AIDS, seizure, diabetes and hypertension may be problematic in women who are being abused. Emerging research shows that women who are abused are less likely to engage in important preventive health care behaviors such as regular mammography.[34] Intimate partner violence is also linked with significant short- and long-term mental health consequences for victims.[35,36,37,38,39]

Female adolescents who reported being sexually or physically abused are more than twice as likely to report smoking, drinking and using illegal drugs as non-abused teens.[40] In addition, 32 percent of teen victims report bingeing and purging, compared to 12 percent of non-abused teens. Adolescent women who are battered are also less likely to attend school and less likely to receive good grades if they are in school.[41]

Adolescents' experiences with sex are also associated with their history of dating violence. A study of adolescents found that those who experienced dating violence were more likely than their non-abused peers to have sexual intercourse before age 15 and to have had three or more sex partners in the past three months.[42] Among young mothers on public assistance, half (51 percent) report birth control sabotage by a dating partner.[43] Additionally, high school girls reporting violence from dating partners are approximately four to six times more likely than their non-abused peers to have ever been pregnant.[44] The experience of interpersonal violence is correlated with rapid repeat pregnancy and higher incidences of miscarriage among low-income adolescents.[45] Finally, abused teens are more likely to enter prenatal care later in their pregnancy: 24 percent of teens identified as abused entered prenatal care in the third trimester compared to only nine percent of non-abused teens.[46]

Overview

Health Effects of Intimate Partner Violence on Children

More than 100 studies have explored the effects of intimate partner violence on children. These studies enumerate both short and long term effects of intimate partner violence on children.[47] The most obvious and potentially dangerous risk for children who live in homes in which there is intimate partner violence is that they become direct victims of abuse. In 30 to 60 percent of families affected by intimate partner violence, children are also directly abused.[48] Young children and adolescents are more vulnerable to the abuse. Very young children cannot get out of harm's way, and adolescents more frequently intervene to stop the violence, thereby putting themselves at greater risk for injury.[49]

Children who are exposed to intimate partner violence, particularly chronic episodes of violence, often show symptoms associated with posttraumatic stress disorder. One study found that exposure to intimate partner violence (without being directly victimized) was sufficiently traumatic to precipitate moderate to severe symptoms of posttraumatic stress in 85 percent of the children.[50]

Children who are exposed to intimate partner violence are more likely to exhibit behavioral and physical health problems including chronic somatic complaints, depression, anxiety and violence towards peers.[51] They are also more likely to attempt suicide, abuse drugs and alcohol, run away from home, engage in teenage prostitution and commit sexual assault crimes.[52] Children who are exposed to intimate partner violence have increased difficulties with learning and school functioning.[53] Symptoms of trauma including sleep difficulties, hyper-vigilance, poor concentration and distractibility which interfere with a child's ability to focus and to complete academic tasks in a school setting.

Intimate partner violence also affects parenting. The emotional consequences of being injured, harassed or terrified may be significant for the parent who is victimized. That parent may be less attuned to children's needs or less emotionally available to the children. However this does not mean that victims of intimate partner violence are inherently abusive or neglectful of their children. Parents who batter are generally less involved with child rearing, more likely to use physical punishment and less able to distinguish or recognize the child's needs as separate from the parent's needs.

Children who grow up with violence in the home learn early and powerful lessons about the use of violence in interpersonal relationships. They learn that violence is an acceptable way to assert one's views, get one's way or to discharge stress. These children also learn that violence may be an inherent part of loving relationships. Exposure to violence thus provides justification for children to use violence in their own relationships. This may be particularly true for adolescents.[54]

Studies demonstrate that children are not equally affected by exposure to intimate partner violence.[55,56,57] Children react in different ways to trauma, and they have a range of strengths and vulnerabilities to cope with this stress. Some children appear to be more resilient; others may be deeply affected. Variables such as age, gender, proximity to the violence and the frequency and severity of the violence affect children's responses. In addition, the response of the caregiver and other characteristics of the family and community affect children's responses.

Working Cross Culturally

Intimate partner violence affects people regardless of race, ethnicity, class, sexual and gender identity, religious affiliation, age, immigration status and ability. The term culture is used in this context to refer to those axes of identification and other shared experiences. Because of the sensitive nature of abuse, providing culturally relevant care is critical when working with victims of abuse. In order to provide care that is accessible and tailored to each patient and their family, providers must consider the multiple issues that victims may deal with simultaneously (including language barriers, limited resources, homophobia, acculturation, accessibility issues and racism) and recognize that each victim of intimate partner violence will experience both the abuse and the health system in culturally specific ways.

Disparities in access to and quality of health care also impact providers ability to help victims of intimate partner violence. For example, women who are members of racial and ethnic minority groups are more likely than white women to experience difficulty communicating with their doctors, and often feel they are treated disrespectfully in the health care setting.[58] English-speaking Latinos, Asians and Blacks report not fully understanding their doctors and feeling like their doctors were not listening to them.[59] People with cognitive or communication disabilities may be dependent on an abusive intimate partner and thus at especially high risk. In addition, some patients may experience abuse from the health care system itself and this may affect their approach to and utilization of the health care system.[60]

Providers also enter health care encounters with their own cultural experiences and perspectives that may differ from those of the victim. In a successful health care interaction within a diverse client population, the provider communicates effectively with the patient, is aware of personal assumptions, asks questions in a culturally sensitive way and provides relevant interventions. Eliciting specific information about the patient's beliefs and experience with abuse, sharing general information about intimate partner violence relevant to that experience and providing culturally accessible resources in the community, improves the quality of care for victims of violence. In addition, having skilled interpreters who are trained to understand intimate partner violence (and not family members, caregivers or children) is crucial when helping non-English speaking patients[61] and their families. Culturally sensitive screening questions for all caretakers and adolescent patients

Overview

can facilitate discussion and help providers offer appropriate and effective interventions.

Identifying and Responding to Abuse Can Make a Difference

The health care system plays an important role in identifying and preventing public health problems. Models developed to identify other chronic health problems may effectively be applied to intimate partner violence. **A primary starting point to improve the medical practice approach to intimate partner violence is routine screening, with a focus on early identification of all families and victims of intimate partner violence whether or not symptoms are immediately apparent.**

Since nearly all young children and teens are seen at some point in a health care setting, these settings present a compelling opportunity to identify teens, mothers and children who may be living with intimate partner violence. A 2001 study in North Carolina found that only 23 percent of women injured by a partner shortly after pregnancy received treatment for their injuries. However, almost all of these women used health care services for their infants, indicating that child health settings are potentially important for identifying intimate partner violence.[62]

Universal and regular face-to-face screening of women in adult health settings by skilled health care providers markedly increases the identification of victims of intimate partner violence, as well as those who are at risk for verbal, physical and sexual partner abuse.[63,64] Expert opinion suggests that such interventions in adult health settings may lead to reduced morbidity and mortality.[65] Screening can assist clinicians in their diagnosis and assure more appropriate care for a victim's health symptoms by treating the underlying problems. Screening also gives victims a valuable opportunity to tell their providers about their experiences with abuse.[66] Battered women report that one of the most important parts of their interactions with their physicians is being listened to about the abuse. *(See Appendix III: Abstracts of selected studies on Provider and Patient Attitudes: Forward Screening for IPV in the Child Health Setting).*

Although there is no research as yet that proves the efficacy of screening in child health settings, it is reasonable to assume that such screening would increase opportunities for identification and intervention within families, thereby enabling pediatric, family practice and primary care providers to assist both victims and their children. When child witnesses of intimate partner violence, victims or those at risk for intimate partner violence are identified early, providers may be able to intervene to help patients understand their options, live more safely within the relationship or safely leave the relationship. The child health care provider's direct discussion about safety at home tells the family that this is an important topic and one that belongs in the realm of pediatric and family practice care. Even if a woman denies that she is being abused, the provider can often lay the groundwork for the possibility of future disclosure or discussion of the issue.

PART 11 | DILEMMAS FACED BY PROVIDERS

A policy of universal and regular screening for intimate partner violence in child health settings presents dilemmas to the providers who conduct the screening that may not exist when screening patients in an adult health setting. Perhaps the fundamental difference lies in the fact that adults are not the primary patients during pediatric visits. This section reviews several major dilemmas and provides specific recommendations for responding. Because these dilemmas present challenging practice and ethical questions for the provider, this panel strongly recommends that child health practices have access to legal consultation, as well as consultation from battered women's service providers, child protection and child mental health. These resources can be helpful in making decisions about how to intervene in ways that do not increase risk for the family or unnecessarily alienate the non-offending parent.

When Does Child Exposure to Intimate Partner Violence Become Child Maltreatment?

Because of the high rate of co-occurrence of intimate partner violence and child abuse, child health providers need to be concerned about the possibility of child abuse whenever intimate partner violence is disclosed. Whenever a child is abused, either intentionally or unintentionally, as a result of intimate partner violence, state law requires health care providers to report this abuse to child protection services. Mandated reporters would also report any high-risk situation of intimate partner violence in which children are at risk.

However, state laws are less clear about whether exposure to domestic violence in the absence of injury or serious risk of injury to the child would require a report to children's protective services.

- In some states, stringent rules/laws require mandated reporters to notify child protection services whenever a child is in the home and has been exposed to a parent's abuse, whether or not the child has been directly abused. Proponents of this definition point to the ample documentation of the overlap between adult intimate partner violence and child abuse and the adverse psychological effects on children who witness intimate partner violence. Opponents of this policy believe it penalizes women for abuse that they have no control over and may discourage women from seeking help.

- In other states, a child's exposure to intimate partner violence does not automatically require a mandatory child protection report. The provider has wider discretion to assess whether a child has been directly involved and what other factors may exist to put the child at risk. In these states, a provider would take into account the existence of direct injury to a child, the potential danger of the situation, and the capacity of the mother to keep her children safe in deciding whether to notify Child Protective Services (CPS).

Dilemmas

Many victim advocates recommend having the victim place a phone call themselves to CPS from the practitioner's office, thus protecting her from charges of "failure to protect" while simultaneously protecting the child and meeting statutory child abuse reporting laws.

Unless a child health care provider is legally required to report all incidences of intimate partner violence to CPS, it is preferable to make this decision based on the specifics of the case and the provider's clinical judgment. In some instances, the children are not in danger; the victim has planned for their safety and is responding adequately to the child's needs or emotional reactions. In these cases, a provider should offer voluntary services and support instead of simply submitting a report to CPS, especially if not mandated.

A policy that automatically defines child exposure to intimate partner violence as neglect or maltreatment assumes that victims are neglectful parents solely because their children witnessed the abuse, implying that somehow the victim could have stopped the abuse. This approach implies that not only are these parents victims of abuse, but that they also bear the responsibility for child neglect. This may be inaccurate and unfair. This policy also makes the assumption that all children are adversely affected by exposure to violence, no matter the circumstances. It ignores the fact that some children are more adversely affected than others and that some families and communities are more able to support children than others. Finally, opponents of this policy allege that mandatory reports also would increase the demands on protective services—a system that is already overburdened and under funded in most states.[67] In addition, the practice of routinely reporting intimate partner violence incidents that involve children to protective services discourages victims from seeking help with intimate partner violence. If a victim believes that children may be removed from her care, she will be less likely to seek help from medical professionals. A mandatory reporting policy also may discourage child health care providers from screening for intimate partner violence because they do not want to involve protective services in their patient's life.

RECOMMENDATIONS:

Know your state's child abuse reporting laws (see **Appendix IX**) and its specific policies on defining child exposure to intimate partner violence as child maltreatment. In a state that requires mandated reporting in all cases of intimate partner violence, the provider should inform the non-offending parent of the obligation to file a report to CPS, assess the safety needs of the victim, and inform CPS about the specifics of the perpetrator, his anticipated response and the potential for danger. In states where more discretion is left to the provider, the provider should assess the specifics of each situation as a means of making a decision about whether it is necessary to make a report. The assessment should include inquiries about injury or abuse to children, the current safety of the home, and whether the perpetrator has made threats to the children. Depending on the answers to these questions, the provider can make a decision about the imminent risk of harm to the child

DILEMMAS

Dilemmas

and victim. If the situation is not currently dangerous, the provider can refer the victim to voluntary services: battered women's services, counseling (preferably with a provider who has worked with victims of intimate partner violence), or child-focused services. If the situation is currently dangerous to the child, a report needs to be filed. Consider involving the mother in filing the report and follow the recommendations above to maximize the protection afforded to the mother during the CPS investigation.

BOX 1

In States with Mandatory Reporting Requirements for Child Exposure to Intimate Partner Violence

PROVIDERS SHOULD:
- Inform the non-offending parent of obligation to report to CPS
- Assess the safety needs of the victim
- Give CPS specific information about the perpetrator, the intimate partner violence, and the potential for danger
- Have resources available for the non-offending parent

In States with Less Specific Reporting Requirements for Child Exposure to Intimate Partner Violence

PROVIDERS SHOULD DECIDE WHETHER TO FILE A REPORT WITH CPS BASED ON:
- An inquiry about direct injury to child
- An assessment of potential for danger (threats, weapons, substance abuse)
- An assessment of mother's ability to plan for children's safety
- An assessment of support and connections to community

If provider decides not to report to CPS, he/she should offer referrals to voluntary services and provide follow-up care.

IF PROVIDER DOES DECIDE TO REPORT:
- Consider asking the mother to file a report herself to avoid charges of "failure to protect"
- Follow all the steps outlined above for reports in mandated states

Dilemmas

Intimate Partner Violence Victimization Reporting Requirements for Health Care Providers

While all states mandate reporting of child abuse or neglect, most states have also enacted general mandatory reporting laws which require the reporting of specified injuries and wounds, suspected abuse or intimate partner violence for individuals being treated by a health care professional. These mandatory reporting laws are distinct from child abuse, elder abuse or vulnerable adult abuse reporting laws, in that the individuals to be protected are not limited to a specific class. These laws pertain to all individuals to whom the health care professional provides treatment or medical care, or who come before the health care facility.

The laws vary from state to state, but generally fall into four categories: 1) states that require reporting of injuries caused by weapons; 2) states that mandate reporting for injuries caused in violation of criminal laws, as a result of violence, or through non-accidental means; 3) states that specifically address reporting in intimate partner violence cases; and 4) states that have no general mandatory reporting laws. *(See **Appendix VII** for state codes on Intimate Partner Violence Victimization Reporting Requirements for Health Care Providers).*

In the majority of states, neither statutory nor case law specifies if a health care provider must report a parent's injuries if they are observed or discovered during a health care visit with that parent's child. Therefore, under a strict reading of most laws, if a child's health care provider is not providing treatment or medical care to the abused parent during the child's visit, the health care provider would not be required to make a report. In family practice situations where the child and parent are the provider's patients, and the current visit appointment is for the child, the same reasoning could be applied, although it is less clear-cut. That is, the health care provider would not be required to report since he or she is not treating the parent for the specified injuries during the appointment. This issue merits further discussion among health care providers, advocates, licensing authorities, and other professionals, as it is uncharted territory. There has been much debate about the benefit of mandatory reporting of intimate partner violence by health care providers. *(A more extensive discussion of these laws, their risks and benefits, and their application to pediatric and family practice providers can be found in **Appendix VI**.)*

RECOMMENDATIONS:

Providers should know their state's intimate partner violence reporting law, including who is required to report and under what conditions. *(**Appendix VIII** contains a chart listing state codes).* In order to maximize patient input regarding law enforcement action, providers should also familiarize themselves with how their local law enforcement agency responds to such reports. Becoming familiar with such procedures will allow the provider

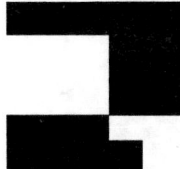

Dilemmas

to better assist the patient in safety planning, and in knowing what to expect. Intimate partner violence reporting responsibilities should be carefully discussed with teens prior to screening for dating violence or intimate partner violence in their homes. Additionally, recent federal privacy regulations require providers to inform patients of health information use and disclosure practices in general, and whenever a specific report has been made. Health care facilities should ensure that their intimate partner violence protocols and training materials address their state reporting laws and federal regulations.

Asking about Intimate Partner Violence with a Child in the Room

Providers differ in their practice of asking sensitive questions to the mother when the child is present. Generally, if the child is under age three, most providers assume that asking a mother about safety or other sensitive issues is appropriate. However, there is not consensus about whether to require that an older child not be present in the room when screening the mother for intimate partner violence. Some providers are concerned about asking questions when older children are present. They assert that having the child in the room will be a barrier to disclosure because parents will avoid discussing it in front of their children. Some say that it would be upsetting for children to hear such conversation or that children may reveal the conversation to the batterer which may endanger the mother and child. Other providers believe that the screening questions about intimate partner violence should be asked regardless of the age of the child. They assert that children generally are aware of the intimate partner violence and that mothers will indicate if they are uncomfortable with the subject, thus giving the provider the opportunity to schedule a more private conversation with the parent.

RECOMMENDATIONS:

It is best to conduct screening without children in the room. Screening should occur regardless of the age of the child. In some practices it is possible to have the child wait in a supervised waiting area or under the supervision of another staff member. In other practice settings, it is not possible to have children leave the exam room. In these situations, providers can ask general questions and should always be sensitive to the comfort level of the parent. If the parent seems uncomfortable, the provider can offer other options for talking more privately, either by telephone or in a follow-up visit. Providers should be aware of the impact of a disclosure on a child, and should ask follow-up questions about the child and family's safety.

Dilemmas

BOX 2

Asking about Intimate Partner Violence with a Child in the Room

Child in the Room
PRACTICAL POINTS:
1. Ask general questions first.
2. Be sensitive to comfort level of parent.
3. If parent is uncomfortable, schedule a time to talk without the child present.

Child not in the Room
PRACTICAL POINTS:
1. Ask during routine parts of visit when child is not in the room: vision screening, immunizations, laboratory work.
2. Have the child wait briefly in a supervised waiting area if possible.

Documentation

There is no consensus over the procedure for documenting the presence of intimate partner violence in a family in a child's chart. If the batterer is the biological or custodial parent, he may have access to the chart and the information about the victim would thus not be confidential. Therefore, putting information about intimate partner violence disclosures in the child's chart may not be advisable. On the other hand, the information is important and other providers who work with the family should know about this risk factor if they read the child's chart. Charting can also be helpful to the victim should custody disputes arise.

RECOMMENDATIONS:

A review of the literature and current practice reveals that recommendations for documentation are contradictory and inconsistent. One recommendation is for the provider to document all screenings for intimate partner violence in the child's chart. The suggested notation, perhaps in the section on anticipatory guidance, is: "The parent was routinely asked about verbal abuse, threats, physical violence in the home and community. If so, the parent was offered information about community resources for safety planning and counseling."[68] This type of routine documentation is recommended for tracking and quality assurance. If possible, the documentation for the outcome of the screening (if positive for abuse) should be placed in the woman's health chart or in social work notes where there is more protection of confidentiality. Some practices use non-specific terms or a code word to indicate the presence of intimate partner violence in a child's chart: for example, "family problems," "difficult home situation" or "+ wtv." Some practices maintain a section of the child's chart that is confidential and is not released when there is a request for medical records. A brief notation of intimate partner violence in this section is appropriate. Intimate partner violence should not be listed as a discharge diagnosis on billing information that is sent home or can otherwise be viewed by the perpetrator.

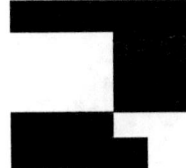

Dilemmas

If the provider is unsure about documentation and its confidentiality from the battering parent, he/she should consult with medical records experts, billing personnel, risk management professionals or attorneys.

BOX 3

Options for Documentation

- Document that inquiry has occurred.
- Document results of inquiry by using non-specific terms or code works: "family problems," "difficult home situation," or "wtv."
- Maintain a section of the child's chart that is confidential (not released with a request for medical records). Document finding of intimate partner violence in this section.
- If possible, document the existence of intimate partner violence in the woman's health chart or in social work notes where there is more confidentiality.

Responding to a Child's Disclosure of Intimate Partner Violence in the Home

Direct disclosures of intimate partner violence occur more frequently with older children or teenagers who see child health providers without their parents. If the parents are unaware of the disclosure, the provider must decide how to inform the parents in a way that protects the child and does not create an unsafe situation in the home. The provider may feel uncomfortable about how to handle this disclosure. Should the provider notify child protective services? What are the consequences for the child who tells someone outside the family about the violence? What are the issues and laws related to confidentiality?

RECOMMENDATIONS:

Find out as much specific information as possible about the abuse and the extent of risk for the child and the adult victim. If the situation is dangerous, notify protective services. Inform the child of your concern about his/her safety and tell the child that you would like to speak to the non-offending parent about the situation. Inform the non-offending parent of the child's concerns, taking care to stress that you are concerned and that you want to be helpful and supportive. Ask if the parent is safe and what types of supports would be helpful. If possible, make a referral to an intimate partner violence support agency or to counseling/social services/mental health. Schedule a follow-up appointment for the next week.

Dilemmas

BOX 4

Responding to Child Disclosure of Intimate Partner Violence

PRACTICAL POINTS:

- Inform the child of your concern about her/his safety and that you intend to speak to the non-offending parent about the situation.
- Inform the non-offending parent of the child's concerns.
- Ask if the parent is safe and what types of supports would be helpful.
- If possible make a referral to an intimate partner violence support agency or to counseling/social services/mental health for the adult or adolescent victim and their children.
- Schedule a follow-up appointment for the next week.
- Notify protective services if there are safety concerns about the child.

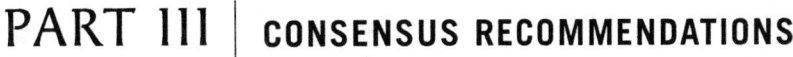

PART III | CONSENSUS RECOMMENDATIONS

SCREENING FOR INTIMATE PARTNER VIOLENCE WHEN YOUR PATIENT IS A CHILD OR ADOLESCENT

All health care providers seeing children and adolescents should provide intimate partner violence screening as part of routine patient care in public health, private practice and managed care settings.

Who and How Often to Screen

- Screen female caregivers/parents who accompany their children during new patient visits; at least once per year at well child visits; and, thereafter, whenever they disclose a new intimate relationship.
- Screen female and male caregivers/parents known to be in same-sex relationships who accompany their children during new patient visits; at least once per year at well-child visits; and, thereafter; whenever they disclose a new intimate relationship.
- Screen adolescents during new patient visits; at health maintenance visits once per year; or whenever they disclose a new intimate relationship.
- Ask pregnant teens at first pre-natal visit; at least once per trimester; and at the postpartum visit.[i]
- Also ask whenever signs and symptoms raise concerns:[ii]
  - Specifically, screen when the child or adolescent has:
    - Obvious physical signs of physical or sexual abuse;
    - Behavioral or emotional problems, such as increased aggression, increased fear or anxiety, difficulty sleeping or eating, or other signs of emotional distress; or
    - Chronic somatic complaints.
  - When adults present with obvious physical injuries or a history of intimate partner violence.

*(See **Appendix IV**: Dilemmas When Screening All Patients for Victimization).*

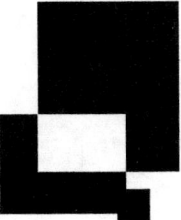

---

[i] Recommended by the American College of Obstetricians and Gynecologists
[ii] See *Appendix V*: Indicators of Abuse.

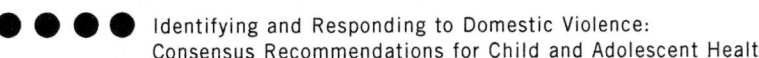

BOX 5

Who and How Often to Screen

TYPE OF VISIT	WHO TO SCREEN	WHEN TO SCREEN
New Born	Caregiver	At postpartum visit
New Patient	Caregiver & Adolescent	At first visit
Well Child:		
Child	Caregiver	At 2, 6 and 12 months, then yearly
Adolescent	Adolescent	Yearly
Prenatal	Adolescent Mother	Once per trimester
Mental Health	Caregiver & Adolescent	At initial visit
Emergency	Caregiver & Adolescent	At every visit
Other Visits	Caregiver or Adolescent	Whenever there are physical or behavioral indicators or chronic somatic complaints

How to Screen

- Direct questions should be asked, whether or not signs or symptoms are present and whether or not the provider suspects abuse has occurred.
- Inform patient about the limits of practitioner/patient confidentiality related to intimate partner violence prior to screening.
- Use language that is direct, specific and easy to understand.
- Conduct screening in a private room.
- For a parent, it should take place without the intimate partner or other adult family members present.
- For adolescents, it should take place without the parent (or partner) in the room.
- Can be included as part of a written health questionnaire or health history, but this should not replace face-to-face screening.
- Should be conducted in a patient's primary language.
- If an interpreter is used, it should not be an acquaintance or relative of the family. Children should never be used as interpreters.

What to Ask[iii]

Intimate partner violence questions can be framed within discussion of other safety issues such as car and bicycle helmet safety, and assessing for guns at home or community violence.

[iii] There are no controlled studies of the efficacy of screening questions in pediatric or family practice settings. The questions we propose are drawn from three sources: Family Violence Prevention Fund, Preventing Domestic Violence: Clinical Guidelines on Routine Screening. San Francisco, October, 1999. Groves, B. (1994). Children who Witness Violence, in Developmental and Behavioral Pediatrics: A Handbook for Primary Care. Parker, S. and Zuckerman, B., eds. Boston, Little Brown & Co. 334-336. McNamara M. (2001). "Clinical guidelines for screening and responding to child and youth exposure to domestic violence for healthcare providers". LINC (Living in a Nonviolent Community), UCSF Department of Pediatrics, November 2001.

Consensus Recommendations

For Adults who Accompany Their Children:

INTRODUCTORY STATEMENTS OR QUESTIONS
- "I have begun to ask all of the women/parents/caregivers in my practice about their family life as it affects their health and safety, and that of their children. May I ask you a few questions?"
- "Violence is an issue that unfortunately effects everyone today and thus I have begun to ask all families in my practice about exposure to violence. May I ask you a few questions?"

INDIRECT QUESTIONS
- "What happens when there is a disagreement with your partner/husband/boyfriend or other adults in your home?"
- "Do you feel safe in your home and in your relationship?"

DIRECT QUESTIONS
- "Have you ever been hurt or threatened by your partner/husband or boyfriend?"
- "Do you ever feel afraid of (or controlled or isolated by) your partner/husband/boyfriend?"[iv]
- "Has your child witnessed a violent or frightening event in your neighborhood or home?"

For Adolescents

INTRODUCTORY STATEMENTS OR QUESTIONS
- "Many teens your age experience threats, name calling, uninvited touching, sex or violence, so I ask all my teen patients about it. May I ask you a few questions?"
- "I don't know if this is a concern for you, but many teens I see are dealing with violence or bullying issues, so I've started asking questions about violence routinely."
- "Sometimes when I see an injury like yours, it's because somebody got hit. How did you get this injury/bruise?"
- "Now I am going to ask you confidential questions. The answers are confidential, unless your health is in immediate danger."
- "How are disagreements handled in your family?"

INDIRECT QUESTIONS
- "Are you in a relationship or seeing anyone?" or "Do you have a boyfriend or girlfriend? What happens when you disagree with them?"
- "How are your parents getting along?"

[iv] In case of same-sex relationships we recommend using "partner" or mirroring the language of the adult being screened. For example, if a parent refers to her same-sex partner as "roommate," use "roommate." If the sexual orientation is unknown, we recommend "partner."

 Identifying and Responding to Domestic Violence:
Consensus Recommendations for Child and Adolescent Health

Consensus Recommendations

• "How often do you have yelling or screaming fights? Do any of them involve pushing or slapping?"

DIRECT QUESTIONS:
• "Sometimes if someone is being hurt in her/his own relationship, they may have seen it happen in their own family. Have you seen anyone get hurt in your home?"
• "Teens see a lot of violence these days. Seeing parents or other adults fight can feel as bad as being hit yourself. Has this happened to you?"
• "We all have disagreements sometimes with family members or friends. Have you ever been hurt or threatened by anyone?"
• "Have you ever been hurt – hit, kicked, slapped, shoved, pushed by a friend or person you know?"
• "Have you ever been forced to do something sexual that you didn't want to do?" —as part of sexual history.
• "Do you ever feel afraid of or controlled by someone you're dating or a friend?"
• "Has anyone hit you at home in the last year?"

QUESTIONS BASED ON INDICATORS:
• "I noticed that you have an injury. Sometimes injuries like that come from someone hurting you. What happened to you?"

Asking about Intimate Partner Violence with a Child in the Room

There are different opinions about whether inquiry about sensitive issues such as intimate partner violence should take place with the child in the room or whether the questions should be asked without the child's presence. For further discussion of this issue, see page 247.

• If it is possible to see the parent without the child, (e.g. the child is old enough to wait alone; the child is in a supervised waiting area; the child is having laboratory work or vision /hearing screening done), questions can be asked in the manner mentioned in the section "What to Ask" on page 252.
• For children under age three, asking the mother questions about safety and relationships in the presence of the child is generally not an issue.

IF THE CHILD IS IN THE ROOM:
• Begin inquiry with an indirect question (see section "What to Ask" (on page 252).
• If parent appears uncomfortable or upset and it is not possible to see the parent alone in this visit, ask if there is another time to speak by telephone or to follow-up.
• If parent appears comfortable with the questions, proceed to ask more specific questions about intimate partner violence.

Who Should Screen

QUESTIONS CAN BE ASKED BY ANY HEALTH CARE PROVIDER WHO IS:
- Educated about the dynamics of intimate partner violence, how children are affected and how to assess safety of children and/or know what resources are available for further assessment and counseling services;
- Trained on how to ask about abuse, how to assess the safety needs of an abuse victim, and how to assist the victim, and who recognizes her autonomy and right to make her own decision or is trained to refer the patient to someone who can assess safety needs and further assist her;
- Sensitive to issues of culture and class in interactions with patients; and
- Knowledgeable about community resources.

RESPONDING TO INTIMATE PARTNER VIOLENCE WHEN YOUR PATIENT IS A CHILD OR ADOLESCENT

If the patient or his/her mother tells you that s/he has been abused, you become an important part of her/his support system. Living with intimate partner violence or making the decision to leave a relationship are ongoing issues for both patient and family that affect their health care. Providers need to respect the integrity and authority of victims of intimate partner violence to make decisions about their own relationships, even if the provider does not agree with those decisions. The health care provider can play an important role in the victim's decision making process by asking the right questions, providing information about the nature of intimate partner violence, giving messages of support, and letting her know about resources available to her. At times it will be appropriate for the health care provider to make recommendations about what to do, but only after understanding the reality of the victim's situation and only with the understanding that, ultimately, the victim must and will make her own choices, not withstanding child abuse laws.

Support the Victim

- Express concern for the patient's or parent's safety.
- If the victim is comfortable, encourage her/him to talk about what has happened.
- Listen without making judgments.
- Tell victims that they are not alone and that you and other people can help them.
- Tell her/him that the violence is not their fault, s/he does not deserve to be abused and that only her/his abuser can stop the abuse, and that there is no excuse for intimate partner violence.
- Make sure s/he knows that there is help available and that there are people s/he can turn to for support.

Consensus Recommendations

- Remind the victim that you are a resource, should s/he need further assistance.
- Inform the attending parent or adolescent of any reporting laws and requirements.

Provide Information on Intimate Partner Violence

- Intimate partner violence is common (among all social strata, educational levels and ethnic groups).
- Most violence continues for a long time and often gets more frequent and more severe.
- Violence happens in all kinds of relationships – including teen relationships and LGBT relationships.
- Violence in the home can harm all family members including children, both physically and emotionally.
- There are resources for families, and this clinic/practice/provider can help find them.
- Intimate partner violence affects victim health and the health of the family.

What to Say to the Child Who has Witnessed Intimate Partner Violence

If a parent discloses intimate partner violence, the provider with the parent's permission can specifically acknowledge the disclosure with the child by saying:

- "What are your worries about the fighting at home?"
- "I am concerned about the safety of people in your home and I am glad your mother told me about this."
- "What is going on in your house is not your fault."
- "You are not responsible for solving these problems. I am going to work with your mother (father, caretaker, etc.) to try to make things better."

The way in which the provider discusses these issues with children will vary by their age and level of cognitive development. For a four-year-old, it is probably sufficient to provide simple acknowledgment and reassurance about safety. For an eight-year-old, it may be appropriate to add more specific reassurances about what steps the parent is taking to handle the situation. For an older child or an adolescent, it may be important to offer the opportunity to talk about their perspectives of the situation at home.

For Adolescents Who are Victims of Violence

- Address the health issues by obtaining a complete history.
- If possible, conduct a complete, unclothed, physical exam. Look for – and document – evidence of current or previous injuries and sexual abuse.
- Ask about medical and psychological effects resulting from abuse, such as chronic pain, worsening of existing medical conditions, psychological distress, anxiety, sleeping and eating disorders, miscarriages or substance abuse.

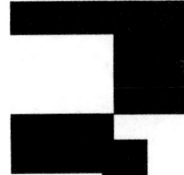

Consensus Recommendations

- Schedule a follow-up appointment, encourage your patient to return and make other appropriate referrals.
- Encourage the patient to talk to his/her parents or trusted adult about dating violence.
- For severe violence, inform adolescents that you must inform their parents or guardian to keep them safe. In this case, you may need to inform state protective service if the caretaker will not protect the child.

Assess and Address Safety Issues

Before your adolescent patient or a parent leaves, talk with her/him about immediate and future safety. These questions can also be asked over time and during subsequent visits.

- Ask her/him about her/his immediate plans. Is s/he going home to the person who hurt her/him? Does s/he have a friend or relative s/he can talk to? If s/he is going to leave, where is s/he going to go?
- Depending on the amount of time the clinician has, the following issues can be pursued to assess current danger:
  - What happened during the latest incident? Is the abuse increasing in frequency or severity?
  - Were weapons involved?
  - Have there been prior incidents?
  - Have you sought any kind of assistance for previous battering? Have you ever left before?
  - Has the abuser ever threatened or physically injured the children?
- Assess for suicidal ideation and risk of homicide:
  - Have you ever considered, threatened or attempted suicide?
  - What injuries did you sustain during the worst incident of violence?
  - Has the violence increased in frequency and/or severity?
  - Has the abuser ever threatened to kill you? Do you believe s/he is capable of killing you? Has the abuser used a weapon or threatened you with a weapon before?
  - Are you planning to leave/divorce him in the near future?
  - Are there firearms or other weapons in the house?
- Help parents think about safety issues for their children. For example:
  - Do the kids usually get involved when a violent incident occurs?
  - What do they do when violence erupts?
  - Do you talk with them about it? What do you say?
  - Children should be taught that their job in a violent situation is to stay safe, not to protect their parents or stop the fighting. They should be taught now to call 911 (where age appropriate).
  - Help the victim think about options and their implications.
- Inquire about the possibility of referring a victim to appropriate services from a

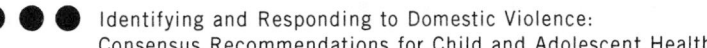

Consensus Recommendations

battered women's shelter or support network and/or other culturally relevant agency such as a community center, church or other organization serving the victim's community. *(See **Appendix X** for a Safety Plan and Instructions).*

Referrals for Adult Parents and Adolescents

Help your patient find culturally appropriate support from a hospital or community-based social worker or advocate who can help the victim with:
• Emergency shelter or permanent housing
• Emergency financial assistance or transportation
• Counseling and/or support groups for victims and their children
• Child care, visitation centers
• Legal assistance
• Mental health and substance abuse treatment
• Social services
• Batterer intervention programs
• Independent living centers

Note: Couples treatment and mediation are not usually recommended[v]

When possible, refer patients to organizations that reflect their cultural background or address their special needs such as organizations with multiple language capacity and those who specialize in working with teen, disabled or LGBT clients.

Allow her/him to use your phone to make calls. If you don't have information about intimate partner violence programs in your area, call the National Domestic Violence Hotline at 800-799-SAFE (800-799-7233 or TDD: 800-787-3224).

---

[v] Mediation and couples counseling imply that both parties are responsible for the perpetrator's violent behavior, a message that blames victims and fails to hold offenders accountable for their crimes. Mediation also presumes that both parties have equal power and can negotiate a mutually agreeable settlement. Where there is domestic violence, sexual assault, or stalking behavior, however, one party has controlled the other through sexual, physical, emotional and/or economic abuse. Even the most skilled mediator or therapist cannot shift the balance of power when one party has abused or assaulted the other, making mediation and joint counseling dangerous and ineffective in such cases.

Consensus Recommendations

Referrals For Children

Children react to witnessing intimate partner violence in many different ways. The family's capacity to support these children also varies, as do their beliefs or ways of seeking help. If the parent is concerned about her child, options for help should be discussed, including a counseling referral, mental health assessment or other support services (such as Big Brother/Big Sister). A referral would be strongly recommended in the following circumstances:

- If the child has witnessed severe violence resulting in injury or hospitalization of either the child, sibling or the parent.
- If the child's symptoms have persisted for more than three months.
- If there has been a change in behavior or an increase in aggression or depression.
- If the caretaker is unable to be emotionally attuned to the child's needs.
- If the violence has resulted in the death of a parent.

Reporting Requirements for Child Abuse and Intimate Partner Violence

Know your state's child abuse and intimate partner violence reporting laws. *(Discussion of the complexity of these issues can be found in **Appendices VIII and IX**).* Contact your local prosecutor or state attorney general, and local law enforcement to interpret the law.

- Before asking about intimate partner violence, you may want to disclose any limits of confidentiality. Since many adolescents who are victimized by an intimate partner do not want their family to know about an intimate relationship, it is important that you understand and explain the limits of confidentiality of both their medical record and reporting before screening.[vi]
- If the child has been injured, or if your state requires mandated reporting in all cases of a child's exposure to intimate partner violence, you must:
- Follow the state guidelines for completing a report.
- Encourage the victim to place a call to CPS themselves from the practitioners office, thus protecting her from charges of "failure to protect" while simultaneously protecting the child and meeting statutory child abuse reporting laws.
- If possible, when making the report yourself, tell the attending parent what you will say in the report and/or allow her to read/hear what you will say.
- When making the report to CPS, inform the screener or intake worker about the specifics of the domestic abuse and give as much information as possible about the risks for safety of the mother and child, the perpetrator, his current location, the anticipated response and the potential for subsequent violence.

[vi] Federal health privacy regulations allow parents of teens to access health information unless the teen is emancipated or legally seeking care without parental consent such as services offered in Title XX, family planning clinics or STD clinics.

Consensus Recommendations

How to Document Intimate Partner Violence

Documentation provides information on the effects of intimate partner violence over time and improves continuity of care. Make sure you are following your institution, state and federal privacy policies.

• Documentation is recommended. However, use caution in documenting intimate partner violence in a child's chart if the abuser is the biological or custodial parent. It may be advantageous to document on a separate form.

• For adolescents, documentation should be handled consistently with documentation of other sensitive issues, such as sexual activity, alcohol or drug use.[vi]

• When documenting, use direct quotes like " Mother/Patient states...". Avoid judgmental terms such as "patient alleges" or "patient claims."

• With permission, photograph or draw picture of any injuries.

What to Do if a Patient Says "No" or Will Not Discuss Abuse

Many victims of intimate partner violence will talk about their experiences if asked to do so in a sensitive and empathetic way. However, some victims may be reluctant to talk about their experiences regardless, because they are embarrassed or ashamed, or afraid that if they tell anyone they may face more severe abuse. There may be financial issues and or immigration concerns. Patients need to decide for themselves about whether they wish to disclose. If you suspect intimate partner violence and the victim remains reluctant to discuss or disclose, let her/him know that should s/he need your assistance in the future, you are available. The goal is not to get the victim to admit to the problem, but to let her/him know that you are a resource should intimate partner violence ever be an issue for them.

PART IV | PREPARING YOUR CHILD HEALTH PRACTICE

It is important that the practice or clinic setting be set up to support the staff in responding effectively and efficiently to disclosures of intimate partner violence. In preparing your practice to begin routine screening for and responding to intimate partner violence, it is advisable to obtain support from the leadership and administration, as well as to solicit staff input.

Physical Environment Should:

- Allow for confidential interviewing.
- Have posters on intimate partner violence that are multicultural and multilingual; that present available resources; and that include information about victims, perpetrators, and/or other family and community members affected by family violence.
- Have brochures/pocket cards for victims and perpetrators and resources that describe the impact of intimate partners violence on children.
- Have brochures placed in exam rooms and private places such as bathrooms.
- Patient materials should include: brochures, discharge instructions, safety planning handouts and referral information on services for on-site or off-site advocacy, counseling, and legal and other community-based services for child witnesses, victims, perpetrators and others affected by intimate partner violence.

*(See **Appendix VIII** for resources or www@endabuse.org for materials).*

Training for Staff Should Include:

- Short- and long-term developmental and behavioral effects of childhood exposure to domestic violence and child abuse.
- Survivors' perspectives.
- Cultural competency.
- Dynamics of victimization and perpetration.
- Skills building—how to screen, assess, intervene supportively and document appropriately.
- Interactive role playing and modeling of screening and response techniques.
- Information on where employees in abusive relationships can access help.

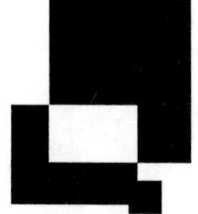

Training should be part of staff orientation; ongoing, repeated and institutionalized; and mandatory for all employees. Providers who will be screening and documenting in the medical record should receive training on dynamics and clinical response. Other staff — including allied health professionals, receptionists and security, who can play an essential role in identifying and protecting victims and their children — should receive general awareness training on intimate partner violence. Interpreters in particular should be trained in advance about the dynamics of intimate partner violence, childhood exposure to violence, the importance of confidentiality and non-judgmental interpretation, and appropriate word choices for translation of routine screening questions.

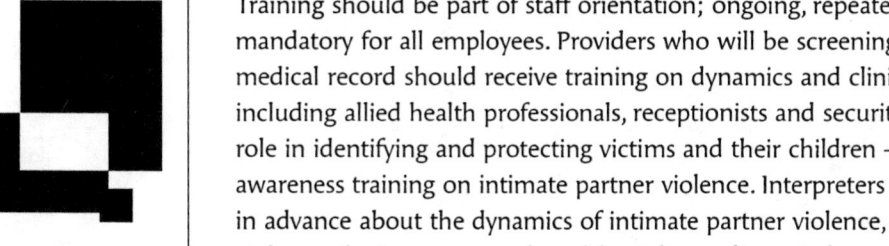
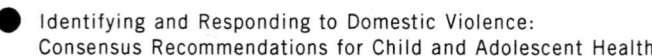

Protocols Should Include:

- Definitions, guiding principles, routine screening, assessment, intervention and documentation strategies, reporting policies and confidentiality rules.
- Roles and responsibilities of staff.

All staff should receive an orientation on the protocol. It should also be updated regularly and informed by new knowledge, laws and policies regarding intimate partner violence. It should be accessible to all staff.

Continuous Quality Improvement (CQI) Program :

- Scheduled audits of medical records to review compliance with the protocol.
- Patient satisfaction surveys.
- Regular discussions during staff meetings regarding functioning of intimate partner violence program.
- Links to other quality improvement efforts.
- Links to medical information system developments.
- CQI goals publicized.

Provider Resources Should Include:

- Chart prompts in the medical record.
- Documentation and assessment forms.
- Posters and practitioner pocket cards.
- Materials that are easily accessible to providers and regularly updated.
- Consultation with on-site or off-site domestic violence advocates, legal and forensic experts, counselors with expertise in trauma treatment, and community experts from diverse communities (LGBT, disability, elder, teen, and ethnic-specific, immigrant, and others).
- Feedback mechanisms for providers.

Employee Assistance or Human Resources Programs (for large facilities) Should:

- Address intimate partner violence victimization and perpetration.
- Be confidential (within legal limits), easily accessible and well publicized.
- Be incorporated into managerial training.
- Include intimate partners violence information in employee publications and alerts.

APPENDIX 1 | POSITION STATEMENTS FROM HEALTH PROFESSIONAL ASSOCIATIONS —EXCERPTS—

AMERICAN ACADEMY OF PEDIATRICS
COMMITTEE ON CHILD ABUSE AND NEGLECT

The Role of the Pediatrician in Recognizing and Intervening on Behalf of Abused Women (RE9748)

ABSTRACT. Pediatricians are in a position to recognize abused women in pediatric settings. Intervening on behalf of battered women is an active form of child abuse prevention. Knowledge of local resources and state laws for reporting abuse are emphasized.

The abuse of women is a pediatric issue. The American Academy of Pediatrics (AAP) and its membership recognize the importance of improving the physician's ability to recognize partner violence as well as child abuse and other forms of family violence. Intervention is crucial because children whose mothers are being assaulted are also likely to be victims. Identifying and intervening on behalf of battered women may be one of the most effective means of preventing child abuse.

Abuse of spouses and intimate partners is a pediatric issue even when children are not being physically assaulted. Pediatricians should be aware of the profound effects family violence has on children who witness it or even overhear it. Witnessing violence in the home can be as traumatic for children as being the victim of physical or sexual abuse. Children whose mothers are abused may experience serious emotional distress and manifest severe behavioral problems as a result. Adolescents who observe abusive relationships at home may repeat that dynamic in dating or other relationships. (Men and older persons of both genders also can be victims of partner and intimate violence, but they are less likely to be seen in pediatric settings).

Abused women are unlikely to seek care for their injuries from pediatricians. However, mothers of children seen by pediatricians may show signs of injury such as facial bruising. They may have other less obvious signs of abuse such as depression, anxiety, failure to keep medical appointments, reluctance to answer questions about discipline in the home, or frequent office visits for complaints not borne out by the medical evaluation of their child. Women may reveal the abuse to the pediatrician if they are questioned in a sympathetic and sensitive manner, in a confidential setting, away from the abuser, and provided some assurance of safety.

Questions about family violence should become part of anticipatory guidance. Pediatricians must understand the dynamics of abusive relationships. Excellent guidelines for managing situations of abuse have been published, and pediatricians need to become familiar with them. There also are increasing numbers of continuing education opportunities available to learn intervention techniques.

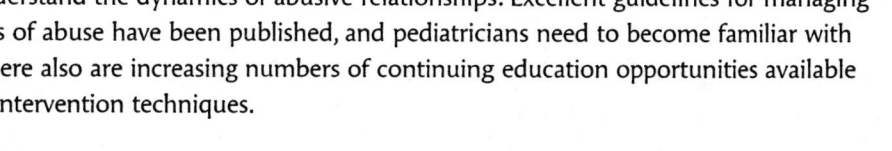

Appendix I

Pediatricians should have a protocol or action plan that has been reviewed with local authorities on domestic violence. Because of time constraints in a busy office practice or emergency room setting, an interdisciplinary approach to family violence may be most appropriate. Pediatricians can call on nurses, social workers or advocacy groups with expertise in assisting and counseling victims. The *AMA's 1996 Diagnostic and Treatment Guidelines on Domestic Violence* state that optimal care for the woman in an abusive relationship depends on the physician's working knowledge of community resources that can provide safety, advocacy, and support. The AMA and many state medical associations provide directories of agencies that provide services or information about all forms of family violence.

Pediatricians can provide education to agencies that deal with battered women about the risk of primary and secondary abuse to children whose mothers are abused. Every effort should be made to secure counseling for children who have been exposed to family violence. Such treatment may be provided in groups or individually, but the focus should be on understanding violence and how to avoid it. There is increasing evidence that children who grow up with violence are prone to violent behavior themselves, and pediatricians are in a position to break the cycle.

THE AAP RECOGNIZES THAT FAMILY AND INTIMATE PARTNER VIOLENCE IS HARMFUL TO CHILDREN. THE AAP RECOMMENDS THAT:

1. Residency training programs and continuing medical education (CME) program leaders incorporate education on family and intimate partner violence and its implications for child health into the curricula of pediatricians and pediatric emergency department physicians;
2. Pediatricians should attempt to recognize evidence of family or intimate partner violence in the office setting;
3. Pediatricians should intervene in a sensitive and skillful manner that maximizes the safety of women and children victims; and
4. Pediatricians should support local and national multidisciplinary efforts to recognize, treat and prevent family and intimate partner violence.

American Academy of Child and Adolescent Psychiatry

This statement has been approved by the Council on Child and Adolescent Health.

The recommendations in this statement do not indicate an exclusive course of treatment or serve as a standard of medical care. Variations, taking into account individual circumstances, may be appropriate.

Copyright © 1998 by the American Academy of Pediatrics.

AMERICAN ACADEMY OF FAMILY PHYSICIANS-Violence (Position Paper)

Family violence permeates our society. It affects us as individuals, family physicians, parents, spouses, educators and citizens. The breadth of the problem is staggering. Public health officials identify family violence as a public health issue of epidemic proportions.

Appendix I

THE FAMILY PHYSICIAN'S ROLE

Family violence will affect at least one third of the patients cared for by family physicians, and the impact of family violence may become evident in the one-on-one relationship of the family physician and the patient. It is imperative that physicians be aware of the prevalence of violence in all sectors of society and be alert for its effects in their encounters with virtually every patient.

Violence against women will be the form of family violence most frequently seen in family practice. Physicians need to recognize that women who are victims of domestic violence will be patients in every family practice in this country because one in every four women has been a victim of domestic violence at some point in her life, and one in seven women has been victimized in the past year. Pregnancy confers no protection. In fact, abuse often begins or escalates during pregnancy. One in six pregnant women is abused during pregnancy and 17 percent of physical or sexual abuse of women occurs during pregnancy. One study reported abuse in 37 percent of obstetric patients and showed that class, race and educational level made no difference.

THE ROLE OF THE FAMILY PHYSICIAN IN THE IDENTIFICATION AND TREATMENT OF FAMILY VIOLENCE

Despite barriers to the diagnosis and treatment of victims of family violence, family physicians are in an ideal position to take on this challenge and are compelled to do so by the sheer magnitude of the problem. Family physicians are better able to identify those at risk because they are trained to care for the whole family and for the individual as a part of the larger community. Because of the continuity of care family physicians provide, they can gain patient confidence over time and can serve as sympathetic listeners and patient advocates. Family physicians can provide early intervention to break the cycle of violence through routine screening and the identification of abuse. They can help by teaching parenting skills and counseling patients on the stress of caring for children or elderly parents. Physicians can talk with women and men about their experiences of previous abuse and can be a central referral source for other resources in the community.

AAFP INITIATIVES TO DECREASE FAMILY VIOLENCE

Among activities for the American Academy of Family Physicians (AAFP) to consider are the following:

1. Developing or adapting teaching modules for members to present to medical students, residents, hospital staff and community groups;
2. Creating an ongoing education program for members on screening, recognition and treatment of violence, including distribution of the American Medical Association's guidelines for history-taking around issues of violence and abuse;
3. Supporting or developing university-, hospital- or office-based protocols and policies about family violence;
4. Publicizing to members the hotline numbers for organizations that help physicians and

Appendix I

patients deal with abuse;

5. Offering continuing medical education for members to increase their skills in screening for, identifying and treating cases of domestic violence;

6. Participating in public policy initiatives and legislative reform to protect victims and rehabilitate batterers and partnering with other organizations committed to decreasing family violence and;

7. Promoting reasonable and responsible control of firearms and other weapons.

AMERICAN COLLEGE OF OBSTETRICIANS AND GYNECOLOGISTS

Division of Women's Health Issues, ACOG Educational Bulletin, No. 257, December 1999
Domestic Violence

DOMESTIC VIOLENCE SCREENING AND IDENTIFICATION

Specific measures can be taken to improve identification and facilitate disclosure of domestic violence. A prefacing statement followed by a few simple, direct questions will identify most women with a history of abuse or assault. The introduction or preface should establish that screening is universal. The screening assessment should follow with direct questioning.

Children in violent homes should be evaluated by a professional who can assess the child's behavioral patterns and help the child address the emotional impact of the violence. Referrals to such resources are essential, because the victim may not be willing or able to do so on her own, especially if she fears removal of the child more than the violence.

Physicians or other health care workers who provide acute or chronic medical care to the older adult may see the older adult on a regular basis and have unique opportunities for screening and assessment. Additionally, an opportunity for screening and recognition exists during all health-related encounters of older individuals, such as routine gynecologic examinations.

SUMMARY

Many physicians, especially in the current managed care environment, are concerned that abuse screening and disclosure will require inordinate amounts of time, but with an established protocol and referral system this important problem can be managed. Screening all patients is the key to identifying abuse. With disclosure of ongoing domestic violence, the physician's responsibility should incude acknowledgement of abuse, making a safety assessment, assisting with a safety plan, providing appropriate referrals, documentation, and continued support. For disclosure of past violence, the responsibilities are similar but generally do not require immediate intervention. Women with a history of past victimization need to have that history identified and acknowledged and may need referral to other professionals to assist with the resolution of their trauma-related issues. Regardless of the types of victimization a woman has experienced, providing a safe setting in which she can discuss the problem and receive support is an important part of her recovery. Through these measures, the health care team can help abused women take the first steps toward ending the violence and achieving a healthy recovery.

APPENDIX II | BIBLIOGRAPHY

Identifying and Responding to Domestic Violence in Child Health Settings

Augustyn M, Parker S, Groves B, Zuckerman B. "Silent victims: Children who witness violence". Contemporary Pediatrics. 1997;12 (8), 35-57.

Carter L, Stevenson C. *The Future of Children: Domestic Violence and Children.* Los Altos, CA: The David and Lucille Packard Foundation;1999;9(3).

Christian CW, Scribiano P, Seidl T, Pinto-Martin JA. "Pediatric injury resulting from family violence". Pediatrics. 1997;99(2).

Cohall A, Cohall R, Bannister H, Northridge M. "Love shouldn't hurt: strategies for health care providers to address adolescent dating violence". J Am Med Women's Association. 1999;54(3):144-148.

Committee on Child Abuse and Neglect, American Academy of Pediatrics. "The role of the pediatrician in recognizing and intervening on behalf of abused women". Pediatrics. 1998;101(6):1091-1092.

Dubowitz H, King H. *Family violence: a child-centered, family-focused approach.* "Pediatic Clinics of North America". Philadelphia, PA: W.B. Saunders Company; 1995;42(1):153-163.

Duffy SJ, McGrath ME, Becker BM, Linakis JG. "Mothers with histories of domestic violence in a pediatric emergency department". Pediatrics. 1999;103(5):1007-1013.

Edelson JL. "Children's witnessing of adult domestic violence." J Interpersonal Violence. 1999;14(8):839-870.

Edelson JL. "The overlap between child maltreatment and women battering." Violence Against Women. 1999;5(2):134-154.

Erickson MJ, Hill TD, Siegel RM. "Barriers to domestic violence screening in the pediatric setting". Pediatrics. 2001;108(1): 98-102.

Family Violence Prevention Fund. *National Consensus Guidelines on Identifying and Responding to Domestic Violence Victimization in Health Care Settings.* San Francisco, CA: Family Violence Prevention Fund; 2002

Fantuzzo J, Boruch R, Beriama, et al. "Domestic violence and children: prevalence and risk in five major U.S. cities". J Am Academy Child Adolesc Psychiatry. 1997;36(1):116-122.

Felitti VJ, Anda RF, Nordenberg D, Williamson DF, Spitz AM, Edwards V, Kiss MP, Marks JS. "Relationship of childhood abuse and household dysfunction to many of the leading causes of death in adults". Am J Prev Med. 1998;14(4):245-258.

Groves BM. *Children Who See Too Much: Lessons from the Child Witness to Violence Project.* Boston: Beacon Press; 2002.

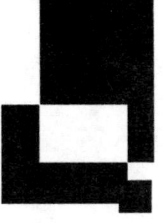

Appendix II
BIBLIOGRAPHY

Groves BM, Zuckerman B, Marans S, Cohen D. "Silent Victims: Children who witness violence". JAMA. 1993; 269(2):262-264.

Jacoby M, et al. "Rapid repeat pregnancy and experiences of interpersonal violence among low-income adolescents". Am J Prev Med. 1999;16(4):318-321.

Jaffe P, Suderman M. "Child witness of women abuse: research and community responses". In Stith S, Straus M. *Understanding partner violence: prevalence, causes, consequences, and solutions.* Families in Focus Services, 2. Minneapolis, MN: National Council on Family Relations; 1995.

Jaffe P, Wolfe,Wilson. *Children of Domestic Violence.* Newbury Park, CA: Sage Publications; 1990.

Kerker BD, Horowitz SM, Leventhal JM, Plichta S, Leaf PJ. "Identification of violence in the home". Arch Pediatr Adolesc Med. 2000;154:457-462.

Kilpatrick KI, Litt M, Williams L. "Post-traumatic stress disorder in child witness to domestic violence". American Journal of Orthopsychiatry. 1997; 67(4):639-644.

King H, Strauss M. Routine Screen for Domestic Violence in Pediatric Practice. Newton, MA: Newton-Wellesley Hospital or online at www.drkingsoffice.com; 2000.

King HS, Strauss M. *Routine Screening for Domestic Violence in Pediatric Practice.* Wellesley, MA: Newton-Wellesley Domestic Violence Prevention Council, 2000.

Knapp JF, Dowd MD. "Family violence: implications for the pediatrician". Pediatrics in Review. 1998;19(9):316-319.

Martin SL, Mackie L, Kupper LL, Buescher PA, Moracco KE. "Physical abuse of women before, during, and after pregnancy". JAMA. 1999;285(12):1581-1584.

McKibben L, Roberts L. "The Pediatric Family Violence Awareness Project: Partner Violence Training for Pediatric Health Care Providers". Working Draft. 1996
Plichta SB, Duncan MM, Plichta L. "Spouse abuse, patient-physician communication, and patient satisfaction". Am J Prev Med. 1996;12(5):297-303.

National Institute of Justice and Centers for Disease Control and Prevention. *Prevalence, Incidence and Consequences of Violence Against Women: Findings from the National Violence Against Women Survey.* Washington, DC: National Institute of Justice and Centers for Disease Control and Prevention; 1998. Parkinson GW, Adams RC, Emerling FG. "Maternal domestic violence screening in an office based pediatric practice". Pediatrics. 2001;108:1-9.

Renzetti C. *Violent betrayal: partner abuse in lesbian relationships.* Newbury Park, CA: Sage Publications; 1998:18.

Richards J. "Battering in a population of adolescent females". J Am Academy Nurse Practitioners. 1991;3(4).

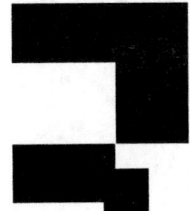

Appendix II

BIBLIOGRAPHY

Siegel RM, Hill TD, Henderson VA, Ernst, HM, Boat BW. "Screening for domestic violence in the community pediatric setting". Pediatrics. 1999;104(4):874-877.

Silverman JG, Raj A, Mucci LA, Hathaway JE. "Dating violence against adolescent girls and associated substance use, unhealthy weight control, sexual behavior, pregnancy, and suicidality". JAMA. 2001; 286(5):572-578.

Spaccarelli S, Coatsworth JD, Bowden BS. "Exposure to serious family violence among incarcerated boys: its association with violent offending and potential mediating variables". Violence and Victims. 1995;10:163-182.

Thompson RS, Krugman R. "Screening mothers for intimate partner abuse at well-baby visits". JAMA. 2001;285(12)

U.S. Department of Justice. *Intimate partner violence.* Washington, DC: U.S. Department of Justice, Bureau of Justice Statistics; 2000.

U.S. Department of Justice. *Violence by intimates: analysis of data on crimes by current or former spouses, boyfriends, and girlfriends.* Washington, DC: U.S. Department of Justice, Bureau of Justice Statistics; 1998.

U.S. Department of Justice. *Violence by intimates: analysis of data on crimes committed by current & former spouses, boyfriends & girlfriends.* Washington, DC: U.S. Department of Justice, Bureau of Justice Statistics;1997.*

Whitney P, Davis L. "Child abuse and domestic violence in Massachusetts: Can practice be integrated in a public child welfare setting?" Child Maltreatment. 1999;4(2):159-166.

Wolfe DA, Wekerle C, Reizel D, Gough R. "Strategies to address violence in the lives of high risk youth". In Peled E, Jaffe PG, Edleson JL (eds). *Ending the Cycle of Violence: Community Responses to Children of Battered Women.* Newbury Park, CA: Sage Publications; 1995.

Wright RJ, Wright RO, Isaac NE. "Response to battered mothers in the pediatric emergency department: a call for an interdisciplinary approach to family violence." Pediatrics. 1997;99(2):186-192.

Zink T. "Should children be in the room when the mother is screened for partner violence?" Journal of Family Practice. 2000; 49(2):130-136.

Zuckerman B, Augustyn M, Groves BM, Parker, S. "Silent victims revisited: the special case of domestic violence." Pediatrics. 1995;96:511.

APPENDIX III | ABSTRACTS OF SELECTED STUDIES ON PROVIDER AND PATIENT ATTITUDES

Knocking Down Walls: Barrier Myths to Screening for Violence in Primary Care

Marilyn Augustyn, Tracy Magee, Mary Duffy Pediatrics, Boston University School of Medicine, Boston, MA; Nursing, Boston College, Boston, MA

BACKGROUND: In 1998 the AAP in a policy statement recommended that "questions about domestic violence (DV) should become part of anticipatory guidance". Since that time, studies have shown that providers are hesitant to follow the recommendation. Barriers have been sited from child presence in the room to fear of offending parents.

OBJECTIVE: This study explored how frequently providers in an urban practice screened for DV, whether children's age and/presence in the room, length of time providers knew the family and how providers perceived parents response influenced screening.

DESIGN/METHODS: At baseline, 24 providers in an urban pediatric practice completed an interview about their current practices of screening for a child's exposure to violence. Over the following 4 weeks, they completed a form at the conclusion of well child care visits (children birth to 12 years) which covered several areas including whether they screened for DV and a Likert scale rating provider perceptions of parents' response to being asked these questions.

RESULTS: The providers were 16 residents, 6 attending pediatricians, 1 nurse practicioner and 1 fellow. Eighty four percent reported they asked screening questions with the child in the room. During the 4 week period of the study, 60% of the providers reported that they screened for DV with 60% also reporting screening for community violence (CV). Ninety three percent of the time, providers asked these questions with the child in the room. Of these encounters, 78% were first visits with the family. Of the 22% that were repeat visits, 80% had known the family more than 6 months. Seventy percent of the providers rated parent response as an 8 or higher on a 10 point scale (10 being most receptive). Controlling for child age and how long the provider knew the family, providers were more likely to screen when the child was older whether or not they had known the family previously.

CONCLUSIONS: Over 3 years after the statement was issued recommending universal screening for DV, providers continue to struggle with several barriers. In this pilot data of an urban practice, only 60% of visits were screened and these primarily were visits among older children. Interestingly, child presence in the room did not appear to be a barrier nor did parent response to the questions. Since the greatest risk for DV is often when children are less than 5 years of age, providers perhaps need to consider alternative methods to screen more effectively.

Appendix III

ABSTRACTS OF SELECTED STUDIES ON PROVIDER AND PATIENT ATTITUDES

Maternal Screening for Domestic Violence during Pediatric Visits: Physicians' Practices and Perspectives
Linda Chamberlain, Ph.D, MPH

OBJECTIVES: Very little is known about how physicians respond to domestic violence in the pediatric setting. Our objectives were to examine physicians' maternal screening and intervention practices for domestic violence and to investigate perceived barriers to screening during child health care visits.

METHODS/DESIGN: A 17-question survey about current screening and intervention practices, training and perspectives on perceived screening barriers was conducted by mail.

SAMPLE STUDIED: All physicians practicing in Alaska who provided health care to children, age 18 or younger.

PRELIMINARY RESULTS: Surveys were completed by 393 (73%) of the 540 eligible physicians, including 208 family practitioners and general practitioners; 70 pediatricians and 48 emergency medicine physicians. Forty-nine percent of physicians had specific training on the effects of domestic violence on children. More than one-quarter (29%) estimated that 1 in 10 children in their practices had lived in a household with domestic violence. The majority of physicians screened often or always for domestic violence when the mother had signs of injury (88%) or when they suspected child abuse (95%). Routine screening was less common at initial pediatric visits (16%), well-child visits (11%), urgent care visits (31%), and when providing counseling/anticipatory guidance to mothers of newborn infants (16%). Commonly reported intervention strategies included providing information on victim services (87%), talking to the mother about safety concerns (81%), and talking to the child alone when appropriate (51%). The majority of physicians did not consider commonly perceived barriers such as inadequate training and concerns about child witness reporting requirements as major barriers to screening. Nearly all (98%) respondents agreed that witnessing domestic violence in an important health issue for children. Eighty-five percent of physicians agreed that they have a responsibility as part of their practice to screen mothers for domestic violence when providing health care to children. There was nearly total agreement (99.5%) among respondents that helping a mother who is being battered can make a difference in the lives of her children.

CONCLUSION: While physicians frequently screen mothers for domestic violence when there is evidence of maternal injury or suspected child abuse, opportunities to screen at other child health care visits are being missed. Most physicians agreed that domestic violence is an important children's health care issue that should be addressed in the pediatric setting. Many commonly perceived barriers to screening may not be predictive of physicians' maternal screening practices.

ABSTRACTS OF SELECTED STUDIES ON PROVIDER AND PATIENT ATTITUDES

Mothers' and Health Care Providers' Perspectives on Screening for Intimate Partner Violence in a Pediatric Emergency Department

M. Denise Dowd, MD, MPH; Christopher Kennedy, MD; Jane F. Knapp, MD
From the Division of Emergency Medicine, Children's Mercy Hospital, Kansas City, MO

NOTE: This abstract with full article will be published in Archives of Pediatric and Adolescent Medicine, August, 2002. For full citation with pages send email to apam@u.washington.edu

OBJECTIVE: To determine the attitudes, feelings and beliefs of mothers and pediatric emergency department health care providers toward routine intimate partner violence screening.

METHODS: This qualitative project employed focus groups of mothers who brought their children to a children's hospital emergency department for care and physicians and nurses who staffed the same department. We held six ethnically homogeneous mother groups: two Caucasian, two African-American, two Latina and four provider groups: two predominately female nurse groups and two physician groups: one male and one female. Professional moderators conducted the sessions using a semi-structured discussion guide. All groups were audio- and videotaped and tapes were reviewed for reoccurring themes.

RESULTS: A total of 59 mothers, 21 nurses and 17 physicians participated. Mothers identified intimate partner violence as a common problem in their communities and most remarked that routine screening for adult intimate partner violence is an appropriate activity for a pediatric emergency department. However, many expressed concern that willingness to disclose might be affected by a fear of being reported to child protective services. They stressed the importance of addressing the child's health problem first, that screening be done in an empathetic way and that immediate assistance be available if needed. Themes identified in the provider groups included concerns about time constraints, fear of offending and concerns that unless immediate intervention was available the victim could be placed in jeopardy. Many said they would feel obligated to notify child protective services upon disclosure of intimate partner violence.

CONCLUSIONS: Intimate partner violence screening protocols in the pediatric emergency department should take into consideration the beliefs and attitudes of both those doing the screening and those being screened. Those developing screening protocols for a pediatric emergency department should consider: 1) Those assigned to screen must demonstrate empathy, warmth and a helping attitude; 2) The importance of addressing the child's medical needs first and a screening process that is minimally disruptive to the emergency department; 3) A defined, organized approach to assessing danger to the child and how and when it is appropriate to notify CPS when a caregiver screens positive; 4) Resources must be available immediately to a victim who requests them.

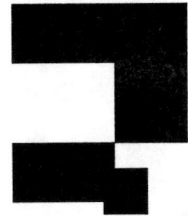

Appendix III

ABSTRACTS OF SELECTED STUDIES ON PROVIDER AND PATIENT ATTITUDES

Pediatrician's Views on the Treatment and Preventions of Violent Injuries to Children

LM Olson, KG O'Connor, H Spivak & MZ Esquivel, American Academy of Pediatrics, Elk Grove Village, IL.
Periodic Survey of Fellows, American Academy of Pediatrics, Division of Health Policy Research from *Pediatric Academic Societies,* May 2001

OBJECTIVE: To assess the portion of pediatricians treating violent injuries and their perceived capacity to address violence in the office setting.

DESIGN: National random sample, mailed survey.

PARTICIPANTS: 574 U.S. members of the American Academy of Pediatrics who provide direct patient care.

RESULTS: Many pediatricians report they treated (in the past 12 months) injuries due to child abuse (61%), domestic violence (43%) or community violence (45%). Substantial numbers of respondents believe that pediatricians should address, in the community and in practice, violence against children. However, while pediatricians generally feel confident about their skills in treating child abuse, they are less likely to feel adequately prepared to treat children at risk for domestic violence.

	Proportion of Pediatricians Indicating Agreement (%)		
	CHILD ABUSE	DOMESTIC VIOL.	COMMUNITY VIOL.
Are confident in ability to identify children at risk for.................	63.7	35.1	32.6
Are confident in ability to manage cases of................................	62.6	43.1	46.4
Have received adequate training in the area of............................	48.5	19.7	15.8

CONCLUSION: Injury from violence is a problem confronting large numbers of pediatric practices. The identified gaps can help shape new training programs and interventions to help practitioners address this critical risk to children.

ABSTRACTS OF SELECTED STUDIES ON PROVIDER AND PATIENT ATTITUDES

Should Children Be in the Room When the Mother Is Screened for Partner Violence?

Zink, Therese MD, MPH

The Journal of Family Practice, © 2000 by Appleton & Lange. All rights reserved.
Volume 49(2) February 2000 pp 130-136

BACKGROUND: The goal of our study was to understand the important issues to consider when screening women for intimate partner violence in front of their children.

METHODS: Interviews and focus groups were conducted with experienced family physicians and pediatricians and family violence experts (child psychologists, social workers, and domestic violence agency directors). Session transcripts were coded and categorized.

RESULTS: Experts disagreed on the appropriateness of general screening for intimate partner violence in front of children older than 2 to 3 years. The majority thought that general questions were appropriate, if the in-depth questioning of the abused parent was done in private. Screening for child abuse when domestic violence is identified (and for domestic violence when child abuse is discovered) was recommended. Documentation about intimate partner violence in the child's medical chart raises questions about confidentiality, since the person committing the abuse may have access, if he or she is a legal guardian. Physicians need more education on the symptoms of children who are exposed to violence between adults.

CONCLUSIONS: More research is needed to understand appropriate questions and methods of screening for intimate partner violence in front of children. The tension is between practical recommendations for routine screening and preserving the safety of the parent and the children. Intimate partner violence screening by physicians is important. Interrupting the cycle of violence may give a child a better chance at maturing into a healthy adult.

APPENDIX IV | DILEMMAS WHEN SCREENING ALL PATIENTS FOR VICTIMIZATION

Routinely screening all parents and caretakers (both female and male) for IPV victimization raises additional policy and practice issues for providers and there is debate in the field about appropriate responses. Those opposed to these policies assert that the risks of alerting perpetrators to protocols identifying and assessing IPV outweigh the benefits. The concerns are that perpetrators may limit their partner's access to health care, may threaten victims who disclose, or may learn about safety planning materials which could ultimately undermine victim safety. Proponents of policies to screen men and women assert that, because men in same-sex relationships experience DV in equal rates as women in heterosexual relationships, and some men in heterosexual couples experience abuse, it is critical to identify and assist as many victims as possible. Proponents also argue that determined perpetrators can already access safety planning materials and that screening all patients offers unparalleled opportunities for abuse prevention. Still others maintain that because the majority of IPV victims are women, providers should begin by screening all female patients and integrate screening for men as a second step, after gaining more experience in screening for victimization and developing policies to address some of the difficult practical concerns that are raised when screening all parents and caretakers. Providers and health facilities should consider the dilemmas and recommendations listed below as they develop their unique protocols.

DILEMMAS

It may be difficult to assess who the victim is. The accounts of one or both parties may lead to significant confusion about the incident.

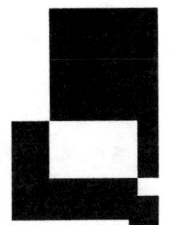

- Male perpetrators often claim victimization to avoid consequences or as a tactic to further control victims.[69] Because the majority of IPV perpetrators are male, screening men increases the likelihood of screening perpetrators who may claim they are victims. There is not sufficient experience with female perpetrators of violence to know if this is also true of them.
- Victims may take the blame for the abuse because they have been told repeatedly by their partners that the problems in the relationship are their fault or because they used violence or other tactics in self-defense.
- Both parties may use physical force in an incident.

Whether the patient is viewed as a victim or perpetrator will influence the health care provider's response and may lead to inappropriate treatment.

- A victim who takes the blame for the abuse might prevent providers from offering them support and information about IPV.
- Perpetrators who falsely claim they are victims might lead providers to share safety-planning strategies with perpetrators, inadvertently colluding with them and undermining victims' safety planning efforts.

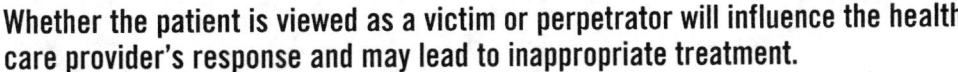

Appendix IV

DILEMMAS WHEN SCREENING ALL PATIENTS
FOR VICTIMIZATION

• What is recorded in the medical record by the health care provider can have legal
  ramifications for the victim particularly in divorce, custody or other legal cases.

While it is not the role of the health care provider to determine if the patient is telling the
truth, the provider should take care in evaluating the patient's information and in identifying
whether or not s/he is a victim of IPV, just as they take care in evaluating other patient's
reports of health concerns. Understanding the definition of IPV and being skilled in
behavioral inquiry assists providers in making accurate identification of victimization.

RECOMMENDATIONS FOR POLICY IMPLEMENTATION

The Family Violence Prevention Fund recommends that providers implement policies to
screen all male and female parents for victimization only after taking precautions to
protect victims whose perpetrators claim to be abused. Training providers on perpetrator
dynamics and responses to LGBT and heterosexual victims is critical for all IPV programs,
including those that target women only. When implementing a policy to screen all
patients, first:

• Contact local DV programs (and batterer's intervention programs that they recommend)
  and explain that you are considering a plan to screen all patients for victimization. This will
  prepare them for referrals and will give them an opportunity to inform the development of
  your protocol.
• Inform all patients that you screen men and women for victimization and make safety
  planning materials available to both, so that victims who are concerned about perpetrators
  sabotaging their safety plan efforts can plan accordingly. Make information available about
  advocates on-site or in the community that can help the victim with these plans, regardless
  of whether the victim discloses abuse.
• Understand and conduct training on IPV prevalence studies. Emerging research
  demonstrates that IPV occurs at similar rates in LGBT adolescent and adult populations[70]
  with higher rates in male same-sex relationships than female.[71] Most studies indicate that
  about 5-10%[72] of all victims are men (an unknown percentage of whom are gay or
  bisexual). Because of this, you should expect to see a fairly small percentage of heterosexual
  male victims in your practice — but should be prepared to respond to all victims.
• Understand and conduct training on the dynamics of IPV: IPV serves the purpose of
  establishing power and control through various tactics. This establishment of an abusive
  imbalance of power and control is fundamentally what distinguishes IPV perpetrators
  from victims. There are multiple indicators of abusive behavior (denying access to
  friends/family, intimidation, etc.) not just physical abuse, and victims' lives generally
  become more limited and controlled.

Appendix IV

DILEMMAS WHEN SCREENING ALL PATIENTS FOR VICTIMIZATION

Recommendations for Clinical Practice

- Do not blame patients or force them to prove their "victimhood."
- Assessments should be handled sensitively and without bias.
- Even if you are unsure if your patient is a victim, document that you screened, the patient's response, and note the details of the abuse and health consequences. Offer the patient educational materials about IPV and referrals.

HEALTH CARE PROVIDER RESPONSE TO LGBT AND HETEROSEXUAL MALE VICTIMS

Lesbian, Gay, Bisexual, and Transgendered Victims of Abuse

Emerging research demonstrates that IPV occurs at similar rates in LGBT adolescent and adult populations as in heterosexual populations[vii] with higher rates in male same-sex relationships than female[viii]. However, it is important to realize that the statistics may be low because those in a same-sex relationships may not be comfortable stating their sexual preference. A policy to screen all patients should include specific recommendations for responding to LGBT victims. Specialized services may be limited in your area so, when unavailable, refer patients to national organizations or the National Domestic Violence Hotline.

PRIOR TO IMPLEMENTING A PROGRAM TO SCREEN ALL PATIENTS, IT IS IMPORTANT TO:

- Beware of your own bias and/or homophobia.
- Call your local IPV program and determine what resources are available for lesbian, gay, bisexual and transgendered clients.
- Call any local programs for LGBT communities and determine what resources they offer for victims of IPV.
- In addition (or if no programs exist in your area), provide LGBT victims with the national DV hotline number for more information or materials.
- Have educational and safety materials available that are appropriate for LGBT victims (for materials, go to the FVPF website www.endabuse.org).
- Refer gay male victims of IPV to Community United Against Violence (San Francisco), Gay Men's Domestic Violence Project (Boston) or other organizations for information and support *(See **Appendix VIII**)*.

[vii] Bureau of Justice Statistics Special Report, Intimate Partner Violence and Age of Victim, 1993-99, United States Department of Justice, October 2001.

[viii] Morrow, Jeanie (April 1994). Identifying and treating battered lesbians. San Francisco Medicine Letellier, Patrick (April 1994). Identifying and treating battered gay men in a medical setting. San Francisco Medicine. Goodenow, Carol. (1998). 1997 Massachusetts Youth Risk Behavior Survey. Malden, MA: Massachusetts Department of Education. Renzetti, C. Violent Betrayal: Partner Abuse in Lesbian Relationships. Sage Publications. 1992, 18.

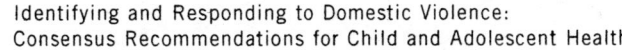

DILEMMAS WHEN SCREENING ALL PATIENTS
FOR VICTIMIZATION

- Refer lesbian and female bisexual victims to the Network for Battered Lesbians and Bisexual Women (Boston), Anti-Violence Project, Community United Against Violence and/or other local organizations for information and support *(See Appendix VIII).*
- Refer transgendered victims to Community United Against Violence *(See Appendix VIII).*

Heterosexual Male Victims

There is limited research on male victims of IPV in heterosexual relationships. Most major studies on male victimization do not clarify if male victims are in gay or heterosexual relationships. However, a policy to screen all patients should include specific recommendations for responding to heterosexual male victims. Services for male victims may be very limited in your area, so be prepared to refer patients to national or international programs and the National Domestic Violence Hotline. Prior to implementing a program it is important to:

- Be aware of your own bias regarding heterosexual male victims of abuse.
- Call your local DV program and learn about their policy on heterosexual male victims.
- Refer patients to any local programs available, the National Domestic Violence Hotline or other resources including: www.vix.com/menmag/batamen.htm or the Easton Alliance for the Prevention of Family Violence at www.geocities.com/heartland/5593.
- Have gender neutral educational materials available about abuse or refer patients to the websites listed in Appendix VIII for more educational materials for battered men.

APPENDIX V | INDICATORS OF ABUSE

Many victims of IPV will talk about their experiences if asked to do so in a sensitive and empathetic way. However, other victims may be reluctant to disclose. They may be embarrassed, ashamed, or afraid that if they tell anyone they may be at risk for more severe abuse. There may be financial issues and/or concerns about immigration status, or they may lack trust in people because trust was violated in their intimate relationship. Below are some of the reasons one might suspect IPV and might ask follow-up questions.

For Adults

- Failure to keep medical appointments, or comply with medical protocols.
- Secrecy or obvious discomfort when interviewed about relationship.
- The presence of a partner who comes into the examining room with the patient and controls or dominates the interview, is overly solicitous and will not leave the patient alone with her/his provider.
- The patient returns repeatedly with vague complaints.
- A patient who presents with health problems associated with abuse.
- Unexplained injuries or injuries inconsistent with the history given.
- Somatic complaints.
- Delay between an injury and seeking medical treatment.
- Injury to the head, neck, chest, breasts, abdomen, or genitals.
- Bilateral or multiple injuries, especially if in different stages of healing.
- Physical injury during pregnancy, especially on the breasts and abdomen.
- Chronic pain without apparent etiology.
- An unusually high number of visits to health care providers.
- High number of STI's, pregnancies, miscarriages, and abortions repeat vaginal and urinary tract infections.

(See Appendix F for others)

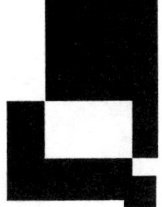

For Children and Adolescents

All of the applicable health problems listed above as well as:
- Age inappropriate injuries, burns, injuries to the genital areas.
- Developmental & behavioral problems.
- Psychological distress such as depression, suicidal ideation or attempts, attachment problems, anxiety, sleeping and/or eating disorders, panic attacks, symptoms of PTSD, and substance use/abuse problems.

If you see any of these indicators, or if you suspect abuse, yet the patient remains reluctant to discuss or disclose, provide the patient with a hotline number and other resources in case they need them in the future. Let the patient know that should s/he ever need it, you are available as a resource. Bring the issue up during the next visit. The goal is not to force the victim to admit to a problem, but to try and anticipate her/his concerns about disclosure and to let her/him know that you can be a resource should this ever be a problem. Encourage her/him to return and schedule a follow-up visit within a short time.

APPENDIX VI | INTIMATE PARTNER VIOLENCE VICTIMIZATION REPORTING REQUIREMENTS: HOW IT AFFECTS CHILD HEALTH SETTINGS

Most states have enacted mandatory reporting laws, which require the reporting of specified injuries and wounds, suspected abuse or domestic violence for individuals being treated by a health care professional, or who come before the health care facility.[ix] Mandatory reporting laws are distinct from elder abuse or vulnerable adult abuse reporting laws,[x] in that the individuals to be protected are not limited to a specific class, but pertain to all individuals[xi] whom the health care professional provides treatment or medical care to, or who come before the health care facility.

The elements that trigger these reports vary, from specific injuries such as gunshot and stab wounds to more broadly described "wounds indicating violence." With few exceptions, these reporting laws were not passed with domestic violence in mind. However, as the health care community became more aware of domestic violence, many asked how mandatory reporting laws should be applied in cases of domestic violence.

THE LAWS VARY FROM STATE TO STATE, BUT GENERALLY FALL INTO FOUR CATEGORIES:

1. States that require reporting of injuries caused by weapons;
2. States that mandate reporting for injuries caused in violation of criminal laws, as a result of violence, or through non-accidental means;
3. States that specifically address reporting in domestic violence cases; and
4. States that have no general mandatory reporting laws.

In a majority of states, existing laws would most likely not apply in those cases when a child health provider is treating a child and screening the child's parent for domestic violence. In the pediatric visit where the parent is not the patient and not seeking treatment, the clinician is generally under no legal obligation to report because the parent does not fall within the purview of the reporting law. However, for family physician visits, the case may be more complicated. The parent may be a patient of the provider, even though she is not seeking treatment during the particular visit. Additionally, if the child is also presenting with injuries, child abuse reporting laws may require the physician to report.

(See page 243: When does child exposure to intimate partner violence become child abuse?)

[ix] Different states have different reporting requirements of various health care professionals, and various health care facilities. Because the differences vary widely, we do not include them in this paper. Please be sure to consult your state law and/or local expert for further information on reporting requirements in your state. A list of the specific codes can be found in Appendix VII.

[x] Elder abuse or vulnerable adult abuse reporting laws seek to protect a specific class of individuals being treated, i.e. the elderly, or mentally or physically incapacitated individuals.

[xi] Please note that all states with general mandatory reporting laws except for California, Georgia, Kentucky, and Wisconsin use the term "person(s)" in the text of the law. Georgia, California, and Wisconsin use the term "patient." Kentucky's general mandatory reporting law is an exception, as it uses the term "adult," rather than "person(s)" or "patient."

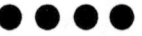

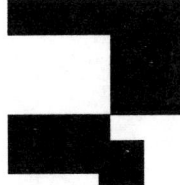

Appendix VI

INTIMATE PARTNER VIOLENCE VICTIMIZATION
REPORTING REQUIREMENTS

There has been much debate about the benefit of mandatory reporting of domestic violence by health care providers. Most advocates and providers support state laws that require reports to law enforcement only in the case of gunshot or other potentially life-threatening assault. However, several laws require reports of any domestic violence assault, regardless of severity or victim preference. The intended goals of these laws include assisting officers in solving crimes, enhancing patient safety, holding batterers accountable, and improving domestic violence data collection and documentation. Opponents argue that there are serious risks created by these laws, including unintentionally endangering victims, deterring victims who do not want or need police involvement from seeking medical care, and reducing victim autonomy, control, and ability to plan for safety for herself and her children.

Providers should know their state's domestic violence reporting law, including who is required to report, and under what conditions. *(Appendices VII contains a chart listing state codes).* In order to maximize patient input regarding law enforcement action, providers should also familiarize themselves with how their local law enforcement agency responds to such reports. Becoming familiar with such procedures will also allow the provider to better assist the patient in safety planning, and in knowing what to expect. Additionally, recent federal privacy regulations require providers to inform patients of health information use and disclosure practices in general, and whenever a specific report has been made. Health care facilities should also ensure that their domestic violence protocols and training materials address their state reporting laws and federal regulations.

How do Mandatory Reporting Laws Apply to the Pediatric and Family Practice Setting?

In the vast majority of states, neither statutory nor case law specifies when or if a health care provider must report a parent's injuries if they are observed or discovered during a health care visit with that parent's child. Therefore, under a strict reading of most laws, if a child's health care provider is not providing treatment or medical care to the abused parent during the child's visit, the health care provider would not be required to make a report. In family practice situations where the child and parent are the provider's patients, and the current visit appointment is for the child, the same reasoning could be applied, although it is less clear-cut. That is, the health care provider would not be required to report since he or she is not treating the parent for the specified injuries during the appointment. This issue merits further discussion among health care providers, advocates, licensing authorities, and other professionals, as it is uncharted territory.

Appendix VI

INTIMATE PARTNER VIOLENCE VICTIMIZATION
REPORTING REQUIREMENTS

Georgia, Kentucky, and Ohio[xii] require reports when a provider believes that an individual has suffered certain injuries, or observes such injuries, but is not necessarily providing treatment or medical care. Since these laws do not specifically require that the individual must be seeking treatment or medical care in order to trigger the reporting requirement, a parent with visible injuries accompanying a child to a child health appointment may fall within the class of individuals the statutes apply to, and reporting would be required.

There are also two states that do not fit either category of laws: Michigan and Pennsylvania. In both of these states, the laws do not mention whether the physician must be providing treatment or medical care in order to trigger the reporting requirement. Additionally, the laws do not contain any language regarding a physician's belief or observance of the specified injuries. Thus, practitioners in these states should consult a local expert regarding further interpretation of these laws

[xii] The Family Violence Prevention Fund opposes laws that specifically mandate health care providers to report all injuries, including those that may not be serious, to law enforcement or to any other authorities. See the paper entitled *Mandatory Reporting of Domestic Violence* by Health Care Providers: A Policy Paper (November, 1997), prepared by Ariella Hyman for the Family Violence Prevention Fund (FVPF), published by the FVPF: (415) 252-8900.

APPENDIX VII

STATE CODES ON INTIMATE PARTNER VIOLENCE VICTIMIZATION REPORTING REQUIREMENTS FOR HEALTH CARE PROVIDERS[xiii]

Current through March 8, 2002

Code Number	States with General Mandatory Reporting Laws	IF ANY OF THE FOLLOWING TYPES OF INJURIES ARE PRESENT, PRACTITIONERS IN THE STATE MUST MAKE A REPORT:								Treatment of Specified Injuries Requires Practitioners to Report[xiv]
		Injuries Resulting from Domestic Violence or Abuse	Injuries Resulting from Criminal Activity	Injuries Resulting from General Violence	Intentionally Inflicted Injuries	Injuries Inflicted by Gun or Firearm	Injuries Inflicted by Knife or Other Sharp Object	Burn Injuries	Injuries Likely to Cause Death	
AL										
AK Alaska Stat. §08.64.369	•					•			•	•
AZ A.R.S. §13-3806	•		•		•	•			•	•
AR A.C.A. §12-12-602	•				•	•				
CA Cal. Pen. Code §11160	•	•	•			•	•	•		•
CO C.R.S. §12-36-135	•	•	•		•	•				•
CT Conn. Gen. Stat §19a-490f	•					•				•
DC D.C. Code §7-2601	•					•				•
DE 24 Del. C. §1762	•				•	•	•			•
FL Fla. Stat. §790.24	•			•	•	•			•	
GA O.C.G.A. §31-7-9	•			•	•	•			•	•
HA HRS §453-14	•					•	•			•
ID Idaho Code §39-1390	•		•		•	•			•	•
IL 20 ILCS 2630/3.2	•		•		•					
IN Ind. Code Ann. §35-47-7-1	•				•	•	•		•	•
IA Iowa Code §147.111	•				•	•	•		•	•
KS K.S.A. §21 – 4213	•				•					•
KY KRS §209.030	•	•								
LA La. R.S. §14:403.4 to 3.5	•				•			•	•	•
ME 17-A M.R.S. §512	•				•	•				•
MD Md. Ann. Code art. 27, §336A	•					•		•		•
MA Ma. Ann. Laws ch. 112, §12A	•		•							
MI MCLS §750.411	•			•	•	•	•		•	•
MN Minn. Stat. §626.52	•		•		•	•				•
MS Miss. Code Ann. §45-9-31	•				•	•	•	•	•	•
MO §578.350 R.S.Mo.	•				•	•				•
MT Mont. Code Anno. §37-2-302	•				•					•

[xiii] This document is intended to provide a cursory overview of mandatory reporting laws. Please be sure to consult the complete set of mandatory reporting laws in your state for further information. If you note any changes or errors on this document, please contact the FVPF at 415-252-8900.

[xiv] Under a strict reading of these laws, practitioners must be providing treatment or medical care to the person with specified injuries in order to trigger the reporting requirement. Therefore, in a pediatric or family practice setting, if an attending parent with injuries is bringing her child in for a health care appointment, the attending parent is not actually receiving treatment or medical care from the practitioner, and thus the practitioner in the state would not be required to report. Further discussion is merited, given the lack of statutory or case law that have been developed around this area.

[xv] The law provides an exception to reporting if the patient is over the age of 18, did not suffer a gunshot wound, and does not consent to reporting.

[xvi] Report is made for medical data collection purposes only, and does not contain identification information.

Prepared by Josephine Yeh, J.D., for the Family Violence Prevention Fund

APPENDIX VII

STATE CODES ON INTIMATE PARTNER VIOLENCE VICTIMIZATION REPORTING REQUIREMENTS FOR HEALTH CARE PROVIDERS[xiii] *Current through March 8, 2002*

	Code Number	States with General Mandatory Reporting Laws	IF ANY OF THE FOLLOWING TYPES OF INJURIES ARE PRESENT, PRACTITIONERS IN THE STATE MUST MAKE A REPORT:								Treatment of Specified Injuries Requires Practitioners to Report[xiv]
			Injuries Resulting from Domestic Violence or Abuse	Injuries Resulting from Criminal Activity	Injuries Resulting from General Violence	Intentionally Inflicted Injuries	Injuries Inflicted by Gun or Firearm	Injuries Inflicted by Knife or Other Sharp Object	Burn Injuries	Injuries Likely to Cause Death.	
NE	R.R.S. Neb. §28-902	•	•	•	•						
NV	Nev. Rev. Stat. Ann. §629.041, §629.045								•	•
NH	RSA §631:6	•	[xv]	•	•		•		•	•	•
NJ	N.J. Stat. §2C:58-8	•					•		•		•
NM											
NY	NY CLS Penal §265.25 to .26	•	•	•	•						
NC	N.C. Gen. Stat. §90-21.20	•	•	•	•		•	•	•	•	•
ND	N.D. Cent. Code, §43-17-41	•		•			•	•			•
OH	ORC Ann. 2921.22	•					•	•	•		•
OK	10 Okl. St. §7104	•		•							
OR	ORS §146.750	•				•	•				•
PA	18 P.A.C.S. §5106	•		•			•				•
RI	R.I. Gen. Laws §11-47-48, §12-29-9	•	[xvi]				•				•
SC	S.C. Code Ann. §16-3-1072	•					•				•
SD	S.D. Codified Laws §23-13-10						•				•
TN	Tenn. Code Ann. §38-1-101	•			•		•	•			•
TX	Texas Health & Safety Code §161.041	•									•
UT	Utah Code Ann. §26-23a-2	•		•			•				•
VT	13 V.S.A. §4012	•					•	•			•
VA	Va. Code Ann. §54.1-2967	•					•	•	•		•
WA											
WV	W. Va. Code §61-2-27	•		•			•				•
WI	Wis. Stat. §146.995	•					•	•	•		•
WY											

xiii This document is intended to provide a cursory overview of mandatory reporting laws. Please be sure to consult the complete set of mandatory reporting laws in your state for further information. If you note any changes or errors on this document, please contact the FVPF at 415-252-8900.

xiv Under a strict reading of these laws, practitioners must be providing treatment or medical care to the person with specified injuries in order to trigger the reporting requirement. Therefore, in a pediatric or family practice setting, if an attending parent with injuries is bringing her child in for a health care appointment, the attending parent is not actually receiving treatment or medical care from the practitioner, and thus the practitioner in the state would not be required to report. Further discussion is merited, given the lack of statutory or case law that have been developed around this area.

xv The law provides an exception to reporting if the patient is over the age of 18, did not suffer a gunshot wound, and does not consent to reporting.

xvi Report is made for medical data collection purposes only, and does not contain identification information.

Prepared by Josephine Yeh, J.D., for the Family Violence Prevention Fund

APPENDIX VIII | RESOURCES AND REFERRALS

HOTLINES FOR VICTIMS OF IPV/DOMESTIC VIOLENCE

National Domestic Violence Hotline 24 hours, 1-800-799-SAFE (7233), 1-800-787-3224 (TTY)
Links individuals to help in their area using a nationwide database that includes detailed
information on DV shelters, other emergency shelters, legal advocacy and assistance programs, and
social service programs. website: *www.ndvh.org*

Rape Abuse & Incest National Network (RAINN) 24 hours, 1-800-656-HOPE
Will automatically transfer the caller to the nearest rape crisis center, anywhere in the nation. It can
be used as a last resort if people cannot find a DV shelter. 635-B Pennsylvania Ave SE, Washington,
DC 20003 phone: 1.800.656.HOPE (4673) ext. 3 fax: (202) 544-3556 e-mail: *rainnmail@aol.com*
website: *www.rainn.org*

Local DV Programs (numbers are listed in the front of your telephone book).
For the list of State Domestic Violence or Sexual Assault Coalitions visit:
www.ojp.usdoj.gov/vawo/state.htm

DOMESTIC VIOLENCE (IPV) ORGANIZATIONS

Family Violence Prevention Fund (FVPF) is a national non-profit organization that focuses on
domestic violence education, prevention and public policy reform; and provides health care specific
materials and information. 383 Rhode Island St., Suite 304, San Francisco, CA 94103-5133 phone:
(415) 252-8900 fax: (415) 252-8991 e-mail: *fund@endabuse.org* website: *www.endabuse.org*

**Pennsylvania Coalition Against Domestic Violence (PCADV) and National Resource Center
on Domestic Violence** is a private, nonprofit membership organization and is dedicated to ending
domestic violence and helping battered women and their children re-establish physical, social, and
economic dignity; PCADV has established health care advocacy programs throughout the state.
6400 Flank Drive, Suite 1300, Harrisburg, PA 17112 phone: (800) 932-4632 fax: (717) 671-
8149 website: *www.pcadv.org*

National Coalition Against Domestic Violence (NCADV) is dedicated to the empowerment of
battered women and their children and is committed to the elimination of personal and societal
violence in the lives of battered women and their children. PO Box 18749, Denver, CO 80218
phone: (303) 839-1852 fax: (303) 831-9251
website: *www.ncadv.org*

National Network to End Domestic Violence is a membership and advocacy organization
of state domestic violence coalitions, allied organizations and supportive individuals and is a
leading voice among domestic violence advocates in public policy. 660 Pennsylvania Ave.,
SE, Suite 303, Washington D.C. phone (202) 543-5566 email: nnedv@bellatlantic.net
website: *www.nnedv.org/who.html*

RESOURCES AND REFERRALS

Sacred Circle: The National Resource Center to End Violence Against Native Women
Dedicated to the actions that promote the sovereignty and safety of women. 722 St. Joseph St. Rapid City, SD 57701 Phone: (605) 341-2050. (877) RED-ROAD (733-7623)

Asian & Pacific Island Institute on Domestic Violence strives to eliminate domestic violence in Asian and Pacific Islander communities by increasing awareness about the extent and depth of the problem making culturally specific issues visible; strengthening community models of prevention and intervention; identifying and expanding resources; informing and promoting research and policy and deepening understanding and analysis of the issues surrounding violence against women. 942 Market Street, Suite 200, San Francisco, CA 94102 phone: (415) 954-9964 fax: (415) 954-9999 website: *www.apiahf.org*

Institute on Domestic Violence in the African American Community provides an interdisciplinary vehicle and forum by which scholars, practitioners, and observers of family violence within the African American community will have the continual opportunity to articulate their perspectives on family violence through research findings, the examination of service delivery and intervention mechanisms, and the identification of appropriate and effective responses to prevent/reduce family violence in the African American community. 290 Peters Hall, 1404 Gortner Avenue St. Paul, MN 55108-6142 phone: (877) NID-VAAC (643-8222) fax: (612) 624-9201 website: *www.dvinstitute.org*

National Latino Alliance for the Elimination of Domestic Violence is a network of nationally recognized Latina and Latino advocates, community activists, practitioners, researchers, and survivors of domestic violence working together to promote understand, sustain dialogue, and generate solutions to move toward the elimination of domestic violence in Latino communities, with an understanding of the sacredness of all relations and communities. P.O. Box 322086 Fort Washington New York, NY 10032 phone: (800) 342-9903 fax: (800) 216-2404 website: *www.dvalianza.org*

CLINICAL MATERIALS FOR THE HEALTH CARE SETTING
The National Health Resource Center on Domestic Violence a project of the FVPF, provides support to thousands of health care professionals, policy makers and domestic violence advocates through its four main program areas: model training strategies, practical tools, technical assistance, and public policy. 383 Rhode Island St, Suite 304, San Francisco, CA 94103 phone: (888) Rx-ABUSE TTY: (800) 595-4889 fax: (415) 252-8991 e-mail: *health@endabuse.org* website: *www.endabuse.org/health*

Physicians for a Violence-free Society (PVS) is a national non-profit organization that helps physicians and other health professionals improve their response to victims of violence, particularly IPV through educational programs, written materials and web-based resources. 160 14th Street, San Francisco, California 94103 phone: (415) 621-3584, fax: (415) 621-3438 e-mail: *pvs@pvs.org* website: *www.pvs.org*.

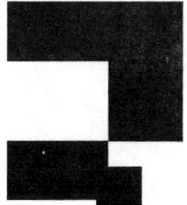

Appendix VIII

RESOURCES AND REFERRALS

The Child Witness to Violence Project at Boston Medical Center provides mental health services to young children exposed to violence. Staff also provide training and technical assistance to a wide range of professionals working with young children and families affected by violence and have published a training curriculum for mental health professionals and victim advocates: "Shelter from the Storm: Clinical Intervention with Young Children Affected by Domestic Violence". phone: (617) 414-4244. website: *www.bostonchildhealth.org/special/CWTV/overview.html*

Alaska Family Violence Prevention Project specializes in training for health care and service providers, has articles, curricula in PowerPoint that can be downloaded and run a clearinghouse of education materials. website: *www.hss.state.ak.us/dph/mcfh/akfvpp*

Howard S. King, MD, MPH and Melinda Strauss, ACSW, LISCW authors of *Routine Screen for Domestic Violence in Pediatric Practice* written to help pediatricians and family practitioners become aware of the problem of domestic violence and to consider screening for it during the routine office visit. View or download this publication at *www.drkingsoffice.com*

The Institute for Safe Families' (ISF) mission is to prevent family violence and to offer an alternative vision for wholeness, healing, family health, and personal empowerment. ISF is conducting a Philadelphia area initiative to address domestic violence within the pediatric setting and has developed a pocket card on what to do, with a variety of materials in development. ISF, 3502 Scotts Lane, Philadelphia, PA 19129, phone: (215) 843-2046 website: *ISF2002@aol.com*

WEBSITES OF INTEREST FOR ADOLESCENTS

The Empower Program works with youth to end the culture of violence. 1312 8th Street, Washington, DC 20001 phone: (202) 882-2800 fax: (202) 234-1901 e-mail: *empower@empowered.org* website: *www.empowered.org*

Girls Incorporated National Resource Center is a national youth organization dedicated to inspiring all girls to be strong, smart and bold. 441 West Michigan Street, Indianapolis, IN 46202 phone: (317) 634-7546 fax: (317) 634-3024 e-mail: *girlsinc@girls-inc.org* website: *www.girlsinc.org*

Liz Claiborne Inc. produces "A Teen's Handbook" and web pages to help teens learn about dating violence by providing facts, guidance and resources. To order a free handbook, phone: (800) 449-STOP (7867) website: *www.lizclaiborne.com/lizinc/lizworks/women/handbook.asp#teen*

LESBIAN, GAY, BISEXUAL, TRANSGENDERED, QUEER (LGBTQ)

Community United Against Violence (CUAV) is a 20-year old multicultural organization working

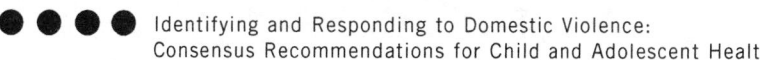

RESOURCES AND REFERRALS

to end violence against and within lesbian, gay, bisexual, transgender and queer/questioning (LGBTQ) communities. The Love & Justice Project aims to lead the discussion on positive communication skills, consensual sexuality, partnership decision making and naming abusive behavior in LGBTQ youth relationships by building bridges and community resources between LGBTQ youth and elders. 973 Market St., #500, San Francisco, CA 94103 phone: (415) 777-5500 Fax: (415) 777-5565 24 Hr. Support Line: (415) 333-HELP (4357) e-mail: *cuav@aol.com* website: *www.cuav.org*

Parents, Families, and Friends of Lesbians and Gays (PFLAG) is a national organization that promotes the health and well-being of gay, lesbian, bisexual and transgendered persons, their families and friends. Their web site provides users with information on local chapters, advocacy and support information and other resources that support the family and friends of gays and lesbians. 1726 M Street, NW, Suite 400, Washington, DC 20036 phone: (202) 467-8180 fax: (202) 467-8194 e-mail: *info@pflag.org* website: *www.pflag.org/pflag.html*

Gay Men's Domestic Violence Project is a grassroots, non-profit organization in Boston providing community education and direct services for clients. GMDVP offers shelter, guidance, and resources to allow gay, bisexual, and transgender men in crisis to remove themselves from violent situations and relationships GMDVP, PMB 131, 955 Mass Ave. Cambridge, MA 02139 phone: (617) 354-6056 crisis: (800) 832-1901 fax: 617 354 6072 toll-free: (800)832-1901 website: *www.gmdvp.org*

Network for Battered Lesbians and Bisexual Women was formed to address battering in lesbian, bisexual women's, and transgender communities. POB 6011 Boston, MA 02114. phone/TTY: (617) 695-0877 hotline]TTY (617) 423-7233 website: *www.thenetworklared.org*

TEEN PREGNANCY

American College of Obstetricians and Gynecologists (ACOG) has a membership of 40,000 physicians and is the nation's leading group of professionals providing health care for women. ACOG's website provides adolescent sexual assault screening tools as well as other teen pregnancy materials. To request free copies of their educational bulletins, call: (202) 638-5577 or e-mail: *violence@acog.org* ACOG, 409 12th Street, SW, PO Box 96920 Washington, DC 20024 phone: (202) 863-2487 fax: (202) 484-3917 e-mail: *adolhlth@acog.org* website: *www.acog.org*

SEXUAL ASSAULT

Center for the Prevention of Sexual and Domestic Violence is an interreligious educational resource addressing issues of sexual and domestic violence whose goal is to engage religious leaders in the task of ending abuse, and to serve as a bridge between

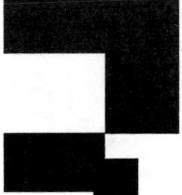

Appendix VIII

RESOURCES AND REFERRALS

religious and secular communities. 936 North 34th St., Suite 200, Seattle, WA 98103
phone: (206) 634-1903 fax: (206) 634-0115
e-mail: *cpsdv@cpsdv.org* website: *www.cpsdv.org*

Rape Abuse & Incest National Network (RAINN) *(see "Hotlines" for further info)*

Sexual Assault Resource Service (SARS) is designed for nursing professionals involved in
providing evaluations of sexually abused victims. SARS' website provides information and technical
assistance to individuals and institutions interested in developing new SANE-SART programs or
improving existing ones. website: *www.sane-sart.com*

OTHER WEBSITES OF INTEREST

American Academy of Pediatrics: *www.aap.org*

American College of Emergency Physicians: *www.acep.org*

American College of Nurse Midwives: *www-acnm.org*

American College of Obstetricians and Gynecologists: *www.acog.org*

American Medical Association: *www.ama-assn.org*

American Medical Women's Association: *www.amwa-doc.org*

American Psychological Association: *www.apa.org*

Association of Traumatic Stress Specialists: *www.atss-hq.com/a/indix.htm*

Battered Women and Their Children: *http://cwolf.uaa.alaska.edu/~afrhm1/*

Child Witness to Violence Project at Boston Medical Center:
www.bostonchildhealth.org/PediatricsDept/ChildWitness/

Family Violence and Sexual Assault Institute: *www.fvsai.org/*

International Association of Forensic Nurses: *www.forensicnurse.org*

Johns Hopkins University School of Nursing: *www.son.jhmi.edu*

Massachusetts Medical Society: *www.massmed.org*

Men Stopping Violence: *www.menstoppingviolence.org*

Nursing Network to End Violence Against Women International: *www.nnvawi.org*

National Sexual Violence Resource Center: *www.nsvor.org*

Physicians for a Violence-Free Society: *www.pvs.org*

Society of Academic Emergency Medicine: *www.saem.org*

APPENDIX IX | CHILD ABUSE AND NEGLECT REPORTING LAWS

WHO MUST REPORT	Dentist	Doctor	Mental Health	Nurse	Social Worker	Standard for Reporting?	Report What?	Report to Whom?	Report How?
Alabama Ala. Code § 26-14-3 (2000)	Y	Y	Y	Y	Y	Knowledge or suspicion	Child Abuse or Neglect	Law enforcement Department of Human resources	Oral and written
Alaska Alaska Stat. § 47.17.020 (Michie 2000)	Y	Y	Y	Y	Y	Reasonable cause to suspect	Harm as a result of child abuse or neglect	Department of Health and Social Services	Not Specified
Arizona Ariz. Rev. Stat. § 13-3620 (2000)	Y	Y	Y	Y	Y	Resonable grounds to believe	Injury, commercial sexual expiation of a minor, sexual exploitation of a minor, incest, child prostitution, death, abuse, or nonaccidental physical neglect	Law enforcement or Child Protective Services	Oral and written
Arkansas Ark. Code Ann. § 12-12-507 (Michie 1999)	Y	Y	Y	Y	Y	Reasonable cause to suspect	Child maltreatment or conditions that will reasonavle result in child maltreatment	Child abuse hotline	Oral
California Cal. [Penal] Code § 11166 (West 2000)	Y	Y	Y	Y	Y	Knowledge or reasonable suspicion	Child abuse	Child protective agency	Oral and written
Colorado Colo. Rev. Stat. § 19-3-304 (1999)	Y	Y	Y	Y	Y	Reasonable cause to know or suspect	Child abuse or neglect	County Department of Human Services or law enforcement	Not Specified
Connecticut Conn. Gen. Stat. §§ 17a-101 to -101b (1999)	Y	Y	Y	Y	Y	Reasonable cause to suspect or believe	Abuse, nonaccidental physical injury, or neglect	Commissioner of Children and families or law enforcement agency	Oral

APPENDIX IX | CHILD ABUSE AND NEGLECT REPORTING LAWS

WHO MUST REPORT	Dentist	Doctor	Mental Health	Nurse	Social Worker	Standard for Reporting?	Report What?	Report to Whom?	Report How?
Delaware Del. Code Ann. Tit.16, §§ 903-904 (1999)	Y	Y	Y	Y	Y	Knowledge or good faith suspicion	Child abuse or neglect	Division of Child Protective Services of Department of Services for Children Youth, and Their Families	Oral and written (if requested)
District of Columbia D.C. Code Ann. § 2-1352 (1999)	Y	Y	Y	Y	Y	Knowledge or reasonable cause to suspect	Immediate danger of physical or mental avuse or neglect	Law enforcement or Child Protective Services	Not Specified
Florida Fla. Stat. ch. 39.201 (1999)	Y	Y	Y	Y	Y	Knowledge or reasonable cause to suspect	Abuse, abandonment, or neglect	Department of Children and Family Services	Oral
Georgia Ga. Code Ann. § 19-7-5 (1999)	Y	Y	Y	Y	Y	Reasonable cause	Abuse	Child welfare agency designated by the Department of Human Resources or law enforcement Commissioner of Children and families or law enforcement agency	Oral and written (if requested)
Hawaii Haw. Rev. Stat. § 350-1.1 (1999)	Y	Y	Y	Y	Y	Reason to believe	Child abuse or neglect or substantial risk of above in reasonably foreseeable future	Department of Human Services and law enforcement	Oral and written
Idaho Idaho Code § 16-1619 (1999)	Y	Y	Y	Y	Y	Reason to believe	Abuse, abandonment, or neglect or conditions that would reasonably result in any of above	Law enforcement or Department of Health and Welfare	Not specfied

APPENDIX IX | CHILD ABUSE AND NEGLECT REPORTING LAWS

WHO MUST REPORT	Dentist	Doctor	Mental Health	Nurse	Social Worker	Standard for Reporting?	Report What?	Report to Whom?	Report How?
Illinois 325 Ill. Comp. Stat. 5/4 (West 2000)	Y	Y	Y	Y	Y	Reasonable cause to believe	Abuse or neglect	Department of Children and Family Services	Not specified
Indiana Ind. Code §§ 31-33-5-1 to -2, -4 (1999)	Y	Y	Y	Y	Y	Reason to believe	Abuse or neglect	Child protective services or law enforcement	Oral
Iowa Iowa Code § 232.69 (1999)	Y	Y	Y	Y	Y	Reasonable belief	Child abuse	Department of Human Services	Oral and written
Kansas Kan. Stat. Ann. § 38-1522 (1999)	Y	Y	Y	Y	Y	Reason to suspect	Injury resulting from physical, mental, or emotional, neglect, or sexual abuse	Department of Social and Rehabilitation Services	Oral and written (if requested)
Kentucky Ky. Rev. Stat. Ann. § 620.030 (Michie 1998)	Y	Y	Y	Y	Y	Knows or has reasonable cause to believe	Dependency, neglect or abuse	Law enforcement, Cabinet for Families and Children, or county attorney	Oral or written
Louisiana La. Civ. Stat. Ann. Art. 603, 609-610 (West 2000)	Y	Y	Y	Y	Y	Cause to believe	Endangerment of child's physical or mental health or welfare due to neglect or abuse	Child Pretection Unit of Department of Social Services	Written
Maine Me. Rev. Stat. Ann. Tit. 22 § 4011 (West 1999)	Y	Y	Y	Y	Y	Knowledge or reasonable cause to suspect	Child likely to be or has been abused or neglected	Department of Human Services	Not Specified
Maryland Md. Code. Ann., [Fam. Law] § 5-704 (1999)	Y	Y	Y	Y	Y	Reason to believe	Abuse or neglect	Department of Social Services or law enforcement	Oral and written

APPENDIX IX | CHILD ABUSE AND NEGLECT REPORTING LAWS

WHO MUST REPORT	Dentist	Doctor	Mental Health	Nurse	Social Worker	Standard for Reporting?	Report What?	Report to Whom?	Report How?
Massachusetts Mass. Gen. Laws ch. 119, § 51A (2000)	Y	Y	Y	Y	Y	Reasonable cause to believe	Physical or emotional injury resulting from abuse which causes harm or substantial risk of harm to child's health or welfare;	Juvenile Court	Oral and written
Michigan Mich. Comp. Laws § 722.623 (1999)	Y	Y	Y	Y	Y	Reasonable cause to suspect	Abuse or neglect	Department of Social Services	Oral and written
Minnesota Minn. Stat. § 626.556 (1999)	Y	Y	Y	Y	Y	Knows or has reason to believe	Neglect, or physical or sexual abuse, currently or within past three years	Welfare agency or law enforcement	Not specified
Mississppi Miss. Code Ann. § 43-21-353 (2000)	Y	Y	Y	Y	Y	Reasonable cause to suspect	Neglect or abuse	Department of Human Services	Oral and written
Missouri Mo. Rev. Stat. § 210.115 (1999)	Y	Y	Y	Y	Y	Reasonable cause to suspect	Child has been or may be subjected to abuse or neglect or is being subjected to conditions that would reasonably result in abuse or neglect	Division of Family Services	Not specified
Montana Mont. Code Ann. § 41-3-201 (1999)	Y	Y	Y	Y	Y	Knows or has reasonable cause to suspect	Abuse or neglect	Department of public Health and Human Services	Not specified
Nebraska Neb. Rev. Stat. § 28-711 (2000)	Y	Y	Y	Y	Y	Reasonable cause to believe	Abuse or neglect or conditions that reasonably would result in abuse or neglect	Law enforcement or Department of Health and Human Services	Oral and written

HEALTH SCIENCES BROOKFIELD LIBRARY CORK

APPENDIX IX | CHILD ABUSE AND NEGLECT REPORTING LAWS

WHO MUST REPORT	Dentist	Doctor	Mental Health	Nurse	Social Worker	Standard for Reporting?	Report What?	Report to Whom?	Report How?
Nevada Nev. Rev. Stat. § 432B.220 (2000)	Y	Y	Y	Y	Y	Knowledge or reasonable cause to believe	Abuse or neglect	Law enforcement or protective services	Not specified
New Hampshire N.H. Rev. Stat. Ann. §§ 169-C:29 to –C:30 (1999)	Y	Y	Y	Y	Y	Reason to suspect	Abuse or neglect	Department of Health and Human Services	Oral and written (if requested)
New Jersey N.J. Stat. Ann. § 9:6–8.10 (west 2000)	Y	Y	Y	Y	Y	Reasonable cause to believe	Abuse	Division of Youth and Family Services	Oral or written
New Mexico N.M. Stat. Ann. § 32A-4-3 (Michie)	Y	Y	Y	Y	Y	Knowledge or reasonable suspicion	Abuse or Neglect	Law enforcement or Department of Children, Youth, and Families or tribal law enforcement (if child resides in Indian country)	Not specified
New York N.Y. [Soc. Serv.] Law § 413 (McKinney 1999)	Y	Y	Y	Y	Y	Reasonable cause to suspect	Abuse or maltreatment	Central register of child abuse and maltreatment	Oral and written
North Carolina N.C. Gen. Stat. § 7B-301 (1999)	Y	Y	Y	Y	Y	Cause to suspect	Abuse, neglect, dependency, or death resulting from maltreatment	Department of Social Services	Oral or written
North Dakota N.D. Cent. Code § 50-25.1-03 (2000)	Y	Y	Y	Y	Y	Knowledge or reasonable cause to suspect	Abuse, neglect, or death resulting from abuse or neglect	Department of Human Services	Not specified

● ● ● ● Family Violence Prevention Fund

APPENDIX IX CHILD ABUSE AND NEGLECT REPORTING LAWS

WHO MUST REPORT	Dentist	Doctor	Mental Health	Nurse	Social Worker	Standard for Reporting?	Report What?	Report to Whom?	Report How?
Ohio Ohio Rev. Code. Ann. § 2151.421 (Anderson 1999)	Y	Y	Y	Y	Y	Knowledge or suspicion	Suffers or faces threat of suffering abuse, neglect, physical or mental wound, injury or diability that reasonably indicates abuse or neglect	Public Children Services Agency or law enforcement	Oral and written (if requested)
Oklahoma Okla. Stat. Tit. 10, § 7103 (1999)	Y	Y	Y	Y	Y	Reason to believe	Abuse or neglect	Department of Human Services	Oral or written
Oregon Or. Rev. Stat. §§ 419B.005, .010-.015 (1997)	Y	Y	Y	Y	Y	Reasonable cause to believe	Abuse	Office for Services to Children and Families or law enforcement	Oral
Pennsylvania 23 Pa. Cons. Stat. § 6311 (1999)	Y	Y	Y	Y	Y	Reasonable cause to suspect	Abuse	Department or appropriate county agency	Oral and written
Rhode Island R.I. Gen. Laws § 40-11-3 (2000)	Y	Y	Y	Y	Y	Reasonable cause to know or suspect	Abuse, neglect, or sexual abuse perpetrated by another child	Department for Children and Their Families	Oral
South Carolina S.C. Code Ann. § 20-7-510 (Law. Co-op. 1999)	Y	Y	Y	Y	Y	Reason to believe	Physical or mental health or welfare has been or may be adversely affected by abuse or neglect	Department of Social Services or law enforcement	Oral
South Dakota S.D. Codified Laws §§ 26-8A-3, -6	Y	Y	Y	Y	Y	Reasonable cause to suspect	Abuse or neglect	State's attorney, Department of Social Services. or law enforcement	Oral

●●●● Identifying and Responding to Domestic Violence:
Consensus Recommendations for Child and Adolescent Health

APPENDIX IX | CHILD ABUSE AND NEGLECT REPORTING LAWS

WHO MUST REPORT	Dentist	Doctor	Mental Health	Nurse	Social Worker	Standard for Reporting?	Report What?	Report to Whom?	Report How?
Tennessee Tenn. Code Ann. § 37-1-403 (1999)	Y	Y	Y	Y	Y	Knowledge or reasonable indication or reasonable appearance	Wound, injury, diability, physical or mental condition caused by brutality, abuse, or neglect	Juvenile court judge, Department of Children's Services, or law enforcement	Oral or written
Texas Tex. [Fam.] Code Ann. §§ 261.101-.103 (West 2000)	Y	Y	Y	Y	Y	Cause to believe	Physical or mental health or welfare adversely affected by abuse or neglect	Law enforcement or Department of Protective and Regulartory Services	Not specified
Utah Utah Code Ann. § 62A-4a-403 (1999)	Y	Y	Y	Y	Y	Observation or has reason to believe	Incest, molestation, sexual exploitation, sexual abuse, physical abuse, neglect, or circumstances reasonably resulting in any of above	Law enforcement or Division of Child and Family Services	Not specified
Vermont Vt. Stat. Ann. Tit. 33, §§ 4913-4914 (2000)	Y	Y	Y	Y	Y	Resonable cause to believe	Abuse or neglect	Commissioner of Social And Rehabilitaiton Services	Oral and written
Virginia Va. Code Ann. § 63.1-248.3 (Michie 1999)	Y	Y	Y	Y	Y	Reason to suspect	Abuse or neglect	Department of Social Services	Oral
Washington Wash. Rev. Code § 26.44.030 (2000)	Y	Y	Y	Y	Y	Observation or reasonable cause to believe	Abuse or neglect or conditions likely to result in neglect or abuse	Law enforcement or Department of Social and Health Services	Not specified
West Virginia W. Va. Code § 49-6A-2 (2000)	Y	Y	Y	Y	Y	Reasonable cause to suspect	Neglect or abuse, or conditions likely to result in neglect or abuse	State Department of Human Services and Division of Public Safety and law enforcement (if serious)	Not specified

●●●● Family Violence Prevention Fund

APPENDIX IX   CHILD ABUSE AND NEGLECT REPORTING LAWS

WHO MUST REPORT	Dentist	Doctor	Mental Health	Nurse	Social Worker	Standard for Reporting?	Report What?	Report to Whom?	Report How?
Wisconsin Wis. Stat. § 48.981 (1999)		Y	Y	Y	Y	Reasonable cause to suspect or reason to believe	Abuse or neglect, or threat of abuse or neglect	Department of Health and Family Services	Oral and written (if requested)
Wyoming Wyo. Stat. Ann. § 14-3 205 (Michie 1999)		Y	Y	Y	Y	Knowledge or reasonable cause to believe or suspect	Abuse or neglect or subjection to conditions that would reasonably result in abuse or neglect	Child protective agency or law enforcement	Not specified

NOTE: Because the term allied health professional is defined variably among different states, this Chart cannot accurately summarize the duties of all persons who might be included in this broad category

Reprinted with permission from *Confronting Chronic Neglect: The Education and Training of Health Professionals on Family Violence.* Copyright 2002 by the National Academy of Sciences. Courtesy of the National Academy Press, Washington, D.C.

● ● ● ● Identifying and Responding to Domestic Violence:
Consensus Recommendations for Child and Adolescent Health

APPENDIX X | SAFETY PLAN AND INSTRUCTIONS

SAFETY PLAN for adult victims living with their abusers

Step 1:

Safety during a violent incident. I can use some or all of the following strategies:

A. If I have/decide to leave my home, I will go _____
B. I can tell _____ (neighbors) about the violence and request they call the police if they hear suspicious noises coming from my house.
C. I can teach my children how to use the telephone to contact the police.
D. I will use _____ as my code word so someone can call for help.
E. I can keep my purse/car keys ready at (place) _____, in order to leave quickly.
F. I will use my judgment and intuition. If the situation is very serious, I can give my partner what he/she wants to calm him/her down. I have to protect myself until I/we are out of danger.

Step 2:

Safety when preparing to leave. I can use some or all of the following safety strategies:

A. I will keep copies important documents, keys, clothes and money at _____.
B. I will open a savings account by _____, to increase my independence.
C. Other things I can do to increase my independence include: _____.
D. I can keep change for my phone calls on me at all times. I understand that if I use my telephone credit card, the telephone bill will show my partner those numbers that I called after I left.
E. I will check with _____ to see who would be able to let me stay with them or lend me some money.
F. If I plan to leave, I won't tell my abuser in advance face-to-face, but I will call or leave a note from a safe place.

Step 3:

Safety in my own residence. Safety measures I can use include:

A. I can change the locks on my doors and windows as soon as possible.
B. I can replace wooden doors with steel/metal doors.
C. I can install additional locks, window bars, poles to wedge against doors, and electronic systems etc.
D. I can install motion lights outside.
E. I will teach my children how to make a collect call to _____ if my partner takes the children.
F. I will tell people who take care of my children that my partner is not permitted to pick up my children.
G. I can inform _____ (neighbor) that my partner no longer resides with me and they should call the police if he is observed near my residence.

Step 4.

Safety with a protection order. The following are steps that help the enforcement of my protection order:

A. Always carry a certified copy with me and keep a photocopy.
B. I will give my protection order to police departments in the community where I work and live.
C. I can get my protection order to specify and describe all guns may partner may own and authorize a search for removal.

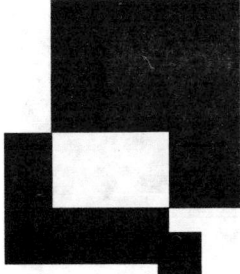

Appendix X

SAFETY PLAN AND INSTRUCTIONS

SAFETY INSTRUCTIONS

If you are currently being abused...

Are you here as a result of someone hitting or threatening you—a spouse, boyfriend, lover, relative or someone you know? Have you been sexually abused by someone you know? As you read this, you may be feeling confused, frightened, sad, angry or ashamed. **You are not alone!** Unfortunately, what happened to you is very common. Domestic violence does not go away on its own. It tends to get worse and more frequent with time. There are people who can help you. If you want to begin talking about the problem, need a safe place to stay or want legal advice—call one of the agencies listed on the back of this instruction sheet today.

While still at the clinic...

• Think about whether it is safe to return home. If not, call one of the resources listed on the back of this instruction sheet or stay with a friend or relative.
• You have received instructions on caring for your injuries and taking medications prescribed. Remember, if you have received tranquilizers they may help you rest but they won't solve the problem of battering.
• Battering is a crime and you have the right to legal intervention. You should consider calling the police for assistance (see information on back of this sheet). You may also obtain a court order prohibiting your partner from contacting you in any way (including in person or by phone). Contact a local DV program or an attorney for more information.
• Ask the doctor or nurse to take photos of your injuries to become part of your medical record.

When you get home...

• Develop an "exit plan" in advance for you and your children. Know exactly where you could go even in the middle of the night—and how to get there.
• Pack an "overnight bag" in case you have to leave home in a hurry. Either hide it yourself or give it to a friend to keep for you.
• Pack toilet articles, medications, an extra set of keys to the house and car, an extra set of clothing for you and your children, and a toy for each child.
• Have extra cash, loose change for phone calls, checkbook, or savings account book hidden or with a friend.
• Pack important papers and financial records (the originals or copies), such as social security cards, birth certificates, green cards, passports, work authorization and any other immigration documents, voter registration cards, medical cards and records, drivers license, rent receipts, title to the car and proof of insurance, etc.
• Notify your neighbors if you think it is safe.

REFERENCES

[1] McFarlane, J, Christoffel K, Bateman L, Miller V, Bullock L. (1991). "Assessing for abuse: self-report versus nurse interview." Public Health Nurs.; 8:242-250.

[2] McFarlane J, Greenberg L, Weltge A, Watson M. (1995). "Identification of abuse in emergency departments; effectiveness of a two-question screening tool." Journal Emergency Nursing. 21:391-394.

[3] McFarlane J, Parker B, Soeken K, Bullock L. (1992). "Assessing for abuse during pregnancy; severity and frequency of injuries and associated entry into prenatal care." Journal of the American Medical Association. 267:3176-3178.

[4] Caralis P, Musialowski R. (1997). "Women's Experiences with Domestic Violence and Their Attitudes and Expectations Regarding Medical Care of Abuse Victims." South Medical Journal, 90:1075-1080.

[5] McCauley J, Yurk R, Jenckes M, Ford D. "Inside 'Pandora's Box': Abused Women's Experiences with Clinicians and Health Services" (1998). Archives of Internal Medicine, 13:549-555.

[6] Friedman L, Samet J, Roberts M, Hudlin M, Hans P. "Inquiry About Victimization Experiences: A Survey of Patient Preferences and Physician Practices." (1992) Archives of Internal Medicine, 152:1186-1190.

[7] Rodriguez M, Quiroga SS, Bauer H. "Breaking the Silence: Battered Women's Perspectives on Medical Care" (1996). Archives of Family Medicine, 5:153-158.

[8] Borowsky IW, Ireland M. (1999). "National Survey of Pediatricians' Violence Prevention Counseling." Archives of Pediatric and Adolescent Medicine," 153: 1170-1176.

[9] American Academy of Pediatrics. Committee on Child Abuse and Neglect. (1998). "The role of the pediatrician in recognizing and intervening on behalf of abused women." Pediatrics, 101 (6), 1091-1092.

[10] Family Violence Prevention Fund (1999). *Preventing Domestic Violence: Clinical Guidelines on Routine Screening.* San Francisco, CA: Family Violence Prevention Fund.

[11] For a complete discussion of children who witness domestic violence, see: Jaffe P, Wolfe, & Wilson. (1990). *Children of Domestic Violence.* Newbury Park CA: Sage Publications.

[12] *Bureau of Justice Statistics Special Report, Intimate Partner Violence and Age of Victim, 1993-99,* United States Department of Justice, October 2001.

[13] National Institute of Justice and Centers for Disease Control and Prevention. *Prevalence, Incidence, and Consequences of Violence Against Women: Findings from the National Violence Against Women Survey.* Washington, DC: National Institute of Justice and Centers for Disease Control and Prevention; 1998.

[14] McCauley J, Kern DE, Kolodner K, Dill L, Schroeder AF, DeChant HK, Ryden J, Bass EB, Derogatis LR. (1995). "The 'battering syndrome': prevalence and clinical characteristics of domestic violence in primary care internal medicine practices." Annals of Internal Medicine; 123:737-746.

[15] Dearwater SR, Coben JH, Campbell JC, Nah G, Glass N, McLoughlin E, Bekemeier B. (1998). "Prevalence of intimate partner abuse in women treated at community hospital emergency departments." Journal of the American Medical Association; 280:433-438.

[16] U.S. Department of Justice. (1998). *Violence by Intimates: Analysis of Data on Crimes by Current or Former Spouses, Boyfriends, and Girlfriends.* Washington, DC: U.S. Department of Justice, Bureau of Justice Statistics.

[17] *U.S. Department of Justice, Intimate Partner Violence, May 2000.* Washington, DC: U.S. Department of Justice, Bureau of Justice Statistics.

[18] Greenfield L.; Rand M.; Craven, D. et al. (1998). "Violence by Intimates: analysis of data on crimes

References

by current or former spouses, boyfriends, and girlfriends." Bureau of Justice Statistics Factbook. Washington, DC: U.S. Department of Justice. Publication NCJ 167237.

[19] Foshee, VA; Linder, GF; Bauman, KE; Langwick, SA; Arriaga, XB; Heath, JL; McMahon, PM; Bangdiwala, S. (1996). "The Safe Dates Project: Theoretical basis, evaluation design, and selected baseline findings." American Journal of Preventive Medicine, 12(5 Suppl):39–47.

[20] Cohall, A; Cohall, R; Bannister, H; Northridge, M. (1999). "Love shouldn't hurt: Strategies for health care providers to address adolescent dating violence." Journal of the American Medical Women's Association, 54 (3):144-8.

[21] Silverman J, Raj A, Mucci L, Hathaway J. (2001). "Dating violence against adolescent girls and associated substance use, unhealthy weight control, sexual risk behavior, pregnancy, and suicidality." Journal of the American Medical Association, 286(5). 572-579.

[22] Rennison, M. (2001). *Intimate Partner Violence and Age of Victim, 1993-1999, Bureau of Justice Statistics: Special Report.* Washington, DC. U.S. Department of Justice. Publication NCJ 187635.

[23] Parker, B., McFarlane, J. (1993). "Physical and Emotional Abuse in Pregnancy: A Comparison of Adult and Teenage Women." Nursing Research, Vol. 42. No. 3, 173-177.

[24] Ibid.

[25] Silverman, Op.Cit.

[26] Goodenow, Carol. (1998). 1997 "Massachusetts Youth Risk Behavior Survey." Malden, MA: Massachusetts Department of Education.

[27] Renzetti, C. *Violent Betrayal: Partner Abuse in Lesbian Relationships.* Sage Publications. 1992, 18.

[28] Edleson JL, (1999). "Children's witnessing of adult domestic violence." Journal of Interpersonal Violence. 14 (8), 839-870.

[29] Fantuzzo J, Boruch R, Beriama A, Atkins M, Marcus S (1997). "Domestic violence and children: Prevalence and risk in five major U.S. cities." Journal of the American Academy of Child and Adolescent Psychiatry, 36 (1), 116-122.

[30] Lenares O, Groves B, Bronfman E, et al. (1999). "Restraining orders: A Frequent marker of adverse maternal health." Pediatrics, 104 (2), 249-256.

[31] Parkinson GW, Adams RC, Emerling FG (2001). "Maternal domestic violence screening in an office-based practice." Pediatrics. 108: 1-9.

[32] Felitti VJ, Anda RF, Nordenberg D, Williamson DF, Spitz AM, Edwards V, Kiss MP, Marks Js. (1998). "Relationship of childhood abuse and household dysfunction to many of the leading causes of death in adults." American Journal of Preventive Medicine, 14 (4), 245-258.

[33] Coker, A., Smith, P., Bethea, L., King, M., McKeown, R. (2000). "Physical Health Consequences of Physical and Psychological Intimate Partner Violence." Archives of Family Medicine, Vol. 9.

[34] Barkan, H., Farley, M., and Minkof, J., "Mammography Screening and Domestic Violence." Abstract presented at the National Conference on Health Care and Domestic Violence. October 2000. Accepted for publication in Women's Health.

[35] Danielson, K., Moffit, T., Caspi, A., and Silva, P. (1998). "Comorbidty Between Abuse of an Adult and DSM-III-R Mental Disorders: Evidence From an Epidemiological Study." American Journal of Psychiatry, 155(1).

[36] Stark, E. and Flitcraft, A.(1995). "Killing the beast within: Woman battering and female suicidality." International Journal of Health Sciences, 25(1)

[37] Housekamp, B.M. and Foy, D.(1991). "The assessment of posttraumatic stress disorder in battered women." Journal of Interpersonal Violence, 6(3).

References
_____

[38] Gelles, R.J. and Harrop, J.W. (1989). "Violence, battering, and psychological distress among women." Journal of Interpersonal Violence, 4(1).

[39] Housekamp and Foy, 1991.

[40] Schoen, C., Davis, K., Collins, K., Greenburg, L., Des Roches, C. Abrams, M., (1997). *The Commonwealth Fund Survey of the Health of Adolescent Girls.* New York, NY: The Commonwealth Fund.

[41] Richards, Julie, RNC, MS, MSN, 1991, "Battering in a population of adolescent females." Journal of the American Academy of Nurse Practitioners, 3 (4).

[42] Silverman, Op.Cit.

[43] Center for Impact Research (2000) *Domestic Violence and Birth Control Sabotage: A Report from the Teen Parent Project.* Chicago, IL: Center for Impact on Research.

[44] Ibid.

[45] Jacoby, M., et. al., (1999). "Rapid repeat pregnancy and experiences of interpersonal violence among low-income adolescents." American Journal of Preventive Medicine, 16 (4), 318-321.

[46] Parker, B., McFarlane, J., Soeken, K., Torres, S., Campbell, D. (1993). "Physical and Emotional Abuse in Pregnancy: A Comparison of Adult and Teenage Women." Nursing Research, Vol. 42 (3): 173-178.

[47] Edleson, 1999. P. 845.

[48] Edleson JL. (1999). "The overlap between child maltreatment and woman battering." Violence Against Women. 5(2). 134-154.

[49] Christian C, Scribano P, Seidl T, Pinto-Martin J. (1997). "Pediatric injury resulting from family violence." Pediatrics, 99 (2): 208-212.

[50] Kilpatrick KI, Litt, M, & Williams L. (1997). "Post-traumatic stress disorder in child witnesses to domestic violence." American Journal of Orthopsychiatry, 67(4), 639-644.

[51] Jaffe, P. and Sudermann, M., "Child Witness of Women Abuse: Research and Community Responses," in Stith, S. and Straus, M., (1995). *Understanding Partner Violence: Prevalence, Causes, Consequences, and Solutions. Families in Focus Services,* Vol. II. Minneapolis, MN: National Council on Family Relations.

[52] Wolfe, D.A., Wekerle, C., Reitzel, D. and Gough, R., "Strategies to address violence in the lives of high risk youth." In Peled, E., Jaffe, P.G. and Edleson, J.L. (eds.), *Ending the Cycle of Violence: Community Responses to Children of Battered Women.* New York: Sage Publications. 1995.

[53] See Rossman R. (1998). "Descartes' error and posttraumatic stress disorder: Cognition and emotion in children who are exposed to parental violence." In Holden, GW, Gefner, RA, Jouriles, EN. (1998). *Children Exposed to Marital Violence: Theory, Research, and Applied Issues.* Washington DC: American Psychological Association. Lieberman, A., Von Horn, P., Grandison, C,, and Pekarsky. J. "Mental health assessment of infants, toddlers and preschoolers in a service program and a treatment outcome research program." Infant Mental Health Journal, (1997) 18,2: 158-170.

[54] Spaccarelli S, Coatsworth JD, & Bowden BS, (1995). "Exposure to serious family violence among incarcerated boys: Its association with violent offending and potential mediating variables." Violence and Victims. 10, 163-182.

[55] Hughes, HM & Luke, DA (1998). "Heterogeneity in adjustment among children of battered women." In GW Holden, R. Geffner & EN Jouriles (Eds), *Children Exposed to Marital Violence,* Washington DC, American Psychological Association.

[56] Grych, JH & Fincham, FD. (1990). "Marital conflict and children's adjustment: A cognitive-contextual framework." Psychological Bulletin, 108, 267-290.

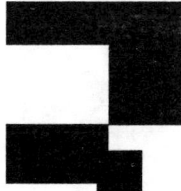

References

[57] Sullivan, CM, Nguyen, H, Allen, N, Bybee, D, Juras, J. (2000). "Beyond searching for deficits: Evidnece that physically and emotionally abused women are nurturing parents." Journal of Emotional Abuse. 2, 51-71.

[58] *The Commonwealth Fund 2001 Health Care Quality Survey.* (2001). New York, NY: The Commonwealth Fund.

[59] *Racial and Ethnic Variations in Patient-Physician Communication and Adherence to Doctor's Advice.* The Commonwealth Fund and Princeton Survey Research Associates, 2001. For more references on cultural disparities in health care see: Campbell, J.C., Pliska, M.J., Taylor, W., & Sheridan, D. (1994). "Battered women's experience in the emergency room." Journal of Emergency Nursing, 20, 280-288. Websdale N, *Rural Women Battering and the Justice System: An Ethnography.* Sage Publication: Thousand Oaks, CA, 1998. Comas-Diaz, L, Greene Be. (Eds) *Women of Color: Integrating Ethnic and Gender Identities in Psychotherapy.* Guildford Press, New York, 1994.

[60] Lucas D'Olivera, AF, Diniz SG, Schraiber LB. "Violence Against Women in Health-care Institutions: An Emerging Problem." The Lancet: Vol 359 May 2002 Pg. 1681.

[61] Title VI Prohibition Against National Origin Discrimination as it Affects Persons with Limited English Proficiency.

[62] Martin, S., Mackie, L, Kupper, L., Buescher, P., & Moracco, K. (2001). "Physical abuse of women before, during, and after pregnancy." The Journal of the American Medical Association, 285 (12).

[63] McFarlane J, Christoffel K, Bateman L, Miller V, Bullock L. (1991). "Assessing for abuse: self-report versus nurse interview." Public Health Nursing. Vol. 8, 242-250.

[64] Koziol-McLain, J. Coates, C., and Lowenstein, S. (2001). "Predictive validity of a screen for partner violence against women." American Journal of Preventative Medicine, 21 (2), 93-100.

[65] Saltzman LE, Salmi, LR, Branche, CM, Bolen, JC. (1997) "Public health screening for intimate violence." Violence Against Women. Vol. 3, 319-331.

[66] Hamberger LK, Ambuel B, Marbella A, Donze J. (1998). "Physician interaction with battered women: the women's perspective." Archives of Family Medicine. Vol. 7, 575-582.

[67] For information about how the perspective of domestic violence is woven into a state child protection agency's policies, see Whitney P. & Davis L. (1999). "Child abuse and domestic violence in Massachusetts: Can practice be integrated in a public child welfare setting?" Child Maltreatment 4 (2), 159-166.

[68] King, H. & Strauss M. (2000). *Routine Screening for Domestic Violence in Pediatric Practice.* Newton-Wellesley Hospital, Wellesley MA.

[69] David Adams, EdD. "Guidelines for Doctors on Identifying and Helping in their Patients who batter." Journal of the American Medical Women's Association. 1996; 51: 123-6. Oriel KA, Fleming MF. "Screening Men for Partner Abuse in a Primary Care setting." Journal of Family Practice. Volume 46 No. 6, 1998.

[70] Goodenow, C. (1998). *1997 Massachusetts Youth Risk Behavior Survey.* Malden, MA: Massachusetts Department of Education; Renzetti, C. (1992). *Violent Betrayal: Partner Abuse in Lesbian Relationships.* Sage Publications. p 18.

[71] Tjaden P., Thoennes N. (November 1998). *Prevalence, Incidence, and Consequences of Violence Against Women: Findings from the National Violence Against Women Survey.* National Institute of Justice, Centers for Disease Control. Bureau of Justice Statistics, 202-633-3047.

[72] Bureau of Justice Statistics Special Report (October 2001). *Intimate Partner Violence and Age of Victim, 1993-99,* United States Department of Justice.

Early Detection of Developmental Dysplasia of the Hip

- *Clinical Practice Guideline*
- *Technical Report Summary*

AMERICAN ACADEMY OF PEDIATRICS

Committee on Quality Improvement, Subcommittee on Developmental Dysplasia of the Hip

Clinical Practice Guideline: Early Detection of Developmental Dysplasia of the Hip

ABSTRACT. *Developmental dysplasia of the hip* is the preferred term to describe the condition in which the femoral head has an abnormal relationship to the acetabulum. Developmental dysplasia of the hip includes frank dislocation (luxation), partial dislocation (subluxation), instability wherein the femoral head comes in and out of the socket, and an array of radiographic abnormalities that reflect inadequate formation of the acetabulum. Because many of these findings may not be present at birth, the term *developmental* more accurately reflects the biologic features than does the term *congenital*. The disorder is uncommon. The earlier a dislocated hip is detected, the simpler and more effective is the treatment. Despite newborn screening programs, dislocated hips continue to be diagnosed later in infancy and childhood,[1-11] in some instances delaying appropriate therapy and leading to a substantial number of malpractice claims. The objective of this guideline is to reduce the number of dislocated hips detected later in infancy and childhood. The target audience is the primary care provider. The target patient is the healthy newborn up to 18 months of age, excluding those with neuromuscular disorders, myelodysplasia, or arthrogryposis.

ABBREVIATIONS. DDH, developmental dysplasia of the hip; AVN, avascular necrosis of the hip.

BIOLOGIC FEATURES AND NATURAL HISTORY

Understanding the developmental nature of developmental dysplasia of the hip (DDH) and the subsequent spectrum of hip abnormalities requires a knowledge of the growth and development of the hip joint.[12] Embryologically, the femoral head and acetabulum develop from the same block of primitive mesenchymal cells. A cleft develops to separate them at 7 to 8 weeks' gestation. By 11 weeks' gestation, development of the hip joint is complete. At birth, the femoral head and the acetabulum are primarily cartilaginous. The acetabulum continues to develop postnatally. The growth of the fibrocartilaginous rim (the labrum) that surrounds the bony acetabulum deepens the socket. Development of the femoral head and acetabulum are intimately related, and normal adult hip joints depend on further growth of these structures. Hip dysplasia may occur in utero, perinatally, or during infancy and childhood.

The acronym DDH includes hips that are unstable, subluxated, dislocated (luxated), and/or have malformed acetabula. A hip is *unstable* when the tight fit between the femoral head and the acetabulum is lost and the femoral head is able to move within (subluxated) or outside (dislocated) the confines of the acetabulum. A *dislocation* is a complete loss of contact of the femoral head with the acetabulum. Dislocations are divided into 2 types: teratologic and typical.[12] *Teratologic dislocations* occur early in utero and often are associated with neuromuscular disorders, such as arthrogryposis and myelodysplasia, or with various dysmorphic syndromes. The *typical dislocation* occurs in an otherwise healthy infant and may occur prenatally or postnatally.

During the immediate newborn period, laxity of the hip capsule predominates, and, if clinically significant enough, the femoral head may spontaneously dislocate and relocate. If the hip spontaneously relocates and stabilizes within a few days, subsequent hip development usually is normal. If subluxation or dislocation persists, then structural anatomic changes may develop. A deep concentric position of the femoral head in the acetabulum is necessary for normal development of the hip. When not deeply reduced (subluxated), the labrum may become everted and flattened. Because the femoral head is not reduced into the depth of the socket, the acetabulum does not grow and remodel and, therefore, becomes shallow. If the femoral head moves further out of the socket (dislocation), typically superiorly and laterally, the inferior capsule is pulled upward over the now empty socket. Muscles surrounding the hip, especially the adductors, become contracted, limiting abduction of the hip. The hip capsule constricts; once this capsular constriction narrows to less than the diameter of the femoral head, the hip can no longer be reduced by manual manipulative maneuvers, and operative reduction usually is necessary.

The hip is at risk for dislocation during 4 periods: 1) the 12th gestational week, 2) the 18th gestational week, 3) the final 4 weeks of gestation, and 4) the postnatal period. During the 12th gestational week, the hip is at risk as the fetal lower limb rotates medially. A dislocation at this time is termed teratologic. All elements of the hip joint develop abnor-

The recommendations in this statement do not indicate an exclusive course of treatment or serve as a standard of medical care. Variations, taking into account individual circumstances, may be appropriate.

The Practice Guideline, "Early Detection of Developmental Dysplasia of the Hip," was reviewed by appropriate committees and sections of the American Academy of Pediatrics (AAP) including the Chapter Review Group, a focus group of office-based pediatricians representing each AAP District: Gene R. Adams, MD; Robert M. Corwin, MD; Diane Fuquay, MD; Barbara M. Harley, MD; Thomas J. Herr, MD, Chair; Kenneth E. Matthews, MD; Robert D. Mines, MD; Lawrence C. Pakula, MD; Howard B. Weinblatt, MD; and Delosa A. Young, MD. The Practice Guideline was also reviewed by relevant outside medical organizations as part of the peer review process. PEDIATRICS (ISSN 0031 4005). Copyright © 2000 by the American Academy of Pediatrics.

mally. The hip muscles develop around the 18th gestational week. Neuromuscular problems at this time, such as myelodysplasia and arthrogryposis, also lead to teratologic dislocations. During the final 4 weeks of pregnancy, mechanical forces have a role. Conditions such as oligohydramnios or breech position predispose to DDH.[13] Breech position occurs in ~3% of births, and DDH occurs more frequently in breech presentations, reportedly in as many as 23%. The frank breech position of hip flexion and knee extension places a newborn or infant at the highest risk. Postnatally, infant positioning such as swaddling, combined with ligamentous laxity, also has a role.

The true incidence of dislocation of the hip can only be presumed. There is no "gold standard" for diagnosis during the newborn period. Physical examination, plane radiography, and ultrasonography all are fraught with false-positive and false-negative results. Arthrography (insertion of contrast medium into the hip joint) and magnetic resonance imaging, although accurate for determining the precise hip anatomy, are inappropriate methods for screening the newborn and infant.

The reported incidence of DDH is influenced by genetic and racial factors, diagnostic criteria, the experience and training of the examiner, and the age of the child at the time of the examination. Wynne-Davies[14] reported an increased risk to subsequent children in the presence of a diagnosed dislocation (6% risk with healthy parents and an affected child, 12% risk with an affected parent, and 36% risk with an affected parent and 1 affected child). DDH is not always detectable at birth, but some newborn screening surveys suggest an incidence as high as 1 in 100 newborns with evidence of instability, and 1 to 1.5 cases of dislocation per 1000 newborns. The incidence of DDH is higher in girls. Girls are especially susceptible to the maternal hormone relaxin, which may contribute to ligamentous laxity with the resultant instability of the hip. The left hip is involved 3 times as commonly as the right hip, perhaps related to the left occiput anterior positioning of most non-breech newborns. In this position, the left hip resides posteriorly against the mother's spine, potentially limiting abduction.

PHYSICAL EXAMINATION

DDH is an evolving process, and its physical findings on clinical examination change.[12,15,16] The newborn must be relaxed and preferably examined on a firm surface. Considerable patience and skill are required. The physical examination changes as the child grows older. No signs are pathognomonic for a dislocated hip. The examiner must look for asymmetry. Indeed, bilateral dislocations are more difficult to diagnose than unilateral dislocations because symmetry is retained. Asymmetrical thigh or gluteal folds, better observed when the child is prone, apparent limb length discrepancy, and restricted motion, especially abduction, are significant, albeit not pathognomonic signs. With the infant supine and the pelvis stabilized, abduction to 75° and adduction to

30° should occur readily under normal circumstances.

The 2 maneuvers for assessing hip stability in the newborn are the Ortolani and Barlow tests. The Ortolani elicits the sensation of the dislocated hip reducing, and the Barlow detects the unstable hip dislocating from the acetabulum. The Ortolani is performed with the newborn supine and the examiner's index and middle fingers placed along the greater trochanter with the thumb placed along the inner thigh. The hip is flexed to 90° but not more, and the leg is held in neutral rotation. The hip is gently abducted while lifting the leg anteriorly. With this maneuver, a "clunk" is felt as the dislocated femoral head reduces into the acetabulum. This is a positive Ortolani sign. The Barlow provocative test is performed with the newborn positioned supine and the hips flexed to 90°. The leg is then gently adducted while posteriorly directed pressure is placed on the knee. A palpable clunk or sensation of movement is felt as the femoral head exits the acetabulum posteriorly. This is a positive Barlow sign. The Ortolani and Barlow maneuvers are performed 1 hip at a time. Little force is required for the performance of either of these tests. The goal is not to prove that the hip can be dislocated. Forceful and repeated examinations can break the seal between the labrum and the femoral head. These strongly positive signs of Ortolani and Barlow are distinguished from a large array of soft or equivocal physical findings present during the newborn period. High-pitched clicks are commonly elicited with flexion and extension and are inconsequential. A dislocatable hip has a rather distinctive clunk, whereas a subluxable hip is characterized by a feeling of looseness, a sliding movement, but without the true Ortolani and Barlow clunks. Separating true dislocations (clunks) from a feeling of instability and from benign adventitial sounds (clicks) takes practice and expertise. This guideline recognizes the broad range of physical findings present in newborns and infants and the confusion of terminology generated in the literature. By 8 to 12 weeks of age, the capsule laxity decreases, muscle tightness increases, and the Barlow and Ortolani maneuvers are no longer positive regardless of the status of the femoral head. In the 3-month-old infant, limitation of abduction is the most reliable sign associated with DDH. Other features that arouse suspicion include asymmetry of thigh folds, a positive Allis or Galeazzi sign (relative shortness of the femur with the hips and knees flexed), and discrepancy of leg lengths. These physical findings alert the examiner that abnormal relationships of the femoral head to the acetabulum (dislocation and subluxation) *may* be present.

Maldevelopments of the acetabulum alone (acetabular dysplasia) can be determined only by imaging techniques. Abnormal physical findings may be absent in an infant with acetabular dysplasia but no subluxation or dislocation. Indeed, because of the confusion, inconsistencies, and misuse of language in the literature (eg, an Ortolani sign called a click by some and a clunk by others), this guideline uses the following definitions.

- A *positive examination* result for DDH is the Barlow or Ortolani sign. This is the clunk of dislocation or reduction.
- An *equivocal examination* or *warning signs* include an array of physical findings that may be found in children with DDH, in children with another orthopaedic disorder, or in children who are completely healthy. These physical findings include asymmetric thigh or buttock creases, an apparent or true short leg, and limited abduction. These signs, used singly or in combination, serve to raise the pediatrician's index of suspicion and act as a threshold for referral. Newborn soft tissue hip clicks are not predictive of DDH[17] but may be confused with the Ortolani and Barlow clunks by some screening physicians and thereby be a reason for referral.

IMAGING

Radiographs of the pelvis and hips have historically been used to assess an infant with suspected DDH. During the first few months of life when the femoral heads are composed entirely of cartilage, radiographs have limited value. Displacement and instability may be undetectable, and evaluation of acetabular development is influenced by the infant's position at the time the radiograph is performed. By 4 to 6 months of age, radiographs become more reliable, particularly when the ossification center develops in the femoral head. Radiographs are readily available and relatively low in cost.

Real-time ultrasonography has been established as an accurate method for imaging the hip during the first few months of life.[15,18-25] With ultrasonography, the cartilage can be visualized and the hip can be viewed while assessing the stability of the hip and the morphologic features of the acetabulum. In some clinical settings, ultrasonography can provide information comparable to arthrography (direct injection of contrast into the hip joint), without the need for sedation, invasion, contrast medium, or ionizing radiation. Although the availability of equipment for ultrasonography is widespread, accurate results in hip sonography require training and experience. Although expertise in pediatric hip ultrasonography is increasing, this examination may not always be available or obtained conveniently. Ultrasonographic techniques include *static evaluation* of the morphologic features of the hip, as popularized in Europe by Graf,[26] and a *dynamic evaluation*, as developed by Harcke[20] that assesses the hip for stability of the femoral head in the socket, as well as static anatomy. Dynamic ultrasonography yields more useful information. With both techniques, there is considerable interobserver variability, especially during the first 3 weeks of life.[7,27]

Experience with ultrasonography has documented its ability to detect abnormal position, instability, and dysplasia not evident on clinical examination. Ultrasonography during the first 4 weeks of life often reveals the presence of minor degrees of instability and acetabular immaturity. Studies[7,28,29] indicate that nearly all these mild early findings, which will not be apparent on physical examination, resolve spontaneously without treatment. Newborn screening with ultrasonography has required a high frequency of reexamination and results in a large number of hips being unnecessarily treated. One study[23] demonstrates that a screening process with higher false-positive results also yields increased prevention of late cases. Ultrasonographic screening of all infants at 4 to 6 weeks of age would be expensive, requiring considerable resources. This practice is yet to be validated by clinical trial. *Consequently, the use of ultrasonography is recommended as an adjunct to the clinical evaluation.* It is the technique of choice for clarifying a physical finding, assessing a high-risk infant, and monitoring DDH as it is observed or treated. Used in this selective capacity, it can guide treatment and may prevent overtreatment.

PRETERM INFANTS

DDH may be unrecognized in prematurely born infants. When the infant has cardiorespiratory problems, the diagnosis and management are focused on providing appropriate ventilatory and cardiovascular support, and careful examination of the hips may be deferred until a later date. The most complete examination the infant receives may occur at the time of discharge from the hospital, and this single examination may not detect subluxation or dislocation. Despite the medical urgencies surrounding the preterm infant, it is critical to examine the entire child.

METHODS FOR GUIDELINE DEVELOPMENT

Our goal was to develop a practice parameter by using a process that would be based whenever possible on available evidence. The methods used a combination of expert panel, decision modeling, and evidence synthesis[30] (see the Technical Report available on *Pediatrics electronic pages* at www.pediatrics.org). The predominant methods recommended for such evidence synthesis are generally of 2 types: a *data-driven* method and a *model-driven*[31,32] method. In data-driven methods, the analyst finds the best data available and induces a conclusion from these data. A model-driven method, in contrast, begins with an effort to define the context for evidence and then searches for the data as defined by that context. Data-driven methods are useful when the quality of evidence is high. A careful review of the medical literature revealed that the published evidence about DDH did not meet the criteria for high quality. There was a paucity of randomized clinical trials.[8] We decided, therefore, to use the model-driven method.

A decision model was constructed based on the perspective of practicing clinicians and determining the best strategy for screening and diagnosis. The target child was a full-term newborn with no obvious orthopaedic abnormalities. We focused on the various options available to the pediatrician* for the detection of DDH, including screening by physical examination, screening by ultrasonography, and episodic screening during health supervision. Because

---

*In this guideline, the term *pediatrician* includes the range of pediatric primary care providers, eg, family practitioners and pediatric nurse practitioners.

the detection of a dislocated hip usually results in referral by the pediatrician, and because management of DDH is not in the purview of the pediatrician's care, treatment options are not included. We also included in our model a wide range of options for detecting DDH during the first year of life if the results of the newborn screen are negative.

The outcomes on which we focused were a dislocated hip at 1 year of age as the major morbidity of the disease and avascular necrosis of the hip (AVN) as the primary complication of DDH treatment. AVN is a loss of blood supply to the femoral head resulting in abnormal hip development, distortion of shape, and, in some instances, substantial morbidity. Ideally, a gold standard would be available to define DDH at any point in time. However, as noted, no gold standard exists except, perhaps, arthrography of the hip, which is an inappropriate standard for use in a detection model. Therefore, we defined outcomes in terms of the *process of care*. We reviewed the literature extensively. The purpose of the literature review was to provide the probabilities required by the decision model since there were no randomized clinical trials. The article or chapter title and the abstracts were reviewed by 2 members of the methodology team and members of the subcommittee. Articles not rejected were reviewed, and data were abstracted that would provide evidence for the probabilities required by the decision model. As part of the literature abstraction process, the evidence quality in each article was assessed. A computer-based literature search, hand review of recent publications, or examination of the reference section for other articles ("ancestor articles") identified 623 articles; 241 underwent detailed review, 118 of which provided some data. Of the 100 ancestor articles, only 17 yielded useful articles, suggesting that our accession process was complete. By traditional epidemiologic standards,[33] the quality of the evidence in this set of articles was uniformly low. There were few controlled trials and few studies of the follow-up of infants for whom the results of newborn examinations were negative. When the evidence was poor or lacking entirely, extensive discussions among members of the committee and the expert opinion of outside consultants were used to arrive at a consensus. No votes were taken. Disagreements were discussed, and consensus was achieved.

The available evidence was distilled in 3 ways.

First, estimates were made of DDH at birth in infants without risk factors. These estimates constituted the baseline risk. Second, estimates were made of the rates of DDH in the children with risk factors. These numbers guide clinical actions: rates that are too high might indicate referral or different follow-up despite negative physical findings. Third, each screening strategy (pediatrician-based, orthopaedist-based, and ultrasonography-based) was scored for the estimated number of children given a diagnosis of DDH at birth, at mid-term (4–12 months of age), and at late-term (12 months of age and older) and for the estimated number of cases of AVN incurred, assuming that all children given a diagnosis of DDH would be treated. These numbers suggest the best strategy, balancing DDH detection with incurring adverse effects.

The baseline estimate of DDH based on orthopaedic screening was 11.5/1000 infants. Estimates from pediatric screening were 8.6/1000 and from ultrasonography were 25/1000. The 11.5/1000 rate translates into a rate for not-at-risk boys of 4.1/1000 boys and a rate for not-at-risk girls of 19/1000 girls. These numbers derive from the facts that the relative risk—the rate in girls divided by the rate in boys across several studies—is 4.6 and because infants are split evenly between boys and girls, so $.5 \times 4.1/1000 + .5 \times 19/1000 = 11.5/1000$.[34,35] We used these baseline rates for calculating the rates in other risk groups. Because the relative risk of DDH for children with a positive family history (first-degree relatives) is 1.7, the rate for boys with a positive family history is $1.7 \times 4.1 = 6.4/1000$ boys, and for girls with a positive family history, $1.7 \times 19 = 32/1000$ girls. Finally, the relative risk of DDH for breech presentation (of all kinds) is 6.3, so the risk for breech boys is $7.0 \times 4.1 = 29/1000$ boys and for breech girls, $7.0 \times 19 = 133/1000$ girls. These numbers are summarized in Table 1.

These numbers suggest that boys without risk or those with a family history have the lowest risk; girls without risk and boys born in a breech presentation have an intermediate risk; and girls with a positive family history, and especially girls born in a breech presentation, have the highest risks. Guidelines, considering the risk factors, should follow these risk profiles. Reports of newborn screening for DDH have included various screening techniques. In some, the screening clinician was an orthopaedist, in

TABLE 1. Relative and Absolute Risks for Finding a Positive Examination Result at Newborn Screening by Using the Ortolani and Barlow Signs

Newborn Characteristics	Relative Risk of a Positive Examination Result	Absolute Risk of a Positive Examination Result per 1000 Newborns With Risk Factors
All newborns	...	11.5
Boys	1.0	4.1
Girls	4.6	19
Positive family history	1.7	
Boys	...	6.4
Girls	...	32
Breech presentation	7.0	
Boys	...	29
Girls	...	133

TABLE 2.   Newborn Strategy*

Outcome	Orthopaedist PE	Pediatrician PE	Ultrasonography
DDH in newborn	12	8.6	25
DDH at ~6 mo of age	.1	.45	.28
DDH at 12 mo of age or more	.16	.33	.1
AVN at 12 mo of age	.06	.1	.1

* PE indicates physical examination. Outcome per 1000 infants initially screened.

others, a pediatrician, and in still others, a physio-therapist. In addition, screening has been performed by ultrasonography. In assessing the expected effect of each strategy, we estimated the newborn DDH rates, the mid-term DDH rates, and the late-term DDH rates for each of the 3 strategies, as shown in Table 2. We also estimated the rate of AVN for DDH treated before 2 months of age (2.5/1000 treated) and after 2 months of age (109/1000 treated). We could not distinguish the AVN rates for children treated between 2 and 12 months of age from those treated later. Table 2 gives these data. The total cases of AVN per strategy are calculated, assuming that all infants with positive examination results are treated.

Table 2 shows that a strategy using pediatricians to screen newborns would give the lowest newborn rate but the highest mid- and late-term DDH rates. To assess how much better an ultrasonography-only screening strategy would be, we could calculate a cost-effectiveness ratio. In this case, the "cost" of ultrasonographic screening is the number of "extra" newborn cases that probably include children who do not need to be treated. (The cost from AVN is the same in the 2 strategies.) By using these cases as the cost and the number of later cases averted as the effect, a ratio is obtained of 71 children treated neo-natally because of a positive ultrasonographic screen for each later case averted. Because this number is high, and because the presumption of better late-term efficacy is based on a single study, we do not recommend ultrasonographic screening at this time.

RECOMMENDATIONS AND NOTES TO ALGORITHM (Fig 1)

1. **All newborns are to be screened by physical examination.** The evidence† for this recommen-dation is good. The expert consensus‡ is strong. Although initial screening by orthopaedists§ would be optimal (Table 2), it is doubtful that if widely practiced, such a strategy would give the same good results as those published from pedi-atric orthopaedic research centers. **It is recom-mended that screening be done by a properly trained health care provider** (eg, physician, pedi-atric nurse practitioner, physician assistant, or physical therapist). (Evidence for this recommen-dation is strong.) A number of studies performed by properly trained nonphysicians report results

indistinguishable from those performed by physi-cians.[36] The examination after discharge from the neonatal intensive care unit should be performed as a newborn examination with appropriate screening. **Ultrasonography of all newborns is not recommended.** (Evidence is fair; consensus is strong.) Although there is indirect evidence to support the use of ultrasonographic screening of all newborns, it is not advocated because it is operator-dependent, availability is questionable, it increases the rate of treatment, and interob-server variability is high. There are probably some increased costs. We considered a strategy of "no newborn screening." This arm is politically inde-fensible because screening newborns is inherent in pediatrician's care. The technical report details this limb through decision analysis. Regardless of the screening method used for the newborn, DDH is detected in 1 in 5000 infants at 18 months of age.[3] The evidence and consensus for newborn screening remain strong.

Newborn Physical Examination and Treatment

2. **If a positive Ortolani or Barlow sign is found in the newborn examination, the infant should be referred to an orthopaedist.** Orthopaedic referral is recommended when the Ortolani sign is un-equivocally positive (a clunk). Orthopaedic refer-ral is not recommended for any softly positive finding in the examination (eg, hip click without dislocation). The precise time frame for the new-born to be evaluated by the orthopaedist cannot be determined from the literature. However, the literature suggests that the majority of "abnor-mal" physical findings of hip examinations at birth (clicks and clunks) will resolve by 2 weeks; therefore, consultation and possible initiation of treatment are recommended by that time. The data recommending that all those with a positive Ortolani sign be referred to an orthopaedist are limited, but expert panel consensus, nevertheless, was strong, because pediatricians do not have the training to take full responsibility and because true Ortolani clunks are rare and their manage-ment is more appropriately performed by the or-thopaedist.

If the results of the physical examination at birth are "equivocally" positive (ie, soft click, mild asym-metry, but neither an Ortolani nor a Barlow sign is present), then a follow-up hip examination by the pediatrician in 2 weeks is recommended. (Evidence is good; consensus is strong.) The available data sug-gest that most clicks resolve by 2 weeks and that these "benign hip clicks" in the newborn period do

† In this guideline, evidence is listed as good, fair, or poor based on the methodologist's evaluation of the literature quality. (See the Technical Report.)
‡ Opinion or consensus is listed as *strong* if opinion of the expert panel was unanimous or *mixed* if there were dissenting points of view.
§ In this guideline, the term *orthopaedist* refers to an orthopaedic surgeon with expertise in pediatric orthopaedic conditions.

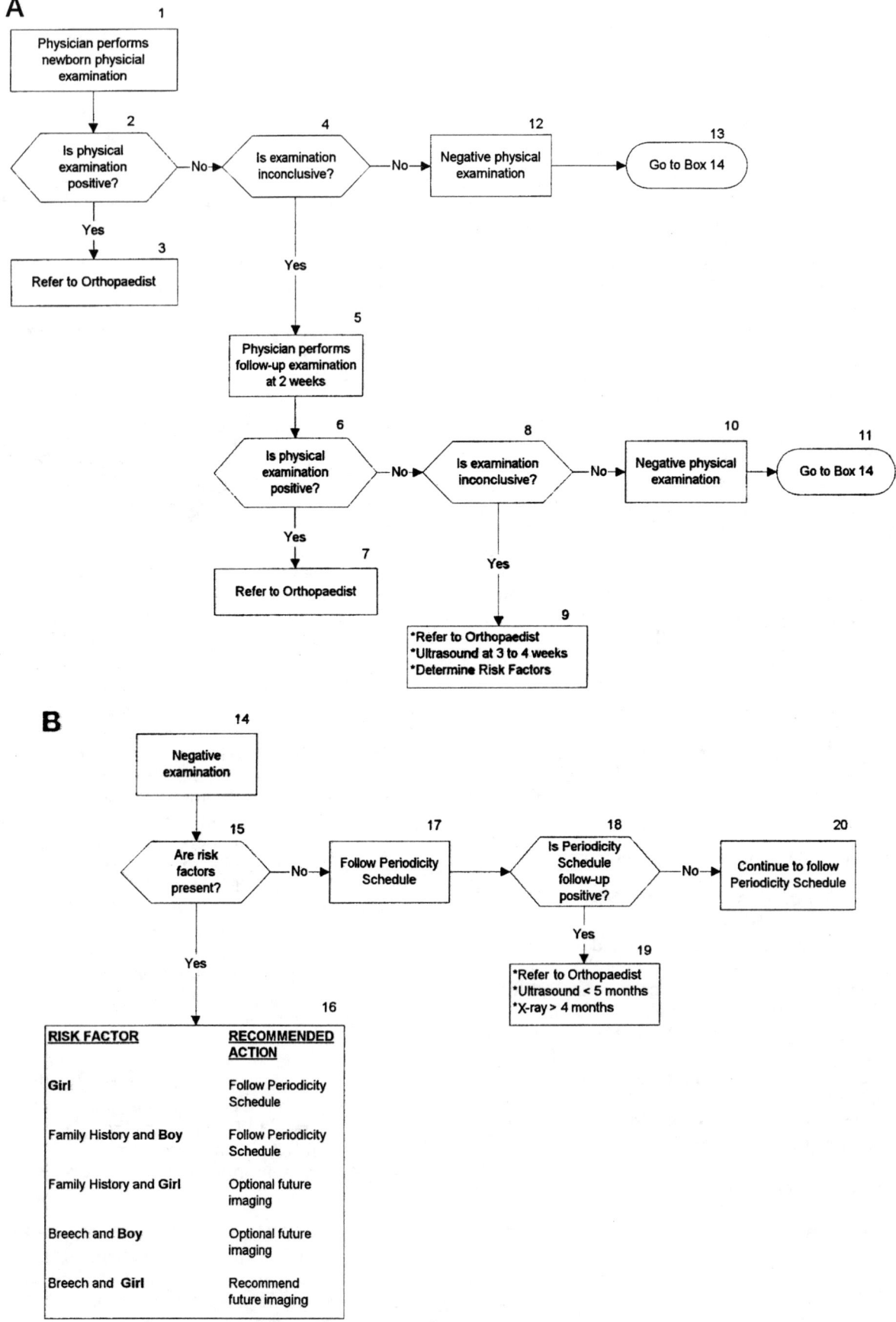

Fig 1. Screening for developmental hip dysplasia—clinical algorithm.

not lead to later hip dysplasia.[9,17,28,37] Thus, for an infant with softly positive signs, the pediatrician should reexamine the hips at 2 weeks before making referrals for orthopaedic care or ultrasonography. We recognize the concern of pediatricians about adherence to follow-up care regimens, but this concern regards all aspects of health maintenance and is not a reason to request ultrasonography or other diagnostic study of the newborn hips.

3. **If the results of the newborn physical examination are positive (ie, presence of an Ortolani or a Barlow sign), ordering an ultrasonographic examination of the newborn is not recommended.** (Evidence is poor; opinion is strong.) Treatment decisions are not influenced by the results of ultrasonography but are based on the results of the physical examination. The treating physician may use a variety of imaging studies during clinical management. **If the results of the newborn physical examination are positive, obtaining a radiograph of the newborn's pelvis and hips is not recommended** (evidence is poor; opinion is strong), because they are of limited value and do not influence treatment decisions.

The use of triple diapers when abnormal physical signs are detected during the newborn period is not recommended. (Evidence is poor; opinion is strong.) Triple diaper use is common practice despite the lack of data on the effectiveness of triple diaper use; and, in instances of frank dislocation, the use of triple diapers may delay the initiation of more appropriate treatment (such as with the Pavlik harness). Often, the primary care pediatrician may not have performed the newborn examination in the hospital. The importance of communication cannot be overemphasized, and triple diapers may aid in follow-up as a reminder that a possible abnormal physical examination finding was present in the newborn.

2-Week Examination

4. **If the results of the physical examination are positive (eg, positive Ortolani or Barlow sign) at 2 weeks, refer to an orthopaedist.** (Evidence is strong; consensus is strong.) Referral is urgent but is not an emergency. Consensus is strong that, as in the newborn, the presence of an Ortolani or Barlow sign at 2 weeks warrants referral to an orthopaedist. An Ortolani sign at 2 weeks may be a new finding or a finding that was not apparent at the time of the newborn examination.

5. **If at the 2-week examination the Ortolani and Barlow signs are absent but physical findings raise suspicions, consider referral to an orthopaedist or request ultrasonography at age 3 to 4 weeks.** Consensus is mixed about the follow-up for softly positive or equivocal findings at 2 weeks of age (eg, adventitial click, thigh asymmetry, and apparent leg length difference). Because it is necessary to confirm the status of the hip joint, the pediatrician can consider referral to an orthopaedist or for ultrasonography if the constellation of physical findings raises a high level of suspicion.

However, if the physical findings are minimal, continuing follow-up by the periodicity schedule with focused hip examinations is also an option, provided risk factors are considered. (See "Recommendations" 7 and 8.)

6. **If the results of the physical examination are negative at 2 weeks, follow-up is recommended at the scheduled well-baby periodic examinations.** (Evidence is good; consensus is strong.)

7. **Risk factors. If the results of the newborn examination are negative (or equivocally positive), risk factors may be considered.**[13,21,38–41] Risk factors are a study of thresholds to act.[42] Table 1 gives the risk of finding a positive Ortolani or Barlow sign at the time of the initial newborn screening. If this examination is negative, the absolute risk of there being a true dislocated hip is greatly reduced. Nevertheless, the data in Table 1 may influence the pediatrician to perform confirmatory evaluations. Action will vary based on the individual clinician. The following recommendations are made (evidence is strong; opinion is strong):

- **Girl** (newborn risk of 19/1000). When the results of the newborn examination are negative or equivocally positive, hips should be reevaluated at 2 weeks of age. If negative, continue according to the periodicity schedule; if positive, refer to an orthopaedist or for ultrasonography at 3 weeks of age.

- **Infants with a positive family history of DDH** (newborn risk for boys of 9.4/1000 and for girls, 44/1000). When the results of the newborn examination in boys are negative or equivocally positive, hips should be reevaluated at 2 weeks of age. If negative, continue according to the periodicity schedule; if positive, refer to an orthopaedist or for ultrasonography at 3 weeks of age. In girls, the absolute risk of 44/1000 may exceed the pediatrician's threshold to act, and imaging with an ultrasonographic examination at 6 weeks of age or a radiograph of the pelvis at 4 months of age is recommended.

- **Breech presentation** (newborn risk for boys of 26/1000 and for girls, 120/1000). **For negative or equivocally positive newborn examinations, the infant should be reevaluated at regular intervals (according to the periodicity schedule) if the examination results remain negative.** Because an absolute risk of 120/1000 (12%) probably exceeds most pediatricians' threshold to act, imaging with an ultrasonographic examination at 6 weeks of age or with a radiograph of the pelvis and hips at 4 months of age is recommended. In addition, because some reports show a high incidence of hip abnormalities detected at an older age in children born breech, this imaging strategy remains an option for all children born breech, not just girls. These hip abnormalities are, for the most part, inadequate development of the acetabulum. Acetabular dysplasia is best found by a radiographic examination at 6 months of age or older. A suggestion of poorly formed acetabula may be observed at 6 weeks of age by ultrasonography, but the best study remains a radiograph performed closer to 6 months of age. Ultrasonographic newborn screening of all breech infants will not eliminate the possibility of later acetabular dysplasia.

8. **Periodicity. The hips must be examined at every well-baby visit according to the recommended periodicity schedule for well-baby examinations (2–4 days for newborns discharged in less than 48 hours after delivery, by 1 month, 2 months, 4 months, 6 months, 9 months, and 12 months of age).** If at any time during the follow-up period DDH is suspected because of an abnormal physical examination or by a parental complaint of difficulty diapering or abnormal appearing legs, the pediatrician must confirm that the hips are stable, in the sockets, and developing normally. Confirmation can be made by a focused physical examination when the infant is calm and relaxed, by consultation with another primary care pediatrician, by consultation with an orthopaedist, by ultrasonography if the infant is younger than 5 months of age, or by radiography if the infant is older than 4 months of age. (Between 4 and 6 months of age, ultrasonography and radiography seem to be equally effective diagnostic imaging studies.)

DISCUSSION

DDH is an important term because it accurately reflects the biologic features of the disorder and the susceptibility of the hip to become dislocated at various times. Dislocated hips always will be diagnosed later in infancy and childhood because not every dislocated hip is detectable at birth, and hips continue to dislocate throughout the first year of life. Thus, this guideline requires that the pediatrician follow *a process of care for the detection of DDH.* The process recommended for early detection of DDH includes the following:

- Screen all newborns' hips by physical examination.
- Examine all infants' hips according to a periodicity schedule and follow-up until the child is an established walker.
- Record and document physical findings.
- Be aware of the changing physical examination for DDH.
- If physical findings raise suspicion of DDH, or if parental concerns suggest hip disease, confirmation is required by expert physical examination, referral to an orthopaedist, or by an age-appropriate imaging study.

When this process of care is followed, the number of dislocated hips diagnosed at 1 year of age should be minimized. However, the problem of late detection of dislocated hips will not be eliminated. The results of screening programs have indicated that 1 in 5000 children have a dislocated hip detected at 18 months of age or older.[3]

TECHNICAL REPORT

The Technical Report is available from the American Academy of Pediatrics from several sources. The Technical Report is published in full-text on *Pediatrics electronic pages.* It is also available in a compendium of practice guidelines that contains guidelines and evidence reports together. The objective was to create a recommendation to pediatricians and other primary care providers about their role as screeners for detecting DDH. The patients are a theoretical cohort of newborns. A model-based method using decision analysis was the foundation. Components of the approach include:

- Perspective: primary care provider
- Outcomes: DDH and AVN
- Preferences: expected rates of outcomes
- Model: influence diagram assessed from the subcommittee and from the methodology team with critical feedback from the subcommittee
- Evidence sources: Medline and EMBase (detailed in "Methods" section)
- Evidence quality: assessed on a custom, subjective scale, based primarily on the fit of the evidence in the decision model

The results are detailed in the "Methods" section. Based on the raw evidence and Bayesian hierarchical meta-analysis,[34,35] estimates for the incidence of DDH based on the type of screener (orthopaedist vs pediatrician); the odds ratio for DDH given risk factors of sex, family history, and breech presentation; and estimates for late detection and AVN were determined and are detailed in the "Methods" section and in Tables 1 and 2.

The decision model (reduced based on available evidence) suggests that orthopaedic screening is optimal, but because orthopaedists in the published studies and in practice would differ in pediatric expertise, the supply of pediatric orthopaedists is relatively limited, and the difference between orthopaedists and pediatricians is statistically insignificant, we conclude that pediatric screening is to be recommended. The place for ultrasonography in the screening process remains to be defined because of the limited data available regarding late diagnosis in ultrasonography screening to permit definitive recommendations.

These data could be used by others to refine the conclusion based on costs, parental preferences, or physician style. Areas for research are well defined by our model-based method. All references are in the Technical Report.

RESEARCH QUESTIONS

The quality of the literature suggests many areas for research, because there is a paucity of randomized clinical trials and case-controlled studies. The following is a list of possibilities:

1. Minimum diagnostic abilities of a screener. Although there are data for pediatricians in general, few, if any, studies evaluated the abilities of an individual examiner. What should the minimum

suggestion of poorly formed acetabula may be observed at 6 weeks of age by ultrasonography, but the best study remains a radiograph performed closer to 6 months of age. Ultrasonographic newborn screening of all breech infants will not eliminate the possibility of later acetabular dysplasia.

8. **Periodicity. The hips must be examined at every well-baby visit according to the recommended periodicity schedule for well-baby examinations (2–4 days for newborns discharged in less than 48 hours after delivery, by 1 month, 2 months, 4 months, 6 months, 9 months, and 12 months of age).** If at any time during the follow-up period DDH is suspected because of an abnormal physical examination or by a parental complaint of difficulty diapering or abnormal appearing legs, the pediatrician must confirm that the hips are stable, in the sockets, and developing normally. Confirmation can be made by a focused physical examination when the infant is calm and relaxed, by consultation with another primary care pediatrician, by consultation with an orthopaedist, by ultrasonography if the infant is younger than 5 months of age, or by radiography if the infant is older than 4 months of age. (Between 4 and 6 months of age, ultrasonography and radiography seem to be equally effective diagnostic imaging studies.)

DISCUSSION

DDH is an important term because it accurately reflects the biologic features of the disorder and the susceptibility of the hip to become dislocated at various times. Dislocated hips always will be diagnosed later in infancy and childhood because not every dislocated hip is detectable at birth, and hips continue to dislocate throughout the first year of life. Thus, this guideline requires that the pediatrician follow *a process of care for the detection of DDH.* The process recommended for early detection of DDH includes the following:

- Screen all newborns' hips by physical examination.
- Examine all infants' hips according to a periodicity schedule and follow-up until the child is an established walker.
- Record and document physical findings.
- Be aware of the changing physical examination for DDH.
- If physical findings raise suspicion of DDH, or if parental concerns suggest hip disease, confirmation is required by expert physical examination, referral to an orthopaedist, or by an age-appropriate imaging study.

When this process of care is followed, the number of dislocated hips diagnosed at 1 year of age should be minimized. However, the problem of late detection of dislocated hips will not be eliminated. The results of screening programs have indicated that 1 in 5000 children have a dislocated hip detected at 18 months of age or older.[3]

TECHNICAL REPORT

The Technical Report is available from the American Academy of Pediatrics from several sources. The Technical Report is published in full-text on *Pediatrics electronic pages.* It is also available in a compendium of practice guidelines that contains guidelines and evidence reports together. The objective was to create a recommendation to pediatricians and other primary care providers about their role as screeners for detecting DDH. The patients are a theoretical cohort of newborns. A model-based method using decision analysis was the foundation. Components of the approach include:

- Perspective: primary care provider
- Outcomes: DDH and AVN
- Preferences: expected rates of outcomes
- Model: influence diagram assessed from the subcommittee and from the methodology team with critical feedback from the subcommittee
- Evidence sources: Medline and EMBase (detailed in "Methods" section)
- Evidence quality: assessed on a custom, subjective scale, based primarily on the fit of the evidence in the decision model

The results are detailed in the "Methods" section. Based on the raw evidence and Bayesian hierarchical meta-analysis,[34,35] estimates for the incidence of DDH based on the type of screener (orthopaedist vs pediatrician); the odds ratio for DDH given risk factors of sex, family history, and breech presentation; and estimates for late detection and AVN were determined and are detailed in the "Methods" section and in Tables 1 and 2.

The decision model (reduced based on available evidence) suggests that orthopaedic screening is optimal, but because orthopaedists in the published studies and in practice would differ in pediatric expertise, the supply of pediatric orthopaedists is relatively limited, and the difference between orthopaedists and pediatricians is statistically insignificant, we conclude that pediatric screening is to be recommended. The place for ultrasonography in the screening process remains to be defined because of the limited data available regarding late diagnosis in ultrasonography screening to permit definitive recommendations.

These data could be used by others to refine the conclusion based on costs, parental preferences, or physician style. Areas for research are well defined by our model-based method. All references are in the Technical Report.

RESEARCH QUESTIONS

The quality of the literature suggests many areas for research, because there is a paucity of randomized clinical trials and case-controlled studies. The following is a list of possibilities:

1. Minimum diagnostic abilities of a screener. Although there are data for pediatricians in general, few, if any, studies evaluated the abilities of an individual examiner. What should the minimum

23. Rosendahl K, Markestad T, Lie RT. Ultrasound screening for developmental dysplasia of the hip in the neonate: the effect on treatment rate and prevalence of late cases. *Pediatrics.* 1994;94:47–52

24. Terjesen T. Ultrasound as the primary imaging method in the diagnosis of hip dysplasia in children aged <2 years. *J Pediatr Orthop B.* 1996;5:123–128

25. Vedantam R, Bell M. Dynamic ultrasound assessment for monitoring of treatment of congenital dislocation of the hip. *J Pediatr Orthop.* 1995;15:725–728

26. Graf R. Classification of hip joint dysplasia by means of sonography. *Arch Orthop Trauma Surg.* 1984;102:248–255

27. Berman L, Klenerman L. Ultrasound screening for hip abnormalities: preliminary findings in 1001 neonates. *Br Med J (Clin Res Ed).* 1986;293:719–722

28. Castelein R, Sauter A, de Vlieger M, van Linge B. Natural history of ultrasound hip abnormalities in clinically normal newborns. *J Pediatr Orthop.* 1992;12:423–427

29. Clarke N. Sonographic clarification of the problems of neonatal hip stability. *J Pediatr Orthop.* 1986;6:527–532

30. Eddy DM. The confidence profile method: a Bayesian method for assessing health technologies. *Operations Res.* 1989;37:210–228

31. Howard RA, Matheson JE. Influence diagrams. In: Matheson JE, ed. *Readings on the Principles and Applications of Decision Analysis.* Menlo Park, CA: Strategic Decisions Group; 1981:720–762

32. Nease RF, Owen DK. Use of influence diagrams to structure medical decisions. *Med Decis Making.* 1997;17:265–275

33. Guyatt GH, Sackett DL, Sinclair JC, Hayward R, Cook DJ, Cook RJ. Users' guide to the medical literature, IX: a method for grading health care recommendations. *JAMA.* 1995;274:1800–1804

34. Gelman A, Carlin JB, Stern HS, Rubin DB. *Bayesian Data Analysis.* London, UK: Chapman and Hall; 1997

35. Spiegelhalter D, Thomas A, Best N, Gilks W. *BUGS 0.5: Bayesian Inference Using Gibbs Sampling Manual, II.* Cambridge, MA: MRC Biostatistics Unit, Institute of Public Health; 1996. Available at: http://www.mrc-bsu.cam.ac.uk/bugs/software/software.html

36. Fiddian NJ, Gardiner JC. Screening for congenital dislocation of the hip by physiotherapists: results of a ten-year study. *J Bone Joint Surg Br.* 1994;76:458–459

37. Dunn P, Evans R, Thearle M, Griffiths H, Witherow P. Congenital dislocation of the hip: early and late diagnosis and management compared. *Arch Dis Child.* 1992;60:407–414

38. Holen KJ, Tegnander A, Terjesen T, Johansen OJ, Eik-Nes SH. Ultrasonographic evaluation of breech presentation as a risk factor for hip dysplasia. *Acta Paediatr.* 1996;85:225–229

39. Jones D, Powell N. Ultrasound and neonatal hip screening: a prospective study of "high risk" babies. *J Bone Joint Surg Br.* 1990;72:457–459

40. Teanby DN, Paton RW. Ultrasound screening for congenital dislocation of the hip: a limited targeted programme. *J Pediatr Orthop.* 1997;17:202–204

41. Tonnis D, Storch K, Ulbrich H. Results of newborn screening for CDH

42. with and without sonography and correlation of risk factors. *J Pediatr Orthop.* 1990;10:145–152

42. Pauker SG, Kassirer JP. The threshold approach to clinical decision making. *N Engl J Med.* 1980;302:1109–1117

43. Bower C, Stanley F, Morgan B, Slattery H, Stanton C. Screening for congenital dislocation of the hip by child-health nurses in western Australia. *Med J Aust.* 1989;150:61–65

44. Franchin F, Lacalendola G, Molfetta L, Mascolo V, Quagliarella L. Ultrasound for early diagnosis of hip dysplasia. *Ital J Orthop Traumatol.* 1992;18:261–269

ADDENDUM TO REFERENCES FOR THE DDH GUIDELINE

New information is generated constantly. Specific details of this report must be changed over time.

New articles (additional articles 1–7) have been published since the completion of our literature search and construction of this Guideline. These articles taken alone might seem to contradict some of the Guideline's estimates as detailed in the article and in the Technical Report. However, taken in context with the literature synthesis carried out for the construction of this Guideline, our estimates remain intact and no conclusions are obviated.

ADDITIONAL ARTICLES

1. Bialik V, Bialik GM, Blazer S, Sujov P, Wiener F, Berant M. Developmental dysplasia of the hip: a new approach to incidence. *Pediatrics.* 1999;103:93–99

2. Clegg J, Bache CE, Raut VV. Financial justification for routine ultrasound screening of the neonatal hip. *J Bone Joint Surg.* 1999;81-B:852–857

3. Holen KJ, Tegnander A, Eik-Nes SH, Terjesen T. The use of ultrasound in determining the initiation in treatment in instability of the hips in neonates. *J Bone Joint Surg.* 1999;81-B:846–851

4. Lewis K, Jones DA, Powell N. Ultrasound and neonatal hip screening: the five-year results of a prospective study in high risk babies. *J Pediatr Orthop.* 1999;19:760–762

5. Paton RW, Srinivasan MS, Shah B, Hollis S. Ultrasound screening for hips at risk in developmental dysplasia: is it worth it? *J Bone Joint Surg.* 1999;81-B:255–258

6. Sucato DJ, Johnston CE, Birch JG, Herring JA, Mack P. Outcomes of ultrasonographic hip abnormalities in clinically stable hips. *J Pediatr Orthop.* 1999;19:754–759

7. Williams PR, Jones DA, Bishay M. Avascular necrosis and the aberdeen splint in developmental dysplasia of the hip. *J Bone Joint Surg.* 1999;81-B:1023–1028

Technical Report Summary:
Developmental Dysplasia of the Hip

Authors:

Harold P. Lehmann, MD, PhD; Richard Hinton, MD, MPH;
Paola Morello, MD; and Jeanne Santoli, MD
in conjunction with the
American Academy of Pediatrics
Subcommittee on Developmental
Dysplasia of the Hip

American Academy of Pediatrics
PO Box 927, 141 Northwest Point Blvd
Elk Grove Village, IL 60009-0927

ABSTRACT

Objective. To create a recommendation for pediatricians and other primary care providers about their role as screeners for detecting developmental dysplasia of the hip (DDH) in children.

Patients. Theoretical cohorts of newborns.

Method. Model-based approach using decision analysis as the foundation. Components of the approach include the following:

Perspective: Primary care provider.

Outcomes: DDH, avascular necrosis of the hip (AVN).

Options: Newborn screening by pediatric examination; orthopaedic examination; ultrasonographic examination; orthopaedic or ultrasonographic examination by risk factors. Intercurrent health supervision-based screening.

Preferences: 0 for bad outcomes, 1 for best outcomes.

Model: Influence diagram assessed by the Subcommittee and by the methodology team, with critical feedback from the Subcommittee.

Evidence Sources: Medline and EMBASE search of the research literature through June 1996. Hand search of sentinel journals from June 1996 through March 1997. Ancestor search of accepted articles.

Evidence Quality: Assessed on a custom subjective scale, based primarily on the fit of the evidence to the decision model.

Results. After discussion, explicit modeling, and critique, an influence diagram of 31 nodes was created. The computer-based and the hand literature searches found 534 articles, 101 of which were reviewed by 2 or more readers. Ancestor searches of these yielded a further 17 articles for evidence abstraction. Articles came from around the globe, although primarily Europe, British Isles, Scandinavia, and their descendants. There were 5 controlled trials, each with a sample size less than 40. The remainder were case series. Evidence was available for 17 of the desired 30 probabilities. Evidence quality ranged primarily between one third and two thirds of the maximum attainable score (median: 10–21; interquartile range: 8–14).

Based on the raw evidence and Bayesian hierarchical meta-analyses, our estimate for the incidence of DDH revealed by physical examination performed by pediatricians is 8.6 per 1000; for orthopaedic screening, 11.5; for ultrasonography, 25. The odds ratio for DDH, given breech delivery, is 5.5; for female sex, 4.1; for positive family history, 1.7, although this last factor is not statistically significant. Postneonatal cases of DDH were divided into mid-term (younger than 6 months of age) and late-term (older than 6 months of age). Our estimates for the mid-term rate for screening by pediatricians is 0.34/1000 children screened; for orthopaedists, 0.1; and for ultrasonography, 0.28. Our estimates for late-term DDH rates are 0.21/1000 newborns screened by pediatricians; 0.08, by orthopaedists; and 0.2 for ultrasonography. The rates of AVN for children referred before 6 months of age is estimated at 2.5/1000 infants referred. For those referred after 6 months of age, our estimate is 109/1000 referred infants.

The decision model (reduced, based on available evidence) suggests that orthopaedic screening is optimal, but because orthopaedists in the published studies and in practice would differ, the supply of orthopaedists is relatively limited, and the difference between orthopaedists and pediatricians is statistically insignificant, we conclude that pediatric screening is to be recommended. The place of ultrasonography in the screening process remains to be defined because there are too few data about postneonatal diagnosis by ultrasonographic screening to permit definitive recommendations. These data could be used by others to refine the conclusions based on costs, parental preferences, or physician style. Areas for research are well defined by our model-based approach. *Pediatrics* 2000;105(4). URL: http://www.pediatrics.org/cgi/content/full/105/4/e57; keywords: *developmental dysplasia of the hip, avascular necrosis of the hip, newborn.*

I. GUIDELINE METHODS

A. Decision Model

The steps required to build the model were taken with the Subcommittee as a whole, with individuals in the group, and with members of the methodology team. Agreement on the model was sought from the Subcommittee as a whole during face-to-face meetings.

1. Perspective

Although there are a number of perspectives to take in this problem (parental, child's, societal, and payer's), we opted for the view of the practicing clinician: What are the clinician's obligations, and what is the best strategy for the clinician? This choice of perspective meant that the focus would be on screening for developmental dysplasia of the hip (DDH) and obviated the need to review the evidence for efficacy or effectiveness of specific strategies.

2. Context

The target child is a full-term newborn with no obvious orthopaedic abnormalities. Children with such findings would be referred to an orthopaedist, obviating the need for a practice parameter.

3. Options

We focused on the following options: screening by physical examination (PE) at birth by a pediatrician, orthopaedist, or other care provider; ultrasonographic screening at birth; and episodic screening during health supervision. Treatment options are not included.

We also included in our model a wide range of options for managing the screening process during the first year of life when the newborn screening was negative.

4. Outcomes

Our focus is on dislocated hips at 1 year of age as the major morbidity of the disease and on avascular necrosis of the hip (AVN), as the primary sentinel complication of DDH therapy.

Ideally, we would have a "gold standard" that would define DDH at any point in time, much as cardiac output can be obtained from a pulmonary-artery catheter. However, no gold standard exists. Therefore, we defined our outcomes in terms of the process of care: a pediatrician and an ultrasonographer perform initial or confirmatory examinations and refer the patient, whereas the orthopaedist treats the patient. It is the treatment that has the greatest effect on post-neonatal DDH or on complications, so we focus on that intermediate outcome, rather than the orthopaedist's stated diagnosis. We operationalized the definitions of these outcomes for use in abstracting the data from articles. A statement that a "click" was found on PE was considered to refer to an intermediate result, unless the authors defined their "click" in terms of our definition of a positive examination. Dynamic ultrasonographic examinations include those of Harcke et al, and static refers primarily to that of Graf. The radiologic focus switches from ultrasonography to plain radiographs after 4 months of age, in keeping with the development of the femoral head.

5. Decision Structure

We used an influence diagram to represent the decision model. In this representation, nodes refer to actions to be taken or to states of the world (the patient) about which we are uncertain. We devoted substantial effort to the construction of a model that balanced the need to represent the rich array of possible screening pathways with the need to be parsimonious. We constructed the master influence diagram and determined its construct validity through consensus by the Subcommittee before data abstraction. However, the available evidence could specify only a portion of the diagram. The missing components suggest research questions that need to be posed.

6. Probabilities

The purpose of the literature review was to provide the probabilities required by the decision model. The initial number of individual probabilities was 55. (Sensitivity and specificity for a single truth-indicator pair are counted as a single probability because they are garnered from the same table.) Although this is a large number of parameters, the structure of the model helped the team of readers. As 1 reader said, referring to the influence diagram, "Because we did the picture together, it was easy to find the parameters." What follows are some operational rules for matching the data to our parameters. The list is not complete. If an orthopaedic clinic worked at case finding, we used our judgment to determine whether to accept such reports as representing a population incidence.

Risk factors were included generally only if a true control group was used for comparison. For post-neonatal diagnoses, no study we reviewed included the examination of all children without DDH, say, 1 year of age, so there is always the possibility of missed cases (false-negative diagnoses) in the screen, which leads to a falsely elevated estimate of the denominator. For studies originating in referral clinics, the data on the reasons for referrals were not usable for our purposes.

7. Preferences

Ideally, we would have cost data for the options, as well as patient data on the human burden of therapy and of DDH itself. We have deferred these assessments to later research. Therefore, we assigned a preference score of 0 to DDH at 1 year of age and 1 to its absence; for AVN, we assigned 0 for presence at 1 year of age and 1 for absence at 1 year of age.

B. Literature Review

For the literature through May 1995, the following sources were searched: Books in Print, CAT-LINE, Current Contents, EMBASE, Federal Research in Progress, Health Care Standards, Health Devices Alerts, Health Planning and Administration, Health Services/Technology Assessment, International Health Technology Assessment, and Medline. Medline and EMBASE were searched through June 1996. The search terms used in all databases included the following: hip dislocation, congenital; hip dysplasia; congenital hip dislocation; developmental dysplasia; ultrasonography/adverse effects; and osteonecrosis. Hand searches of leading orthopaedic journals were performed for the issues from June 1996 to March 1997. The bibliographies of journals accepted for use in formulating the practice parameter also were perused.

The titles and the abstracts were then reviewed by 2 members of the methodology team to determine whether to accept or reject the articles for use. Decisions were reviewed by the Subcommittee, and conflicts were adjudicated. Similarly, articles were read by pairs of reviewers; conflicts were resolved in discussion.

The focus of the data abstraction process was on data that would provide evidence for the probabilities required by the decision model.

As part of the literature abstraction process, the evidence quality in each article was assessed. The scoring process was based on our decision model and involved traditional epidemiologic concerns, like outcome definition and bias of ascertainment, as well as influence–diagram-based concerns, such as how well the data fit into the model.

Cohort definition: Does the cohort represented by the denominator in the study match a node in our influence diagram? Does the cohort represented by the numerator match a node in our influence diagram? The closer the match, the more confident we are that the reported data provide good evidence of the conditional probability implied by the arrow between the corresponding nodes in the influence diagram.

Path: Does the implied path from denominator to numerator lead through 1 or more nodes of the influence diagram? The longer the path, the more likely that uncontrolled biases entered into the study, making us less confident about accepting the raw data as a conditional probability in our model. Assignment and comparison: Was there a control group? How was assignment made to experimental or control arms? A randomized, controlled study provides the best quality evidence.

Follow-up: Were patients with positive and negative initial findings followed up? The best studies should have data on both.

Outcome definition: Did the language of the outcome definitions (PE, orthopaedic examination, ultrasonography, and radiography) match ours, and, in particular, were PE findings divided into 3 categories or 2? The closer the definition to ours, the more we could pool the data. Studies with only 2 categories do not help to distinguish clicks from "clunks."

Ascertainment: When the denominator represented more than 1 node, to what degree was the denominator a mix of nodes? The smaller the contamination, the more confident we were that the raw data represented a desired conditional probability.

Results: Did the results fill an entire table or were data missing? This is related to the follow-up category but is more general.

C. Synthesis of Evidence

There are 3 levels of evidence synthesis.

1. Listing evidence for individual probabilities
2. Summarizing evidence across probabilities
3. Integrating the pooled evidence for individual probabilities into the decision model

A list of evidence for an individual probability (or arc) is called an *evidence table* and provides the reader a look at the individual pieces of data. The probabilities are summarized in 3 ways: by averaging, by averaging weighted by sample size (pooled), and by meta-analysis. We chose Bayesian meta-analytic techniques, which allow the representation of *prior belief* in the evidence and provide an explicit portrayal of the uncertainty of our conclusions. The framework we used was that of a hierarchical Bayesian model, similar to the random effects model in traditional meta-analysis. In this hierarchical model, each study has its own parameter, which, in turn, is sampled from a wider population parameter. Because there are 2 stages (ie, population to sample and sample to observation), and, therefore, the population parameter of interest is more distant from the data, the computed estimates in the population parameters are, in general, less certain (wider confidence interval) than simply pooling the data across studies. This lower certainty is appropriate in the DDH content area because the studies vary so widely in their raw estimates because of the range in time and geography over which they were performed. In the Bayesian model, the observations were assumed to be Poisson distributed, given the study DDH rates. Those rates, in turn, were assumed to be Gamma distributed, given the population rate. The prior belief on that rate was set as Gamma $(\propto, \beta)$, with mean $\propto / \beta$, and variance $\propto / \beta^2$ (as defined in the BUGS software). In this parameterization, $\propto$ has the semantics closest to that of location, and β has the semantics of certainty: the higher its value, the narrower the distribution and the more certain we are of the estimate. The parameter, $\propto$, was modeled as Exponential (1), and β, as Gamma (0.01, 1), with a mean of 0.01. Together, these correspond to a prior belief in the rate of a mean of 100 per 1000, and a standard deviation (SD) of 100, representing ignorance of the true rate.

As an example of interpretation, for pediatric newborn screening, the posterior $\propto$ was 1.46, and the posterior β was 0.17, to give a posterior rate of 8.6/1000, with a variance of 50, or an SD of 7.1. The value of β rose from 0.01 to 0.17, indicating a higher level of certainty.

The Bayesian confidence interval is the narrowest interval that contains 95% of the area under the posterior-belief curve. The confidence interval for the prior curve is 2.53 to 370. The confidence interval for the posterior curve is 0.25 to 27.5, a significant shrinking and increase in certainty but still broad.

The model for the odds ratios is more complicated and is based on the Oxford data set and analysis in the BUGS manual.

D. Thresholds

In the course of discussions about results, the Subcommittee was surveyed about the acceptable risks of DDH for different levels of interventions.

E. Recommendations

Once the evidence and thresholds were obtained, a decision tree was created from the evidence available and was reviewed by the Subcommittee. In parallel, a consensus guideline (flowchart) was created. The Subcommittee evaluated whether evidence was available for links within the guidelines, as well as their strength of consensus. The decision tree was evaluated to check consistency of the evidence with the conclusions.

F. "Cost"-Effectiveness Ratios

To integrate the results, we defined cost-effectiveness ratios, in which cost was excess neonatal referrals or excess cases of AVNs, and *effectiveness* was a decrease in the number of later cases. The decision tree from section E ("Recommendations") was used to calculate the expected outcomes for each of pediatric, orthopaedic, and ultrasonographic strategies. Pediatric strategy was used as the baseline, because its neonatal screening rate was the lowest. The cost-effectiveness ratios then were calculated as the quotient of the difference in cost and the difference in effect.

RESULTS

A. Articles

The peak number of articles is for 1992, with 10 articles. The articles are from sites all over the world, although the Nordic, Anglo-Saxon, and European communities and their descendants are the most represented.

B. Evidence

By traditional epidemiologic standards, the quality of evidence in this set of articles is uniformly low. There are few controlled trials and few studies in which infants with negative results on their newborn examinations are followed up. (A number of studies attempted to cover all possible places where an affected child might have been ascertained.)

We found data on all chance nodes, for a total of 298 distinct tables. *Decision* nodes were poorly represented: beyond the neonatal strategy, there were almost no data clarifying the paths for the diagnosis children after the newborn period. Thus, although communities like those in southeast Norway have a postnewborn screening program, it is unclear what the program was, and it was unclear how many examination results were normal before a child was referred to an orthopaedist.

The mode is a score of 10, achieved in 16 articles. The median is 9.9, with an interquartile range of 8 to 14, suggesting that articles with scores below 8 are poor sources of evidence. Note that the maximum achievable quality score is 21, so half the articles do not achieve half the maximum quality score.

Graphing evidence quality against publication year suggests an improvement in quality over time, as shown in Fig 9, but the linear fit through the data is statistically indistinguishable from a flat line. (A nonparametric procedure yields the same conclusion).

The studies include 5 in which a comparative arm was designed into the study. The remainder are divided between prospective and retrospective studies. Surprisingly, the evidence quality is not higher in the former than in the latter (data not shown).

Of the 298 data tables, half the data tables relate to the following:

• probabilities of DDH in different screening strategies
• relative risk of DDH, given risk factors
• the incidence of postneonatal DDH, and
• the incidence of AVN.

The remainder of our discussion will focus on these probabilities.

C. Evidence Tables

The evidence table details are found in the appendix of the full technical report.

1. Newborn Screening

a. Pediatric Screening

There were 51 studies, providing 57 arms, for pediatric screening. However, of these, 17 were unclear on how the intermediate examinations were handled, and, unsurprisingly, their observed rates of positivity (clicks) were much higher than the studies that distinguished 3 categories, as we had specified. Therefore, we included only the 34 studies that used 3 categories.

For pediatric screening, the rate is about 8 positive cases per 1000 examinations. The rates are distributed almost uniformly between 0 and 20 per 1000. All studies represent a large experience: a total of 2 149 972 subjects. Although their methods may not have been the best, the studies demand attention simply because of their size.

In looking for covariates or confounding variables, we studied the relationship between positivity rate and the independent variables, year of publication, evidence quality, and sample size. Year and evidence quality show a positive effect: the higher the year (slope: 0.2; P 5 .018) or evidence quality (slope: 0.6; P 5 .046), the higher the observed rate. A model with both factors has evidence that suggests that most of the effect is in the factor, year (slope for year: 0.08; P 5 .038; slope for quality of evidence: 0.49; P 5 .09). Note that a regression using evidence quality is improper, because our evidence scale is not properly ratio (eg, the distance between 6 and 7 is not necessarily equivalent to the distance between 14 and 15), but the regression is a useful exploratory device.

b. Orthopaedic Screening

Evidence was found in 25 studies. Three studies provided 2 arms each.

The positivity rate for orthopaedic screening is between 7 and 11/1000. One outlier study, with an observed rate of more than 300/1000, skews the unweighted and meta-analytic averages. The estimate (between 7.1 and 11) is just below that of pediatric screening and is statistically indistinguishable. Note, however, that a fair number of studies have rates near 22/1000 or higher.

Unlike with pediatric screening, there are no correlations with other factors.

c. Ultrasonographic Screening

Evidence was found in 17 studies, each providing a single arm.

The rate for ultrasonographic screening is 20/1000 or more. Although the estimates are sensitive to pooling and to the outlier, the positivity rate is clearly higher than in either PE strategy. There are no correlating factors. In particular, studies that use the Graf method 2 or those that use the method of Harcke et al show comparable rates.

2. Postneonatal Cases

We initially were interested in all postneonatal diagnoses of DDH. However, the literature did not provide data within the narrow time frames initially specified for our model. Based on the data that were available, we considered 3 classes of postneonatal DDH: DDH diagnosed after 12 months of age ("late-term"), DDH diagnosed between 6 and 12 months of age ("mid-term"), and DDH diagnosed before 6 months of age. There were few data for the latter group, which often was combined with the newborn screening programs. Therefore, we collected data on only the first 2 groups.

a. After Pediatric Screening

Evidence was found in 24 studies. The study by Dunn and O'Riordan provided 2 arms. It is difficult to discern an estimate rate for mid-term DDH, because the study by Czeizel et al is such an outlier, with a rate of 3.73/1000, and because the weighted and unweighted averages also differ greatly. The meta-analytic estimate of 0.55/1000 seems to be an upper limit.

The late-term rate is easier to estimate at ~0.3/1000. Although it is intuitive that the late-term rate should be lower than the mid-term rate, our data do not allow us to draw that conclusion.

b. After Orthopaedic Screening

There were only 4 studies. The rates were comparable for mid- and late-term: 0.1/1000 newborns. A meta-analytic estimate was not calculated.

c. After Ultrasonographic Screening

Only 1 study, by Rosendahl et al is available; it reported rates for infants with and without initial risk factors (eg, family history and breech presentation). The mid-term rate was 0.28/1000 newborns in the non-risk group, and the late-term rate was 0/1000 in the same group.

3. AVN After Treatment

For these estimates, we grouped together all treatments, because from the viewpoint of the referring primary care provider, orthopaedic treatment is a "black box:" A literature synthesis that teased apart the success and complications of particular *therapeutic* strategies is beyond the scope of the present study.

The complication rate should depend only on the age of the patient at time of orthopaedic referral and on the type of treatment received. We report on the complication rates for children treated before and after 12 months of age.

a. After Early Referral

There were 17 studies providing evidence. Infants were referred to orthopaedists during the newborn period in each study except 2. In the study by Pool et al, infants were referred during the newborn period and before 2 months of age; in the study by Sochart and Paton, infants were referred between 2 weeks and 2 months of age.

The range of AVN rates per 1000 infants referred was huge, from 0 to 123. The largest rate occurred in the study by Pool et al, a sample-based study that included later referrals. Its evidence quality was 8, within the 7 to 13 interquartile range of the other studies in this group. As in earlier tables, the meta-analytic estimate lies between the average and weighted (pooled) average of the studies.

b. After Later Referral

Evidence was obtained from 6 studies. Some of the studies included children referred during the newborn period or during the 2-week to 2-month period, but even in these, the majority of infants were referred later during the first year of life.

There were no outlier rates, although the highest rate (216/1000 referred children) occurred in the study with the oldest referred children in the sample with children referred who were older than 12 months of age. One study contributed 5700 patients to the analysis, more than half of the 9270 total, so its AVN rate of 27/1000 brought the unweighted rate of 116/1000 to 54. A meta-analytic estimate was not computed.

4. Risk Factors

A number of factors are known to predispose infants to DDH. We sought evidence for 3 of these: sex, obstetrical position at birth, and family history. Studies were included in these analyses only if a control group could be ascertained from the available study data.

The key measure is the odds ratio, an estimate of the relative risk. The meaning of the odds ratio is that if the DDH rate for the control group is known, then the DDH rate for the at-risk group is the product of the control-group DDH rate and the odds ratio for the risk factor. An odds ratio statistically significantly greater than 1 indicates that the factor is a risk factor.

The Bayesian meta-analysis produces estimates between the average of the odds ratios and the pooled odds ratio and is, therefore, the estimate we used in our later analyses.

a. Female

The studies were uniform in discerning a risk to girls ~4 times that of boys for being diagnosed with DDH. This risk was seen in all 3 screening environments.

b. Breech

The studies for breech also were confident in finding a risk for breech presentation, on the order of five-fold. One study found breech presentation to be protective, but the study was relatively small and used ultrasonography rather than PE as its outcome measure.

c. Family History

Although some studies found family history to be a risk factor, the range was wide. The confidence intervals for the pooled odds ratio and for the Bayesian analysis contained 1.0, suggesting that family history is *not* an independent risk factor for DDH. However, because of traditional concern with this risk factor, we kept it in our further considerations.

D. Evidence Summary and Risk Implications

To bring all evidence tables together, we constructed a summary table, which contains the estimates we chose for our recommendations. The intervals are asymmetric, in keeping with the intuition that rates near zero cannot be negative, but certainly can be very positive.

Risk factors are based on the pediatrician population rate of 8.6 labeled cases of DDH per 1000 infants screened. In the Subcommittee's discussion, 50/1000 was a cutoff for automatic referral during the newborn period. Hence, girls born in the breech position are classified in a separate category for newborn strategies than infants with other risk factors.

If we use the orthopaedists' rate as our baseline, numbers suggest that boys without risks or those with a family history have the lowest risk; girls without risks and boys born in the breech presentation have an intermediate risk; and girls with a positive family history, and especially girls born in the breech presentation, have the highest risks. Guidelines that consider risk factors should follow these risk profiles.

E. Decision Recommendations

With the evidence synthesized, we can estimate the expected results of the target newborn strategies for postneonatal DDH and AVN.

If a case of DDH is observed in an infant with an initially negative result of screening by an orthopaedist in a newborn screening program, that case is "counted" against the orthopaedist strategy.

The numbers are combined using a simple decision tree, which is not the final tree represented by our influence diagram but is a tree that is supported by our evidence. The results show that pediatricians diagnose fewer newborns with DDH and perhaps have a higher postneonatal DDH rate than orthopaedists but one that is comparable to ultrasonography (acknowledging that our knowledge of postneonatal DDH revealed by ultrasonographic screening is limited). The AVN rates are comparable with pediatrician and ultrasonographic screening and less than with orthopaedist screening.

F. Cost-Effectiveness Ratios

In terms of excess neonatal referrals, the ratios suggest that there is a trade-off: for every case that these strategies detect beyond the pediatric strategy, they require more than 7000 or 16 000 extra referrals, respectively.

DISCUSSION

A. Summary

We derived 298 evidence tables from 118 studies culled from a larger set of 624 articles. Our literature review captured most in our model-based approach, if not all, of the past literature on DDH that was usable. The decision model (reduced based on available evidence) suggests that orthopaedic screening is optimal, but because orthopaedists in the published studies and in practice would differ, the supply of orthopaedists is relatively limited, and the difference between orthopaedists and pediatricians is relatively small, we conclude that pediatric screening is to be recommended. The place of ultrasonography in the screening process remains to be defined because there are too few data about postneonatal diagnosis by ultrasonographic screening to permit definitive recommendations.

Our conclusions are tempered by the uncertainties resulting from the wide range of the evidence. The confidence intervals are wide for the primary parameters. The uncertainties mean that, even with all the evidence collected from the literature, we are left with large doubts about the values of the different parameters.

Our data do not bear directly on the issue about the earliest point that any patient destined to have DDH will show signs of the disease. Our use of the terms *mid-term* and *late-term* DDH addresses that ignorance.

Our conclusions about other areas of the full decision model are more tentative because of the paucity of data about the effectiveness of periodicity examinations. Even the studies that gave data on mid-term and late-term case findings by pediatricians were sparse in their details about how the screening was instituted, maintained, or followed up.

Our literature search was weakest in addressing the European literature, where results about ultrasonography are more prevalent. We found, however, that many of the seminal articles were republished in English or in a form that we could assess.

B. Specific Issues

1. Evidence Quality

Our measure of evidence quality is unique, although it is based on solid principles of study design and decision modeling. In particular, our measure was based on the notion that if the data conform poorly to how we need to use it, we downgrade its value.

However, throughout the analyses, there was never a correlation with the results of a study (in terms of the values of outcomes) and with evidence quality, so we never needed to use the measure for weighting the values of the outcome or for culling articles from our review. Had this been so, the measures would have needed further scrutiny and validation.

2. Outliers

Perhaps the true surrogates for study quality were the outlying values of outcomes. In general, however, there were few cases in which the outliers were clearly the result of poor-quality studies. One example is that of the outcomes of pediatric screening (1→3), in which the DDH rates in studies using only 2 categories were generally higher than those that explicitly specified 3 levels of outcomes.

Our general justification for using estimates that excluded outliers is that the outliers so much drove the results that they dominated the conclusion out of

proportion to their sample sizes. As it is, our estimates have wide ranges.

3. Newborn Screening

The set of studies labeled "pediatrician screening" includes studies with a variety of examiners. We could not estimate the sensitivity and specificity of pediatricians' examinations versus those of other primary care providers versus orthopaedists. There are techniques for extracting these measures from agreement studies, but they are beyond the scope of the present study. It is intuitive that the more cases that one examines, the better an examiner one will be, regardless of professional title.

We were surprised that the results did not show a clear difference in results between the Graf and Harcke et al ultrasonographic examinations. Our data make no statement about the relative advantages of these methods for following up children or in addressing treatment.

4. Postneonatal Cases

As mentioned, our data cannot say when a postneonatal case is established or, therefore, the best time to screen children. We established our initial age categories for postneonatal cases based on biology, treatment changes, and optimal imaging and examination strategies. It is frustrating that the data in the literature are not organized to match this pathophysiological way of thinking about DDH. Similarly, as mentioned, the lack of details by authors on the methods of intercurrent screening means that we cannot recommend a preferred method for mid-term or late-term screening.

5. AVN

We used AVN as our primary marker for treatment morbidity. We acknowledge that the studies we grouped together may reflect different philosophies and results of orthopaedic practice. The hierarchical meta-analysis treats every study as an individual case, and the wide range in our confidence intervals reflects the uncertainty that results in grouping disparate studies together.

C. Comments on Methods

This study is unique in its strong use of decision modeling at each step in the process. In the end, our results are couched in traditional terms (estimated rates of disease or morbidity outcomes), although the context is relatively nontraditional: attaching the estimates to strategies rather than to treatments. In this, our study is typical of an *effectiveness* study, which studied results in the real world, rather than of an *efficacy* study, which examines the biological effects of a treatment.

We made strong and recurrent use of the Bayesian hierarchical meta-analysis. A review of the tables will confirm that the Bayesian results were in the same "ballpark" as the average and pooled average estimates and had a more solid grounding.

The usual criticism of using Bayesian methods is that they depend on prior belief. The usual response is to show that the final estimates are relatively insensitive to the prior belief. In fact, for the screening strategies, a wide range of prior beliefs had no effect on the estimate. However, the prior belief used for the screening strategies—with a mean of 100 cases/1000 with a variance of 100—was too broad for the postneonatal case and AVN analyses; when data were sparse, the prior belief overwhelmed the data. For instance, in late-term DDH revealed by orthopaedic screening (53 30), in an analysis not shown, the posterior estimate from the 4 studies was a rate of 0.345 cases per 1000, despite an average and a pooled average on the order of 0.08. Four studies were insufficient to overpower a prior belief of 100.

D. Research Issues

The place of ultrasonography in DDH screening needs more attention, as does the issue of intercurrent pediatrician screening. In the latter case, society and health care systems must assess the effectiveness of education and the "return on investment" for educational programs. The place of preferences—of the parents, of the clinician—must be established.

We hope that the framework we have delineated—of a decision model and of data—can be useful in these future research endeavors.

Recommendations for Using Fluoride to Prevent and Control Dental Caries in the United States

The following guideline for recommendations for using fluoride to prevent and control dental caries in the United States, developed by the Centers for Disease Control and Prevention, has been endorsed by the American Academy of Pediatrics.

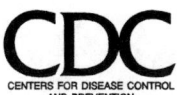

August 17, 2001 / Vol. 50 / No. RR-14

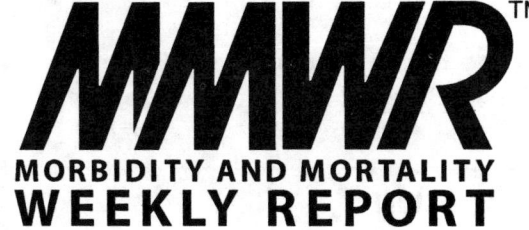

MORBIDITY AND MORTALITY
WEEKLY REPORT

Recommendations
and
Reports

Inside: **Continuing Education Examination**

Recommendations for Using Fluoride to Prevent and Control Dental Caries in the United States

U.S. DEPARTMENT OF HEALTH AND HUMAN SERVICES
Centers for Disease Control and Prevention (CDC)
Atlanta, GA 30333

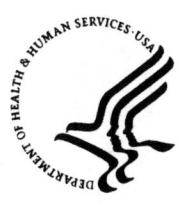

The *MMWR* series of publications is published by the Epidemiology Program Office, Centers for Disease Control and Prevention (CDC), U.S. Department of Health and Human Services, Atlanta, GA 30333.

SUGGESTED CITATION

Centers for Disease Control and Prevention. Recommendations for using fluoride to prevent and control dental caries in the United States. MMWR 2001;50(No. RR-14):[inclusive page numbers].

Centers for Disease Control and Prevention .... Jeffrey P. Koplan, M.D., M.P.H.
                                                                       Director

The material in this report was prepared for publication by
  National Center for Chronic Disease Prevention
    and Health Promotion .... James S. Marks, M.D., M.P.H.
                                                                       Director

    Division of Oral Health .... William R. Maas, D.D.S., M.P.H.
                                                                       Director

This report was produced as an *MMWR* serial publication in

  Epidemiology Program Office .... Stephen B. Thacker, M.D., M.Sc.
                                                                       Director

    Office of Scientific and Health Communications .... John W. Ward, M.D.
                                                                       Director
                                                                   Editor, MMWR *Series*

        Recommendations and Reports .... Suzanne M. Hewitt, M.P.A.
                                                                       Managing Editor

                                                                   Amanda Crowell
                                                                   Elizabeth L. Hess
                                                                   Project Editors

                                                                   Martha F. Boyd
                                                                   Visual Information Specialist

                                                                   Michele D. Renshaw
                                                                   Erica R. Shaver
                                                                   Information Technology Specialists

Fluoride Recommendations Work Group

Steven M. Adair, D.D.S., M.S.
School of Dentistry
Medical College of Georgia
Augusta, Georgia

William H. Bowen, Ph.D.
Caries Research Center
University of Rochester
Rochester, New York

Brian A. Burt, B.D.S., M.P.H., Ph.D.
School of Public Health
University of Michigan
Ann Arbor, Michigan

Jayanth V. Kumar, D.D.S., M.P.H.
New York Department of Health
Albany, New York

Steven M. Levy, D.D.S., M.P.H.
College of Dentistry
University of Iowa
Iowa City, Iowa

David G. Pendrys, D.D.S., Ph.D.
School of Dental Medicine
University of Connecticut
Farmington, Connecticut

R. Gary Rozier, D.D.S., M.P.H.
School of Public Health
University of North Carolina
Chapel Hill, North Carolina

Robert H. Selwitz, D.D.S., M.P.H.
National Institute of Dental and Craniofacial
    Research
Bethesda, Maryland

John W. Stamm, D.D.S., D.D.P.H.
School of Dentistry
University of North Carolina
Chapel Hill, North Carolina

George K. Stookey, Ph.D., D.D.S.
School of Dentistry
Indiana University
Indianapolis, Indiana

Gary M. Whitford, Ph.D., D.M.D.
School of Dentistry
Medical College of Georgia
Augusta, Georgia

Fluoride Recommendations Reviewers

Myron Allukian, Jr., D.D.S., M.P.H.
Director of Oral Health
Boston Public Health Commission
Boston, Massachusetts

John P. Brown, B.D.S., Ph.D.
Department of Community Dentistry
University of Texas Health Science Center
San Antonio, Texas

Joseph A. Ciardi, Ph.D.
National Institute of Dental and Craniofacial
  Research
Bethesda, Maryland

D. Christopher Clark, D.D.S., M.P.H.
Faculty of Dentistry
University of British Columbia
North Vancouver, Canada

Stephen B. Corbin, D.D.S., M.P.H.
Oral Health America
Brookeville, Maryland

Michael W. Easley, D.D.S., M.P.H.
School of Dental Medicine
State University of New York
Buffalo, New York

Caswell A. Evans, D.D.S., M.P.H.
County Dental Director
Los Angeles, California

Lawrence J. Furman, D.D.S., M.P.H.
National Institute of Dental and Craniofacial
  Research
Bethesda, Maryland

Stanley B. Heifetz, D.D.S., M.P.H.
Department of Dental Medicine
  and Public Health
School of Dentistry
University of Southern California
Los Angeles, California

Keith E. Heller, D.D.S., Dr.P.H.
School of Public Health
University of Michigan
Ann Arbor, Michigan

Amid I. Ismail, D.D.S., Dr.P.H.
School of Dentistry
University of Michigan
Ann Arbor, Michigan

David W. Johnston, B.D.S., M.P.H.
School of Dentistry
University of Western Ontario
London, Canada

John V. Kelsey, D.D.S., M.B.A.
US Food and Drug Administration
Rockville, Maryland

James A. Lalumandier, D.D.S., M.P.H.
School of Dentistry
Case Western Reserve University
Hudson, Ohio

Stephen J. Moss, D.D.S., M.S.
College of Dentistry
New York University
New York, New York

Ernest Newbrun, D.M.D., Ph.D.
School of Dentistry
University of California, San Francisco
San Francisco, California

Kathy R. Phipps, Dr.P.H.
School of Dentistry
Oregon Health Sciences University
Portland, Oregon

Mel L. Ringelberg, D.D.S., Dr.P.H.
State Dental Director
State of Florida Department of Health
Tallahassee, Florida

Jay D. Shulman, D.M.D., M.S.P.H.
Baylor College of Dentistry
Dallas, Texas

Phillip A. Swango, D.D.S., M.P.H.
Private dental consultant
Albuquerque, New Mexico

Gerald R. Vogel, Ph.D.
ADA Health Foundation Paffenbarger
  Research Center
Gaithersburg, Maryland

James S. Wefel, Ph.D.
College of Dentistry
University of Iowa
Iowa City, Iowa

B. Alex White, D.D.S., Dr.P.H.
Kaiser-Permanente, Inc.
Portland, Oregon

The following CDC staff members prepared this report:

William G. Kohn, D.D.S.
William R. Maas, D.D.S., M.P.H.
Dolores M. Malvitz, Dr. P.H.
Scott M. Presson, D.D.S., M.P.H.
Kerald K. Shaddix, D.D.S., M.P.H.
Division of Oral Health
National Center for Chronic Disease Prevention and Health Promotion

Recommendations for Using Fluoride to Prevent and Control Dental Caries in the United States

Summary

Widespread use of fluoride has been a major factor in the decline in the prevalence and severity of dental caries (i.e., tooth decay) in the United States and other economically developed countries. When used appropriately, fluoride is both safe and effective in preventing and controlling dental caries. All U.S. residents are likely exposed to some degree to fluoride, which is available from multiple sources. Both health-care professionals and the public have sought guidance on selecting the best way to provide and receive fluoride. During the late 1990s, CDC convened a work group to develop recommendations for using fluoride to prevent and control dental caries in the United States. This report includes these recommendations, as well as a) critical analysis of the scientific evidence regarding the efficacy and effectiveness of fluoride modalities in preventing and controlling dental caries, b) ordinal grading of the quality of the evidence, and c) assessment of the strength of each recommendation.

Because frequent exposure to small amounts of fluoride each day will best reduce the risk for dental caries in all age groups, the work group recommends that all persons drink water with an optimal fluoride concentration and brush their teeth twice daily with fluoride toothpaste. For persons at high risk for dental caries, additional fluoride measures might be needed. Measured use of fluoride modalities is particularly appropriate during the time of anterior tooth enamel development (i.e., age <6 years).

The recommendations in this report guide dental and other health-care providers, public health officials, policy makers, and the public in the use of fluoride to achieve maximum protection against dental caries while using resources efficiently and reducing the likelihood of enamel fluorosis. The recommendations address public health and professional practice, self-care, consumer product industries and health agencies, and further research. Adoption of these recommendations could further reduce dental caries in the United States and save public and private resources.

INTRODUCTION

Dental caries (i.e., tooth decay) is an infectious, multifactorial disease afflicting most persons in industrialized countries and some developing countries (1). Fluoride reduces the incidence of dental caries and slows or reverses the progression of existing lesions (i.e., prevents cavities). Although pit and fissure sealants, meticulous oral hygiene, and appropriate dietary practices contribute to caries prevention and control, the most effective and widely used approaches have included fluoride use. Today, all U.S. residents are exposed to fluoride to some degree, and widespread use of fluoride has been a major factor in the decline in the prevalence and severity of dental caries in the United States and other economically developed countries (1). Although this decline is a major public health achievement, the burden of disease is still considerable in all age groups. Because many fluoride modalities are effective, inexpensive, readily available, and can be used in both private and public health settings, their use is likely to continue.

Fluoride is the ionic form of the element fluorine, the 13th most abundant element in the earth's crust. Fluoride is negatively charged and combines with positive ions (e.g., calcium or sodium) to form stable compounds (e.g., calcium fluoride or sodium fluoride). Such fluorides are released into the environment naturally in both water and air. Fluoride compounds also are produced by some industrial processes that use the mineral apatite, a mixture of calcium phosphate compounds. In humans, fluoride is mainly associated with calcified tissues (i.e., bones and teeth) because of its high affinity for calcium.

Fluoride's ability to inhibit or even reverse the initiation and progression of dental caries is well documented. The first use of adjusted fluoride in water for caries control began in 1945 and 1946 in the United States and Canada, when the fluoride concentration was adjusted in the drinking water supplying four communities (2–5). The U.S. Public Health Service (PHS) developed recommendations in the 1940s and 1950s regarding fluoride concentrations in public water supplies. At that time, public health officials assumed that drinking water would be the major source of fluoride for most U.S. residents. The success of water fluoridation in preventing and controlling dental caries led to the development of fluoride-containing products, including toothpaste (i.e., dentifrice), mouthrinse, dietary supplements, and professionally applied or prescribed gel, foam, or varnish. In addition, processed beverages, which constitute an increasing proportion of the diets of many U.S. residents (6,7), and food can contain small amounts of fluoride, especially if they are processed with fluoridated water. Thus, U.S. residents have more sources of fluoride available now than 50 years ago.

Much of the research on the efficacy and effectiveness of individual fluoride modalities in preventing and controlling dental caries was conducted before 1980, when dental caries was more common and more severe. Modalities were usually tested separately and with the assumption that the method would provide the main source of fluoride. Thus, various modes of fluoride use have evolved, each with its own recommended concentration, frequency of use, and dosage schedule. Health-care professionals and the public have sought guidance regarding selection of preventive modalities from among the available options. The United States does not have comprehensive recommendations for caries prevention and control through various combinations of fluoride modalities. Adoption of such recommendations could further reduce dental caries while saving public and private resources and reducing the prevalence of enamel fluorosis, a generally cosmetic developmental condition of tooth enamel.

This report presents comprehensive recommendations on the use of fluoride to prevent and control dental caries in the United States. These recommendations were developed by a work group of 11 specialists in fluoride research or policy convened by CDC during the late 1990s and reviewed by an additional 23 specialists. Although the recommendations were developed specifically for the United States, aspects of this report could be relevant to other countries. The recommendations guide health-care providers and the public on efficient and appropriate use of fluoride modalities, direct attention to fluoride intake among children aged <6 years to decrease the risk for enamel fluorosis, and suggest areas for further research. This report focuses on critical analysis of the scientific evidence regarding the efficacy and effectiveness of each fluoride modality in preventing and controlling dental caries and on the use of multiple sources of fluoride.

The safety of fluoride, which has been documented comprehensively by other scientific and public health organizations (e.g., PHS [8], National Research Council [9], World Health Organization [10], and Institute of Medicine [11]) is not addressed.

HOW FLUORIDE PREVENTS AND CONTROLS DENTAL CARIES

Dental caries is an infectious, transmissible disease in which bacterial by-products (i.e., acids) dissolve the hard surfaces of teeth. Unchecked, the bacteria can penetrate the dissolved surface, attack the underlying dentin, and reach the soft pulp tissue. Dental caries can result in loss of tooth structure, pain, and tooth loss and can progress to acute systemic infection.

Cariogenic bacteria (i.e., bacteria that cause dental caries) reside in dental plaque, a sticky organic matrix of bacteria, food debris, dead mucosal cells, and salivary components that adheres to tooth enamel. Plaque also contains minerals, primarily calcium and phosphorus, as well as proteins, polysaccharides, carbohydrates, and lipids. Cariogenic bacteria colonize on tooth surfaces and produce polysaccharides that enhance adherence of the plaque to enamel. Left undisturbed, plaque will grow and harbor increasing numbers of cariogenic bacteria. An initial step in the formation of a carious lesion takes place when cariogenic bacteria in dental plaque metabolize a substrate from the diet (e.g., sugars and other fermentable carbohydrates) and the acid produced as a metabolic by-product demineralizes (i.e., begins to dissolve) the adjacent enamel crystal surface (Figure 1). Demineralization involves the loss of calcium, phosphate, and carbonate. These minerals can be captured by surrounding plaque and be available for reuptake by the enamel surface. Fluoride, when present in the mouth, is also retained and concentrated in plaque.

Fluoride works to control early dental caries in several ways. Fluoride concentrated in plaque and saliva inhibits the demineralization of sound enamel and enhances the remineralization (i.e., recovery) of demineralized enamel (12,13). As cariogenic bacteria metabolize carbohydrates and produce acid, fluoride is released from dental plaque in response to lowered pH at the tooth-plaque interface (14). The released fluoride and the fluoride present in saliva are then taken up, along with calcium and phosphate, by demineralized enamel to establish an improved enamel crystal structure. This improved structure is more acid resistant and contains more fluoride and less carbonate (12,15–19) (Figure 1). Fluoride is more readily taken up by demineralized enamel than by sound enamel (20). Cycles of demineralization and remineralization continue throughout the lifetime of the tooth.

Fluoride also inhibits dental caries by affecting the activity of cariogenic bacteria. As fluoride concentrates in dental plaque, it inhibits the process by which cariogenic bacteria metabolize carbohydrates to produce acid and affects bacterial production of adhesive polysaccharides (21). In laboratory studies, when a low concentration of fluoride is constantly present, one type of cariogenic bacteria, *Streptococcus mutans*, produces less acid (22–25). Whether this reduced acid production reduces the cariogenicity of these bacteria in humans is unclear (26).

Saliva is a major carrier of topical fluoride. The concentration of fluoride in ductal saliva, as it is secreted from salivary glands, is low — approximately 0.016 parts per million (ppm) in areas where drinking water is fluoridated and 0.006 ppm in nonfluoridated areas (27). This concentration of fluoride is not likely to affect cariogenic activity. However, drinking fluoridated water, brushing with fluoride toothpaste, or using other fluoride

FIGURE 1. The demineralization and remineralization processes lead to remineralized enamel crystals with surfaces rich in fluoride and lower in solubility

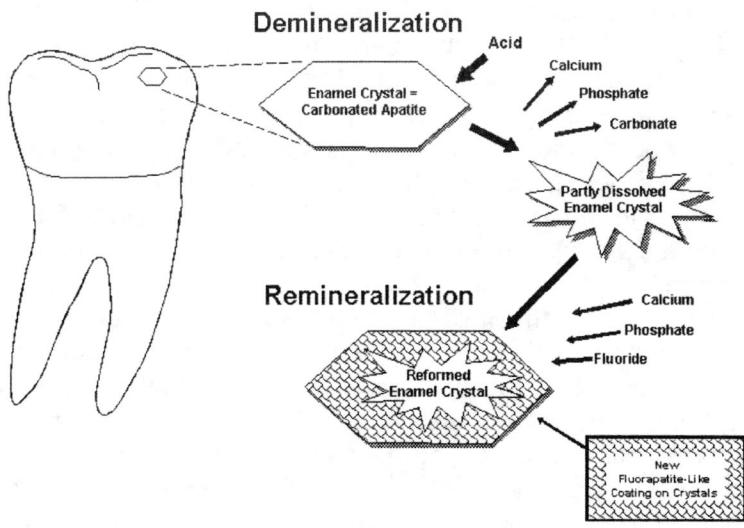

Source: Adapted from Featherstone JDB. Prevention and reversal of dental caries: role of low level fluoride. Community Dent Oral Epidemiol 1999;27:31–40. Reprinted with permission from Munksgaard International Publishers Ltd., Copenhagen, Denmark.

dental products can raise the concentration of fluoride in saliva present in the mouth 100- to 1,000-fold. The concentration returns to previous levels within 1–2 hours but, during this time, saliva serves as an important source of fluoride for concentration in plaque and for tooth remineralization (28).

Applying fluoride gel or other products containing a high concentration of fluoride to the teeth leaves a temporary layer of calcium fluoride-like material on the enamel surface. The fluoride in this material is released when the pH drops in the mouth in response to acid production and is available to remineralize enamel (29).

In the earliest days of fluoride research, investigators hypothesized that fluoride affects enamel and inhibits dental caries only when incorporated into developing dental enamel (i.e., preeruptively, before the tooth erupts into the mouth) (30,31). Evidence supports this hypothesis (32–34), but distinguishing a true preeruptive effect after teeth erupt into a mouth where topical fluoride exposure occurs regularly is difficult. However, a high fluoride concentration in sound enamel cannot alone explain the marked reduction in dental caries that fluoride produces (35,36). The prevalence of dental caries in a population is not inversely related to the concentration of fluoride in enamel (37), and a higher concentration of enamel fluoride is not necessarily more efficacious in preventing dental caries (38).

The laboratory and epidemiologic research that has led to the better understanding of how fluoride prevents dental caries indicates that fluoride's predominant effect is posteruptive and topical and that the effect depends on fluoride being in the right amount in the right place at the right time. Fluoride works primarily after teeth have erupted, especially when small amounts are maintained constantly in the mouth, specifically in dental plaque and saliva (37). Thus, adults also benefit from fluoride, rather than only children, as was previously assumed.

RISK FOR DENTAL CARIES

The prevalence and severity of dental caries in the United States have decreased substantially during the preceding 3 decades (*39*). National surveys have reported that the prevalence of any dental caries among children aged 12–17 years declined from 90.4% in 1971–1974 to 67% in 1988–1991; severity (measured as the mean number of decayed, missing, or filled teeth) declined from 6.2 to 2.8 during this period (*40–43*).

These decreases in caries prevalence and severity have been uneven across the general population; the burden of disease now is concentrated among certain groups and persons. For example, 80% of the dental caries in permanent teeth of U.S. children aged 5–17 years occurs among 25% of those children (*43*). To develop and apply appropriate and effective caries prevention and control strategies, identification and assessment of groups and persons at high risk for developing new carious lesions is essential (*44*). Caries risk assessment is difficult because it attempts to account for the complex interaction of multiple factors. Although various methods for assessing risk exist, no single model predominates in this emerging science. Models that take multiple factors into account predict the risk more accurately, especially for groups rather than persons. However, for persons in a clinical setting, models do not improve on a dentist's perception of risk after examining a patient and considering the personal circumstances (*45*).

Populations believed to be at increased risk for dental caries are those with low socioeconomic status (SES) or low levels of parental education, those who do not seek regular dental care, and those without dental insurance or access to dental services (*45–47*). Persons can be at high risk for dental caries even if they do not have these recognized factors. Individual factors that possibly increase risk include active dental caries; a history of high caries in older siblings or caregivers; root surfaces exposed by gingival recession; high levels of infection with cariogenic bacteria; impaired ability to maintain oral hygiene; malformed enamel or dentin; reduced salivary flow because of medications, radiation treatment, or disease; low salivary buffering capacity (i.e., decreased ability of saliva to neutralize acids); and the wearing of space maintainers, orthodontic appliances, or dental prostheses. Risk can increase if any of these factors are combined with dietary practices conducive to dental caries (i.e., frequent consumption of refined carbohydrates). Risk decreases with adequate exposure to fluoride (*44,45*).

Risk for dental caries and caries experience* exists on a continuum, with each person at risk to some extent; 85% of U.S. adults have experienced tooth decay (*48*). Caries risk can vary over time — perhaps numerous times during a person's lifetime — as risk factors change. Because caries prediction is an inexact, developing science, risk is dichotomized as low and high in this report. If these two categories of risk were applied to the U.S. population, most persons would be classified as low risk at any given time.

Children and adults who are at low risk for dental caries can maintain that status through frequent exposure to small amounts of fluoride (e.g., drinking fluoridated water and using fluoride toothpaste). Children and adults at high risk for dental caries might benefit from additional exposure to fluoride (e.g., mouthrinse, dietary supplements, and professionally applied products). All available information on risk factors should be considered before a group or person is identified as being at low or high risk for dental caries. However, when classification is uncertain, treating a person as high risk is prudent until further information or experience allows a more accurate assessment. This assumption

---

*For this report, the term "caries experience" is used to mean the sum of filled and unfilled cavities, along with any missing teeth resulting from tooth decay.

increases the immediate cost of caries prevention or treatment and might increase the risk for enamel fluorosis for children aged <6 years, but reduces the risk for dental caries for groups or persons misclassified as low risk.

RISK FOR ENAMEL FLUOROSIS

The proper amount of fluoride helps prevent and control dental caries. Fluoride ingested during tooth development can also result in a range of visually detectable changes in enamel opacity (i.e., light refraction at or below the surface) because of hypomineralization. These changes have been broadly termed enamel fluorosis, certain extremes of which are cosmetically objectionable (49). (Many other developmental changes that affect the appearance of enamel are not related to fluoride [50].) Severe forms of this condition can occur only when young children ingest excess fluoride, from any source, during critical periods of tooth development. The occurrence of enamel fluorosis is reported to be most strongly associated with cumulative fluoride intake during enamel development, but the severity of the condition depends on the dose, duration, and timing of fluoride intake. The transition and early maturation stages of enamel development appear to be most susceptible to the effects of fluoride (51); these stages occur at varying times for different tooth types. For central incisors of the upper jaw, for example, the most sensitive period is estimated at age 15–24 months for boys and age 21–30 months for girls (51,52).

Concerns regarding the risk for enamel fluorosis are limited to children aged ≤8 years; enamel is no longer susceptible once its preeruptive maturation is complete (11). Fluoride sources for children aged ≤8 years are drinking water, processed beverages and food, toothpaste, dietary supplements that include fluoride (tablets or drops), and other dental products. This report discusses the risk for enamel fluorosis among children aged <6 years. Children aged ≥6 years are considered past the age that fluoride ingestion can cause cosmetically objectionable fluorosis because only certain posterior teeth are still at a susceptible stage of enamel development, and these will not be readily visible. In addition, the swallowing reflex has developed sufficiently by age 6 years for most children to be able to control inadvertent swallowing of fluoride toothpaste and mouthrinse.

The very mild and mild forms of enamel fluorosis appear as chalklike, lacy markings across a tooth's enamel surface that are not readily apparent to the affected person or casual observer (53). In the moderate form, >50% of the enamel surface is opaque white. The rare, severe form manifests as pitted and brittle enamel. After eruption, teeth with moderate or severe fluorosis might develop areas of brown stain (54). In the severe form, the compromised enamel might break away, resulting in excessive wear of the teeth. Even in its severe form, enamel fluorosis is considered a cosmetic effect, not an adverse functional effect (8,11,55,56). Some persons choose to modify this condition with elective cosmetic treatment.

The benefits of reduced dental caries and the risk for enamel fluorosis are linked. Early studies that examined the cause of "mottled enamel" (now called moderate to severe enamel fluorosis) led to the unexpected discovery that fluoride in community drinking water inhibits dental caries (57). Historically, a low prevalence of the milder forms of enamel fluorosis has been accepted as a reasonable and minor consequence balanced against the substantial protection from dental caries from drinking water containing an optimal concentration of fluoride, either naturally occurring or through adjustment (*11,53*). When enamel fluorosis was first systematically investigated during the 1930s and 1940s, its prevalence was 12%–15% for very mild and mild forms and zero for moderate and severe forms among children who lived in communities with drinking water that naturally contained 0.9–1.2 ppm fluoride (*53*). Although the prevalence of this condition in the United States has since increased (*8,58,59*), most fluorosis today is of the mildest form, which affects neither cosmetic appearance nor dental function. The increased prevalence in areas both with and without fluoridated community drinking water (*8*) indicates that, during the first 8 years of life (i.e., the window of time when this condition can develop), the total intake of fluoride from all sources has increased for some children.

The 1986–1987 National Survey of Dental Caries in U.S. School Children (the most recent national estimates of enamel fluorosis prevalence) indicated that the prevalence of any enamel fluorosis among children was 22%–23% (range: 26% of children aged 9 years to 19% of those aged 17 years) (*60,61*). Almost all cases reported in the survey were of the very mild or mild form, but some cases of the moderate (1.1%) and severe (0.3%) forms were observed. Cases of moderate and severe forms occurred even among children living in areas with low fluoride concentrations in the drinking water (*61*). Although this level of enamel fluorosis is not considered a public health problem (*53*), prudent public health practice should seek to minimize this condition, especially moderate to severe forms. In addition, changes in public perceptions of what is cosmetically acceptable could influence support for effective caries-prevention measures. Research into the causes of enamel fluorosis has focused on identifying risk factors (*62–65*). Adherence to the recommendations in this report regarding appropriate use of fluoride for children aged ≤6 years will reduce the prevalence and severity of enamel fluorosis.

NATIONAL GUIDELINES FOR FLUORIDE USE

PHS recommendations for fluoride use include an optimally adjusted concentration of fluoride in community drinking water to maximize caries prevention and limit enamel fluorosis. This concentration ranges from 0.7 ppm to 1.2 ppm depending on the average maximum daily air temperature of the area (*66–68*). In 1991, PHS also issued policy and research recommendations for fluoride use (*8*). The U.S. Environmental Protection Agency (EPA), which is responsible for the safety and quality of drinking water in the United States, sets a maximum allowable limit for fluoride in community drinking water at 4 ppm and a secondary limit (i.e., nonenforceable guideline) at 2 ppm (*69,70*). The U.S. Food and Drug Administration (FDA) is responsible for approving prescription and over-the-counter fluoride products marketed in the United States and for setting standards for labeling bottled water (*71*) and over-the-counter fluoride products (e.g., toothpaste and mouthrinse) (*72*).

Nonfederal agencies also have published guidelines on fluoride use. The American Dental Association (ADA) reviews fluoride products for caries prevention through its voluntary Seal of Acceptance program; accepted products are listed in the *ADA Guide to Dental Therapeutics* (*73*). A dosage schedule for fluoride supplements for infants and children aged ≤16 years, which is scaled to the fluoride concentration in the community drinking water, has been jointly recommended by ADA, the American Academy of Pediatric Dentistry (AAPD), and the American Academy of Pediatrics (AAP) (Table 1) (*44,74,75*). In 1997, the Institute of Medicine published age-specific recommendations for total dietary intake of fluoride (Table 2). These recommendations list adequate intake to prevent dental caries and tolerable upper intake, defined as a level unlikely to pose risk for adverse effects in almost all persons.

TABLE 1. Recommended dietary fluoride supplement* schedule

Age	Fluoride concentration in community drinking water[†]		
	<0.3 ppm	0.3–0.6 ppm	>0.6 ppm
0–6 months	None	None	None
6 months–3 years	0.25 mg/day	None	None
3–6 years	0.50 mg/day	0.25 mg/day	None
6–16 years	1.0 mg/day	0.50 mg/day	None

* Sodium fluoride (2.2 mg sodium fluoride contains 1 mg fluoride ion).

† 1.0 parts per million (ppm) = 1 mg/L.

Sources:

Meskin LH, ed. Caries diagnosis and risk assessment: a review of preventive strategies and management. J Am Dent Assoc 1995;126(suppl):1S–24S.

American Academy of Pediatric Dentistry. Special issue: reference manual 1994–95. Pediatr Dent 1995;16(special issue):1–96.

American Academy of Pediatrics Committee on Nutrition. Fluoride supplementation for children: interim policy recommendations. Pediatrics 1995;95:777.

TABLE 2. Recommended total dietary fluoride intake

Age	Reference weight*		Adequate intake[†]	Tolerable upper intake[§]
	kg	lb	mg/day	mg/day
0–6 months	7	16	0.01	0.7
6–12 months	9	20	0.5	0.9
1–3 years	13	29	0.7	1.3
4–8 years	22	48	1.1	2.2
≥9 years	40–76	88–166	2.0–3.8	10.0

* Values based on data collected during 1988–1994 as part of the third National Health and Nutrition Examination Survey.

† Intake that maximally reduces occurrence of dental caries without causing unwanted side effects, including moderate enamel fluorosis.

§ Highest level of nutrient intake that is likely to pose no risks for adverse health effects in almost all persons.

Source: Adapted from Institute of Medicine. Fluoride. In: Dietary reference intakes for calcium, phosphorus, magnesium, vitamin D, and fluoride. Washington, DC: National Academy Press, 1997:288–313.

FLUORIDE SOURCES AND THEIR EFFECTS

Fluoridated community drinking water and fluoride toothpaste are the most common sources of fluoride in the United States and are largely responsible for the low risk for dental caries for most persons in this country. Persons at high risk for dental caries might require more frequent or more concentrated exposure to fluoride and might benefit from use of other fluoride modalities (e.g., mouthrinse, dietary supplements, and topical gel, foam, or varnish). The effects of each of these fluoride sources on dental caries and enamel fluorosis are described.

Fluoridated Drinking Water and Processed Beverages and Food

Fluoridated drinking water contains a fluoride concentration effective for preventing dental caries; this concentration can occur naturally or be reached through water fluoridation, which is the controlled addition of fluoride to a public water supply. When fluoridated water is the main source of drinking water, a low concentration of fluoride is routinely introduced into the mouth. Some of this fluoride is taken up by dental plaque; some is transiently present in saliva, which serves as a reservoir for plaque fluoride; and some is loosely held on the enamel surfaces (76). Frequent consumption of fluoridated drinking water and beverages and food processed in fluoridated areas maintains the concentration of fluoride in the mouth.

Estimates of fluoride intake among U.S. and Canadian adults have ranged from ≤1.0 mg fluoride per day in nonfluoridated areas to 1–3 mg fluoride per day in fluoridated areas (77–80). The average daily dietary fluoride intake for both children and adults in fluoridated areas has remained relatively constant for several years (11). For children who live in optimally fluoridated areas, this average is approximately 0.05 mg/kg/day (range: 0.02–0.10); for children who live in nonfluoridated areas, the average is approximately half (11). In a survey of four U.S. cities with different fluoride concentrations in the drinking water (range: 0.37–1.04 ppm), children aged 2 years ingested 0.41–0.61 mg fluoride per day and infants aged 6 months ingested 0.21–0.54 mg fluoride per day (81,82).

In the United States, water and processed beverages (e.g., soft drinks and fruit juices) can provide approximately 75% of a person's fluoride intake (83). Many processed beverages are prepared in locations where the drinking water is fluoridated. Foods and ingredients used in food processing vary in their fluoride content (11). As consumption of processed beverages by children increases, fluoride intake in communities without fluoridated water will increase whenever the water source for the processed beverage is fluoridated (84). In fluoridated areas, dietary fluoride intake has been stable because processed beverages have been substituted for tap water and for beverages prepared in the home using tap water (11).

A study of Iowa infants estimated that the mean fluoride intake from water during different periods during the first 9 months of life, either consumed directly or added to infant formula or juice, was 0.29–0.38 mg per day, although estimated intake for some infants was as high as 1.73 mg per day (85). As foods are added to an infant's diet, replacing some of the formula prepared with fluoridated water, the amount of fluoride the infant receives typically decreases (86). The Iowa study also reported that infant formula and processed baby food contained variable amounts of fluoride. Since 1979, U.S. manufacturers of infant formula have voluntarily lowered the fluoride concentration of their products, both ready-to-feed and concentrates, to <0.3 ppm fluoride (87).

Drinking Water

Community Water. During the 1940s, researchers determined that 1 ppm fluoride was the optimal concentration in community drinking water for climates similar to the Chicago area (88,89). This concentration would substantially reduce the prevalence of dental caries, while allowing an acceptably low prevalence (i.e., 10%–12%) of very mild and mild enamel fluorosis and no moderate or severe enamel fluorosis. Water fluoridation for caries control began in 1945 and 1946, when the fluoride concentration was adjusted in the drinking water supplying four communities in the United States and Canada (*2–5*). This public health approach followed a long period of epidemiologic research into the effects of naturally occurring fluoride in drinking water (*53,57,88,89*).

Current federal fluoridation guidelines, maintained by the PHS since 1962, state that community drinking water should contain 0.7–1.2 ppm fluoride, depending on the average maximum daily air temperature of the area. These temperature-related guidelines are based on epidemiologic studies conducted during the 1950s that led to the development of an algebraic formula for determining optimal fluoride concentrations (*67,90–92*). This formula determined that a lower fluoride concentration was appropriate for communities in warmer climates because persons living in warmer climates drank more tap water. However, social and environmental changes since 1962 (e.g., increased use of air conditioning and more sedentary lifestyles) have reduced the likelihood that persons in warmer regions drink more tap water than persons in cooler regions (*7*).

By 1992, fluoridated water was reaching 144 million persons in the United States (56% of the total population and 62% of those receiving municipal water supplies) (*93*). Approximately 10 million of these persons were receiving water containing naturally occurring fluoride at a concentration of $\geq$0.7 ppm. In 11 states and the District of Columbia, >90% of the population had such access, whereas <5% received this benefit in two states. In 2000, a total of 38 states and the District of Columbia provided access to fluoridated public water supplies to $\geq$50% of their population (CDC, unpublished data, 2000) (Figure 2).

FIGURE 2. Percentage of state populations with access to fluoridated water through public water systems

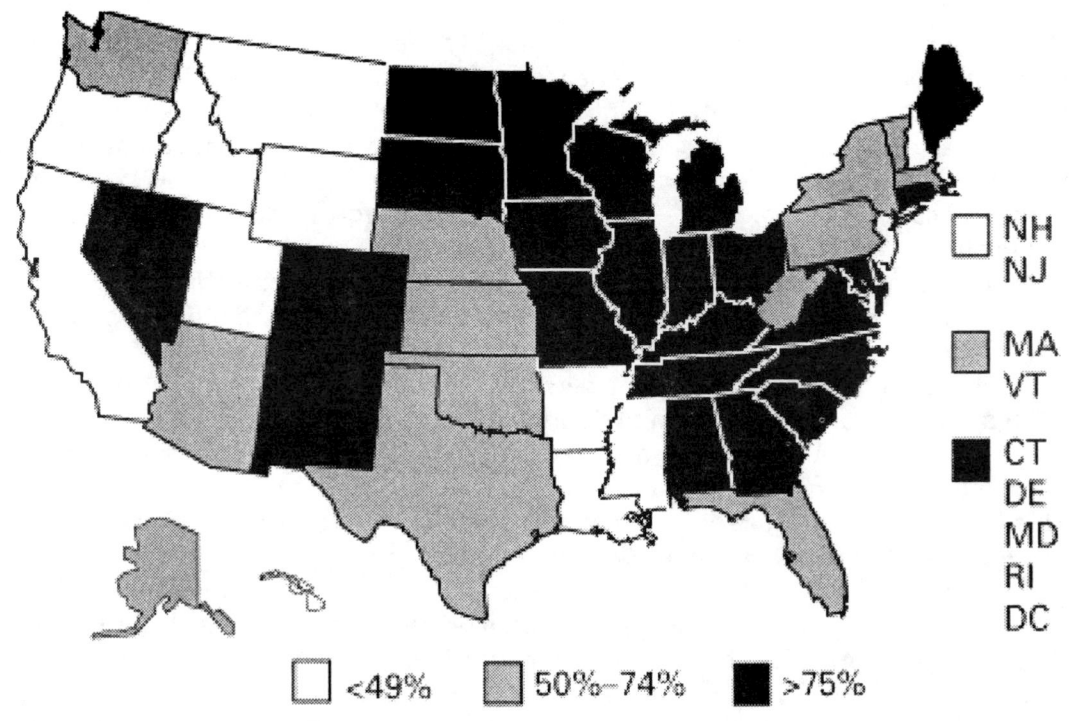

Source: CDC, unpublished data, 2000.

Initial studies of community water fluoridation demonstrated that reductions in child-hood dental caries attributable to fluoridation were approximately 50%–60% (*94–97*). More recent estimates are lower — 18%–40% (*98,99*). This decrease in attributable benefit is likely caused by the increasing use of fluoride from other sources, with the widespread use of fluoride toothpaste probably the most important. The diffusion or "halo" effect of beverages and food processed in fluoridated areas but consumed in nonfluoridated areas also indirectly spreads some benefit of fluoridated water to nonfluoridated communities. This effect lessens the differences in caries experience among communities (*100*).

Quantifying the benefits of water fluoridation among adults is more complicated be-cause adults are rarely surveyed, their fluoride histories are potentially more varied, and their tooth loss or restorations might be caused by dental problems other than caries (e.g., trauma or periodontal diseases). Nevertheless, adults are reported to receive caries-preventive benefits from community water fluoridation (*99,101–103*). These ben-efits might be particularly advantageous for adults aged >50 years, many of whom are at increased risk for dental caries. Besides coronal caries, older adults typically experience gingival recession, which results in teeth with exposed root surfaces. Unlike the crowns of teeth, these root surfaces are not covered by enamel and are more susceptible to caries. Because tooth retention among older age groups has increased in recent decades in the United States (*39*), these groups' risk for caries will increase as the country's population ages. Older adults also frequently require multiple medications for chronic conditions, and many of these medications can reduce salivary output (*104*). Drinking water containing an optimal concentration of fluoride can mitigate the risk factors for caries among older adults. Studies have reported that the prevalence of root caries among adults is inversely related to fluoride concentration in the community drinking water (*105–107*).

Water fluoridation also reduces the disparities in caries experience among poor and nonpoor children (*108–111*). Caries experience is considerably higher among persons in low SES strata than among those in high SES strata (*39,46,112*). The reasons for this discrepancy are not well understood; perhaps persons in low SES strata have less knowl-edge of oral diseases, have less access to dental care, are less likely to follow recom-mended self-care practices, or are harder to reach through traditional approaches, including public health programs and private dental care (*48*). Thus, these persons might receive more benefit from fluoridated community water than persons from high SES strata. Regardless of SES, water fluoridation is the most effective and efficient strategy to reduce dental caries (*112*).

Enamel fluorosis occurs among some persons in all communities, even in communi-ties with a low natural concentration of fluoride. During 1930–1960, U.S. studies docu-mented that, in areas with a natural or adjusted concentration of fluoride of approximately 1.0 ppm in the community drinking water, the permanent teeth of 7%–16% of children with lifetime residence in those areas exhibited very mild or mild forms of enamel fluoro-sis (*53,113,114*). Before 1945, when naturally fluoridated drinking water was virtually the only source of fluoride, the moderate and severe forms of this condition were not observed unless the natural fluoride concentration was $\geq$2 ppm (*53*). The likelihood of a child developing the mild forms of enamel fluorosis might be higher in a fluoridated area than in a nonfluoridated area, but prevalence might not change in every community (*115,116*). The most recent national study of this condition indicated that its prevalence had increased in both fluoridated and nonfluoridated areas since the 1940s, with the relative increase higher in nonfluoridated areas. In communities with drinking water containing 0.7–1.2 ppm fluoride, the prevalence was 1.3% for the moderate form of enamel fluorosis and zero for the severe form; thus, few cases of enamel fluorosis were likely to be of cosmetic consequence (8,61). Because combined fluoride intake from drinking water and processed beverages and food by children in fluoridated areas has reportedly remained stable since the 1940s, the increase in fluoride intake resulting in increased enamel fluorosis almost certainly stems from use of fluoride-containing dental products by children aged <6 years (11).

Two studies reported that extended consumption of infant formula beyond age 10–12 months was a risk factor for enamel fluorosis, especially when formula concentrate was mixed with fluoridated water (62,63). These studies examined children who used pre-1979 formula (with higher fluoride concentrations). Whether fluoride intake from formula that exceeds the recommended amount during only the first 10–12 months of life contributes to the prevalence or severity of enamel fluorosis is unknown.

Fluoride concentrations in drinking water should be maintained at optimal levels, both to achieve effective caries prevention and because changes in fluoride concentration as low as 0.2 ppm can result in a measurable change in the prevalence and severity of enamel fluorosis (52,117). Since the late 1970s, CDC has provided guidelines and recommendations for managers of fluoridated water supply systems at state and local levels to help them establish and maintain appropriate fluoride concentrations. CDC periodically updates these guidelines; the most recent revision was published in 1995 (68).

School Water Systems. In some areas of the United States where fluoridating a community's drinking water was not feasible (e.g., rural areas), the alternative of fluoridating a school's public water supply system was promoted for many years. This method was used when a school had its own source of water and was not connected to a community water supply system (i.e., stand-alone systems). Because children are at school only part of each weekday, a fluoride concentration of 4.5 times the optimal concentration for a community in the same geographic area was recommended (118) to compensate for the more limited consumption of fluoridated water. At the peak of this practice in the early 1980s, a total of 13 states had initiated school water fluoridation in 470 schools serving 170,000 children (39). Since then, school water fluoridation has been phased out in several states; the current extent of this practice is not known.

Studies of the effects of school water fluoridation in the United States reported that this practice reduced caries among schoolchildren by approximately 40% (118–122). A more recent study indicated that this effect might no longer be as pronounced (123).

Several concerns regarding school water fluoridation exist. Operating and maintaining small fluoridation systems (i.e., those serving <500 persons) create practical and logistical difficulties (68). These difficulties have occasionally caused higher than recommended fluoride concentrations in the school drinking water, but no lasting effects among children have been observed (124–126). In schools that enroll preschoolers in day care programs, children aged <6 years might receive more than adequate fluoride.

Bottled Water. Many persons drink bottled water, replacing tap water partially or completely as a source of drinking water. Water is classified as "bottled water" if it meets all applicable federal and state standards, is sealed in a sanitary container, and is sold for human consumption. Although some bottled waters marketed in the United States contain an optimal concentration of fluoride (approximately 1.0 ppm), most contain <0.3 ppm fluoride (127–129). Thus, a person substituting bottled water with a low fluoride concentration for fluoridated community water might not receive the full benefits of community water fluoridation (*130*). For water bottled in the United States, current FDA regulations require that fluoride be listed on the label only if the bottler adds fluoride during processing; the concentration of fluoride is regulated but does not have to be stated on the label (Table 3). Few bottled water brands have labels listing the fluoride concentration.

TABLE 3. U.S. Food and Drug Administration (FDA) fluoride requirements for bottled water packaged in the United States

Annual average of maximum daily air temperature (F) where the bottled water is sold at retail	Maximum fluoride concentration (mg/L) allowed in bottled water	
	No fluoride added to bottled water	Fluoride added to bottled water
≤53.7	2.4	1.7
53.8–58.3	2.2	1.5
58.4–63.8	2	1.3
63.9–70.6	1.8	1.2
70.7–79.2	1.6	1
79.3–90.5	1.4	0.8

Note: FDA regulations require that fluoride be listed on the label only if the bottler adds fluoride during processing; the bottler is not required to list the fluoride concentration, which might or might not be optimal. FDA does not allow imported bottled water with no added fluoride to contain >1.4 mg fluoride/L or imported bottled water with added fluoride to contain >0.8 mg fluoride/L.
Source: US Department of Health and Human Services, Food and Drug Administration. 21 CFR Part 165.110. Bottled water. Federal Register 1995;60:57124–30.

Determining Fluoride Concentration. Uneven geographic coverage of community water fluoridation throughout the United States, wide variations in natural fluoride concentrations found in drinking water, and almost nonexistent labeling of fluoride concentration in bottled water make knowing the concentration of fluoride in drinking water difficult for many persons. Persons in nonfluoridated areas can mistakenly believe their water contains an optimal concentration of fluoride. To obtain the fluoride concentration of community drinking water, a resident can contact the water supplier or a local public health authority, dentist, dental hygienist, physician, or other knowledgeable source. EPA requires that all community water supply systems provide each customer an annual report on the quality of water, including the fluoride concentration (*131*). Testing for private wells is available through local and state public health departments as well as some private laboratories. If the fluoride concentration is not listed on the label of bottled water, the bottler can be contacted directly to obtain this information.

Fluoride Toothpaste

Fluoride is the only nonprescription toothpaste additive proven to prevent dental caries. When introduced into the mouth, fluoride in toothpaste is taken up directly by dental plaque (*132–134*) and demineralized enamel (*135,136*). Brushing with fluoride toothpaste also increases the fluoride concentration in saliva 100- to 1,000-fold; this concentration returns to baseline levels within 1–2 hours (*137*). Some of this salivary fluoride is taken up by dental plaque. The ambient fluoride concentration in saliva and plaque can increase during regular use of fluoride toothpaste (*132,133*).

By the 1990s, fluoride toothpaste accounted for >90% of the toothpaste market in the United States, Canada, and other developed countries (*138*). Because water fluoridation is not available in many countries, toothpaste might be the most important source of fluoride globally (*1*).

Studies of 2–3 years duration have reported that fluoride toothpaste reduces caries experience among children by a median of 15%–30% (*139–148*). This reduction is modest compared with the effect of water fluoridation, but water fluoridation studies usually measured lifetime — rather than a few years' — exposure. Regular lifetime use of fluoride toothpaste likely provides ongoing benefits that might approach those of fluoridated water. Combined use of fluoride toothpaste and fluoridated water offers protection above either used alone (*99,149,150*).

Few studies evaluating the effectiveness of fluoride toothpaste, gel, rinse, and varnish among adult populations are available. Child populations have typically been used for studies on caries prevention because of perceived increased caries susceptibility and logistical reasons. However, teeth generally remain susceptible to caries throughout life, and topically applied fluorides could be effective in preventing caries in susceptible patients of any age (*151,152*).

Most persons report brushing their teeth at least once per day (*153,154*), but more frequent use can offer additional protection (*139,141,155–158*). Brushing twice a day is a reasonable social norm that is both effective and convenient for most persons' daily routines, and this practice has become a basic recommendation for caries prevention. Whether increasing the number of daily brushings from two to three times a day results in lower dental caries experience is unclear. Because the amount and vigor of rinsing after toothbrushing affects fluoride concentration in the mouth and reportedly affects caries experience (*157–160*), persons aged ≥6 years can retain more fluoride in the mouth by either rinsing briefly with a small amount of water or not at all.

In the United States, the standard concentration of fluoride in fluoride toothpaste is 1,000–1,100 ppm. Toothpaste containing 1,500 ppm fluoride has been reported to be slightly more efficacious in reducing dental caries in U.S. and European studies (*161–164*). Products with this fluoride concentration have been marketed in the United States, but are not available in all areas. These products might benefit persons aged ≥6 years at high risk for dental caries.

Children who begin using fluoride toothpaste at age <2 years are at higher risk for enamel fluorosis than children who begin later or who do not use fluoride toothpaste at all (*62,63,165–170*). Because studies have not used the same criteria for age of initiation, amount of toothpaste used, or frequency of toothpaste use, the specific contribution of each factor to enamel fluorosis among this age group has not been established.

Fluoride toothpaste contributes to the risk for enamel fluorosis because the swallowing reflex of children aged <6 years is not always well controlled, particularly among children aged <3 years (*171,172*). Children are also known to swallow toothpaste deliberately when they like its taste. A child-sized toothbrush covered with a full strip of toothpaste holds approximately 0.75–1.0 g of toothpaste, and each gram of fluoride toothpaste, as formulated in the United States, contains approximately 1.0 mg of fluoride. Children aged <6 years swallow a mean of 0.3 g of toothpaste per brushing (*11*) and can inadvertently swallow as much as 0.8 g (*138,173–176*). As a result, multiple brushings with fluoride toothpaste each day can result in ingestion of excess fluoride (*177*). For this reason, high-fluoride toothpaste (i.e., containing 1,500 ppm fluoride) is generally contraindicated for children aged <6 years.

Use of a pea-sized amount (approximately 0.25 g) of fluoride toothpaste ≤2 times per day by children aged <6 years is reported to sharply reduce the importance of fluoride toothpaste as a risk factor for enamel fluorosis (65). Since 1991, manufacturers of fluoride toothpaste marketed in the United States have, as a requirement for obtaining the ADA Seal of Acceptance, placed instructions on the package label stating that children aged <6 years should use only this amount of toothpaste. Toothpaste labeling requirements mandated by FDA in 1996 (72) also direct parents of children aged <2 years to seek advice from a dentist or physician before introducing their child to fluoride toothpaste.

The propensity of young children to swallow toothpaste has led to development of "child-strength" toothpaste with lower fluoride concentrations (176). Such a product would be a desirable alternative to currently available products for many young children. Clinical trials outside the United States have reported that toothpaste containing 250 ppm fluoride is less effective than toothpaste containing 1,000 ppm fluoride in preventing dental caries (178,179). However, toothpaste containing 500–550 ppm fluoride might be almost as efficacious as that containing 1,000 ppm fluoride (180). A British study reported that the prevalence of diffuse enamel opacities (an indicator of mild enamel fluorosis) in the upper anterior incisors was substantially lower among children who used toothpaste containing 550 ppm fluoride than among those who used toothpaste containing 1,050 ppm fluoride (181). Toothpaste containing 400 ppm fluoride has been available in Australia and New Zealand for approximately 20 years, but has not been tested in clinical trials, and no data are available to assess whether toothpaste at this concentration has reduced the prevalence of enamel fluorosis in those countries. A U.S. clinical trial of the efficacy of toothpaste with lower fluoride concentrations, required by FDA before approval for marketing and distribution, has not been conducted (182).

Fluoride Mouthrinse

Fluoride mouthrinse is a concentrated solution intended for daily or weekly use. The fluoride from mouthrinse, like that from toothpaste, is retained in dental plaque and saliva to help prevent dental caries (183). The most common fluoride compound used in mouthrinse is sodium fluoride. Over-the-counter solutions of 0.05% sodium fluoride (230 ppm fluoride) for daily rinsing are available for use by persons aged >6 years. Solutions of 0.20% sodium fluoride (920 ppm fluoride) are used in supervised, school-based weekly rinsing programs. Throughout the 1980s, approximately 3 million children in the United States participated in school-based fluoride mouthrinsing programs (39). The current extent of such programs is not known.

Studies indicating that fluoride mouthrinse reduces caries experience among schoolchildren date mostly from the 1970s and early 1980s (184–191). In one review, the average caries reduction in nonfluoridated communities attributable to fluoride mouthrinse was 31% (191). Two studies reported benefits of fluoride mouthrinse approximately 2.5 and 7 years after completion of school-based mouthrinsing programs (192,193), but a more recent study did not find such benefits 4 years after completion of a mouthrinsing program (194). The National Preventive Dentistry Demonstration Program (NPDDP), a large project conducted in 10 U.S. cities during 1976–1981 to compare the cost and effectiveness of combinations of caries-prevention procedures, reported that fluoride mouthrinse had little effect among schoolchildren, either among first-grade students with high and low caries experience (195) or among all second- and fifth-grade students (*196*). NPDDP documented only a limited reduction in dental caries attributable to fluoride mouthrinse, especially when children were also exposed to fluoridated water.

Although no studies of enamel fluorosis associated with use of fluoride mouthrinse have been conducted, studies of the amount of fluoride swallowed by children aged 3–5 years using such rinses indicated that some young children might swallow substantial amounts (*191*). Use of fluoride mouthrinse by children aged ≥6 years does not place them at risk for cosmetically objectionable enamel fluorosis because they are generally past the age that fluoride ingestion might affect their teeth.

Dietary Fluoride Supplements

Dietary fluoride supplements in the form of tablets, lozenges, or liquids (including fluoride-vitamin preparations) have been used throughout the world since the 1940s. Most supplements contain sodium fluoride as the active ingredient. Tablets and lozenges are manufactured with 1.0, 0.5, or 0.25 mg fluoride. To maximize the topical effect of fluoride, tablets and lozenges are intended to be chewed or sucked for 1–2 minutes before being swallowed. For infants, supplements are available as a liquid and used with a dropper.

In 1986, an estimated 16% of U.S. children aged <2 years used fluoride supplements (*197*). All fluoride supplements must be prescribed by a dentist or physician. The prescription should be consistent with the 1994 dosage schedule developed by ADA, AAPD, and AAP (Table 1). Because fluoride supplements are intended to compensate for fluoride-deficient drinking water, the dosage schedule requires knowledge of the fluoride content of the child's primary drinking water; consideration should also be given to other sources of water (e.g., home, child care settings, school, or bottled water) and to other sources of fluoride (e.g., toothpaste or mouthrinse), which can complicate the prescribing decision.

The evidence for using fluoride supplements to mitigate dental caries is mixed. Use of fluoride supplements by pregnant women does not benefit their offspring (*198*). Several studies have reported that fluoride supplements taken by infants and children before their teeth erupt reduce the prevalence and severity of caries in teeth (*98,199–207*), but several other studies have not (*19,208–212*). Among children aged 6–16 years, fluoride supplements taken after teeth erupt reduce caries experience (*213–215*). Fluoride supplements might be beneficial among adults who have limitations with toothbrushing, but this use requires further study.

A few studies have reported no association between supplement use by children aged <6 years and enamel fluorosis (*208,216*), but most have reported a clear association (*19,62,64,165,170,199–201,209,210,212,217–222*). In one study, the risk for this condition was high when supplements were used in fluoridated areas (odds ratio = 23.74; 95% confidence interval = 3.43–164.30) (*62*), a use inconsistent with the supplement schedule. Reports of the frequency of supplement use in fluoridated areas have ranged from 7% to 35% (*223–228*). In response to the accumulated data on fluoride intake and the prevalence of enamel fluorosis, the supplement dosage schedule for children aged <6 years was markedly reduced in 1994 when ADA, AAPD, and AAP jointly established the current schedule (Table 1) (*73*). The risk for enamel fluorosis among children this age attributable to fluoride supplements could be lower, but not enough information is available yet to evaluate the effects of this change.

When prescribing any pharmaceutical agent, dentists and physicians should attempt to maximize benefit and minimize harm (*229*). For infants and children aged <6 years, both a benefit of dental caries prevention and a risk for enamel fluorosis are possible. Although the primary (i.e., "baby") teeth of children aged 1–6 years would benefit from fluoride's posteruptive action, and some preeruptive benefit for developing permanent teeth could exist, fluoride supplements also could increase the risk for enamel fluorosis at this age (*138,223*).

Professionally Applied Fluoride Compounds

In the United States, dentists and dental hygienists have been applying high-concentration fluoride compounds directly to patients' teeth for approximately 50 years. Application procedures were developed on the assumption that the fluoride would be incorporated into the crystalline structure of the dental enamel and develop a more acid-resistant enamel. To maximize this reaction, a professional tooth cleaning was considered mandatory before the application. However, subsequent research has demonstrated that high-concentration fluoride compounds (e.g., those in gel or varnish) do not directly enter the enamel's crystalline structure (*230*). The compound forms a calcium fluoride-like material on the enamel's surface that releases fluoride for remineralization when the pH in the mouth drops. Thus, professional tooth cleaning solely to prepare the teeth for application of a fluoride compound is unnecessary; toothbrushing and flossing appear equally effective in improving the efficacy of high-concentration fluoride compounds (*231*).

Fluoride Gel and Foam

Because an early study reported that fluoride uptake by dental enamel increased in an acidic environment (*232*), fluoride gel is often formulated to be highly acidic (pH of approximately 3.0). Products available in the United States include gel of acidulated phosphate fluoride (1.23% [12,300 ppm] fluoride), gel or foam of sodium fluoride (0.9% [9,040 ppm] fluoride), and self-applied (i.e., home use) gel of sodium fluoride (0.5% [5,000 ppm] fluoride) or stannous fluoride (0.15% [1,000 ppm] fluoride) (*73*).

Clinical trials conducted during 1940–1970 demonstrated that professionally applied fluorides effectively reduce caries experience in children (*233*). In more recent studies, semiannual treatments reportedly caused an average decrease of 26% in caries experience in the permanent teeth of children residing in nonfluoridated areas (*191,234–236*). The application time for the treatments was 4 minutes. In clinical practice, applying fluoride gel for 1 minute rather than 4 minutes is common, but the efficacy of this shorter application time has not been tested in human clinical trials. In addition, the optimal schedule for repeated application of fluoride gel has not been adequately studied to support definitive guidelines, and studies that have examined the efficacy of various gel application schedules in preventing and controlling dental caries have reported mixed results. On the basis of the available evidence, the usual recommended frequency is semiannual (*151,237,238*).

Because these applications are relatively infrequent, generally at 3- to 12-month intervals, fluoride gel poses little risk for enamel fluorosis, even among patients aged <6 years. Proper application technique reduces the possibility that a patient will swallow the gel during application.

Fluoride Varnish

High-concentration fluoride varnish is painted directly onto the teeth. Fluoride varnish is not intended to adhere permanently; this method holds a high concentration of fluoride in a small amount of material in close contact with the teeth for many hours. Fluoride varnish has practical advantages (e.g., ease of application, a nonoffensive taste, and use of smaller amounts of fluoride than required for gel applications). Such varnishes are available as sodium fluoride (2.26% [2,600 ppm] fluoride) or difluorsilane (0.1% [1,000 ppm] fluoride) preparations.

Fluoride varnish has been widely used in Canada and Europe since the 1970s to prevent dental caries (152,239). FDA's Center for Devices and Radiological Health has cleared fluoride varnish as a medical device to be used as a cavity liner (i.e., to provide fluoride at the junction of filling material and tooth) and root desensitizer (i.e., to reduce sensitivity to temperature and touch that sometimes occurs on root surfaces exposed by receding gingiva) (240); FDA has not yet approved this product as an anticaries agent. Caries prevention is regarded as a drug claim, and companies would be required to submit appropriate clinical trial evidence for review before this product could be marketed as an anticaries agent. However, a prescribing practitioner can use fluoride varnish for caries prevention as an "off-label" use, based on professional judgement (241).

Studies conducted in Canada (242) and Europe (243–246) have reported that fluoride varnish is efficacious in preventing dental caries in children. Applied semiannually, this modality is as effective as professionally applied fluoride gel (247). Some researchers advocate application of fluoride varnish as many as four times per year to achieve maximum effect, but the evidence of benefits from more than two applications per year remains inconclusive (240,246,248). Other studies have reported that three applications in 1 week, once per year, might be more effective than the more conventional semiannual regimen (249,250).

European studies have reported that fluoride varnish prevents decalcification (i.e., an early stage of dental caries) beneath orthodontic bands (251) and slows the progression of existing enamel lesions (252). Studies examining the effectiveness of varnish in controlling early childhood caries are being conducted in the United States. Research on fluoride varnish (e.g., optimal fluoride concentration, the most effective application protocols, and its efficacy relative to other fluoride modalities) is likely to continue in both Europe and North America.

No published evidence indicates that professionally applied fluoride varnish is a risk factor for enamel fluorosis, even among children aged <6 years. Proper application technique reduces the possibility that a patient will swallow varnish during its application and limits the total amount of fluoride swallowed as the varnish wears off the teeth over several hours.

Fluoride Paste

Fluoride-containing paste is routinely used during dental prophylaxis (i.e., cleaning). The abrasive paste, which contains 4,000–20,000 ppm fluoride, might restore the concentration of fluoride in the surface layer of enamel removed by polishing, but it is not an adequate substitute for fluoride gel or varnish in treating persons at high risk for dental caries (151). Fluoride paste is not accepted by FDA or ADA as an efficacious way to prevent dental caries.

Combinations of Fluoride Modalities

Studies comparing various combinations of fluoride modalities have generally reported that their effectiveness in preventing dental caries is partially additive. That is, the percent reduction in the prevalence or severity of dental caries from a combination of modalities is higher than the percent reduction from each modality, but less than the sum of the percent reduction of the modalities combined. Attempts to use a formula to apply sequentially the percent reduction of an additional modality to the estimated remaining caries increment have overestimated the effect (*151,253*). For example, if the first modality reduces caries by 40% and the second modality reduces caries by 30%, then the calculation that caries will be reduced by a total of 58% (i.e., 40% plus 18% [30% of the 60% decay remaining after the first modality]) will likely be an overestimate.

QUALITY OF EVIDENCE FOR DENTAL CARIES PREVENTION AND CONTROL

Members of the work group convened by CDC identified the published research in their areas of expertise and evaluated the quality of scientific evidence for each fluoride modality in preventing and controlling dental caries. Evidence was drawn from the most relevant English-language, peer-reviewed scientific publications regarding the current effectiveness of fluoride modalities. Additional references were suggested by reviewers. Members used their own methods for critically analyzing articles. A formal protocol for duplicate review was not followed, but members collectively agreed on the grade reflecting the quality of evidence regarding each fluoride modality. Criteria used to grade the quality of scientific evidence (i.e., ordinal grading) was adapted from the U.S. Preventive Services Task Force (Box 1) (*254*). Grades range from I to III.

BOX 1. Grading system used for determining the quality of evidence for a fluoride modality

Grade	Criteria
I	Evidence obtained from one or more properly conducted randomized clinical trials (i.e., one using concurrent controls, double-blind design, placebos, valid and reliable measurements, and well-controlled study protocols).
II-1	Evidence obtained from one or more controlled clinical trials without randomization (i.e., one using systematic subject selection, some type of concurrent controls, valid and reliable measurements, and well-controlled study protocols).
II-2	Evidence obtained from one or more well-designed cohort or case-control analytic studies, preferably from more than one center or research group.
II-3	Evidence obtained from cross-sectional comparisons between times and places; studies with historical controls; or dramatic results in uncontrolled experiments (e.g., the results of the introduction of penicillin treatment in the 1940s).
III	Opinions of respected authorities on the basis of clinical experience, descriptive studies or case reports, or reports of expert committees.

Source: US Preventive Services Task Force. Guide to clinical preventive services. 2nd ed. Alexandria, VA: International Medical Publishing, 1996.

Community Water Fluoridation

Studies on the effectiveness of adjusting fluoride in community water to the optimal concentration cannot be designed as randomized clinical trials. Random allocation of study subjects is not possible when a community begins to fluoridate the water because all residents in a community have access to and are exposed to this source of fluoride. In addition, clinical studies cannot be conducted double-blind because both study subjects and researchers usually know whether a community's water has been fluoridated. Efforts to blind the examiners by moving study subjects to a neutral third site for clinical examinations, using radiographs of teeth without revealing where the subjects live, or including transient residents as study subjects have not fully resolved these inherent limitations. Early studies that led to the unexpected discovery that dental caries was less prevalent and severe among persons with mottled enamel (subsequently identified as a form of enamel fluorosis) were conducted before the caries-preventive effects of fluoride were known (*255*). In those studies, researchers did not have an a priori reason to suspect they would find either reduced or higher levels of dental caries experience in communities with low levels of mottled enamel. Researchers also had no reason to believe that patients selected where they lived according to their risk for dental caries. In that regard, these studies were randomized, and examiners were blinded.

Despite the strengths of early studies of the efficacy of naturally occurring fluoride in community drinking water, the limitations of these studies make summarizing the quality of evidence on community water fluoridation as Grade I inappropriate (Table 1). The quality of evidence from studies on the effectiveness of adjusting fluoride concentration in community water to optimal levels is Grade II-1. Research limitations are counterbalanced by broadly similar results from numerous well-conducted field studies by other investigators that included thousands of persons throughout the world (*256,257*).

School Water Fluoridation

Field trials on the effect of school water fluoridation were not blindly conducted and had no concurrent controls (*118*). Thus, the quality of evidence for this modality is Grade II-3.

Fluoride Toothpaste

Studies that have demonstrated the efficacy of fluoride toothpaste in preventing and controlling dental caries include all of the essential features of well-conducted clinical trials. These include randomized groups, double-blind designs, placebo controls, and meticulous procedural protocols. Taken together, the trials on fluoride toothpaste provide solid evidence that fluoride is efficacious in controlling caries (*144*). The quality of evidence for toothpaste is Grade I.

Fluoride Mouthrinse

Early studies of the efficacy of fluoride mouthrinse in reducing dental caries experience were randomized clinical trials (*184,185*) or studies that used historical control groups rather than concurrent control groups (*186–189*). The quality of evidence for fluoride mouthrinse is Grade I.

Dietary Fluoride Supplements

The only randomized controlled trial to assess fluoride supplements taken by pregnant women provides Grade I evidence of no benefit for their children. Many studies of the effectiveness of fluoride supplements in preventing dental caries among children aged <6 years have been flawed in design and conduct. Problems included self-selection into test and control groups, absence of concurrent controls, high attrition rates, and nonblinded examiners. Because of these flaws, the quality of evidence to support use of fluoride supplements by children aged <6 years is Grade II-3. The well-conducted randomized clinical trials on the effects of fluoride supplements on dental caries among children aged 6–16 years in programs conducted in schools provide Grade I evidence.

Fluoride Gel

The quality of evidence for using fluoride gel to prevent and control dental caries in children is Grade I. However, data were gathered when dental caries was more prevalent and severe than today. Subjects in earlier studies were probably more representative of persons who now would be characterized as being at high risk for caries.

Fluoride Varnish

The quality of evidence for the efficacy of high-concentration fluoride varnish in preventing and controlling dental caries in children is Grade I. Although the randomized controlled clinical studies that established Grade I evidence were conducted in Europe, U.S. results should be the same.

COST-EFFECTIVENESS OF FLUORIDE MODALITIES

Documented effectiveness is the most basic requirement for providing a health-care service and an important prerequisite for preventive services (e.g., caries-preventive modalities). However, effectiveness alone is not a sufficient reason to initiate a service. Other factors, including cost, must be considered (*254*). A modality is more cost-effective when deemed a less expensive way, from among competing alternatives, of meeting a stated objective (*258*). In public health planning, determination of the most cost-effective alternative for prevention is essential to using scarce resources efficiently. Dental-insurance carriers are also interested in cost-effectiveness so they can help purchasers use funds efficiently. Because half of dental expenditures are out of pocket (*259*), this topic interests patients and their dentists as well. Potential improvement to quality of life is also a consideration. The contribution of a healthy dentition to quality of life at any age has not been quantified, but is probably valued by most persons.

Although solid data on the cost-effectiveness of fluoride modalities alone and in combination are needed, this information is scarce. In 1989, the Cost Effectiveness of Caries Prevention in Dental Public Health workshop, which was attended by health economists, epidemiologists, and dental public health professionals, attempted to assess the cost-effectiveness of caries-preventive approaches available in the United States (*260*).

All other things being equal, fluoride modalities are most cost-effective for persons at high risk for dental caries. Because persons at low risk develop little dental caries, limited benefit is gained by adding caries-preventive modalities to water fluoridation and fluoride toothpaste, even those demonstrated to be effective among populations at high risk.

Members of the CDC work group reached consensus regarding the populations for which each modality would be expected to have the necessary level of cost-effectiveness to warrant its use.

Community Water Fluoridation

Health economists at the 1989 workshop on cost-effectiveness of caries prevention calculated that the average annual cost of water fluoridation in the United States was $0.51 per person (range: $0.12–$5.41) (*260*). In 1999 dollars,* this cost would be $0.72 per person (range: $0.17–$7.62). Factors reported to influence the per capita cost included

- size of the community (the larger the population reached, the lower the per capita cost);

- number of fluoride injection points in the water supply system;

- amount and type of system feeder and monitoring equipment used;

- amount and type of fluoride chemical used, its price, and its costs of transportation and storage; and

- expertise of personnel at the water plant.

When the effects of caries are repaired, the price of the restoration is based on the number of tooth surfaces affected. A tooth can have caries at >1 location (i.e., surface), so the number of surfaces saved is a more appropriate measure in calculating cost-effectiveness than the number of teeth with caries. The 1989 workshop participants concluded that water fluoridation is one of the few public health measures that results in true cost savings (i.e., the measure saves more money than it costs to operate); in the United States, water fluoridation cost an estimated average of $3.35 per carious surface saved ($4.71 in 1999 dollars*) (*260*). Even under the least favorable assumptions in 1989 (i.e., cities with populations <10,000, higher operating costs, and effectiveness projected at the low end of the range), the cost of a carious surface saved because of community water fluoridation ranged from $8 to $12 ($11–$17 in 1999 dollars*) (*260*), which is still lower than the fee for a one-surface restoration ($54 in 1995 or $65 in 1999 dollars†) (*261*).

A Scottish study conducted in 1980 reported that community water fluoridation resulted in a 49% saving in dental treatment costs for children aged 4–5 years and a 54% saving for children aged 11–12 years (*262*). These savings were maintained even after the secular decline in the prevalence of dental caries was recognized (*263*). The effect of community water fluoridation on the costs of dental care for adults is less clear. This topic cannot be fully explored until the generations who grew up drinking optimally fluoridated water are older.

---

*US$ 1988 converted to US$ 1999 using the Consumer Price Index for All Urban Customers (CPI-Urban) (all items). More information is available at the U.S. Department of Labor, Bureau of Labor Statistics website at <http://stats.bls.gov/cpihome.htm>. Accessed June 25, 2001.
†US$ 1995 converted to US$ 1999 using CPI-Urban (dental services). More information is available at the U.S. Department of Labor, Bureau of Labor Statistics website at <http://stats.bls.gov/cpihome.htm>. Accessed June 25, 2001.

School Water Fluoridation

Costs for school water fluoridation are similar to those of any public water supply system serving a small population (i.e., <1,000 persons). In 1988, the average annual cost of school water fluoridation was $4.52 per student per year (range: $0.81–$9.72) (264). In 1999 dollars,* this cost would be $6.37 per person (range: $1.14–$13.69). Use of this modality must be carefully weighed in the current environment of low caries prevalence, widespread use of fluoride toothpaste, and availability of other fluoride modalities that can be delivered in the school setting.

Fluoride Toothpaste

Fluoride toothpaste is widely available, no more expensive than nonfluoride toothpaste, and periodically improved. Use of a pea-sized amount (0.25 g) twice per day requires approximately two tubes of toothpaste per year, for an estimated annual cost of $6–$12, depending on brand, tube size, and retail source (265). Persons who brush and use toothpaste regularly to maintain periodontal health and prevent stained teeth and halitosis (i.e., bad breath) incur no additional cost for the caries-preventive benefit of fluoride in toothpaste. Because of its multiple benefits, most persons consider fluoride toothpaste a highly cost-effective caries-preventive modality.

Fluoride Mouthrinse

Public health programs of fluoride mouthrinsing have long been presumed to be cost-effective, especially when teachers can supervise weekly rinsing in classrooms at no direct cost to the program. In other programs, volunteers or hourly workers provide supervision. Under these circumstances, administrators of fluoride mouthrinsing programs have claimed annual program costs of approximately $1 per child ($1.41 in 1999 dollars*) (264). This figure likely is an underestimate because indirect costs are not included (196,266). Fluoride mouthrinsing is a reasonable procedure for groups and persons at high risk for dental caries, but its cost-effectiveness as a universal, population-wide strategy in the modern era of widespread fluoride exposure is questionable (267).

Dietary Fluoride Supplements

Dietary fluoride supplements prescribed to persons cost an estimated $37 per year. Fluoride supplements in school programs have direct costs of approximately $2.50 per child ($3.52 in 1999 dollars*) for the tablet or lozenge (264); program administrative costs and considerations are similar to those in school mouthrinsing programs.

Professionally Applied Fluoride Compounds

High-concentration fluoride gel and varnish are effective in preventing dental caries, but because application requires professional expertise, they are inherently more expensive than self-applied methods (e.g., drinking fluoridated water or brushing with fluoride toothpaste). For groups and persons at low risk for dental caries, professionally applied methods are unlikely to be cost-effective (268,269). In the NPDDP study, prophy-

---

*US$ 1988 converted to US$ 1999 using CPI-Urban (all items). More information is available at the U.S. Department of Labor, Bureau of Labor Statistics website at <http://stats.bls.gov/cpihome.htm>. Accessed June 25, 2001.

lactic cleaning and gel application costs were $23 per year ($66 in 1999 dollars*) for semiannual applications, which prevented 0.03–0.26 decayed surfaces per year (*196*). A Swedish study claimed that fluoride varnish was cost-effective, but few supporting data were presented (*270*). Varnish might be cost-effective in Scandinavian school dental services, in which dental professionals regularly examine and treat each student, but the cost-effectiveness of fluoride varnish in public health programs in the United States remains undocumented. Whether fluoride varnish or gel would be most efficiently used in clinical programs targeting groups at high risk for dental caries or should be reserved for individual patients at high risk is unclear.

Combinations of Fluoride Modalities

Because the caries-preventive effects of a combination of fluoride modalities are only partially additive, estimates of the cost-effectiveness when adding a modality (e.g., fluoride mouthrinse for a group already drinking fluoridated water and using fluoride toothpaste) should take into account these smaller, incremental reductions in caries. This consideration is particularly relevant for groups and persons at low risk for caries (*253*). The scarcity of research on the cost-effectiveness of combinations limits the ability to draw more detailed conclusions.

RECOMMENDATIONS

In developing the recommendations for specific fluoride modalities that address public health and clinical practice and self-care, the CDC work group considered the quality of evidence of each modality's effect on dental caries, its association with enamel fluorosis, and its cost-effectiveness. The strength of the recommendation for each fluoride modality was determined by the work group, which adapted a coding system used by the U.S. Preventive Services Task Force (Box 2). The work group considered these factors when determining the population for which each recommendation applies (Table 4). The work

BOX 2. Coding system used to classify recommendations for use of specific fluoride modalities to control dental caries

Code	Criteria
A	Good evidence to support the use of the modality.
B	Fair evidence to support the use of the modality.
C	Lack of evidence to develop a specific recommendation (i.e., the modality has not been adequately tested) or mixed evidence (i.e., some studies support the use of the modality and some oppose it).
D	Fair evidence to reject the use of the modality.
E	Good evidence to reject the use of the modality.

Source: US Preventive Services Task Force. Guide to clinical preventive services. 2nd ed. Alexandria, VA: International Medical Publishing, 1996.

---

*US$ 1981 converted to US$ 1999 using CPI-Urban (dental services). More information is available at the U.S. Department of Labor, Bureau of Labor Statistics website at <http://stats.bls.gov/cpihome.htm>. Accessed June 25, 2001.

group recognized that some recommendations can only be addressed by health-care industries or agencies and that additional research is required to resolve some questions regarding fluoride modalities.

Before promoting a fluoride modality or combination of modalities, the dental-care or other health-care provider must consider a person's or group's risk for dental caries, current use of other fluoride sources, and potential for enamel fluorosis. Although these recommendations are based on assessments of caries risk as low or high, the health-care provider might also differentiate among patients at high risk and provide more intensive interventions as needed. Also, a risk category can change over time; the type and frequency of preventive interventions should be adjusted accordingly.

TABLE 4. Quality of evidence, strength of recommendation, and target population of recommendation for each fluoride modality to prevent and control dental caries

Modality*	Quality of evidence (grade)	Strength of recommendation (code)	Target population[†]
Community water fluoridation	II-1	A	All areas
School water fluoridation	II-3	C	Rural, nonfluoridated areas
Fluoride toothpaste	I	A	All persons
Fluoride mouthrinse	I	A	High risk[§]
Fluoride supplements			
Pregnant women	I	E	None
Children aged <6 years	II-3	C	High risk
Children aged 6–16 years	I	A	High risk
Persons aged >16 years	¶	C	High risk
Fluoride gel	I	A	High risk
Fluoride varnish	I	A	High risk

* Modalities are assumed to be used as directed in terms of dosage and age of user.

[†] Quality of evidence for targeting some modalities to persons at high risk is grade III (i.e., representing the opinion of respected authorities) and is based on considerations of cost-effectiveness that were not included in the studies establishing efficacy or effectiveness.

[§] Populations believed to be at increased risk for dental caries are those with low socioeconomic status or low levels of parental education, those who do not seek regular dental care, and those without dental insurance or access to dental services. Individual factors that possibly increase risk include active dental caries; a history of high caries experience in older siblings or caregivers; root surfaces exposed by gingival recession; high levels of infection with cariogenic bacteria; impaired ability to maintain oral hygiene; malformed enamel or dentin; reduced salivary flow because of medications, radiation treatment, or disease; low salivary buffering capacity (i.e., decreased ability of saliva to neutralize acids); and the wearing of space maintainers, orthodontic appliances, or dental prostheses. Risk can increase if any of these factors are combined with dietary practices conducive to dental caries (i.e., frequent consumption of refined carbohydrates). Risk decreases with adequate exposure to fluoride.

¶ No published studies confirm the effectiveness of fluoride supplements in controlling dental caries among persons aged >16 years.

Public Health and Clinical Practice

Continue and Extend Fluoridation of Community Drinking Water

Community water fluoridation is a safe, effective, and inexpensive way to prevent dental caries. This modality benefits persons in all age groups and of all SES, including those difficult to reach through other public health programs and private dental care. Community water fluoridation also is the most cost-effective way to prevent tooth decay among populations living in areas with adequate community water supply systems. Continuation of community water fluoridation for these populations and its adoption in additional U.S. communities are the foundation for sound caries-prevention programs.

In contrast, the appropriateness of fluoridating stand-alone water systems that supply individual schools is limited. Widespread use of fluoride toothpaste, availability of other fluoride modalities that can be delivered in the school setting, and the current environment of low caries prevalence limit the appropriateness of fluoridating school drinking water at 4.5 times the optimal concentration for community drinking water. Decisions to initiate or continue school fluoridation programs should be based on an assessment of present caries risk in the target school(s), alternative preventive modalities that might be available, and periodic evaluation of program effectiveness.

Counsel Parents and Caregivers Regarding Use of Fluoride Toothpaste by Young Children, Especially Those Aged <2 Years

Fluoride toothpaste is a cost-effective way to reduce the prevalence of dental caries. However, for children aged <6 years, especially those aged <2 years, an increased risk for enamel fluorosis exists because of inadequately developed control of the swallowing reflex. Parents or caregivers should be counseled regarding self-care recommendations for toothpaste use for young children (i.e., limit the child's toothbrushing to ≤2 times a day, apply a pea-sized amount to the toothbrush, supervise toothbrushing, and encourage the child to spit out excess toothpaste).

For children aged <2 years, the dentist or other health-care provider should consider the fluoride level in the community drinking water, other sources of fluoride, and factors likely to affect susceptibility to dental caries when weighing the risk and benefits of using fluoride toothpaste.

Target Mouthrinsing to Persons at High Risk

Because fluoride mouthrinse has resulted in only limited reductions in caries experience among schoolchildren, especially as their exposure to other sources of fluoride has increased, its use should be targeted to groups and persons at high risk for caries (see Risk for Dental Caries). Children aged <6 years should not use fluoride mouthrinse without consultation with a dentist or other health-care provider because enamel fluorosis could occur if such mouthrinses are repeatedly swallowed.

Judiciously Prescribe Fluoride Supplements

Fluoride supplements can be prescribed for children at high risk for dental caries and whose primary drinking water has a low fluoride concentration. For children aged <6 years, the dentist, physician, or other health-care provider should weigh the risk for caries without fluoride supplements, the caries prevention offered by supplements, and the potential for enamel fluorosis. Consideration of the child's other sources of fluoride, especially drinking water, is essential in determining this balance. Parents and caregivers should be informed of both the benefit of protection against dental caries and the possibility of enamel fluorosis. The prescription dosage of fluoride supplements should be consistent with the schedule established by ADA, AAPD, and AAP. Supplements can be prescribed for persons as appropriate or used in school-based programs. When practical, supplements should be prescribed as chewable tablets or lozenges to maximize the topical effects of fluoride.

Apply High-Concentration Fluoride Products to Persons at High Risk for Dental Caries

High-concentration fluoride products can play an important role in preventing and controlling dental caries among groups and persons at high risk. Dentists and other health-care providers must consider the risk status and age of the patient to determine the appropriate intensity of treatment. Routine use of professionally applied fluoride gel or foam likely provides little benefit to persons not at high risk for dental caries, especially those who drink fluoridated water and brush daily with fluoride toothpaste.

If FDA approves use of fluoride varnish to prevent and control dental caries, its indications for use will be similar to those of fluoride gel. Such varnishes have practical advantages for children aged <6 years at high risk.

Self-Care

Know the Fluoride Concentration in the Primary Source of Drinking Water

All persons should know whether the fluoride concentration in their primary source of drinking water is below optimal, optimal, or above optimal. This knowledge is the basis for all individual and professional decisions regarding use of other fluoride modalities (e.g., mouthrinse or supplements). Parents and caregivers of children, especially children aged <6 years, must know the fluoride concentration in their child's drinking water when considering whether to alter the child's fluoride intake. For example, in nonfluoridated areas where the natural fluoride concentration is below optimal, fluoride supplements might be considered, whereas in areas where the natural fluoride concentration is >2 ppm, children should use alternative sources of drinking water. Knowledge of the water's fluoride concentration is also key in public policy discussions regarding community water fluoridation.

Frequently Use Small Amounts of Fluoride

All persons should receive frequent exposure to small amounts of fluoride, which minimizes dental caries by inhibiting demineralization of tooth enamel and facilitating tooth remineralization. This exposure can be readily accomplished by drinking water with an optimal fluoride concentration and brushing with a fluoride toothpaste twice daily.

Supervise Use of Fluoride Toothpaste Among Children Aged <6 Years

Children's teeth should be cleaned daily from the time the teeth erupt in the mouth. Parents and caregivers should consult a dentist or other health-care provider before introducing a child aged <2 years to fluoride toothpaste. Parents and caregivers of children aged <6 years who use fluoride toothpaste should follow the directions on the label, place no more than a pea-sized amount (0.25 g) of toothpaste on the toothbrush, brush the child's teeth (recommended particularly for preschool-aged children) or supervise the toothbrushing, and encourage the child to spit excess toothpaste into the sink to minimize the amount swallowed. Indiscriminate use can result in inadvertent swallowing of more fluoride than is recommended.

Consider Additional Measures for Persons at High Risk for Dental Caries

Persons at high risk for dental caries might require additional fluoride or other preventive measures to reduce development of caries. This additional fluoride can come from daily use of another fluoride product at home or from professionally applied, topical fluoride products. Other preventive measures might include dental sealants and targeted antimicrobial therapies. Parents and caregivers should not provide additional fluoride to children aged <6 years without consulting a dentist or other health-care provider regarding the associated benefits and potential for enamel fluorosis. Persons should seek professional advice regarding their risk status or that of their children.

Use an Alternative Source of Water for Children Aged ≤8 Years Whose Primary Drinking Water Contains >2 ppm Fluoride

In some regions in the United States, community water supply systems and home wells contain a natural concentration of fluoride >2 ppm. At this concentration, children aged ≤8 years are at increased risk for developing enamel fluorosis, including the moderate and severe forms, and should have an alternative source of drinking water, preferably one containing fluoride at an optimal concentration.

In areas where community water supply systems contain >2 ppm but <4 ppm fluoride, EPA requires that each household be notified annually of the desirability of using an alternative source of water for children aged ≤8 years. For families receiving water from home wells, testing is necessary to determine the natural fluoride concentration.

Consumer Product Industries and Health Agencies

Label the Fluoride Concentration of Bottled Water

Producers of bottled water should label the fluoride concentration of their products. Such labeling will allow consumers to make informed decisions and dentists, dental hygienists, and other health-care professionals to appropriately advise patients regarding fluoride intake and use of fluoride products.

Promote Use of Small Amounts of Fluoride Toothpaste Among Children Aged <6 Years

Labels and advertisements for fluoride toothpaste should promote use of a pea-sized amount (0.25 g) of toothpaste on a child-sized toothbrush for children aged <6 years. Efforts to educate parents and caregivers and to encourage supervised use of fluoride toothpaste among young children can reduce inadvertent swallowing of excess toothpaste.

Develop a Low-Fluoride Toothpaste for Children Aged <6 Years

Manufacturers are encouraged to develop a dentifrice for children aged <6 years that is effective in preventing dental caries but alleviates the risk for enamel fluorosis. A "child-strength" toothpaste with a fluoride concentration lower than current products could reduce the risk for cosmetic concerns associated with inadvertent swallowing of toothpaste.

Collaborate to Educate Health-Care Professionals and the Public

Professional health-care organizations, public health agencies, and suppliers of oral-care products should collaborate to educate health-care professionals and trainees and the public regarding the recommendations in this report. Broad collaborative efforts to educate health-care professionals and the public and to encourage behavior change can promote improved, coordinated use of fluoride modalities.

Further Research

Continue Metabolic Studies of Fluoride

Metabolic studies with animals and humans to determine the influence of environmental, physiological, and pathological conditions on the pharmacokinetics and effects of fluoride should continue. Research in these areas will enhance the knowledge base concerning fluoride use, thereby resulting in more effective and efficient use of fluoride.

Identify Biomarkers of Fluoride

As an alternative to direct fluoride intake measurement, biomarkers (i.e., distinct biological indicators) should be identified to estimate a person's fluoride intake and the amount of fluoride in the body. Identification of such biomarkers could allow more efficient research.

Reevaluate the Method of Determining Optimal Fluoride Concentration of Community Drinking Water

The current method of determining the optimal concentration of fluoride in community drinking water, which depends on the average maximum annual ambient air temperature, should be reevaluated because of the social and environmental changes that have occurred since it was adopted in 1962. Research into current consumption patterns of water, processed beverages, and processed foods is also needed. Such research will either validate the current method for determining optimal fluoride concentration in community drinking water or indicate improved methods.

Evaluate the Effect of Fluoride Mouthrinse, Fluoride Supplements, and Other Fluoride Modalities on Dental Caries

Additional clinical trials are needed to evaluate the current effect of fluoride mouthrinse, supplements, and other modalities on dental caries both individually and in combination. Cohorts of particular interest are groups and persons at high risk for dental caries, including older adults (i.e., those aged >50 years). Such research, as well as studies to determine the effects of new fluoride modalities and various combinations among groups and persons at high risk, could lead to more effective and efficient use of these interventions.

Study the Current Cost-Effectiveness of Fluoride Modalities

The increasing availability of multiple fluoride modalities and the lower caries prevalence in the United States indicate a need for current cost-effectiveness studies of fluoride modalities, especially logical combinations of regimens in populations with different caries risks. Such research will allow both more efficient use of resources and a better understanding of the additive effects of combined modalities.

Conduct Descriptive and Analytic Epidemiologic Studies

Descriptive and analytic epidemiologic studies should be conducted to determine the association between dental caries and fluoride exposure from several sources, as well as the current role of community water fluoridation in preventing coronal and root caries among adults. Studies should assess the effect of interruption or discontinuation of water fluoridation; the prevalence of fluorosis associated with different patterns of fluoride use and intake among various populations; and the relationship between objectively measured fluorosis and the aesthetic perceptions of persons, parents, and dentists and other health-care professionals. Studies are needed to refine methods of caries risk assessment. As appropriate, studies should use national, state, and local data. Research addressing these questions will improve understanding of the relationships between fluoride modalities and the benefits and unintended effects of their use.

Identify Effective Strategies to Promote Adoption of Recommendations for Using Fluoride

Effective strategies should be identified to promote adherence by parents, caregivers, children, adults, and health-care providers to recommendations regarding fluoride use. Such research could result in more effective behavior change, more efficient use of resources, improved caries prevention, and less enamel fluorosis.

CONCLUSION

When used appropriately, fluoride is a safe and effective agent that can be used to prevent and control dental caries. Fluoride has contributed profoundly to the improved dental health of persons in the United States and other countries. Fluoride is needed regularly throughout life to protect teeth against tooth decay. To ensure additional gains in oral health, water fluoridation should be extended to additional communities, and fluoride toothpaste should be used widely. Adoption of these and other recommendations in this report could lead to considerable savings in public and private resources without compromising fluoride's substantial benefit of improved dental health.

References
1. Bratthall D, Hänsel Petersson G, Sundberg H. Reasons for the caries decline: what do the experts believe? Eur J Oral Sci 1996;104:416–22.
2. Blaney JR, Tucker WH. The Evanston Dental Caries Study. II. Purpose and mechanism of the study. J Dent Res 1948;27:279–86.
3. Ast DB, Finn SB, McCaffrey I. The Newburgh-Kingston Caries Fluorine Study. I. Dental findings after three years of water fluoridation. Am J Public Health 1950;40:716–24.
4. Dean HT, Arnold FA, Jay P, Knutson JW. Studies on mass control of dental caries through fluoridation of the public water supply. Public Health Rep 1950;65:1403–8.
5. Hutton WL, Linscott BW, Williams DB. The Brantford fluorine experiment: interim report after five years of water fluoridation. Can J Public Health 1951;42:81–7.

6. Pao EM. Changes in American food consumption patterns and their nutritional significance. Food Technol 1981;35:43–53.

7. Heller KE, Sohn W, Burt BA, Eklund SA. Water consumption the United States in 1994–1996 and implications for water fluoridation policy. J Public Health Dent 1999;59:3–11.

8. Public Health Service Committee to Coordinate Environmental Health and Related Programs. Review of fluoride: benefits and risk. Washington, DC: US Department of Health and Human Services, Public Health Service, 1991.

9. National Research Council Committee on Toxicology. Health effects of ingested fluoride. Washington, DC: National Academy Press, 1993.

10. World Health Organization. Environmental health criteria 36: fluorine and fluorides. Geneva: World Health Organization, 1984.

11. Institute of Medicine. Fluoride. In: Dietary reference intakes for calcium, phosphorus, magnesium, vitamin D, and fluoride. Washington, DC: National Academy Press, 1997:288–313.

12. Featherstone JDB. Prevention and reversal of dental caries: role of low level fluoride. Community Dent Oral Epidemiol 1999;27:31–40.

13. Koulourides T. Summary of session II: fluoride and the caries process. J Dent Res 1990;69(special issue):558.

14. Tatevossian A. Fluoride in dental plaque and its effects. J Dent Res 1990;69(special issue):645–52.

15. Chow LC. Tooth-bound fluoride and dental caries. J Dent Res 1990;69(special issue):595–600.

16. Ericsson SY. Cariostasis mechanisms of fluorides: clinical observations. Caries Res 1977;11(suppl 1):2–23.

17. Kidd EAM, Thylstrup A, Fejerskov O, Bruun C. Influence of fluoride in surface enamel and degree of dental fluorosis on caries development in vitro. Caries Res 1980;14:196–202.

18. Thylstrup A. Clinical evidence of the role of pre-eruptive fluoride in caries prevention. J Dent Res 1990;69(special issue):742–50.

19. Thylstrup A, Fejerskov O, Bruun C, Kann J. Enamel changes and dental caries in 7-year-old children given fluoride tablets from shortly after birth. Caries Res 1979;13:265–76.

20. White DJ, Nancollas GH. Physical and chemical considerations of the role of firmly and loosely bound fluoride in caries prevention. J Dent Res 1990;69(special issue):587–94.

21. Hamilton IR. Biochemical effects of fluoride on oral bacteria. J Dent Res 1990;69(special issue):660–7.

22. Bowden GHW. Effects of fluoride on the microbial ecology of dental plaque. J Dent Res 1990;69(special issue):653–9.

23. Bowden GHW, Odlum O, Nolette N, Hamilton IR. Microbial populations growing in the presence of fluoride at low pH isolated from dental plaque of children living in an area with fluoridated water. Infect Immun 1982;36:247–54.

24. Marquis RE. Diminished acid tolerance of plaque bacteria caused by fluoride. J Dent Res 1990;69(special issue):672–5.

25. Rosen S, Frea JI, Hsu SM. Effect of fluoride-resistant microorganisms on dental caries. J Dent Res 1978;57:180.

26. Van Loveren C. The antimicrobial action of fluoride and its role in caries inhibition. J Dent Res 1990;69(special issue):676–81.

27. Oliveby A, Twetman S, Ekstrand J. Diurnal fluoride concentration in whole saliva in children living in a high- and a low-fluoride area. Caries Res 1990;24:44–7.

28. Rölla G, Ekstrand J. Fluoride in oral fluids and dental plaque. In: Fejerskov O, Ekstrand J, Burt BA, eds. Fluoride in dentistry. 2nd ed. Copenhagen: Munksgaard, 1996:215–29.

29. LeGeros RZ. Chemical and crystallographic events in the caries process. J Dent Res 1990;69(special issue):567–74.

30. Dean HT, Dixon RM, Cohen C. Mottled enamel in Texas. Public Health Rep 1935;50:424–42.

31. McClure FJ, Likins RC. Fluorine in human teeth studied in relation to fluorine in the drinking water. J Dent Res 1951;30:172–6.

32. Marthaler TM. Fluoride supplements for systemic effects in caries prevention. In: Johansen E, Taves DR, Olsen TO, eds. Continuing evaluation of the use of fluorides. Boulder, CO: Westview, 1979:33–59. (American Assocation for the Advancement of Science selected symposium no. 11).

33. Murray JJ. Efficacy of preventive agents for dental caries. Systemic fluorides: water fluoridation. Caries Res 1993;27(suppl 1):2–8.

34. Groeneveld A, Van Eck AAMJ, Backer Dirks O. Fluoride in caries prevention: is the effect pre- or post-eruptive? J Dent Res 1990;69(special issue):751–5.

35. Levine RS. The action of fluoride in caries prevention: a review of current concepts. Br Dent J 1976;140:9–14.

36. Margolis HC, Moreno EC. Physicochemical perspectives on the cariostatic mechanisms of systemic and topical fluorides. J Dent Res 1990;69(special issue):606–13.

37. Clarkson BH, Fejerskov O, Ekstrand J, Burt BA. Rational use of fluorides in caries control. In: Fejerskov O, Ekstrand J, Burt BA, eds. Fluorides in dentistry. 2nd ed. Copenhagen: Munksgaard, 1996:347–57.

38. Arends J, Christoffersen J. Nature and role of loosely bound fluoride in dental caries. J Dent Res 1990;69(special issue):601–5.

39. Burt BA, Eklund SA. Dentistry, dental practice, and the community. 5th ed. Philadelphia, PA: W.B. Saunders, 1999.

40. National Institute of Dental Research. The prevalence of dental caries in United States children, 1979–1980. Bethesda, MD: U.S. Public Health Service, Department of Health and Human Services, National Institutes of Health, 1981; NIH publication no. 82-2245.

41. Kelly JE, Harvey CR. Basic dental examination findings of persons 1–74 years. In: Basic data on dental examination findings of persons 1–74 years, United States, 1971–1974. Hyattsville, MD: US Department of Health, Education, and Welfare, Public Health Service, Office of Health Research, Statistics, and Technology, National Center for Health Statistics, 1979; DHEW publication no. (PHS) 79-1662. (Vital and health statistics data from the National Health Interview Survey; series 11, no. 214).

42. National Institute of Dental Research. Oral health of United States children. The National Survey of Dental Caries in U.S. School Children: 1986–1987. National and regional findings. Bethesda, MD: US Department of Health and Human Services, Public Health Service, National National Institutes of Health, National Institute of Dental Research, 1989; NIH publication no. 89-2247.

43. Kaste LM, Selwitz RH, Oldakowski RJ, Brunelle JA, Winn DM, Brown LJ. Coronal caries in the primary and permanent dentition of children and adolescents 1–17 years of age: United States, 1988–1991. J Dent Res 1996;75(special issue):631–41.

44. Meskin LH, ed. Caries diagnosis and risk assessment: a review of preventive strategies and management. J Am Dent Assoc 1995;126(suppl):1S–24S.

45. Pitts NB. Risk assessment and caries prediction. J Dent Educ 1998;62:762–70.

46. Vargas CM, Crall JJ, Schneider DA. Sociodemographic distribution of pediatric dental caries: NHANES III, 1988–1994. J Am Dent Assoc 1998;129:1229–38.

47. Edelstein BL. The medical management of dental caries. J Am Dent Assoc 1994;125(suppl):31–9.

48. US Department of Health and Human Services. Oral health in America: a report of the Surgeon General. Rockville, MD: US Department of Health and Human Services, National Institute of Dental and Craniofacial Research, National Institutes of Health, 2000:63, 74–94, 245–74.

49. Fejerskov O, Manji F, Baelum V. The nature and mechanisms of dental fluorosis in man. J Dent Res 1990;69(special issue):692–700.
50. Avery JK. Agents affecting tooth and bone development. In: Avery JK, ed. Oral development and histology. 2nd ed. New York, NY: Theime Medical Publishers, 1994:130–41.
51. DenBesten PK, Thariani H. Biological mechanisms of fluorosis and level and timing of systemic exposure to fluoride with respect to fluorosis. J Dent Res 1992;71:1238–43.
52. Evans RW, Stamm JW. Dental fluorosis following downward adjustment of fluoride in drinking water. J Public Health Dent 1991;51:91–8.
53. Dean HT. The investigation of physiological effects by the epidemiological method. In: Moulton FR, ed. Fluorine and dental health. Washington, DC: American Association for the Advancement of Science, 1942;19:23–31.
54. Fejerskov O, Manji F, Baelum V, Møller IJ. Dental fluorosis—a handbook for health workers. Copenhagen: Munksgaard, 1988.
55. Kaminsky LS, Mahoney MC, Leach J, Melius J, Miller MJ. Fluoride: benefits and risks of exposure. Crit Rev Oral Biol Med 1990;1:261–81.
56. Clark DC, Hann HJ, Williamson MF, Berkowitz J. Aesthetic concerns of children and parents in relation to different classifications of the Tooth Surface Index of Fluorosis. Community Dent Oral Epidemiol 1993;21:360–4.
57. Dean HT. Endemic fluorosis and its relation to dental caries. Public Health Rep 1938;53:1443–52.
58. Clark DC. Trends in prevalence of dental fluorosis in North America. Community Dent Oral Epidemiol 1994;22:148–52.
59. Szpunar SM, Burt BA. Trends in the prevalence of dental fluorosis in the United States: a review. J Public Health Dent 1987;47:71–9.
60. Brunelle JA. The prevalence of dental fluorosis in U.S. children, 1987. J Dent Res 1989;68(special issue):995.
61. Heller KE, Eklund SA, Burt BA. Dental caries and dental fluorosis at varying water fluoride concentrations. J Public Health Dent 1997;57:136–43.
62. Pendrys DG, Katz RV, Morse DR. Risk factors for enamel fluorosis in a fluoridated population. Am J Epidemiol 1994;140:461–71.
63. Osuji OO, Leake JL, Chipman ML, Nikiforuk G, Locker D, Levine N. Risk factors for dental fluorosis in a fluoridated community. J Dent Res 1988;67:1488–92.
64. Pendrys DG, Katz RV. Risk for enamel fluorosis associated with fluoride supplementation, infant formula, and fluoride dentifrice use. Am J Epidemiol 1989;130:1199–208.
65. Pendrys DG. Risk for fluorosis in a fluoridated population: implications for the dentist and hygienist. J Am Dent Assoc 1995;126:1617–24.
66. US Department of Health, Education, and Welfare. Public Health Service drinking water standards, revised 1962. Washington, DC: US Public Health Service, Department of Health, Education, and Welfare, 1962; PHS publication no. 956.
67. Galagan DJ, Vermillion JR. Determining optimum fluoride concentrations. Public Health Rep 1957;72:491–3.
68. CDC. Engineering and administrative recommendations for water fluoridation, 1995. MMWR 1995;44(No. RR-13):1–40.
69. US Environmental Protection Agency. 40 CFR Part 141.62. Maximum contaminant levels for inorganic contaminants. Code of Federal Regulations 1998:402.
70. US Environmental Protection Agency. 40 CFR Part 143. National secondary drinking water regulations. Code of Federal Regulations 1998;514–7.
71. US Department of Health and Human Services, Food and Drug Administration. 21 CFR Part 165.110. Bottled water. Federal Register 1995;60:57124–30.
72. US Food and Drug Administration. 21 CFR Part 355. Anticaries drug products for over-the-counter human use. Code of Federal Regulations 1999:280–5.

73. American Dental Association. ADA guide to dental therapeutics. 1st ed. Chicago, IL: American Dental Association, 1998.

74. American Academy of Pediatric Dentistry. Special issue: reference manual 1995. Pediatr Dent 1994–95;16(special issue):1–96.

75. American Academy of Pediatrics Committee on Nutrition. Fluoride supplementation for children: interim policy recommendations. Pediatrics 1995;95:777.

76. Singer L, Jarvey BA, Venkateswarlu P, Armstrong WD. Fluoride in plaque. J Dent Res 1970;49:455.

77. Dabeka RW, McKenzie AD, Lacroix GMA. Dietary intakes of lead, cadmium, arsenic and fluoride by Canadian adults: a 24-hour duplicate diet study. Food Addit Contam 1987;4:89–102.

78. Kramer L, Osis D, Wiatrowski E, Spencer H. Dietary fluoride in different areas of the United States. Am J Clin Nutr 1974;27:590–4.

79. Osis D, Kramer L, Wiatrowski E, Spencer H. Dietary fluoride intake in man. J Nutr 1974;104:1313–8.

80. Singer L, Ophaug RH, Harland BF. Fluoride intake of young adult males in the United States. Am J Clin Nutr 1980;33:328–32.

81. Ophaug RH, Singer L, Harland BF. Estimated fluoride intake of average two-year-old children in four dietary regions of the United States. J Dent Res 1980;59:777–81.

82. Ophaug RH, Singer L, Harland BF. Estimated fluoride intake of 6-month-old infants in four dietary regions of the United States. Am J Clin Nutr 1980;33:324–7.

83. Singer L, Ophaug RH, Harland BF. Dietary fluoride intake of 15-19-year-old male adults residing in the United States. J Dent Res 1985;64:1302–5.

84. Pang DTY, Phillips CL, Bawden JW. Fluoride intake from beverage consumption in a sample of North Carolina children. J Dent Res 1992;71:1382–8.

85. Levy SM, Kohout FJ, Guha-Chowdhury N, Kiritsy MC, Heilman JR, Wefel JS. Infants' fluoride intake from drinking water alone, and from water added to formula, beverages, and food. J Dent Res 1995;74:1399–407.

86. Levy SM, Kiritsy MC, Warren JJ. Sources of fluoride intake in children. J Public Health Dent 1995;55:39–52.

87. Johnson J Jr, Bawden JW. The fluoride content of infant formulas available in 1985. Pediatr Dent 1987;9:33–7.

88. Dean HT, Jay P, Arnold FA Jr, Elvove E. Domestic water and dental caries. II. A study of 2,832 white children, aged 12–14 years, of 8 suburban Chicago communities, including *Lactobacillus acidophilus* studies of 1,761 children. Public Health Rep 1941;56:761–92.

89. Dean HT, Arnold FA Jr, Elvove E. Domestic water and dental caries. V. Additional studies of the relation of fluoride domestic water to dental caries experience in 4,425 white children, aged 12 to 14 years, of 13 cities in 4 states. Public Health Rep 1942;57:1155–79.

90. Galagan DJ. Climate and controlled fluoridation. J Am Dent Assoc 1953;47:159–70.

91. Galagan DJ, Lamson GG Jr. Climate and endemic dental fluorosis. Public Health Rep 1953;68:497–508.

92. Galagan DJ, Vermillion JR, Nevitt GA, Stadt ZM, Dart RE. Climate and fluid intake. Public Health Rep 1957;72:484–90.

93. CDC. Fluoridation census 1992 summary. Atlanta, GA: US Department of Health and Human Services, Public Health Service, CDC, 1993.

94. Arnold FA Jr, Likins RC, Russell AL, Scott DB. Fifteenth year of the Grand Rapids Fluoridation Study. J Am Dent Assoc 1962;65:780–5.

95. Ast DB, Fitzgerald B. Effectiveness of water fluoridation. J Am Dent Assoc 1962;65:581–7.

96. Blayney JR, Hill IN. Fluorine and dental caries. J Am Dent Assoc 1967;74(special issue):225–302.

97. Hutton WL, Linscott BW, Williams DB. Final report of local studies on water fluoridation in Brantford. Can J Public Health 1956;47:89–92.

98. Brunelle JA, Carlos JP. Recent trends in dental caries in U.S. children and the effect of water fluoridation. J Dent Res 1990;69(special issue):723–7.

99. Newbrun E. Effectiveness of water fluoridation. J Public Health Dent 1989;49(special issue):279–89.

100. Ripa LW. A half-century of community water fluoridation in the United States: review and commentary. J Public Health Dent 1993;53:17–44.

101. Grembowski D, Fiset L, Spadafora A. How fluoridation affects adult dental caries: systemic and topical effects are explored. J Am Dent Assoc 1992;123:49–54.

102. Wiktorsson A-M, Martinsson T, Zimmerman M. Salivary levels of lactobacilli, buffer capacity and salivary flow rate related to caries activity among adults in communities with optimal and low water fluoride concentrations. Swed Dent J 1992;16:231–7.

103. Eklund SA, Burt BA, Ismail AI, Calderone JJ. High-fluoride drinking water, fluorosis, and dental caries in adults. J Am Dent Assoc 1987;114:324–8.

104. Sreebny LM, Schwartz SS. A reference guide to drugs and dry mouth—2nd ed. Gerodontology 1997;14:33–47.

105. Burt BA, Ismail AI, Eklund SA. Root caries in an optimally fluoridated and a high-fluoride community. J Dent Res 1986;65:1154–8.

106. Stamm JS, Banting DW, Imrey PB. Adult root caries survey of two similar communities with contrasting natural water fluoride levels. J Am Dent Assoc 1990;120:143–9.

107. Brustman B. Impact of exposure to fluoride-adequate water on root surface caries in elderly. Gerodontics 1986;2:203–7.

108. Jones CM, Taylor GO, Whittle JG, Evans D, Trotter DP. Water fluoridation, tooth decay in 5 year olds, and social deprivation measured by the Jarman score: analysis of data from British dental surveys. BMJ 1997;315:514–7.

109. Provart SJ, Carmichael CL. The relationship between caries, fluoridation, and material deprivation in five-year-old children in County Durham. Community Dent Health 1995;12:200–3.

110. Slade GD, Spencer AJ, Davies MJ, Stewart JF. Influence of exposure to fluoridated water on socioeconomic inequalities in children's caries experience. Community Dent Oral Epidemiol 1996;24:89–100.

111. Kumar JV, Swango PA, Lininger LL, Leske GS, Green EL, Haley VB. Changes in dental fluorosis and dental caries in Newburgh and Kingston, New York. Am J Public Health 1998;88:1866–70.

112. Graves RC, Bohannan HM, Disney JA, Stamm JW, Bader JD, Abernathy JR. Recent dental caries and treatment patterns in US children. J Public Health Dent 1986;46:23–9.

113. Ast DB, Smith DJ, Wachs B, Cantwell KT. Newburgh-Kingston caries-fluorine study. XIV. Combined clinical and roentgenographic dental findings after ten years of fluoride experience. J Am Dent Assoc 1956;52:314–25.

114. Russell AL. Dental fluorosis in Grand Rapids during the seventeenth year of fluoridation. J Am Dent Assoc 1962;65:608–12.

115. Lewis DW, Banting DW. Water fluoridation: current effectiveness and dental fluorosis. Community Dent Oral Epidemiol 1994;22:153–8.

116. Kumar JV, Swango PA. Fluoride exposure and dental fluorosis in Newburgh and Kingston, New York: policy implications. Community Dent Oral Epidemiol 1999;27:171–80.

117. Szpunar SM, Burt BA. Dental caries, fluorosis, and fluoride exposure in Michigan schoolchildren. J Dent Res 1988;67:802–6.

118. Horowitz HS. School fluoridation for the prevention of dental caries. Int Dent J 1973;23:346–53.

119. Horowitz HS, Law FE, Pritzker T. Effect of school water fluoridation on dental caries, St. Thomas, V.I. Public Health Rep 1965;80:381–8.

120. Horowitz HS, Heifetz SB, Law FE, Driscoll WS. School fluoridation studies in Elk Lake, Pennsylvania, and Pike County, Kentucky—results after eight years. Am J Public Health 1968;58:2240–50.

121. Horowitz HS, Heifetz SB, Law FE. Effect of school water fluoridation on dental caries: final results in Elk Lake, PA, after 12 years. J Am Dent Assoc 1972;84:832–8.

122. Heifetz SB, Horowitz HS, Brunelle JA. Effect of school water fluoridation on dental caries: results in Seagrove, NC, after 12 years. J Am Dent Assoc 1983;106:334–7.

123. King RS, Iafolla TJ, Rozier RG, Satterfield WC, Spratt CJ. Effectiveness of school water fluoridation and fluoride mouthrinses. J Dent Res 1995;74(special issue):192.

124. CDC. Acute fluoride poisoning—North Carolina. MMWR 1974;23:199.

125. Hoffman R, Mann J, Calderone J, Trumbull J, Burkhart M. Acute fluoride poisoning in a New Mexico elementary school. Pediatrics 1980;65:897–900.

126. Vogt RL, Witherell L, LaRue D, Klaucke DN. Acute fluoride poisoning associated with an on-site fluoridator in a Vermont elementary school. Am J Public Health 1982;72:1168–9.

127. Stannard J, Rovero J, Tsamtsouris A, Gavris V. Fluoride content of some bottled waters and recommendations for fluoride supplementation. J Pedod 1990;14:103–7.

128. Weinberger SJ. Bottled drinking waters: are the fluoride concentrations shown on the label accurate? Int J Paediatr Dent 1991;1:143–6.

129. Van Winkle S, Levy SM, Kiritsy MC, Heilman JR, Wefel JS, Marshall T. Water and formula fluoride concentrations: significance for infants fed formula. Pediatr Dent 1995;17:305–10.

130. Mark AM. Americans taking to the bottle: loss of important fluoride source may be result. ADA News 1998;29:12.

131. US Environmental Protection Agency. 40 CFR Part 141 Subpart O. Consumer confidence reports. Federal Register 1998;63:44526–36.

132. Duckworth RM, Morgan SN, Burchell CK. Fluoride in plaque following use of dentifrices containing sodium monofluorophosphate. J Dent Res 1989;68:130–3.

133. Duckworth RM, Morgan SN. Oral fluoride retention after use of fluoride dentifrices. Caries Res 1991;25:123–9.

134. Sidi AD. Effect of brushing with fluoride toothpastes on the fluoride, calcium, and inorganic phosphorus concentrations in approximal plaque of young adults. Caries Res 1989;23:268–71.

135. Reintsema H, Schuthof J, Arends J. An in vivo investigation of the fluoride uptake in partially demineralized human enamel from several different dentifrices. J Dent Res 1985;64:19–23.

136. Stookey GK, Schemehorn BR, Cheetham BL, Wood GD, Walton GV. In situ fluoride uptake from fluoride dentifrices by carious enamel. J Dent Res 1985;64:900–3.

137. Bruun C, Givskov H, Thylstrup A. Whole saliva fluoride after toothbrushing with NaF and MFP dentifrices with different F concentrations. Caries Res 1984;18:282–8.

138. Levy SM. Review of fluoride exposures and ingestion. Community Dent Oral Epidemiol 1994;22:173–80.

139. Horowitz HS, Law FE, Thompson MB, Chamberlin SR. Evaluation of a stannous fluoride dentifrice for use in dental public health programs. I. Basic findings. J Am Dent Assoc 1966;72:408–22.

140. James PMC, Anderson RJ. Clinical testing of a stannous fluoride-calcium pyrophosphate dentifrice in Buckinghamshire school children. Br Dent J 1967;123:33–9.

141. Jordan WA, Peterson JK. Caries-inhibiting value of a dentifrice containing stannous fluoride: final report of a two year study. J Am Dent Assoc 1959;58:42–4.

142. Muhler JC. Effect of a stannous fluoride dentifrice on caries reduction in children during a three-year study period. J Am Dent Asoc 1962;64:216–24.

143. Stookey GK. Are all fluoride dentifrices the same? In: Wei SHY, ed. Clinical uses of fluorides: a state of the art conference on the uses of fluorides in clinical dentistry: May 11 and 12, 1984, Holiday Inn, Union Square, San Francisco, California. Philadelphia, PA: Lea & Febiger, 1985:105–31.

144. Clarkson JE, Ellwood RP, Chandler RE. A comprehensive summary of fluoride dentifrice caries clinical trials. Am J Dent 1993;6(special issue):59–106.

145. Stamm JW. The value of dentifrices and mouthrinses in caries prevention. Int Dent J 1993;43:517–27.

146. Mellberg JR, Ripa LW. Fluoride dentifrices. In: Mellberg JR, Ripa LW. Fluoride in preventive dentistry: theory and clinical applications. Chicago, IL: Quintessence Publishing Co., 1983:215–41.

147. Mellberg JR. Fluoride dentifrices: current status and prospects. Int Dent J 1991;41:9–16.

148. Richards A, Banting DW. Fluoride toothpastes. In: Fejerskov O, Ekstrand J, Burt BA, eds. Fluoride in dentistry. 2nd ed. Copenhagen: Munksgaard, 1996:328–46.

149. Lind OP, von der Fehr FR, Joost Larsen M, Möller IJ. Anti-caries effect of a 2% Na_2PO_3F-dentifrice in a Danish fluoride area. Community Dent Oral Epidemiol 1976;4:7–14.

150. O'Mullane DM, Clarkson J, Holland T, O'Hickey S, Whelton H. Effectiveness of water fluoridation in the prevention of dental caries in Irish children. Community Dent Health 1988;5:331–44.

151. Stookey GK, Beiswanger BB. Topical fluoride therapy. In: Harris NO, Christen AG, eds. Primary preventive dentistry. 4th ed. Stamford, CT: Appleton & Lang, 1995:193–233.

152. Horowitz HS, Ismail AI. Topical fluorides in caries prevention. In: Fejerskov O, Ekstrand J, Burt BA, eds. Fluorides in dentistry. 2nd ed. Copenhagen: Munksgaard, 1996:311–27.

153. Ronis DL, Land WP, Passow E. Tooth brushing, flossing, and preventive dental visits by Detroit-area residents in relation to demographic and socioeconomic factors. J Public Health Dent 1993;53:138–45.

154. Wagener DK, Nourjah P, Horowitz AM. Trends in childhood use of dental care products containing fluoride: United States, 1983–89. Hyattsville, MD: U.S. Department of Health and Human Services, Public Health Service, CDC, 1992. (Advanced data from vital health statistics; no. 219).

155. Peffley GE, Muhler JC. The effect of a commercially available stannous fluoride dentifrice under controlled brushing habits on dental caries incidence in children: preliminary report. J Dent Res 1960;39:871–5.

156. Bixler D, Muhler JC. Experimental clinical human caries test design and interpretation. J Am Dent Assoc 1962;65:482–90.

157. Chesters RK, Huntington E, Burchell CK, Stephen KW. Effect of oral care habits on caries in adolescents. Caries Res 1992;26:299–304.

158. Chesnutt IG, Schafer F, Jacobson APM, Stephen KW. The influence of toothbrushing frequency and post-brushing rinsing on caries experience in a caries clinical trial. Community Dent Oral Epidemiol 1998;26:406–11.

159. Duckworth RM, Knoop DTM, Stephen KW. Effect of mouthrinsing after toothbrushing with a fluoride dentifrice on human salivary fluoride levels. Caries Res 1991;25:287–91.

160. Sjögren K, Birkhed D, Ruben J, Arends J. Effect of post-brushing water rinsing on caries-like lesions at approximal and buccal sites. Caries Res 1995;9:337–42.

161. Conti AJ, Lotzkar S, Daley R, Cancro L, Marks RG, McNeal DR. A 3-year clinical trial to compare efficacy of dentifrices containing 1.14% and 0.76% sodium monofluorophosphate. Community Dent Oral Epidemiol 1988;16:135–8.

162. Fogels HR, Meade JJ, Griffith J, Miragliuolo R, Cancro LP. A clinical investigation of a high-level fluoride dentifrice. J Dent Child 1988;55:210–5.

163. Hanachowicz L. Caries prevention using a 1.2% sodium monofluorophosphate dentifrice in an aluminum oxide trihydrate base. Community Dent Oral Epidemiol 1984;12:10–6.

164. O'Mullane DM, Kavanagh D, Ellwood RP, et al. A three-year clinical trial of a combination of trimetaphosphate and sodium fluoride in silica toothpastes. J Dent Res 1997;76:1776–81.

165. Lalumandier JA, Rozier RG. The prevalence and risk factors of fluorosis among patients in a pediatric dental practice. Pediatr Dent 1995;17:19–25.

166. Mascarenhas AK, Burt BA. Fluorosis risk from early exposure to fluoride toothpaste. Community Dent Oral Epidemiol 1998;26:241–8.
167. Milsom K, Mitropoulos CM. Enamel defects in 8-year-old children in fluoridated and non-fluoridated parts of Cheshire. Caries Res 1990;24:286–9.
168. Riordan PJ. Dental fluorosis, dental caries and fluoride exposure among 7-year-olds. Caries Res 1993;27:71–7.
169. Skotowski MC, Hunt RJ, Levy SM. Risk factors for dental fluorosis in pediatric dental patients. J Public Health Dent 1995;55:154–9.
170. Pendrys DG, Katz RV, Morse DE. Risk factors for enamel fluorosis in a nonfluoridated population. Am J Epidemiol 1996;143:808–15.
171. Nacacche H, Simard PL, Trahan L, et al. Factors affecting the ingestion of fluoride dentrifice by children. J Public Health Dent 1992;52:222–6.
172. Simard PL, Naccache H, Lachapelle D, Brodeur JM. Ingestion of fluoride from dentifrices by children aged 12 to 24 months. Clin Pediatr 1991;30:614–7.
173. Barnhart WE, Hiller LK, Leonard GJ, Michaels SE. Dentifrice usage and ingestion among four age groups. J Dent Res 1974;53:1317–22.
174. Baxter PM. Toothpaste ingestion during toothbrushing by school children. Br Dent J 1980;148:125–8.
175. Hargreaves JA, Ingram GS, Wagg BJ. A gravimetric study of the ingestion of toothpaste by children. Caries Res 1972;6:236–43.
176. Beltrán ED, Szpunar SM. Fluoride in toothpastes for children: suggestion for change. Pediatr Dent 1988;10:185–8.
177. Levy SM. A review of fluoride intake from fluoride dentifrice. J Dent Child 1993;61:115–24.
178. Koch G, Petersson L-G, Kling E, Kling L. Effect of 250 and 1000 ppm fluoride dentifrice on caries: a three-year clinical study. Swed Dent J 1982;6:233–8.
179. Mitropoulos CM, Holloway PJ, Davies TGH, Worthington HV. Relative efficacy of dentifrices containing 250 or 1000 ppm F⁻ in preventing dental caries—report of a 32-month clinical trial. Community Dent Health 1984;1:193–200.
180. Winter GB, Holt RD, Williams BF. Clinical trial of a low-fluoride toothpaste for young children. Int Dent J 1989;39:227–35.
181. Holt RD, Morris CE, Winter GB, Downer MC. Enamel opacities and dental caries in children who used a low fluoride toothpaste between 2 and 5 years of age. Int Dent J 1994;44:331–41.
182. Horowitz HS. The need for toothpastes with lower than conventional fluoride concentrations for preschool-aged children. J Public Health Dent 1992;52:216–21.
183. Zero DT, Raubertas RF, Fu J, Pedersen AM, Hayes AL, Featherstone JDB. Fluoride concentrations in plaque, whole saliva, and ductal saliva after application of home-use topical fluorides. J Dent Res 1992;71:1768–75.
184. Horowitz HS, Creighton WE, McClendon BJ. The effect on human dental caries of weekly oral rinsing with a sodium fluoride mouthwash: a final report. Arch Oral Biol 1971;16:609–16.
185. Rugg-Gunn AJ, Holloway PJ, Davies TGH. Caries prevention by daily fluoride mouthrinsing: report of a three-year clinical trial. Br Dent J 1973;135:353–60.
186. DePaola PF, Soparkar P, Foley S, Bookstein F, Bakhos Y. Effect of high-concentration ammonium and sodium fluoride rinses in dental caries in schoolchildren. Community Dent Oral Epidemiol 1977;5:7–14.
187. Leverett DH, Sveen OB, Jensen ØE. Weekly rinsing with a fluoride mouthrinse in an unfluoridated community: results after seven years. J Public Health Dent 1985;45:95–100.
188. Ripa LW, Leske GS, Sposato A, Rebich T. Supervised weekly rinsing with a 0.2 percent neutral NaF solution: final results of a demonstration program after six school years. J Public Health Dent 1983;43:53–62.
189. Ripa LW, Leske GS, Sposato AL, Rebich T Jr. Supervised weekly rinsing with a 0.2% neutral NaF solution: results after 5 years. Community Dent Oral Epidemiol 1983;11:1–6.

190. Ripa LW, Leske G. Effect on the primary dentition of mouthrinsing with a 0.2 percent neutral NaF solution: results from a demonstration program after four school years. Pediatr Dent 1981;3:311–5.
191. Ripa LW. A critique of topical fluoride methods (dentifrices, mouthrinses, operator-, and self-applied gels) in an era of decreased caries and increased fluorosis prevalence. J Public Health Dent 1991;51:23–41.
192. Haugejorden O, Lervik T, Riordan PJ. Comparison of caries prevalence 7 years after discontinuation of school-based fluoride rinsing or toothbrushing in Norway. Community Dent Oral Epidemiol 1985;13:2–6.
193. Leske GS, Ripa LW, Green E. Posttreatment benefits in a school-based fluoride mouthrinsing program: final results after 7 years of rinsing by all participants. Clin Prev Dent 1986;8:19–23.
194. Holland TJ, Whelton H, O'Mullane DM, Creedon P. Evaluation of a fortnightly school-based sodium fluoride mouthrinse 4 years following its cessation. Caries Res 1995;29:431–4.
195. Disney JA, Graves RC, Stamm JW, Bohannan HM, Abernathy JR. Comparative effects of a 4-year fluoride mouthrinse program on high and low caries forming grade 1 children. Community Dent Oral Epidemiol 1989;17:139–43.
196. Klein SP, Bohannan HM, Bell RM, Disney JA, Foch CB, Graves RC. The cost and effectiveness of school-based preventive dental care. Am J Public Health 1985;75:382–91.
197. Nourjah P, Horowitz AM, Wagener DK. Factors associated with the use of fluoride supplements and fluoride dentifrice by infants and toddlers. J Public Health Dent 1994;54:47–54.
198. Leverett DH, Adair SM, Vaughan BW, Proskin HM, Moss ME. Randomized clinical trial of the effect of prenatal fluoride supplements in preventing dental caries. Caries Res 1997;31:174–9.
199. Aasenden R, Peebles TC. Effects of fluoride supplementation from birth on human deciduous and permanent teeth. Arch Oral Biol 1974;19:321–6.
200. de Liefde B, Herbison GP. The prevalence of developmental defects of enamel and dental caries in New Zealand children receiving differing fluoride supplementation in 1982 and 1985. N Z Dent J 1989;85:2–8.
201. D'Hoore W, Van Nieuwenhuysen J-P. Benefits and risks of fluoride supplementation: caries prevention versus dental fluorosis. Eur J Pediatr 1992;151:613–6.
202. Allmark C, Green HP, Linney AD, Wills DJ, Picton DCA. A community study of fluoride tablets for school children in Portsmouth: results after six years. Br Dent J 1982;153:426–30.
203. Fanning EA, Cellier KM, Somerville CM. South Australian kindergarten children: effects of fluoride tablets and fluoridated water on dental caries in primary teeth. Aust Dent J 1980;25:259–63.
204. Marthaler TM. Caries-inhibiting effect of fluoride tablets. Helv Odont Acta 1969;13:1–13.
205. Widenheim J, Birkhed D. Caries-preventive effect on primary and permanent teeth and cost-effectiveness of an NaF tablet preschool program. Community Dent Oral Epidemiol 1991;19:88–92.
206. Widenheim J, Birkhed D, Granath L, Lindgren G. Preeruptive effect of NaF tablets on caries in children from 12 to 17 years of age. Community Dent Oral Epidemiol 1986;14:1–4.
207. Margolis FJ, Reames HR, Freshman E, Macauley JC, Mehaffey H. Fluoride: ten-year prospective study of deciduous and permanent dentition. Am J Dis Child 1975;129:794–800.
208. Bagramian RA, Narendran S, Ward M. Relationship of dental caries and fluorosis to fluoride supplement history in a non-fluoridated sample of schoolchildren. Adv Dent Res 1989;3:161–7.

209. Holm A-K, Andersson R. Enamel mineralization disturbances in 12-year-old children with known early exposure to fluorides. Community Dent Oral Epidemiol 1982;10:335–9.

210. Awad MA, Hargreaves JA, Thompson GW. Dental caries and fluorosis in 7–9 and 11–14 year old children who received fluoride supplements from birth. J Can Dent Assoc 1994;60:318–22.

211. Friis-Hasché E, Bergmann J, Wenzel A, Thylstrup A, Pedersen KM, Petersen PE. Dental health status and attitudes to dental care in families participating in a Danish fluoride tablet program. Community Dent Oral Epidemiol 1984;12:303–7.

212. Kalsbeek H, Verrips GH, Backer Dirks O. Use of fluoride tablets and effect on prevalence of dental caries and dental fluorosis. Community Dent Oral Epidemiol 1992;20:241–5.

213. DePaola PF, Lax M. The caries-inhibiting effect of acidulated phosphate-fluoride chewable tablets: a two-year double-blind study. J Am Dent Assoc 1968;76:554–7.

214. Driscoll WS, Heifetz SB, Korts DC. Effect of chewable fluoride tablets on dental caries in schoolchildren: results after six years of use. J Am Dent Assoc 1978;97:820–4.

215. Stephen KW, Campbell D. Caries reduction and cost benefit after 3 years of sucking fluoride tablets daily at school: a double-blind trial. Br Dent J 1978;144:202–6.

216. Stephen KW, McCall DR, Gilmour WH. Incisor enamel mottling in child cohorts which had or had not taken fluoride supplements from 0–12 years of age. Proc Finn Dent Soc 1991;87:595–605.

217. Larsen MJ, Kirkegaard E, Poulsen S, Fejerskov O. Dental fluorosis among participants in a non-supervised fluoride tablet program. Community Dent Oral Epidemiol 1989;17:204–6.

218. Riordan PJ, Banks JA. Dental fluorosis and fluoride exposure in Western Australia. J Dent Res 1991;70:1022–8.

219. Suckling GW, Pearce EIF. Developmental defects of enamel in a group of New Zealand children: their prevalence and some associated etiological factors. Community Dent Oral Epidemiol 1984;12:177–84.

220. Wöltgens JHM, Etty EJ, Nieuwland WMD. Prevalence of mottled enamel in permanent dentition of children participating in a fluoride programme at the Amsterdam dental school. J Biol Buccale 1989;17:15–20.

221. Woolfolk MW, Faja BW, Bagramian RA. Relation of sources of systemic fluoride to prevalence of dental fluorosis. J Public Health Dent 1989;49:78–82.

222. Ismail AI, Brodeur J-M, Kavanagh M, Boisclair G, Tessier C, Picotte L. Prevalence of dental caries and dental fluorosis in students, 11–17 years of age, in fluoridated and non-fluoridated cities in Quebec. Caries Res 1990;24:290–7.

223. Margolis FJ, Burt BA, Schork A, Bashshur RL, Whittaker BA, Burns TL. Fluoride supplements for children: a survey of physicians' prescription practices. Am J Dis Child 1980;134:865–8.

224. Szpunar SM, Burt BA. Fluoride exposure in Michigan schoolchildren. J Public Health Dent 1990;50:18–23.

225. Levy SM, Muchow G. Provider compliance with recommended dietary fluoride supplement protocol. Am J Public Health 1992;82:281–3.

226. Pendrys DG, Morse DE. Use of fluoride supplementation by children living in fluoridated communities. J Dent Child 1990;57:343–7.

227. Pendrys DG, Morse DE. Fluoride supplement use by children in fluoridated communities. J Public Health Dent 1995;55:160–4.

228. Jackson RD, Kelly SA, Katz BP, Hull JR, Stookey GK. Dental fluorosis and caries prevalence in children residing in communities with different levels of fluoride in the water. J Public Health Dent 1995;55:79–84.

229. Lasagna L. Balancing risks versus benefits in drug therapy decisions. Clin Ther 1998;20(suppl C):72–9.

230. Dijkman TG, Arends J. The role of 'CaF$_2$-like' material in topical fluoridation of enamel in situ. Acta Odontol Scand 1988;46:391–7.

231. Houpt M, Koenigsberg S, Shey Z. The effect of prior toothcleaning on the efficacy of topical fluoride treatment: two-year results. Clin Prev Dent 1983;5:8–10.

232. Brudevold F, Savory A, Gardner DE, Spinelli M, Speirs R. A study of acidulated fluoride solutions. I. In vitro effects on enamel. Arch Oral Biol 1963;8:167–77.

233. Ripa LW. Professionally (operator) applied topical fluoride therapy: a critique. Int Dent J 1981;31:105–20.

234. Wei SHY, Yiu CKY. Evaluation of the use of topical fluoride gel. Caries Res 1993;27(suppl I):29–34.

235. Hagen PP, Rozier RG, Bawden JW. The caries-preventive effect of full- and half-strength topical acidulated phosphate fluoride. Pediatr Dent 1985;7:185–91.

236. Ripa LW. An evaluation of the use of professional (operator-applied) topical fluorides. J Dent Res 1990;69(special issue):786–96.

237. Horowitz HS, Doyle J. The effect on dental caries of topically applied acidulated phosphate-fluoride: results after three years. J Am Dent Assoc 1971;82:359–65.

238. Johnston DW, Lewis DW. Three-year randomized trial of professionally applied topical fluoride gel comparing annual and biannual application with/without prior prophylaxis. Caries Res 1995;29:331–6.

239. Petersson LG. Fluoride mouthrinses and fluoride varnishes. Caries Res 1993;27(suppl 1):35–42.

240. Mandel ID. Fluoride varnishes—a welcome addition [Editorial]. J Public Health Dent 1994;54:67.

241. Wakeen LM. Legal implications of using drugs and devices in the dental office. J Public Health Dent 1992;52:403–8.

242. Clark DC, Stamm JW, Tessier C, Robert G. The final results of the Sherbrooke-Lac Mégantic fluoride varnish study. J Can Dent Assoc 1987;53:919–22.

243. de Bruyn H, Arends J. Fluoride varnishes—a review. J Biol Buccale 1987;15:71–82.

244. Helfenstein U, Steiner M. Fluoride varnishes (Duraphat): a meta-analysis. Community Dent Oral Epidemiol 1994;22:1–5.

245. Twetman S, Petersson LG, Pakhomov GN. Caries incidence in relation to salivary mutans streptococci and fluoride varnish applications in preschool children from low- and optimal-fluoride areas. Caries Res 1996;30:347–53.

246. Seppä L. Studies of fluoride varnishes in Finland. Proc Finn Dent Soc 1991;87:541–7.

247. Seppä L, Leppänen T, Hausen H. Fluoride varnish versus acidulated phosphate fluoride gel: a 3-year clinical trial. Caries Res 1995;29:327–30.

248. Seppä L, Tolonen T. Caries preventive effect of fluoride varnish applications performed two or four times a year. Scand J Dent Res 1990;98:102–5.

249. Petersson LG, Arthursson L, Östberg C, Jönsson P, Gleerup A. Caries-inhibiting effects of different modes of Duraphat varnish reapplication: a 3-year radiographic study. Caries Res 1991;25:70–3.

250. Sköld L, Sundquist B, Eriksson B, Edeland C. Four-year study of caries inhibition of intensive Duraphat application in 11–15-year-old children. Community Dent Oral Epidemiol 1994;22:8–12.

251. Adriaens ML, Dermaut LR, Verbeeck RMH. The use of 'Fluor Protector,' a fluoride varnish, as a caries prevention method under orthodontic molar bands. Eur J Orthod 1990;12:316–9.

252. Peyron M, Matsson L, Birkhed D. Progression of approximal caries in primary molars and the effect of Duraphat treatment. Scand J Dent Res 1992;100:314–8.

253. Marthaler TM. Cariostatic efficacy of the combined use of fluorides. J Dent Res 1990;69(special issue):797–800.

254. US Preventive Services Task Force. Guide to clinical preventive services. 2nd ed. Alexandria, VA: International Medical Publishing, 1996.
255. McKay FS. Relation of mottled enamel to caries. J Am Dent Assoc 1928;15:1429–37.
256. Clark DC, Hann HJ, Williamson MF, Berkowitz J. Effects of lifelong consumption of fluoridated water or use of fluoride supplements on dental caries prevalence. Community Dent Oral Epidemiol 1995;23:20–4.
257. Murray JJ, Rugg-Gunn AJ. Fluorides in caries prevention. 2nd ed. Boston, MA: Wright-PSG, 1982. (Dental practitioner handbook no. 20).
258. Warner KE, Luce BR. Cost-benefit and cost-effectiveness analysis in health care: principles, practice, and potential. Ann Arbor, MI: Health Administration Press, 1982.
259. Manski RJ, Moeller JF, Maas WR. Dental services: use, expenditures and sources of payment, 1987. J Am Dent Assoc 1999;130:500–8.
260. Burt BA, ed. Proceedings for the workshop: Cost-effectiveness of caries prevention in dental public health, Ann Arbor, Michigan, May 17–19, 1989. J Public Health Dent 1989;49(special issue):331–7.
261. Brown LJ, Lazar V. Dental procedure fees 1975 through 1995: how much have they changed? J Am Dent Assoc 1998;129:1291–5.
262. Downer MC, Blinkhorn AS, Attwood D. Effect of fluoridation on the cost of dental treatment among urban Scottish schoolchildren. Community Dent Oral Epidemiol 1981;9:112–6.
263. Attwood D, Blinkhorn AS. Reassessment of the effect of fluoridation on cost of dental treatment among Scottish schoolchildren. Community Dent Oral Epidemiol 1989;17:79–82.
264. Garcia AI. Caries incidence and costs of prevention programs. J Public Health Dent 1989:49(special issue):259–71.
265. Anonymous. Which toothpaste is right for you? Consumer Reports 1998;August:11–4.
266. Doherty NJG, Brunelle JA, Miller AJ, Li S-H. Costs of school-based mouthrinsing in 14 demonstration programs in USA. Community Dent Oral Epidemiol 1984;12:35–8.
267. Leverett DH. Effectiveness of mouthrinsing with fluoride solutions in preventing coronal and root caries. J Public Health Dent 1989;49(special issue):310–6.
268. van Rijkom HM, Truin GJ, van 't Hof MA. A meta-analysis of clinical studies on the caries-inhibiting effect of fluoride gel treatment. Caries Res 1998;32:83–92.
269. Eklund SA, Pittman JL, Heller KE. Professionally applied topical fluoride and restorative care in insured children. J Public Health Dent 2000;60:33–8.
270. Petersson LG, Westerberg I. Intensive fluoride varnish program in Swedish adolescents: economic assessment of a 7-year follow-up study on proximal caries incidence. Caries Res1994;28:59–63.

Use of trade names and commercial sources is for identification only and does not imply endorsement by the U.S. Department of Health and Human Services.

References to non-CDC sites on the Internet are provided as a service to *MMWR* readers and do not constitute or imply endorsement of these organizations or their programs by CDC or the U.S. Department of Health and Human Services. CDC is not responsible for the content of pages found at these sites.

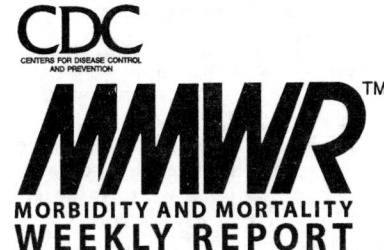

August 17, 2001 / Vol. 50 / No. RR-14

Recommendations
and
Reports

Continuing Education Activity
Sponsored by CDC

Recommendations for Using Fluoride to Prevent and Control Dental Caries in the United States

EXPIRATION — August 17, 2002

You must complete and return the response form electronically or by mail by **August 17, 2002**, to receive continuing education credit. If you answer all of the questions, you will receive an award letter for 2.0 hours Continuing Medical Education (CME) credit, 0.2 Continuing Education Units (CEUs), or 2.6 contact hours Continuing Nursing Education (CNE) credit. If you return the form electronically, you will receive educational credit immediately. If you mail the form, you will receive educational credit in approximately 30 days. No fees are charged for participating in this continuing education activity.

INSTRUCTIONS
By Internet
1. Read this *MMWR* (Vol. 50, RR-14), which contains the correct answers to the questions beginning on the next page.
2. Go to the *MMWR* Continuing Education Internet site at <http://www.cdc.gov/mmwr/cme/conted.html>.
3. Select which exam you want to take and select whether you want to register for CME, CEU, or CNE credit.
4. Fill out and submit the registration form.
5. Select exam questions. To receive continuing education credit, you must answer all of the questions. Questions with more than one correct answer will instruct you to "Indicate all that apply."
6. Submit your answers no later than **August 17, 2002**.
7. Immediately print your Certificate of Completion for your records.

By Mail or Fax
1. Read this *MMWR* (Vol. 50, RR-14), which contains the correct answers to the questions beginning on the next page.
2. Complete all registration information on the response form, including your name, mailing address, phone number, and e-mail address, if available.
3. Indicate whether you are registering for CME, CEU, or CNE credit.
4. Select your answers to the questions, and mark the corresponding letters on the response form. To receive continuing education credit, you must answer all of the questions. Questions with more than one correct answer will instruct you to "Indicate all that apply."
5. Sign and date the response form or a photocopy of the form and send no later than **August 17, 2002**, to
   Fax: 404-639-4198   Mail: MMWR CE Credit
                                     Office of Scientific and Health Communications
                                     Epidemiology Program Office, MS C-08
                                     Centers for Disease Control and Prevention
                                     1600 Clifton Rd, N.E.
                                     Atlanta, GA 30333
6. Your Certificate of Completion will be mailed to you within 30 days.

ACCREDITATION

Continuing Medical Education (CME). CDC is accredited by the Accreditation Council for Continuing Medical Education (ACCME) to provide continuing medical education for physicians. CDC designates this educational activity for a maximum of 2.0 hours in category 1 credit toward the AMA Physician's Recognition Award. Each physician should claim only those hours of credit that he/she actually spent in the educational activity.

Continuing Education Unit (CEU). CDC has been approved as an authorized provider of continuing education and training programs by the International Association for Continuing Education and Training and awards 0.2 Continuing Education Units (CEUs).

Continuing Nursing Education (CNE). This activity for 2.6 contact hours is provided by CDC, which is accredited as a provider of continuing education in nursing by the American Nurses Credentialing Center's Commission on Accreditation.

GOAL AND OBJECTIVES

This *MMWR* provides recommendations regarding the use of fluoride to prevent and control dental caries in the United States. These recommendations were prepared by CDC staff members and a work group of specialists in fluoride research or policy. This goal of this report is to increase appropriate use of fluoride modalities in preventing and controlling dental caries through improved professional understanding and practice. Upon completion of this continuing educational activity, the reader should be able to a) list the factors used in the decision to prescribe fluoride supplements; b) describe the recommendations for counseling patients on the use of fluoride products in oral self-care practices, especially for children aged <6 years; c) list the sources for determining the current level of fluoride delivered by a community water system; d) identify the factors used to assess caries risk; e) explain how fluoride prevents dental caries; f) describe the recommendations for choosing the appropriate fluoride modalities for patients; and g) list the risk factors for enamel fluorosis.

To receive continuing education credit, please answer all of the following questions.

1. **Which of the following statements are true?** (*Indicate all that apply.*)

   A. The U.S. Environmental Protection Agency requires all community water systems to provide each customer an annual report that includes the fluoride concentration of their water.

   B. Fluoridated community drinking water and toothpaste containing fluoride are the most common sources for fluoride in the United States.

   C. A person at high risk for dental caries will not require more frequent exposure to fluoride than persons at low risk.

   D. Water and other beverages provide <50% of a person's fluoride intake in the United States.

2. **Which of the following persons are believed to be at greater risk for dental caries?** (*Indicate all that apply.*)

   A. Persons who do not seek dental treatment on a regular basis.

   B. Persons with dental insurance.

   C. Persons living in families with incomes below the poverty level.

   D. Children with an older brother/sister having a history of high levels of dental decay.

3. **Which of the following are risk factors for enamel fluorosis for children aged <6 years?** (*Indicate all that apply.*)

   A. Taking fluoride supplements in an area with fluoridated drinking water.

   B. Not being allowed to deliberately swallow toothpaste.

   C. Using a pea-sized amount of toothpaste no more than twice a day.

   D. Ingesting too much fluoride from any source during critical periods of tooth development.

4. **What is the most cost-effective measure to prevent dental caries in the United States?**

   A. Fluoridation of individual school water systems.

   B. Use of a pea-sized amount of fluoride toothpaste twice a day.

   C. Adding fluoride to the community water system.

   D. Giving fluoride supplements to schoolchildren.

5. **Which of the following statements regarding effective fluoride use are true?** (*Indicate all that apply.*)

    A. Community water fluoridation should be continued as a safe and inexpensive method to prevent dental caries.

    B. Parents and caregivers should be provided information on use of fluoride toothpaste for children aged <6 years.

    C. Other fluoride modalities (e.g., mouthrinse and professionally applied gels) should be targeted to patients at high risk for dental caries.

    D. Fluoride supplements should be provided to children whose primary drinking water has a low fluoride concentration and who are at high risk for dental caries.

6. **Enamel fluorosis is . . .**

    A. hypermineralization of the dentin.

    B. hypomineralization of the enamel.

    C. demineralization of the enamel.

    D. demineralization of the dentin.

7. **At what age should a fluoride supplement first be prescribed to a child at high risk for dental caries living in a community where the level of fluoride is below the optimal level?**

    A. Birth.

    B. 3 months.

    C. 6 months.

    D. 9 months.

8. **For which children at high risk should fluoride mouthrinses be used?**

    A. Those aged ≥2 years.

    B. Those attending Head Start programs.

    C. Those aged ≥6 years.

    D. Those aged ≥2 years living in rural areas.

9. **Currently, how many persons in the United States have access to fluoridated water in their communities?**

    A. 104 million.

    B. 114 million.

    C. 134 million.

    D. 144 million.

10. **What is the optimal concentration of fluoride in community water systems in the United States?**

    A. 0.7 parts per million (ppm).

    B. 0.7–0.9 ppm.

    C. 0.7–1.0 ppm.

    D. 0.7–1.2 ppm.

11. **Indicate your work setting.**

   A. State/local health department.
   B. Other public health agency.
   C. Hospital clinic/private practice.
   D. Managed care organization.
   E. Academic institution.
   F. Other.

12. **Which best describes your professional activities?**

   A. Family practice.
   B. Pediatrics.
   C. Nursing.
   D. General dentistry.
   E. Pediatric dentistry.
   F. Dental hygiene.

13. **I plan to use these recommendations as the basis for . . .** (*Indicate all that apply.*)

   A. health education materials.
   B. insurance reimbursement policies.
   C. local practice guidelines.
   D. public policy
   E. other.

14. **Each month, approximately how many patients do you counsel regarding fluoride use?**

   A. None.
   B. 1–5.
   C. 6–15.
   D. 16–24.
   E. 25.

15. **How much time did you spend reading this report and completing the exam?**

   A. 2–2.5 hours.
   B. More than 2.5 hours but fewer than 3 hours.
   C. 3–3.5 hours.
   D. More than 3.5 hours but fewer than 4 hours.
   E. More than 4 hours.

16. **After reading this report, I am confident I can list the factors used in the decision to prescribe fluoride supplements.**

   A. Strongly agree.
   B. Agree.
   C. Neither agree or disagree.
   D. Disagree.
   E. Strongly disagree.

17. After reading this report, I am confident I can describe the recommendations for counseling patients on the use of fluoride products in oral self-care practices, especially for children aged <6 years.

   A. Strongly agree.
   B. Agree.
   C. Neither agree or disagree.
   D. Disagree.
   E. Strongly disagree.

18. After reading this report, I am confident I can list the sources for determining the current level of fluoride delivered by a community water system.

   A. Strongly agree.
   B. Agree.
   C. Neither agree or disagree.
   D. Disagree.
   E. Strongly disagree.

19. After reading this report, I am confident I can identify the factors used to assess caries risk.

   A. Strongly agree.
   B. Agree.
   C. Neither agree or disagree.
   D. Disagree.
   E. Strongly disagree.

20. After reading this report, I am confident I can explain how fluoride prevents dental caries.

   A. Strongly agree.
   B. Agree.
   C. Neither agree or disagree.
   D. Disagree.
   E. Strongly disagree.

21. After reading this report, I am confident I can describe the recommendations for choosing the appropriate fluoride modalities for patients.

   A. Strongly agree.
   B. Agree.
   C. Neither agree or disagree.
   D. Disagree.
   E. Strongly disagree.

22. After reading this report, I am confident I can list the risk factors for enamel fluorosis.

   A. Strongly agree.
   B. Agree.
   C. Neither agree or disagree.
   D. Disagree.
   E. Strongly disagree.

23. **The objectives are relevant to the goal of this report.**

   A.   Strongly agree.
   B.   Agree.
   C.   Neither agree nor disagree.
   D.   Disagree.
   E.   Strongly disagree.

24. **The figures, tables, and boxes are useful.**

   A.   Strongly agree.
   B.   Agree.
   C.   Neither agree nor disagree.
   D.   Disagree.
   E.   Strongly disagree.

25. **Overall, the presentation of the report enhanced my ability to understand the material.**

   A.   Strongly agree.
   B.   Agree.
   C.   Neither agree nor disagree.
   D.   Disagree.
   E.   Strongly disagree.

26. **These recommendations will affect my practice.**

   A.   Strongly agree.
   B.   Agree
   C.   Neither agree nor disagree.
   D.   Disagree.
   E.   Strongly disagree.

27. **How did you learn about this continuing education activity?**

   A.   Internet.
   B.   Advertisement (e.g., fact sheet, *MMWR* cover, newsletter, or journal).
   C.   Coworker/supervisor.
   D.   Conference presentation.
   E.   *MMWR* subscription.
   F.   Other.

Correct answers for questions 1–10

1. A,B; 2. A,C,D; 3. A,D; 4. C; 5. A,B,C,D; 6. B; 7. C; 8. C; 9. D; 10. D.

Vol. 50 / No. RR-14   MMWR   CE-7

MMWR Response Form for Continuing Education Credit
August 17, 2001/Vol. 50/No. RR-14

Recommendations for Using Fluoride to Prevent and Control Dental Caries in the United States

To receive continuing education credit, you must
1. *provide your contact information;*
2. *indicate your choice of CME, CEU, or CNE credit;*
3. *answer all of the test questions;*
4. *sign and date this form or a photocopy;*
5. *submit your answer form by August 17, 2002.*
Failure to complete these items can result in a delay or rejection of your application for continuing education credit.

Detach or photocopy.

Last Name   First Name

Street Address or P.O. Box

Apartment or Suite

City   State   ZIP Code

Phone Number   Fax Number

E-Mail Address

Check One
- [ ] *CME Credit*
- [ ] *CEU Credit*
- [ ] *CNE Credit*

Fill in the appropriate blocks to indicate your answers. Remember, you must answer all of the questions to receive continuing education credit!

1. [ ] A [ ] B [ ] C [ ] D
2. [ ] A [ ] B [ ] C [ ] D
3. [ ] A [ ] B [ ] C [ ] D
4. [ ] A [ ] B [ ] C [ ] D
5. [ ] A [ ] B [ ] C [ ] D
6. [ ] A [ ] B [ ] C [ ] D
7. [ ] A [ ] B [ ] C [ ] D
8. [ ] A [ ] B [ ] C [ ] D
9. [ ] A [ ] B [ ] C [ ] D
10. [ ] A [ ] B [ ] C [ ] D
11. [ ] A [ ] B [ ] C [ ] D [ ] E [ ] F
12. [ ] A [ ] B [ ] C [ ] D [ ] E [ ] F
13. [ ] A [ ] B [ ] C [ ] D [ ] E
14. [ ] A [ ] B [ ] C [ ] D [ ] E

15. [ ] A [ ] B [ ] C [ ] D [ ] E
16. [ ] A [ ] B [ ] C [ ] D [ ] E
17. [ ] A [ ] B [ ] C [ ] D [ ] E
18. [ ] A [ ] B [ ] C [ ] D [ ] E
19. [ ] A [ ] B [ ] C [ ] D [ ] E
20. [ ] A [ ] B [ ] C [ ] D [ ] E
21. [ ] A [ ] B [ ] C [ ] D [ ] E
22. [ ] A [ ] B [ ] C [ ] D [ ] E
23. [ ] A [ ] B [ ] C [ ] D [ ] E
24. [ ] A [ ] B [ ] C [ ] D [ ] E
25. [ ] A [ ] B [ ] C [ ] D [ ] E
26. [ ] A [ ] B [ ] C [ ] D [ ] E
27. [ ] A [ ] B [ ] C [ ] D [ ] E [ ] F

Signature   *Date I Completed Exam*

The *Morbidity and Mortality Weekly Report (MMWR)* Series is prepared by the Centers for Disease Control and Prevention (CDC) and is available free of charge in electronic format and on a paid subscription basis for paper copy. To receive an electronic copy on Friday of each week, send an e-mail message to *listserv@listserv.cdc.gov*. The body content should read *SUBscribe mmwr-toc*. Electronic copy also is available from CDC's World-Wide Web server at *http://www.cdc.gov/mmwr/* or from CDC's file transfer protocol server at *ftp://ftp.cdc.gov/pub/Publications/mmwr/*. To subscribe for paper copy, contact Superintendent of Documents, U.S. Government Printing Office, Washington, DC 20402; telephone (202) 512-1800.

Data in the weekly *MMWR* are provisional, based on weekly reports to CDC by state health departments. The reporting week concludes at close of business on Friday; compiled data on a national basis are officially released to the public on the following Friday. Address inquiries about the *MMWR* Series, including material to be considered for publication, to: Editor, *MMWR* Series, Mailstop C-08, CDC, 1600 Clifton Rd., N.E., Atlanta, GA 30333; telephone (888) 232-3228.

All material in the *MMWR* Series is in the public domain and may be used and reprinted without permission; citation as to source, however, is appreciated.

☆U.S. Government Printing Office: 2001-633-173/48246 Region IV

Foster Care Mental Health Values

• •

The following guideline for foster care mental health values, developed by the American Academy of Child and Adolescent Psychiatry, has been endorsed by the American Academy of Pediatrics.

AACAP/CWLA Values and Principles for Mental Health and Substance Abuse Services and Supports for Children in Foster Care

PREAMBLE

In the past few years, significant attention has been given to the growing number of children who suffer needlessly because their emotional, behavioral, and developmental needs are not being met. All of us are urged to take seriously the task of preventing mental health or substance abuse problems and providing services and supports for treating mental illness or substance abuse in children.

The Surgeon General's *Report on Children's Mental Health* and the United Nations Convention on the Rights of the Child have emphasized that treatment should be considered a basic right for children and families that suffer from a mental health or substance abuse problem. President Bush issued an executive order, the New Freedom Initiative (NFI) of June 18th, 2001, to remove barriers to community living for persons with disabilities, including children with severe emotional disturbances. NFI highlights the fact that there is no "wrong door" for accessing services and creating opportunity for children to receive community-based services within their local service systems. The president's announced plan to establish a National Commission on Mental Health will further support addressing the emotional/mental health needs of children.

Children served by the foster care system are coping with the events that precipitated their coming into care and enduring the grief and trauma that accompany the loss of a family. Currently, more than 500,000 children reside in foster care in the United States, and 85% of them are estimated to have an emotional disorder and/or substance abuse problem. The American Academy of Child and Adolescent Psychiatry (AACAP) and the Child Welfare League of America (CWLA) began an initiative in March 2001 to improve the design, delivery, and outcomes of the mental health and substance abuse services provided to children in foster care and their families. AACAP and CWLA have been joined by more than 30 consumer and professional organizations, which have contributed their expertise and resources to this initiative.

The seriousness, intensity, prevalence, and urgency of the unmet needs of these children and their families substantiates our commitment to this initiative. Drawing on the values and principles already developed through such efforts as the systems of care, which focused on service delivery to children with serious emotional disturbances, the values and principles delineated in this document will guide efforts to improve policies and practices in the systems that serve children in foster care and their families. We believe such values and principles will drive practice in addressing the mental health and substance abuse needs of children and their families. This will lead to other reforms in how local communities and formal systems intersect on mental health, substance abuse, and child welfare issues to ensure the well-being of children in foster care and their families.

Our mutual interest is the emotional/mental health of children and their families. We must develop innovative and evidence-based assessment tools to identify children's emotional and/or behavioral problems as early as possible and to ensure that all children and their families have access to and receive evidence-based, effective, mental health and substance abuse prevention and treatment services and supports. It is our professional responsibility to provide the most timely, appropriate, and effective prevention/treatment services and supports to children and their families to ensure the best outcomes.

To this end, we support and advocate for providing mental health and substance abuse prevention strategies, assessments, treatments, services, and supports designed for children in the foster care system and their families that abide by the following five **VALUES:**

1. Child-focused mental health and substance abuse services and supports

2. Family-driven mental health and substance abuse services and supports

3. Integration, collaboration, and coordination of community-based mental health and substance abuse services and supports with the foster care system

4. Culturally competent, relevant, and strength-based services and supports provided by knowledgeable, skilled service providers who understand the cultural diversity of the community.

5. Timely, effective, evidence-based, outcome-driven mental health and substance abuse services and supports

Further discussion of the values appears in the appendix.

PRINCIPLES GENERATED BY THE VALUES

The principles outlined here are infused by the core values mentioned above and provide greater detail for how they are to be implemented.

Service Coordination and Case/Care Management

- Coordination among mental health, substance abuse, physical health, developmental disability, legal, educational, and child welfare services is essential.

- Children in foster care deserve services that are designed, assessed, and delivered as part of their foster care services plan.

- System coordination can ensure the most appropriate use of limited resources and eliminate fragmentation experienced with different funding streams for the needed services and supports.

- Many children and youth in foster care have co-occurring mental health and substance abuse issues. Service coordination ensures that their substance abuse and mental health services and supports are provided concurrently.

- Coordination must include services children and family members are receiving.
- Information must be shared on a regular basis among organizations providing services and support to the child and family. Barriers must be eliminated while complying with the confidentiality requirements in HIPAA. This information should follow the child from placement to placement.

Prevention and Early Identification

- Prevention and early identification programs and supports for potential mental health and substance abuse issues are vital to children in the foster care system and their families.
- Children from birth to age 3 are of particular concern, given they are a significant percentage of the population of children in foster care. Prevention and early intervention programs should be targeted to them.
- Assessments for children entering the foster care system should include screening for potential mental health and substance abuse issues. Children should be reassessed for mental health and substance abuse problems at specific intervals (minimally, EPSDT timeframes) so prevention and treatment services can be provided as early as possible. A referral should be made for a mental health and substance abuse assessment by a trained professional.

Planned and Coordinated Transitions Among Agencies and Providers and Between Children, Families, and Adult Systems

- Children and families suffer significant negative effects when transitions and discharges are not successful. Therefore, coordination and effective planning are necessary whenever children are involved in changing providers and/or agencies, returning home, changing levels of care, changing placements, transitioning to self-sufficiency, or being transferred to another service system.
- Youth making the transition to self-sufficiency may need services provided by the adult system, such as mental health, substance abuse, housing, financial, health, dental, educational, and/or employment assistance. Effective coordination must take place between child and adult serving systems.
- Each child leaving the system must have a developmentally appropriate transition and/or discharge plan. Planning must provide skills that allow young people to transition to adulthood and provide for their own permanency, safety, and well-being.
- Transition can significantly affect the child and family. It is important that the child's needs and wishes take precedence over the system's needs whenever possible. If a child experiences more than two placements, the child welfare system should have a process in place to review the reasons and ensure attachment issues and the child's mental health and substance abuse needs are being considered.

- To minimize the negative effect of turnover in workers, training should be provided to workers on the affect of removal from home and/or transitions on children and their ability to form attachments, effective interventions for dealing with attachment trauma, and signs that a child should be referred for mental health and substance abuse treatment.

Human Rights and Responsibilities Regarding Protection and Advocacy

- All children in foster care have the right to express their views through their words and behavior to the extent that is developmentally appropriate or be represented by an adult who offers the child's perspective on the following:
  1. Access to quality mental health and substance abuse services and supports.
  2. Which mental health and substance abuse services assist them based on their strengths and needs.
  3. The development, monitoring, and revision of their mental health and substance abuse treatment plan, which is in keeping with their permanency and family service plan.
  4. What mental health and substance abuse services and supports work for them.
  5. Refusal of mental health and substance abuse services and supports unless their refusal would put them at risk of harm.
  6. Provision of services and supports in the least intrusive environment possible.
  7. Their constitutional rights when placed in foster care.
  8. The affect of placement decisions on their mental health.
  9. When very young or developmentally immature, consideration of the effect of placement decisions on their mental health.
  10. Frequent, ongoing contact with siblings and other family members when the family cannot be maintained as a single unit.
- All families with children in foster care (except when parental rights are terminated or other legal decisions take precedence) have the right to:
  1. Participate in the mental health and substance abuse treatment services and supports that will assist them and their child based on their strengths and needs.
  2. Participate in the development, monitoring, and revision of their child's mental health and substance abuse treatment plan.
  3. Decide which mental health and substance abuse services and supports work for them.
  4. Refuse mental health and substance abuse services and supports, when their refusal does not put their child at risk of harm.
  5. Have access to quality mental health and substance abuse services and supports.
  6. Be provided services and supports in the least intrusive environment possible.
  7. Retain their constitutional rights when their child is placed in foster care.

- Through a release of information form, emancipated youth and family members can provide consent on who gets information about them.
- Children and their families have the right to be treated in compliance with federal, state, and local policies and standards.
- Children and their families have the right to seek advocacy support.
- Children and their families have the right to raise concerns about the mental health and substance abuse services and supports that they receive without retribution. All agencies should have a defined process for how such concerns can be addressed.
- Children and their families have the right to receive services that are culturally competent and to choose providers who value their language, culture, and beliefs.
- Children and their families have the right to access the courts to address concerns about the mental health and substance abuse services they are receiving or believe they should be receiving.

Nondiscrimination in Access to Services for Children in Care

- There should be no discrimination on the basis of race, religion, ethnicity, language, gender, age, sexual orientation, marital status, or disability.
- Providers should deliver services and supports in compliance with the Americans with Disabilities Act.
- Public and private providers must ensure services are accessible without discrimination, including interpreters if needed.

A Comprehensive and Accessible Array of Services

- Given the complexity of serving children and families, it is crucial to have a comprehensive array of services. This includes traditional, faith-based, nontraditional, formal, and informal supports and services.
- This service array should be appropriate to address treatment needs of children and families.
- Services chosen from the array should be age and developmentally appropriate.
- This service array should support children and their families in the community if possible.
- This service array should take into account the ongoing developing strengths of children and their families.

Individualized Service Planning

- Service planning to address the mental health and substance abuse needs of children should be individualized and include the following:
  1. Focus on the strengths, desires, values, and goals of the child and family,
  2. Assessment of the specific needs of the child and the services and supports the family requires to support a child with these mental health and substance abuse needs,
  3. Measures to address issues of emotional distress arising from transitions,
  4. Consistency between the child's permanency plan and the family service plan,

  5. Informal and formal mental health and substance abuse services and supports, and
  6. Measurable goals identified by the child and family.
- This individualized service plan should include the continuation of treatment when the child is reunified with his or her family. If a child is not receiving services or supports at the time of reunification, it is important to initiate any treatment services that are needed as part of the reintegration process.
- The individualized service plan should be developed in partnership with the child and family and other professionals working with them.
- The individualized service plan should be reviewed and updated to reflect the progress of the child, with input from the child and family when appropriate.
- The individualized service plan should include the discharge and transition plans.

Services in the Least Intrusive Community-Based Environment

- Service planning should focus on providing services and supports for children and families at the appropriate level and intensity and in the least intrusive environment to increase the child's functioning and physical stability.
- Every effort should be made to keep children in their community whenever possible. Risk to the child takes precedence over the placement that is least intrusive.
- There should be an easily accessed array of community-based services that support children receiving treatment. This might be over a widespread region, particularly in rural areas where it is not financially feasible to have all services in each community.
- When services are being designed, family and community input should be part of the process.
- When children need to be placed outside the home community, it is essential that treatment be provided to maintain the family connection.

Family Participation in All Aspects of Planning, Service Delivery, and Evaluation

- The family should be part of the engagement process at all levels of planning, service delivery, and evaluation.
- The family should be involved in activities involving the child when possible.
- Families should be given the choice to participate or not.
- Family choices should be considered in all planning for the child outside of situations that put the child at risk of harm.
- Families should be treated with respect and provided advocacy and representation.

Integrated Services with Coordinated Planning Across the Child-Serving System

- Children in the foster care system with mental health and substance abuse issues are often involved with multiple organizations and systems. They require well-coordinated planning and integration of services.

- To ensure the most effective service delivery, services should be coordinated across the child-serving system.

- Often, children in the foster care system initially access services through primary care. The EPSDT screening process should facilitate coordination of services to meet needs.

- When funding streams cannot be combined, there is greater potential for integrating services when planning is coordinated across systems. Integrated planning makes better use of limited dollars and reduces potential duplication of services while increasing the availability of services and supports for the child and family.

- Consistency in planning across systems is important to ensure the child and/or family does not hear conflicting messages or has treatment approaches that are contraindicated. All systems must work to mitigate the burden caused by uncoordinated planning between agencies and families.

- The goal is one document in which the plans of various child-serving systems are incorporated into the foster care system case plan. The plan should be reasonable, useful, and respectful.

APPENDIX

Glossary of Terms

Child—Any child placed in out-of-home care.

Child-focused—When both the physical and emotional well-being of the child is central to all levels of decision-making and a process is in place for resolving conflicts between these two domains. The child's own views are expressed, where possible, directly through the child's words and behaviors or, as required, through an adult whose offers the child's perspective along with the viewpoint of members of the child's family.

Child safety—A child is considered safe when an analysis concludes that the child is not in immediate danger of serious harm and no safety interventions are necessary.

Cultural competence—A system is considered culturally competent when there is professional, formalized competence throughout the system in policies, procedures, outreach, advocacy efforts, and training. Cultural competence, sensitivity, and relevance is demonstrated through the array of services, delivery, framework, and recognition of the importance of community-based, informal support networks such as churches, extended kinship networks, and social organizations. Cultural competence is demonstrated when there are skilled staff who are aware of cultural issues within the community and who understand the diversity of the community.

Family—Families can include birthparents, foster and adoptive parents, grandparents, as well as kinship caregivers and others who have primary responsibility for providing love, guidance, food, shelter, clothing, supervision, and protection for children and adolescents. It is the extent of daily interaction with and responsibility for a child, not a legal construct, that identifies a family member.

Family-driven—A system is family-driven when the family is involved in all decisionmaking. Identification and engagement of the family receiving services is required so that the family's experiences and perspectives drive the planning and outcomes for the foster child. This moves the system beyond being centered and focused on the family to having service delivery be more family-driven.

Prevention and early intervention—

Primary prevention: Efforts to avert mental health and substance abuse problems altogether. For children, these efforts include interventions directed at parents or professionals involved with children.

Secondary prevention: Efforts to detect mental health and/or substance abuse problems in their early stages of development and to apply techniques to reduce the severity and duration of incipient problems.

Tertiary prevention: Attempts to arrest further deterioration in individuals who already suffer from severe mental health and/or substance abuse problems. Treatment is tertiary prevention.

System of care—A system of mental health, substance abuse, social services, education, medical, physical health, primary care, juvenile justice, and other organizations, and formal and informal services that work with the family to meet the child's needs.

Substance Abuse—Refers to the use of alcohol or illicit drugs and the misuse of prescription drugs.

VALUES DISCUSSION POINTS

1. **Child-Focused Mental Health and Substance Abuse Services and Supports**

   - Attachment issues are significant to the mental health of children in all placement decisions. The trauma children endure when moved from placement to placement is not conducive to normal development. When placing children outside the home, it is essential to help them create meaningful new attachments while maintaining existing attachments if possible.

   - Children's views of how their mental health will be affected by placement decisions should be represented in all proceedings, in keeping with the age and maturity of the child.

   - The current child welfare system tends to focus on the physical safety of the child while not adequately considering the effect of removal on the child's emotional/mental health.

   - Practice guidelines must be established to address not only safety issues but also children's emotional, mental, and behavioral health needs.

   - Foster care providers need resources to address the mental health and substance abuse needs of the children they serve. Ensuring that services are delivered in a timely, appropriate manner is necessary.

   - The child and birthfamily should maintain contact while the child is in care. Assessment decisions need to be made to determine if the birthfamily can be in immediate and continuing contact to decrease the severity of separation trauma. Whenever possible, the birthparents and foster parents or other agency caregivers should communicate with each other to maximize continuity and mutuality in accomplishing therapeutic goals.

- Providing mental health intervention at the time of the initial placement and while in care helps prevent attachment disorders and/or the progression of already existing mental health and substance abuse problems.

- Reunification with the family of origin may not always be the best option for the child. Other options must be considered to ensure the child's well-being.

2. **Family-Driven Mental Health and Substance Abuse Services and Supports**

- For child welfare services, a family-driven policy that does not compromise the child's safety is necessary.

- The foster care system is currently focused on the child. To really meet the child's needs, it should place greater emphasis on the family of origin. This family-centered approach could result in a major change of mindset within the child welfare system.

- The child welfare system is concerned with safety, permanency, and well-being. Every child should have a safe home as soon as possible, but not necessarily with the family of origin.

- To every extent possible, the birth family should be involved even when it is not the custodial family.

3. **Integration, Collaboration and Coordination of Community-Based Mental Health and Substance Abuse Services and Supports with the Foster Care System**

- Best practices in mental and behavioral health services and supports should be available to children in foster care and their families.

- Mental and behavioral health care providers must have a clear and defined role, driven by professional expertise and values, in treating children and families.

- To ensure child safety and achieve quality services and supports for children and families, it is crucial to increase the input of community members and professionals.

- There may be differences in how states define *safety*. How local communities participate in setting the community standards further affects the differences in definition.

- The child's comprehensive health assessment must include the elements of the EPSDT screening and assessment, such as physical, dental, substance abuse, mental health, and comorbidity evaluations.

- Foster parents must be provided with effective ways their child's needs can be met.

4. **Culturally Competent, Relevant, and Strengths-Based Services and Supports Provided by Knowledgeable, Skilled Service Providers Who Understand the Cultural Diversity of the Community**

- Assessment tools and mental health and substance abuse services and supports must be culturally competent, be culturally sensitive, and take into account the strengths of children and families. They should take into account the cultural status, economic status, and diversity of the population being served.

- There should be culturally competent policies and professional competence in procedures, outreach, advocacy, and training throughout the service delivery system.

- To facilitate rapport and successful outcomes, the team delivering services and supports to children and families should, if possible, represent the diversity of the population.

5. **Timely, Effective, Evidence-Based, Outcome-Driven Mental Health and Substance Abuse Services and Supports**

- The trauma children experience when they are placed in the foster care system must be taken into account when assessing their needs and providing services and supports. An initial mental health and substance abuse screening should be done within 24 hours of placement. The mental health and substance abuse screen identifies children in urgent need of emergency services. This screening assesses internalized and externalized levels of distress in the child regarding separation from their family of origin. A triage intervention to address the child's feelings and help the child cope should be provided as quickly as possible.

- All children in foster care and their families must have a comprehensive mental health and substance abuse assessment once the child is stabilized, minimally within the timeframes of EPSDT. The assessments should always address the child's attachment issues and be done in a timely fashion, especially when there is transition between placements.

- The child welfare system must take into account the difference between a child having a mental disorder and/or substance abuse problem and a child requiring mental health and substance abuse intervention to prevent a future disorder. Currently, a mental health and/or substance abuse assessment is often not done until there is a crisis.

- Just as it is necessary for periodic reviews to be done on individual case plans, it is necessary for systems and providers to perform evidence-based, outcome-driven reviews of results to demonstrate progress in achieving the goals for children and families.

- To provide compassionate, relevant services, it is essential to reach for and use feedback from children and families about service effectiveness.

Mental Health and Substance Use Screening and Assessment of Children in Foster Care

The following guideline for mental health and substance use screening and assessment of children in foster care, developed by the American Academy of Child and Adolescent Psychiatry, has been endorsed by the American Academy of Pediatrics.

AACAP/CWLA Policy Statement on Mental Health and Substance Use Screening and Assessment of Children in Foster Care

I. INTRODUCTION

Children who are removed from their primary caregivers because of suspected child abuse, neglect, or caregiver impairment have compelling and urgent mental health and are at risk for substance abuse disorders. The American Academy of Child and Adolescent Psychiatry (AACAP) and the Child Welfare League of America (CWLA) urge that these children receive immediate mental health and substance use screening followed by a comprehensive mental health and substance use assessment and periodic reassessments. This screening and assessment is to assure that these children receive prompt and appropriate mental health and substance use care. In order to achieve this, the screening and assessment should be:

II. COMPLETED IN A TIMELY WAY BY TRAINED AND QUALIFIED PROFESSIONALS

An initial mental health and substance use screening should be conducted within 24 hours of a child's placement in the care of the child welfare agency. The mental health and substance use screening is intended to identify children in urgent need of emergency mental health and substance use services, including youth whose behavior may pose a danger to themselves or others. Appropriate training should be provided on the screening protocol, and the individual administering the screening should have on-site or readily accessible mental health and substance use consultation. Ideally, the mental health and substance use screening will take place as part of a child's health examination upon entry into care and be conducted by a health professional with expertise in the developmental and mental health and substance use needs of children in foster care.[3]

Children who are removed from their family may require an intervention to address their separation issues immediately. The screening process should assess the internalized and externalized levels of distress the child is in regarding the separation and identify and support the child's strengths and successful coping strategies. Based on the outcome of the individualized screen the child minimally should be provided a triage intervention to address the child's feelings regarding the separation, the needs of the new placement, and to provide support for the child around the separation. It is recommended that the process be monitored to ensure all children receive the mental health and substance use screen and appropriate intervention based on their individualized needs.

Children entering foster care and their families should receive a comprehensive mental health and substance use assessment within 60 days of placement, or sooner based on the severity of the child's needs as identified in the screening process.

Assessments should be conducted by qualified mental health and substance use providers and include the active involvement of a child and adolescent psychiatrist. The comprehensive assessment should incorporate use of developmentally appropriate techniques and tools, be conducted in a comfortable and accessible setting, and address the child and family's strengths as well as needs. Informed consent should be obtained from the party or parties legally responsible for the child. Where indicated, the child or adolescent ought to be directly involved with procedures such as informed assent and be made partner to all assessments and treatment.

III. CHILD-FOCUSED

This process should include support for the child that acknowledges and addresses that removal from primary caregivers usually constitutes a psychological and social crisis for the child and family. The initial screening should be developmentally sensitive and seek to understand the child's internal experience of the placement and the nature of the child's attachments.

Placement often suddenly separates a child from everything familiar, including places (home, neighborhood, school) and people (primary caregivers, birth family, other family members, friends). This sudden and complete loss may result in unrecognized experiences of trauma and bereavement, which in turn can interfere with making new attachments and with the success of placement. New caregivers may need immediate advice on how to help the child make a positive adjustment. Children may need mental health and substance use services to cope with the trauma of placement, even in the absence of symptoms that constitute a psychiatric diagnosis. Children with internalizing problems, such as depression and anxiety, should receive the same consideration for mental health and substance use care as those with externalizing problems such as disruptive behavior. A child's wishes about placement and visitation should be ascertained and given as much weight as possible.

Children and adolescents should be assessed individually, and adequate time and preparation must be devoted to the assessment so that every child and adolescent has the opportunity to freely express his or her concerns.

IV. FAMILY-CENTERED

Approximately 80% of children placed outside of the home are returned to their family of origin. In order to achieve successful reunification, whenever possible, we must consider the family of origin including siblings in assessments and services/supports for children placed in out-of-home care. Assessment and services/supports should be both child-focused and family-centered. The definition of family includes biological, foster and adoptive parents, grandparent and their partners, as well as kinship caregivers and others who have primary responsibility for providing love, guidance, food, shelter, clothing, supervision, and protection for children and adolescents (National Peer Technical Assistance Network, 1997). Finally, other persons may be considered members of the family for purposes of assessment and services/supports depending on the family of origin, their culture, ethnicity, language and the culture of their community.

Professionals are expected to work in partnership with the family to:

- assess the individual strengths and needs of the children;
- assess the parents/families strengths and needs to effectively deal with their children's emotional/mental health and substance use needs;
- identify ways to effectively provide the appropriate mental health and substance use services/supports to children and their family; to determine the level of involvement required with the foster family to successfully return the child home; and
- determine the level/type of relationship which is needed between the foster parents and the birth parents to ensure the emotional/mental health and substance use needs of the child are met.

Some specific decisions need to be made early because they have a strong impact on a child's experience while in foster care. These include the following:

- if a child and his birth family can be in immediate and continuing contact (face-to-face visitation and/or by telephone) to decrease the trauma of separation; and
- if the birth parents and foster parents can be expected to communicate with each other to maximize continuity and mutuality in accomplishing therapeutic goals.

Initial assessments and follow up assessments should address these questions as well.

Family members, as defined above, should be considered essential partners for successful treatment unless there is evidence to the contrary. Unless mandated otherwise by the courts, there should always be family involvement in the assessment and reassessment process, the development of the individualized treatment plan and the treatment/support process. All treatment plans should be individualized for the child and family and include family treatment services and supports as part of the plan unless the courts have restricted access/contact due to safety issues or there is evidence to the contrary. The treatment plan should also be in keeping with the permanency plan for the child as well as the family service plan. When parents are mandated to not have contact and/or are not available to have contact with the child, the initial assessment and reassessments must address the impact of this loss upon the child and recommend effective interventions.

Placing a child in out-of-home care automatically expands the definition of their family, at least temporarily, to include the foster parents. This means including the foster parents' input in the ongoing assessment and treatment/support process. With family-centered practice, when indicated, families are supported and empowered to be an advocate for the needs of their child and for the services which will facilitate the family being successful in dealing with the emotional/mental health and substance use needs of their child. Other key components of family-centered practice include:

- focusing on the whole family as the unit of attention;
- organizing assistance in accord with the family's strengths while acknowledging but not emphasizing deficits;
- except where a child's safety is at risk, service planning and delivery should take family priorities into consideration;
- structuring treatment/support service delivery to ensure accessibility, minimal disruption of family integrity and routine; and
- sharing results of assessments/reassessments with the birth family when a child is returning home (should this not have been done for some reason during out-of-home care) or the adoptive families when a child is being adopted.

V.   **CULTURALLY SENSITIVE AND ADMINISTERED IN A CULTURALLY COMPETENT MANNER**
The assessment and reassessment of children and their families must take into account the influence of each family's heritage. This includes culture, ethnicity and religion and consists of-but is not limited to race, religion, gender, socioeconomic status, language, sexual orientation, geographic origin and location and their immigration status.

Clinicians and/or staff who perform assessments should develop specialized knowledge and understanding about the history, tradition, values, family systems, perceptions, communication styles and artistic expressions of major client groups that they serve (NASW, 2001). Acquiring this knowledge should be accompanied by a regular assessment of their own personal values, beliefs, and biases in an effort to inform their practice and increase the quality of relationships they have with the children and families they serve (NASW, 2001).

This cross-cultural knowledge and personal awareness should be considered and applied to all approaches, skills, and techniques when working with children and families (NASW, 2001). This kind of approach is necessary to understand the stigma and shame that many cultures associate with mental health and substance use issues. This insight will help clinicians and/or staff to better understand the kind of help people seek, the types of coping and communication styles, social supports needed and the level of resistance to treatment that can be expected from the children and families they serve (DHHS, 2001).

In all circumstances, special consideration should be given to ensure that there are adequate numbers of clinicians and staff who speak the language(s) of the client groups served and when not available that there are procedures in place for obtaining translation and/or interpreter services.

In addition, it is necessary to ensure that all screening tools, protocols, instruments and approaches used in the mental health and substance use screening, assessment, reassessment and treatment process are tailored for the population being served.

This commitment to cultural competence is essential to adequately assess and treat the mental health and substance use needs of children and families in the foster care system. It is recommended that there be a monitoring process to ensure this takes place (DHHS, 2001).

VI. PERIODICALLLY REPEATED WITH STANDARDIZED COLLECTION OF HEALTH INFORMATION

Since all foster children are at serious risk for mental health and/or substance use problems, they need individualized reassessment. The appropriate intervals depend on the severity of the child's disturbance and the family's needs and must be determined on a case-by-case basis that is consistent with requirements for case planning.

Children who are found at initial screening to have mental health and/or substance use problems need to be treated and reassessed at regular intervals as recommended by guidelines from AACAP, the American Academy of Pediatrics and/or CWLA. Reassessments should collect standardized information needed to ensure continuity of care.

Children who need psychotropic medications, including psychostimulants, should be reassessed following the AACAP Policy Statement, "Prescribing Psychoactive Medications for Children and Adolescents." During the initial stabilization period, children should be reassessed frequently and have immediate access to a psychiatrist if they experience any difficulty adjusting to their medication. Once the child is stabilized on a standard dose of medication, he or she should be reassessed in a face-to-face interview no less than every three months. When children are moved to a new placement, all medications should be turned over to the caregiver at the next placement to ensure continuity of care. Once a child has settled into his or her new placement, all medications should be reassessed to determine if any adjustments are needed. It is crucial that this assessment and reassessment process include clear and regular communication between the clinical service provider and the caregiver(s) where the child is living.

Children and families who are adjusting well to foster care and are in no apparent need of mental health and substance use intervention should also be reassessed in face-to-face interviews at regular intervals-no less than every 12 months or as requested by the child or family. Given the level of vulnerability of children and the potential to be re-victimized/traumatized, professionals must assess and reassess to ensure the ongoing safety and well-being of children in out-of-home care.

Children about to leave the system whether moving to self-sufficiency or returning home should be reassessed. Recognition should be given that children moving into self-sufficiency may still require assistance in dealing with issues related to their family and their individual mental health and substance use needs. Those who need, or desire further mental health and substance use services should have adequate referral and follow-up plans in place to assure proper continuity of care. All parties involved in the child's care should be notified of any follow-up appointments. The clinician should follow the standard procedures (locale specific) that are in place to document summary reports and to assure that the child's health data is conveyed to the next provider or caregiver.

VII. CONCLUSION

These most vulnerable and traumatized of children need and deserve appropriate screening, comprehensive assessment and reassessments, effective mental health and substance use treatment services/supports provided by appropriately trained individuals, including the active involvement, when indicated, of a child and adolescent psychiatrist. We urge local, state and federal authorities to work together with the mental health, substance use and child welfare professions and other relevant child and family serving systems to assure that these children's mental health and substance use needs are met and that the children have the skills, capacities, and support necessary to thrive.

REFERENCES

American Academy of Child and Adolescent Psychiatrists. (2001, September). *Psychiatric care of children in the foster care system.* Retrieved from www.aacap.org/publications/policy/ps45.htm

Child Welfare League of America. (1988). *CWLA Standards for health care service for children in out of home care.* Washington, DC. Author.

National Peer Technical Assistance Network's Partnership for Children's Mental Health. (1997). *Family-professional relationships: Moving forward together.* Alexandria, VA: Federation of Families for Children's Mental Health.

National Association of Social Workers. (2001, June). *Standards for cultural competence in social work practice.* In Standard 3: Cross-cultural knowledge. Retrieved from www.naswdc.org/pubs/standards/cultural.htm #Standard 2

U. S. Department of Health and Human Services. (2001). Mental health: Culture, race, and ethnicity-a supplement to mental health: A report of the surgeon general. (DHHS Publication No. SMA-01-3613). Rockville, MD: DHHS, Substance Abuse and Mental Health Services Administration, Center for Mental Health Services.

American Academy of Pediatrics. (2000). *Developmental Issues for Young Children in Foster Care.* Washington DC. Pediatrics Vol. 106 No.5. Pg. 1145-1150.

American Academy of Pediatrics. (2002). *Health Care of Young Children in Foster Care.* Washington DC. Pediatrics Vol. 109 No. 3. Pg. 536-541.

The Management of Acute Gastroenteritis in Young Children

• •

- *Clinical Practice Guideline*
- *Technical Report Summary*

Readers of this clinical practice guideline are urged to review the technical report to enhance the evidence-based decision-making process. The full technical report is available on the enclosed CD-ROM.

AMERICAN ACADEMY OF PEDIATRICS

Subcommittee on Acute Gastroenteritis, Provisional Committee on Quality Improvement

Clinical Practice Guideline: The Management of Acute Gastroenteritis in Young Children

ABSTRACT

This practice parameter formulates recommendations for health care providers about the management of acute diarrhea in children ages 1 month to 5 years. It was developed through a comprehensive search and analysis of the medical literature. Expert consensus opinion was used to enhance or formulate recommendations where data were insufficient.

The Provisional Committee on Quality Improvement of the American Academy of Pediatrics (AAP) selected a subcommittee composed of pediatricians with expertise in the fields of gastroenterology, infectious diseases, pediatric practice, and epidemiology to develop the parameter. The subcommittee, the Provisional Committee on Quality Improvement, a review panel of practitioners, and other groups of experts within and outside the AAP reviewed and revised the parameter. Three specific management issues were considered: (1) methods of rehydration, (2) refeeding after rehydration, and (3) the use of antidiarrheal agents. Main outcomes considered were success or failure of rehydration, resolution of diarrhea, and adverse effects from various treatment options. A comprehensive bibliography of literature on gastroenteritis and diarrhea was compiled and reduced to articles amenable to analysis.

Oral rehydration therapy was studied in depth; inconsistency in the outcomes measured in the studies interfered with meta-analysis but allowed for formulation of strong conclusions. Oral rehydration was found to be as effective as intravenous therapy in rehydrating children with mild to moderate dehydration and is the therapy of first choice in these patients. Refeeding was supported by enough comparable studies to permit a valid meta-analysis. Early refeeding with milk or food after rehydration does not prolong diarrhea; there is evidence that it may reduce the duration of diarrhea by approximately half a day and is recommended to restore nutritional balance as soon as possible. Data on antidiarrheal agents were not sufficient to demonstrate efficacy; therefore, the routine use of antidiarrheal agents is not recommended, because many of these agents have potentially serious adverse effects in infants and young children.

This practice parameter is not intended as a sole source of guidance in the treatment of acute gastroenteritis in children. It is designed to assist pediatricians by providing an analytic framework for the evaluation and treatment of this condition. It is not intended to replace clinical judgment or to establish a protocol for all patients with this condition. It rarely will provide the only appropriate approach to the problem. A technical report describing the analyses used to prepare this guideline and a patient education brochure are available through the American Academy of Pediatrics.

BACKGROUND

Although most children with gastroenteritis who live in developed countries have mild symptoms and little or no dehydration, a substantial number will have more severe disease. In the United States, an average of 220 000 children younger than 5 years are hospitalized each year with gastroenteritis, accounting for more than 900 000 hospital days. Approximately 9% of all hospitalizations of children younger than 5 years are because of diarrhea.[1] In addition, approximately 300 children younger than 5 years die each year of diarrhea and dehydration (R. I. Glass, written communication, February 1995). Clinicians should be aware that young infants who were premature and children of teenaged mothers who have not completed high school, had little or no prenatal care, and belong to minority groups are at higher risk of death caused by diarrhea (R. I. Glass, written communication, February 1995).

In the United States, the incidence of diarrhea in children younger than 3 years has been estimated to be 1.3 to 2.3 episodes per child per year; rates in children attending day care centers are higher.[2] Hospitalization and outpatient care for pediatric diarrhea result in direct costs of more than $2.0 billion per year.[3–5] There are also indirect costs to families. Surveys show that many health care providers do not follow recommended procedures for management of this disorder.[6] This practice parameter is intended to present current knowledge about the optimal treatment of children with diarrhea.

Children Covered by the Parameter

In this practice parameter, acute gastroenteritis is defined as diarrheal disease of rapid onset, with or without accompanying symptoms and signs, such as nausea, vomiting, fever, or abdominal pain. Although the emphasis of this parameter is on diarrhea, vomiting can be an important component of gastroenteritis and is addressed specifically below. These recommendations apply to children 1 month to 5 years of age who live in developed countries and who have no previously diagnosed disorders, including immunodeficiency, affecting major organ systems. Episodes of diarrhea lasting longer than 10 days, diarrhea accompanying failure to thrive, and vomiting with no accompanying diarrhea are not addressed. Although most patients meeting the criteria of this parameter will have viral or self-limited bacterial diarrhea, children with bacterial dysentery or protozoal disease can be treated according to the principles presented herein but may benefit from specific antimicrobial therapy.

Outcomes Studied

The major outcomes studied in this analysis of management options were success or failure of rehydration, resolution of diarrhea, and adverse effects of antidiarrheal agents.

Target Audience and Settings

This parameter was designed to aid physicians, nurse practitioners, physician assistants, nurses, and other health care providers who care for children with acute diarrheal disease in outpatient and inpatient settings. It is meant to guide treatment of such children; clinical judgment guided by the special circumstances of each situation will determine the ultimate care of any individual child and may vary from the management outlined herein.

Sources of Information

Ideally, medical information and recommendations are derived from well-designed, properly analyzed scientific studies. When such data are not available on a given subject, consensus may be obtained from experts in the field. In this parameter, three specific topics have received in-depth analysis: rehydration, reintroduction of feeding, and the use of medications designed to influence diarrhea and to provide symptomatic relief. These issues were chosen because of their importance in the management of diarrhea, because there is evidence that practitioners need more information in these areas, and because data are available for study.

In researching these key aspects of the management of acute gastroenteritis, references were identified through MEDLINE searches using the terms *gastroenteritis, diarrhea,* and *diarrhea, infantile* to provide an initial, broad database of articles. In addition, specific MEDLINE searches were conducted for various antidiarrheal agents. To supplement the MEDLINE results, articles also were obtained from a number of other sources, including personal files of subcommittee members, bibliographies of articles identified through the computer search, the Centers for Disease Control and Prevention report on management of acute diarrhea in children,[7] the *Federal Register* notice,[8] and a petition to the Food and Drug Administration from the consumer group Public Citizen (written communication, January 1993). More than 4000 articles were included on the original list; after evaluation for relevance and validity, 230 articles were selected for complete review.

Sufficient randomized trials with similar outcomes performed in developed countries were available on early refeeding to allow the combining of results for meta-analysis. Many controlled studies on oral rehydration therapy (ORT) in developed countries were available, but the outcomes of these studies varied; it was not possible to combine their results quantitatively. Many trials on ORT performed in developing countries were available but were not included in this analysis. Few studies on specific antidiarrheal agents were available, although the committee examined reports on drug therapy from developing as well as developed countries. Recommendations have been drawn from analysis of available literature and have been augmented by expert consensus opinion. The sources and validity of data underlying the committee's conclusions are indicated. Further details on the literature review and analyses are available in the technical report. A summary of the technical report follows this practice parameter.

Other clinical decisions must be addressed when treating children with gastroenteritis, eg, when to obtain stool cultures, the appropriate use of antibiotics, and the prevention of diarrhea. Extensive evaluation of these issues has not been included as part of this parameter. For additional information, the reader is referred to the general review articles that address many of these issues in detail.

REHYDRATION AND REFEEDING: SCIENTIFIC BACKGROUND

ORT

Recommendation. **ORT is the preferred treatment of fluid and electrolyte losses caused by diarrhea in children with mild to moderate dehydration** (based on evaluation of controlled clinical trials documenting the effectiveness of ORT; an explanation of what constitutes a recommendation can be found in the technical report).

Replacement of fluid and electrolyte losses is the critical central element of effective treatment of acute diarrhea. Beginning with initial studies conducted 150 years ago, investigators have demonstrated that stool losses of water, sodium, potassium, chloride, and base must be restored to ensure effective rehydration.[9–11] Approximately 60 years ago, intravenous (IV) therapy became the first successful routine method of administration of fluid and electrolytes and was widely accepted as the standard form of rehydration therapy.[12] The treatment of diarrhea was advanced further in the mid-1960s with the discovery of coupled transport of sodium and glucose (or other small, organic molecules), providing scientific justification for ORT as an alternative to IV therapy.[12]

ORT has obvious potential advantages over IV therapy; it is less expensive and can be administered in many settings, including at home by family members. The first studies comparing oral glucose-electrolyte solutions with standard IV therapy were conducted successfully in patients with cholera in Bangladesh and India in the late 1960s.[13,14] The solutions used were similar to the oral rehydration salt solution recommended by the World Health Organization and the United Nations Children's Fund that has been used successfully throughout the world for more than 20 years.

During the past decade, a series of studies from developed countries has proved the effectiveness of ORT compared with IV therapy in children with diarrhea from causes other than cholera.[15–19] These studies evaluated glucose-electrolyte ORT solutions with sodium concentrations ranging from 50 to 90 mmol/L compared with rapidly administered IV therapy. These ORT solutions successfully rehydrated more than 90% of dehydrated children and had lower complication rates than those for IV therapy.[15] The cost of ORT, when hospitalization can be spared, is substantially less than that of IV therapy,[17] but the frequency of stools, duration of diarrhea, and rate of weight gain are similar with both therapies.[15–19]

A variety of oral solutions are available in the United States (Table 1). Those most readily available commercially and used most commonly have sodium concentrations ranging from 45 to 50 mmol/L, which is at or just less than the lower concentration of the solutions studied. Although these products are best suited for use as maintenance solutions, they can rehydrate satisfactorily otherwise healthy

TABLE 1. Composition of Representative Glucose-Electrolyte Solutions*

Solution	CHO, mmol/L	Na, mmol/L	K, mmol/L	Base, mmol/L	Osmolality
Naturalyte (unlimited beverage)	140	45	20	48	265
Pediatric electrolyte (NutraMax)	140	45	20	30	250
Pedialyte (Ross)	140	45	20	30	250
Infalyte (formerly Ricelyte; Mead Johnson)	70	50	25	30	200
Rehydralyte (Ross)	140	75	20	30	310
WHO/UNICEF oral rehydration salts†	111	90	20	30	310

* Adapted from Snyder J. The continuing evolution of oral therapy for diarrhea. *Semin Pediatr Infect Dis.* 1994;5:231–235. CHO, carbohydrate; Na, sodium; K, potassium; WHO, World Health Organization; UNICEF, United Nations Children's Fund.

† Available from Jaianas Bros Packaging Co, 2533 SW Blvd, Kansas City, MO 64108.

children who are mildly or moderately dehydrated.[15,16,20] Glucose-electrolyte solutions such as these, which are formulated on physiologic principles, must be distinguished from other popular but nonphysiologic liquids that have been used inappropriately to treat children with diarrhea (Table 2). These beverages have inappropriately low electrolyte concentrations for ORT use and are hypertonic, owing to their high carbohydrate content.[6] Parents should be discouraged from using nonphysiologic solutions to treat children with diarrhea.

Although glucose-electrolyte ORT is extremely effective in replacing fluid and electrolyte losses, it has no effect on stool volume or the duration of diarrhea. To address this limitation, investigators have administered cereal-based solutions that include naturally occurring food polymers from starch, simple proteins, and a variety of other substrates. Starch and simple proteins provide more cotransport molecules with little osmotic penalty, thus increasing fluid and electrolyte uptake by enterocytes and reducing stool losses.[21,22] The best studied of these solutions contain rice, 50 g/L, instead of glucose. These solutions are not the same as rice water, which has a low concentration of glucose and glucose polymers and is used inappropriately in some parts of the United States, nor are they the same as a commercial product that derives its carbohydrates from glucose polymers purified from rice. Cereal-based ORT can reduce stool volume by more than 30% in children with toxicogenic diarrhea and by close to 20% in those with nontoxicogenic diarrhea.[22] Cereal- or rice powder–based solutions are not presently available commercially; early refeeding, however, can provide similar benefits (see following text).

Hypo-osmolar solutions containing glucose polymers to supply transport molecules also have been developed (Table 1). These solutions have shown no appreciable additional benefit compared with the standard glucose-electrolyte oral solution.[23]

Early Feeding of Appropriate Foods

Recommendation. **Children who have diarrhea and are not dehydrated should continue to be fed age-appropriate diets. Children who require rehydration should be fed age-appropriate diets as soon as they have been rehydrated** (based on evaluation of controlled clinical studies documenting the benefits of early feeding of liquid and solid foods).

Optimal oral therapy regimens have incorporated early feeding of age-appropriate foods as an integral component. When used with glucose-electrolyte ORT, early feeding can reduce stool output as much as cereal-based ORT can.[24,25] A variety of early feeding regimens have been studied, including human milk,[26–29] diluted and full-strength animal milk and animal milk formulas,[26,27,29–31] diluted and full-strength lactose-free formulas,[26,32,33] and staple food diets with milk.[28,30,31,34–37] These studies have demonstrated that unrestricted diets do not worsen the course or symptoms of mild diarrhea[27,28] and can decrease stool output[32,36,37] compared with ORT or IV therapy alone. The literature from developed countries on early refeeding[27,32,34,35] allows for meta-analysis, which shows that the duration of diarrhea may be reduced by 0.43 days (95% confidence interval, –0.74 to –0.12). Although these beneficial effects are modest,

TABLE 2. Composition of Representative Clear Liquids Not Appropriate for Oral Rehydration Therapy*

Liquid	CHO, mmol/L	Na, mmol/L	K, mmol/L	Base, mmol/L	Osmolality
Cola	700 (F,G)	2	0	13	750
Apple juice	690 (F,G,S)	3	32	0	730
Chicken broth	0	250	8	0	500
Sports beverage	255 (S,G)	20	3	3	330

* Adapted from Snyder J. The continuing evolution of oral therapy for diarrhea. *Semin Pediatr Infect Dis.* 1994;5:231–235. CHO, carbohydrate; F, fructose; G, glucose; K, potassium; Na, sodium; S, sucrose.

of major importance is the added benefit of improved nutrition with early feeding.[32,33]

A meta-analysis was performed to evaluate the use of lactose-containing feedings in children with diarrhea and concluded that 80% or more of children with acute diarrhea can tolerate full-strength milk safely.[38] Although reduction in intestinal brush-border lactase levels is often associated with diarrhea,[39] most infants with decreased lactase levels will not have clinical signs or symptoms of malabsorption.[7,39] Infants fed human milk can be nursed safely during episodes of diarrhea.[26] Full-strength animal milk or animal milk formula usually is well tolerated by children who have mild, self-limited diarrhea.[27,38] The combination of milk with staple foods, such as cereal, is an appropriate and well-tolerated regimen for children who are weaned.[28,30,34–37] In the past, the American Academy of Pediatrics (AAP) recommended gradual reintroduction of milk-based formulas or cow's milk in the management of acute diarrhea, beginning with diluted mixtures.[40] This recommendation has been reevaluated in light of recent data. If children are monitored to identify the few in whom signs of malabsorption develop, a regular age-appropriate diet, including full-strength milk, can be used safely.

The question of which foods are best for refeeding has been an issue of continuing study. Although agreement is not universal, clinical experience based on controlled clinical trials suggests that certain foods, including complex carbohydrates (rice, wheat, potatoes, bread, and cereals), lean meats, yogurt, fruits, and vegetables, are better tolerated.[24,25,36,37] Fatty foods or foods high in simple sugars (including tea, juices, and soft drinks) should be avoided.[7] Note that this is not the classic BRAT diet, which consists of bananas, rice, applesauce, and toast. Although these foods can be tolerated, this limited diet is low in energy density, protein, and fat.

REHYDRATION AND REFEEDING: MANAGEMENT GUIDELINES

The following therapeutic recommendations are based on the evaluation of available literature augmented by expert opinion, as described in previous sections. These recommendations are presented in schematic form in the algorithm.

General Considerations

Evaluation of Dehydration

Available published data have provided rigorous justification for the principles of ORT for diarrhea. Successful implementation of ORT starts with an evaluation of the child's degree of dehydration. Guidelines for assessment of dehydration and rehydration are listed in Table 3. If an accurate recent weight is available, determination of the percentage of weight lost is an objective measure of dehydration. Capillary refill time can be a helpful adjunctive measure to determine the degree of dehydration.[41] Although refill can be affected by fever, ambient temperature, and age,[42] the clinician should consider delayed capillary refill to be a sign of significant dehydration until proven otherwise. Urinary output and specific gravity are helpful measures to confirm the degree of dehydration and to determine that rehydration has been achieved. Parents should be taught the natural history of diarrhea and the signs of dehydration.

Electrolyte Measurement

Most episodes of dehydration caused by diarrhea are isonatremic, and serum electrolyte determinations are unnecessary. Electrolyte levels should be measured in moderately dehydrated children whose histories or physical findings are inconsistent with straightforward diarrheal episodes and in all severely dehydrated children. Clinicians should be aware of the features of hypernatremic dehydration, which can lead to neurologic damage and which requires special rehydration techniques. This condition can result from ingestion of hypertonic liquids (boiled milk and homemade solutions to which salt is added) or the loss of hypotonic fluids in the stool or urine. Irritability and fever may be present, and a doughy feel to the skin is a distinctive feature. The typical loose skin and tenting of the skin associated with the more common isotonic and hypotonic dehydration may not be present. In children receiving IV therapy, electrolyte levels should be measured initially and as therapy progresses. ORT can be used effectively in the treatment of both hypernatremic and hyponatremic dehydration, as well as isonatremic dehydration.

Vomiting

Vomiting occurs frequently in the course of acute gastroenteritis and sometimes may be the only manifestation. Almost all children who have vomiting and dehydration can be treated with ORT.[7] The key to therapy is to administer small volumes of a glucose-electrolyte solution frequently. Studies have indicated that therapy can be initiated with 5-mL (1-teaspoon) aliquots given every 1 to 2 minutes. Although this technique is labor intensive, it can be done by a parent and will deliver 150 to 300 mL/h.

As dehydration and electrolyte imbalance are corrected by the repeated administration of small amounts of the solution, vomiting often decreases in frequency. As the vomiting lessens, larger amounts of the solution can be given at longer intervals. When rehydration is achieved, other fluids, including milk, as well as food, may be introduced.

The use of a nasogastric tube is another option in a child with frequent vomiting; continuous rather than bolus infusion of ORT solution can result in improved absorption of fluid and electrolytes. Nasogastric infusion also can be used as a temporary expedient while IV access is being sought; however, nasogastric infusion should not be used in a comatose patient or in a child who may have ileus or an intestinal obstruction.

The committee did not evaluate the use of antiemetic drugs. Consensus opinion is that antiemetic drugs are not needed. Physicians who feel that antiemetic therapy is indicated in a given situation should be aware of potential adverse effects.

If vomiting continues despite efforts to administer an oral rehydrating solution, IV hydration is indicated, with return to the oral route when vomiting abates.

Refusal to Take an Oral Rehydrating Solution

Experience gained from more than 25 years of ORT use indicates that children who are dehydrated rarely refuse ORT; however, those who are not dehydrated may refuse the solution because of its salty taste. Children with mild diarrhea and no dehydration should be fed regular diets and do not require glucose-electrolyte solutions. As long as it is clear to the physician and parents that the child is not

TABLE 3. Assessment of Dehydration*

Variable	Mild, 3%–5%	Moderate, 6%–9%	Severe, ≥10%
Blood pressure	Normal	Normal	Normal to reduced
Quality of pulses	Normal	Normal or slightly decreased	Moderately decreased
Heart rate	Normal	Increased	Increased†
Skin turgor	Normal	Decreased	Decreased
Fontanelle	Normal	Sunken	Sunken
Mucous membranes	Slightly dry	Dry	Dry
Eyes	Normal	Sunken orbits	Deeply sunken orbits
Extremities	Warm, normal capillary refill	Delayed capillary refill	Cool, mottled
Mental status	Normal	Normal to listless	Normal to lethargic or comatose
Urine output	Slightly decreased	<1 mL/kg/h	<<1 mL/kg/h
Thirst	Slightly increased	Moderately increased	Very thirsty or too lethargic to indicate

* Adapted from Duggan et al.[7] See text regarding hypernatremic dehydration. The percentages of body weight reduction that correspond to different degrees of dehydration will vary among authors. The critical factor in assessment is the determination of the patient's hemodynamic and perfusion status. If a clinician is unsure of the category into which a patient falls, it is recommended that therapy for the more severe category be used.

† Bradycardia may appear in severe cases.

dehydrated and is in stable condition or showing improvement, special solutions need not be added to the regular feeding routine; however, young children should be given more fluids than usual during an episode of diarrhea.

Some practical techniques exist to induce reluctant children to drink glucose-electrolyte solutions. Administering the solution in small amounts at first may allow the child to get accustomed to the taste. Some commercial solutions have flavors added that do not alter their basic composition but may make them more palatable. Glucose-electrolyte solutions can be frozen into an ice-pop form, which may appeal to some children.

IV Therapy

Clinical studies strongly emphasize ORT; yet the clinician must know when and how to administer IV therapy, which maintains an important role in the treatment of children with diarrhea. All children who are severely dehydrated and in a state of shock or near shock require immediate and vigorous IV therapy. Children who are moderately dehydrated and who cannot retain oral liquids because of persistent vomiting also should receive fluids by the IV route, as should children who are unconscious or have ileus. Administration of ORT is labor intensive, requiring care givers who can administer small amounts of fluid at frequent intervals. If such personnel are not available, IV therapy is indicated.

Clinicians must evaluate a child's condition in light of the circumstances. If staff are skilled in IV administration and are unable to devote time to oral rehydration, and if reliable parents are not available, insertion of an IV line will be more expedient. Facility in IV therapy should not lead automatically to its use. Because children may show considerable improvement after periods of IV therapy, a child who is not severely dehydrated may be able to go home and complete rehydration orally, if proper follow-up is available, after receiving IV fluids for several hours in an emergency department or a similar facility.

The committee emphasizes the need for clinicians to recognize the advantages and disadvantages of both ORT and IV therapy in selecting the best treatment for an individual patient in a specific setting.

Costs

The major factor affecting the cost of rehydrating a child is the setting in which therapy occurs, with the expense increasing as one moves from home to office to emergency department or hospital ward. Oral rehydration is better suited to less-intensive levels of care, but clinicians must be certain that adequate assistance and supervision are available to provide effective therapy. If appropriate assistance is not available, a child may require hospital care for ORT. Clinicians should document the requirements of these patients to justify the need for such services to insurers.

Specific Therapy

The treatment of a child with diarrhea is directed primarily by the degree of dehydration present.

No Dehydration

ORT. Although ORT has been used to replace ongoing stool losses in children with mild diarrhea and no dehydration by giving 10 mL/kg for each stool,[7] these children are the least likely to take ORT, in part because of the salty taste of the solutions. If the stool output remains modest, a supplemental glucose-electrolyte solution may not be required if age-appropriate feeding is continued and fluid consumption is encouraged.

Feeding. Continued age-appropriate feeding, with the foods discussed above and increased fluid intake, may be the only therapy required if hydration is normal, which is the case in most US children with diarrhea. Infants should continue to drink human milk or regular strength formula. Older children may continue to drink milk.

Mild Dehydration (3% to 5%)

ORT. Dehydration should be corrected by giving 50 mL/kg ORT plus replacement of continuing losses during a 4-hour period.[7] Replacement of continuing losses from stool and emesis is accomplished by giving 10 mL/kg for each stool;[7] also, emesis volume is estimated and replaced. Reevaluation of hydration and replacement of losses should occur at least every 2 hours.

Feeding. As soon as dehydration is corrected, feeding should begin and should follow the guidelines given above.

Moderate Dehydration (6% to 9%)

ORT. Dehydration is corrected by giving 100 mL/kg ORT plus replacement of continuing losses during a 4-hour period. Rapid restoration of the circulating volume helps correct acidosis and improves tissue perfusion, which aids the early refeeding process. At the end of each hour of rehydration, hydration should be assessed, and continuing stool and emesis losses should be calculated with the total added to the amount remaining to be given. This task may be accomplished best in a supervised setting, such as an emergency department, urgent-care facility, or physician's office.

Feeding. When rehydration is complete, feeding should be resumed and should follow the guidelines given above.

Severe Dehydration (≥10%)

Severe dehydration causes shock or a near-shock condition and is a medical emergency. The key to the treatment of the severely dehydrated child is bolus IV therapy with a solution such as normal saline or Ringer's lactate. A common recommendation is to give 20 mL/kg of body weight during a 1-hour period; however, larger quantities and much shorter periods of administration may be required.

Electrolyte levels must be determined in children with severe dehydration. Frequent clinical reevaluation is critical. If the patient does not respond to rapid bolus rehydration, the clinician should consider the possibility of an underlying disorder, including, but not limited to, septic shock, toxic shock syndrome, myocarditis, myocardiopathy, or pericarditis.

For appropriate guidance in treating these critically ill patients, the reader is referred to comprehensive reviews.[43–45]

ORT. When the patient's condition has stabilized and mental status is satisfactory, ORT may be instituted, with the IV line kept in place until it is certain that IV therapy is no longer needed.

Feeding. When rehydration is complete, feeding should be resumed and should follow the guidelines given above.

THERAPY WITH ANTIDIARRHEAL COMPOUNDS

Drugs are used to alter the course of diarrhea by decreasing stool water and electrolyte losses, shortening the course of illness, or relieving discomfort. Passage of a formed stool is not in itself a measure of successful therapy, because water can remain high in formed stools. Such cosmetic changes may give patients or their families a false sense of security, causing a delay in seeking more effective therapy.

A variety of pharmacologic agents have been used to treat diarrhea. These compounds may be classified by their mechanisms of action, which include: (1) alteration of intestinal motility, (2) alteration of secretion, (3) adsorption of toxins or fluid, and (4) alteration of intestinal microflora. Some agents may have more than one mechanism of action. Many of the agents have systemic toxic effects that are augmented in infants and children or in the presence of diarrheal disease; most are not approved for children younger than 2 or 3 years. Few published data are available to support the use of most antidiarrheal agents to treat acute diarrhea, especially in children. For the purposes of this review, these drugs have been grouped for analysis by their proposed mechanisms of action. Agents for which there are

sufficient available data are considered individually. Table 4 lists generic and brand names of the drugs commonly used to treat persons with diarrhea.

Recommendation. **As a general rule, pharmacologic agents should not be used to treat acute diarrhea** (based on limited studies and strong committee consensus).

Drugs That Alter Intestinal Motility

Loperamide

Loperamide is a piperadine derivative, chemically related to meperidine, which decreases transit velocity and may increase the ability of the gut to retain fluid. Loperamide also may inhibit calmodulin, a protein involved in intestinal transport. Loperamide is more specific for the μ-opiate receptors of the gut and thus has fewer of the effects on the central nervous system associated with other opiates.[46] Under certain controlled conditions, it also has been shown to have antisecretory properties, but this effect was not seen in an adult volunteer model of acute gastroenteritis.[47] Well-designed clinical trials in both adults and children have demonstrated some beneficial effects of loperamide in the treatment of acute diarrhea.[47–49] Loperamide, when used in conjunction with oral rehydration, reduced the volume of stool losses and shortened the course of disease in children 3 months to 3 years of age. These effects, although statistically significant, were not clinically significant, and the small number of studies makes it difficult to combine them in a meaningful way. In addition, many of the studies and case reports involving children have shown unacceptably high rates of side effects, including lethargy, ileus, respiratory depression, and coma, especially in infants.[7,48,50–55] Death also has been associated with loperamide therapy.[51]

Recommendation. **Loperamide is not recommended to treat acute diarrhea in children** (based on limited scientific evidence that the risks of adverse effects of loperamide outweigh its limited benefits in reducing stool frequency, and on strong committee consensus).

Other Opiates

Few data support the use of other opiate analogues or opiate and atropine combinations (Table 4) to treat diarrhea in children. The potential for toxic side effects is a major con-

---

TABLE 4. Medications Used to Relieve Symptoms in Patients With Acute Diarrhea*

Alteration of intestinal motility
  Opiates
    Loperamide (Imodium, Imodium-AD, Maalox Antidiarrhea, Pepto Diarrhea Control)
    Difenoxin and atropine (Motofen)†
    Diphenoxylate and atropine (Lomotil)†
    Tincture of opium (paregoric)†
Alteration of secretion
  Bismuth subsalicylate (Pepto-Bismol)
Adsorption of toxins and water
  Attapulgite (Diasorb, Donnagel, Kaopectate, Rheaban)
Alteration of intestinal microflora
  Lactobacillus (Pro-Bionate, Superdophilus)

* The actual formulations marketed under these trade names change frequently. More changes are anticipated in the near future based on Food and Drug Administration rulings. Other medications with similar mechanisms of action may be available.
† Requires prescription.

cern.[49,56–59] Opiates can produce respiratory depression, altered mental status, and ileus. These drugs pose an additional danger to individuals with fever, toxemia, or bloody stools, because they have been shown to worsen the course of diarrhea in patients with shigellosis,[60] antimicrobial-associated colitis,[61] and diarrhea caused by *Escherichia coli* 0157:H7.[62]

Recommendation. **Opiates as well as opiate and atropine combination drugs are contraindicated in the treatment of acute diarrhea in children** (based on limited scientific evidence and strong committee consensus).

Anticholinergic Agents

Parasympatholytic agents have been used in the treatment of acute gastroenteritis to decrease the cramping associated with diarrhea. They exert their effect on gastrointestinal tract smooth muscle by decreasing motility and reducing tone. Few data are available to document the efficacy of these agents in children with diarrhea. A placebo-controlled trial of the drug mepenzolate bromide in adults failed to demonstrate a positive effect, and many anticholinergic side effects were reported.[63] A dry mouth, the most frequently observed side effect, may alter the clinical evaluation of dehydration. Infants and young children are especially susceptible to the toxic effects of anticholinergic drugs.[64] Coma, respiratory depression, and paradoxical hyperexcitability have been reported.[64]

Recommendation. **Anticholinergic agents are not recommended in the management of diarrhea in children** (based on limited scientific evidence and strong committee consensus).

Alteration of Secretion

Bismuth Subsalicylate

Bismuth subsalicylate, as well as bismuth subnitrate and bismuth subgallate, has been used as adjunctive therapy for acute diarrhea. The mechanism of action of these compounds is uncertain, although laboratory studies have shown that bismuth subsalicylate inhibits intestinal secretion caused by enterotoxicogenic *E coli* and cholera toxins.[65] Controlled trials have demonstrated that bismuth subsalicylate reduced the frequency of unformed stools and increased stool consistency in adults with traveler's diarrhea[66] and in volunteers receiving the Norwalk virus.[67] A controlled clinical trial in children with acute diarrhea demonstrated that the administration of bismuth subsalicylate was associated with a decreased duration of diarrhea and a decreased frequency of unformed stools.[68] A second controlled trial in children receiving only oral therapy for acute diarrhea found that bismuth subsalicylate administration was associated with a shorter duration of diarrhea, decreased total stool output, decreased need for intake of an oral rehydration solution, and reduced hospitalization,[69] although criteria for hospital discharge were not standardized in this study. Overall, the beneficial effects have been modest, and the treatment regimen involves a dose every 4 hours for 5 days. Salicylate absorption after ingestion of a bismuth subsalicylate compound has been reported in adults[70] and children.[71] Insufficient data exist as to the risk of Reye syndrome associated with this compound; such a risk is of at least theoretical concern. Bismuth-associated encephalopathy and other toxic effects have been reported

after the long-term ingestion of high doses of bismuth-containing compounds.[72]

Recommendation. **The routine use of bismuth subsalicylate is not recommended in the treatment of children with acute diarrhea** (based on limited scientific evidence that the benefit of bismuth subsalicylate is modest in most children with diarrhea because of concerns about toxic effects, and on committee consensus; further studies may demonstrate a therapeutic role for this agent).

Adsorption of Fluid and Toxins

Adsorbents

Several antidiarrheal compounds are reported to work by adsorbing bacterial toxins and by binding water to reduce the number of bowel movements and to improve stool consistency. Kaolin-pectin, fiber, and activated charcoal are classified in this category, but the only such agent currently used widely is attapulgite. No conclusive evidence is available to show that these agents reduce the duration of diarrhea, stool frequency, or stool fluid losses.[50] Disadvantages include adsorption of nutrients, enzymes, and antibiotics in the intestine.[73]

Recommendation. **Adsorbents are not recommended for the treatment of diarrhea in children** (based on limited scientific evidence and committee consensus; efficacy has not been shown, although major toxic effects are not a concern).

Alteration of Intestinal Microflora

Lactobacillus

Lactobacillus is administered to patients with acute diarrhea to alter the composition of the intestinal flora.[74] Normally, saccharolytic bacteria in the intestine ferment dietary carbohydrates that have not been absorbed completely, causing a decrease in pH that produces short-chain fatty acids and deters intestinal pathogens. The short-chain fatty acids are absorbed through the colonic mucosa and facilitate absorption of water. When a patient has diarrhea, the fecal flora are diminished, production of short-chain fatty acids is reduced, and colonic absorption of water is impaired.[75] There is no consistent evidence that administration of *Lactobacillus*-containing compounds alters the course of diarrhea.[76,77] The supplementation of infant formula with *Bifidobacterium bifidum* and *Streptococcus thermophilus* has been shown to reduce the incidence of acute diarrhea and rotavirus shedding in hospitalized infants.[78] Two studies of young children demonstrated a reduction in the duration of diarrhea caused by rotavirus associated with the administration of *Lactobacillus GG*.[79,80] Additional research is needed in the area of bacterial interference using *Lactobacillus*-containing compounds.[77]

Recommendation. **Lactobacillus-containing compounds currently are not recommended in the treatment of acute diarrhea in children** (based on limited scientific evidence and committee consensus; efficacy has not been shown, although toxic effects are not a concern).

Newer Treatments for Diarrhea

Several medications have shown promise in the treatment of acute diarrhea on an experimental basis, mostly in studies involving adults. These include derivatives of berberine,[81] nicotinic acid, clonidine,[82] chloride channel blockers,[83] calmodulin inhibitors,[84] octreotide acetate,[85] and nonsteroidal anti-inflammatory drugs. All of these agents must be considered experimental at this time.

Other Agents

A variety of drugs not discussed herein are used in clinical practice to treat diarrhea. Little evidence exists regarding their safety or efficacy; therefore, they cannot be recommended.

RESEARCH ISSUES

In developing this practice parameter, the committee reviewed a large body of literature, but only a fraction was amenable to rigorous scientific analysis. Only the issue of refeeding was supported by a sufficient number of comparable studies to allow meta-analysis. The systematic evaluation of the evidence for the remaining questions points to areas that need more research. In particular, the usefulness of drug therapy for acute gastroenteritis needs to be examined more closely. In developed countries, studies of ORT that focus on factors such as barriers to implementation, costs, and acceptability to parents and health care providers would help facilitate its use.

The practice parameter, "The Management of Acute Gastroenteritis in Young Children," was reviewed by the appropriate committees and sections of the AAP, including the Chapter Review Group, a focus group of office-based pediatricians representing each AAP district: Gene R. Adams, MD; Robert M. Corwin, MD; Lawrence C. Pakula, MD; Barbara M. Harley, MD; Howard B. Weinblatt, MD; Thomas J. Herr, MD; Kenneth E. Mathews, MD; Diane Fuquay, MD; Robert D. Mines, MD; and Delosa A. Young, MD. Comments also were solicited from relevant outside medical organizations. The clinical algorithm was developed by James R. Cooley, MD, Harvard Community Health Plan.

References

1. Cicirello HG, Glass RI. Current concepts of the epidemiology of diarrheal diseases. *Semin Pediatr Infect Dis*. 1994;5:163–167
2. Pickering LK, Hadler SC. Management and prevention of infectious diseases in day care. In: Feigin RD, Cherry JC, eds. *Textbook of Pediatric Infectious Diseases*. Philadelphia: WB Saunders; 1992:2308–2334
3. Glass RI, Ho MS, Lew J, Lebaron CW, Ing D. Cost-benefit studies of rotavirus vaccine in the United States. In: Sack DA, Freij L, eds. *Prospects for Public Health Benefits in Developing Countries From New Vaccines Against Enteric Infections*. Swedish Agency Research Cooperation With Developing Countries; 1990;2:102–107. Conference Report
4. Avendano P, Matson DO, Long J, Whitney S, Matson CC, Pickering LK. Costs associated with office visits for diarrhea in infants and toddlers. *Pediatr Infect Dis J*. 1993;12:897–902
5. Matson DO, Estes MK. Impact of rotavirus infection at a large pediatric hospital. *J Infect Dis*. 1990;162:598–604
6. Snyder JD. Use and misuse of oral therapy for diarrhea: comparison of US practices with American Academy of Pediatrics' recommendations. *Pediatrics*. 1991;87:28–33
7. Duggan C, Santosham M, Glass RI. The management of acute diarrhea in children: oral rehydration, maintenance, and nutritional therapy. *MMWR*. 1992;41(RR-16):1–20
8. 51.83 *Federal Register* 16138
9. Pratt EL. Development of parenteral fluid therapy. *J Pediatr*. 1984;104:581–584
10. Powers GF. A comprehensive plan of treatment for the so-called intestinal intoxication of children. *Am J Dis Child*. 1926;32:232–257
11. Darrow DC, Pratt EL, Flett J Jr, et al. Disturbances of water and electrolytes in infantile diarrhea. *Pediatrics*. 1949;3:129–156
12. Hirschhorn NJ. The treatment of acute diarrhea in children: an historical and physiological perspective. *Am J Clin Nutr*. 1980;33:637–663
13. Hirschhorn NJ, Kinzie JL, Sachar DB, et al. Decrease in net stool output in cholera during intestinal perfusion with glucose-containing solutions. *N Engl J Med*. 1968;279:176–181
14. Pierce NF, Sack RB, Mitra RC, et al. Replacement of water and electrolyte losses in cholera by an oral glucose-electrolyte solution. *Ann Intern Med*. 1969;70:1173–1181
15. Santosham M, Daum RS, Dillman L, et al. Oral rehydration therapy of infantile diarrhea: a controlled study of well-nourished children hospitalized in the United States and Panama. *N Engl J Med*. 1982;306:1070–1076
16. Tamer AM, Friedman LB, Maxwell SR, Cynamon HA, Perez HN, Cleveland WW. Oral rehydration of infants in a large urban US medical center. *J Pediatr*. 1985;107:14–19
17. Listernick R, Zieserl E, Davis AT. Outpatient oral rehydration in the United States. *Am J Dis Child*. 1986;140:211–215
18. Vesikari T, Isolauri E, Baer M. A comparative trial of rapid oral and intravenous rehydration in acute diarrhoea. *Acta Paediatr Scand*. 1987;76:300–305
19. MacKenzie A, Barnes G. Randomized controlled trial comparing oral and intravenous rehydration therapy in children with diarrhoea. *Br Med J*. 1991;303:393–396
20. Santosham M, Burns B, Nadkami V, et al. Oral rehydration therapy for acute diarrhea in ambulatory children in the United States: a double-blind comparison of four different solutions. *Pediatrics*. 1985;76:159–166
21. Carpenter CC, Greenough WB, Pierce NF. Oral rehydration therapy: the role of polymeric substrates. *N Engl J Med*. 1988;319:1346–1348
22. Gore SM, Fontaine O, Pierce NF. Impact of rice based oral rehydration solution of stool output and duration of diarrhoea: meta-analysis of 13 clinical trials. *Br Med J*. 1992;304:287–291
23. Pizarro D, Posada G, Sandi L, Moran JR. Rice-based oral electrolyte solutions for the management of infantile diarrhea. *N Engl J Med*. 1991;324:517–521
24. Santosham M, Fayad I, Hashem M, et al. A comparison of rice-based oral rehydration solution and "early feeding" for the treatment of acute diarrhea in infants. *J Pediatr*. 1990;116:868–875
25. Fayad IM, Hashem M, Duggan C, Refat M, Bakir M, Fontaine O. Comparative efficacy of rice-based and glucose-based oral rehydration salts plus early reintroduction of food. *Lancet*. 1993;342:772–775
26. Khin MU, Nyunt-Nyunt W, Myokhin AJ, et al. Effect of clinical outcome of breast feeding during acute diarrhoea. *Br Med J*. 1985;290:587–589
27. Margolis PA, Litteer T. Effects of unrestricted diet on mild infantile diarrhea: a practice-based study. *Am J Dis Child*. 1990;144:162–164
28. Gazala E, Weitzman S, Weitzman Z, et al. Early versus late refeeding in acute infantile diarrhea. *Isr J Med Sci*. 1988;24:175–179
29. Fox R, Leen CL. Acute gastroenteritis in infants under 6 months old. *Arch Dis Child*. 1990;65:936–938
30. Rees L, Brook CGD. Gradual reintroduction of full-strength milk after acute gastroenteritis in children. *Lancet*. 1979; 1:770–771

31. Placzek M, Walker-Smith JA. Comparison of two feeding regimens following acute gastroenteritis in infancy. *J Pediatr Gastroenterol Nutr.* 1984;3:245–248

32. Santosham M, Foster S, Reid R, et al. Role of soy-based, lactose-free formula during treatment of acute diarrhea. *Pediatrics.* 1985;76:292–298

33. Brown KH, Gastanaduy AS, Saaverdra JM, et al. Effect of continued oral feeding on clinical and nutritional outcomes of acute diarrhea in children. *J Pediatr.* 1988;112:191–200

34. Hjelt K, Paerregaard A, Petersen W, Christiansen L, Krasilnikoff PA. Rapid versus gradual refeeding in acute gastroenteritis in childhood: energy intake and weight gain. *J Pediatr Gastroenterol Nutr.* 1989;8:75–80

35. Isolauri E, Vesikari T. Oral rehydration, rapid refeeding and cholestyramine for treatment of acute diarrhoea. *J Pediatr Gastroenterol Nutr.* 1985;4:366–374

36. Brown KH, Perez F, Gastanaduy AS. Clinical trial of modified whole milk, lactose-hydrolyzed whole milk, or cereal-milk mixtures for the dietary management of acute childhood diarrhea. *J Pediatr Gastroenterol Nutr.* 1991;12:340–350

37. Alarcon P, Montoya R, Perez F, Dongo JW, Peerson JM, Brown KH. Clinical trial of home available, mixed diets versus a lactose-free, soy-protein formula for the dietary management of acute childhood diarrhea. *J Pediatr Gastroenterol Nutr.* 1991;12:224–232

38. Brown KH, Peerson JM, Fontaine O. Use of nonhuman milks in the dietary management of young children with acute diarrhea: a meta-analysis of clinical trials. *Pediatrics.* 1994;93:17–27

39. Sunshine P, Kretchmer N. Studies of small intestine during development, III: infantile diarrhea associated with intolerance to disaccharides. *Pediatrics.* 1964;34:38–50

40. American Academy of Pediatrics, Committee on Nutrition. Use of oral fluid therapy and post-treatment feeding following enteritis in children in a developed country. *Pediatrics.* 1985;75:358–361

41. Saavedra JM, Harris GD, Li S, Finberg L. Capillary refilling (skin turgor) in the assessment of dehydration. *Am J Dis Child.* 1991;145:296–298

42. Schriger DL, Baraff L. Defining normal capillary refill: variation with age, sex, and temperature. *Ann Emerg Med.* 1988;17:932–935

43. Shaw KN. Dehydration. In: Fleisher GR, Ludwig R, eds. *Textbook of Pediatric Emergency Medicine.* 3rd ed. Baltimore, MD: Williams & Wilkins; 1993:147–151

44. Silverman BK, ed. *Advanced Pediatric Life Support.* 2nd ed. Elk Grove Village, IL: American Academy of Pediatrics, American College of Emergency Physicians; 1993

45. Chameides L, ed. *Textbook of Pediatric Advanced Life Support.* Dallas: American Heart Association, American Academy of Pediatrics; 1990

46. Schiller LR, Santa Ana CA, Morawski SG, Fordtran JS. Mechanism of the antidiarrheal effect of loperamide. *Gastroenterology.* 1984;85:1475–1483

47. Diarrhoeal Diseases Study Group (UK). Loperamide in acute diarrhoea in childhood: results of a double-blind, placebo controlled multicentre clinical trial. *Br Med J.* 1984;289:1263–1267

48. Motala C, Hill ID. Effect of loperamide on stool output and duration of acute infectious diarrhea. *J Pediatr.* 1990;117:467–471

49. Prakash P, Saxena S, Sareen DK. Loperamide versus diphenoxylate in the diarrhea of infants and children. *Indian J Pediatr.* 1980;47:303–306

50. World Health Organization. *The Rational Use of Drugs in the Management of Acute Diarrhoea in Children.* Geneva: World Health Organization; 1990

51. Bhutta TI, Tahir KI. Loperamide poisoning in children. *Lancet.* 1990;335:363

52. Chow CB, Li SH, Leung NK. Loperamide associated necrotizing enterocolitis. *Acta Pediatr Scand.* 1986;75:1034–1036

53. Minton NA, Smith PGD. Loperamide toxicity in a child after a single dose. *Br Med J.* 1987;294:1383

54. Herranz J, Luzuriaga C, Sarralle R, Florez J. Neurological symptoms precipitated by loperamide. *Anales Espanoles Pediatr.* 1980;13:1117–1120

55. Schwartz RH, Rodriguez WJ. Toxic delirium possibly caused by loperamide. *J Pediatr.* 1991;118:656–657

56. Ginsberg CM. Lomotil (diphenoxylate and atropine) intoxication. *Am J Dis Child.* 1973;125:241–242

57. Rumack BH, Temple AP. Lomotil poisoning. *Pediatrics.* 1974;53:495–500

58. Curtis JAQ, Goel KM. Lomotil poisoning in children. *Arch Dis Child.* 1979;54:222–225

59. Bala K, Khandpur S, Gujral V. Evaluation of efficacy and safety of lomotil in acute diarrheas in children. *Indian Pediatr.* 1979;16:903–907

60. DuPont HL, Hornick RB. Adverse effect of lomotil therapy in shigellosis. *JAMA.* 1973;226:1525–1528

61. Novak E, Lee JG, Seckman CE, Phillips JP, Disanto AR. Unfavorable effect of atropine-diphenoxylate (Lomotil) therapy in linomycin-caused diarrhea. *JAMA.* 1976;235:1451–1454

62. Pickering LK, Obrig TG, Stapleton FB. Hemolytic uremic syndrome and enterohemorrhagic *E coli. Pediatr Infect Dis J.* 1994;13:459–475

63. Reves R, Bass P, DuPont HL, Sullivan P, Mendiola J. Failure to demonstrate effectiveness of an anticholinergic drug in the symptomatic treatment of acute traveler's diarrhea. *J Clin Gastroenterol.* 1983;5:223–227

64. US Pharmacopeia. *Anticholinergic/Antispasmodics System.* Rockville, MD: US Pharmacopeia Dispensing Information; 1992;1:312

65. Ericsson CD, Evans DG, DuPont HL, Evans DJ Jr, Pickering LK. Bismuth subsalicylate inhibits activity of crude toxins of *Escherichia coli* and *Vibrio cholerae. J Infect Dis.* 1977;136:693–696

66. DuPont HL, Ericsson CD, Johnson PG, et al. Prevention of traveler's diarrhea by the tablet formulation of bismuth subsalicylate. *JAMA.* 1987;257:1347–1350

67. Steinhoff MC, Douglas RG Jr, Greenberg HB, Callahan DR. Bismuth subsalicylate therapy of viral gastroenteritis. *Gastroenterology.* 1980;78:1495–1499

68. Soriano-Brucher H, Avendano P, O'Ryan M, et al. Bismuth subsalicylate in the treatment of acute diarrhea in children: a clinical study. *Pediatrics.* 1991;87:18–27

69. Figueroa-Quintanilla D, Salazar-Lindo E, Sack RB, et al. A controlled trial of bismuth subsalicylate in infants with acute watery diarrheal disease. *N Engl J Med.* 1993;328:1653–1658

70. Feldman S, Chen SL, Pickering LK, Cleary TG, Ericsson CD, Hulse M. Salicylate absorption from a bismuth subsalicylate preparation. *Clin Pharmacol Ther.* 1981;29:788–792

71. Pickering LK, Feldman S, Ericsson CD, Cleary TG. Absorption of salicylate and bismuth from a bismuth subsalicylate-containing compound (Pepto-Bismol). *J Pediatr.* 1981;99:654–656

72. Mendelowitz PC, Hoffman RS, Weber S. Bismuth absorption and myoclonic encephalopathy during bismuth subsalicylate therapy. *Ann Intern Med.* 1990;112:140–141

73. Parpia SH, Nix DE, Hejmanowski LG, Goldstein HR, Wilton JH, Schentag JJ. Sucralfate reduces the gastrointestinal absorption of norfloxacin. *Antimicrob Agents Chemother.* 1989;33:99–102

74. Lidbeck A, Nord CE. Lactobacilli and the normal human anaerobic microflora. *Clin Infect Dis.* 1993;16(suppl 4): S181–S187

75. Ramakrishna BS, Mathan VI. Colonic dysfunction in acute diarrhoea: the role of luminal short chain fatty acids. *Gut.* 1993;34:1215–1218

76. Clements ML, Levine MM, Black RE, et al. *Lactobacillus* prophylaxis for diarrhea due to enterotoxigenic *Escherichia coli.* *Antimicrob Agents Chemother.* 1981;20:104–108

77. Reid G, Bruce AW, McGroorty JA, et al. Is there a role for lactobacilli in prevention of urogenital and intestinal infections? *Clin Microbiol Rev.* 1993;3:335–344

78. Saavedra JM, Bauman NA, Oung I, Perman JA, Yolken RH. Feeding *Bifidobacterium bifidum* and *Streptococcus thermophilus* to infants in hospital for prevention of diarrhoea and shedding of rotavirus. *Lancet.* 1994;334:1046–1049

79. Isolauri E, Juntunen M, Rautanen T, Sillanaukee P, Koivula T. A human *Lactobacillus* strain (*Lactobacillus casei*, sp strain GG) promotes recovery from acute diarrhea in children. *Pediatrics.* 1991;88:90–97

80. Kaila M, Isolauri E, Soppi E, Virtanen E, Laine S, Arvilommi H. Enhancement of the circulating antibody secreting cell response in human diarrhea by a human *Lactobacillus* strain. *Pediatr Res.* 1992;32:141–144

81. Donowitz M, Levine S, Watson A. New drug treatments for diarrhoea. *J Intern Med Suppl.* 1990;228:155–163

82. Schiller LR, Santa Ana CA, Morawski SG, Fordtran JS. Studies of the antidiarrheal action of clonidine: effects on motility and intestinal absorption. *Gastroenterology.* 1985; 89:982–988

83. Bridges RJ, Worrell RT, Frizzell RA, Benos DJ. Stilbene disulfonate blockade of colonic secretory Cl-channels in planar lipid bilayers. *Am J Physiol.* 1989;256:907–912

84. DuPont HL, Ericsson CD, Mathewson JJ, Marani S, Knellwolf-Cousin AL, Martinez-Sandoval FG. Zalaride maleate, an intestinal calmodulin inhibitor, in the therapy of traveler's diarrhea. *Gastroenterology.* 1993;104:709–715

85. Cook DJ, Kelton JG, Stanisz AM, Collins SM. Somatostatin treatment for cryptosporidial diarrhea in a patient with the acquired immunodeficiency syndrome (AIDS). *Ann Intern Med.* 1988;108:708–709

General References

Duggan C, Santosham M, Glass RI. The management of acute diarrhea in children: oral rehydration, maintenance, and nutritional therapy. *MMWR.* 1992;41(RR-16):1–20

Pickering LK, Cleary TG. Approach to patients with gastrointestinal tract infections and food poisoning. In: Feigin RD, Cherry JC, eds. *Textbook of Pediatric Infectious Disease.* 3rd ed. Philadelphia: WB Saunders; 1992:565–596

Cohen MB, Balistreri WF. Diagnosing and treating diarrhea. *Contemp Pediatr.* 1989;6:89–114

Grisanti KA, Jaffe DM. Dehydration syndromes: oral rehydration and fluid replacement. *Emerg Med Clin North Am.* 1991;9:565–588

Management of acute diarrheal disease. Proceedings of a symposium, 1990. *J Pediatr.* 1991;118:S25–S138

Guerrant RL, Bobak DA. Bacterial and protozoal gastroenteritis. *N Engl J Med.* 1991;325:327–340

Pickering LK, Matson DO. Therapy for diarrheal illness in children. In: Blaser MJ, Smith PD, Ravdin JI, Greenburg HB, Guerrant RL, eds. *Infections of the Gastrointestinal Tract.* New York: Raven Press; 1995

Northrup RS, Flanigan TP. Gastroenteritis. *Pediatr Rev.* 1994;15:461–472

The Management of Acute Gastroenteritis in Young Children Algorithm

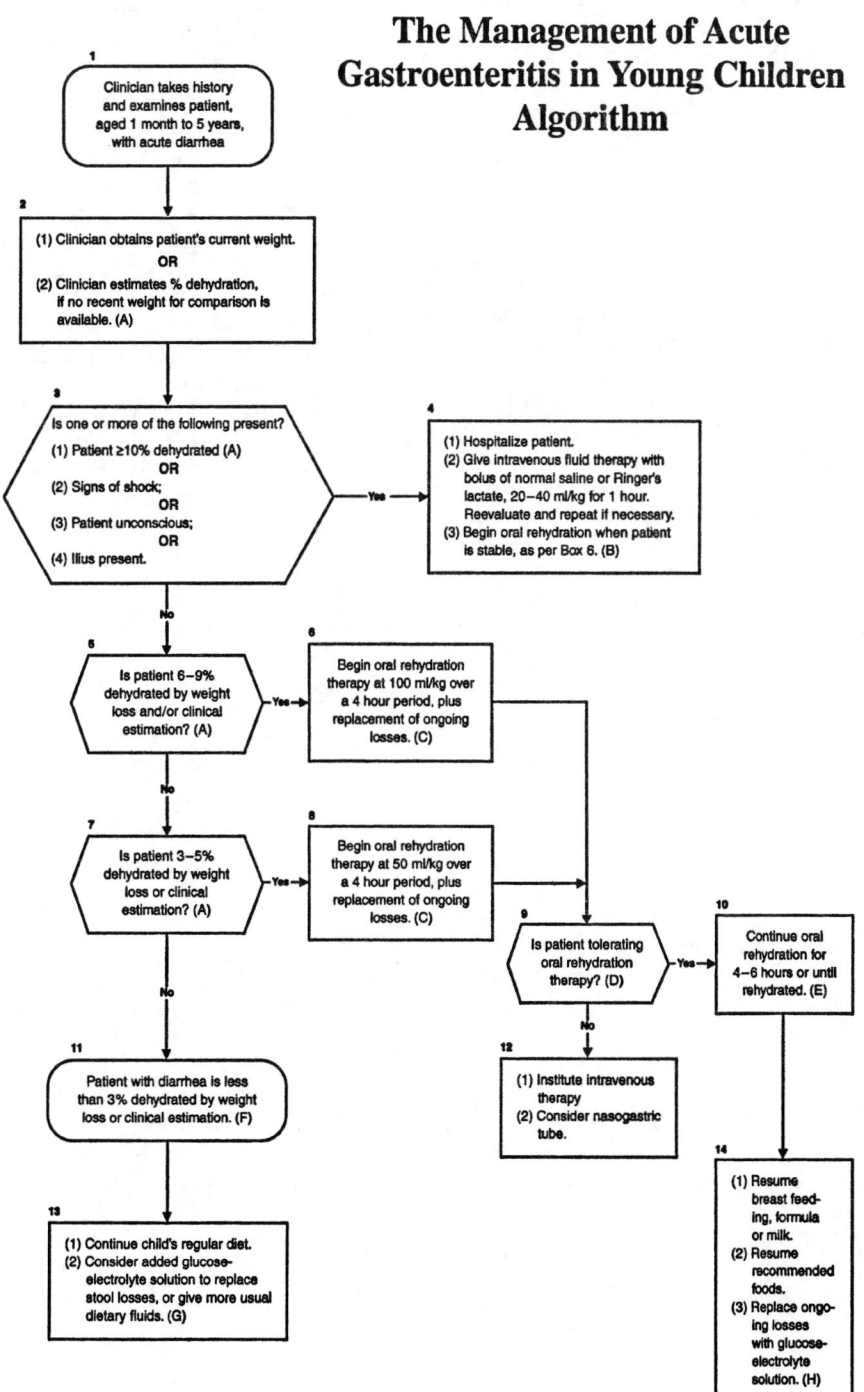

1 Clinician takes history and examines patient, aged 1 month to 5 years, with acute diarrhea

2
(1) Clinician obtains patient's current weight.
OR
(2) Clinician estimates % dehydration, if no recent weight for comparison is available. (A)

3 Is one or more of the following present?
(1) Patient ≥10% dehydrated (A)
OR
(2) Signs of shock;
OR
(3) Patient unconscious;
OR
(4) Ilius present.

4
(1) Hospitalize patient.
(2) Give intravenous fluid therapy with bolus of normal saline or Ringer's lactate, 20–40 ml/kg for 1 hour. Reevaluate and repeat if necessary.
(3) Begin oral rehydration when patient is stable, as per Box 6. (B)

5 Is patient 6–9% dehydrated by weight loss and/or clinical estimation? (A)

6 Begin oral rehydration therapy at 100 ml/kg over a 4 hour period, plus replacement of ongoing losses. (C)

7 Is patient 3–5% dehydrated by weight loss or clinical estimation? (A)

8 Begin oral rehydration therapy at 50 ml/kg over a 4 hour period, plus replacement of ongoing losses. (C)

9 Is patient tolerating oral rehydration therapy? (D)

10 Continue oral rehydration for 4–6 hours or until rehydrated. (E)

11 Patient with diarrhea is less than 3% dehydrated by weight loss or clinical estimation. (F)

12
(1) Institute intravenous therapy
(2) Consider nasogastric tube.

13
(1) Continue child's regular diet.
(2) Consider added glucose-electrolyte solution to replace stool losses, or give more usual dietary fluids. (G)

14
(1) Resume breast feeding, formula or milk.
(2) Resume recommended foods.
(3) Replace ongoing losses with glucose-electrolyte solution. (H)

Annotations for the Management of Acute Gastroenteritis in Young Children

Rehydration and Refeeding Algorithm

A. See Table 3 for guidance in the assessment of the degree of dehydration.

B. Restoration of cardiovascular stability is critical and is accomplished by giving bolus IV therapy with normal saline or Ringer's lactate solution (see text). In the patient who does not respond, consider the possibility of an underlying disorder, such as myocarditis, myocardiopathy, pericarditis, septic shock, or toxic shock syndrome. When the patient is in stable condition and has achieved satisfactory mental status, ORT can be used according to the ORT guidelines.

C. Solutions containing 45 to 90 mmol/L sodium should be given in a volume of 100 mL/kg for moderate dehydration and 50 mL/kg for mild dehydration. Giving the child these volumes requires patience and persistence, and progress must be monitored frequently.

D. Intractable, severe vomiting, unconsciousness, and ileus are contraindications to ORT. Persistent refusal to drink may require a trial of IV therapy.

E. The rehydration phase usually can be completed in 4 hours; reevaluation should occur every 1 to 2 hours. See text for guidance to decide when rehydration has been achieved.

F. The type and intensity of therapy will vary with the individual clinical situation.

G. Often, a child has diarrhea but remains adequately hydrated. The parent can be reassured but should be taught to assess hydration and to identify a worsening condition. If the stool output remains modest, ORT might not be required if early, age-appropriate feeding is instituted and increased consumption of usual dietary fluids is encouraged. More significant stool losses can be replaced with an oral rehydrating solution at the rate of 10 mL/kg for each stool.

H. Breastfeeding should be resumed. Nonlactose formula, milk-based formula, or milk may be given, although a small percentage of children will not tolerate lactose-containing fluids. Lactose-containing solutions seem to be tolerated better when combined with complex carbohydrates in weaned children. Children who are eating foods may resume eating, although certain foods are tolerated better than others. Recommended foods include complex carbohydrates (rice, wheat, potatoes, bread, and cereals), lean meats, yogurt, fruits, and vegetables. Avoid fatty foods and foods high in simple sugars (including juices and soft drinks). Supplement feeding with an oral electrolyte solution, 10 mL/kg for each diarrheal stool and the estimated amount vomited for each emesis.

Technical Report Summary:
Acute Gastroenteritis

Authors:
Gail Brown, MD, MPH
Peter Margolis, MD, PhD

The University of North Carolina at Chapel Hill

Epidemiologic Consultants to the Subcommittee on Gastroenteritis

American Academy of Pediatrics
PO Box 927, 141 Northwest Point Blvd
Elk Grove Village, IL 60009-0927

SUBCOMMITTEE ON ACUTE GASTROENTERITIS
1992 – 1995
Lawrence F. Nazarian, MD, Chairman

James H. Berman, MD

Gail Brown, MD, MPH

Peter A. Margolis, MD, PhD

David O. Matson, MD, PhD

Juhling McClung, MD

Larry K. Pickering, MD

John D. Snyder, MD

PROVISIONAL COMMITTEE ON QUALITY IMPROVEMENT
1993 – 1995
David A. Bergman, MD, Chairman

Richard D. Baltz, MD

James R. Cooley, MD

John B. Coombs, MD

Lawrence F. Nazarian, MD

Thomas A. Riemenschneider, MD

Kenneth B. Roberts, MD

Daniel W. Shea, MD

Liaison Representatives:

Michael J. Goldberg, MD
  Section Liaison

Charles J. Homer, MD, MPH
  Section on Epidemiology

Thomas F. Tonniges, MD
  AAP Board of Directors

INTRODUCTION

The practice parameter on acute gastroenteritis is intended to present current knowledge about optimal treatment of children with diarrhea. This technical report details the process followed in its development, and presents the evidence used to formulate the final recommendations.

METHODS

The approach to developing this guideline was based on the principles for guideline development outlined by Eddy and Woolf.

Development of the Evidence Model

Definitions

In this report and in the practice parameter, acute gastroenteritis is defined as diarrheal disease of rapid onset of 10 days' duration or less. Episodes of diarrhea may or may not be accompanied by other signs and symptoms, such as vomiting, fever, or pain.

The parameter applies to children aged 1 month to 5 years who live in developed countries and who have no previously diagnosed disorders affecting major organ systems, including immunodeficiency. Not addressed are episodes of diarrhea lasting longer than 10 days, diarrhea accompanying failure to thrive, or vomiting with no accompanying diarrhea. The practice parameter is not intended to apply to chronic intestinal disorders, inflammatory bowel disease, or other previously diagnosed chronic conditions affecting major organ systems. Children with dysentery can be treated according to the principles presented here but may benefit from specific antimicrobial therapy.

Target Audience

The intended users of the practice parameter include pediatricians, family physicians, general practitioners, emergency physicians, public health nurses and nurse practitioners, physician assistants, and staff members of nutritional support groups (eg, Supplemental Feeding Program for Women, Infants, and Children [WIC]), and other individuals or organizations interested in the nutrition of children.

The practice settings targeted are the offices of private pediatricians and family physicians, hospital outpatient departments, emergency departments, acute inpatient facilities, acute care ambulatory facilities, public health clinics, and WIC programs and other nutritional support programs.

Interventions

Diagnostic interventions discussed by the subcommittee (but not necessarily included in the parameter) included tests designed to determine the severity of the patient's condition (including urinalysis), the likely cause (stool pattern and microscopic examination), and positive identification of the organism (stool culture, blood culture, sensitivities, microscopic examination for ova and parasites, and rapid identification tests). Therapeutic interventions considered included hospital vs home therapy, rehydration/restoration of electrolyte balance (oral or intravenous [IV]) adjunctive drug therapy for symptom relief or hastening of recovery, empirical antimicrobial therapy, and restoration of normal nutritional status (when to resume feeding, what foods, progression of foods, timetable of pro-

gression of foods, etc). Public health interventions considered included the primary prevention of disease through appropriate day care procedures, including hand washing, diapering, and breastfeeding.

Outcomes

The subcommittee listed the following health outcomes as potentially related to the parameter:

1. Restoration of function: return to normal functioning and state of well-being, return to normal nutritional status, and return to normal daily activities (eg, day care/school).
2. Prevention of adverse health events: hospitalization, inappropriate emergency department visits, acute complications of acute gastroenteritis (eg, shock, acute renal failure, sagittal sinus thrombosis, and seizures), severe electrolyte imbalance, cardiac arrhythmias, and death.
3. Prevention of iatrogenic complications: worsening of dehydration, electrolyte imbalance, seizures, adverse-drug effects, and emergence of antibiotic-resistant organisms.
4. Avoidance of long-term complications of acute gastroenteritis: intractable diarrhea, prolonged carrier state of infectious organisms, and transmission of disease.
5. Improved patient (parental) satisfaction.
6. Cost.

Clinical outcomes used to measure improved status were expected to be state of hydration and electrolyte balance (weight, blood chemistry levels, and urine output); severity and duration of diarrhea, change in stool patterns, patient functioning (days in the hospital, and number of days out of school or day care), and the presence or absence of infectious organisms in the stool.

Although all of these outcomes were considered by the subcommittee in the initial stages of work on the parameter, not all were addressed in the parameter because of limitations in the available data.

Evidence Model

Each subcommittee member was asked to prepare a draft evidence model to help the subcommittee consider the aspects of the problem for which evidence would be required. After consideration of their models, the subcommittee chose three clinical management issues on which to focus. The three specific questions were as follows:

1. Is oral rehydration therapy (ORT) as effective as IV therapy for dehydration secondary to acute gastroenteritis?
2. For children without dehydration, or after a rehydration phase, does altering diet hasten the resolution of the disease?
3. Does drug therapy improve the course of diarrhea?

Literature Review

A literature search was conducted by staff at the American Academy of Pediatrics via the National Library of Medicine database using the terms *gastroenteritis* and *diarrhea, infantile*. The list of resulting articles was selectively reviewed by limiting studies to those involving human subjects and children older than 1 month and to the English-language literature.

For symptomatic drug therapy, staff performed a literature search using the terms *gastroenteritis* and *diarrhea*. Additional terms added to the search included *antacids, laxatives, digestants, antiemetics, bismuth, loperamide, attapulgite, diphenoxylate, scopolamine, hyoscyamine, lactobacillus, kaolin, pectin, hydroxyquinolones, toxiferine, dicyclomine, mepenzolate, donnatal, propantheline,* and *clidinium*. Addition of the term *parasympathetics* yielded no additional information. The resulting list of articles was selectively reviewed by limiting studies to those involving human subjects, and children older than 1 month, and to the English-language literature.

Additional articles were identified by subcommittee member input, bimonthly manual searches of current pediatric journals available in the American Academy of Pediatrics' library, comparison with bibliographies from other reviews, including The Public Citizen's group report to the Food and Drug Administration, *The Federal Register* notice, and the *MMWR* Recommendations and Reports on "The Management of Acute Diarrhea in Children: Oral Rehydration, Maintenance, and Nutritional Therapy." The subcommittee's literature database was compared with that in Current World Literature (sections on gastroenterology and nutrition, pathophysiology and physiology of carbohydrate absorption, and normal growth and nutrition). The two reference lists contained compatible information. This process produced no unpublished original studies.

Article Selection

Based on titles and abstract review, subcommittee members selected articles for full review. The reviewers were asked to include any article that reported outcomes of interests, specifically duration of disease, complications of therapy, parental satisfaction, and cost. Committee members were also asked to consider articles most useful if the population studied was comparable to the US population. To address the question of ORT vs IV therapy, only randomized clinical trials were considered.

A literature review form developed for this project was used by the subcommittee members to review all selected articles (Appendix). Reviewers classified articles by study type and study question. If the reviewers decided that an article did not meet the criteria listed above, it was no longer included as part of the data. If reviewers determined that an article was appropriate for inclusion, then the reviewer went on to summarize the population studied, methods, and outcomes. The form took less than an hour to complete.

The methodologists sorted the forms and articles as to clinical question and compared outcomes. Articles were incorporated into evidence tables, which formed the basis for discussion of the guidelines and also served as the background for decision making when studies could not be combined statistically.

Statistical Methods

When sufficient studies were available, the effectiveness of therapy was summarized by pooling data across studies. The difference between treatment and control groups was used as the measure of the relative benefit of one form of therapy over another. The overall impact of a therapy was calculated as the weighted average of the outcome measure across all studies (eg, mean duration and proportion of treatment failures). Pooled 95% confidence intervals (CIs) were calculated for each trial and for the combined data.

The similarity of data from different studies was assessed by reviewing plots of the data and by performing a test of homogeneity. Sensitivity analyses were performed to assess the importance of individual studies on overall conclusions.

Recommendations and Level of Evidence

Recommendations are made based on the quality of scientific evidence. In the absence of high-quality scientific evidence, subcommittee consensus or a combination of evidence and consensus is used as the basis for recommendations.

Clinical Options are actions for which the subcommittee failed to find compelling evidence to support or refute. A health care provider might or might not wish to implement clinical options in the treatment of a given child.

No recommendation is made when scientific evidence is lacking and there is no compelling reason to make an expert judgment.

RESULTS

The literature search identified 230 articles that could potentially be included in the parameter. Of these, 88 compared ORT with IV therapy for dehydration, 46 compared different refeeding strategies, and 76 reported the effects of symptomatic drug therapy. An additional 20 articles contained potentially useful general information.

ORT vs IV Therapy

Of the 88 articles initially accepted by the reviewers, five contained primary data concerning the outcomes of interest in children in developed countries. Unfortunately, these articles reported different outcomes. Outcomes reported in the studies included duration of diarrhea, weight gain, length of hospital stay, stool volume, costs, time to rehydration, stool frequency, electrolyte balance, and sodium intake. It was not possible to pool the estimates of effect across studies.

Complications of ORT and IV therapy were discussed in the five articles with original data. Two studies measured duration of illness, and two studies measured weight gain at hospital discharge. One of these studies found a statistically significant reduction in the duration of diarrhea among children receiving ORT. The other study of duration showed no difference between treatment groups. Neither study showed a significant difference in weight gain.

Although it was not possible to combine statistically the results of the five studies with original data, the tables were presented to all of the subcommittee members. These summaries, as well as data in the articles themselves, provided the basis for the recommendations. Based on an evaluation of the randomized trials documenting the effectiveness of ORT, the subcommittee recommended the use of ORT as the preferred treatment of fluid and electrolyte losses due to diarrhea in children with mild to moderate dehydration.

Refeeding

Of the 46 articles reviewed that dealt with early refeeding, 10 were combined into an evidence table. The other articles had outcomes that were not comparable or did not present original data. Four of the studies were conducted in developing countries, and six were conducted in developed countries. The studies used a variety of early refeeding regimens, including: breastfeeding, dilute soy, cow's milk formula, and rice-based formula. Because all of the studies compared dilute formula with undiluted formula and gradual reintroduction of feeding with reinstitution of normal feedings upon rehydration and used a comparable outcome measurement (duration of diarrhea), the results of the 10 studies were pooled. Data were insufficient to combine other outcomes, such as weight gain, stool output, or length of hospital stay.

The difference in the duration of diarrhea between dilute and undiluted feeding was used as the measure of effectiveness of the therapy. Combined data from all 10 studies revealed that in children who received full-strength feedings, diarrhea lasted 0.3 days (95% CI, −0.53, −0.07) less than in those in whom feedings were gradually reintroduced. However, a test of homogeneity yielded significant results (P=.011), indicating that the effectiveness of the therapy was not uniform among studies. A plot of the data from the studies suggested that studies from developing countries were associated with less of an effect of early refeeding than studies from developed countries. The plot also suggested that the study by Santosham et al might be influencing the results substantially.

Sensitivity analyses were performed to examine the impact in different studies on the duration of diarrhea. When studies from developing countries were excluded from the analysis, early refeeding was associated with 0.67 fewer days of diarrhea (95% CI, −0.96, −0.38) compared with gradual refeeding. However, the results of a test for homogeneity remained significant (P<.001). When the study by Santosham et al was excluded, the duration of diarrhea was 0.43 days less (95% CI, −0.74, −0.12), and the results of a test for homogeneity were not significant (P=.14). Exclusion of the study by Santosham et al from the original group of studies also resulted in nonsignificant results of a test of homogeneity. However, the observed reduction in the number of days of diarrhea also became nonsignificant.

In summary, these results suggest that early refeeding may be associated with a small reduction in the duration of diarrhea when studies from developed and developing countries are combined. When studies from only developed countries are considered, there is a reduction in the duration of diarrhea of about half a day. There is no evidence that early refeeding prolongs diarrhea over gradual refeeding. Based on this statistical analysis, the subcommittee observed that early refeeding appears to be associated with a clinically meaningful reduction in the duration of diarrhea and recommended the return to full-strength formula or normal feeding during an episode of diarrhea as soon as rehydration has been achieved.

Pharmacologic Therapy for Diarrhea

The literature search identified 76 articles that considered drug therapy for diarrhea. The search was not limited to studies performed in developed countries.

Four clinical trials of loperamide contained primary data and were compared in a table. The complications of these four trials were considered by the subcommittee. In addition, the four trials were combined in an evidence table that compared the duration of diarrhea in the study vs control groups. The subcommittee was impressed with the number of reports of toxic effects, especially in infants, and decided that the risks of adverse effects outweighed the limited benefits of loperamide, thus recommending that it not be used in children.

Four trials considered diphenoxylate in the treatment of acute diarrhea, but various outcomes, including duration of diarrhea, the proportion of patients responding, stool frequency, and water content of stools, were measured. Only two studies, which were summarized in an evidence table, reported duration of diarrhea. Complications reported in two studies ranged from sedation to poisoning. In light of the evidence, the subcommittee decided not to recommend the use of opiates in the management of acute diarrhea in childhood.

Two trials measured the effectiveness of bismuth subsalicylate in diarrheal disease in children. Both studies showed a decrease in duration of diarrhea in the treatment groups. However, the subcommittee observed that the benefit of bismuth subsalicylate would be minimal in most children and that there were no data about potential toxic effects. The subcommittee did not recommend the routine use of bismuth subsalicylate but recognized that future studies may demonstrate a role for this agent.

The remaining studies dealt with other pharmacologic agents or case reports of the agents mentioned above. There was not enough information on any one agent to recommend its routine use in children with diarrhea.

DISCUSSION

The parameter contains the following subcommittee recommendations:

1. Oral rehydration therapy is recommended as the preferred treatment of fluid and electrolyte losses due to diarrhea in children with mild to moderate dehydration.

2. Appropriate diets are recommended during an episode of diarrhea as soon as rehydration has been achieved.

3. Pharmacologic agents are not recommended to treat acute childhood diarrhea.

Oral rehydration therapy was studied in-depth, but variation in measured outcomes prevented pooling of results across studies. Refeeding was covered by enough comparable studies to perform a meta-analysis and to use these data in forming recommendations. Insufficient data were available on specific drugs to demonstrate their efficacy.

The step-by-step method followed in the development of the practice parameter outlined in this technical report helped to define the questions to be addressed and to arrive at consensus opinion. Ultimately, only the question of refeeding lent itself to meta-analysis. However, the systematic evaluation of the evidence for the remaining questions points to areas needing more research. In particular, the usefulness of drug therapy for acute gastroenteritis and the use of oral rehydration in developed countries need to be examined more closely.

Guideline for Evaluation and Treatment of Gastroesophageal Reflux in Infants and Children

- *Clinical Practice Guideline*

JPGN

Volume 32
Supplement 2
2001

JOURNAL OF PEDIATRIC GASTROENTEROLOGY AND NUTRITION

The Official Journal of
European Society of Paediatric Gastroenterology, Hepatology and Nutrition
and the
North American Society for Pediatric Gastroenterology and Nutrition

CONTENTS

(Continued on next page)

Listed in Index Medicus/Medline, Current Contents/Clinical Medicine/Life Science, Excerpta Medica, Biosis, and PASCAL/CNRS.
Articles and issue photocopies and 16 mm microfilm, 35 mm microfilm, and 105 mm microfiche are available from University
Microfilms International (UMI), 300 North Zeeb Road, Ann Arbor, MI 48106-1346, U.S.A.

    Journal of Pediatric Gastroenterology and Nutrition (ISSN 0277-2116) is published monthly except June and December in two volumes per year by Lippincott Williams & Wilkins, at 16522 Hunters Green Parkway, Hagerstown, MD 21740-2116. Business and production offices are located at 530 Walnut Street, Philadelphia, PA 19106-3621. Periodicals postage paid at Hagerstown, MD and at additional mailing offices. Copyright © 2001 by Lippincott Williams & Wilkins.
    Address for subscription information, orders, or change of address (except Japan, India, Bangladesh, Sri Lanka, Nepal and Pakistan): 16522 Hunters Green Parkway, Hagerstown, MD 21740-2116; phone 1-800-638-3030; fax 301-223-2400; in Maryland, call collect 301-223-2300. In Japan, contact LWW Igaku-Shoin Ltd., 3-23-14 Hongo, Bunkyo-ku, Tokyo 113-0033, Japan; phone: 81-3-5689-5400; fax: 81-3-5689-5402. In India, Bangladesh, Sri Lanka, Nepal and Pakistan, contact Globe Publication Pvt. Ltd. B-13, 3rd FL, A Block, Shopping Complex, Naraina Vihar, Ring Road, New Delhi 110028, India; phone: 91-11-579-3211; fax; 91-11-579-8876.
    Annual subscription rates worldwide: $317.00 Individual Domestic, $336.00 Individual International, $605.00 Institutional Domestic, $706.00 Institutional International, $159.00 Students/Residents Domestic, $159.00 Students/Residents International. (The Canadian GST tax of 7% will be added to the subscription price of all orders shipped to Canada. Lippincott Williams & Wilkins' GST Identification Number is 895524239. Publications Mail Agreement #0617695.) Subscriptions outside the United States must be prepaid. Subscriptions outside North America must add $13.00 for airfreight delivery. Prices subject to change without notice. Copies will be replaced without charge if the publisher receives a request within 90 days of the mailing date, both in the U.S. and worldwide. Visit us on-line at www.lww.com.
    Website: www.jpgn.org
    Postmaster: Send address changes to *Journal of Pediatric Gastroenterology and Nutrition*, P.O. Box 1550, Hagerstown, MD 21740.

CONTENTS

Lippincott Williams & Wilkins, Inc., cannot be held responsible for errors or for any consequences arising from the use of the information contained in this journal. The appearance of advertising in this journal does not constitute an endorsement or approval by Lippincott Williams & Wilkins, Inc. of the quality or value of the product advertised or of the claims made for it by its manufacturer.

When citing this journal, abbreviate as *J Pediatr Gastroenterol Nutr.*

Permission to reproduce copies of articles for noncommercial use may be obtained from the Copyright Clearance Center, 222 Rosewood Drive, Danvers, MA 01923; (978) 750-8400, FAX: (978) 750-4470, www.copyright.com.

Abstract

Gastroesophageal reflux (GER), defined as passage of gastric contents into the esophagus, and GER disease (GERD), defined as symptoms or complications of GER, are common pediatric problems encountered by both primary and specialty medical providers. Clinical manifestations of GERD in children include vomiting, poor weight gain, dysphagia, abdominal or substernal pain, esophagitis and respiratory disorders. The GER Guideline Committee of the North American Society for Pediatric Gastroenterology and Nutrition has formulated a clinical practice guideline for the management of pediatric GER. The GER Guideline Committee, consisting of a primary care pediatrician, two clinical epidemiologists (who also practice primary care pediatrics) and five pediatric gastroenterologists, based its recommendations on an integration of a comprehensive and systematic review of the medical literature combined with expert opinion. Consensus was achieved through Nominal Group Technique, a structured quantitative method.

The Committee examined the value of diagnostic tests and treatment modalities commonly used for the management of GERD, and how those interventions can be applied to clinical situations in the infant and older child. The guideline provides recommendations for management by the primary care provider, including evaluation, initial treatment, follow-up management and indications for consultation by a specialist. The guideline also provides recommendations for management by the pediatric gastroenterologist.

This document represents the official recommendations of the North American Society for Pediatric Gastroenterology and Nutrition on the evaluation and treatment of gastroesophageal reflux in infants and children. The American Academy of Pediatrics has also endorsed these recommendations. The recommendations are summarized in a synopsis within the article. This review and recommendations are a general guideline and are not intended as a substitute for clinical judgment or as a protocol for the management of all patients with this problem.

SYNOPSIS

This clinical practice guideline was developed to assist the primary and specialist medical provider in the evaluation and management of gastroesophageal reflux in infants and children. Recommendations are based on an integration of a comprehensive and systematic review of the medical literature combined with expert opinion. The guideline is not intended for the management of neonates less than 72 hours old, premature infants or infants and children with either neurologic impairments or anatomic disorders of the upper gastrointestinal tract. The recommendations are a general guideline and are not intended as a substitute for clinical judgment or as a protocol for the management of all patients with this problem.

Gastroesophageal reflux (GER), defined as the passage of gastric contents into the esophagus, and GER disease (GERD), defined as symptoms or complications of GER, are common pediatric problems. Clinical manifestations of GERD in children include vomiting, poor weight gain, dysphagia, abdominal or substernal pain, esophagitis and respiratory disorders. The following section summarizes the conclusions and recommendations of the GER Guideline Committee of the North American Society for Pediatric Gastroenterology and Nutrition on the value of diagnostic tests and treatment modalities commonly used for the management of GERD, and how those interventions can be applied to clinical situations in the infant and older child.

Diagnostic Approaches

History and Physical Examination. In most infants with vomiting, and in most older children with regurgitation and heartburn, a history and physical examination are sufficient to reliably diagnose GER, recognize complications, and initiate management.

Upper GI Series. The upper gastrointestinal (GI) series is neither sensitive nor specific for the diagnosis of GER, but is useful for the evaluation of the presence of anatomic abnormalities, such as pyloric stenosis, malrotation and annular pancreas in the vomiting infant, as well as hiatal hernia and esophageal stricture in the older child.

Esophageal pH Monitoring. Esophageal pH monitoring is a valid and reliable measure of acid reflux. Esophageal pH monitoring is useful to establish the presence of abnormal acid reflux, to determine if there is a temporal association between acid reflux and frequently occurring symptoms, and to assess the adequacy of therapy in patients who do not respond to treatment with acid suppression. Esophageal pH monitoring may be normal in some patients with GERD, particularly those with respiratory complications.

Endoscopy and Biopsy. Endoscopy with biopsy can assess the presence and severity of esophagitis, strictures and Barrett's esophagus, as well as exclude other disorders, such as Crohn's disease and eosinophilic or infectious esophagitis. A normal appearance of the esophagus during endoscopy does not exclude histopathological esophagitis; subtle mucosal changes such as erythema and pallor may be observed in the absence of esophagitis. Esophageal biopsy is recommended when endoscopy is performed to detect microscopic esophagitis and to exclude causes of esophagitis other than GER.

Empiric Medical Therapy. A trial of time-limited medical therapy for GER is useful for determining if GER is causing a specific symptom.

Treatment Options

Diet Changes in the Infant. There is evidence to support a one-to two-week trial of a hypoallergenic formula in formula fed infants with vomiting. Milk-thickening agents do not improve reflux index scores but do decrease the number of episodes of vomiting.

Positioning in the Infant. Esophageal pH monitoring has demonstrated that infants have significantly less GER when placed in the prone position than in the supine position. However, prone positioning is associated with a higher rate of the sudden infant death syndrome (SIDS). In infants from birth to 12 months of age with GERD, the risk of SIDS generally outweighs the potential benefits of prone sleeping. Therefore, non-prone positioning during sleep is generally recommended. Supine positioning confers the lowest risk for SIDS and is preferred. Prone positioning during sleep is only considered in unusual cases where the risk of death from complications of GER outweighs the potential increased risk of SIDS. When prone positioning is necessary, it is particularly important that parents be advised not to use soft bedding, which increases the risk of SIDS in infants placed prone.

Positioning in the Child & Adolescent. In children older than one year it is likely that there is a benefit to left side positioning during sleep and elevation of the head of the bed.

Lifestyle Changes in the Child & Adolescent. It is recommended that children and adolescents with GERD avoid caffeine, chocolate and spicy foods that provoke symptoms. Obesity, exposure to tobacco smoke and alcohol are also associated with GER. It is not known whether lifestyle changes have an additive benefit in patients receiving pharmacological therapy.

Acid-suppressant Therapy. Histamine-2 receptor antagonists (H2RAs) produce relief of symptoms and mucosal healing. Proton pump inhibitors (PPIs), the most effective acid suppressant medications, are superior to H2RAs in relieving symptoms and healing esophagitis. Chronic antacid therapy is generally not recommended since more convenient and safe alternatives (H2RAs and PPIs) are available.

Prokinetic Therapy. Cisapride is available in the USA only through a limited-access program. Cisapride reduces the frequency of symptoms, including regurgitation and vomiting. However, because of concerns about the potential for serious cardiac arrhythmias in patients receiving cisapride, appropriate patient selection and monitoring as well as proper use, including correct dosage (0.2 mg/kg/dose QID) and avoidance of co-administration of contraindicated medications, are important. Other prokinetic agents have not been shown to be effective in the treatment of GERD in children.

Surgical Therapy. Case series indicate that surgical therapy generally results in favorable outcomes. The potential risks, benefits and costs of successful prolonged medical therapy versus fundoplication have not been well studied in infants or children in various symptom presentations.

Evaluation and Management of Infants and Children with Suspected GERD

The approach to the evaluation and management of infants and children with GERD depends upon the presenting symptoms or signs. Below is a summary of conclusions and recommendations derived from an integration of the research evidence with clinical experience for various clinical presentations. Where there are no randomized studies, the recommendations are based on the consensus opinion of the GER Guideline Committee.

The Infant with Recurrent Vomiting. In the infant with recurrent vomiting, a thorough history and physical examination, with attention to warning signals, is generally sufficient to allow the clinician to establish a diagnosis of uncomplicated GER (the "happy spitter"). An upper GI series is not required unless there are signs of gastrointestinal obstruction. Other diagnostic tests may be indicated if there are symptoms of poor weight gain, excessive crying, irritability, disturbed sleep, feeding or respiratory problems. In the infant who has uncomplicated GER, parental education, reassurance and anticipatory guidance are recommended. Generally no other intervention is necessary. Thickening of formula and a brief trial of a hypoallergenic formula are other treatment options. If symptoms worsen or do not improve by 18 to 24 months of age, re-evaluation for complications of GER is recommended. Generally this includes an upper GI series and consultation with a pediatric gastroenterologist.

The Infant with Recurrent Vomiting and Poor Weight Gain. In the infant with vomiting and poor weight gain it is recommended that the adequacy of calories and the effectiveness of swallowing be assessed. If there is poor weight gain despite adequate caloric intake, a diagnostic evaluation to uncover other causes of vomiting or weight loss is generally indicated. Tests may include a complete blood count, electrolytes, bicarbonate, urea nitrogen, creatinine, alanine aminotransferase, ammonia, glucose, urinalysis, urine ketones and reducing substances, and a review of newborn screening tests. An upper GI series to evaluate anatomy is also recommended. Treatment options include thickening of formula, a trial of a hypoallergenic formula, increasing the caloric density of the formula, acid suppression therapy, prokinetic therapy and, in selected cases, prone positioning. Further management options include endoscopy with biopsy, hospitalization, tube feedings and rarely surgical therapy. Careful follow-up is necessary to assure adequate weight gain.

The Infant with Recurrent Vomiting and Irritability. Normal infants typically fuss or cry intermittently for an average of two hours daily, which may be perceived as excessive by some parents. A symptom diary may be useful to determine the extent to which the infant is irritable and has disturbed sleep. As in all infants with vomiting, other causes of vomiting need to be excluded. Expert opinion suggests two diagnostic and treatment strategies. Empiric treatment with either a sequential or simultaneous two-week trial of a hypoallergenic formula and acid suppression may be initiated. If there is no improvement, either esophageal pH monitoring to determine the adequacy of therapy or upper endoscopy with biopsy to diagnose esophagitis may be performed. If there is no response to therapy and these studies are normal, it is unlikely that GER is contributing to symptoms. Alternatively, evaluation could begin with esophageal pH monitoring to determine if episodes of irritability and sleep disturbance are temporally associated with acid reflux.

The Child or Adolescent with Recurrent Vomiting or Regurgitation. In otherwise normal children who have recurrent vomiting or regurgitation after the age of 2 years, management options include an upper GI series, upper endoscopy with biopsy, and prokinetic therapy.

Heartburn in the Child or Adolescent. For the treatment of heartburn in children or adolescents, lifestyle changes accompanied by a two- to four-week therapeutic trial of an H_2RA or PPI are recommended. If symptoms persist or recur, the child can be re-

ferred to a pediatric gastroenterologist for upper endoscopy with biopsy and in some cases long-term therapy.

Esophagitis. In the infant or child with esophagitis, initial treatment consists of lifestyle changes and H_2RA or PPI therapy. In patients with only histopathological esophagitis, the efficacy of therapy can be monitored by the degree of symptom relief. In patients with erosive esophagitis, repeat endoscopy is recommended to assure healing.

Dysphagia or Odynophagia. In the child with dysphagia (difficulty swallowing) or odynophagia (painful swallowing), a barium esophagram is recommended. If the initial history is suggestive of esophagitis, upper endoscopy may be performed as the initial diagnostic test. Treatment without prior diagnostic evaluation is not recommended. In the infant with feeding refusal, because a large variety of disorders may contribute to infant feeding difficulties, empiric therapy for GER is generally not recommended. However, if there are other signs or symptoms suggestive of GERD then a time-limited course of medical therapy can be considered.

Apnea or Apparent Life-threatening Events (ALTE). In patients with ALTEs recurrent regurgitation or emesis is common. However, investigations in unselected patients with ALTE have not demonstrated a convincing temporal relationship between esophageal acidification and apnea or bradycardia. There are no randomized studies to evaluate the usefulness of esophageal pH monitoring in infants with ALTE. In patients with frequent ALTE in which the role of GER is uncertain, esophageal pH monitoring may be useful to determine if there is a temporal association of acid reflux with ALTE. The evidence suggests that infants with ALTE and GER may be more likely to respond to anti-reflux therapy when there is gross emesis or oral regurgitation at the time of the ALTE, when episodes occur in the awake infant, and when the ALTE is characterized by obstructive apnea. Therapeutic options include thickened feedings and prokinetic and acid suppressant therapy. Since most infants improve with medical management, surgery is considered only in severe cases.

Asthma. In patients where symptoms of asthma and GER coexist, and in infants and toddlers with chronic vomiting or regurgitation and recurrent episodes of cough and wheezing, a three-month trial of vigorous acid suppressant therapy of GER is recommended. In patients with persistent asthma without symptoms of GER, esophageal pH monitoring is recommended in selected patients who are more likely to benefit from GER therapy. These include patients with radiographic evidence of recurrent pneumonia; patients with nocturnal asthma more than once a week; and patients requiring either continuous oral corticosteroids, high-dose inhaled corticosteroids, more than two bursts per year of oral corticosteroids or those with persistent asthma unable to wean medical management. If esophageal pH monitoring demonstrates an increased frequency or duration of esophageal acid exposure, a trial of prolonged medical therapy for GER is recommended.

Recurrent Pneumonia. GER can cause recurrent pneumonia in the absence of esophagitis or when esophageal pH monitoring is normal. There is insufficient evidence to provide recommendations for a uniform approach to diagnosis and treatment. Diagnostic evaluation may include flexible bronchoscopy with pulmonary lavage for lipid-laden macrophages, nuclear scintigraphy and assessment of airway protective mechanisms during swallowing.

Upper Airway Symptoms. Hoarseness, chronic cough, stridor and globus sensation can be associated with GER in infants and children. There is insufficient evidence to provide recommendations for diagnosis and treatment.

1. Background

Gastroesophageal reflux (GER), defined as passage of gastric contents into the esophagus, is a normal physiologic process that occurs throughout the day in healthy infants, children, and adults (1–4). Most episodes of reflux are brief and asymptomatic, not extending above the distal esophagus. Regurgitation is defined as passage of refluxed gastric contents into the oral pharynx. Vomiting is defined as expulsion of the refluxed gastric contents from the mouth. GER occurs during episodes of transient relaxation of the lower esophageal sphincter or inadequate adaptation of the sphincter tone to changes in abdominal pressure (5,6). The strength of the lower esophageal sphincter, the primary antireflux barrier, is normal in the vast majority of children with GER (5,6).

Gastroesophageal reflux disease (GERD) occurs when gastric contents reflux into the esophagus or oropharynx and produce symptoms (Table 1). The pathogenesis of GERD is multifactorial and complex, involving the frequency of reflux, gastric acidity, gastric emptying, esophageal clearing mechanisms, the esophageal mucosal barrier, visceral hypersensitivity, and airway responsiveness. To date no medical treatment targets the primary mechanism of GER, transient relaxation of the lower esophageal sphincter. The primary goals of therapy are to relieve the patient's symptoms, promote normal weight gain and growth, heal inflammation caused by refluxed gastric contents (esophagitis), and prevent respiratory and other complications associated with chronic reflux of gastric contents.

During infancy GER is common and is most often manifest as vomiting. Recurrent vomiting occurs in 50% of infants in the first three months of life, in 67% of four month old infants, and in 5% of 10 to 12 month old infants (7). Vomiting resolves spontaneously in nearly all

TABLE 1. *Complications of gastroesophageal reflux*

Symptoms
    Recurrent vomiting
    Weight loss or poor weight gain
    Irritability in infants
    Regurgitation
    Heartburn or chest pain
    Hematemesis
    Dysphagia or feeding refusal
    Apnea or ALTE
    Wheezing or stridor
    Hoarseness
    Cough
    Abnormal neck posturing (Sandifer syndrome)

Findings
    Esophagitis
    Esophageal stricture
    Barrett's esophagus
    Laryngitis
    Recurrent pneumonia
    Hypoproteinemia
    Anemia

of these infants (8). Parents do not usually perceive vomiting as a problem when it occurs no more often than once daily, but they are more likely to be concerned when vomiting is more frequent, the volume of vomitus is large, or when the infant cries frequently or with vomiting.

A small minority of infants develop GERD with symptoms including anorexia, dysphagia (difficulty swallowing), odynophagia (painful swallowing), arching of the back during feedings, irritability, hematemesis, anemia or failure to thrive. GER is one of the causes of apparent life-threatening events (ALTE) in infants and has been associated with chronic respiratory disorders including reactive airways disease, recurrent stridor, chronic cough and recurrent pneumonia in infants.

In preschool age children GER may manifest as intermittent vomiting. Older children are more likely to have the adult-type pattern of chronic heartburn or regurgitation with reswallowing. Esophagitis in older children may present as dysphagia or food impaction. Rarely, esophageal pain causes stereotypical, repetitive stretching and arching movements that are mistaken for atypical seizures or dystonia (Sandifer syndrome) (9,10). More severe inflammation may cause chronic blood loss with anemia, hematemesis, hypoproteinemia or melena (11). If the inflammation is untreated, circumferential scarring or strictures may form. Chronic inflammation may also result in replacement of distal esophageal mucosa with a metaplastic potentially malignant specialized epithelium known as a Barrett's mucosa (12). GER is common in children with asthma, but recurrent aspiration pneumonia due to GER is uncommon except in the neurologically impaired child. Hoarseness has also been associated with GER in children.

Little is known about the prevalence or natural history of GERD in children and adolescents. Numerous disorders can present with the same symptoms and signs as GER or GERD. Diagnostic and therapeutic approaches vary with the age of the patient and the presenting sign or symptom. Although GER is a common pediatric problem, no evidence-based guidelines for its evaluation and treatment currently exist. Therefore, the GER Guideline Committee was formed by the North American Society for Pediatric Gastroenterology and Nutrition (NASPGN) to develop a clinical practice guideline for the management of GER and GERD in infants and children.

The GER Guideline Committee consists of a primary care pediatrician, two clinical epidemiologists who are also primary care pediatricians and five pediatric gastroenterologists. This clinical practice guideline is designed to assist primary care providers, pediatric gastroenterologists, pediatric surgeons, pediatric pulmonologists and pediatric otolaryngologists in the management of children with GER in both inpatient and outpatient settings. The guideline is not intended for the management of neonates less than 72 hours old, premature infants or infants and children with either neurologic impairments or anatomic disorders of the upper gastrointestinal tract. The management of infants less than two years of age was considered separately from the management of children and adolescents two to 18 years of age. The desirable outcome of optimal management was defined as improvement or resolution of the presenting symptoms and complications of GER, with interventions that have few or no adverse effects, and with resultant resumption of functional health. Cost effectiveness was not considered because of a lack of information in pediatric patients.

This document represents the official recommendations of the North American Society for Pediatric Gastroenterology and Nutrition on the evaluation and treatment of gastroesophageal reflux in infants and children. The American Academy of Pediatrics has also endorsed these recommendations. This review and recommendations are a general guideline and are not intended as a substitute for clinical judgment or as a protocol for the management of all patients with this problem.

2. Methods

In order to develop an evidence-based guideline the following search strategy was used. Articles on diagnosis, treatment, and complications were searched separately. Articles published in English between January 1966 and March 1999 on GER in children were searched using Ovid and PubMed. Letters, abstracts, editorials, case reports, reviews, and articles related to premature infants and children with neurological impairments were excluded. The search strategies for diagnosis yielded 169 articles, 129 articles after exclusion criteria were applied, while the search strategy for treatment yielded 770 articles. After exclusion criteria were applied, there were 23 articles related to non-pharmacological treatment (positioning and dietary changes), 42 to pharmacological treatment (prokinetics and acid-suppressants) and 70 to surgical treatment (fundoplication). Searches on specific complications of GER yielded the following: 140 before and 20 after application of exclusion criteria for apnea and apparent life-threatening events; 91 before and 27 after exclusion criteria for asthma; 18 before and 9 after exclusion criteria for eosinophilic esophagitis; and 83 before and 34 after exclusion criteria for pulmonary disease. Subsequently, additional articles were identified and reviewed. When the pediatric literature was insufficient, the adult literature was also considered.

Articles were evaluated using published criteria (13,14). To evaluate inter-rater reliability, both clinical epidemiologists independently reviewed twenty-nine of the therapy articles on respiratory complications. Concordance using the criteria was 48% with all differences attributable to case series (Level IIa) and descriptive studies (Level III) evidence. If case series and large case reports were considered equivalent, the concordance was 100%. The Committee based its recommendations on

integration of the literature review with expert opinion. Consensus was achieved through Nominal Group Technique, a structured, quantitative method (15). Using the methods of the Canadian Preventive Services Task Force (16), the quality of evidence of each of the recommendations made by the GER Guideline Committee was determined and is summarized in the Appendix.

In the following sections we examine the effectiveness of diagnostic tests and treatment modalities commonly utilized for the management of GERD. Subsequent sections indicate how those interventions can be applied to various clinical situations in the infant and older child.

3. Diagnostic Approaches

Although many tests have been used for the diagnosis of GER, few objective studies compare the various diagnostic approaches. More importantly, it is not known whether tests can predict when an individual patient will improve with either medical or surgical therapy for GERD. A test may be useful to document the occurrence of GER, to detect complications of GER, to establish a causal relationship between GER and symptoms, to evaluate therapy or to exclude other causes of symptoms. Since each test is designed to answer a particular question, it is valuable only when used in the appropriate clinical situation.

3.1 History and Physical Examination

A review of the medical literature found no reports comparing the history and physical examination to diagnostic tests. In two pediatric studies of persistent GER there was no relationship between symptoms and the presence of esophagitis (17,18). Nonetheless, based upon expert opinion, in most infants with vomiting and most older children with regurgitation and heartburn, a history and physical examination are sufficient to reliably diagnose GER, recognize complications, and initiate management.

3.2 Barium Contrast Radiography

The upper gastrointestinal (GI) series is useful to detect anatomic abnormalities, such as pyloric stenosis, malrotation, hiatal hernia and esophageal stricture. When compared to esophageal pH monitoring, the upper GI series is neither sensitive nor specific for the diagnosis of GER. The sensitivity, specificity and positive predictive value of the upper GI series range from 31% to 86%, 21% to 83%, and 80% to 82% respectively when compared to esophageal pH monitoring (19–24). The brief duration of the upper GI series results in false negative results, while the frequent occurrence of non-pathological reflux results in false positive results. Thus, the upper GI series is not a useful test to reliably determine the presence or absence of GER.

3.3 Esophageal pH Monitoring

Esophageal pH monitoring, used widely as an index of esophageal acid exposure, measures the frequency and duration of episodes of acid reflux (25). The test is performed by the transnasal placement of a microelectrode into the lower esophagus, which measures and records intraesophageal pH. Most clinicians utilize computerized devices that record intraesophageal pH every 4 to 8 seconds (26,27). Computerized analysis calculates the number and duration of reflux episodes (28). An episode of acid reflux is usually defined as esophageal pH <4 for a specified minimum duration, usually 15 to 30 seconds (29).

The recording device, diet, position and activity during the study affect the measurement of esophageal pH. Location of the probe sensor also affects the results; the distal esophagus is normally exposed to more acid than the proximal esophagus. There is technical and biological variability on sequential 24-hour pH monitoring studies, but this variability appears to affect the interpretation of results in only a small number of patients (30–32). Abbreviated studies of fewer than 12 hours are less reproducible than longer studies (33,34).

Asymptomatic episodes of acid reflux occur in normal infants, children, adolescents and adults. In a study of 509 normal infants, 0 to 11 months of age, there were 31 ± 21 episodes of acid reflux per day; the upper limit of normal was 73 episodes daily (2). In three studies of 48 children, 0 to 9 years of age, the mean upper limit of normal was 25 daily (29,35,36) and in 50 normal adults it was 45 daily (37). The mean upper limit of normal for the number of episodes of acid reflux lasting 5 minutes or longer was 9.7 in infants, 6.8 in children and 3.2 in adults. The percentage of the total time that the esophageal pH is <4, also called the reflux index, is considered the most valid measure of reflux because it reflects the cumulative exposure of the esophagus to acid. The mean upper limit of normal of the reflux index was 11.7% in infants 0 to 11 months (2), 5.4% in children 0 to 9 years old (29,35,36), and approximately 6% in 432 normal adults (38). These studies indicate that acid reflux is a physiologic process that is more common in normal infants in the first year of life than it is in normal older children and adults. Based on the above studies, it is recommended that the upper limit of normal of the reflux index be defined as up to 12% in the first year of life and up to 6% thereafter.

The presence of endoscopic and histopathological esophagitis is strongly associated with abnormal esophageal pH monitoring. In pediatric patients with endoscopic esophagitis (ulcerations or erosions) or biopsy proven esophagitis, approximately 95% will have an abnormal reflux index (39–41). However, not all patients with GER have esophagitis. In the selected populations of patients reported, esophagitis is present in 50% of patients with positive esophageal pH monitoring studies (39–41) and the severity of esophagitis does not correlate with the reflux index (42). Proximal esophageal and pharyngeal pH monitoring have not been proven to be more useful than lower esophageal pH monitoring alone for determining which patients are at risk for upper airway complications of GER (3,43,44).

Esophageal pH monitoring can be used to detect abnormal acid reflux in selected clinical situations. Esophageal pH monitoring can determine if a patient's symptom is temporally associated with acid reflux by calculating the symptom index. The symptom index is the ratio of the number of episodes of a symptom (e.g., heartburn) that occur concurrent with acid reflux divided by the total number of episodes of that symptom. In adults, symptom index scores ≥0.5 suggest a relationship between heartburn and gastroesophageal reflux; in these cases, symptoms have successfully been controlled with acid suppression therapy (45). One study using the symptom index in infants compared behavior with episodes of acid reflux (46). Esophageal pH monitoring is also useful to assess the adequacy of the dosage of acid suppression therapy in children being treated with a proton pump inhibitor (47) and may be useful to determine if a patient may be at increased risk for airway complications of GER. For example, approximately 60% of children with asthma, poorly responsive to conventional treatment, had abnormal esophageal pH monitoring studies (48–50).

Esophageal pH monitoring does not detect non-acidic reflux episodes such as occur post-prandially in infants. In some patients, esophageal pH monitoring may be within the range of normal but brief episodes of GER may cause complications such as ALTE, cough or aspiration pneumonia.

In summary, esophageal pH monitoring is a valid and reliable measure of acid reflux. Esophageal pH monitoring establishes the presence of abnormal acid reflux, to determine if there is a temporal association between acid reflux and frequently occurring symptoms, and to assess the adequacy of therapy in patients who do not respond to treatment with acid suppressants

3.4 Endoscopy and Biopsy

Endoscopy enables both visualization and biopsy of the esophageal epithelium. Endoscopy and biopsy can determine the presence and severity of esophagitis, strictures and Barrett's esophagus, as well as exclude other disorders, such as Crohn's disease, webs and eosinophilic or infectious esophagitis. A normal appearance of the esophagus during endoscopy does not exclude histopathological esophagitis. The subtle mucosal changes of erythema and pallor may be observed in the absence of esophagitis (18,42,51). Endoscopic visualization of esophageal erosions or ulceration correlates with histopathological esophagitis, but the severity of endoscopic and histopathological changes may not correlate since the lesion can be patchy and biopsies sample only a small portion of the mucosal surface. Endoscopic grading systems for the severity of erosive esophagitis, such as the Los Angeles criteria (52), have not yet been validated in pediatric patients but may provide more uniform definitions of severity, if applied. Other findings, such as the presence of vertical lines (53) also correlate with histopathological esophagitis in children. Because there is a poor correlation between endoscopic appearance and histopathology, esophageal biopsy is recommended when diagnostic endoscopy is performed.

In normal infants and children, eosinophils and neutrophils are not present in the esophageal epithelium (40,54). Basal zone hyperplasia (>20% to 25% of total epithelial thickness) and increased papillary length (>50% to 75% of epithelial thickness) have been found to correlate with increased acid exposure (40,55). The available pediatric data suggest that intraepithelial eosinophils or neutrophils as well as morphometric measures of basal cell layer thickness and papillary height are valid indicators of reflux esophagitis. It has been proposed that a high number of eosinophils in the esophageal epithelium (>7 to 24 per high power field) suggest the diagnosis of eosinophilic esophagitis (56,57).

3.5 Scintigraphy

A nuclear scintiscan is performed by the oral ingestion or instillation of technetium-labeled formula or food into the stomach. The areas of interest, the stomach, esophagus and lungs, are scanned for evidence of GER and aspiration. Unlike esophageal pH monitoring, the nuclear scan can demonstrate reflux of non-acidic gastric contents. Scintigraphy also provides information about gastric emptying, which may be delayed in children with GERD (58–60). However, a lack of standardized techniques and the absence of age-specific normative data limit the value of this test. Episodes of aspiration may be detected during a one-hour study or on images obtained up to 24 hours after the feeding is administered (61). A negative test does not exclude the possibility of infrequently occurring aspiration (62).

The reported sensitivity and specificity of the nuclear scan for the diagnosis of GER are 15% to 59% and 83% to 100%, respectively, when compared to esophageal pH monitoring (19,63–65). This lack of correlation most likely reflects the difference in techniques of the two tests. Scintigraphy measures both acid and non-acid reflux in the initial postprandial period, whereas esophageal pH monitoring measures acid reflux for prolonged periods up to 24 hours and protocols used for analysis often exclude the postprandial recording times (64,66). The role of nuclear scintigraphy in the diagnosis and management of GERD in infants and children is unclear.

3.6 Empiric Therapy

A trial of time-limited medical therapy for GER is useful for determining if GER is causing a specific symptom. Empiric therapy is widely used (67) but has not been validated for any symptom presentation in pediatric patients. Empiric treatment trials with omeprazole have been reported for cough (68,69), heartburn (70,71), non-cardiac chest pain (72) and dyspepsia (73) in adult patients.

4. Treatment Options

Treatment options are classified as lifestyle changes and pharmacological or surgical therapies. Lifestyle changes for infants include alterations in formula composition and sleep positioning. Lifestyle changes in adolescents include dietary modifications, altered sleep position, weight reduction and smoking cessation (74). Medications buffer gastric acid, reduce gastric acid secretion or alter gastrointestinal motility. Surgical therapy includes operative techniques that reduce or eliminate GER.

4.1 Lifestyle Changes

4.1.1 Feeding Changes in Infants. In most infants, symptoms of GER do not decrease when there is a change from one milk formula to another. However, a subset of infants with vomiting has cow's milk protein allergy (75). In these infants, elimination of cow's milk protein from the diet resulted in decreased vomiting within 24 hours. Two successive, blind challenges corroborated the diagnosis of cow's milk protein allergy-induced vomiting in infants (76,77). A similar study found that IgG anti-ß-lactoglobulin, a major antigenic determinant in cow's milk, was present in infants allergic to cow's milk protein with symptom reduction following the elimination of cow's milk (78,79). There is, therefore, evidence to support a one to two week trial of a hypoallergenic formula in formula fed infants with vomiting. There are no studies that evaluate the therapeutic value of a soy-protein formula for this indication, nor are there studies that evaluate whether sensitization to soy proteins causes vomiting. Similarly, there are no studies that examine whether sensitization to maternal dietary proteins passed into human breast milk leads to vomiting in breast fed infants. The role of breast feeding versus formula feeding in the treatment of GERD is uncertain. One study (80) measured esophageal acidification in breast-fed and formula-fed healthy term neonates aged 2 to 8 days during various sleep states. During active sleep, but not other sleep states, formula fed infants had an increased number of reflux episodes and increased esophageal acid exposure compared to breast fed infants.

Milk-thickening agents do not improve reflux index scores (81,82) but do decrease the number of episodes of vomiting (81–83). In the United States of America (USA), thickening is usually achieved with the addition of rice cereal to formula (83). When thickening an infant formula with a caloric density of 20 kcal per ounce, the addition of one tablespoonful of rice cereal per ounce of formula increases the caloric density to approximately 34 kcal per ounce, whereas the addition of one tablespoonful of rice cereal per two ounces of formula increases the caloric density to approximately 27 kcal per ounce. When formula is thickened it is necessary to cross-cut the nipple to allow for adequate flow. Thickened formula may increase coughing during feedings (84). Newer formulas that contain carob flour or locust bean gum as thickening agents are now available in Europe. These formulas have been reported to decrease vomiting and esophageal acid exposure when compared with unthickened formula (85) and formula thickened with rice cereal (86). A formula with added rice starch is now available in the USA and Canada but there are no published studies regarding its efficacy for the treatment of GERD in infants.

Infants who are underweight due to GERD may gain weight when the caloric density of their feedings is increased. Some infants require more aggressive intervention such as overnight nasogastric tube feeding to promote weight gain (87). Rarely, patients require nasojejunal tube feeding to promote growth and prevent vomiting or aspiration. Although these approaches to therapy of GERD are widely utilized, there are no controlled studies comparing these treatment approaches to pharmacological or surgical treatments.

4.1.2 Positioning Therapy for Infants. Esophageal pH monitoring has demonstrated that infants have significantly less GER when placed in the prone position than in the supine position. In a study of 79 infants and children (11.6 ± 27 months old) with symptomatic GER, the reflux index during sleep was 24% in the supine position and 8% in the prone position (88). In a study of 60 asymptomatic newborns (1 to 10 days old) kept in one position for 17 hours, the reflux index was 5% when supine and 1% when prone (89). In a randomized crossover design study of 24 infants <5 months of age, each infant was evaluated in each of four positions (prone, supine, left, right) in both horizontal and 30 degree upright positions. The reflux index was significantly higher in the supine (15%) than in the prone (7%) position (90). There is conflicting evidence whether there is less reflux in infants placed prone at a 30-degree angle compared to prone flat (88–91). The amount of reflux is similar in the supine 30-degree angle and in the supine flat positions (88,90). The prone position is superior to semi-supine positioning in an infant seat, which exacerbates GER (92).

One sudy of 60 asymptomatic newborns showed similar reflux in the left, right and supine positions, which was more reflux than in the prone position (89). In contrast, in a study of 24 infants <5 months old, the left side position was similar to the prone position and led to less reflux than the right side and supine positions (90). In adults reflux occurs less often in the left lateral decubitus

(left side down) than in the right lateral decubitus (right side down) position (93,94).

Prone positioning has been recommended for the treatment and prevention of GER in infants. However, this advice conflicts with the recent recognition that prone positioning is associated with a higher rate of the sudden infant death syndrome (SIDS). The Nordic epidemiological SIDS study demonstrated that the odds ratio of SIDS mortality was 13.9 for the prone position and 3.5 for the side position when compared to the supine position (95). Another study demonstrated that the SIDS mortality per 1000 live births was 4.4 in the prone position and <0.1 for the non-prone position (96). In California the SIDS rate declined from 1.2 to 0.7 per 1000 live births after a public health campaign to promote back sleeping (97). Evidence suggests that universal use of the supine position would likely markedly reduce SIDS (98). The side position appears to be unstable, because infants turn during sleep from side to prone. Prone sleeping results in longer uninterrupted sleep periods, and supine sleeping in more arousability, frequent awakening and crying during the night.

In view of the recent evidence describing the successful prevention of SIDS with supine positioning, it is now appropriate to modify the earlier advocacy of prone positioning for GERD. In infants from birth to 12 months with GERD, the risk of SIDS generally outweighs the potential benefits of prone sleeping. Therefore, consistent with the new recommendations of the American Academy of Pediatrics, non-prone positioning during sleep is recommended (99). Supine positioning confers the lowest risk for SIDS and is preferred. Prone positioning is acceptable while the infant is awake, particularly in the postprandial period. Prone positioning during sleep is only considered in unusual cases where the risk of death from complications of GER outweighs the potential increased risk of SIDS. When prone positioning is necessary, it is particularly important that parents be advised not to use soft bedding, which increases the risk of SIDS in infants placed prone (odds ratio 1.7) (100,101).

The efficacy of positioning therapy in children older than one year has not been studied. It is likely that there is a benefit to left side positioning and elevation of the head of the bed, as in adults (102–104).

4.1.3 Lifestyle Changes in Children and Adolescents. Lifestyle changes are often recommended to adults with gastroesophageal reflux. These include dietary modification, avoidance of alcohol, weight loss, and cessation of smoking. Most of the studies investigating these factors have been performed in adults; thus, their applicability to children remains indeterminate. A review of the pediatric and adult literature may be summarized as follows. The current evidence does not support a recommendation to decrease fat intake to treat GER (105–112). However, the limited evidence available supports the recommendation that children and adolescents with GERD avoid caffeine, chocolate and spicy foods that provoke symptoms (113–124). Similarly there is evidence that obesity, exposure to tobacco smoke and alcohol are associated with GER (125–148). It is not known whether lifestyle changes have an additive benefit in patients receiving pharmacological therapy.

4.2 Pharmacological Therapies

The purpose of the two major pharmacological treatments for GERD, acid suppressants and prokinetic agents, is to reduce the amount of acid refluxate to which the esophagus or respiratory tract is exposed, thereby preventing symptoms and promoting healing. The aim of acid suppressants is to reduce esophageal acid exposure by either neutralizing gastric acid or decreasing secretion. The aim of prokinetic agents is to reduce the amount of refluxate by improving contractility of the body of the esophagus, increasing pressure in the lower esophageal sphincter, decreasing the frequency of transient lower esophageal sphincter relaxations and accelerating gastric emptying.

Studies of pharmacological therapies for the treatment of GERD in children are difficult to compare because of heterogeneous patient populations, variable drug doses and duration of therapy, and a lack of standard outcome variables. The majority of studies published to date have used two outcome assessments: symptom responses and change in results of esophageal pH monitoring. Many studies are confounded by multiple treatments including lifestyle changes and other drugs. For purposes of this guideline, double blind single drug studies or randomized comparison studies of pharmacological therapies were reviewed. When no such studies were available, other studies were considered. Recommended drug doses and the common adverse effects of these medications are listed in Table 2.

4.2.1 Acid Suppressants. Acid suppressants act to decrease esophageal acid exposure by reducing the quantity of gastric acid. The antisecretory agents, histamine-2 receptor antagonists (H_2RAs) and proton pump inhibitors (PPIs), reduce the secretion of gastric acid, whereas antacids neutralize gastric acid. Because of their superior efficacy and convenience, antisecretory agents have largely superceded antacids and surface agents in the treatment of GERD. Generally PPIs produce a greater reduction in acid secretion and have a longer duration of action than H_2RAs.

4.2.1.1 Histamine-2 Receptor Antagonists. H_2RAs act to decrease acid secretion by inhibiting the histamine-$_2$ receptor on the gastric parietal cell. In one study in infants ranitidine treatment, 2 mg per kg per dose BID, reduced by 44% the duration that gastric pH was <4, and with TID dosing the reduction was 90% (149). Ranitidine 5 mg/kg per dose orally has been shown to increase gastric pH for 9 to 10 hours in infants (150). Tolerance to intravenous ranitidine and escape from its acid inhibitory effect within six weeks has been observed (151).

Numerous randomized controlled trials in adults have demonstrated that cimetidine, ranitidine and famotidine

TABLE 2. *Drugs demonstrated to be effective in gastroesophageal reflux disease*

Type of medication	Recommended oral dosage	Adverse effects/precautions
Histamine$_2$ receptor antagonists		
Cimetidine	40mg/kg/day divided TID or QID (adult dose: 800–1200 mg/dose BID or TID)	rash, bradycardia, dizziness, nausea, vomiting, hypotension, gynecomastia, reduces hepatic metabolism of theophylline and other medications, neutropenia, thrombocytopenia, agranulocytosis, doses should be decreased with renal insufficiency
Nizatidine	10 mg/kg/day divided BID. (adult dose: 150 mg BID or 300 mg qhs)	headaches, dizziness, constipation, diarrhea, nausea, anemia, urticaria, doses should be decreased with renal insufficiency
Ranitidine	5 to 10 mg/kg/day divided TID (Adult dose: 300mg BID)	headache, dizziness, fatigue, irritability, rash, constipation, diarrhea, thrombocytopenia, elevated transaminases, doses should be decreased with renal insufficiency
Famotidine	1 mg/kg/day divided BID (adult dose: 20 mg BID)	headaches, dizziness, constipation, diarrhea, nausea, doses should be decreased with renal insufficiency
Proton pump inhibitors		
Omeprazole	1.0 mg/kg/day divided qd or BID (adult dose 20 mg qd)	headache, diarrhea, abdominal pain, nausea, rash, constipation, vitamin B12 deficiency
Lanzoprazole	No pediatric dose available (adult dose: 15–30 mg qd)	headache, diarrhea, abdominal pain, nausea, elevated transaminase, proteinuria, angina, hypotension
Pantoprazole	No pediatric dose available. (adult dose: 40 mg qd)	headache, diarrhea, abdominal pain, nausea
Rabeprazole	No pediatric dose available (adult dose: 20 mg qd)	headache, diarrhea, abdominal pain, nausea
Prokinetic		
Cisapride	0.8 mg/kg/day divided QID. (adult dose: 10–20 mg QID)	rare cases of serious cardiac arrhythmia (FDA recommends ECG before administration) beware of drug interactions do not use in patients with liver, cardiac or electrolyte abnormalities (FDA recommends K+, Ca++, Mg++ and creatinine before administration)

are superior to placebo for relief of symptoms and healing of esophageal mucosa (152–154). However, the efficacy of H$_2$RAs is much greater for mild esophagitis than for severe esophagitis (155). One randomized placebo-controlled trial in infants and children with erosive esophagitis demonstrated the efficacy of H$_2$RA therapy (156) in 32 children who received either cimetidine 30–40 mg/kg per day or placebo. The cimetidine treated group had significant improvement in clinical and histopathology scores, but there was no improvement in the placebo group. Another randomized placebo controlled study in 24 children with mild to moderate esophagitis demonstrated that nizatidine 10 mg/kg per day was more effective than placebo for the healing of esophagitis and symptom relief (157). There are case series that provide additional support for the efficacy of H$_2$RAs in infants and children (158–161). Although no randomized controlled studies in children demonstrate the efficacy of ranitidine or famotidine for the treatment of esophagitis, expert opinion is that these agents appear to be as effective as cimetidine and nizatidine.

4.2.1.2 Proton Pump Inhibitors. Proton pump inhibitors (PPIs), the most effective acid suppressant medications, covalently bond and deactivate the H+, K+ –ATPase pumps (162). To be activated PPIs require acid in the parietal cell canaliculus, and they are most effective when the parietal cell is stimulated by a meal following a fast (162). Optimal effectiveness is achieved when the PPI is administered one–half hour before breakfast so that peak plasma concentrations coincide with the mealtime. If given twice daily, the second dose is best administered one–half hour before the evening meal. Concomittant administration of H$_2$RAs can inhibit efficacy. A steady state of acid suppression is not achieved for several days. There are limited data on the pharmacology of PPIs in infants and children. In one study, doses of omeprazole of 10 to 60 mg (0.7 to 3.3 mg/kg) daily were required to normalize esophageal pH monitoring, and a starting dose of 0.7 mg/kg per day was recommended (47). In other case series reporting successful omeprazole treatment of esophagitis, doses of 0.5 or 0.6 mg/kg daily were administered for 6 to 13 weeks (163–166).

Numerous randomized controlled trials in adults have demonstrated that PPIs are superior to H$_2$RAs in relieving symptoms and healing esophagitis (152). PPIs are effective in patients with esophagitis refractory to high–dose H$_2$RA therapy (167,168), and are more effective than H$_2$RAs in maintaining remission of erosive esophagitis (169). There are currently no reported placebo controlled trials of PPIs in infants or children. However, one randomized controlled trial of 25 infants and children with reflux esophagitis found comparable effectiveness of omeprazole (40 mg per 1.73 m^2 surface area) and very high dose ranitidine (20 mg/kg/day) in reducing symptoms and improving histopathology and esophageal pH monitoring (170). In addition, in multiple case series of

pediatric patients refractory to previous treatment regimens including H$_2$RAs, omeprazole appeared to be highly effective in the treatment of severe esophagitis, resulting in both symptomatic and endoscopic improvement while on treatment (47,163–166). Other proton pump inhibitors, lansoprazole, pantoprazole and rabeprazole, have been introduced recently but studies of their efficacy in infants and children have not yet been reported. Esophageal pH monitoring can be performed to assess the adequacy of the dosage but target values for either esophageal acid exposure or gastric pH that assure therapeutic efficacy are not known. Long term safety studies in adults treated with omeprazole for a mean of 6.5 years (range 1.4 to 11.2 years) show omeprazole is highly effective and safe for the control of reflux esophagitis in adults (171). Despite omeprazole therapy, 12% of the patients who did not have Barrett's esophagus at baseline developed Barrett's metaplasia during follow–up. Similar studies of the efficacy and safety of long term treatment have not been performed in pediatric patients.

One approach to acid reducing therapy, called *step-up* therapy, is to begin treatment with an H$_2$RA at standard dosage, following with a PPI at standard dosage and then a PPI at higher dosage if necessary to achieve improvement (47). An alternative approach, called *step-down* therapy, is to begin treatment with a PPI at higher dosage to achieve improvement, following with a PPI at standard dosage and then an H$_2$RA to maintain improvement. Studies in adults indicate that the step-down approach may be more cost effective (171) and has been recommended in a recently published evidence-based guideline for adult patients (172), but there are no published studies comparing these two strategies in children.

The current evidence supports the recommendation to use antisecretory therapy for the treatment of reflux esophagitis. The effectiveness of acid reducing therapy for other manifestations of GERD is not well documented in children. However, since these agents reduce esophageal acid exposure they are likely to be a useful treatment of GER-related respiratory disorders (see sections 5.5 to 5.9).

4.2.1.3 Antacids. The aim of antacids, which act by neutralizing gastric acid, is to reduce esophageal acid exposure and thereby reduce symptoms of heartburn, alleviate esophagitis and prevent acid-triggered respiratory symptoms. Intensive high-dose antacid therapy (magnesium hydroxide and aluminum hydroxide; 700 mmol/1.73 m2/day) has been shown to be as effective as cimetidine for the treatment of peptic esophagitis in children aged 2 to 42 months (173,174). However, treatment with aluminum-containing antacids significantly increases plasma aluminum levels in infants (175,176). Plasma aluminum levels measured in infants receiving these agents approach levels previously noted to cause osteopenia, microcytic anemia, and neurotoxicity in pediatric patients (177–179). There are no published studies evaluating the efficacy or safety of commercially available antacids containing either magnesium hydroxide alone or calcium carbonate. Antacid therapy is commonly used for the short-term relief of intermittent symptoms of GER in children and adolescents. Although there appears to be little risk to this approach, it has not been formally studied. Because more convenient and safe alternatives are available, chronic antacid therapy is generally not recommended.

4.2.2 Prokinetic Therapy. Transient lower esophageal sphincter relaxations, which are prolonged relaxations unaccompanied by a swallow, are considered the most important pathophysiological mechanism of GER. Other mechanisms are free reflux and strain-induced reflux, when abdominal pressure exceeds the pressure of the lower esophageal sphincter. Although prokinetic agents appear to increase lower esophageal sphincter pressure, a number of studies have failed to demonstrate that prokinetic agents reduce the frequency of episodes of acid reflux, suggesting that they do not reduce the frequency of transient relaxations of the lower esophageal sphincter. The rationale for prokinetic therapy in the treatment of GERD is based on evidence it enhances esophageal peristalsis and accelerates gastric emptying.

Since regurgitation and vomiting are common symptoms in infants and children with reflux, even in the absence of erosive esophagitis, prokinetic agents may have a special role in the treatment of GER in infants and children with conditions where acid suppressants are unlikely to be helpful. Double blind single drug studies and randomized comparison studies of cisapride, metoclopramide, bethanecol and domperidone have been performed in infants and children with GER. Cisapride appears to be a marginally effective prokinetic agent for the treatment of GERD, whereas the effectiveness in children of other prokinetic agents is unproven.

Cisapride is a mixed serotonergic agent that facilitates the release of acetylcholine at synapses of the myenteric plexus. Six randomized controlled trials of cisapride therapy in infants less than two years of age have demonstrated improvement in symptoms or esophageal pH monitoring or both when compared to placebo (180–185). Modest improvement in clinical symptoms, with a reduction in the frequency and volume of vomiting, has been reported in four of five studies where duration of therapy was at least four weeks (180–182,184,186). Improvement occurred more often in infants who regurgitated or vomited after every meal or more than six times daily (182,184,186). One study reported complete resolution of vomiting in less than 20 percent of treated infants (182). In all studies a significant percentage of patients receiving placebo also improved, and in one study vomiting resolved in 14 percent of placebo-treated patients (182).

Randomized controlled trials using prolonged esophageal pH monitoring have demonstrated that cisapride therapy is superior to placebo in reducing esophageal acid exposure and enhancing esophageal acid clearance

following reflux. All studies reported statistically significant improvement compared to baseline measurements of one or more of the following parameters: reflux index (percentage of the time that esophageal pH was less than 4), mean duration of reflux episodes, and number of episodes longer than 5 minutes (180–187). Cisapride improved symptom scores, esophageal histopathology, and pulmonary function in patients with reflux esophagitis and respiratory complications (50,180,181). This may be due to reduced esophageal acid exposure and enhanced esophageal acid clearance.

Metoclopramide is an antidopaminergic agent with cholinomimetic and mixed serotonergic effects. In adults the effects of metoclopramide on esophageal motility and clinical efficacy have been equivocal (188) and the addition of metoclopramide to ranitidine therapy for treatment of GERD resulted in no better efficacy and increased the number of adverse events (189). Four randomized controlled studies of at least two weeks duration on the efficacy of metoclopramide in the treatment of GER in children have been reported. Two of four studies reported a decrease in the frequency and volume of vomiting (190,191), whereas in two other studies metoclopramide was no better or worse than placebo (192,193). The reported effects on esophageal pH monitoring of acute and steady-state dosing of metoclopramide have also been contradictory, with both positive (187,194,195) and negative results (192,193,196). Adverse effects of metoclopramide, which are not uncommon, include central nervous system complications such as parkinsonian reactions and tardive dyskinesia, which may be irreversible (197).

Bethanechol, a direct cholinergic agonist, has been studied in two controlled trials of 6 weeks duration. In one study bethanechol was superior to placebo in reducing the frequency and volume of vomiting, but prolonged esophageal pH monitoring was not performed (198). The other study, which compared bethanechol to antacids, found no difference between the two treatments in clinical outcome or esophageal pH monitoring (199). Of three reports regarding domperidone therapy, one study found improvement in both clinical symptoms and pH score following two weeks of therapy (191), while two studies reported no improvement in either outcome measure following four and eight weeks of therapy (200,201).

In conclusion, there is evidence to support the use of cisapride when a prokinetic is indicated for the treatment of GERD in infants and children. However, because of concerns about the potential for serious cardiac arrhythmias in patients receiving cisapride, appropriate patient selection and monitoring as well as proper use, including correct dosage and avoidance of co-administration of contraindicated medications, are important (202). Despite these concerns, the use of cisapride can be considered for the treatment of selected infants with vomiting and poor weight gain, ALTE or asthma who have failed lifestyle and antisecretory therapy. In some children over

2 years of age with asthma or with recurrent vomiting that is adversely affecting lifestyle cisapride therapy may also be considered. Cisapride recently was withdrawn from the USA market due to these safety concerns and therefore in order to receive cisapride patients must be enrolled in a limited access protocol that requires repeated venipuncture and electrocardiograms, making the use of cisapride a less practical option. There is insufficient evidence that other prokinetic agents are effective in the treatment of GERD in infants and children.

4.2.3 Surface Agents. Sodium alginate forms a surface gel that decreases the regurgitation of gastric contents into the esophagus and protects the esophageal mucosa. Randomized comparison studies have demonstrated conflicting outcomes for both symptoms (203,204) and esophageal pH monitoring (205,206). The formulation utilized for most published studies is not available in the USA.

Sucralfate gel acts by adhering to peptic lesions, and protects the esophageal mucosal surface. In adults sucralfate (1 g po QID) decreases symptoms and promotes healing in patients with non-erosive esophagitis (207). The only randomized comparison study in children demonstrated that sucralfate is as effective as cimetidine for treatment of esophagitis (208). Sucralfate is an aluminum complex, and the potential adverse effects of aluminum in infants and children need to be considered. The available data are inadequate for determining the safety or efficacy of sucralfate in the treatment of GERD in children.

4.3 Surgical Treatment for GERD

Surgery is often considered for the child with GERD who has persistence of symptoms following medical management or who is unable to be weaned from medical therapy. The Nissen fundoplication is the most popular of the many surgical procedures that have been used. Recently experience with laparoscopic procedures has been reported. Results and complication rates do not appear to vary by procedure.

The literature concerning surgical treatment of GERD in children consists of a large number of descriptive papers composed of case series (209–221). The methodology for patient selection and outcome was not always well defined. Patients usually had surgery for failed medical management. There are no published randomized controlled trials. Because most series extended over many years, medical management in earlier patients was often limited to life style changes such as positional therapy and thickened feedings. Some patients received H$_2$RAs but few if any patients received PPIs. Most did not receive a prokinetic agent and those that did often received metoclopramide. Thus many of the patients did not receive optimal medical therapy by today's standards. Outcome measures were often vague or unspeci-

fied. The groups were heterogeneous without adjustment for co-morbid conditions. Many (if not most) of the surgically treated patients were neurologically impaired. A variety of surgical procedures were used. The addition of a pyloroplasty was variable. The outcome was sometimes defined by symptoms and at other times by postoperative tests.

Success rates (complete relief of symptoms) from 57% to 92% have been reported. Mortality related to operation in large series has ranged from 0% to 4.7%. Unrelated death rates from co-morbid conditions were 0% to 21%. The reported overall complication rates have varied between 2.2% and 45%. The most commonly reported complications include breakdown of the wrap (0.9% to 13%), small bowel obstruction (1.3% to 11%), gas bloat syndrome (1.9% to 8%), infection (1.2% to 9%), atelectasis or pneumonia (4.3% to 13%), perforation (2% to 4.3%), persistent esophageal stricture (1.4% to 9%) and esophageal obstruction (1.4% to 9%). Other complications not reported in enough detail to estimate complication rates include dumping syndrome (222,223), incisional hernia and gastroparesis. Reoperation rates were 3% to 18.9%. The results of pediatric series of laparoscopic fundoplications suggest that the results and complication rates are similar to those of the open procedure, but hospitalization is shortened (224,225).

These case series indicate overall favorable outcomes. The potential risks, benefits and costs of successful prolonged medical therapy versus surgical therapy have not been well-studied in infants or children with various symptom presentations. If chronic esophagitis is the primary indication for possible GERD surgery, an upper endoscopy with biopsy and prolonged esophageal pH monitoring study is recommended to demonstrate conclusively that esophagitis is due to GER, rather than other etiologies, such as eosinophilic esophagitis. If airway symptoms are the primary indication for surgery, review of diagnostic studies including radiographic studies, bronchoalveolar lavage, esophageal pH monitoring studies and swallowing studies may all impact on the decision to proceed with surgery, which may be beneficial in some patients even when esophageal pH monitoring is normal (226).

5. Evaluation and Management of Infants and Children with Suspected GERD

The approach to evaluation and management of infants and children with GERD depends upon the presenting symptoms or signs. The following sections discuss the evidence that supports a relationship between a particular clinical disorder and GER in pediatric patients. The approach to determining if GER is causing disease in a patient and the management of pediatric patients with specific symptom presentations is then reviewed. Recommendations are based upon the available evidence and the consensus opinion of the GER Guidelines Guideline Committee.

5.1 Recurrent Vomiting

The diagnostic challenge for the practitioner is to distinguish between vomiting due to GER and vomiting caused by other disorders. Numerous disorders can present with recurrent vomiting that mimics GERD (see Table 3). Laboratory and radiographic investigation may be necessary to exclude other causes of vomiting. The infant with recurrent vomiting is discussed separately from the older child with recurrent vomiting.

5.1.1 The Infant with Recurrent Vomiting. In the infant with recurrent vomiting, a thorough history and physical examination (Table 4), with attention to warning signals that suggest other diagnosis (Table 5), is generally sufficient to allow the clinician to establish a diagnosis of uncomplicated GER (Figure 1). An upper GI series or other diagnostic test is not required unless gastrointestinal obstruction is suspected. Other diagnostic tests may be indicated if there are symptoms of poor weight gain, excessive crying, irritability, disturbed sleep, feeding or respiratory problems.

5.1.2 The Infant with Uncomplicated GER (Figure 1). The classical presentation of uncomplicated GER in infants is effortless, painless vomiting in a well appearing child with normal growth, often referred to as the "happy spitter'. Generally, only parental education, reassurance and anticipatory guidance are necessary for management of the infant who has uncomplicated GER. Parents are advised about potential complications, including poor weight gain, excessive crying, and feeding or respiratory problems. Some infants with cow milk allergy have symptoms that are indistinguishable from GER. Therefore, a one to two week trial of a hypoallergenic formula may be reasonable (section 4.1.1). Thickening of formula may also be considered as an option for therapy. Continuation of supine positioning is recommended. There is no evidence that pharmacological therapy affects the natural history of uncomplicated GER in infants.

Recurrent vomiting due to GER generally decreases in frequency over the first year of life and resolves by 12 months of age (8). If symptoms worsen or do not improve by 18 to 24 months of age, further evaluation is recommended, including an upper GI series and consultation with a pediatric gastroenterologist is recommended (see section 5.1.5).

5.1.3 The Infant with Recurrent Vomiting and Poor Weight Gain (Figure 2). The infant with recurrent vomiting and poor weight gain is a distinct clinical entity that is not to be confused with the happy spitter. While the history and physical examination, as well as the detection of warning signals, is identical to that described for the infant with recurrent vomiting (section 5.1.1), the

TABLE 3. *Differential diagnosis of vomiting in infants and children*

Gastrointestinal obstruction
    pyloric stenosis
    malrotation with intermittent volvulus
    intermittent intussusception
    intestinal duplication
    Hirschsprung disease
    antral/duodenal web
    foreign body
    incarcerated hernia

Gastrointestinal disorders
    achalasia
    gastroparesis
    gastroenteritis
    peptic ulcer disease
    gastroesophageal reflux
    eosinophilic esophagitis/ gastroenteritis
    food allergy or intolerance
    inflammatory bowel disease
    pancreatitis
    appendicitis

Neurologic
    hydrocephalus
    subdural hematoma
    intracranial hemorrhage
    mass lesion

Infectious
    sepsis
    meningitis
    urinary tract infection
    pneumonia
    otitis media
    hepatitis

Metabolic/endocrine
    galactosemia
    hereditary fructose intolerance
    urea cycle defects
    amino and organic acidemias
    congenital adrenal hyperplasia
    maple syrup urine disease

Renal
    obstructive uropathy
    renal insufficiency

Toxic
    lead
    iron
    Vitamin A or D
    medications (ipecac, digoxin, theophylline, etc.)

Cardiac
    congestive heart failure

finding of growth failure is a crucial factor that alters clinical management. No well-controlled studies of diagnostic or therapeutic strategies for these infants are available, and the following approach is based on expert opinion. Other causes of poor weight gain are first considered. It is recommended that the adequacy of calories being offered and ingested be assessed, by careful evaluation of the dietary history, approach to formula preparation and effectiveness of swallowing. If problems are

TABLE 4. *History in the child with suspected gastroesophageal reflux disease*

Feeding history
    Amount/frequency (overfeeding)
    Type (preparation errors)
    Changes
    Position/burping
    Behavior during feedings
        choking, gagging, coughing, arching
        discomfort, feeding refusal

Pattern of vomiting
    Frequency/amount
    Painful
    Forceful
    Hematemesis
    Association with fever, lethargy, diarrhea

Past medical history
    Prematurity
    Growth and development (MR/CP/Dev Delay)
    Surgery
    Hospitalization
    Newborn screen (galactosemia, maple sugar urine disease,
        congenital adrenal hyperplasia)
    Recurrent illness (croup/stridor, pneumonia, wheeze, hoarseness,
        excessive fussiness/crying, hiccups)
    Apnea
    Inadequate weight gain

Psycho-social history
    Stress

Family history
    Significant Illness
    GI (familial pattern to obstructive disorders, celiac)
    Other (metabolic, allergy)

Growth chart
    Length, weight
        Head circumference

Warning signs (see Table 5)

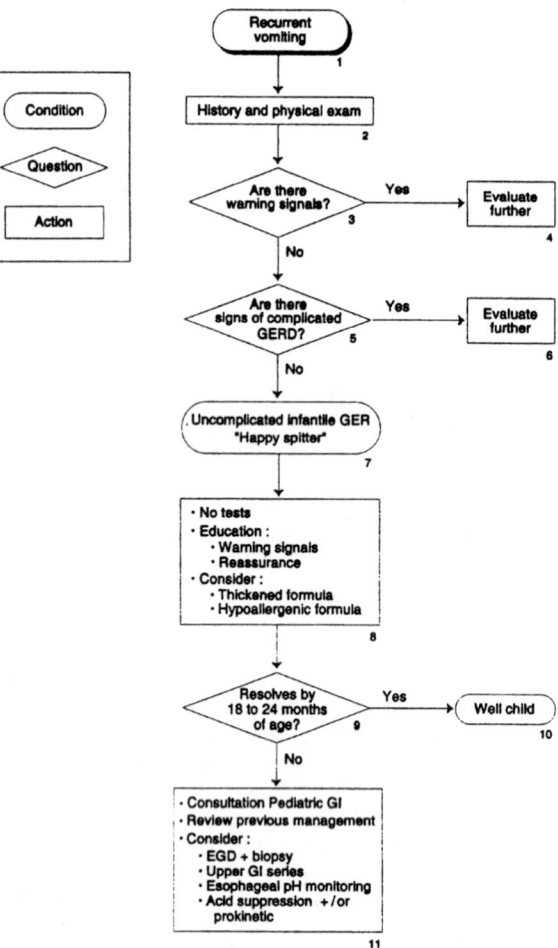

FIG. 1. An algorithm for the management of an infant with uncomplicated GER (the "happy spitter"). (Pediatric GI = pediatric gastroenterologist; EGD = esophagogastroduodenoscopy; UGI = upper gastrointestinal series radiography).

identified, these are addressed such that adequate caloric intake is assured. Parents may need to be instructed to not limit formula intake. If problems are identified and ameliorated, close follow-up will determine if further

TABLE 5. *Warning signals in the vomiting infant*

    Bilious vomiting
    GI bleeding: hematemesis, hematochezia
    Forceful vomiting
    Onset of vomiting after 6 months of life
    Failure to thrive
    Diarrhea
    Constipation
    Fever
    Lethargy
    Hepatosplenomegaly
    Bulging fontanelle
    Macro/microcephaly
    Seizures
    Abdominal tenderness, distention
    Genetic disorders (eg: Trisomy 21)
    Other chronic disorders (eg: HIV)

evaluation is indicated. See section 5.4 regarding the infant who is unable or refuses to ingest formula.

If an infant with vomiting is not gaining weight despite ingesting adequate calories then further diagnostic evaluation is necessary. Tests to uncover other causes of vomiting (such as a complete blood count, electrolytes, bicarbonate, urea nitrogen, creatinine, alanine aminotransferase, ammonia, glucose, urinalysis, urine ketones and reducing substances, and review of newborn screening for galactosemia and maple sugar urine disease) are considered. An upper GI series to evaluate anatomy is also recommended.

When no abnormalities are found, management options include medical therapy, observation in the hospital and endoscopy with biopsy. Initial medical therapeutic options include thickening of the formula, a trial of a hypoallergenic formula, acid suppression therapy, prokinetic therapy and consideration of prone positioning. Hospitalization to observe the parent-child interaction

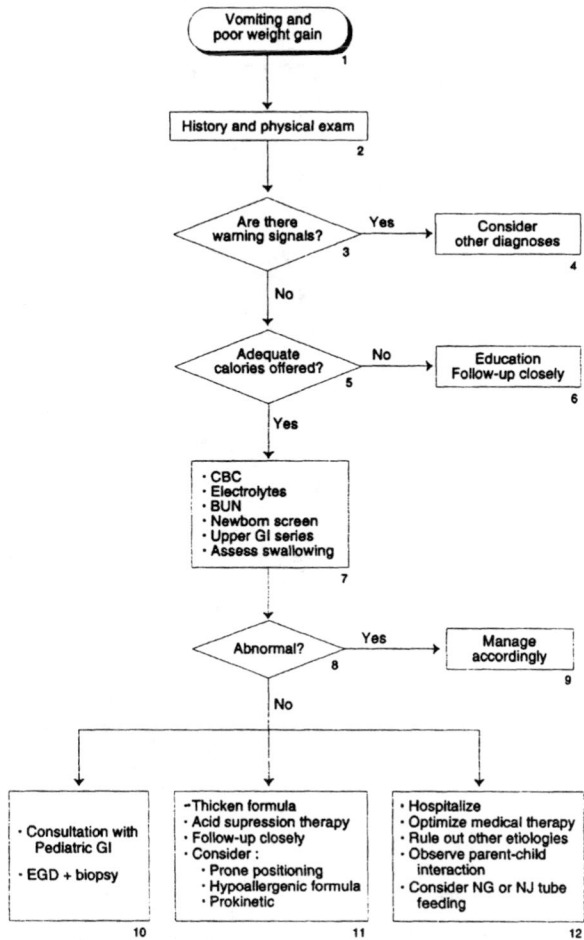

FIG. 2. An algorithm for the management of an infant with vomiting and poor weight gain. (CBC = complete blood count; BUN = blood urea nitrogen; NG = nasogastric; NJ = nasojejunal).

and to optimize medical management may be indicated in more severe cases. Endoscopy with biopsy may be useful to determine if esophagitis is present and to delineate other causes of vomiting or poor weight gain. Other options to improve caloric intake in the infant with vomiting include increasing the caloric density of the formula, and nasogastric or transpyloric tube feedings (87). Rarely surgical therapy may be indicated. Careful follow-up is necessary to assure adequate weight gain (85). If weight gain is sustained, the patient can be expected to have decreasing requirements for interventions as the amount of vomiting and regurgitation decrease with age.

5.1.4 The Infant with Recurrent Vomiting and Irritability. Vomiting, irritability and disturbed sleep in a child less than one year of age may be due to GERD. These non-specific symptoms also occur in normal infants and are associated with a wide range of conditions. Although crying is a quantifiable measure of irritability, normal infants typically fuss or cry intermittently for an

average of two hours daily. Substantial individual variation occurs; some infants cry as much as six hours per day. The duration of crying typically peaks at six weeks of age (227). One parent may consider crying to be normal while another would describe the same behavior as extreme irritability. Similarly, the sleeping patterns of infants show individual and maturational variation as does the parental perceptions of normal infant sleep patterns (228).

Evidence supporting the theory that reflux causes esophageal pain and hence irritability or sleep disturbance in infancy is largely extrapolated from studies in adults (45,229,230). Very few pediatric studies address this issue. Using simultaneous video and esophageal pH monitoring, one study (46) showed an association between grimacing and reflux episodes. However, another pediatric study showed no correlation between excessive crying and esophagitis (18) and another noted no increase in irritability or back arching in infants with pathologic reflux (231). In two small studies, an association between excessive irritability and sleep disturbance in infants with abnormal pH probe studies was observed. One study found more nighttime waking, delayed onset of sleeping and greater daytime sleeping in infants with GER as compared to population norms but not when compared to a control group of infants with normal pH probe findings (232). Another study demonstrated no increase in sleep disturbances in those infants with pathologic reflux (231). One study of five infants with colic and esophagitis showed that treatment with cimetidine decreased crying from 3.7 to 1.2 hours after a week of treatment, which was significantly different from 13 children with colic who did not have esophagitis and who were not treated (233).

No studies address the best approach to evaluation of infants with vomiting and irritability or disturbed sleep. As in all infants with vomiting, other causes of vomiting need to be excluded (section 5.1.1 and Table 3). A symptom diary (234) may be useful to determine the extent to which the infant is irritable and has disturbed sleep. In addition, it is important to assure that the infant is receiving adequate feedings, since hunger may also result in irritability. Expert opinion suggests two diagnostic and treatment strategies, neither of which has been validated. The first approach is to empirically treat potential etiologies, beginning with a simultaneous or sequential two-week trial of a hypoallergenic formula and/or acid suppression (Section 5.1). If neither therapy succeeds in reducing symptoms, either esophageal pH monitoring to determine the adequacy of acid suppression (see section 3.3) or upper endoscopy with biopsy to diagnose esophagitis (see section 3.4) may be performed. If these studies are normal, and no response to empiric therapy has occurred, it is unlikely that GER is contributing to the symptoms. An alternative approach is to perform esophageal pH monitoring to determine if episodes of irritability or sleep disturbance are temporally associated with acid reflux by calculating a symptom index (see section 3.3). One study suggested that simultaneous video monitoring was helpful (46). Time limited therapy can be initiated if episodes of GER provoke symptoms.

5.1.5 Management of the Child Over 2 Years of Age with Recurrent Regurgitation or Vomiting. No published studies describe the management of a group of otherwise normal children who have recurrent regurgitation or vomiting after the age of 2 years. These children usually vomit, or regurgitate and reswallow, between once a day and once a week. The vomiting is not associated with pain or discomfort, is not posttussive, and is non-bloody and non-bilious. Often the vomiting occurs postprandially or with exertion. This type of vomiting can be a nuisance or in some instances may disrupt a child's normal participation in childhood activities. Expert opinion suggests that in most patients an upper GI series be performed to exclude an anatomic abnormality. Some experts also recommend upper endoscopy with biopsy, although in many cases there will be no abnormalities. If vomiting persists and the child remains otherwise asymptomatic, a therapeutic trial of a prokinetic agent may be considered. If a good response to the prokinetic agent occurs, long-term therapy is an option. The small risks must be balanced with the potential improved quality of life in the individual and the family. In very unusual circumstances where the vomiting does not improve with pharmacological therapy and produces serious adverse effects on the patient's lifestyle, surgical therapy is a consideration.

5.2 Management of the Child with Heartburn or Chest Pain (Figure 3)

Heartburn or substernal burning pain may be caused by GER in the presence or absence of esophagitis (235). Other causes of chest pain include cardiac, respiratory, musculoskeletal, medication induced or infectious etiologies. In older children and adolescents the description and localization of esophageal pain is similar to adults, but in younger children symptom description and localization may be atypical. Regurgitation of sour fluid into the mouth may be present. No randomized, placebo-controlled studies evaluating the efficacy of either lifestyle or pharmacological therapy for the treatment of heartburn in children or adolescents have been published. Expert opinion suggests the use of management approaches similar to those described in adult patients. Initial interventions of lifestyle changes, avoidance of precipitating factors, accompanied by a two to four week therapeutic trial of an H₂RA or PPI are recommended (172,236–238). If no improvement occurs, the child can be referred to a pediatric gastroenterologist for upper endoscopy with biopsy. If the child improves, therapy can be administered for two to three months. If symptoms recur as therapy is discontinued, referral for upper

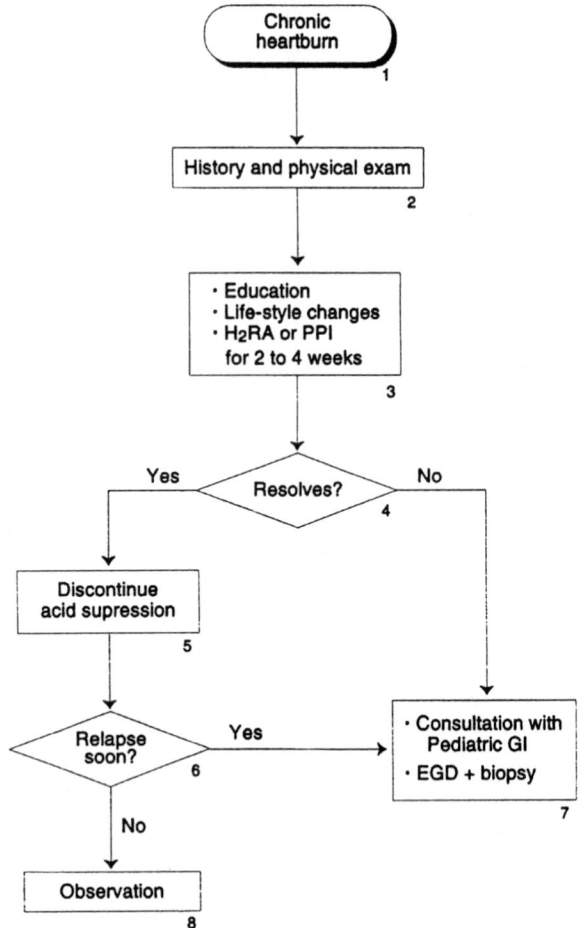

FIG. 3. An algorithm for the management of a child or adolescent with chronic heartburn. (H₂RA = histamine-₂ receptor antagonist; PPI = proton pump inhibitor).

endoscopy to determine the presence and severity of esophagitis is recommended. Because persistent symptoms of heartburn may have a substantial negative impact on a patient's quality of life, long-term therapy can be continued with either a PPI or H₂RA to provide relief from symptoms even in the absence of esophagitis (70,239). Episodic meal-induced heartburn in older children may be treated with antacids or an H₂RA, as in adults (240).

5.3 The Infant or Child with Esophagitis (Figure 4)

The typical features of reflux esophagitis are described in section 3.5. Initial treatment consists of lifestyle changes and H₂RA or PPI therapy Initialtherapy. Initial treatment with a PPI results in a more rapid rate of symptom relief and healing compared to treatment with an H₂RA (152). If patients have previously been treated for GERD, medical therapy can be optimized by either the

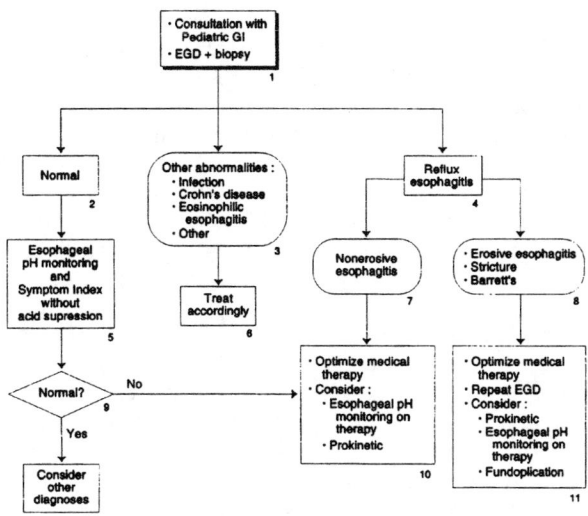

FIG. 4. An algorithm for the continued management of a child or adolescent with esophagitis.

addition of a PPI or a higher dose of PPI (47,241). In one pediatric study, cisapride alone was effective for treatment of histologic esophagitis (181). However, in adults a comparison of the efficacy of a PPI alone versus a combination of a PPI and cisapride did not show a statistically significant difference (169).

Expert opinion suggests that in infants and children with only histologic esophagitis, the efficacy of therapy can be monitored by the degree of symptom relief, whereas in patients with erosive esophagitis, repeat endoscopy is recommended to assure healing. Complete healing may prevent complications including esophageal stricture, Barrett's esophagus or esophageal adenocarcinoma, although no data are available to support this contention. High dose, long-term PPI therapy or surgical therapy may be considered when Barrett's esophagus or esophageal stricture is also present.

If patients do not respond to therapy there are two potential explanations to explore: either the diagnosis is incorrect or treatment is inadequate. The possibility of another diagnosis, such as eosinophilic esophagitis may be considered (56,57). If the clinical presentation and histopathology are consistent with a diagnosis of reflux esophagitis, then the evaluation of adherence to and adequacy of therapy is recommended. Esophageal pH monitoring while the patient is *on therapy* will determine if higher doses of acid reducing medications are needed. If the diagnosis is uncertain, esophageal pH monitoring while the patient is *off therapy* may be useful since a normal study would suggest that esophagitis is less likely to be due to GER.

When surgical therapy is considered, the potential complications of anti-reflux surgery are balanced with the nuisance, risks, effectiveness and cost of long-term pharmacological therapy. There are no studies compar-

ing long term outcomes of medical versus surgical therapy in infants and children since the introduction of PPIs.

5.4 The Infant with Feeding Refusal or the Child with Dysphagia

Esophagitis may cause discomfort or pain (odynophagia) or difficulty (dysphagia) with eating in infants, children and adults. The older child or adult is able to describe sensations that aid in discriminating between oropharyngeal disorders and esophageal disorders. Mouth or pharyngeal pain, poor coordination of bolus formation, coughing or apnea during feeding suggests oropharyngeal anatomical or functional problems. Complaints of chest pain or food being stuck in the chest generally indicate that there is an esophageal disorder, although the sensory discrimination of the site of obstruction is often inaccurate. Reflux esophagitis appears to be one of the more common causes of these symptoms in children, being diagnosed in 12 of 16 children reported in one retrospective series (242).

In the older child or adolescent with symptoms suggestive of an esophageal cause of dysphagia or odynophagia, diagnostic evaluation usually begins with a radiographic contrast study (barium esophagram) to identify anatomic abnormalities, such as strictures or vascular rings, and motility disorders, such as achalasia. Upper endoscopy with biopsy is also usually performed. If esophagitis is present, treatment of the underlying cause of esophagitis (e.g., reflux esophagitis, pill esophagitis or eosinophilic esophagitis) generally leads to symptom resolution. There are no studies evaluating this proposed diagnostic approach in older children or adolescents; however, in a study of young adults (243), the barium esophagram revealed a cause of symptoms in 70% of patients. If the initial history is suggestive of esophagitis, upper endoscopy may be performed as the initial diagnostic test. Treatment without prior diagnostic evaluation is generally not recommended.

In infants, although case series have described an association of feeding difficulties with signs and symptoms of GER (244–246), none has demonstrated that GER is causally related to the feeding difficulties or that feeding improves following treatment. Because a large variety of disorders may contribute to infant feeding difficulties (247), empiric therapy for GER is generally not recommended in children with feeding difficulties. However, if there are other signs or symptoms suggestive of GERD (section 5.1.1) then a time-limited course of medical therapy can be considered.

5.5 The Infant with Apnea or ALTE

An apparent life-threatening event (ALTE) is defined as an episode occurring in an infant that is frightening to the observer and characterized by a combination of apnea, change in color (cyanosis, pallor, rubor, plethora), change in muscle tone (limpness, stiffness), or choking and gagging that requires intervention by the caretaker (248). The first event usually occurs between one and two months, and rarely after 8 months of age (249,250). There is evidence that ALTEs can recur (250–252), and that infants with an ALTE are at risk for a subsequent sudden death (252–258). ALTEs can be caused by intentional suffocation, cardiac, central nervous system and infectious disorders, and can be due to upper airway obstruction or central apnea as well as GER.

In patients with ALTEs the prevalence of recurrent regurgitation or emesis is 60% to 70% (249,252), and 40% to 80% of patients have abnormal esophageal pH monitoring (259–261). Case reports have described ALTEs triggered by overt regurgitation into the oropharynx or by aspiration of refluxed gastric contents (262–264). Gross emesis or oral regurgitation has been correlated with either prolonged apnea (>20 seconds), or with shorter apnea and bradycardia, but the majority of prolonged apnea episodes in these patients were not associated with regurgitation (265). The first report of simultaneous recordings of esophageal pH, heart rate, chest wall movement and nasal airflow demonstrated that reflux could precede apnea (262). In selected patients with a history of ALTE, esophageal acid infusion has been shown to induce obstructive apnea (262) or oxygen desaturation (259), suggesting that one mechanism by which GER may trigger an ALTE is acid stimulation of laryngeal, pharyngeal, or esophageal chemoreceptors with resultant laryngospasm.

Despite these early reports and the demonstrated potential for GER to cause apnea, subsequent investigations in unselected patients with ALTE have not demonstrated a convincing temporal relationship between esophageal acidification and apnea or bradycadia (260, 261, 266–272). Although several studies reported an occasional correlation of GER with short mixed central apneas (5 to 15 sec) (266,269,271), all of the patients reported also had episodes of apnea which were unrelated to episodes of GER, suggesting a primary impairment in the regulation of respiration. The most convincing relationship between GER and episodes of obstructive or mixed apnea has been in infants in whom the episodes occurred while the patient was awake, supine and within one hour of a feeding. One study performed simultaneous recording of esophageal pH, heart rate, chest wall movement and nasal airflow to demonstrate a relationship between GER and obstructive or mixed apnea in 8 of 15 such patients (273).

At present there is no evidence that the characteristics of an ALTE or polysomnographic diagnostic study can predict which infants are at risk for future life-threatening episodes or sudden death. In one study of 182 infants with ALTE followed for two months, the coexistence of GER and ALTE did not predict the risk for a subsequent episode of prolonged apnea or bradycardia. SIDS has rarely been reported to occur in patients with a previous ALTE and documented GER (261,274); in none of these patients was a previous correlation between esophageal acidification and a cardiopulmonary event recorded.

Similarly there are no randomized studies to evaluate the usefulness of esophageal pH monitoring in infants with ALTE. In patients with frequent ALTE in which the role of GER is uncertain, esophageal pH monitoring may be useful to determine if there is a temporal association of acid reflux with ALTE. For adequate interpretation of esophageal pH monitoring in this situation, simultaneous recording of heart rate, chest wall impedance, nasal airflow and oxygen saturation is necessary to detect obstructive apnea.

The evidence suggests that infants with ALTE and GER may be more likely to respond to anti-reflux therapy when there is gross emesis or oral regurgitation at the time of the ALTE, when episodes occur in the awake infant, and when the ALTE is characterized by obstructive apnea. The effectiveness of medical therapy of GER-associated ALTEs has not been adequately studied. To reduce overt emesis and inhibit acid reflux, therapeutic options include thickened feedings and prokinetic and acid suppressant therapy. Surgical therapy has been reported to be effective in preventing recurrent ALTE and death in heterogeneous groups of patients (263,274), but there are no studies comparing surgery to medical management. Since most infants improve with medical management, surgery is considered only in severe cases. Caution should be exercised when diagnosing and treating GER as a presumptive cause of ALTE. Antireflux surgery has been performed for GER in infants with ALTE that was subsequently determined to be due to repetitive intentional suffocation (275).

5.6 The Infant or Child with Asthma (Figure 5)

Asthma affects an estimated 4.8 million children (276), 5% of whom have persistent asthma, defined as a frequency greater than 2 or 3 times weekly. Although a direct causal relationship between GER and asthma is rare, a number of animal and human studies have suggested that GER may contribute to asthma severity. Proposed pathogenetic mechanisms include direct aggravation of airway inflammation by aspiration of gastric contents, or airway hyperresponsiveness triggered by aspiration of minute amounts of acid into the lower airway (277–279). Esophageal acidification as an independent variable has minimal effect on pulmonary function (277). However, esophageal acid exposure in asthmatic patients may contribute to airway hyperresponsiveness and variable airflow obstruction (280).

Symptoms of GER are common in children with asthma (281). A high percentage of children with persis-

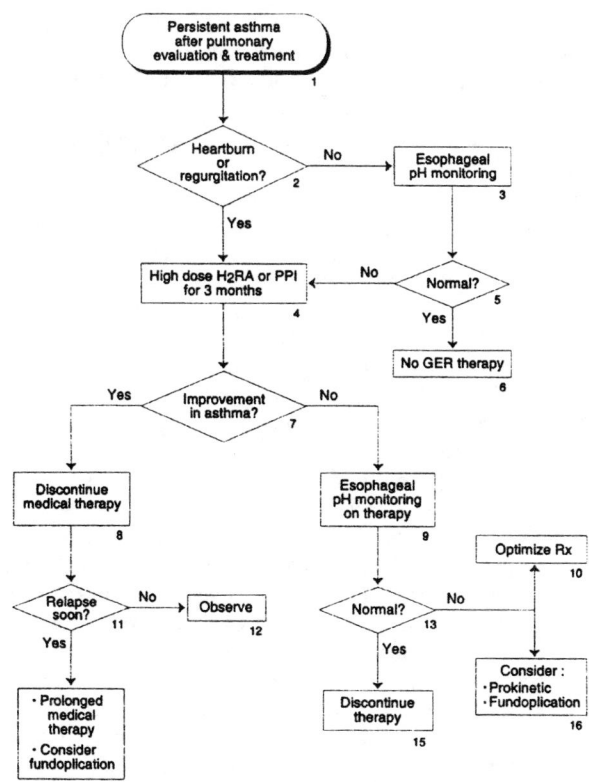

FIG. 5. An algorithm for the management of a child or adolescent with persistent asthma and suspected GER. See also Figure 3. (Rx = therapy).

tent asthma have gastroesophageal reflux detectable by abnormal esophageal pH monitoring. The reported prevalence ranges from 25% to 75%. Of 668 patients studied in 13 series, 407 or 61% were reported to have abnormal pH studies utilizing a variety of scoring techniques (48–50,65,282–290). There was a similar prevalence of GER (53%) in three studies of infants less than 2 years of age (49,282,283). Approximately 50% of patients with persistent asthma and abnormal esophageal pH monitoring have no or minimal clinical symptoms of GER, such as vomiting, regurgitation, or heartburn (48, 50,282,284,288). There is no consistent evidence that specific asthma symptoms or response to asthma therapy correlates with abnormal esophageal pH monitoring.

A number of cohort comparisons have been performed in patients with GER symptoms or positive esophageal pH probe monitoring. These studies demonstrate that prolonged medical treatment of GER improves clinical symptoms of persistent asthma and reduces required doses of bronchodilator and anti-inflammatory medications. From four case series reporting on a total of 168 patients, 63% had clinical improvement or reduced dosages of bronchodilator and anti-inflammatory medications following a variety of medical approaches (50,284, 288,291). Improvement of respiratory variables has been

described in infants less than one year of age (291) and older children with or without atopy (50). Reported successful therapies have included positional therapy and thickened formula without medication (284,288), cisapride (50), and H_2RA (292). There are no studies of combined prokinetic and antisecretory therapy to treat GER in patients with asthma. Adult studies suggest that duration of therapy is very important, and aggressive acid suppression for at least 3 months may be necessary to reduce respiratory symptoms (68) (293,294). No studies address the empiric treatment of asthma in patients without GER symptoms or with normal esophageal pH monitoring.

More striking results have been reported following antireflux surgery. Eighty-five percent of 258 patients reported in 6 case series improved clinically as assessed by decreased frequency and severity of asthmatic attacks and reduced dosages of bronchodilator and anti-inflammatory medications (213,284,288,291,295,296). Although details were often not provided, it appears that all the patients had severe persistent asthma requiring frequent oral steroids or high dose inhaled steroid prior to surgery. The diagnosis of GER was most often confirmed by esophageal pH monitoring. Indications for antireflux surgery included evidence of recurrent pneumonia, failed time-limited medical antireflux management, dependence on aggressive medical management, and non-respiratory complications (persistent vomiting, vomiting with growth retardation, severe esophagitis). Subjective improvement in asthma after fundoplication was correlated with a clear history of reflux symptoms preceding the onset of asthma symptoms, a positive response to medical therapy prior to surgery, a history of recurrent pneumonia, and nocturnal attacks of asthma. Failure of medical antireflux management did not preclude a favorable response to surgical antireflux management. Adult surgical series have shown similar improvements in symptoms and reductions of medication use following surgery but without dramatic improvement in pulmonary function tests (297).

Thus there is substantial published evidence that GER is a potential contributor to symptoms of persistent asthma. The true incidence of GER in children with asthma is not known, as the reported data is from selected referred groups of patients with persistent asthma. The available evidence does not support therapy of GER in all patients with persistent asthma who fail to respond to standard asthma therapy. However, a trial of vigorous, prolonged medical therapy of GER is recommended for children when symptoms of asthma and GERD (e.g., heartburn, regurgitation) co-exist, and in infants and toddlers with chronic vomiting or regurgitation and recurrent episodes of cough and wheezing.

If a patient with persistent asthma does not have symptoms of GER, esophageal pH monitoring is recommended in selected patients who are more likely to benefit from GER therapy. This includes patients with radiographic evidence of recurrent pneumonia; patients with nocturnal asthma more than once a week; and patients requiring either continuous oral corticosteroids, high-dose inhaled corticosteroids, more than two bursts per year of oral corticosteroids or those with persistent asthma unable to wean medical management. If esophageal pH monitoring demonstrates an increased frequency or duration of esophageal acid exposure, a trial of prolonged medical therapy for GER is recommended.

Currently there is insufficient pediatric evidence to establish the optimal medical therapy for GER in patients with asthma. It is recommended that a three month trial of vigorous antisecretory therapy and possibly cisapride be considered. It is recommended that outcome variables be determined prior to initiating therapy and be monitored during therapy. Outcome variables include heartburn and regurgitation; frequency of asthma symptoms (coughing, dyspnea, wheezing, and chest tightness); frequency and severity of acute exacerbations; frequency of nocturnal symptoms and breathlessness; symptom scores; quick-relief beta2-agonist use; changes in spirometry measurements (FEV1, FVC, FEV1/FVC) in older children; and subjective measures of quality of life. Antireflux surgery is considered in patients with persistent asthma and recurrent pneumonia, patients requiring prolonged medical therapy and patients with nonrespiratory complications of GER such as persistent vomiting, vomiting with growth retardation and severe esophagitis.

5.7 Recurrent Pneumonia and GER

GER-related aspiration pneumonia may arise in the absence of esophagitis. The incidence of GER and recurrent pneumonia in otherwise normal infants and children (288,290) (298) is difficult to establish due to the heterogeneity of the patients in reported studies, which include a large number of children with neurological disabilities and anatomic disorders of the upper intestinal tract. Several reports show that pediatric patients with recurrent pneumonia and GER improve after receiving medical or surgical GER therapy (296,299). In addition, many patients with idiopathic pulmonary fibrosis have GER (300), suggesting that repeated small episodes of aspiration of gastric contents can eventually cause severe compromise of pulmonary function. These clinical reports as well as clinical experience indicate that GER can cause recurrent pneumonia and chronic pulmonary fibrosis.

Before considering GER as a potential cause of recurrent pneumonia, it is important to exclude other causes, such as an anatomic abnormality, aspiration during swallowing, foreign body, cystic fibrosis or immunodeficiency (301). Determining whether GER is causing recurrent pneumonia in an individual patient is difficult but certain patient populations are prone to aspiration. The presence

of neuromuscular disease (302) or a history of esophageal or laryngeal anatomic abnormalities increases the risk of aspiration during swallowing and following episodes of GER. The incidence of GER-related recurrent aspiration in otherwise normal infants and children is unknown but it appears to be rare.

Normal esophageal pH monitoring does not exclude GER as a cause of aspiration pneumonia. The addition of an upper esophageal or pharyngeal pH recording does not improve the ability of pH monitoring to determine which patients are at risk for aspiration as a complication of GER (43). Presumably, patients with even rare episodes of reflux of gastric contents into the pharynx are at risk for aspiration if airway protective reflexes are abnormal. A variety of tests may be useful to evaluate these protective mechanisms.

Flexible bronchoscopy with pulmonary lavage for lipid laden alveolar macrophages has been utilized to detect aspiration (303,304). However, lipid-laden macrophages may be present in normal individuals so their presence in pulmonary lavage lacks sensitivity and specificity for determining if the cause of pulmonary disease is aspiration. Recent efforts to improve the sensitivity and specificity utilize careful protocols that score the lipid content of over 100 macrophages, but considerable overlap exists between normal controls, patients with other causes of pulmonary disease and those with a history consistent with aspiration (305–308). If bronchoscopy with pulmonary lavage demonstrates a large percentage of lipid-laden macrophages, aspiration is more likely, but this test does not discriminate between aspiration that occurs during swallowing and that following GER. The lack of specificity of the test requires that the results be interpreted in the context of other clinical findings.

Nuclear scintigraphy can detect episodes of aspiration when follow-up images are obtained up to 24 hours after the feeding is administered. A positive test demonstrates that aspiration occurred but a negative test does not exclude the possibility that GER with aspiration occurs infrequently (section 3.5). Despite the potential utility of scintigraphy, no data are available regarding its predictive value in management of children or adults with suspected aspiration pneumonia.

Evaluation of airway protection mechanisms during feeding may also be helpful since patients who aspirate during feedings are also likely to aspirate refluxate. One study in neurologically disabled children showed that recurrent pneumonia was more likely in those with an abnormal swallowing study (309). Thus, a videofluoroscopic swallowing study (VSS) or fiberendoscopic swallowing evaluation (FEEST), particularly with neurosensory testing, may help identify at risk patients (310–313).

Often the clinician must make management decisions based on inconclusive information. If the patient has severely impaired lung function, it may be necessary to proceed with antireflux surgery in an attempt to prevent further pulmonary damage, despite a lack of definitive proof that GER is causing pulmonary disease in the individual patient. The potential benefits of surgery are balanced with the recognition of potential complications (section 4.3). Alternatively, if minimal pulmonary disease is present, consideration of medical therapy with careful follow-up of pulmonary function can be considered. No controlled studies demonstrate the benefits of any medical therapy in preventing progression of chronic pulmonary disease caused by GER in children, but lifestyle and pharmacological agents are options.

5.8 The Infant or Child with Upper Airway Symptoms or Signs

Airway symptoms of hoarseness (314), chronic cough (315,316) and globus sensation (the sensation of a lump in the throat) (317,318) have been associated with GER in adult patients. Characteristic reflux-induced findings of airway erythema, edema, nodularity, ulceration, granuloma and cobblestoning have been described (319,320). The sensitivity and specificity of descriptive laryngoscopic findings for the identification of GER-induced disease are unknown in both pediatric and adult patients. These symptoms or signs usually occur in the absence of classical symptoms of GER such as heartburn or chest pain. In adult GER patients, increased acid exposure in the proximal esophagus (321) and pharynx (322) has been observed in those with airway symptoms of cough or frequent throat clearing. Gastropharyngeal reflux was more prevalent in a small study of children with recurrent laryngotracheitis compared to control patients (323). An increased frequency of episodes of awake GER in children with hoarseness has been suggested in one pediatric case series (324). One case report documents a temporal association of GER episodes and cough in an infant (325). Another case series suggests that GER may contribute to either the pathogenesis of subglottic stenosis or may compromise surgical results (326), while another notes increased pharyngeal reflux in children with laryngomalacia (44).

Several uncontrolled treatment studies in adults have demonstrated improvements in laryngeal symptoms and findings following aggressive medical therapy for GER, with recurrence of symptoms when treatment was discontinued (68,69,320,327,328). Improvement in symptoms of hoarseness after GER therapy was reported in one child (329). Another uncontrolled case series describes improvement in a variety of upper airway symptoms in pediatric patients following treatment of GER with a variety of therapies (330). One study demonstrates a marked reduction in cough symptoms in adults with GER following laparoscopic fundoplication (331). There are no randomized placebo controlled treatment trials evaluating the efficacy of GER therapy of laryngeal symptoms in adults or children. Adult data suggest that if a therapeutic trial is considered, it must be prolonged (longer than three months) to adequately assess efficacy (68). If there is clinical improvement, followed by a recurrence off therapy, it is reasonable to suspect a role for GER in the pathogenesis of symptoms in an individual patient.

In summary, several studies describe the presence of GER in children with either chronic or recurrent laryngeal symptoms. The evaluation of suspected GER-associated laryngeal symptoms is complicated by a lack of a uniform interpretation of laryngeal findings. Nonetheless laryngoscopy is generally indicated to rule out potential anatomic abnormalities of airway protection such as a laryngeal cleft. At this time, there is insufficient evidence and experience in children to provide recommendations for a uniform approach to diagnosis and treatment.

5.9 Other Disorders Potentially Associated with GER

Multiple case reports suggest an association between GER and a variety of other disorders. One study suggested that adolescents with GER had an increased incidence of erosion of enamel on the lingual surfaces of their teeth (332). However, another study showed no increased incidence of dental erosions in adolescents with abnormal esophageal pH monitoring (333).

GER has been suggested as a potential contributing factor in recurrent sinus disease, pharyngitis and otitis media. One uncontrolled case series of children with chronic sinusitis suggested that treatment of GER dramatically reduced the need for sinus surgery in children (334). Another demonstrated that in children with recurrent rhinopharyngitis, there was an increased number of episodes with the pharyngeal pH falling to below 6 in affected patients compared to controls (335). However, the occurrences of ear and sinus infections were similar in infants with or without GER (8). No data demonstrate an association of otitis media and GER. However, otalgia has been associated with GER in children and was reported to improve with treatment of GER (336).

Authors

Colin D. Rudolph, MD, PhD
Cincinnati, OH

Lynnette J. Mazur, MD
Houston, TX

Gregory S. Liptak, MD
Rochester, NY

Robert D. Baker, MD, PhD
Buffalo, NY

John T. Boyle, MD
Greenville, SC

Richard B. Colletti, MD
Burlington, VT

William T. Gerson, MD
Burlington, VT

Steven L. Werlin, MD
Milwaukee, WI

REFERENCES

1. Vandenplas Y, Sacre-Smits L. Continuous 24-hour esophageal pH monitoring in 285 asymptomatic infants 0-15 months old. *J Pediatr Gastroenterol Nutr* 1987;6:220–4.

2. Vandenplas Y, Goyvaerts H, Helven R, et al. Gastroesophageal reflux, as measured by 24-hour pH monitoring, in 509 healthy infants screened for risk of sudden infant death syndrome. *Pediatrics* 1991;88:834–40.

3. Gustafsson PM, Tibbling L. 24-hour oesophageal two-level pH monitoring in healthy children and adolescents. *Scand J Gastroenterol* 1988;23:91–4.

4. Nelson SP, Chen EH, Syniar GM, et al. Prevalence of symptoms of gastroesophageal reflux during childhood: a pediatric practice-based survey. Pediatric Practice Research Group. *Arch Pediatr Adolesc Med* 2000;154:150–4.

5. Werlin SL, Dodds WJ, Hogan WJ, et al. Mechanisms of gastroesophageal reflux in children. *J Pediatr* 1980;97:244–9.

6. Kawahara H, Dent J, Davidson G. Mechanisms responsible for gastroesophageal reflux in children [see comments]. *Gastroenterology* 1997;113:399–408.

7. Nelson SP, Chen EH, Syniar GM, et al. Prevalence of symptoms of gastroesophageal reflux during infancy. A pediatric practice-based survey. Pediatric Practice Research Group. *Arch Pediatr Adolesc Med* 1997;151:569–72.

8. Nelson SP, Chen EH, Syniar GM, et al. One-year follow-up of symptoms of gastroesophageal reflux during infancy. Pediatric Practice Research Group. *Pediatrics* 1998;102:E67.

9. Werlin SL, D'Souza BJ, Hogan WJ, et al. Sandifer syndrome: an unappreciated clinical entity. *Dev Med Child Neurol* 1980;22:374–8.

10. Gorrotxategi P, Reguilon MJ, Arana J, et al. Gastroesophageal reflux in association with the Sandifer syndrome. *Eur J Pediatr Surg* 1995;5:203–5.

11. Herbst JJ, Johnson DG, Oliveros MA. Gastroesophageal reflux with protein-losing enteropathy and finger clubbing. *Am J Dis Child* 1976;130:1256–8.

12. Hassall E. Barrett's esophagus: new definitions and approaches in children. *J Pediatr Gastroenterol Nutr* 1993;16:345–64.

13. Sackett DL, Richardson WS, Rosenberg W, et al. Evidence-based Medicine: How to Practice and Teach EBM. 1998, Edinburgh: Churchill Livingston.

14. Sackett DL, Haynes B, Tugwell P. Clinical Epidemiology: A Basic Science for Clinical Medicine. 2nd ed. 1991, Boston: Little Brown.

15. McMurray AR. Three decision-making aids: brainstorming, nominal group, and Delphi technique. J Nurs Staff Dev 1994;10:62–5.

16. Examination CTFotPH, The periodic health examination. *Can Med Assoc J* 1979;121:119.

17. Hyams JS, Ricci A, Jr, Leichtner AM. Clinical and laboratory correlates of esophagitis in young children. *J Pediatr Gastroenterol Nutr* 1988;7:52–6.

18. Chadwick LM, Kurinczuk JJ, Hallam LA, et al. Clinical and endoscopic predictors of histological oesophagitis in infants. *J Paediatr Child Health* 1997;33:388–93.

19. Seibert JJ, Byrne WJ, Euler AR, et al. Gastroesophageal reflux–the acid test: scintigraphy or the pH probe? *AJR Am J Roentgenol* 1983;140:1087–90.

20. Stephen TC, Younoszai MK, Massey MP, et al. Diagnosis of gastroesophageal reflux in pediatrics. *J Ky Med Assoc* 1994; 92: 188–91.

21. Meyers WF, Roberts CC, Johnson DG, et al. Value of tests for evaluation of gastroesophageal reflux in children. *J Pediatr Surg* 1985;20:515–20.

22. Thompson JK, Koehler RE, Richter JE. Detection of gastroesophageal reflux: value of barium studies compared with 24-hr pH monitoring [see comments]. *AJR Am J Roentgenol* 1994;162:621–6.

23. Gupta JP, Kumar A, Jain AK, et al. Gastro-esophageal reflux disease (GERD): an appraisal of different tests for diagnosis. *J Assoc Physicians India* 1990;38 Suppl 1:699–702.

24. Chen MY, Ott DJ, Sinclair JW, Wu WC, et al. Gastroesophageal reflux disease: correlation of esophageal pH testing and radiographic findings. *Radiology* 1992;185:483–6.

25. Colletti RB, Christie DL, Orenstein SR. Statement of the North American Society for Pediatric Gastroenterology and Nutrition (NASPGN). Indications for pediatric esophageal pH monitoring. *J Pediatr Gastroenterol Nutr* 1995;21:253–62.

26. Newman LJ, Berezin S, San Filippo JA, et al. A new ambulatory system for extended esophageal pH monitoring. *J Pediatr Gastroenterol Nutr* 1985;4:707–10.

27. A standardized protocol for the methodology of esophageal pH monitoring and interpretation of the data for the diagnosis of gastroesophageal reflux. Working Group of the European Society of Pediatric Gastroenterology and Nutrition. *J Pediatr Gastroenterol Nutr* 1992;14:467–71.

28. Tappin DM, King C, Paton JY. Lower oesophageal pH monitoring–a useful clinical tool. *Arch Dis Chil* 1992;67:146–8.

29. Euler AR , Byrne WJ. Twenty-four-hour esophageal intraluminal pH probe testing: a comparative analysis. *Gastroenterology* 198;80:957–61.

30. Mahajan L, Wyllie R, Oliva L, et al. Reproducibility of 24-hour intraesophageal pH monitoring in pediatric patients. *Pediatrics* 1998;101:260–3.

31. Hampton FJ, MacFadyen UM, Simpson H. Reproducibility of 24 hour oesophageal pH studies in infants. *Arch Dis Child* 1990;65:1249–54.

32. Vandenplas Y, Helven R, Goyvaerts H, et al. Reproducibility of continuous 24 hour oesophageal pH monitoring in infants and children [see comments]. *Gut* 1990;31:374–7.

33. Friesen CA, Hodge C, Roberts CC. Accuracy and reproducibility of 12-h esophageal pH monitoring. *J Pediatr Gastroenterol Nutr* 1991;12:166–8.

34. Barabino A, Costantini M, Ciccone MO, et al. Reliability of short-term esophageal pH monitoring versus 24-hour study [see comments]. *J Pediatr Gastroenterol Nut,* 1995;21:87–90.

35. Sondheimer JM. Continuous monitoring of distal esophageal pH: a diagnostic test for gastroesophageal reflux in infants. *J Pediatr* 1980;96:804–7.

36. Boix-Ochoa J, Lafuenta JM, Gil-Vernet JM. Twenty-four hour exophageal pH monitoring in gastroesophageal reflux. *J Pediatr Surg* 1980;15:74–8.

37. Jamieson JR, Stein HJ, DeMeester TR, et al. Ambulatory 24-h esophageal pH monitoring: normal values, optimal thresholds, specificity, sensitivity, and reproducibility [see comments]. *Am J Gastroenterol* 1992;87:1102–11.

38. Quigley EM. 24-h pH monitoring for gastroesophageal reflux disease: already standard but not yet gold? [editorial]. *Am J Gastroenterol* 1992;87:1071–5.

39. Vandenplas Y, Franckx-Goossens A, Pipeleers-Marichal M, et al. Area under pH 4: advantages of a new parameter in the interpre-

tation of esophageal pH monitoring data in infants. *J Pediatr Gastroenterol Nutr* 1989;9:34–9.

40. Black DD, Haggitt RC, Orenstein SR, et al. Esophagitis in infants. Morphometric histological diagnosis and correlation with measures of gastroesophageal reflux. *Gastroenterology* 1990; 98: 1408–14.

41. Cucchiara S, Staiano A, Gobio Casali L, et al. Value of the 24 hour intraoesophageal pH monitoring in children. *Gut* 1990;31: 129–33.

42. Biller JA, Winter HS, Grand RJ, et al. Are endoscopic changes predictive of histologic esophagitis in children? *J Pediatr* 1983; 103:215–8.

43. Cucchiara S, Santamaria F, Minella R, et al. Simultaneous prolonged recordings of proximal and distal intraesophageal pH in children with gastroesophageal reflux disease and respiratory symptoms. *Am J Gastroenterol* 1995;90:1791–6.

44. Matthews BL, Little JP, McGuirt WJ, et al. Reflux in infants with laryngomalacia: results of 24-hour double-probe pH monitoring. *Otolaryngol Head Neck Surg* 1999;120:860–4.

45. Katzka DA, Paoletti V, Leite L, et al. Prolonged ambulatory pH monitoring in patients with persistent gastroesophageal reflux disease symptoms: testing while on therapy identifies the need for more aggressive anti-reflux therapy [see comments]. *Am J Gastroenterol* 1996;91:2110–3.

46. Feranchak AP, Orenstein SR, Cohn JF. Behaviors associated with onset of gastroesophageal reflux episodes in infants. Prospective study using split-screen video and pH probe. *Clin Pediatr (Phila)* 1994;33:654–62.

47. Gunasekaran TS, Hassall EG. Efficacy and safety of omeprazole for severe gastroesophageal reflux in children [see comments]. *J Pediatr* 1993;123:148–54.

48. Buts JP, Barudi C, Moulin D, Claus D, et al. Prevalence and treatment of silent gastro-oesophageal reflux in children with recurrent respiratory disorders. *Eur J Pediatr* 1986;145:396–400.

49. Malfroot A, Vandenplas Y, Verlinden M, et al. Gastroesophageal reflux and unexplained chronic respiratory disease in infants and children. *Pediatr Pulmonol* 1987;3:208–13.

50. Tucci F, Resti M, Fontana R, et al. Gastroesophageal reflux and bronchial asthma: prevalence and effect of cisapride therapy [see comments]. *J Pediatr Gastroenterol Nutr* 1993;17:265–70.

51. Leape LL, Ramenofsky ML. Surgical treatment of gastroesophageal reflux in children. Results of Nissen's fundoplication in 100 children. *Am J Dis Child* 1980;134:935–8.

52. Lundell LR, Dent J, Bennett JR, et al. Endoscopic assessment of oesophagitis: clinical and functional correlates and further validation of the Los Angeles classification. *Gut* 1999;45:172–80.

53. Gupta SK, Fitzgerald JF, Chong SK, et al. Vertical lines in distal esophageal mucosa (VLEM): a true endoscopic manifestation of esophagitis in children? *Gastrointest Endosc* 1997;45:485–9.

54. Shub MD, Ulshen MH, Hargrove CB, et al. Esophagitis: a frequent consequence of gastroesophageal reflux in infancy. *J Pediatr* 1985;107:881–4.

55. Winter HS, Madara JL, Stafford RJ, et al. Intraepithelial eosinophils: a new diagnostic criterion for reflux esophagitis. *Gastroenterology* 1982.83:818–23.

56. Liacouras CA, Wenner WJ, Brown K, et al. Primary eosinophilic esophagitis in children: successful treatment with oral corticosteroids [see comments]. *J Pediatr Gastroenterol Nutr* 1998;26: 380–5.

57. Ruchelli E, Wenner W, Voytek T, et al. Severity of esophageal eosinophilia predicts response to conventional gastroesophageal reflux therapy. *Pediatr Dev Pathol* 1999;2:15–8.

58. Di Lorenzo C, Piepsz A, Ham H, et al. Gastric emptying with gastro-oesophageal reflux. *Arch Dis Child* 1987;62:449–53.

59. Papaila JG, Wilmot D, Grosfeld JL, et al. Increased incidence of delayed gastric emptying in children with gastroesophageal reflux. A prospective evaluation. *Arch Surg* 1989;124:933–6.

60. Hillemeier AC, Lange R, McCallum R, et al. Delayed gastric

emptying in infants with gastroesophageal reflux. *J Pediatr* 1981; 98:190–3.

61. McVeagh P, Howman-Giles R, Kemp A. Pulmonary aspiration studied by radionuclide milk scanning and barium swallow roentgenography. *Am J Dis Child* 1987;141:917–21.

62. Fawcett HD, Hayden CK, Adams JC, et al. How useful is gastroesophageal reflux scintigraphy in suspected childhood aspiration? *Pediatr Radiol* 1988;18:311–3.

63. Arasu TS, Wyllie R, Fitzgerald JF, et al. Gastroesophageal reflux in infants and children comparative accuracy of diagnostic methods. *J Pediatr* 1980;96:798–803.

64. Tolia V, Kauffman RE. Comparison of evaluation of gastroesophageal reflux in infants using different feedings during intraesophageal pH monitoring. *J Pediatr Gastroenterol Nutr* 1990; 10:426–9.

65. Balson BM, Kravitz EK, McGeady SJ. Diagnosis and treatment of gastroesophageal reflux in children and adolescents with severe asthma. *Ann Allergy Asthma Immunol* 1998;81:159–64.

66. Orenstein SR, Klein HA, Rosenthal MS. Scintigraphy versus pH probe for quantification of pediatric gastroesophageal reflux: a study using concurrent multiplexed data and acid feedings. *J Nucl Med* 1993;34:1228–34.

67. van Pinxteren B, Numans ME, Bonis PA, et al. Short-term treatment with proton pump inhibitors, H2-receptor antagonists and prokinetics for gastro-oesophageal reflux disease-like symptoms and endoscopy negative reflux disease. *Cochrane Database Syst Rev* 2000;2.

68. Ours TM, Kavuru MS, Schilz RJ, et al. A prospective evaluation of esophageal testing and a double-blind, randomized study of omeprazole in a diagnostic and therapeutic algorithm for chronic cough [see comments]. *Am J Gastroenterol* 1999;94:3131–8.

69. Wo JM, Grist WJ, Gussack G, et al. Empiric trial of high-dose omeprazole in patients with posterior laryngitis: a prospective study [see comments]. *Am J Gastroenterol* 1997;92:2160–5.

70. Havelund T, Lind T, Wiklund I, et al. Quality of life in patients with heartburn but without esophagitis: effects of treatment with omeprazole [see comments]. *Am J Gastroenterol* 1999;94: 1782–9.

71. Lind T, Havelund T, Lundell L, et al. On demand therapy with omeprazole for the long-term management of patients with heartburn without oesophagitis–a placebo-controlled randomized trial. *Ailment Pharmacol Ther* 1999;13:907–14.

72. Fass R, Fennerty MB, Ofman JJ, et al. The clinical and economic value of a short course of omeprazole in patients with noncardiac chest pain [see comments . *Gastroenterology* 1998;115:42–9.

73. Johnsson F, Weywadt L, Solhaug JH, et al. One-week omeprazole treatment in the diagnosis of gastro-oesophageal reflux disease. *Scand J Gastroenterol* 1998;33:15–20.

74. Oliveria SA, Christos PJ, Talley NJ, et al. Heartburn risk factors, knowledge, and prevention strategies: a population-based survey of individuals with heartburn. *Arch Intern Med* 1999;159:1592–8.

75. Forget P, Arends JW. Cow's milk protein allergy and gastrooesophageal reflux. *Eur J Pediatr* 1985;144:298–300.

76. Iacono G, Carroccio A, Cavataio F, et al. Gastroesophageal reflux and cow's milk allergy in infants: a prospective study. *J Allergy Clin Immunol* 1996;97:822–7.

77. Hill DJ, Cameron DJ, Francis DE, et al. Challenge confirmation of late-onset reactions to extensively hydrolyzed formulas in infants with multiple food protein intolerance. *J Allergy Clin Immunol* 1995;96:386–94.

78. Cavataio F, Iacono G, Montalto G, et al. Gastroesophageal reflux associated with cow's milk allergy in infants: which diagnostic examinations are useful? *Am J Gastroenterol* 1996;91:1215–20.

79. Cavataio F, Iacono G, Montalto G, et al. Clinical and pH-metric characteristics of gastro-oesophageal reflux secondary to cows' milk protein allergy [see comments]. *Arch Dis Child* 1996;75: 51–6.

80. Heacock HJ, Jeffery HE, Baker JL, et al. Influence of breast versus formula milk on physiological gastroesophageal reflux in

healthy, newborn infants. *J Pediatr Gastroenterol Nutr* 1992;14:
41–6.

81. Vandenplas Y, Sacre L. Milk-thickening agents as a treatment for
gastroesophageal reflux [published erratum appears in *Clin Pediatr (Phila)* 1987 Mar;26(3):148]. *Clin Pediatr (Phila)* 1987;26:
66–8.

82. Bailey DJ, Andres JM, Danek GD, et al. Lack of efficacy of
thickened feeding as treatment for gastroesophageal reflux. *J Pediatr* 1987;110:187–9.

83. Orenstein SR, Magill HL, Brooks P. Thickening of infant feedings for therapy of gastroesophageal reflux. *J Pediatr* 1987;110:
181–6.

84. Orenstein SR, Shalaby TM, Putnam PE. Thickened feedings as a
cause of increased coughing when used as therapy for gastroesophageal reflux in infants. *J Pediatr* 1992;121:913–5.

85. Vandenplas Y, Hachimi-Idrissi S, Casteels A, et al. A clinical trial
with an "anti-regurgitation" formula. *Eur J Pediatr* 1994;153:
419–23.

86. Borrelli O, Salvia G, Campanozzi A, et al. Use of a new thickened
formula for treatment of symptomatic gastrooesophageal reflux in
infants. *Ital J Gastroenterol Hepatol* 1997;29:237–42.

87. Ferry GD, Selby M, Pietro TJ. Clinical response to short-term
nasogastric feeding in infants with gastroesophageal reflux and
growth failure. *J Pediatr Gastroenterol Nutr* 1983;2:57–61.

88. Meyers WF, Herbst JJ. Effectiveness of positioning therapy for
gastroesophageal reflux. *Pediatrics* 1982;69:768–72.

89. Vandenplas Y, Sacre-Smits L. Seventeen-hour continuous esophageal pH monitoring in the newborn: evaluation of the influence
of position in asymptomatic and symptomatic babies. *J Pediatr
Gastroenterol Nutr* 1985;4:356–61.

90. Tobin JM, McCloud P, Cameron DJ. Posture and gastro-
oesophageal reflux: a case for left lateral positioning. *Arch Dis
Child* 1997;76:254–8.

91. Orenstein SR. Prone positioning in infant gastroesophageal reflux: is elevation of the head worth the trouble? *J Pediatr* 1990;
117:184–7.

92. Orenstein SR, Whitington PF, Orenstein DM. The infant seat as
treatment for gastroesophageal reflux. *N Engl J Med* 1983;309:
760–3.

93. Katz LC, Just R, Castell DO. Body position affects recumbent
postprandial reflux. J Clin Gastroenterol 1994;18:280–3.

94. Khoury RM, Camacho-Lobato L, Katz PO, et al. Influence of
spontaneous sleep positions on nighttime recumbent reflux in
patients with gastroesophageal reflux disease. *Am J Gastroenterol*
1999;94:2069–73.

95. Oyen N, Markestad T, Skaerven R, et al. Combined effects of
sleeping position and prenatal risk factors in sudden infant death
syndrome: the Nordic Epidemiological SIDS Study. *Pediatrics*
1997;100:613–21.

96. Skadberg BT, Morild I, and Markestad T. Abandoning prone
sleeping: effect on the risk of sudden infant death syndrome [see
comments]. *J Pediatr* 1998;132:340–3.

97. Adams EJ, Chavez GF, Steen D, et al. Changes in the epidemiologic profile of sudden infant death syndrome as rates decline
among California infants:1990–1995. *Pediatrics* 1998;102:1445–
51.

98. Jeffery HE, Megevand A, Page M. Why the prone position is a
risk factor for sudden infant death syndrome. *Pediatr* 1999;104:
263–269.

99. Changing concepts of sudden infant death syndrome: implications for infant sleeping environment and sleep position. American Academy of Pediatrics. Task Force on Infant Sleep Position
and Sudden Infant Death Syndrome. *Pediatrics* 2000;105:650–6.

100. Mitchell EA, Thompson JM, Ford RP, et al. Sheepskin bedding
and the sudden infant death syndrome. New Zealand Cot Death
Study Group. *J Pediatr* 1998;133:701–4.

101. Mitchell EA, Thompson JMD, Ford RPK, et al. Softness and
potential to cause rebreathing: differences in bedding used by

infants at high risk for sudden infant death syndrome. *J Pediatr*
1998;133:701–4.

102. Stanciu C, Bennett JR. Effects of posture on gastro-oesophageal
reflux. *Digestion* 1977;15:104–9.

103. Johnson LF, DeMeester TR Evaluation of elevation of the head of
the bed, bethanechol, and antacid form tablets on gastroesophageal reflux. *Dig Dis Sci* 1981;26:673–80.

104. Hamilton JW, Boisen RJ, Yamamoto DT, et al. Sleeping on a
wedge diminishes exposure of the esophagus to refluxed acid.
Dig Dis Sci 1988;33:518–22.

105. Vandenplas Y, Sacre L, Loeb H. Effects of formula feeding on
gastric acidity time and oesophageal pH monitoring data. *Eur J
Pediatr* 1988;148:152–4.

106. Casaubon PR, Dahlstrom KA, Vargas J, et al. Intravenous fat
emulsion (intralipid) delays gastric emptying, but does not cause
gastroesophageal reflux in healthy volunteers. *J Parenter Enteral
Nutr* 1989;13:246–8.

107. Becker DJ, Sinclair J, Castell DO, et al. A comparison of high and
low fat meals on postprandial esophageal acid exposure. *Am J
Gastroenterol* 1989;84:782–6.

108. Iwakiri K, Kobayashi M, Kotoyori M, et al. Relationship between
postprandial esophageal acid exposure and meal volume and fat
content. *Dig Dis Sci* 1996;41:926–30.

109. Noeser A, Gelineck J, Funch-Jensen P, et al. The incidence of
gastro-oesophageal reflux after solid and semi-solid meal. *Ront-
genblatter* 1989;42:530–1.

110. Penagini R, Mangano M, Bianchi PA. Effect of increasing the fat
content but not the energy load of a meal on gastro-oesophageal
reflux and lower oesophageal sphincter motor function [see com-
ments]. *Gut* 1998; 42:330–3.

111. Pehl C, Waizenhoefer A, Wendl B, et al. Effect of low and high
fat meals on lower esophageal sphincter motility and gastroesophageal reflux in healthy subjects. *Am J Gastroenterol* 1999;
94:1192–6.

112. Ruhl CE, Everhart JE. Overweight, but not high dietary fat intake,
increases risk of gastroesophageal reflux disease hospitalization:
the NHANES I Epidemiologic Followup Study. First National
Health and Nutrition Examination Survey. *Ann Epidemiol* 1999;
9:424–35.

113. Vandenplas Y, De Wolf D, Sacre L. Influence of xanthines on
gastroesophageal reflux in infants at risk for sudden infant death
syndrome. *Pediatrics* 1986;77:807–10.

114. Pehl C, Pfeiffer A, Wendl B, et al. The effect of decaffeination of
coffee on gastro-oesophageal reflux in patients with reflux disease. *Aliment Pharmacol Ther* 1997;11:483–6.

115. Wendl B, Pfeiffer A, Pehl C, et al. Effect of decaffeination of
coffee or tea on gastro-oesophageal reflux. *Aliment Pharmacol
Ther* 1994;8:283–7.

116. Brazer SR, Onken JE, Dalton CB, et al. Effect of different coffees
on esophageal acid contact time and symptoms in coffee-sensitive
subjects. *Physiol Behav* 1995;57:563–7.

117. Chang CS, Poon SK, Lien HC, et al. The incidence of reflux
esophagitis among the Chinese. *Am J Gastroenterol* 1997;92:
668–71.

118. Castiglione F, Emde C, Armstrong D, et al. Oesophageal pH-
metry: should meals be standardized? *Scand J Gastroenterol*
1992;27:350–4.

119. Murphy DW, Castell DO. Chocolate and heartburn: evidence of
increased esophageal acid exposure after chocolate ingestion. *Am
J Gastroenterol* 1988;83:633–6.

120. Wright LE, Castell DO. The adverse effect of chocolate on lower
esophageal sphincter pressure. *Am J Dig Dis* 1975;20:703–7.

121. Bartlett DW, Evans DF, Smith BG. Oral regurgitation after reflux
provoking meals: a possible cause of dental erosion? *J Oral Rehabil* 1997;24:102–8.

122. Nebel OT, Fornes MF, Castell DO. Symptomatic gastroesophageal reflux: incidence and precipitating factors. *Am J Dig Dis*
1976;21:953–6.

123. Allen ML, Mellow MH, Robinson MG, et al. The effect of raw

onions on acid reflux and reflux symptoms [see comments]. *Am J Gastroenterol* 1990;85:377–80.

124. Bulat R, Fachnie E, Chauhan U, et al. Lack of effect of spearmint on lower oesophageal sphincter function and acid reflux in healthy volunteers. *Aliment Pharmacol Ther* 1999;13:805–12.

125. Fisher BL, Pennathur A, Mutnick JL, et al. Obesity correlates with gastroesophageal reflux. *Dig Dis Sci* 1999;44:2290–4.

126. Wilson LJ, Ma W, Hirschowitz BI. Association of obesity with hiatal hernia and esophagitis. Am J *Gastroenterol* 1999;94:2840–4.

127. Fraser-Moodie CA, Norton B, Gornall C, et al. Weight loss has an independent beneficial effect on symptoms of gastro-oesophageal reflux in patients who are overweight. *Scand J Gastroenterol* 1999;34:337–40.

128. Kjellin A, Ramel S, Rossner S, et al. Gastroesophageal reflux in obese patients is not reduced by weight reduction. *Scand J Gastroenterol* 1996;31:1047–51.

129. Mathus-Vliegen LM, Tytgat GN. Twenty-four-hour pH measurements in morbid obesity: effects of massive overweight, weight loss and gastric distension [see comments]. *Eur J Gastroenterol Hepatol* 1996;8:635–40.

130. Alaswad B, Toubas PL, Grunow JE. Environmental tobacco smoke exposure and gastroesophageal reflux in infants with apparent life-threatening events. *J Okla State Med Assoc* 1996;89:233–7.

131. Blecker U, de Pont SM, Hauser B, et al. The role of "occult" gastroesophageal reflux in chronic pulmonary disease in children. *Acta Gastroenterol Belg* 1995;58:348–52.

132. Trudgill NJ, Smith LF, Kershaw J, et al. Impact of smoking cessation on salivary function in healthy volunteers. *Scand J Gastroenterol* 1998;33:568–71.

133. Kahrilas PJ, Gupta RR. The effect of cigarette smoking on salivation and esophageal acid clearance. *J Lab Clin Med* 1989;114:431–8.

134. Chattopadhyay DK, Greaney MG, Irvin TT. Effect of cigarette smoking on the lower oesophageal sphincter. *Gut* 1977;18:833–5.

135. Locke GR, Talley NJ, Fett SL, et al. Risk factors associated with symptoms of gastroesophageal reflux. *Am J Med* 1999;106:642–9.

136. Romero Y, Cameron AJ, Locke GR, et al. Familial aggregation of gastroesophageal reflux in patients with Barrett's esophagus and esophageal adenocarcinoma. *Gastroenterology* 1997;113:1449–56.

137. Kadakia SC, Kikendall JW, Maydonovitch C, et al. Effect of cigarette smoking on gastroesophageal reflux measured by 24-h ambulatory esophageal pH monitoring. *Am J Gastroenterol* 1995;90:1785–90.

138. Schindlbeck NE, Heinrich C, Dendorfer A, et al. Influence of smoking and esophageal intubation on esophageal pH-metry. *Gastroenterology* 1987;92:1994–7.

139. Waring JP, Eastwood TF, Austin JM, et al. The immediate effects of cessation of cigarette smoking on gastroesophageal reflux. *Am J Gastroenterol* 1989;84:1076–8.

140. Pehl C, Pfeiffer A, Wendl B, et al. Effect of smoking on the results of esophageal pH measurement in clinical routine. *J Clin Gastroenterol* 1997;25:503–6.

141. Rahal PS, Wright RA. Transdermal nicotine and gastroesophageal reflux. *Am J Gastroenterol* 1995;90:919–21.

142. Environmental tobacco smoke: a hazard to children. American Academy of Pediatrics Committee on Environmental Health [see comments]. *Pediatrics* 1997;99:639–42.

143. Dybing E , Sanner T. Passive smoking, sudden infant death syndrome (SIDS) and childhood infections. *Hum Exp Toxicol* 1999;18:202–5.

144. Cook DG, Strachan DP, Health effects of passive smoking-10: Summary of effects of parental smoking on the respiratory health of children and implications for research. *Thorax* 1999;54:357–66.

145. Banciu T, Sorian E. Gastroesophageal reflux in chronic alcohol-

ics. Endoesophageal pH determinations using Heidelberg tele-metring capsule. *Med Interne* 1989;27:279–82.

146. Vitale GC, Cheadle WG, Patel B, et al. The effect of alcohol on nocturnal gastroesophageal reflux. *Jama* 1987;258:2077–9.

147. Pehl C, Pfeiffer A, Wendl B, et al. Different effects of white and red wine on lower esophageal sphincter pressure and gastroesophageal reflux. *Scand J Gastroenterol* 1998;33:118–22.

148. Pehl C, Wendl B, Pfeiffer A, et al. Low-proof alcoholic beverages and gastroesophageal reflux. *Dig Dis Sci* 1993;38:93–6.

149. Sutphen JL, Dillard VL. Effect of ranitidine on twenty-four-hour gastric acidity in infants. *J Pediatr* 1989;114:472–4.

150. Mallet E, Mouterde O, Dubois F, et al. Use of ranitidine in young infants with gastro-oesophageal reflux. *Eur J Clin Pharmacol* 1989;36:641–2.

151. Hyman PE, Garvey TQd, Abrams CE. Tolerance to intravenous ranitidine. *J Pediatr* 1987;110:794–6.

152. Chiba N, De Gara CJ, Wilkinson JM, et al. Speed of healing and symptom relief in grade II to IV gastroesophageal reflux disease: a meta-analysis. *Gastroenterology* 1997;112:1798–810.

153. McCarty-Dawson D, Sue SO, Morrill B, et al. Ranitidine versus cimetidine in the healing of erosive esophagitis. *Clin Ther* 1996;18:1150–60.

154. Stacey JH, Miocevich ML, Sacks GE The effect of ranitidine (as effervescent tablets) on the quality of life of GORD patients. *Br J Clin Pract* 1996;50:190-4,196.

155. Sabesin SM, Berlin RG, Humphries TJ, et al. Famotidine relieves symptoms of gastroesophageal reflux disease and heals erosions and ulcerations. Results of a multicenter, placebo-controlled, dose-ranging study. USA Merck Gastroesophageal Reflux Disease Study Group [see comments]. *Arch Intern Med* 1991;151:2394–400.

156. Cucchiara S, Gobio-Casali L, Balli F, et al. Cimetidine treatment of reflux esophagitis in children: an Italian multicentric study. *J Pediatr Gastroenterol Nutr* 1989;8:150–6.

157. Simeone D, Caria MC, Miele E, et al. Treatment of childhood peptic esophagitis: a double-blind placebo-controlled trial of nizatidine. *J Pediatr Gastroenterol Nutr* 1997;25:51–5.

158. Kelly DA. Do H2 receptor antagonists have a therapeutic role in childhood? [see comments]. *J Pediatr Gastroenterol Nutr* 1994;19:270–6.

159. Berezin S, Medow MS, Glassman M, et al. Use of the intraesophageal acid perfusion test in provoking nonspecific chest pain in children. *J Pediatr* 1989;115:709–12.

160. Minella R, Basile P, Stalano A, et al. Ranitidine treatment in pediatry. *Med Univ,* 1989.2:1–5.

161. DeAngelis G and Banchini G, Ranitidine in paediatric patients, a personal experience. *Clin Trials J* 1989;26:370–5.

162. Wolfe MM, Sachs G. Acid suppression: Optimizing therapy for gastroduodenal ulcer healing, gastroesophageal reflux disease, and stress-related erosive syndrome. *Gastroenterology* 2000;118 (suppl 1):S9-S31.

163. Kato S, Ebina K, Fujii K, et al. Effect of omeprazole in the treatment of refractory acid-related diseases in childhood: endoscopic healing and twenty-four-hour intragastric acidity. *J Pediatr* 1996;128:415–21.

164. De Giacomo C, Bawa P, Franceschi M, et al. Omeprazole for severe reflux esophagitis in children. *J Pediatr Gastroenterol Nutr* 1997;24:528–32.

165. Alliet P, Raes M, Bruneel E, et al. Omeprazole in infants with cimetidine-resistant peptic esophagitis. *J Pediatr* 1998;132:352–4.

166. Strauss RS, Calenda KA, Dayal Y, et al. Histological esophagitis: clinical and histological response to omeprazole in children. *Dig Dis Sci* 1999;44:134–9.

167. Klinkenberg-Knol EC, Jansen JM, Festen HP, et al. Double-blind multicentre comparison of omeprazole and ranitidine in the treatment of reflux oesophagitis. *Lancet* 1987;1:349–51.

168. Sontag SJ. The medical management of reflux esophagitis. Role

of antacids and acid inhibition. *Gastroenterol Clin North Am* 1990;19:683–712.

169. Vigneri S, Termini R, Leandro G, et al. A comparison of five maintenance therapies for reflux esophagitis [see comments]. *N Engl J Med* 1995;333:1106–10.

170. Cucchiara S, Minella R, Iervolino MR, et al. Omeprazole and high dose ranitidine in the treatment of refractory reflux oesophagitis. *Arch Dis Child* 1993;69:655–9.

171. Klinkenberg-Knol EC, Nelis F, Dent J, et al. Long-term omeprazole treatment in resistant gastroesophageal reflux disease: efficacy, safety, and influence on gastric mucosa [see comments]. *Gastroenterology* 2000;118:661–9.

172. Dent J, Brun J, Fendrick AM, et al. An evidence-based appraisal of reflux disease management– the Genval workshop report. *Gut* 1999;44(suppl 2):S1-S16.

173. Cucchiara S, Staiano A, Romaniello G, et al. Antacids and cimetidine treatment for gastro-oesophageal reflux and peptic oesophagitis. *Arch Dis Child* 1984;59:842–7.

174. Iacono G, Carroccio A, Montalto G, et al. Magnesium hydroxide and aluminum hydroxide in the treatment of gastroesophageal reflux. *Minerva Pediatr* 1991;43:797–800.

175. Tsou VM, Young RM, Hart MH, et al. Elevated plasma aluminum levels in normal infants receiving antacids containing aluminum. *Pediatrics* 1991;87:148–51.

176. Woodard-Knight L, Fudge A, Teubner J, et al. Aluminium absorption and antacid therapy in infancy. *J Paediatr Child Health* 1992;28:257–9.

177. Sedman A. Aluminum toxicity in childhood. *Pediatr Nephrol* 1992;6:383–93.

178. Aluminum toxicity in infants and children. American Academy of Pediatrics, Committee on Nutrition. Pediatrics 1996;97:413–6.

179. Klein GL. Metabolic bone disease of total parenteral nutrition. *Nutrition* 1998;14:149–52.

180. Cucchiara S, Staiano A, Boccieri A, et al. Effects of cisapride on parameters of oesophageal motility and on the prolonged intraoesophageal pH test in infants with gastro-oesophageal reflux disease. *Gut* 1990;31:21–5.

181. Cucchiara S, Staiano A, Capozzi C, et al. Cisapride for gastro-oesophageal reflux and peptic oesophagitis. *Arch Dis Child* 1987; 62:454–7.

182. Vandenplas Y, de Roy C, Sacre L. Cisapride decreases prolonged episodes of reflux in infants. *J Pediatr Gastroenterol Nutr* 1991; 12:44–7.

183. Saye ZN, Forget PP, Geubelle F. Effect of cisapride on gastro-esophageal reflux in children with chronic bronchopulmonary disease: a double-blind cross-over pH-monitoring study. *Pediatr Pulmonol* 1987;3:8–12.

184. Scott RB, Ferreira C, Smith L, et al. Cisapride in pediatric gastroesophageal reflux. *J Pediatr Gastroenterol Nutr* 1997;25:499–506.

185. Cohen RC, O'Loughlin EV, Davidson GP, et al. Cisapride in the control of symptoms in infants with gastroesophageal reflux: a randomized, double-blind, placebo-controlled trial [see comments]. *J Pediatr* 1999;134:287–92.

186. Van Eygen M, Van Ravensteyn H. Effect of cisapride on excessive regurgitation in infants. *Clin Ther* 1989;11:669–77.

187. Rode H, Stunden RJ, Millar AJ, et al. Esophageal pH assessment of gastroesophageal reflux in 18 patients and the effect of two prokinetic agents: cisapride and metoclopramide. *J Pediatr Surg* 1987;22:931–4.

188. Grande L, Lacima G, Ros E, et al. Lack of effect of metoclopramide and domperidone on esophageal peristalsis and esophageal acid clearance in reflux esophagitis. A randomized, double-blind study. *Dig Dis Sci* 1992;37:583–8.

189. Richter JE, Sabesin SM, Kogut DG, et al. Omeprazole versus ranitidine or ranitidine/metoclopramide in poorly responsive symptomatic gastroesophageal reflux disease. *Am J Gastroenterol* 1996;91:1766–72.

190. Leung C, Lai W. Use of metoclopramide for the treatment of

gastroesophageal reflux in infants and children. *Curr Ther Res* 1984;36:911–15.

191. De Loore I, Van Ravensteyn H, Ameryckx L Domperidone drops in the symptomatic treatment of chronic paediatric vomiting and regurgitation. A comparison with metoclopramide. *Postgrad Med J* 1979;55:40–2.

192. Machida HM, Forbes DA, Gall DG, et al. Metoclopramide in gastroesophageal reflux of infancy. *J Pediatr* 1988;112:483–7.

193. Bellissant E, Duhamel JF, Guillot M, et al. The triangular test to assess the efficacy of metoclopramide in gastroesophageal reflux. *Clin Pharmacol Ther* 1997;61:377–84.

194. Kearns GL, Butler HL, Lane JK, Carchman SH, and Wright GJ, Metoclopramide pharmacokinetics and pharmacodynamics in infants with gastroesophageal reflux. *J Pediatr Gastroenterol Nutr* 1988;7:823–9.

195. Tolia V, Calhoun J, Kuhns L, et al. Randomized, prospective double-blind trial of metoclopramide and placebo for gastroesophageal reflux in infants [see comments]. *J Pediatr* 1989;115: 141–5.

196. Pons G, Duhamel JF, Guillot M, et al. Dose-response study of metoclopramide in gastroesophageal reflux in infancy. *Fundam Clin Pharmacol* 1993;7:161–6.

197. Putnam PE, Orenstein SR, Wessel HB, et al. Tardive dyskinesia associated with use of metoclopramide in a child. *J Pediatr* 1992; 121:983–5.

198. Euler AR. Use of bethanechol for the treatment of gastroesophageal reflux. *J Pediatr* 1980;96:321–4.

199. Levi P, Marmo F, Saluzzo C, et al. Bethanechol versus antacids in the treatment of gastroesophageal reflux. *Helv Paediatr Acta* 1985;40:349–59.

200. Bines JE, Quinlan JE, Treves S, et al. Efficacy of domperidone in infants and children with gastroesophageal reflux. *J Pediatr Gastroenterol Nutr* 1992;14:400–5.

201. Carroccio A, Iacono G, Montalto G, et al. Domperidone plus magnesium hydroxide and aluminum hydroxide: a valid therapy in children with gastroesophageal reflux. A double-blind randomized study versus placebo. *Scand J Gastroenterol* 1994;29:300–4.

202. Shulman RJ, Boyle JT, Colletti RB, et al. The use of cisapride in children. The North American Society for Pediatric Gastroenterology and Nutrition. *J Pediatr Gastroenterol Nutr* 1999;28:529–33.

203. Poynard T, Vernisse B, Agostini H. Randomized, multicentre comparison of sodium alginate and cisapride in the symptomatic treatment of uncomplicated gastro-oesophageal reflux. *Aliment Pharmacol Ther* 1998;12:159–65.

204. Greally P, Hampton FJ, MacFadyen UM, et al. Gaviscon and Carobel compared with cisapride in gastro-oesophageal reflux. *Arch Dis Child* 1992;67:618–21.

205. Buts JP, Barudi C, Otte JB. Double-blind controlled study on the efficacy of sodium alginate (Gaviscon) in reducing gastroesophageal reflux assessed by 24 h continuous pH monitoring in infants and children. *Eur J Pediatr* 1987;146:156–8.

206. Forbes D, Hodgson M, Hill R. The effects of gaviscon and metoclopramide in gastroesophageal reflux in children. *J Pediatr Gastroenterol Nutr* 1986;5:556–9.

207. Simon B, Ravelli GP, Goffin H. Sucralfate gel versus placebo in patients with non-erosive gastro- oesophageal reflux disease. *Aliment Pharmacol Ther* 1996;10:441–6.

208. Arguelles-Martin F, Gonzalez-Fernandez F, Gentles MG. Sucralfate versus cimetidine in the treatment of reflux esophagitis in children. *Am J Med* 1989;86:73–6.

209. Dalla Vecchia LK, Grosfeld JL, West KW, et al. Reoperation after Nissen fundoplication in children with gastroesophageal reflux: experience with 130 patients. *Ann Surg* 1997;226:315-21;discussion 321-3.

210. Veit F, Schwagten K, Auldist AW, et al. Trends in the use of fundoplication in children with gastro-oesophageal reflux. *J Paediatr Child Health* 1995;31:121–6.

211. Randolph J. Experience with the Nissen fundoplication for cor-

rection of gastroesophageal reflux in infants. *Ann Surg* 1983;198: 579–84.

212. Bensoussan AL, Yazbeck S, Carceller-Blanchard A. Results and complications of Toupet partial posterior wrap: 10 years' experience. *J Pediatr Surg* 1994;29:1215–7.

213. Ahrens P, Heller K, Beyer P, et al. Antireflux surgery in children suffering from reflux-associated respiratory diseases. *Pediatr Pulmonol* 1999;28:89–93.

214. Bergmeijer JH, Harbers JS, Molenaar JC. Function of pediatric Nissen-Rossetti fundoplication followed up into adolescence and adulthood. *J Am Coll Surg* 1997;184:259–61.

215. Blane CE, Turnage RH, Oldham KT, et al. Long-term radiographic follow-up of the Nissen fundoplication in children. *Pediatr Radiol* 1989;19:523–6.

216. Bliss D, Hirschl R, Oldham K, et al. Efficacy of anterior gastric fundoplication in the treatment of gastroesophageal reflux in infants and children. *J Pediatr Surg* 1994;29:1071-4;discussion 1074-5.

217. Caniano DA, Ginn-Pease ME, et al. The failed antireflux procedure: analysis of risk factors and morbidity. *J Pediatr Surg* 1990; 25:1022-5;discussion 1025-6.

218. Fonkalsrud EW, Ashcraft KW, Coran AG, et al. Surgical treatment of gastroesophageal reflux in children: a combined hospital study of 7467 patients [see comments]. *Pediatrics* 1998;101:419–22.

219. Fonkalsrud EW, Bustorff-Silva J, Perez CA, et al. Antireflux surgery in children under 3 months of age. *J Pediatr Surg* 1999; 34:527–31.

220. Weber TR. Toupet fundoplication for gastroesophageal reflux in childhood. *Arch Surg* 1999;134:717-20; discussion 720-1.

221. Spillane AJ, Currie B, Shi E. Fundoplication in children: experience with 106 cases. *Aust N Z J Surg* 1996; 66:753–6.

222. Samuk I, Afriat R, Horne T, et al. Dumping syndrome following Nissen fundoplication, diagnosis, and treatment. *J Pediatr Gastroenterol Nutr* 1996;23:235–40.

223. Khoshoo V, Roberts PL, Loe WA, et al. Nutritional management of dumping syndrome associated with antireflux surgery. *J Pediatr Surg* 1994;29:1452–4.

224. Tovar JA, Olivares P, Diaz M, et al. Functional results of laparoscopic fundoplication in children. *J Pediatr Gastroenterol Nutr* 1998;26:429–31.

225. Rothenberg SS. Experience with 220 consecutive laparoscopic Nissen fundoplications in infants and children. *J Pediatr Surg* 1998;33:274–8.

226. Tovar JA, Angulo JA, Gorostiaga L, et al. Surgery for gastroesophageal reflux in children with normal pH studies. *J Pediatr Surg* 1991;26:541–5.

227. Hunziker UA, Barr RG. Increased carrying reduces infant crying: a randomized controlled trial. *Pediatrics* 1986;77:641–8.

228. Armstrong KL, Quinn RA, Dadds MR. The sleep patterns of normal children. *Med J Aust* 1994;161:202–6.

229. Singh S, Richter JE, Bradley LA, et al. The symptom index. Differential usefulness in suspected acid-related complaints of heartburn and chest pain [see comments]. *Dig Dis Sci* 1993;38: 1402–8.

230. Wiener GJ, Richter JE, Copper JB, et al. The symptom index: a clinically important parameter of ambulatory 24- hour esophageal pH monitoring. *Am J Gastroenterol* 1988;83:358–61.

231. Heine RG, Jaquiery A, Lubitz L, et al. Role of gastro-oesophageal reflux in infant irritability. *Arch Dis Child* 1995;73:121–5.

232. Ghaem M, Armstrong KL, Trocki O, et al. The sleep patterns of infants and young children with gastro- oesophageal reflux. *J Paediatr Child Health* 1998;34:160–3.

233. Berezin S, Glassman MS, Bostwick H, et al. Esophagitis as a cause of infant colic. *Clin Pediatr (Phila)* 1995;34:158–9.

234. Barr RG, Rotman A, Yaremko J, et al. The crying of infants with colic: a controlled empirical description. *Pediatrics* 1992;90:14–21.

235. Castell DO. A practical approach to heartburn [In Process Citation]. *Hosp Pract (Off Ed)* 1999;34:89-94, 97-8.

236. Richter JE, Kovacs TO, Greski-Rose PA, et al. Lansoprazole in the treatment of heartburn in patients without erosive oesophagitis. *Aliment Pharmacol Ther* 1999;13:795–804.

237. Venables TL, Newland RD, Patel AC, et al. Omeprazole 10 milligrams once daily, omeprazole 20 milligrams once daily, or ranitidine 150 milligrams twice daily, evaluated as initial therapy for the relief of symptoms of gastro-oesophageal reflux disease in general practice. *Scand J Gastroenterol* 1997;32:965–73.

238. DeVault KR, Castell DO. Updated guidelines for the diagnosis and treatment of gastroesophageal reflux disease. The Practice Parameters Committee of the American College of Gastroenterology. *Am J Gastroenterol* 1999;94:1434–42.

239. Revicki DA, Crawley JA, Zodet MW, et al. Complete resolution of heartburn symptoms and health-related quality of life in patients with gastro-oesophageal reflux disease. *Aliment Pharmacol Ther* 1999;13:1621–30.

240. Pappa KA, Williams BO, Payne JE, et al. A double-blind, placebo-controlled study of the efficacy and safety of nonprescription ranitidine 75 mg in the prevention of meal-induced heartburn. *Aliment Pharmacol Ther* 1999;13:467–73.

241. Holloway RH, Dent J, Narielvala F, et al. Relation between oesophageal acid exposure and healing of oesophagitis with omeprazole in patients with severe reflux oesophagitis [see comments]. *Gut* 1996;38:649–54.

242. Catto-Smith AG, Machida H, Butzner JD, et al. The role of gastroesophageal reflux in pediatric dysphagia. *J Pediatr Gastroenterol Nutr* 1991;12:159–65.

243. Lundquist A, Olsson R, Ekberg O. Clinical and radiologic evaluation reveals high prevalence of abnormalities in young adults with dysphagia. *Dysphagia* 1998;13:202–7.

244. Dellert SF, Hyams JS, Treem WR, et al. Feeding resistance and gastroesophageal reflux in infancy. *J Pediatr Gastroenterol Nutr* 1993;17:66–71.

245. Shepherd RW, Wren J, Evans S, et al. Gastroesophageal reflux in children. Clinical profile, course and outcome with active therapy in 126 cases. *Clin Pediatr (Phila)* 1987;26:55–60.

246. Mathisen B, Worrall L, Masel J, et al. Feeding problems in infants with gastro-oesophageal reflux disease: a controlled study. *J Paediatr Child Health* 1999;35:163–9.

247. Rudolph CD. Feeding disorders in infants and children. *J Pediatr* 1994;125:S116-24.

248. National Institutes of Health Consensus Development Conference on Infantile Apnea and Home Monitoring, Sept 29 to Oct 1, 1986. *Pediatrics* 1987;79:292–9.

249. Tirosh E, Kessel A, Jaffe M, et al. Outcome of idiopathic apparent life-threatening events: infant and mother perspectives. *Pediatr Pulmonol* 1999;28:47–52.

250. Steinschneider A, Richmond C, Ramaswamy V, et al. Clinical characteristics of an apparent life-threatening event (ALTE) and the subsequent occurrence of prolonged apnea or prolonged bradycardia. *Clin Pediatr (Phila)* 1998;37:223–9.

251. Cote A, Hum C, Brouillette RT, et al. Frequency and timing of recurrent events in infants using home cardiorespiratory monitors [see comments]. *J Pediatr* 1998;132:783–9.

252. Rosen CL, Frost JD, Jr, Harrison GM. Infant apnea: polygraphic studies and follow-up monitoring. *Pediatrics* 1983;71:731–6.

253. Burchfield DJ, Rawlings DJ. Sudden deaths and apparent life-threatening events in hospitalized neonates presumed to be healthy [see comments]. *Am J Dis Child* 1991;145:1319–22.

254. Kahn A, Blum D, Rebuffat E, et al. Polysomnographic studies of infants who subsequently died of sudden infant death syndrome. *Pediatrics* 1988;82:721–7.

255. Kelly DH, Golub H, Carley D, et al. Pneumograms in infants who subsequently died of sudden infant death syndrome. *J Pediatr* 1986;109:249–54.

256. Kelly DH, Shannon DC, O'Connell K. Care of infants with near-miss sudden infant death syndrome. *Pediatrics* 1978;61:511–4.

257. Oren J, Kelly D, Shannon DC. Identification of a high-risk group for sudden infant death syndrome among infants who were resuscitated for sleep apnea. Pediatrics 1986;77:495–9.

258. Steinschneider A, Weinstein SL, Diamond E. The sudden infant death syndrome and apnea/obstruction during neonatal sleep and feeding. *Pediatrics* 1982;70:858–63.

259. Friesen CA, Streed CJ, Carney LA, et al. Esophagitis and modified Bernstein tests in infants with apparent life- threatening events. *Pediatrics* 1994;94:541–4.

260. Newman LJ, Russe J, Glassman MS, et al. Patterns of gastroesophageal reflux (GER) in patients with apparent life-threatening events. *J Pediatr Gastroenterol Nutr* 1989;8:157–60.

261. Veereman-Wauters G, Bochner A, Van Caillie-Bertrand M. Gastroesophageal reflux in infants with a history of near-miss sudden infant death. *J Pediatr Gastroenterol Nutr* 1991;12:319–23.

262. Herbst JJ, Minton SD, Book LS. Gastroesophageal reflux causing respiratory distress and apnea in newborn infants. *J Pediatr* 1979; 95:763–8.

263. Leape LL, Holder TM, Franklin JD, et al. Respiratory arrest in infants secondary to gastroesophageal reflux. *Pediatrics* 1977;60: 924–8.

264. Herbst JJ, Book LS, Bray PF. Gastroesophageal reflux in the "near miss" sudden infant death syndrome. *J Pediatr* 1978;92: 73–5.

265. Menon AP, Schefft GL, Thach BT. Apnea associated with regurgitation in infants. *J Pediatr* 1985;106:625–9.

266. Sacre L, Vandenplas Y. Gastroesophageal reflux associated with respiratory abnormalities during sleep. *J Pediatr Gastroenterol Nutr* 1989;9:28–33.

267. Ariagno RL. Evaluation and management of infantile apnea. *Pediatr Ann* 1984;13:210-3, 216-7.

268. Kahn A, Rebuffat E, Sottiaux M, et al. Lack of temporal relation between acid reflux in the proximal oesophagus and cardiorespiratory events in sleeping infants. *Eur J Pediatr* 1992;151:208–12.

269. Paton JY, Nanayakkara CS, Simpson H. Observations on gastro-oesophageal reflux, central apnoea and heart rate in infants. *Eur J Pediatr* 1990;149:608–12.

270. Paton JY, Macfadyen U, Williams A, et al. Gastro-oesophageal reflux and apnoeic pauses during sleep in infancy– no direct relation. *Eur J Pediatr* 1990;149:680–6.

271. Walsh JK, Farrell MK, Keenan WJ, et al. Gastroesophageal reflux in infants: relation to apnea. *J Pediatr* 1981;99:197–201.

272. Suys B, De Wolf D, Hauser B, et al. Bradycardia and gastroesophageal reflux in term and preterm infants: is there any relation? *J Pediatr Gastroenterol Nutr* 1994;19:187–90.

273. Spitzer AR, Boyle JT, Tuchman DN, et al. Awake apnea associated with gastroesophageal reflux: a specific clinical syndrome. *J Pediatr* 1984;104:200–5.

274. Jolley SG, Halpern LM, Tunell WP, et al. The risk of sudden infant death from gastroesophageal reflux [see comments]. *J Pediatr Surg* 1991;26:691–6.

275. Meadow R. Suffocation, recurrent apnea, and sudden infant death. *J Pediatr* 1990;117:351–7.

276. Expert Panel Report II. Guidelines for the Diagnosis and Management of Asthma. 1997: National Institute of Health, Bethesda, MD.

277. Field SK. A critical review of the studies of the effects of simulated or real gastroesophageal reflux on pulmonary function in asthmatic adults. *Chest* 1999;115:848–56.

278. Boyle JT, Tuchman DN, Altschuler SM, et al. Mechanisms for the association of gastroesophageal reflux and bronchospasm. *Am Rev Respir Dis* 1985;131:S16-20.

279. Malfroot A, Dab I. Pathophysiology and mechanisms of gastroesophageal reflux in childhood asthma. *Pediatr Pulmonol Suppl* 1995;11:55–6.

280. Herve P, Denjean A, Jian R, et al. Intraesophageal perfusion of acid increases the bronchomotor response to methacholine and to isocapnic hyperventilation in asthmatic subjects. *Am Rev Respir Dis* 1986;134:986–9.

281. Nelson HS. Gastroesophageal reflux and pulmonary disease. *J Allergy Clin Immunol* 1984;73:547–56.

282. Sheikh S, Goldsmith LJ, Howell L, et al. Lung function in infants with wheezing and gastroesophageal reflux [see comments]. *Pediatr Pulmonol* 1999;27:236–41.

283. Vijayaratnam V, Lin CH, Simpson P, et al. Lack of significant proximal esophageal acid reflux in infants presenting with respiratory symptoms [see comments]. *Pediatr Pulmonol* 1999;27: 231–5.

284. Andze GO, Brandt ML, St. Vil D, et al. Diagnosis and treatment of gastroesophageal reflux in 500 children with respiratory symptoms: the value of pH monitoring. *J Pediatr Surg* 1991;26:295-9;discussion 299-300.

285. Gustafsson PM, Kjellman NI, Tibbling L. Bronchial asthma and acid reflux into the distal and proximal oesophagus. *Arch Dis Child* 1990;65:1255–8.

286. Wilson NM, Charette L, Thomson AH, et al. Gastro-oesophageal reflux and childhood asthma: the acid test. *Thorax* 1985;40: 592–7.

287. Martin ME, Grunstein MM, Larsen GL. The relationship of gastroesophageal reflux to nocturnal wheezing in children with asthma. *Ann Allergy* 1982;49:318–22.

288. Berquist WE, Rachelefsky GS, Kadden M, et al. Gastroesophageal reflux-associated recurrent pneumonia and chronic asthma in children. *Pediatrics* 1981;68:29–35.

289. Shapiro GG, Christie DL. Gastroesophageal reflux in steroid-dependent asthmatic youths. *Pediatrics* 1979;63:207–12.

290. Euler AR, Byrne WJ, Ament ME, et al. Recurrent pulmonary disease in children: a complication of gastroesophageal reflux. *Pediatrics* 1979;63:47–51.

291. Eid NS, Shepherd RW, Thomson MA. Persistent wheezing and gastroesophageal reflux in infants. *Pediatr Pulmonol* 1994;18: 39–44.

292. Gustafsson PM, Kjellman NI, Tibbling L. A trial of ranitidine in asthmatic children and adolescents with or without pathological gastro-oesophageal reflux. *Eur Respir J* 1992;5:201–6.

293. Harding SM, Richter JE, Guzzo MR, et al. Asthma and gastroesophageal reflux: acid suppressive therapy improves asthma outcome. *Am J Med* 1996;100:395–405.

294. Harding SM. Nocturnal asthma: role of nocturnal gastroesophageal reflux. *Chronobiol Int* 1999;16:641–62.

295. Rothenberg SS, Bratton D, Larsen G, et al. Laparoscopic fundoplication to enhance pulmonary function in children with severe reactive airway disease and gastroesophageal reflux disease. *Surg Endosc* 1997;11:1088–90.

296. Foglia RP, Fonkalsrud EW, Ament ME, et al. Gastroesophageal fundoplication for the management of chronic pulmonary disease in children. *Am J Surg* 1980;140:72–9.

297. Field SK, Gelfand GA, McFadden SD. The effects of antireflux surgery on asthmatics with gastroesophageal reflux. *Chest* 1999; 116:766–74.

298. Carre IJ. Pulmonary infections in children with a partial thoracic stomach ('hiatus hernia'). *Arch Dis Child* 1960;35:481–4.

299. Chen PH, Chang MH, Hsu SC. Gastroesophageal reflux in children with chronic recurrent bronchopulmonary infection. *J Pediatr Gastroenterol Nutr* 1991;13:16–22.

300. Mays EE, Dubois JJ, Hamilton GB. Pulmonary fibrosis associated with tracheobronchial aspiration. A study of the frequency of hiatal hernia and gastroesophageal reflux in interstitial pulmonary fibrosis of obscure etiology. *Chest* 1976;69:512–5.

301. Regelmann WE. Diagnosing the cause of recurrent and persistent pneumonia in children. *Pediatr Ann* 1993;22:561–8.

302. Wilkinson JD, Dudgeon DL, Sondheimer JM. A comparison of medical and surgical treatment of gastroesophageal reflux in severely retarded children. *J Pediatr* 1981;99:202–5.

303. Nussbaum E, Maggi JC, Mathis R, et al. Association of lipid-laden alveolar macrophages and gastroesophageal reflux in children. *J Pediatr* 1987;110:190–4.

304. Staugas R, Martin AJ, Binns G, et al. The significance of fat-filled

macrophages in the diagnosis of aspiration associated with gastro-oesophageal reflux. *Aust Paediatr J* 1985;21:275–7.

305. Colombo JL, Hallberg TK. Recurrent aspiration in children: lipid-laden alveolar macrophage quantitation. *Pediatr Pulmonol* 1987;3:86–9.
306. Ahrens P, Noll C, Kitz R, et al. Lipid-laden alveolar macrophages (LLAM): a useful marker of silent aspiration in children [see comments]. *Pediatr Pulmonol* 1999;28:83–8.
307. Bauer ML, Lyrene RK. Chronic aspiration in children: evaluation of the lipid-laden macrophage index [see comments]. *Pediatr Pulmonol* 1999;28:94–100.
308. Knauer-Fischer S, Ratjen F. Lipid-laden macrophages in bronchoalveolar lavage fluid as a marker for pulmonary aspiration. *Pediatr Pulmonol* 1999;27:419–22.
309. Morton RE, Wheatley R, Minford J. Respiratory tract infections due to direct and reflux aspiration in children with severe neurodisability. *Dev Med Child Neurol* 1999;41:329–34.
310. Taniguchi MH, Moyer RS. Assessment of risk factors for pneumonia in dysphagic children: significance of videofluoroscopic swallowing evaluation. *Dev Med Child Neurol* 1994;36:495–502.
311. Arvedson J, Rogers B, Buck G, et al. Silent aspiration prominent in children with dysphagia. *Int J Pediatr Otorhinolaryngol* 1994;28:173–81.
312. Aviv JE, Kim T, Sacco RL, et al. FEESST: a new bedside endoscopic test of the motor and sensory components of swallowing. *Ann Otol Rhinol Laryngol* 1998;107:378–87.
313. Link DT, Willging JP, Miller CK, et al. Pediatric laryngopharyngeal sensory testing during FEES: Feasible and Correlative. *Ann Otol Rhinol Laryngol* 2000;XX: XX-XX.
314. Koufman JA. The otolaryngologic manifestations of gastroesophageal reflux disease (GERD): a clinical investigation of 225 patients using ambulatory 24- hour pH monitoring and an experimental investigation of the role of acid and pepsin in the development of laryngeal injury. *Laryngoscope* 1991;101:1–78.
315. Fitzgerald JM, Allen CJ, Craven MA, et al. Chronic cough and gastroesophageal reflux. *Cmaj* 1989;140:520–4.
316. Ing AJ, Ngu MC, Breslin AB. Chronic persistent cough and gastro-oesophageal reflux. *Thorax* 1991;46:479–83.
317. Woo P, Noordzij P, Ross JA. Association of esophageal reflux and globus symptom: comparison of laryngoscopy and 24-hour pH manometry. *Otolaryngol Head Neck Surg* 1996;115:502–7.
318. Curran AJ, Barry MK, Callanan V, et al. A prospective study of acid reflux and globus pharyngeus using a modified symptom index. *Clin Otolaryngol* 1995;20:552–4.
319. Wilson JA, White A, von Haacke NP, et al. Gastroesophageal reflux and posterior laryngitis. *Ann Otol Rhinol Laryngol* 1989;98:405–10.
320. Shaw GY, Searl JP. Laryngeal manifestations of gastroesopha-

geal reflux before and after treatment with omeprazole. *South Med J* 1997;90:1115–22.
321. Jacob P, Kahrilas PJ, Herzon G. Proximal esophageal pH-metry in patients with 'reflux laryngitis'. *Gastroenterology* 1991;100:305–10.
322. Shaker R, Milbrath M, Ren J, et al. Esophagopharyngeal distribution of refluxed gastric acid in patients with reflux laryngitis. *Gastroenterology* 1995;109:1575–82.
323. Contencin P, Narcy P. Gastropharyngeal reflux in infants and children. A pharyngeal pH monitoring study. *Arch Otolaryngol Head Neck Surg* 1992;118:1028–30.
324. Gumpert L, Kalach N, Dupont C, et al. Hoarseness and gastroesophageal reflux in children. *J Laryngol Otol* 1998;112:49–54.
325. Corrado G, D'Eufemia P, Pacchiarotti C, et al. Irritable oesophagus syndrome as cause of chronic cough. *Ital J Gastroenterol* 1996;28:526–30.
326. Halstead LA. Gastroesophageal reflux: a critical factor in pediatric subglottic stenosis. *Otolaryngol Head Neck Surg* 1999;120:683–8.
327. Kamel PL, Hanson D, Kahrilas PJ. Omeprazole for the treatment of posterior laryngitis [see comments]. *Am J Med* 1994;96:321–6.
328. Hanson DG, Kamel PL, Kahrilas PJ. Outcomes of antireflux therapy for the treatment of chronic laryngitis. *Ann Otol Rhinol Laryngol* 1995;104:550–5.
329. Putnam PE, Orenstein SR. Hoarseness in a child with gastroesophageal reflux. *Acta Paediatr* 1992;81:635–6.
330. Conley SF, Werlin SL, Beste DJ. Proximal pH-metry for diagnosis of upper airway complications of gastroesophageal reflux. *J Otolaryngol* 1995;24:295–8.
331. Allen CJ, Anvari M. Gastro-oesophageal reflux related cough and its response to laparoscopic fundoplication. *Thorax* 1998;53:963–8.
332. Bartlett DW, Coward PY, Nikkah C, et al. The prevalence of tooth wear in a cluster sample of adolescent schoolchildren and its relationship with potential explanatory factors [see comments]. *Br Dent J* 1998;184:125–9.
333. O'Sullivan EA, Curzon ME, Roberts GJ, et al. Gastroesophageal reflux in children and its relationship to erosion of primary and permanent teeth. *Eur J Oral Sci* 1998;106:765–9.
334. Bothwell MR, Parsons DS, Talbot A, et al. Outcome of reflux therapy on pediatric chronic sinusitis. *Otolaryngol Head Neck Surg* 1999;121:255–62.
335. Contencin P, Narcy P. Nasopharyngeal pH monitoring in infants and children with chronic rhinopharyngitis. *Int J Pediatr Otorhinolaryngol* 1991;22:249–56.
336. Gibson WS, Jr, Cochran W. Otalgia in infants and children–a manifestation of gastroesophageal reflux. *Int J Pediatr Otorhinolaryngol* 1994;28:213–8.

Appendix A. *Summary of recommendations for diagnostic approaches and the quality of the evidence*

Section	Recommendations	Quality of evidence*
	Diagnostic approaches	
3.1	In most cases a history and physical examination are sufficient to reliably diagnose GER and initiate management.	III
3.2	The upper GI series is neither sensitive nor specific for the diagnosis of GER, but is useful for the evaluation of the presence of anatomic abnormalities, such as pyloric stenosis, malrotation and annular pancreas in the vomiting infant, as well as hiatal hernia and esophageal stricture in the older child.	III
3.3	Esophageal pH monitoring is a valid and reliable measure of acid reflux.	II-2
3.4	Endoscopy and biopsy can determine the presence and severity of esophagitis, strictures and Barrett's esophagus, as well as exclude other disorders. Esophageal biopsy is recommended when endoscopy is performed to detect inapparent esophagitis and to exclude causes of esophagitis other than GER.	II-2
3.5	The role of nuclear scintigraphy (milk scan) in the diagnosis and management of GERD in infants and children is unclear.	III
3.6	A trial of time–limited medical therapy for GER is useful for determining if GER is causing a specific symptom.	III

* Categories of the Quality of Evidence [16]
I   Evidence obtained from at least one properly designed randomized controlled study.
II-1 Evidence obtained from well–designed cohort or case–controlled trials without randomization.
II-2 Evidence obtained from well–designed cohort or case–control analytic studies, preferably from more than one center or research group.
II-3 Evidence obtained from multiple time series with or without the intervention. Dramatic results in uncontrolled experiments (such as the results of the introduction of penicillin treatment in the 1940's) could also be regarded as this type of evidence.
III Opinions of respected authorities, based on clinical experience, descriptive studies, or reports of expert committees.

Appendix B. *Summary of recommendations for treatment options and the quality of the evidence*

Section	Recommendation	Quality of evidence*
	Treatment options	
4.1.1	There is evidence to support a one to two week trial of a hypoallergenic formula in formula fed infants with vomiting.	I
4.1.1	Milk–thickening agents do not improve reflux index scores but do decrease the number of episodes of vomiting.	I
4.1.2	Esophageal pH monitoring has demonstrated that infants have significantly less GER when placed in the prone position than in the supine position.	I
4.1.2	Prone positioning is associated with a higher rate of the sudden infant death syndrome (SIDS). In infants from birth to 12 months of age with GERD, the risk of SIDS generally outweighs the potential benefits of prone sleeping. Therefore, non–prone positioning during sleep is generally recommended.	I
4.1.2	In children older than one year it is likely that there is a benefit to left side positioning and elevation of the head of the bed.	I
4.1.3	It is recommended that children and adolescents with GERD avoid caffeine, chocolate and spicy foods that provoke symptoms. Obesity, exposure to tobacco smoke and alcohol are also associated with GER.	III
4.2.1.1	Histamine–$_2$ receptor antagonists (H$_2$RAs) produce relief of symptoms and mucosal healing. Proton pump inhibitors (PPIs), the most effective acid suppressant medications, are superior to H$_2$RAs in relieving symptoms and healing esophagitis.	I
4.2.1.3	Since more convenient and safe alternatives are available (H$_2$RAs and PPIs), chronic antacid therapy is generally not recommended.	III
4.2	Cisapride reduces the frequency of regurgitation and vomiting. However, because of concerns about the potential for serious cardiac arrhythmias in patients receiving cisapride, appropriate patient selection and monitoring as well as proper use, including correct dosage (0.2 mg/kg/dose QID) and avoidance of co–administration of contraindicated medications, are important. Cisapride is available in the USA only through a limited–access program. Other prokinetic agents have not been shown to be effective in the treatment of GERD in children.	I
4.3	Case series indicate that surgical therapy generally results in favorable outcomes. The potential risks, benefits and costs of successful prolonged medical therapy versus fundoplication have not been well studied in infants or children with varying symptom presentations.	II-3 III

Appendix C. *Summary of recommendations for the evaluation and management of infants and children with suspected GERD and the quality of the evidence*

Section	Recommendation	Quality of evidence*
	Evaluation and management of infants and children with possible GERD	
5.1.1	In the infant with recurrent vomiting, a thorough history and physical examination with attention to warning signals is generally sufficient to allow the clinician to establish a diagnosis of uncomplicated GER.	III
5.1.2	In the infant who has uncomplicated GER, parental education, reassurance and anticipatory guidance are recommended. Generally, no other intervention is necessary. Thickening of formula and a short trial of a hypoallergenic formula are other treatment options. If symptoms worsen or do not improve by 18 to 24 months of age, re–evaluation for complications of GER is recommended.	III
5.1.3	In the vomiting infant with poor weight gain in whom adequate calories are being offered, it is recommended that tests be performed to uncover other causes of vomiting, including an upper GI series to evaluate anatomy and swallowing. Management options include thickening the formula, increasing the caloric density of the formula, acid suppression therapy, prokinetic therapy and, in selected cases, prone positioning. Further management options include endoscopy with biopsy, hospitalization, tube feedings and rarely surgical therapy.	III
5.1.4	In infants with vomiting and irritability, potentially harmful interventions are undertaken with caution because pathological findings are so infrequent. One approach to management is initial empiric therapy; an alternate approach is initial diagnostic evaluation.	III
5.1.5	In otherwise normal children who have recurrent vomiting after the age of 2 years, management options include an upper GI series and upper endoscopy with biopsy.	II-2
	Prokinetic therapy is also an option.	III
5.2	For the treatment of heartburn in children or adolescents, lifestyle changes accompanied by a two– to four–week therapeutic trial of an H_2RA or PPI are recommended. If symptoms persist or recur, the child can be referred to a pediatric gastroenterologist for upper endoscopy with biopsy and in some cases long–term therapy.	III
5.3	In the infant or child with esophagitis, initial treatment consists of lifestyle changes and H_2RA or PPI therapy. In patients with only histologic esophagitis, the efficacy of therapy can be monitored by the degree of symptom relief. In patients with erosive esophagitis, repeat endoscopy is recommended to assure healing.	I
5.4	In the child with dysphagia or odynophagia, a barium esophagram is recommended. If the initial history is suggestive of esophagitis, upper endoscopy may be performed as the initial diagnostic test. Treatment without prior diagnostic evaluation is not recommended. In the infant with feeding refusal, because a large variety of disorders may contribute to infant feeding difficulties, empiric therapy for GER is generally not recommended. However, if there are other signs or symptoms suggestive of GERD then a time–limited course of medical therapy can be considered.	III
5.5	In the infant with apnea or an apparent life–threatening event, if symptoms occur frequently and the role of GER is uncertain, esophageal pH monitoring may be useful to determine if there is a temporal association of acid reflux with ALTE.	II-2
	Therapeutic options include thickened feedings and prokinetic and acid suppressant therapy. Since most infants improve with medical management, surgery is considered only in severe cases.	III
5.6	In patients where symptoms of asthma and esophagitis co–exist, and in infants and toddlers with chronic vomiting or regurgitation and recurrent episodes of cough and wheezing, a three–month trial of vigorous acid suppressant therapy of GER is recommended. If patients with persistent asthma do not have symptoms of GER, esophageal pH monitoring is recommended in selected patients who are more likely to benefit from GER therapy.	III

Prevention of Perinatal Group B Streptococcal Disease

• •

The following guideline for prevention of perinatal group B streptococcal disease, developed by the Centers for Disease Control and Prevention, has been endorsed by the American Academy of Pediatrics.

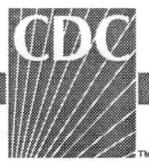

MMWR™

Morbidity and Mortality Weekly Report

Recommendations and Reports　　　　　August 16, 2002 / Vol. 51 / No. RR-11

Prevention of Perinatal Group B Streptococcal Disease

Revised Guidelines from CDC

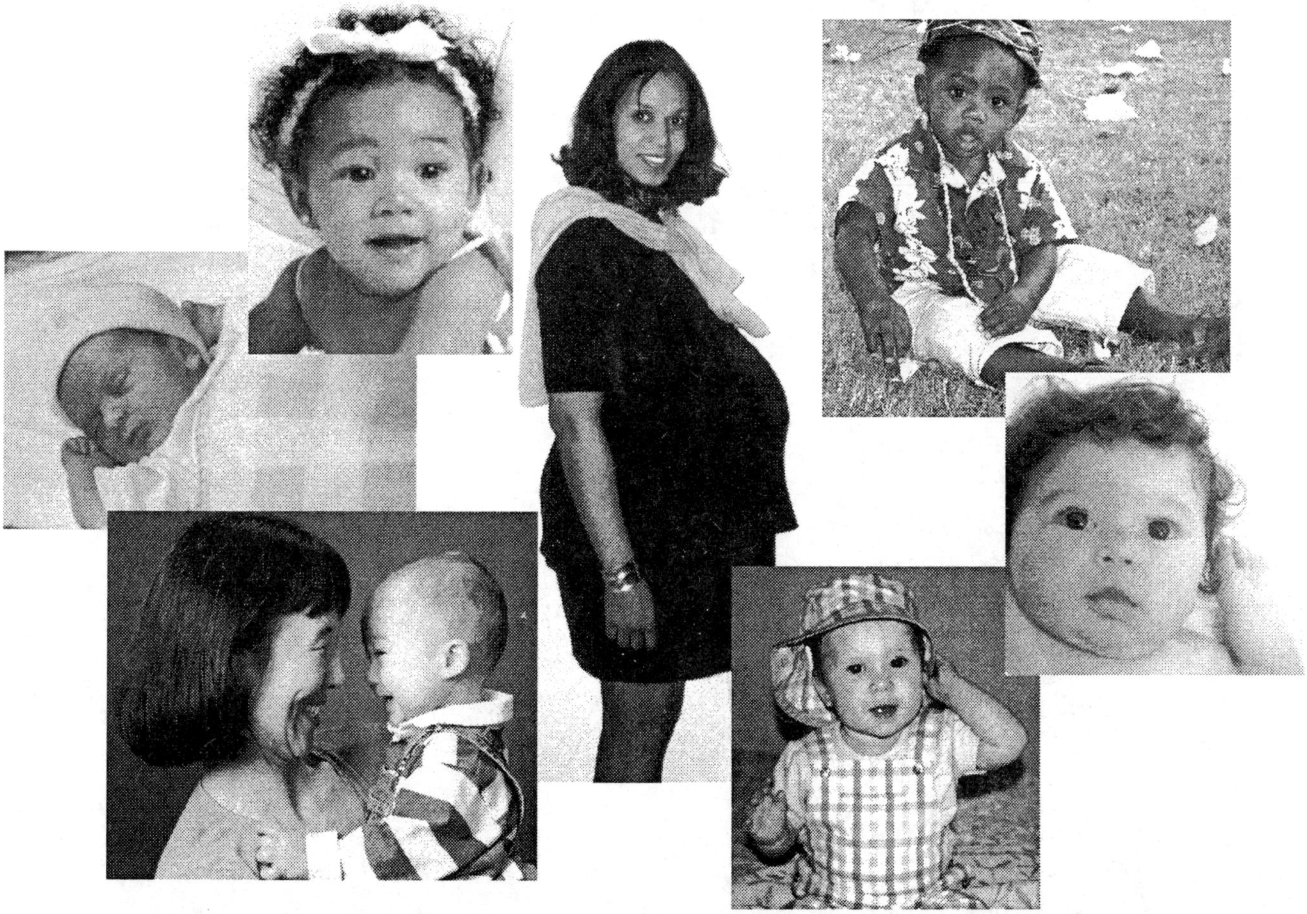

CENTERS FOR DISEASE CONTROL AND PREVENTION

SAFER • HEALTHIER • PEOPLE™

The *MMWR* series of publications is published by the Epidemiology Program Office, Centers for Disease Control and Prevention (CDC), U.S. Department of Health and Human Services, Atlanta, GA 30333.

SUGGESTED CITATION

Centers for Disease Control and Prevention. Prevention of Perinatal Group B Streptococcal Disease. MMWR 2002;51(No. RR-11):[inclusive page numbers].

Centers for Disease Control and Prevention

Julie L. Gerberding, M.D., M.P.H.
Director

David W. Fleming, M.D.
Deputy Director for Science and Public Health

Dixie E. Snider, Jr., M.D., M.P.H.
Associate Director for Science

Epidemiology Program Office

Stephen B. Thacker, M.D., M.Sc.
Director

Office of Scientific and Health Communications

John W. Ward, M.D.
Director
Editor, MMWR Series

Suzanne M. Hewitt, M.P.A.
Managing Editor

Lynne McIntyre, M.A.L.S.
Project Editor

Lynda G. Cupell
Malbea A. Heilman
Beverly J. Holland
Visual Information Specialists

Quang M. Doan
Erica R. Shaver
Information Technology Specialists

CONTENTS

Prevention of Perinatal Group B Streptococcal Disease
Revised Guidelines from CDC

Prepared by
Stephanie Schrag, D. Phil.
Rachel Gorwitz, M.D.
Kristi Fultz-Butts, M.P.H.
Anne Schuchat, M.D.
Division of Bacterial and Mycotic Diseases
National Center for Infectious Diseases

Summary

Group B streptococcus (GBS) remains a leading cause of serious neonatal infection despite great progress in perinatal GBS disease prevention in the 1990s. In 1996, CDC, in collaboration with other agencies, published guidelines for the prevention of perinatal group B streptococcal disease (CDC. Prevention of perinatal group B streptococcal disease: a public health perspective. MMWR 1996;45[RR-7]:1–24). *Data collected after the issuance of the 1996 guidelines prompted reevaluation of prevention strategies at a meeting of clinical and public health representatives in November 2001. This report replaces CDC's 1996 guidelines. The recommendations are based on available evidence and expert opinion where sufficient evidence was lacking. Although many of the recommendations in the 2002 guidelines are the same as those in 1996, they include some key changes:*

- *Recommendation of universal prenatal screening for vaginal and rectal GBS colonization of all pregnant women at 35–37 weeks' gestation, based on recent documentation in a large retrospective cohort study of a strong protective effect of this culture-based screening strategy relative to the risk-based strategy*
- *Updated prophylaxis regimens for women with penicillin allergy*
- *Detailed instruction on prenatal specimen collection and expanded methods of GBS culture processing, including instructions on antimicrobial susceptibility testing*
- *Recommendation against routine intrapartum antibiotic prophylaxis for GBS-colonized women undergoing planned cesarean deliveries who have not begun labor or had rupture of membranes*
- *A suggested algorithm for management of patients with threatened preterm delivery*
- *An updated algorithm for management of newborns exposed to intrapartum antibiotic prophylaxis*

Although universal screening for GBS colonization is anticipated to result in further reductions in the burden of GBS disease, the need to monitor for potential adverse consequences of intrapartum antibiotic use, such as emergence of bacterial antimicrobial resistance or increased incidence or severity of non-GBS neonatal pathogens, continues, and intrapartum antibiotics are still viewed as an interim strategy until GBS vaccines achieve licensure.

Introduction

Group B streptococcus (GBS) emerged as the leading infectious cause of neonatal morbidity and mortality in the United States in the 1970s (*1–4*). Initial case series reported case-fatality ratios as high as 50%. In the early 1980s, clinical trials demonstrated that administering antibiotics during labor to women at risk of transmitting GBS to their newborns could prevent invasive disease in the first week of life (i.e., early-onset disease) (*5*). As a result of the collaborative efforts of clinicians, researchers, professional organizations, parent advocacy groups, and the public health community in the 1990s, recommendations for intrapartum prophylaxis to prevent perinatal GBS disease were issued in 1996 by the American College of Obstetricians and Gynecologists (ACOG) (*6*) and CDC (*7*), and in 1997 by the American Academy of Pediatrics (*8*).

Those guidelines recommended the use of one of two prevention methods, a risk-based approach or a culture-based screening approach. Providers using the risk-based method identify candidates for intrapartum chemoprophylaxis according to the presence of any of the following intrapartum risk factors associated with early-onset disease: delivering at <37 weeks' gestation, having an intrapartum temperature $\geq 100.4°F$ ($\geq 38.0°C$), or rupture of membranes for ≥ 18 hours. The screening-based method recommends screening of all pregnant women for vaginal and rectal GBS colonization between 35 and 37 weeks' gestation. Colonized women are then offered intrapartum antibiotics at the time of labor. Under both strategies, women with GBS bacteriuria during their current

The material in this report was prepared by the National Center for Infectious Diseases, James M. Hughes, M.D., Director; Division of Bacterial and Mycotic Diseases, Mitchell L. Cohen, M.D., Director.

pregnancy, or who previously gave birth to an infant with early-onset GBS disease are candidates for intrapartum antibiotic prophylaxis.

Before active prevention was initiated, an estimated 7,500 cases of neonatal GBS disease occurred annually (9). Despite striking declines in disease incidence coinciding with increased prevention activities in the 1990s, GBS disease remains a leading infectious cause of morbidity and mortality among newborns in the United States (10,11). Moreover, since the release of the 1996 guidelines, new data are available to evaluate the effectiveness of the screening approach relative to the risk-based approach and to resolve some of the clinical challenges of implementing prevention.

In light of these new data, in November 2001, CDC consulted with multiple partners to revise the 1996 guidelines for the prevention of perinatal group B streptococcal disease, using an evidence-based approach where possible and scientific opinion when sufficient data were lacking (Table 1). These updated guidelines replace CDC's 1996 guidelines. They are intended for the following groups: providers of prenatal, obstetric, and pediatric care; supporting microbiology laboratories, hospital administrators and managed care organizations; childbirth educators; public health authorities; and expectant parents and their advocates.

Differences and similarities between current and previous guidelines

Following are major differences in the new guidelines:
- Recommendation of universal prenatal culture-based screening for vaginal and rectal GBS colonization of all pregnant women at 35–37 weeks' gestation
- Updated prophylaxis regimens for women with penicillin allergy

- Detailed instruction on prenatal specimen collection and expanded methods of GBS culture processing, including instructions on susceptibility testing
- Recommendation against routine intrapartum antibiotic prophylaxis for GBS-colonized women undergoing planned cesarean deliveries who have not begun labor or had rupture of membranes
- A suggested algorithm for management of patients with threatened preterm delivery
- An updated algorithm for management of newborns exposed to intrapartum antibiotic prophylaxis

Although important changes have been instituted, many recommendations remain the same:
- Penicillin remains the first-line agent for intrapartum antibiotic prophylaxis, with ampicillin an acceptable alternative.
- Women whose culture results are unknown at the time of delivery should be managed according to the risk-based approach; the obstetric risk factors remain unchanged (i.e., delivery at <37 weeks' gestation, duration of membrane rupture $\geq$18 hours, or temperature $\geq$100.4°F [$\geq$38.0°C]).
- Women with negative vaginal and rectal GBS screening cultures within 5 weeks of delivery do not require intrapartum antimicrobial prophylaxis for GBS even if obstetric risk factors develop (i.e., delivery at <37 weeks' gestation, duration of membrane rupture $\geq$18 hours, or temperature $\geq$100.4°F [$\geq$38.0°C]).
- Women with GBS bacteriuria in any concentration during their current pregnancy or who previously gave birth to an infant with GBS disease should receive intrapartum antimicrobial prophylaxis.
- In the absence of GBS urinary tract infection, antimicrobial agents should not be used before the intrapartum period to treat asymptomatic GBS colonization.

TABLE 1. Evidence-based rating system used to determine strength of recommendations

Category	Definition	Recommendation
Strength of recommendation		
A	Strong evidence for efficacy and substantial clinical benefit	Strongly recommended
B	Strong or moderate evidence for efficacy, but only limited clinical benefit	Generally recommended
C	Insufficient evidence for efficacy; or efficacy does not outweigh possible adverse consequences	Optional
D	Moderate evidence against efficacy or for adverse outcome	Generally not recommended
E	Strong evidence against efficacy or for adverse outcome	Never recommended
Quality of evidence supporting recommendation		
I	Evidence from at least one well-executed randomized, controlled trial or one rigorously designed laboratory-based experimental study that has been replicated by an independent investigator	
II	Evidence from at least one well-designed clinical trial without randomization; cohort or case-controlled analytic studies (preferably from more than one center); multiple time-series studies; dramatic results from uncontrolled studies; or some evidence from laboratory experiments	
III	Evidence from opinions of respected authorities based on clinical or laboratory experience, descriptive studies, or reports of expert committees	

Source: Adapted from CDC, 1999 USPHS/IDSA guidelines for the prevention of opportunistic infections in persons infected with human immunodeficiency virus. MMWR 1999; 48(RR-10):1-66.

Background

Early Infancy and Pregnancy-Related Infections

GBS causes severe invasive disease in young infants. The majority of infections in newborns occur within the first week of life and are designated early-onset disease. Late-onset infections occur in infants aged >1 week, with most infections evident in the first 3 months of life. Young infants with invasive GBS disease usually present with sepsis or pneumonia, and less often contract meningitis, osteomyelitis, or septic arthritis. The proportion of infants with meningitis is higher among those with late-onset infections. When neonatal infections caused by GBS appeared in the 1970s, as many as 50% of patients died. During the 1990s, the case-fatality ratio of early- and late-onset disease was 4% (10) because of advances in neonatal care.

Intrauterine infection of the fetus results from ascending spread of GBS from the vagina of a colonized woman who is typically asymptomatic. Fetal aspiration of infected amniotic fluid can lead to stillbirth, neonatal pneumonia, or sepsis. Infants can also become infected with GBS during passage through the birth canal, although the majority of infants who are exposed to the organism through this route become colonized on skin or mucous membranes but remain asymptomatic.

In pregnant women, GBS can cause clinical infections, but most women have no symptoms associated with genital tract colonization. Urinary tract infections caused by GBS complicate 2%–4% of pregnancies (12,13). During pregnancy or the postpartum period, women can contract amnionitis, endometritis, sepsis, or rarely, meningitis caused by GBS (14–19). Fatalities among women with pregnancy-associated GBS disease are extremely rare.

GBS Colonization

The gastrointestinal tract serves as the natural reservoir for GBS and is the likely source of vaginal colonization. Vaginal colonization is unusual in childhood but becomes more common in late adolescence (20). Approximately 10% to 30% of pregnant women are colonized with GBS in the vagina or rectum (21). GBS colonization can be transient, chronic, or intermittent. Maternal intrapartum GBS colonization is a major risk factor for early-onset disease in infants, and vertical transmission of GBS from mother to fetus primarily occurs after the onset of labor or membrane rupture. However, colonization early in pregnancy is not predictive of neonatal sepsis (22). Culture screening of both the vagina and rectum for GBS late in gestation during prenatal care can detect women who are likely to be colonized with GBS at the time of delivery and are thus at higher risk of perinatal transmission of the organism (23).

Classic epidemiologic studies conducted during the 1980s revealed that women with prenatal GBS colonization were >25 times more likely than women with negative prenatal cultures to deliver infants with early-onset GBS disease (24). Researchers used prenatal cultures as the basis for identifying candidates for intrapartum antimicrobial chemoprophylaxis; clinical trials identified reductions in vertical transmission of the organism, as measured by infant colonization (25,26) or by protection against early-onset disease (5,27). Heavy colonization, defined as culture of GBS from direct plating rather than only from selective broth, is associated with higher risk for early-onset disease. GBS identified in clean-catch urine specimens is considered a surrogate for heavy maternal colonization and also is associated with a higher risk for early-onset GBS disease (12,13); it has been included among indications for intrapartum antibiotic prophylaxis.

GBS Culture-Based Screening Methods

Numerous studies have documented that the accuracy of prenatal screening cultures in identifying intrapartum colonization status can be enhanced by careful attention to the timing of cultures, the anatomic sites swabbed, and the precise microbiologic methods used for culture and detection of organisms (Box 1). Collection of cultures between 35 and 37 weeks' gestation is recommended to improve the sensitivity and specificity of detection of women who remain colonized at the time of delivery (23,28). Swabbing both the lower vagina and rectum (i.e., through the anal sphincter) increases the yield substantially compared with sampling the cervix or sampling the vagina without also swabbing the rectum (29). Studies have indicated that when women in the outpatient clinic setting collect their own screening specimens, with appropriate instruction, GBS yield is similar to when specimens are collected by a health-care provider (30). Although swabbing both sites is recommended and use of two swabs can be justified, both swabs should be placed in a single broth culture medium because the site of isolation is not important for clinical management and laboratory costs can thereby be minimized. Because vaginal and rectal swabs are likely to yield diverse bacteria, use of selective enrichment broth is recommended (Box 1) to maximize the isolation of GBS and avoid overgrowth of other organisms. When direct agar plating is used instead of selective enrichment broth, as many as 50% of women who are GBS carriers have false-negative culture results (31).

BOX 1. Procedures for collecting and processing clinical specimens for group B streptococcal culture and performing susceptibility testing to clindamycin and erythromycin

Procedure for collecting clinical specimens for culture of group B streptococcus at 35–37 weeks' gestation

- Swab the lower vagina (vaginal introitus), followed by the rectum (i.e., insert swab through the anal sphincter) using the same swab or two different swabs. Cultures should be collected in the outpatient setting by the healthcare provider or the patient herself, with appropriate instruction. Cervical cultures are not recommended and a speculum should not be used for culture collection.
- Place the swab(s) into a nonnutritive transport medium. Appropriate transport systems (e.g., Amies or Stuart's without charcoal) are commercially available. If vaginal and rectal swabs were collected separately, both swabs can be placed into the same container of medium. Transport media will maintain GBS viability for up to 4 days at room temperature or under refrigeration.
- Specimen labels should clearly identify that specimens are for group B streptococcal culture. If susceptibility testing is ordered for penicillin-allergic women (Box 2), specimen labels should also identify the patient as penicillin allergic and should specify that susceptibility testing for clindamycin and erythromycin should be performed if GBS is isolated.

Procedure for processing clinical specimens for culture of group B streptococcus

- Remove swab(s) from transport medium.* Inoculate swab(s) into a recommended selective broth medium, such as Todd-Hewitt broth supplemented with either gentamicin (8 µg/ml) and nalidixic acid (15 µg/ml), or with colistin (10 µg/ml) and nalidixic acid (15 µg/ml). Examples of appropriate commercially available options include Trans-Vag broth supplemented with 5% defibrinated sheep blood or LIM broth.[†]
- Incubate inoculated selective broth for 18–24 hours at 35°–37°C in ambient air or 5% CO_2. Subculture the broth to a sheep blood agar plate (e.g., tryptic soy agar with 5% defibrinated sheep blood).

- Inspect and identify organisms suggestive of GBS (i.e., narrow zone of beta hemolysis, gram-positive cocci, catalase negative). Note that hemolysis may be difficult to observe, so typical colonies without hemolysis should also be further tested. If GBS is not identified after incubation for 18–24 hours, reincubate and inspect at 48 hours to identify suspected organisms.
- Various streptococcus grouping latex agglutination tests or other tests for GBS antigen detection (e.g., genetic probe) may be used for specific identification, or the CAMP test may be employed for presumptive identification.

Procedure for clindamycin and erythromycin disk susceptibility testing of isolates, when ordered for penicillin-allergic patients[§]

- Use a cotton swab to make a suspension from 18–24-hour growth of the organism in saline or Mueller-Hinton broth to match a 0.5 McFarland turbidity standard.
- Within 15 minutes of adjusting the turbidity, dip a sterile cotton swab into the adjusted suspension. The swab should be rotated several times and pressed firmly on the inside wall of the tube above the fluid level. Use the swab to inoculate the entire surface of a Mueller-Hinton sheep blood agar plate. After the plate is dry, use sterile forceps to place a clindamycin (2 µg) disk onto half of the plate and an erythromycin (15 µg) disk onto the other half.
- Incubate at 35°C in 5% CO_2 for 20–24 hours.
- Measure the diameter of the zone of inhibition using a ruler or calipers. Interpret according to NCCLS guidelines for *Streptococcus* species other than *S. pneumoniae* (2002 breakpoints:[§] clindamycin: $\geq$19 mm = susceptible, 16–18 = intermediate, $\leq$15 = resistant; erythromycin: $\geq$21 mm = susceptible, 16–20 = intermediate, $\leq$15 = resistant).

---

* Before inoculation step, some laboratories may choose to roll swab(s) on a single sheep blood agar plate or CNA sheep blood agar plate. This should be done only in addition to, and not instead of, inoculation into selective broth. The plate should be streaked for isolation, incubated at 35–37°C in ambient air or 5% CO_2 for 18–24 hours and inspected for organisms suggestive of GBS as described above. If suspected colonies are confirmed as GBS, the broth can be discarded, thus shortening the time to obtaining culture results.

† **Source:** Fenton, LJ, Harper MH. Evaluation of colistin and nalidixic acid in Todd-Hewitt broth for selective isolation of group B streptococci. J Clin Microbiol 1979;9:167–9. Although Trans-Vag medium is often available without sheep blood, direct comparison of medium with and without sheep blood has shown higher yield when blood is added. LIM broth may also benefit from the addition of sheep blood, although the improvement in yield is smaller and sufficient data are not yet available to support a recommendation.

§ **Source:** NCCLS. Performance standard for antimicrobial suceptibility testing, M100-S12, Table 2H, Wayne, Pa.: NCCLS, 2002. NCCLS recommends disk diffusion (M-2) or broth microdilution testing (M-7) for susceptibility testing of GBS. Commercial systems that have been cleared or approved for testing of streptococci other than *S. pneumoniae* may also be used. Penicillin susceptibility testing is not routinely recommended for GBS because penicillin-resistant isolates have not been confirmed to date.

Additional Risk Factors for Perinatal GBS Disease

In addition to colonization with GBS, other factors increase the risk for early-onset disease. These include gestational age <37 completed weeks, longer duration of membrane rupture, intraamniotic infection, young maternal age, black race, Hispanic ethnicity, and low maternal levels of anticapsular antibody (32–37). In a 1985 report of predictors of early-onset disease (24), women with gestation <37 weeks, membrane rupture of >12 hours, or intrapartum temperature >99.5°F (37.5°C) had 6.5 times the risk of having an infant with early-onset GBS disease compared with women with none of those factors. Of note, women who had one of these risk factors but who had negative prenatal screening cultures were at relatively low risk for early-onset GBS disease (attack rate 0.9 per 1,000 births) compared with women who were colonized prenatally but had none of the risk factors (attack rate 5.1 per 1,000 births) (24). In a risk-based strategy promoted during the 1990s as an alternative to prenatal culture-based screening approaches, prematurity (gestation <37 weeks), intrapartum fever (temperature ≥100.4°F or 38°C), or duration of membrane rupture >18 hours were used as clinical indications for intrapartum prophylaxis. Previous delivery of an infant with invasive GBS disease may increase the risk of early-onset disease in subsequent deliveries (38,39), and intrapartum treatment of such women in subsequent pregnancies has been promoted. By contrast, colonization with GBS in a previous pregnancy is not considered an indication for intrapartum prophylaxis in subsequent pregnancies; rather, women require evaluation for prenatal colonization in each pregnancy. Because colonization is transient, the predictive value of culture-based screening is too low to be clinically useful when performed more than 5 weeks before delivery (28); thus, many women with GBS colonization during one pregnancy will no longer be colonized during subsequent pregnancies.

Impact and Implementation of the 1996 Guidelines

Declines in Perinatal GBS Disease Incidence in the Era of Chemoprophylaxis

Before the widespread use of intrapartum antibiotics, the incidence of invasive neonatal GBS disease ranged from 2 to 3 cases per 1,000 live births (9,40). Active, population-based surveillance in selected states in 1990, when GBS prevention was still rarely implemented, projected an incidence of 1.8

cases per 1,000 live births in the United States (early-onset disease: 1.5/1,000; late-onset: 0.35/1,000) (9).

Coinciding with active prevention efforts in the 1990s, the incidence of early-onset disease declined by 70% to 0.5 cases per 1,000 live births in 1999 (Figure 1). Projections from active surveillance data for 1999 from the Active Bacterial Core surveillance/Emerging Infections Program Network (ABCs)(41) estimate that intrapartum antibiotics prevented nearly 4,500 early-onset cases and 225 deaths that year (10,11). Other countries that have adopted perinatal GBS disease prevention guidelines similar to the United States have seen comparable declines in early-onset disease incidence (42–44). Recent estimates of early-onset disease incidence in the United States suggest a slight increase in incidence from 1999 to 2000, consistent with a plateau in the impact of prevention efforts (Figure 1).

The incidence of invasive GBS infections among pregnant women in the United States declined by 21% from 0.29 per 1,000 live births in 1993 to 0.23 in 1998 (10), suggesting that increased use of intrapartum antibiotics also prevented some cases of maternal GBS amnionitis and endometritis. In contrast, the rate of late-onset disease remained fairly constant throughout the 1990s (Figure 1). Although intrapartum chemoprophylaxis for women with heavy GBS colonization may prevent a portion of late-onset disease, the stable incidence of late-onset disease during a period when use of intrapartum antibiotics was increasing suggests that this intervention is not effective against late-onset disease.

FIGURE 1. Incidence of early- and late-onset invasive group B streptococcal disease—selected Active Bacterial Core surveillance areas, 1989–2000, and activities for prevention of group B streptococcal disease

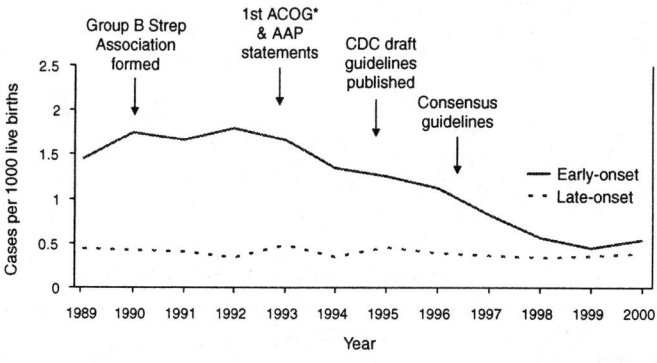

* ACOG, American College of Obstetricians and Gynecologists; AAP, American Academy of Pediatrics. **Source:** Adapted from CDC. Early-onset group B streptococcal disease, United States, 1998–1999. MMWR 2000;49:793–6; and Schrag SJ, Zywicki S, Farley MM, et al. Group B streptococcal disease in the era of intrapartum antibiotic prophylaxis. N Engl J Med 2000;342:15–20.

Implementation of Chemoprophylaxis Strategies After the Release of the 1996 Guidelines

Declines in perinatal GBS disease incidence in the 1990s suggest that prevention strategies have been implemented successfully. Several studies have explored directly the challenges of implementation and extent of compliance with recommendations. Surveys of prenatal care providers in Connecticut and Minnesota in 1998 found that over 80% had a GBS prevention policy (Connecticut, 95%; Minnesota, 85%) (45). In Minnesota, family physicians were less likely to have a policy than were obstetrician/gynecologists and certified nurse midwives (45). A national survey of ACOG members in 2000 found that 98% of respondents had a GBS prevention policy; 75% of respondents reported using a version of the culture-based screening approach (46). Providers in all three surveys scored well on questions about their knowledge of the screening and risk-based strategies (45,46).

In hospitals that established or revised policies for GBS prevention shortly after the release of the 1996 guidelines, rates of early-onset GBS disease declined by 1997 (47). By 1999, although only 63% of hospitals in a multistate survey of hospitals in the ABCs areas had a formal GBS prevention policy (48), having a hospital policy was no longer associated with changes in incidence of GBS disease, likely because a high proportion of individual practitioners had adopted policies by this time.

Several studies of single institutions or health maintenance organizations have evaluated adherence of hospital personnel to GBS guidelines (Table 2). Among hospitals with a risk-based policy, intrapartum antibiotics were administered in 40%–80% of preterm deliveries or deliveries with prolonged rupture of membranes (Table 2) (49–53). Among hospitals with a culture-based screening policy, close to 90% of delivering women had documented GBS screening, and close to 90% of GBS-positive women received intrapartum antibiotics (Table 2) (42,51,54–59).

Correct laboratory processing of culture specimens (Box 1) plays a critical role in successful implementation of the screening policy. A survey of clinical laboratories in selected counties of three states in 1997–1998 found that only a proportion of laboratories were using the recommended selective broth media to process GBS cultures (Georgia, 39% of laboratories; Minnesota, 42%; Connecticut, 62%), suggesting that this may be an area in need of improvement (31).

Although surveys of practitioners and laboratories and reports from single hospitals help monitor implementation of GBS prevention guidelines, a recent CDC-sponsored review of labor and delivery records in selected counties of eight states in the ABCs areas in 1998 and 1999 sheds light on actual provider practices 2 to 3 years after the release of the 1996 guidelines (60). In this population, GBS screening was documented in 52% of deliveries, although this varied widely, from 24% in selected counties of Oregon to 70% in Maryland.

TABLE 2. Institutional-level compliance with 1996 perinatal group B streptococcal disease prevention recommendations

Type of population sampled (ref.)	Deliveries receiving intrapartum antibiotics, %*	Deliveries with prolonged ROM* receiving intrapartum antibiotics, %*	Preterm deliveries receiving intrapartum antibiotics, %*	Women screened overall, %	GBS culture-positive women receiving intrapartum antibiotics, %*
Risk-based strategy evaluated					
2 HMO* hospitals, California (49)	–†	88	81	N/A†	N/A
University hospital, Florida (50)	–	20 in 1992	13 in 1992		
		72 in 1995	42 in 1995	N/A	N/A
Single hospital, Vienna, Austria (51)	11.9	–	–	N/A	N/A
Single hospital, Massachusetts (52)	–	81	–	N/A	N/A
Connecticut (statewide), 1996 (53)	15.2	45	53	N/A	N/A
Screening-based strategy evaluated					
Community hospital, New York (54)	–	N/A	76	91	86
University hospital, North Carolina (55)	12.9 for GBS prophylaxis	N/A	–	98	92
Single hospital, Sydney, Australia (42)	–	N/A	–	90	–
Single hospital, Vienna, Austria (51)	14.5	N/A	96	98.6	91
University hospital, New Mexico (56)	–	N/A	–	81	72
Single hospital, California (59)	26.3	N/A	91	89.8	94.4
Single hospital, Pennsylvania (57)	–	N/A	–	92	86
2 HMO hospitals, Washington State (58)	–	N/A	53	91	74 (automated data)
					87 (chart review)
Single hospital, Massachusetts (52)	–	N/A	–	N/A	100
Connecticut (statewide), 1996 (53)	15.2	N/A	–	(36% of Connecticut births)	78

* Given for any reason.
† ROM, rupture of membranes; HMO, health maintenance organization; –, data not available; N/A, not applicable.

Among screened women, 24% were GBS positive, consistent with carriage rates reported in earlier studies; 89% of GBS-positive women received intrapartum antibiotics. The median time of GBS culture collection was at 35.6 weeks' gestation, consistent with the recommendation of 35–37 weeks' gestation. Among unscreened women, 24% had at least one intrapartum risk factor; however, only 61% of women with at least one risk factor received intrapartum antibiotics. Preterm delivery (<37 weeks' gestation) was the most common indication for which intrapartum antibiotics were not administered. Thus, this multistate record review confirmed trends in adherence identified in reports from single hospitals (Table 2).

Maximizing Prevention by Chemoprophylaxis

Effectiveness of the Risk-Based Approach Versus the Screening Approach

Despite dramatic declines in GBS incidence in the United States in the 1990s, GBS remains a leading cause of newborn morbidity and mortality, resulting in an estimated 1,600 early-onset cases and 80 deaths annually. Although alternatives to intrapartum antibiotics such as a vaccine may become available in the future, intrapartum chemoprophylaxis remains the most effective available intervention against perinatal GBS disease. However, debate about the most effective strategy for identifying candidates for intrapartum chemoprophylaxis continues.

When the 1996 guidelines were issued, data regarding the relative effectiveness of the risk-based and screening approaches were not available. Theoretical predictions based on population estimates of the proportion of early-onset GBS cases without obstetric risk factors (approximately 45% in the preprevention era [61]) suggested that the screening-based approach would lead to greater declines in disease incidence than the risk-based approach (61,62). However, because implementation of the risk-based approach has been viewed as simpler than the screening-based approach, which requires correct specimen collection at the prenatal clinic, appropriate laboratory processing, and timely reporting of results to delivery staff, the actual effectiveness of these strategies is unknown. Consequently, since 1996, both approaches have been recommended as equally acceptable pending further data (6–8).

Although observational data are now available suggesting that each strategy can lead to reduced incidence of early-onset GBS disease (49,50,63–65), the strategies have not been directly compared by clinical trial because of the large sample

size required. A series of single hospital analyses finding benefits of screening over the risk-based approach (51,56,59,66) were limited by sequential use of the strategies and inability to control for potential confounders. A recent CDC-sponsored multistate study provided the first large-scale direct comparison of the strategies (60). By incorporating population-based surveillance for early-onset GBS disease into a sample survey of a population of over 600,000 live births, this analysis found that the screening approach was >50% more effective than the risk-based approach at preventing perinatal GBS disease.

The protective effect of the screening approach was robust and persisted after controlling for risk factors associated with early-onset GBS disease (e.g., preterm delivery, prolonged membrane rupture, young maternal age, black race). The benefit of screening stemmed from two main factors. First, by identifying GBS-colonized women who did not present with obstetric risk factors, screening reached more of the population at risk than did the risk-based approach. Among the cohort of screened women, 18% of all deliveries were to mothers who were colonized with GBS but did not have obstetric risk factors. The efficacy of intrapartum antibiotics in preventing early-onset GBS disease among infants in this cohort was close to 90%, suggesting that chemoprophylaxis of GBS-positive women without obstetric risk factors resulted in significant prevention of early-onset disease.

Women who were GBS positive in the screening cohort were also more likely to receive intrapartum antibiotics than were women with obstetric risk factors in the risk cohort. Although improvements in implementation of the risk-based approach would lead to further decline in disease, this would not be as great as with universal screening (60).

Finally, because the effectiveness of screening in this study was based on actual implementation of this strategy in clinical practice in 1998 and 1999, further improvements in screening implementation (e.g., improvements in specimen collection and the methods used for processing cultures) are expected to result in further benefits.

Rationale for a Universal Prenatal Screening Strategy to Detect GBS Status

The new availability of category II evidence (Table 1) for a large protective effect of prenatal GBS screening compared with the risk-based approach provides the foundation for a recommendation of universal prenatal GBS screening (Figure 2). Statewide prevention activities in some ABCs areas further demonstrate that culture-based screening can be successfully implemented in a variety of settings and institutions. For example, a health department-led survey of clinical

FIGURE 2. Indications for intrapartum antibiotic prophylaxis to prevent perinatal GBS disease under a universal prenatal screening strategy based on combined vaginal and rectal cultures collected at 35–37 weeks' gestation from all pregnant women

Vaginal and rectal GBS screening cultures at 35–37 weeks' gestation for **ALL** pregnant women (unless patient had GBS bacteriuria during the current pregnancy or a previous infant with invasive GBS disease)

Intrapartum prophylaxis indicated

- Previous infant with invasive GBS disease
- GBS bacteriuria during current pregnancy
- Positive GBS screening culture during current pregnancy (unless a planned cesarean delivery, in the absence of labor or amniotic membrane rupture, is performed)
- Unknown GBS status (culture not done, incomplete, or results unknown) and any of the following:
  - Delivery at <37 weeks' gestation*
  - Amniotic membrane rupture ≥18 hours
  - Intrapartum temperature ≥100.4°F (≥38.0°C)[†]

Intrapartum prophylaxis not indicated

- Previous pregnancy with a positive GBS screening culture (unless a culture was also positive during the current pregnancy)
- Planned cesarean delivery performed in the absence of labor or membrane rupture (regardless of maternal GBS culture status)
- Negative vaginal and rectal GBS screening culture in late gestation during the current pregnancy, regardless of intrapartum risk factors

* If onset of labor or rupture of amniotic membranes occurs at <37 weeks' gestation and there is a significant risk for preterm delivery (as assessed by the clinician), a suggested algorithm for GBS prophylaxis management is provided (Figure 3).
[†] If amnionitis is suspected, broad-spectrum antibiotic therapy that includes an agent known to be active against GBS should replace GBS prophylaxis.

laboratories in Connecticut followed by rapid feedback of survey results found that the proportion of laboratories in Connecticut using the correct media for processing GBS screening cultures increased from 62% in 1997 to 92% in 1998 (*67*) and 100% in 2000. Moreover, coinciding with an active prevention campaign launched by the state health department that advocated the screening-based approach, the incidence of early-onset GBS disease in Connecticut declined from 0.6 cases per 1,000 live births in 1996 (*68*) to 0.2 cases per 1,000 live births in 1999.

From the standpoint of implementation, universal screening has two additional benefits over the dual recommendations of 1996. Communication of the public health messages associated with a single strategy is simpler than communicating and educating about multiple strategies. Additionally, screening has clear indicators that facilitate evaluation of implementation (e.g., documentation of GBS test, timing of test, rates of GBS positivity) (*58*) compared with the risk-based approach, in which evidence of prevention implementation cannot be assessed for approximately 75% of deliveries because they have no intrapartum risk factors.

Cost-effectiveness analyses of the screening- and risk-based strategies (*62,69–73*) have indicated that although the initial costs associated with specimen collection and processing make the screening strategy more expensive than the risk-based

approach, the overall cost savings due to disease prevention do not differ importantly between strategies. Additionally, multistate review of labor and delivery records in 1998 and 1999 suggests that perfect implementation of the screening- or risk-based strategies will result in a comparable proportion of deliveries in which women receive intrapartum antibiotic prophylaxis for GBS (24% for both strategies) (*60,74*). Thus, the strategies cannot be distinguished in terms of the proportion of deliveries that will be exposed to intrapartum antibiotics.

Adverse Effects and Unintended Consequences of Chemoprophylaxis

Potential adverse or unintended effects of GBS prevention efforts that have raised concern include allergic or anaphylactic reactions to agents used for intrapartum antibiotic prophylaxis, emergence of GBS strains resistant to standard therapies, and increasing incidence of serious neonatal infections caused by pathogens other than GBS, including antimicrobial-resistant strains. Because of the increasing emergence of bacterial resistance to antimicrobial agents in both nosocomial and community settings, assessment of the impact and continued effectiveness of interventions based on antimicrobial prophylaxis is critical.

Antibiotic Allergies Including Anaphylaxis

Anaphylaxis associated with GBS chemoprophylaxis occurs but is sufficiently rare that any morbidity associated with anaphylaxis is greatly offset by reductions in the incidence of maternal and neonatal invasive GBS disease. Anaphylaxis-related mortality is likely to be a rare event since women receiving intrapartum antibiotics will be in hospital settings where rapid intervention is readily available. Estimates of the rate of anaphylaxis caused by penicillin range from 4/10,000 to 4/100,000 recipients. Additionally, as many as 10% of the adult population have less severe allergic reactions to penicillin (75). Anaphylaxis associated with GBS prophylaxis was reported in the early 1990s (76); since the release of the 1996 guidelines, an additional report of a nonfatal case of anaphylaxis associated with GBS chemoprophylaxis has been published (77). In a CDC multistate sample of over 5,000 live births, a single, nonfatal anaphylactic reaction was noted among the 27% of deliveries in which intrapartum antibiotics were administered (60). In that case, a single dose of penicillin was administered approximately 4 hours before a preterm cesarean delivery, and an anaphylactic reaction occurred shortly after the mother received a single dose of a cephalosporin following umbilical cord clamping.

Resistance in GBS

GBS isolates with confirmed resistance to penicillin or ampicillin have not been observed to date (78–83). Penicillin remains the agent of choice for intrapartum antibiotic prophylaxis. Ampicillin is an acceptable alternative, but penicillin is preferred because it has a narrower spectrum of antimicrobial activity and may be less likely to select for resistant organisms. The efficacy of both penicillin (27) and ampicillin (5) as intrapartum agents for the prevention of early-onset neonatal GBS disease has been demonstrated in clinical trials. Although the intramuscular route of administration for penicillin has been evaluated (25), intravenous administration is the only route of administration recommended for intrapartum chemoprophylaxis to prevent perinatal GBS disease, regardless of the antimicrobial agent used, because of the higher intraamniotic concentrations achieved with this method.

In contrast, the proportions of GBS isolates with in vitro resistance to clindamycin and erythromycin have increased since 1996. The prevalence of resistance among invasive GBS isolates in the United States and Canada ranged from 7% to 25% for erythromycin and from 3% to 15% for clindamycin in reports published between 1998 and 2001(79–81,84). Resistance to erythromycin is frequently but not always associated with clindamycin resistance. Resistance of GBS isolates

to cefoxitin, a second-generation cephalosporin sometimes used as a component of broad-spectrum coverage for chorioamnionitis, has also been reported (85); cefoxitin resistance has similarly been observed among invasive GBS isolates collected from 1996 to 2000 as part of CDC's active surveillance. Whether in vitro resistance of GBS has direct clinical implications remains unclear (86). Despite emerging resistance to some drug classes, minimum inhibitory concentrations of cefazolin, a first-generation cephalosporin available in an intravenous formulation, were low ($\leq$0.5 µg/ml) among a sample of invasive U.S. isolates from 1996 to 2000 (87), suggesting that GBS isolates are currently susceptible to this agent. Although NCCLS guidelines do not specify susceptibility breakpoints for cefazolin, they recommend that all isolates susceptible to penicillin be considered susceptible to cefazolin (88).

In light of the increasing prevalence of resistance to clindamycin, erythromycin, or both, recommended strategies for providing intrapartum antibiotic prophylaxis to penicillin-allergic women are updated (Box 2). Because the efficacy of recommended alternatives to penicillin or ampicillin has not been measured in controlled trials, and because some of the recommended alternatives have a broad spectrum of activity and may be more complicated and costly to administer, verification of a reported history of penicillin allergy is important. Patients with reported penicillin allergy should then be assessed to determine their risk for anaphylaxis. Persons at high risk for anaphylaxis are those who have had immediate hypersensitivity reactions to penicillin (e.g., anaphylaxis, angioedema, or urticaria) or who have a history of asthma or other conditions that would make anaphylaxis more dangerous (89,90). An estimated 10% of persons with penicillin allergy also have immediate hypersensitivity reactions to cephalosporins (90). Among penicillin-allergic women not at high risk for anaphylaxis, cefazolin, because of its narrow spectrum of activity and ability to achieve high intraamniotic concentrations, is the agent of choice for intrapartum chemoprophylaxis.

For penicillin-allergic women at high risk for anaphylaxis, testing of GBS isolates from prenatal screening for susceptibility to clindamycin and erythromycin is recommended if feasible (Box 1). One of these agents should be employed for intrapartum GBS prophylaxis if the screening isolate is susceptible to both agents.

Vancomycin should be reserved for penicillin-allergic women at high risk for beta-lactam anaphylaxis when clindamycin or erythromycin are not options because of in vitro resistance or unknown susceptibility of a prenatal isolate. Vancomycin use is generally restricted because of emerging vancomycin resistance among some gram-positive organisms (e.g., vancomycin-resistant enterococcus and vancomycin-resistant *Staphylococcus*

BOX 2. Recommended regimens for intrapartum antimicrobial prophylaxis for perinatal GBS disease prevention*

Recommended	Penicillin G, 5 million units IV initial dose, then 2.5 million units IV every 4 hours until delivery
Alternative	Ampicillin, 2 g IV initial dose, then 1 g IV every 4 hours until delivery
If penicillin allergic[†]	
Patients not at high risk for anaphylaxis	Cefazolin, 2 g IV initial dose, then 1 g IV every 8 hours until delivery
Patients at high risk for anaphylaxis[§]	
GBS susceptible to clindamycin and erythromycin[¶]	Clindamycin, 900 mg IV every 8 hours until delivery
	OR
	Erythromycin, 500 mg IV every 6 hours until delivery
GBS resistant to clindamycin or erythromycin or susceptibility unknown	Vancomycin,** 1 g IV every 12 hours until delivery

* Broader-spectrum agents, including an agent active against GBS, may be necessary for treatment of chorioamnionitis.

† History of penicillin allergy should be assessed to determine whether a high risk for anaphylaxis is present. Penicillin-allergic patients at high risk for anaphylaxis are those who have experienced immediate hypersensitivity to penicillin including a history of penicillin-related anaphylaxis; other high-risk patients are those with asthma or other diseases that would make anaphylaxis more dangerous or difficult to treat, such as persons being treated with beta-adrenergic–blocking agents.

§ If laboratory facilities are adequate, clindamycin and erythromycin susceptibility testing (Box 1) should be performed on prenatal GBS isolates from penicillin-allergic women at high risk for anaphylaxis.

¶ Resistance to erythromycin is often but not always associated with clindamycin resistance. If a strain is resistant to erythromycin but appears susceptible to clindamycin, it may still have inducible resistance to clindamycin.

** Cefazolin is preferred over vancomycin for women with a history of penicillin allergy other than immediate hypersensitivity reactions, and pharmacologic data suggest it achieves effective intraamniotic concentrations. Vancomycin should be reserved for penicillin-allergic women at high risk for anaphylaxis.

aureus). An estimated 13.8 million hospitalized patients received vancomycin therapy in 1998 (*91*). If penicillin allergy occurs in approximately 10% of adults, and 25% of parturients are colonized with GBS prenatally, approximately 100,000 of the 4 million annual deliveries would require prophylaxis with vancomycin in the absence of clindamycin and erythromycin susceptibility testing of GBS prenatal isolates. This represents a 7% increase in the number of patients exposed to vancomycin. The total grams of vancomycin used annually would increase by less than 1% if all penicillin-allergic colonized women received vancomycin prophylaxis.

Increased Incidence or Resistance in Non-GBS Pathogens

Decreases in the incidence of early-onset GBS sepsis have not usually been accompanied by increases in incidence of early-onset sepsis caused by other pathogens, including those that are antibiotic resistant. Most studies, including population-based multicenter studies, have found stable (*59,92,93*) or decreasing (*43*) rates of non-GBS early-onset sepsis during a period of increasing use of intrapartum antibiotic prophylaxis for GBS (Table 3). This is true both for overall non-GBS sepsis and for neonatal sepsis caused by *Escherichia coli*, the second leading bacterial cause of neonatal sepsis after GBS (*93,94*). Some single hospital studies have found increased rates or case counts of neonatal sepsis caused by *E. coli*, gram-negative organisms in general, or ampicillin-resistant pathogens (*64,94,95*), but these increases appear to be limited to preterm or low-birth-weight infants. An increasing proportion of *E. coli* neonatal sepsis cases caused by ampicillin-resistant organisms was observed in two studies (*92,94*), but again was limited to preterm or low-birth-weight infants. Furthermore, the proportion of community-acquired *E. coli* infections that are ampicillin resistant has been increasing (*96*), suggesting that trends in antimicrobial resistance should not be attributed to GBS prophylaxis.

An association between intrapartum antibiotic exposure and ampicillin resistance in cases of *E. coli* or other non-GBS early-onset sepsis has been observed in several studies (*36,94,95, 97,98*). These reports established that infections caused by antibiotic-resistant organisms were more frequently preceded by antibiotic use than were infections caused by susceptible organisms, and that more doses or longer duration of antibiotics before delivery increased the chance that a neonatal infection, if it occurred, would be caused by an antibiotic-resistant organism. These studies, however, were not designed to assess whether intrapartum antibiotic use increased the rate of antibiotic-resistant infections. Moreover, findings from these studies are consistent with intrapartum antibiotics inducing

TABLE 3. Trends in neonatal sepsis incidence in the era of perinatal GBS disease prevention

Study site	Total births	Cause of early-onset sepsis	Number of cases (rate per 1,000 live births)						p-value
Illinois (1 hospital) (94)	61,498		1982–1987	1988–1993					
		E. coli	12 (0.37)	18 (0.62)					NS*
		E. coli (among low-birth-weight† infants)	2 (0.64)	8 (2.63)					0.05
California (1 hospital) (95)	29,897		1991	1992	1993	1994	1995	1996	
		GBS	5 (0.93)	3 (0.6)	2 (0.41)	2 (0.41)	2 (0.42)	1 (0.21)	NS
		Non-GBS	3 (0.56)	4 (0.8)	3 (0.61)	4 (0.81)	5 (1.04)	8 (1.65)	NS
		E. coli	0 (0)	1 (0.2)	1 (0.2)	2 (0.41)	2 (0.42)	5 (1.03)	0.001
Illinois (1 hospital) (64)	20,981		1992–1996	1997					
		GBS	30 (1.7)	0 (0)					0.02
		All causes	–§ (2.7)	– (2.1)					NS
		All gram negative	5 (0.29)	5 (1.3)					0.02
Connecticut (19 hospitals) (92)	140,923		1996	1997	1998	1999			
		GBS	20 (0.56)	17 (0.49)	20 (0.56)	8 (0.23)			0.01
		Non-GBS	24 (0.68)	23 (0.66)	24 (0.68)	23 (0.65)			NS
		E. coli	5 (0.14)	12 (0.35)	14 (0.39)	8 (0.23)			NS
Australia (multiple hospitals) (43)	172,947		1991–1993	1993–1995	1995–1997				
		GBS	33 (1.4)	68 (0.9)	27 (0.4)				<0.0001
		Non-GBS	30 (1.3)	63 (0.8)	29 (0.4)				<0.0001
California (1 hospital) (59)	29,403		1992–1993	1994–1996	1997–1998	1999–2000			
		GBS	8 (1.2)	15 (1.1)	0 (0)	2 (0.2)			0.001
		Non-GBS	11 (1.6)	14 (1.1)	7 (0.8)	6 (0.6)			NS
Ohio (1 hospital) (93)	41,738		1986–1991	1992–1997					
		GBS	24 (1.1)	11 (0.54)					0.04
		Non-GBS	28 (1.3)	29 (1.4)					NS

* NS = not statistically significant.
† Low birth weight defined as 1,501–2,500 g.
§ Data not available.

resistance among initially susceptible organisms, but also with intrapartum antibiotics preventing antibiotic-susceptible infections and having no impact on antibiotic-resistant infections, resulting in a net decrease in the total rate of infection.

The reported increases in antibiotic-resistant early-onset infections in a few studies are not of sufficient magnitude to outweigh the benefits of intrapartum antibiotic prophylaxis to prevent perinatal GBS disease. However, to assure early detection of increases in the rate of disease or deaths caused by organisms other than GBS, continued surveillance of neonatal sepsis caused by organisms other than GBS is needed.

Clinical Challenges

GBS Bacteriuria During Pregnancy

The presence of GBS bacteriuria in any concentration in a pregnant woman is a marker for heavy genital tract colonization. Therefore, women with any quantity of GBS bacteriuria during pregnancy should receive intrapartum chemoprophylaxis. Vaginal and rectal screening at 35–37 weeks is not necessary for these women. GBS can cause both symptomatic and asymptomatic urinary tract infections, which should be diagnosed and treated according to current standards of care for urinary tract infections in pregnancy. Women with GBS urinary tract infections during pregnancy should receive appropriate treatment at the time of diagnosis as well as intrapartum GBS prophylaxis. Laboratory personnel should report any presence of GBS bacteriuria in specimens obtained from pregnant women. For this to occur, labeling of urine specimens to indicate that they were obtained from a pregnant woman is imperative.

Planned Cesarean Delivery

Because GBS can cross intact amniotic membranes, a cesarean delivery does not prevent mother-to-child transmission of GBS. Moreover, because cesarean delivery itself is associated with health risks for mother and newborn, GBS colonization of the mother is not an indication for cesarean delivery, and cesarean delivery should not be used as an alternative to intrapartum antibiotic prophylaxis for GBS prevention.

However, although a risk does exist for transmission of GBS from a colonized mother to her infant during a planned cesarean delivery performed before onset of labor in a woman with intact amniotic membranes, it is extremely low, based on a retrospective study at a single hospital (99) and a review of CDC active, population-based surveillance data from the 1990s. Thus, in this specific circumstance, in which the risk for disease is extremely low, the individual risks to a mother and her infant from receiving intrapartum antibiotic prophylaxis may balance or outweigh the benefits. Intrapartum antibiotic prophylaxis to prevent perinatal GBS disease is, therefore, not recommended as a routine practice for women undergoing planned cesarean deliveries in the absence of labor or amniotic membrane rupture, regardless of the GBS colonization status of the mother. Patients expected to undergo planned cesarean deliveries should nonetheless still undergo routine vaginal and rectal screening for GBS at 35–37 weeks because onset of labor or rupture of membranes may occur before the planned cesarean delivery. In rare situations in which patients or providers opt for intrapartum prophylaxis before planned cesarean deliveries, administration of antibiotics at the time of incision rather than at least 4 hours before delivery may be reasonable (100).

Threatened Preterm Delivery

Because preterm (at <37 weeks' gestation) delivery is an important risk factor for early-onset GBS disease, and because timing of delivery can be difficult to assess, management of intrapartum prophylaxis for women with threatened preterm delivery can be challenging. Assessing the need for intrapartum prophylaxis for these women can also be difficult because GBS screening is recommended at 35 to 37 weeks' gestation, and culture results are not always available when labor or rupture of membranes occur preterm.

A suggested approach to GBS chemoprophylaxis in the context of threatened preterm delivery is outlined (Figure 3). Because insufficient data are available to suggest a single course of management, other management strategies developed

by individual physicians or institutions may be appropriate alternatives. The algorithm suggests that if GBS screening culture results from the current pregnancy are not available and if onset of labor or rupture of membranes occurs before 37 weeks' gestation with a substantial risk for preterm delivery (as assessed by the woman's health-care provider), intrapartum antibiotic prophylaxis for GBS should be provided pending culture results. For women not yet screened for GBS, a vaginal and rectal specimen for GBS culture should be obtained if time permits. If a negative culture result within the previous 4 weeks is on record, or if the clinician determines that labor can be successfully arrested and preterm delivery averted, antibiotics for GBS prophylaxis should not be initiated. Because recent clinical trials suggest that antibiotics administered during pregnancy may be associated with adverse neonatal outcomes, such as necrotizing enterocolitis or increased need for supplementary oxygen, without evident benefit for preterm labor or preterm premature rupture of membranes (101,102), antibiotics should be reserved for instances in which a significant risk for preterm delivery is present.

No data are available on which to recommend a specific duration of antibiotic administration for GBS-positive women with threatened preterm delivery when delivery is successfully postponed. Management strategies based on scientific opinion

FIGURE 3. Sample algorithm for GBS prophylaxis for women with threatened preterm delivery. This algorithm is not an exclusive course of management. Variations that incorporate individual circumstances or institutional preferences may be appropriate.

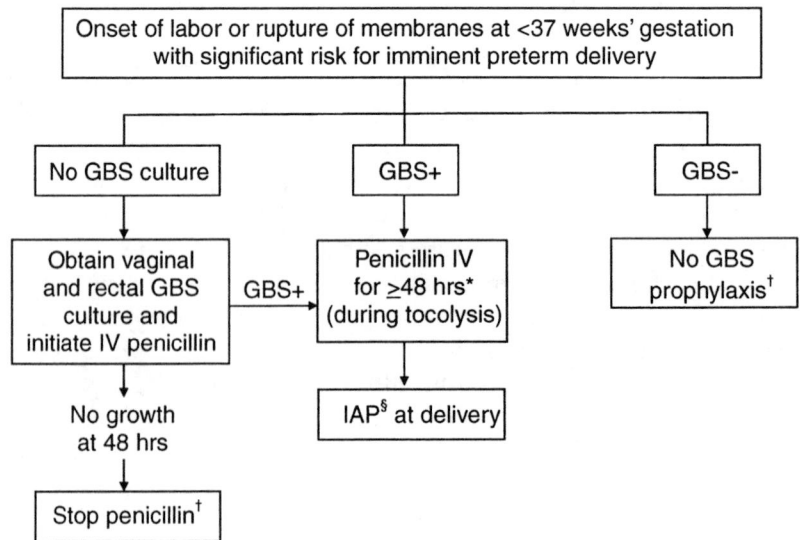

* Penicillin should be continued for a total of at least 48 hours, unless delivery occurs sooner. At the physician's discretion, antibiotic prophylaxis may be continued beyond 48 hours in a GBS culture-positive woman if delivery has not yet occurred. For women who are GBS culture positive, antibiotic prophylaxis should be reinitiated when labor likely to proceed to delivery occurs or recurs.
† If delivery has not occurred within 4 weeks, a vaginal and rectal GBS screening culture should be repeated and the patient should be managed as described, based on the result of the repeat culture.
§ Intrapartum antibiotic prophylaxis.

have been proposed (*100*); without further data, the management approach is left to the discretion of the individual provider. Regardless of management strategy chosen, these women should also receive intrapartum antibiotic chemoprophylaxis for GBS when labor likely to proceed to delivery occurs or recurs.

Previous data (*28*) suggest that the accuracy of GBS screening cultures in predicting colonization status at delivery is greatest if the cultures are collected within 5 weeks of delivery. Therefore, if a woman is screened early for GBS because of threatened preterm delivery but does not deliver within 4 weeks, she should be screened again for GBS colonization and managed according to the result of the repeated screening culture (Figure 3).

Obstetric Procedures for GBS-Colonized Women

Questions have arisen regarding whether certain obstetric procedures, such as digital vaginal examinations, intrauterine fetal monitoring, and membrane stripping or sweeping to hasten the onset of labor, should be performed on GBS-colonized women. Asymptomatic GBS colonization is not an indication to perform any of these procedures. When such procedures are indicated for other reasons, evidence is currently not sufficient to recommend that particular procedures should be avoided because of increased risk of peripartum or perinatal infection. Although some obstetric procedures (frequent vaginal examinations after onset of labor or membrane rupture [*17,36,103–105*], intrauterine fetal monitoring [*104,106,107*], and mechanical cervical ripening devices [*108*]) have been significantly associated with peripartum or perinatal infectious outcomes, most studies to date have been limited by an inability to randomly allocate women to treatment groups and have yielded conflicting results. Moreover, because many studies were performed before GBS prevention was widely implemented, GBS colonization status was often not known and intrapartum chemoprophylaxis was less common. A meta-analysis of available studies examining the use of membrane stripping among women of undetermined GBS colonization status (*109*) found no significant increases in overall peripartum or perinatal infection rates among women who underwent this procedure and their infants compared with those who did not.

Management of Newborns Exposed to Intrapartum Prophylaxis

On the basis of information available since the publication of the 1996 guidelines, a modified approach for empiric management of newborns born to women who receive intrapartum antibiotics to prevent early-onset GBS disease or to treat suspected chorioamnionitis is provided (Figure 4). Variations in the algorithm that incorporate individual circumstances or institutional preferences may be appropriate. The modified approach contains the following changes:

- If a woman receives intrapartum antibiotics for treatment of suspected chorioamnionitis, her newborn should have a full diagnostic evaluation and empiric therapy pending

FIGURE 4. Sample algorithm for management of a newborn whose mother received intrapartum antimicrobial agents for prevention of early-onset group B streptococcal disease* or suspected chorioamnionitis. This algorithm is not an exclusive course of management. Variations that incorporate individual circumstances or institutional preferences may be appropriate.

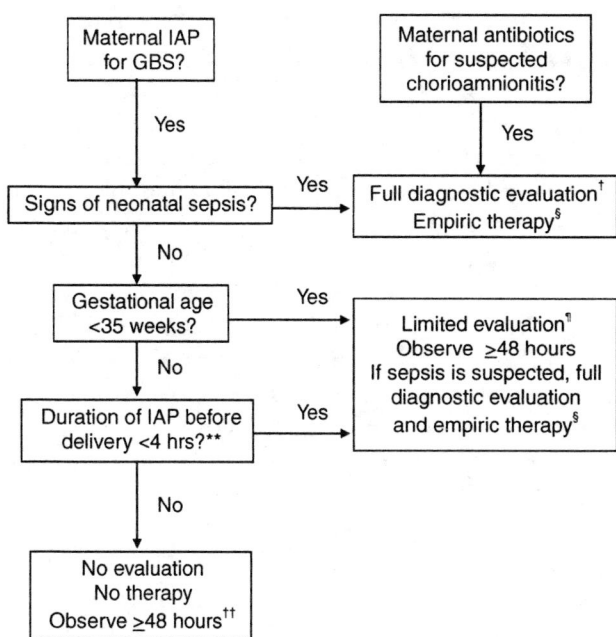

* If no maternal intrapartum prophylaxis for GBS was administered despite an indication being present, data are insufficient on which to recommend a single management strategy.

† Includes complete blood cell count and differential, blood culture, and chest radiograph if respiratory abnormalities are present. When signs of sepsis are present, a lumbar puncture, if feasible, should be performed.

§ Duration of therapy varies depending on results of blood culture, cerebrospinal fluid findings, if obtained, and the clinical course of the infant. If laboratory results and clinical course do not indicate bacterial infection, duration may be as short as 48 hours.

¶ CBC with differential and blood culture.

** Applies only to penicillin, ampicillin, or cefazolin and assumes recommended dosing regimens (Box 2)

†† A healthy-appearing infant who was ≥38 weeks' gestation at delivery and whose mother received ≥4 hours of intrapartum prophylaxis before delivery may be discharged home after 24 hours if other discharge criteria have been met and a person able to comply fully with instructions for home observation will be present. If any one of these conditions is not met, the infant should be observed in the hospital for at least 48 hours and until criteria for discharge are achieved.

culture results, regardless of clinical condition at birth, duration of maternal antibiotic therapy before delivery, or gestational age at delivery (*110*). Empiric therapy for the infant should include antimicrobial agents active against GBS as well as other organisms that might cause neonatal sepsis (e.g., ampicillin and gentamicin).

- When clinical signs in the infant suggest sepsis, a full diagnostic evaluation should include a lumbar puncture, if feasible. Blood cultures can be sterile in as many as 15% of newborns with meningitis (*111–113*), and the clinical management of an infant with abnormal cerebrospinal fluid (CSF) findings differs from that of an infant with normal CSF. If a lumbar puncture has been deferred for a neonate receiving empiric antibiotic therapy, and the therapy is continued beyond 48 hours because of clinical instability, CSF should be obtained for cell count, glucose, protein, and culture.

- In addition to penicillin or ampicillin, initiation of intrapartum antibiotic prophylaxis with cefazolin at least 4 hours before delivery can be considered adequate, based on achievable amniotic fluid concentrations of cefazolin (*114*). Although other agents may be substituted for penicillin if the woman has a history of penicillin allergy (Box 2), the effectiveness of these agents in preventing early-onset GBS disease has not been studied and no data are available to suggest the durations before delivery of these regimens that can be considered adequate.

- Based on the demonstrated effectiveness of intrapartum antibiotic prophylaxis at preventing early-onset GBS disease (*65*) and data indicating that clinical onset occurs within the first 24 hours of life in over 90% of infants who contract early-onset GBS disease (*115*), hospital discharge as early as 24 hours after delivery may be reasonable under certain circumstances. Specifically, a healthy-appearing infant who is ≥38 weeks' gestation at delivery and whose mother received ≥4 hours of intrapartum antibiotic prophylaxis before delivery may be discharged home as early as 24 hours after delivery, assuming that other discharge criteria have been met and that a person able to comply fully with instructions for home observation will be present. A key component of following instructions is the ability of the person observing to communicate with health-care providers by telephone and to transport the child promptly to an appropriate health-care facility if clinical signs of sepsis develop. If these conditions are not met, the infant should remain in the hospital for at least 48 hours of observation and until criteria for discharge are achieved.

Investigations since 1996 lend additional support to several components of the algorithm. A retrospective study of over 250,000 live births (*115*) found that administration of intrapartum antibiotic prophylaxis did not change the clinical spectrum of neonatal illness or delay the onset of clinical signs among infants who contracted GBS disease despite prophylaxis. Thus, the algorithm targets infants born to mothers with suspected chorioamnionitis and infants with signs of sepsis for full diagnostic evaluation and empiric therapy. Also, new evidence indicates that 4 or more hours of intrapartum ampicillin or penicillin administered according to recommended dosing intervals (Box 2) significantly reduces vertical transmission of GBS (*116*) and risk of early-onset GBS disease (*65*). Thus, although the American Academy of Pediatrics 1997 guidelines suggested 2 or more doses as a threshold for prophylaxis adequacy for infants ≥35 weeks' gestation (*8*), the revised algorithm continues to use ≥4 hours, administered according to recommended dosing intervals, as the benchmark for optimal prevention of early-onset GBS disease. Moreover, a review of pregnancies at a West Coast health maintenance organization using the GBS culture-based screening strategy found that among women who received intrapartum antibiotic prophylaxis, 50% received prophylaxis at least 4 hours before delivery, whereas only 14% received at least 2 doses of intrapartum antibiotics (*58*); this indicates that duration of prophylaxis is a more practical target than number of doses, in addition to being associated with efficacy.

One objective of developing an algorithm for management of newborns was to minimize unnecessary evaluation and antimicrobial treatment of infants whose mothers received intrapartum prophylaxis. Although early provider surveys indicated that pediatricians and neonatologists were more likely to conduct diagnostic evaluations and initiate empiric antibiotics for an infant whose mother received intrapartum antibiotic prophylaxis (*117–119*), more recent data indicate that implementation of GBS prevention strategies has not resulted in increased use of health services for neonates (*120*), and in some circumstances, when GBS prophylaxis increased a decrease occurred in the proportion of neonates who received laboratory evaluations (*58*).

Intrapartum antibiotic prophylaxis is the method of choice for preventing neonatal early-onset GBS disease. In the event that intrapartum antibiotics are not given despite an indication (e.g., delivery occurred precipitously before antibiotics could be administered to a GBS-positive woman), sufficient data are not available on which to recommend a single management strategy for the newborn. Some centers provide intramuscular penicillin to asymptomatic infants within 1 hour of birth, based on results of observational studies showing declines in early-onset GBS disease coincident with a policy of universal administration of intramuscular penicillin to all newborns (*121*).

Future Prevention Technology

Rapid Tests to Detect GBS Colonization Status

Rapid tests for detection of GBS colonization at the time of onset of labor or rupture of amniotic membranes might obviate the need for prenatal culture-based screening if their sensitivity and specificity are comparable to culture in selective broth media and they yield results rapidly enough to permit administration of adequate intrapartum antibiotic prophylaxis to women detected as carriers. Currently available rapid tests detect GBS antigen from swab specimens. These tests are insufficiently sensitive to detect light colonization, and therefore are not adequate to replace culture-based prenatal screening (*122,123*) or to use in place of the risk-based approach when culture results are unknown at the time of labor. An adequate rapid intrapartum test must be as sensitive as culture (minimally 85% compared with culture of vaginal and rectal swabs inoculated into selective broth media), rapid so that results are available to clinicians in time for antibiotics to be given before delivery, and convenient for integration into routine laboratory use. Even a highly sensitive rapid detection test would not be adequate if results were not available to clinicians 24 hours a day, 7 days a week. Alternatives to culturing vaginal and rectal swab specimens at 35–37 weeks' gestation using recommended procedures should be validated to show sensitivity similar to recommended culture methods.

A rapid intrapartum test possessing the attributes described above offers the advantage of ascertaining GBS colonization status before delivery among women who have had no prenatal care. Although such tests might initially be introduced selectively in certain facilities with sufficient demand and capability, a general recommendation for their use would require the capacity for effective implementation in a wide range of hospital settings. Drawbacks of rapid tests include delays in administration of intrapartum antibiotic prophylaxis while test results are pending and lack of an isolate for susceptibility testing, which is of particular concern for penicillin-allergic women. Additionally, until rapid tests are universally used, missed opportunities for GBS screening may occur among women who receive prenatal care at institutions relying on intrapartum rapid tests but who deliver at institutions where such tests are not yet available.

In a study of 112 pregnant women at an academic hospital in Quebec, a new, not yet commercially available fluorogenic polymerase chain reaction assay was 97% sensitive and 100% specific when compared with vaginal and rectal cultures collected at admission for delivery. Test results in this study were available within 45 minutes of specimen collection (*124*). Further studies are needed to determine whether this type of test can be adapted for use outside the research setting. If appropriate techniques for rapid detection of GBS become commercially available, they may be integrated into the currently recommended screening strategy.

Vaccines To Prevent GBS Disease

Improved use of intrapartum antimicrobial prophylaxis has resulted in a substantial reduction in early-onset GBS disease, but it is unlikely to prevent most late-onset neonatal infections, GBS-related stillbirths, or prematurity, and does not address GBS disease in nonpregnant adults. Immunization of women during or before pregnancy could prevent peripartum maternal disease and protect infants from perinatally acquired infection by transplacental transfer of protective IgG antibodies (*125,126*). This would eliminate the need for prenatal GBS screening and intrapartum antimicrobial prophylaxis, along with associated costs and concerns regarding the potential adverse effects of intrapartum antibiotic use discussed previously.

Serotype-specific antibodies to GBS capsular polysaccharide, although rare in populations of unvaccinated women, have been shown to protect against disease (*32,127*). Phase 1 and 2 clinical trials among healthy, nonpregnant adults of monovalent protein-conjugate vaccines containing capsular polysaccharide antigens of GBS disease-associated serotypes have shown these vaccines to be well tolerated and immunogenic (*128–130*). One challenge of demonstrating vaccine efficacy in preventing early-onset GBS disease is that the sample size required for clinical trials may be prohibitively large. Identification of surrogate immunologic measures of clinical efficacy may thus be important (*131,132*). Surrogate information on clinical vaccine efficacy may also be gained by measuring the impact of multivalent conjugate vaccines on vaginal GBS colonization (*132,133*).

Anticipated difficulties in making vaccine available to pregnant women have resulted in consideration of other target populations for vaccine administration, including adolescent girls (*134*), women of childbearing age, and infants (*135*). The duration of protection that could be afforded by vaccination is unknown; one or more booster doses might be required, potentially complicating vaccine delivery. Shifts in the GBS serotypes causing disease have provided an additional challenge to vaccine development (*133*) and may necessitate modification of vaccine serotype composition over time.

Research Priorities and Tools To Aid Prevention

Technological advances that aid the implementation of a universal screening strategy will further prevention efforts. In addition to development of reliable rapid tests that can be performed in a wide range of labor and delivery settings, methods of simplifying prenatal culture procedures, e.g., the development of media with a reliable color indicator to signal presence of GBS, might improve accuracy of prenatal culture results and facilitate prenatal culture processing at clinical laboratories with limited technical capacity. Media that have been developed for this purpose, such as Granada (*136,137*) or GBS medium (*138*), should be further evaluated to determine if sensitivity and specificity are comparable to recommended methods, which consist of culture in selective broth media followed by GBS-specific identification.

Although universal prenatal GBS culture-based screening is likely to result in substantial further declines in the incidence of early-onset disease, intrapartum chemoprophylaxis is not a permanent or comprehensive strategy for GBS disease prevention. Because vaccines under development hold promise to prevent a larger portion of the burden of GBS disease with a simpler and sustainable intervention, further work on GBS vaccine development and support of phase 3 clinical trials are warranted (*139*).

Until a safe, effective, and economical vaccine achieves licensure, it will be important to continue to monitor for potential adverse effects of chemoprophylaxis, with an emphasis on tracking key sentinel events signaling a need for revision of the guidelines. Such sentinel events include the emergence of penicillin resistance among GBS, which to date has not been detected, and an increase in the incidence of disease or deaths due to neonatal pathogens other than GBS that offsets the burden of early-onset disease prevented by chemoprophylaxis. Monitoring for the latter will require long-term surveillance of a large population of term and preterm births (*140*).

Because GBS carriage is common among delivering women in the United States, continued surveillance for GBS disease and evaluation of prevention implementation remains important to minimize missed opportunities for prevention. States are encouraged to monitor incidence of GBS disease, to promote activities that enhance perinatal GBS disease prevention and education, and to assess progress toward national objectives for disease reduction, such as Healthy People 2010,

which sets a target of reducing the incidence of early-onset GBS disease in all racial and ethnic groups to 0.5 cases per 1,000 live births (*141*). Practical tools to assist with monitoring for missed opportunities for perinatal GBS prevention within hospitals have been published (*142*); additional prevention information and tools for providers, patients and clinical microbiologists are available at http://www.cdc.gov/groupbstrep, http://www.acog.org, http://sales.acog.com, http://www.aap.org, and http://www.health.state.mn.us/divs/dpc/ades/invbact/strepb.htm.

Recommendations

The following updated recommendations for the prevention of GBS disease are based on critical appraisal of multistate population-based observational data and several studies from individual institutions that have been completed since publication of previous CDC (*7*), ACOG (*6*), and AAP (*8*) recommendations. They replace previous recommendations from CDC. The strength (indicated by a letter) and quality (indicated by a roman numeral) of evidence supporting each recommendation are shown in parentheses, according to the evidence-based rating system outlined in Table 1.

Obstetric-care practitioners, in conjunction with supporting laboratories and labor and delivery facilities, should adopt the following strategy for the prevention of perinatal GBS disease based on prenatal screening for GBS colonization. The risk-based approach is no longer an acceptable alternative except for circumstances in which screening results are not available before delivery (AII).

- All pregnant women should be screened at 35–37 weeks' gestation for vaginal and rectal GBS colonization (Figure 2) (AII). At the time of labor or rupture of membranes, intrapartum chemoprophylaxis should be given to all pregnant women identified as GBS carriers (AII). Colonization during a previous pregnancy is not an indication for intrapartum prophylaxis in subsequent deliveries. Screening to detect GBS colonization in each pregnancy will determine the need for prophylaxis in that pregnancy.
- Women with GBS isolated from the urine in any concentration (e.g., 10^3) during their current pregnancy should receive intrapartum chemoprophylaxis because such women usually are heavily colonized with GBS and are at increased risk of delivering an infant with early-onset GBS disease (BII). Labels on urine specimens from prenatal patients should clearly state the patient's pregnancy status to assist laboratory processing and reporting of results. Prenatal culture-based screening at 35–37 weeks' gestation is not necessary for women with GBS bacteriuria. Women with symptomatic or asymptomatic GBS urinary

tract infection detected during pregnancy should be treated according to current standards of care for urinary tract infection during pregnancy.

- Women who have previously given birth to an infant with invasive GBS disease should receive intrapartum chemoprophylaxis; prenatal culture-based screening is not necessary for these women (BII).

- If the result of GBS culture is not known at the onset of labor, intrapartum chemoprophylaxis should be administered to women with any of the following risk factors: gestation <37 weeks, duration of membrane rupture $\geq$18 hours, or a temperature of $\geq$100.4° F ($\geq$38.0°C) (AII). Women with known negative results from vaginal and rectal GBS screening cultures within 5 weeks of delivery do not require prophylaxis to prevent GBS disease even if any of the intrapartum risk factors develop.

- Women with threatened preterm (<37 weeks' gestation) delivery should be assessed for need for intrapartum prophylaxis to prevent perinatal GBS disease. An algorithm for management of women with threatened preterm delivery is provided (Figure 3). Other management approaches, developed by individual physicians or institutions, may be appropriate (CIII).

- Culture techniques that maximize the likelihood of GBS recovery are required for prenatal screening (Box 1). Collection of specimens for culture may be conducted in the outpatient clinic setting by either the patient, with appropriate instruction, or health-care provider (BII). This involves swabbing the lower vagina and rectum (i.e., through the anal sphincter). Because lower vaginal as opposed to cervical cultures are recommended, cultures should not be collected by speculum examination. Specimens should be placed in a nonnutritive transport medium (e.g., Amies or Stuart's without charcoal). Specimen labels should clearly identify that specimens are for group B streptococcal culture. If susceptibility testing is ordered for penicillin-allergic women (Box 2), specimen labels should also identify the patient as penicillin allergic and should specify that if GBS is isolated, it should be tested for susceptibility to clindamycin and erythromycin. Specimens should be inoculated into a selective broth medium (examples of appropriate commercially available media include Trans-Vag Broth supplemented with 5% defibrinated sheep blood or LIM broth), incubated overnight, and subcultured onto solid blood agar medium (AII). Methods of testing prenatal isolates from penicillin-allergic women for susceptibility to clindamycin and erythromycin are outlined (Box 1). Laboratories should report culture results (positive and negative) and susceptibility testing results to the anticipated site of delivery (when known) and to the health-care provider who ordered the test.

- Health-care providers should inform women of their GBS screening test result and the recommended interventions. In the absence of GBS urinary tract infection, antimicrobial agents should not be used before the intrapartum period to treat GBS colonization. Such treatment is not effective in eliminating carriage or preventing neonatal disease and may cause adverse consequences (DI).

- GBS-colonized women who have a planned cesarean delivery performed before rupture of membranes and onset of labor are at low risk for having an infant with early-onset GBS disease. These women should not routinely receive intrapartum chemoprophylaxis for perinatal GBS disease prevention (CII).

- For intrapartum chemoprophylaxis, the following regimen is recommended for women without penicillin allergy (Box 2): penicillin G, 5 million units intravenously initial dose, then 2.5 million units intravenously every 4 hours until delivery (AII). Because of its narrow spectrum of activity, penicillin is the preferred agent. An alternative regimen is ampicillin, 2 g intravenously initial dose, then 1 g intravenously every 4 hours until delivery (AI).

- Intrapartum chemoprophylaxis for penicillin-allergic women takes into account increasing resistance to clindamycin and erythromycin among GBS isolates (Box 2). During prenatal care, history of penicillin allergy should be assessed to determine whether a patient is at high risk for anaphylaxis, i.e., has a history of immediate hypersensitivity reactions to penicillin (e.g., anaphylaxis, angioedema, or urticaria) or history of asthma or other conditions that would make anaphylaxis more dangerous (89). Women who are not at high risk for anaphylaxis should be given cefazolin, 2 g intravenously initial dose, then 1 g intravenously every 8 hours until delivery (BIII). For women at high risk for anaphylaxis, clindamycin and erythromycin susceptibility testing, if available, should be performed on isolates obtained during GBS prenatal carriage screening. Women with clindamycin- and erythromycin-susceptible isolates should be given either clindamycin, 900 mg intravenously every 8 hours until delivery; OR erythromycin, 500 mg intravenously every 6 hours until delivery. If susceptibility testing is not possible, susceptibility results are not known, or isolates are resistant to erythromycin or clindamycin, the following regimen can be used for women with immediate penicillin hypersensitivity: vancomycin, 1 g intravenously every 12 hours until delivery (CIII).

- Routine use of antimicrobial prophylaxis for newborns whose mothers received intrapartum chemoprophylaxis for GBS infection is not recommended. However, therapeutic use of these agents is appropriate for infants with clinically suspected sepsis. An updated algorithm for management of infants born to mothers who received intrapartum chemoprophylaxis for GBS infection is provided (Figure 4). This revised algorithm is not an exclusive approach to management; variation that incorporates individual circumstances or institutional preferences may be appropriate (CIII).
- Local and state public health agencies, in conjunction with appropriate groups of hospitals, are encouraged to establish surveillance for early-onset GBS disease and to take other steps to promote perinatal GBS disease prevention and education to reduce the incidence of early-onset GBS disease in their states. Efforts to monitor the emergence of perinatal infections caused by other organisms are also encouraged.

Before full implementation of this strategy can be expected in all health-care settings, all members of the health-care team will need to improve protocols for isolation and reporting of GBS culture results, to improve information management to ensure communication of screening results, and to educate medical and nursing staff responsible for prenatal and intrapartum care. Within institutions, such efforts may take several months.

Even with ideal implementation, cases of early-onset GBS disease will continue to occur. Tools to help promote prevention and educate parents of infants with early-onset GBS disease are available at http://www.cdc.gov/groupbstrep. Additional tools available to assist with prevention implementation are available at http://www.acog.org, http://sales.acog.com, http://www.aap.org and http://www.health.state.mn.us/divs/dpc/ades/invbact/strepb.htm Multiple copies of educational materials published by CDC are available at the Public Health Foundation, 1220 L St., NW Suite 350, Washington, DC 20005, telephone 877-252-1200, or online at http://www.phf.org.

References

1. Baker CJ, Barrett FF, Gordon RC, Yow MD. Suppurative meningitis due to streptococci of Lancefield group B: a study of 33 infants. J Pediatr 1973;82:724–9.
2. Barton LL, Feigin RD, Lins R. Group B beta hemolytic streptococcal meningitis in infants. J Pediatr 1973;82:719–23.
3. Franciosi RA, Knostman JD, Zimmerman RA. Group B streptococcal neonatal and infant infections. J Pediatr 1973;82:707–18.
4. McCracken GH. Group B streptococci: the new challenge in neonatal infections. J Pediatr 1973;82:703–6.
5. Boyer KM, Gotoff SP. Prevention of early-onset neonatal group B streptococcal disease with selective intrapartum chemoprophylaxis. N Engl J Med 1986;314:1665–9.
6. American College of Obstetricians and Gynecologists, Committee on Obstetric Practice. Prevention of early-onset group B streptococcal disease in newborns [Opinion 173]. Washington, D. C: American College of Obstetricians and Gynecologists, 1996.
7. CDC. Prevention of perinatal group B streptococcal disease: a public health perspective. MMWR 1996;45 (RR-7):1–24.
8. American Academy of Pediatrics, Committee on Infectious Diseases/Committee on Fetus and Newborn. Revised guidelines for prevention of early-onset group B streptococcal (GBS) disease. Pediatrics 1997;99:489–96.
9. Zangwill KM, Schuchat A, Wenger JD. Group B streptococcal disease in the United States, 1990: report from a multistate active surveillance system. MMWR 1992;41(SS-6):25–32.
10. Schrag SJ, Zywicki S, Farley MM, et al. Group B streptococcal disease in the era of intrapartum antibiotic prophylaxis. N Engl J Med 2000;342:15–20.
11. CDC. Early-onset group B streptococcal disease, United States, 1998–1999. MMWR 2000;49:793–6.
12. Persson K, Christensen KK, Christensen P, Forsgren A, Jorgensen C, Persson PH. Asymptomatic bacteriuria during pregnancy with special reference to group B streptococci. Scand J Infect Dis 1985;17:195–9.
13. Wood EG, Dillon HC. A prospective study of group B streptococcal bacteriuria in pregnancy. Am J Obstet Gynecol 1981;140:515–20.
14. Pass MA, Gray BM, Dillon HC. Puerperal and perinatal infections with group B streptococci. Am J Obstet Gynecol 1982;143:147–52.
15. Bobitt JR, Ledger WJ. Amniotic fluid analysis: its role in maternal and neonatal infection. Obstet Gynecol 1978;51:56–62.
16. Braun TI, Pinover W, Sih P. Group B streptococcal meningitis in a pregnant woman before the onset of labor. Clin Infect Dis 1995;21:1042–3.
17. Yancey MK, Duff P, Clark P, Kurtzer T, Frentzen BH, Kubilis P. Peripartum infection associated with vaginal group B streptococcal colonization. Obstet Gynecol 1994;84:816–9.
18. Fox BC. Delayed-onset postpartum meningitis due to group B streptococcus [letter]. Clin Infect Dis 1994;19:350.
19. Aharoni A, Potasman I, Levitan Z, Golan D, Sharf M. Postpartum maternal group B streptococcal meningitis. Rev Infect Dis 1990;12:273–6.
20. Hammerschlag MR, Baker CJ, Alpert S, et al. Colonization with group B streptococci in girls under 16 years of age. Pediatrics 1977;60:473–6.
21. Regan JA, Klebanoff MA, Nugent RP, Vaginal Infections and Prematurity Study Group. The epidemiology of group B streptococcal colonization in pregnancy. Obstet Gynecol 1991;77:604–10.
22. Regan JA, Klebanoff MA, Nugent RP, et al. Colonization with group B streptococci in pregnancy and adverse outcome. Am J Obstet Gynecol 1996;174:1354–60.
23. Boyer KM, Gadzala CA, Kelly PD, Burd LI, Gotoff SP. Selective intrapartum chemoprophylaxis of neonatal group B streptococcal early-onset disease. II. Predictive value of prenatal cultures. J Infect Dis 1983;148:802–9.
24. Boyer KM, Gotoff SP. Strategies for chemoprophylaxis of GBS early-onset infections. Antibiot Chemother 1985;35:267–80.
25. Easmon CS, Hastings MJ, Deeley J, Bloxham B, Rivers RP, Marwood R. The effect of intrapartum chemoprophylaxis on the vertical transmission of group B streptococci. Br J Obstet Gynaecol 1983;90:633–5.

26. Matorras R, Garcia-Perea A, OmeZaca F, Diez-Enciso M, Madero R, Usandizaga JA. Intrapartum chemoprophylaxis of early-onset group B streptococcal disease. Eur J Obstet Gynecol Reprod Biol 1991;40:57–62.

27. Garland SM, Fliegner JR. Group B streptococcus (GBS) and neonatal infections: the case for intrapartum chemoprophylaxis. Aust NZ J Obstet Gynaecol 1991;31:119–22.

28. Yancey MK, Schuchat A, Brown LK, Ventura VL, Markenson GR. The accuracy of late antenatal screening cultures in predicting genital group B streptococcal colonization at delivery. Obstet Gynecol 1996;88:811–5.

29. Badri MS, Zawaneh S, Cruz AC, et al. Rectal colonization with group B streptococcus: relation to vaginal colonization of pregnant women. J Infect Dis 1977;135:308–12.

30. Mercer BM, Taylor MC, Fricke JL, Baselski VS, Sibai BM. The accuracy and patient preference for self-collected group B streptococcus cultures. Am J Obstet Gynecol 1995;173:1325–8.

31. CDC. Laboratory practices for prenatal group B streptococcal screening and reporting—Connecticut, Georgia, and Minnesota, 1997–1998. MMWR 1999;48:426–8.

32. Baker CJ, Edwards MS, Kasper DL. Role of antibody to native type III polysaccharide of group B streptococcus in infant infection. Pediatrics 1981;68:544–9.

33. Boyer KM, Gadzala CA, Burd LI, Fisher DE, Paton JB, Gotoff SP. Selective intrapartum chemoprophylaxis of neonatal group B streptococcal early-onset disease. I. Epidemiologic rationale. J Infect Dis 1983;148:795–801.

34. Schuchat A, Oxtoby M, Cochi S, et al. Population-based risk factors for neonatal group B streptococcal disease: results of a cohort study in metropolitan Atlanta. J Infect Dis 1990;162:672–7.

35. Schuchat A, Deaver-Robinson K, Plikaytis BD, Zangwill KM, Mohle-Boetani J, Wenger JD. Multistate case-control study of maternal risk factors for neonatal group B streptococcal disease. Pediatr Infect Dis J 1994;13:623–9.

36. Schuchat A, Zywicki S, Dinsmoor MJ, et al. Risk factors and opportunities for prevention of early-onset neonatal sepsis: a multicenter case-control study. Pediatrics 2000;105:21–6.

37. Zaleznik DF, Rench MA, Hillier S, et al. Invasive disease due to group B streptococcus in pregnant women and neonates from diverse population groups. Clin Infect Dis 2000;30:276–81.

38. Christensen KK, Dahlander K, Linden V, Svenningsen N, Christensen P. Obstetrical care in future pregnancies after fetal loss in group B streptococcal septicemia. A prevention program based on bacteriological and immunological follow-up. Eur J Obstet Gynecol Reprod Biol 1981;12:143–50.

39. Faxelius G, Bremme K, Kvist-Christensen K, Christensen P, Ringertz S. Neonatal septicemia due to group B streptococci—perinatal risk factors and outcome of subsequent pregnancies. J Perinat Med 1988;16:423–30.

40. Baker CJ, Edwards MS. Group B streptococcal infections. In: Remington J, Klein JO, eds. Infectious diseases of the fetus and newborn infant. Philadelphia: W.B. Saunders, 1990:742–811.

41. Schuchat A, Hilger T, Zell E, et al. Active Bacterial Core Surveillance of the Emerging Infections Program Network. Emerg Infect Dis 2001;7:92–9.

42. Jeffery HE, Lahra MM. Eight-year outcome of universal screening and intrapartum antibiotics for maternal group B streptococcal carriers. Pediatrics 1998;101:(1). Available at http://www.pediatrics.org/cgi/content/full/101/1/e2.

43. Isaacs D, Royle JA, Australasian Study Group for Neonatal Infections. Intrapartum antibiotics and early onset neonatal sepsis caused by group B *Streptococcus* and by other organisms in Australia. Pediatr Infect Dis J 1999;18:524–8.

44. Davies HD, Adair CE, Schuchat A, Low DE, Sauve RS, McGeer A. Physicians' prevention practices and incidence of neonatal group B streptococcal disease in 2 Canadian regions. CMAJ 2001;164:479–85.

45. CDC. Adoption of perinatal group B streptococcal disease prevention recommendations by prenatal-care providers—Connecticut and Minnesota, 1998. MMWR 2000;49:228–32.

46. Watt JP, Schuchat A, Erickson K, Honig JE, Gibbs R, Schulkin J. Group B streptococcal disease prevention practices of obstetrician-gynecologists. Obstet Gynecol 2001;98:7–13.

47. Factor SH, Whitney CG, Zywicki S, Schuchat A, the Active Bacterial Core Surveillance Team. Effects of hospital policies based on 1996 group B streptococcal disease consensus guidelines. Obstet Gynecol 2000;95:377–82.

48. CDC. Hospital-based policies for prevention of perinatal group B streptococcal disease—United States, 1999. MMWR 2000;49:936–40.

49. Lieu TA, Mohle-Boetani JC, Ray GT, Ackerson LM, Walton DL. Neonatal group B streptococcal infection in a managed care population. Obstet Gynecol 1998;92:21–7.

50. Factor SH, Levine OS, Nassar A, et al. Impact of a risk-based prevention policy on neonatal group B streptococcal disease. Am J Obstet Gynecol 1998;179:1568–71.

51. Hafner E, Sterniste W, Rosen A, et al. Group B streptococci during pregnancy: a comparison of two screening and treatment protocols. Am J Obstet Gynecol 1998;179:677–81.

52. Riley L, Apollon M, Haider S, et al. "Real world" compliance with strategies to prevent early-onset GBS. Presented at the Infectious Diseases Society for Obstetrics and Gynecology Annual Scientific Meeting. Aug. 9–11, 2001, Quebec City, Canada.

53. Schuchat A, Roome A, Zell E, Linardos H, Zywicki S, O'Brien KL. Integrated monitoring of a new group B streptococcal disease prevention program and other perinatal infections. Matern Child Health J 2002;6:107–14.

54. Cheon-Lee E, Amstey MS. Compliance with the Centers for Disease Control and Prevention antenatal culture protocol for preventing group B streptococcal neonatal sepsis. Am J Obstet Gynecol 1998;179:77–9.

55. Katz VL, Moos M-K, Cefalo RC, Thorp JM, Bowes WA, Wells SD. Group B streptococci: results of a protocol of antepartum screening and intrapartum treatment. Am J Obstet Gynecol 1994;170:521–6.

56. Gilson GJ, Christensen F, Bekes K, Silva L, Qualls CR. Prevention of group B streptococcus early-onset neonatal sepsis: comparison of the Centers for Disease Control and Prevention screening-based protocol to a risk-based protocol in infants at greater than 37 weeks' gestation. J Perinatol 2000;20:491–5.

57. Brozanski BS, Jones JG, Krohn MA, Sweet RL. Effect of a screening-based prevention policy on prevalence of early-onset group B streptococcal sepsis. Obstet Gynecol 2000;95:496–501.

58. Davis RL, Hasselquist MB, Cardenas V, et al. Introduction of the new Centers for Disease Control and Prevention group B streptococcal prevention guideline at a large West Coast health maintenance organization. Am J Obstet Gynecol 2001;184:603–10.

59. Main EK, Slagle T. Prevention of early-onset invasive neonatal group B streptococcal disease in a private hospital setting: the superiority of culture-based protocols. Am J Obstet Gynecol 2000;182:1344–54.

60. Schrag SJ, Zell ER, Lynfield R, et al. A population-based comparison of strategies to prevent early-onset group B streptococcal disease in neonates. N Engl J Med 2002;347:233–9.

61. Rosenstein NE, Schuchat A. Opportunities for prevention of perinatal group B streptococcal disease: a multistate surveillance analysis. Obstet Gynecol 1997;90:901–6.

62. Rouse DJ, Goldenberg RL, Cliver SP, Cutter GR, Mennemeyer ST, Fargason CA, Jr. Strategies for the prevention of early-onset neonatal group B streptococcal sepsis: a decision analysis. Obstet Gynecol 1994;83:483–94.

63. Reisner DP, Haas MJ, Zingheim RW, Williams MA, Luthy D. Performance of a group B streptococcal prophylaxis protocol combining high-risk treatment and low-risk screening. Am J Obstet Gynecol 2000;182:1335–43.

64. Levine EM, Ghai V, Barton JJ, Strom CM. Intrapartum antibiotic prophylaxis increases the incidence of gram-negative neonatal sepsis. Infect Dis Obstet Gynecol 1999;7:210–13.

65. Lin FYC, Brenner RA, Johnson YR, et al. The effectiveness of risk-based intrapartum chemoprophylaxis for the prevention of early-onset neonatal group B streptococcal disease. Am J Obstet Gynecol 2001;184:1204–10.

66. Locksmith GJ, Clark P, Duff P. Maternal and neonatal infection rates with three different protocols for prevention of group B streptococcal disease. Am J Obstet Gynecol 1999;180:416–22.

67. CDC. Laboratory practices for prenatal group B streptococcal screening and reporting—Connecticut, Georgia and Minnesota, 1997–1998. MMWR 1999;48:426–8.

68. CDC. Adoption of hospital policies for prevention of perinatal group B streptococcal disease—United States, 1997. MMWR 1998;47:665–70.

69. Mohle-Boetani JC, Schuchat A, Plikaytis BD, Smith JD, Broome CV. Comparison of prevention strategies for neonatal Group B streptococcal infection: a population-based economic approach. JAMA 1993;270:1442–8.

70. Mohle-Boetani JC, Lieu TA, Ray GT, Escobar G. Preventing neonatal group B streptococcal disease: cost-effectiveness in a health maintenance organization and the impact of delayed hospital discharge for newborns who received intrapartum antibiotics. Pediatrics 1999;103:703–10.

71. Gotoff SP, Boyer KM. Prevention of early-onset neonatal group B streptococcal disease. Pediatrics 1997;99:866–9.

72. Benitz WE, Gould JB, Druzin ML. Antimicrobial prevention of early-onset group B streptococcal sepsis: estimates of risk reduction based on a critical literature review. Pediatrics 1999;103:e78. Available at http://www.pediatrics.org/cgi/content/full/103/6/e78.

73. Fargason CA, Peralta-Carcelen M, Rouse DJ, Cutter GR, Goldenberg RL. The pediatric costs of strategies for minimizing the risk of early-onset group B streptococcal disease. Obstet Gynecol 1997;90:347–52.

74. Schrag SJ, Arnold KE, Roome A, et al. Intrapartum antibiotic exposure in the era of perinatal group B streptococcal disease prevention [Abstract G-1824]. In: Program and abstracts of the 41st Annual Interscience Conference on Antimicrobial Agents and Chemotherapy. Washington, DC: American Society for Microbiology, 2001.

75. Goodman LS, Gilman A, Gilman AG. Goodman and Gilman's The pharmacologic basis of therapeutics, Tenth edition. New York: Pergamon Press, 1990:1825.

76. Pylipow M, Gaddis M, Kinney JS. Selective intrapartum prophylaxis for group B streptococcus colonization: management and outcome of newborns. Pediatrics 1994;93:631–5.

77. Dunn AB, Blomquist J, Khouzami V. Anaphylaxis in labor secondary to prophylaxis against group B streptococcus: a case report. J Reprod Med 1999;44:381–4.

78. Aitmhand R, Moustaoui N, Belabbes H, Elmdaghri N, Benbachir M. Serotypes and antimicrobial susceptibility of group B streptococcus isolated from neonates in Casablanca. Scand J Infect Dis 2000;32:339–40.

79. Andrews JJ, Diekema DJ, Hunter SK, et al. Group B streptococci causing neonatal bloodstream infection: antimicrobial susceptibility and serotyping results from SENTRY centers in the Western Hemisphere. Am J Obstet Gynecol 2000;183:859–62.

80. Fernandez M, Hickman ME, Baker CJ. Antimicrobial susceptibilities of group B streptococci isolated between 1992 and 1996 from patients with bacteremia or meningitis. Antimicrob Agents Chemother 1998;42:1517–9.

81. Lin FYC, Azimi PH, Weisman LE, et al. Antibiotic susceptibility profiles for group B streptococci isolated from neonates, 1995–1998. Clin Infect Dis 2000;31:76–9.

82. Morales WJ, Dickey SS, Bornick P, Lim DV. Change in antibiotic resistance of group B streptococcus: impact on intrapartum management. Am J Obstet Gynecol 1999;181:310–4.

83. Silverman NS, Morgan M, Nichols WS. Antibiotic resistance patterns of group B streptococcus in antenatal genital cultures. J Reprod Med 2000;45:979–82.

84. Bland ML, Vermillion ST, Soper DE, Austin M. Antibiotic resistance patterns of group B streptococci in late third-trimester rectovaginal cultures. Am J Obstet Gynecol 2001;184:1125–6.

85. Berkowitz K, Regan JA, Greenberg E. Antibiotic resistance patterns of group B streptococci in pregnant women. J Clin Microbiol 1990;28:5–7.

86. Pearlman MD, Pierson CL, Faix RG. Frequent resistance of clinical group B streptococci isolates to clindamycin and erythromycin. Obstet Gynecol 1998;92:258–61.

87. Castor ML, Whitney C, Facklam R, et al. Antimicrobial susceptibility and serotype patterns of invasive group B *Streptococcus* isolates from Georgia, Minnesota, New York and Oregon, 1996–2000 [Abstract]. International Conference on Emerging Infectious Diseases 2002, program and abstract book. Atlanta: 2002, 132.

88. NCCLS. Performance Standard for Antimicrobial Suceptibility Testing, M100-S12. Table 2H. Wayne, PA, USA: NCCLS, 2002.

89. CDC. Sexually transmitted diseases treatment guidelines, 2002. MMWR 2002;51 (No. RR-6):28–9.

90. Kelkar PS, Li JT. Cephalosporin allergy. N Engl J Med 2001;345:804–9.

91. Lavin BS. Antibiotic cycling and marketing into the 21st century: a perspective from the pharmaceutical industry. Infect Control Hosp Epidemiol 2000;21:S32–5.

92. Baltimore RS, Huie SM, Meek JI, Schuchat A, O'Brien KL. Early-onset neonatal sepsis in the era of group B streptococcal prevention. Pediatrics 2001;108:1094–8.

93. Cordero L, Sananes M, Ayers LW. Bloodstream infections in a neonatal intensive-care unit: 12 years' experience with an antibiotic control program. Infect Control Hosp Epidemiol 1999;20:242–6.

94. Joseph TA, Pyati SP, Jacobs N. Neonatal early-onset *Escherichia coli* disease: the effect of intrapartum ampicillin. Arch Pediatr Adolesc Med 1998;152:35–40.

95. Towers CV, Carr MH, Padilla G, Asrat T. Potential consequences of widespread antepartal use of ampicillin. Am J Obstet Gynecol 1998;179:879–83.

96. Gupta K, Scholes D, Stamm WE. Increasing prevalence of antimicrobial resistance among uropathogens causing acute uncomplicated cystitis in women. JAMA 1999;282:325–6.

97. Mercer BM, Carr TL, Beazley DD, Crouse DT, Sibai BM. Antibiotic use in pregnancy and drug-resistant infant sepsis. Am J Obstet Gynecol 1999;181:816–21.

98. Terrone DA, Rinehart BK, Einstein MH, Britt LB, Martin JN, Perry KG. Neonatal sepsis and death caused by resistant *Escherichia coli*: possible consequences of extended maternal ampicillin administration. Am J Obstet Gynecol 1999;180:1345–8.

99. Ramus RM, McIntire DD, Wendel GD, Jr. Antibiotic chemoprophylaxis for group B strep is not necessary with elective cesarean section at term [Abstract]. Am J Obstet Gynecol 1999;180:S85.

100. Hager WD, Schuchat A, Gibbs R, Sweet R, Mead P, Larsen JW. Prevention of perinatal group B streptococcal infection: current controversies. Obstet Gynecol 2000;96:141–5.

101. Kenyon SL, Taylor DJ, Tarnow-Mordi W, ORACLE Collaborative Group. Broad-spectrum antibiotics for preterm, prelabour rupture of fetal membranes: the ORACLE I randomised trial. Lancet 2001;357:979–88.

102. Kenyon SL, Taylor DJ, Tarnow-Mordi W, ORACLE Collaborative Group. Broad-spectrum antibiotics for spontaneous preterm labour: the ORACLE II randomised trial. Lancet 2001;357:989–94.

103. Gibbs RS, Jones PM, Wilder CJY. Internal fetal monitoring and maternal infection following cesarean section: a prospective study. Obstet Gynecol 1978;52:193–7.

104. Soper DE, Mayhall CG, Froggatt JW. Characterization and control of intraamniotic infection in an urban teaching hospital. Am J Obstet Gynecol 1996;175:304–10.

105. Seaward P, Gareth MB, Hannah ME, et al. International multicentre term prelabor rupture of membranes study: evaluation of predictors of clinical chorioamnionitis and postpartum fever in patients with prelabor rupture of membranes at term. Am J Obstet Gynecol 1997;177:1024–29.

106. Newton ER, Prihoda TJ, Gibbs RS. Logistic regression analysis of risk factors for intra-amniotic infection. Obstet Gynecol 1989;73:571–5.

107. Yancey MK, Duff P, Kubilis P, Clark P, Frentzen BH. Risk factors for neonatal sepsis. Obstet Gynecol 1996;87:188–94.

108. Hibbard JU, Shashoua A, Adamczyk C, Ismail M. Cervical ripening with prostaglandin gel and hygroscopic dilators. Infect Dis Obstet Gynecol 1998;6:18–24.

109. Boulvain M, Stan C, Irion O. Membrane sweeping for induction of labour (Cochrane Review). In: The Cochrane Library, Issue 4. Oxford: 2001.

110. Escobar GJ, Li D, Armstrong MA, et al. Neonatal sepsis workups in infants ≥2000 grams at birth: a population-based study. Pediatrics 2000;106:256–63.

111. Wiswell TE, Baumgart S, Gannon CM, Spitzer AR. No lumbar puncture in the evaluation for early neonatal sepsis: will meningitis be missed? Pediatrics 1995;95:803–6.

112. Visser VE, Hall RT. Lumbar puncture in the evaluation of suspected neonatal sepsis. J Pediatr 1980;96:1063–7.

113. Hristevea L, Booy R, Bowler I, Wilkinson AR. Prospective surveillance of neonatal meningitis. Arch Dis Child 1993;69:14–8.

114. Mitchell TF, Pearlman MD, Chapman RL, Bhatt-Mehta V, Faix RG. Maternal and transplacental pharmacokinetics of cefazolin. Obstet Gynecol 2001;98:1075–9.

115. Bromberger P, Lawrence JM, Braun D, Saunders B, Contreras R, Petitti DB. The influence of intrapartum antibiotics on the clinical spectrum of early-onset group B streptococcal infection in term infants. Pediatrics 2000;106:244–50.

116. de Cueto M, Sanchez M-J, Sampedro A, Miranda J-A, Herruzo A-J, Rosa-Fraile M. Timing of intrapartum ampicillin and prevention of vertical transmission of group B streptococcus. Obstet Gynecol 1998;91:112–4.

117. Wiswell TE, Stoll BJ, Tuggle JM. Management of asymptomatic, term gestation neonates born to mothers treated with intrapartum antibiotics. Pediatr Infect Dis J 1990;9:826–31.

118. Mercer BM, Ramsey RD, Sibai BM. Prenatal screening for group B streptococcus. II. Impact of antepartum screening and prophylaxis on neonatal care. Am J Obstet Gynecol 1995;173:842–6.

119. Peralta-Carcelen M, Fargasan CA, Jr, Cliver SP, Cutter GR, Gigante J, Goldenberg RL. Impact of maternal group B streptococcal screening on pediatric management in full-term newborns. Arch Pediatr Adolesc Med 1996;150:802–8.

120. Balter S, Zell E, O'Brien K, et al. Evaluating the impact of intrapartum antibiotics to prevent group B streptococcus on the care and work-up of the neonate [Abstract]. In: Program and Abstracts of the 40th Interscience Conference on Antimicrobial Agents and Chemotherapy. Washington DC: American Society for Microbiology, 2000:460.

121. Siegel JD, Cushion NB. Prevention of early-onset group B streptococcal disease: another look at single-dose penicillin at birth. Obstet Gynecol 1996;87:692–8.

122. Yancey MK, Armer T, Clark P, Duff P. Assessment of rapid identification tests for genital carriage of group B streptococci. Obstet Gynecol 1992;80:1038–47.

123. Walker CK, Crombleholme WR, Ohm-Smith MJ, Sweet RL. Comparison of rapid tests for detection of group B streptococcal colonization. Am J Perinatol 1992;9:304–8.

124. Bergeron MG, Ke D, Menard C, et al. Rapid detection of group B streptococci in pregnant women at delivery. N Engl J Med 2000;343:175–9.

125. Baker CJ, Rench MA, Edwards MS, Carpenter RJ, Hays BM, Kasper DL. Immunization of pregnant women with a polysaccharide vaccine of group B streptococcus. N Engl J Med 1988;319:1180–5.

126. Schuchat A, Wenger JD. Epidemiology of group B streptococcal disease: risk factors, prevention strategies and vaccine development. Epidemiol Rev 1994;16:374–402.

127. Baker CJ, Kasper DL. Correlation of maternal antibody deficiency with susceptibility to neonatal group B streptococcal infection. N Engl J Med 1976;294:753–6.

128. Baker CJ, Paoletti LC, Rench MA, et al. Use of capsular polysaccharide–tetanus toxoid conjugate vaccine for type II group B streptococcus in healthy women. J Infect Dis 2000;182:1129–38.

129. Baker CJ, Paoletti LC, Wessels MR, et al. Safety and immunogenicity of capsular polysaccharide–tetanus toxoid conjugate vaccines for group B streptococcal types Ia and Ib. J Infect Dis 1999;179:142–50.

130. Kasper DL, Paoletti LC, Wessels MR, et al. Immune response to type III group B streptococcal polysaccharide–tetanus toxoid conjugate vaccine. J Clin Invest 1996;98:2308–14.

131. Lin F-Y, Philips JB, III, Azimi PH, et al. Level of maternal antibody required to protect neonates against early-onset disease caused by group B Streptococcus type Ia: a multicenter, seroepidemiology study. J Infect Dis 2001;184:1022–8.

132. Davies HD, Adair C, McGeer A, et al. Antibodies to capsular polysaccharides of group B Streptococcus in pregnant Canadian women: relationship to colonization status and infection in the neonate. J Infect Dis 2001;184:285–91.

133. Schuchat A. Group B streptococcus. Lancet 1999;353:51–6.

134. Schuchat A. Epidemiology of group B streptococcal disease in the United States: shifting paradigms. Clin Microbiol Rev 1998;11: 497–513.

135. Robbins JB, Schneerson R, Vann WF, Bryla DA, Fattom A. Prevention of systemic infections caused by group B streptococcus and *Staphylococcus aureus* by multivalent polysaccharide–protein conjugate vaccines. Ann NY Acad Sci 1995;754:68–82.

136. Rosa-Fraile M, Rodriguez-Granger J, Cueto-Lopez M, et al. Use of Granada medium to detect group B streptococcal colonization in pregnant women. J Clin Microbiol 1999;37:2674–7.

137. Gil EG, Rodriguez MC, Bartolome R, Berjano B, Cabero L, Andreu A. Evaluation of the Granada agar plate for detection of vaginal and rectal group B streptococci in pregnant women. J Clin Microbiol 1999;37:2648–51.

138. Votava M, Tejkalová M, Drábková M, Unzeitig V, Braveny I. Use of GBS media for rapid detection of group B streptococci in vaginal and rectal swabs from women in labor. Eur J Clin Microbiol Infect Dis 2001;20:120–2.

139. Stratton KR, Durch JS, Lawrence RS. Vaccines for the 21st Century: A tool for decisionmaking. Washington, DC: Institute of Medicine, National Academy Press, 1999.

140. Stoll BJ, Hansen N, Fanaroff AA, et al. Changes in pathogens causing early-onset sepsis in very-low-birth-weight infants. N Engl J Med 2002;347:240–7.

141. U. S. Department of Health and Human Services. Healthy People 2010: understanding and improving health. 2nd ed. Washington, DC: US Government Printing Office, 2000. Available at http://www.health.gov/healthypeople.

142. Schrag SJ, Whitney CG, Schuchat A. Neonatal group B streptococcal disease: how infection control teams can contribute to prevention efforts. Infect Control Hosp Epidemiol 2000;21:473–83.

Consultants

Kathryn Arnold, M.D., Georgia Division of Public Health, Atlanta, Georgia; Carol Baker, M.D., American Academy of Pediatrics/ Committee on Infectious Diseases, Elk Grove Village, Illinois; Gina Burns, M.S., Group B Strep Association, Chapel Hill, North Carolina; Richard Facklam, Ph.D., CDC, Atlanta, Georgia; Monica Farley, M.D., Infectious Diseases Society of America, Alexandria, Virginia; Theodore G. Ganiats, M.D., American Academy of Family Physicians, Leawood, Kansas; Ronald Gibbs, M.D., Infectious Diseases Society of Obstetricians and Gynecologists, Washington, D.C.; Paul Heath, M.D., U.K. GBS Prevention Working Group, London, England; James H. Jorgensen, Ph.D., Health Science Center at San Antonio, University of Texas, San Antonio, Texas; William Kanto, M.D., American Academy of Pediatrics/Committee on Fetus and Newborn, Elk Grove Village, Illinois; Shelene Keith, Jesse Cause Foundation–Saving the Babies from Group B Strep, Port Huenme, California; Tekoa King, M.P.H., American College of Nurse Midwives, Washington, D.C.; Feng Ying Lin, M.D., National Institute of Child Health and Development, National Institutes of Health, Bethesda, Maryland; Ruth Lynfield, M.D., Minnesota Department of Health, Minneapolis, Minnesota; Martin McCaffrey, M.D., Naval Medical Center, San Diego, California; Elliot Philipson, M.D., Cleveland Clinic, Cleveland, Ohio; Lisa Porter, M.Ed., Jacksonville, Florida; Laura Riley, M.D., American College of Obstetricians and Gynecologists, Washington, D.C.; Donna Russell, M.S., Washington Department of Health, Renton, Washington; Pam Sims, Pharm. D., Samford University, Birmingham, Alabama; Carol A. Spiegel, Ph.D., University of Wisconsin, Madison, Wisconsin; Barbara Stoll, M.D., Emory University School of Medicine, Atlanta, Georgia; Beth H. Stover, Healthcare Infection Control Practices Advisory Committee, CDC, Atlanta, Georgia; Cynthia Whitney, M.D., CDC, Atlanta, Georgia; Michael K. Yancey, M.D., Tripler Army Medical Center, Honolulu, Hawaii; Elizabeth Zell, M.Stat., CDC, Atlanta, Georgia

All *MMWR* references are available on the Internet at http://www.cdc.gov/mmwr. Use the search function to find specific articles.

Use of trade names and commercial sources is for identification only and does not imply endorsement by the U.S. Department of Health and Human Services.

References to non-CDC sites on the Internet are provided as a service to *MMWR* readers and do not constitute or imply endorsement of these organizations or their programs by CDC or the U.S. Department of Health and Human Services. CDC is not responsible for the content of these sites. URL addresses listed in *MMWR* were current as of the date of publication.

The *Morbidity and Mortality Weekly Report (MMWR)* series is prepared by the Centers for Disease Control and Prevention (CDC) and is available free of charge in electronic format and on a paid subscription basis for paper copy. To receive an electronic copy each week, send an e-mail message to *listserv@listserv.cdc.gov*. The body content should read *SUBscribe mmwr-toc*. Electronic copy also is available from CDC's Internet server at *http://www.cdc.gov/mmwr* or from CDC's file transfer protocol server at *ftp://ftp.cdc.gov/pub/publications/mmwr*. To subscribe for paper copy, contact Superintendent of Documents, U.S. Government Printing Office, Washington, DC 20402; telephone 202-512-1800.

Data in the weekly *MMWR* are provisional, based on weekly reports to CDC by state health departments. The reporting week concludes at close of business on Friday; compiled data on a national basis are officially released to the public on the following Friday. Address inquiries about the *MMWR* series, including material to be considered for publication, to Editor, *MMWR* Series, Mailstop C-08, CDC, 1600 Clifton Rd., N.E., Atlanta, GA 30333; telephone 888-232-3228.

All material in the *MMWR* series is in the public domain and may be used and reprinted without permission; however, citation of the source is appreciated.

☆U.S. Government Printing Office: 2002-733-100/69047 Region IV

Helicobacter pylori Infection in Children: Recommendations for Diagnosis and Treatment

●●

- *Clinical Practice Guideline*

Medical Position Statement: The North American Society for Pediatric Gastroenterology and Nutrition

Helicobacter pylori Infection in Children: Recommendations for Diagnosis and Treatment

*Benjamin D. Gold, †Richard B. Colletti, ‡Myles Abbott, §Steven J. Czinn, ‖Yoram Elitsur, ¶Eric Hassall, #Colin Macarthur, **John Snyder, and ††Philip M. Sherman

*Division of *Pediatric Gastroenterology and Nutrition, Department of Pediatrics, Emory University School of Medicine, Atlanta, Georgia; †Pediatric Gastroenterology, University of Vermont, Fletcher Allen Health Center, Burlington, Vermont; ‡Berkeley California; §Pediatric Gastroenterology, Rainbow Babies and Children's Hospital, Cleveland, Ohio; ‖Division of Gastroenterology, Marshall University School of Medicine, Huntington, West Virginia; ¶Division of Gastroenterology, BC Children's Hospital, Vancouver, British Columbia, Canada; Divisions of #General Pediatrics and ††Gastroenterology and Nutrition, The Hospital for Sick Children, Toronto, Ontario, Canada; and **Pediatric Gastroenterology, University of California San Francisco, San Francisco, California, U.S.A.*

Helicobacter pylori infects at least 50% of the world's human population (1). However, most individuals infected with *H. pylori* do not experience symptoms or have signs of recognizable disease. In most children, the presence of *H. pylori* infection does not lead to clinically apparent disease, even when the organism colonizing the gastric mucosa causes chronic active gastritis (2). Knowledge about *H. pylori* infection is evolving, particularly in the pediatric age group for which there are still large gaps in knowledge.

Additional multicenter, randomized, placebo-controlled treatment trials in children infected by *H. pylori* are critically needed to definitively characterize the effect of *H. pylori* eradication treatment during childhood on symptoms and gastroduodenal mucosal disease.

There is compelling evidence that this organism is associated with a significant proportion of duodenal ulcers and, to a lesser extent, with gastric ulcers in children (3). There are epidemiologic data linking chronic *H. pylori* infection, probably beginning in childhood, with the development of gastric adenocarcinoma and gastric lymphoma (4). Findings in recently reported animal models support the role of *H. pylori* in the pathogenesis of gastric cancers (5).

There are many studies describing the prevalence of *H. pylori* infection. Most epidemiologic studies of *H. pylori* infection have been performed in adults who had

been infected for many years before clinical symptoms appeared (6). The incidence of *H. pylori* infection in industrialized countries is estimated to be approximately 0.5% of the susceptible population per year. In contrast, there is a significantly higher estimated incidence of *H. pylori* infection in developing countries of approximately 3% to 10% per year (7). The limited data on the incidence of *H. pylori* infection in children consist largely of retrospective seroprevalence studies.

Humans appear to be the primary natural reservoir of *H. pylori* infection. Other reservoirs that have been proposed include water, domestic cats, and houseflies (8–10). The risk factors described for acquiring infection include residence in a developing country, poor socioeconomic conditions, family overcrowding, and possibly an ethnic or genetic predisposition. In North America, the prevalence rates of *H. pylori* among Asian-Americans, African-Americans and Hispanics are similar to those of residents of developing countries (11). The route of transmission of *H. pylori* in humans is not known but is postulated to be fecal-oral, gastric-oral (in vomitus), or oral-oral (12).

Although *H. pylori* infection may be acquired during childhood, there are limited guidelines regarding its diagnosis and treatment in children and adolescents. Such evidence-based consensus guidelines are needed for both primary care and specialty medical providers to ensure judicious use of diagnostic testing and appropriate therapeutic regimens for the management of children with *H. pylori* infection. Therefore, the North American Society for Pediatric Gastroenterology and Nutrition (NASPGN) appointed the *Helicobacter pylori* Infection Guideline Committee to develop a clinical practice guideline for the child with *H. pylori* infection.

Received and accepted September 8, 2000.

Address correspondence and reprint requests to Dr. Benjamin Gold, Emory University School of Medicine, 2040 Ridgewood Drive, NE, Atlanta, GA 30322, U.S.A.; or to Dr. Richard B. Colletti, University of Vermont, Department of Pediatrics, A-121 Given Medical Building, Burlington, VT 05405-5557, U.S.A.

These clinical practice guidelines are designed to assist primary care physicians, nurse practitioners, physician assistants, and pediatric gastroenterologists in the evaluation and treatment of suspected or diagnosed *H. pylori*–associated disease. The desired outcomes of these recommendations are the detection of children and adolescents with *H. pylori* who need treatment. These recommendations are applicable to children in developed countries where the prevalence of infection is low but may not be directly relevant to children living in communities where there is a higher frequency of gastric colonization by *H. pylori*. These recommendations have been endorsed by the Executive Council of NASPGN and by the American Academy of Pediatrics. They are general guidelines to assist medical care providers in the diagnosis and treatment of *H. pylori* infection in children. They are not intended as a substitute for clinical judgment or as a protocol for the management of all patients.

In its deliberations, the committee addressed four issues about *H. pylori* infection in children: How reliable are tests to detect *H. pylori*? When is testing for *H. pylori* indicated? When is treatment of *H. pylori* infection indicated? What is the preferred treatment of *H. pylori*? A summary of the recommendations of the *H. pylori* Infection Guideline Committee is presented in Table 1.

METHODS

The *H. pylori* Infection Guideline Committee consisted of a primary care pediatrician, a clinical epidemiologist, and seven pediatric gastroenterologists. To develop evidence-based guidelines, articles published in English from January 1966 through May 1999 on *H. pylori* in children were searched. Articles on diagnosis and treatment were sought separately. Letters, editorials, case reports, abstracts, and reviews were excluded. Evidence tables were prepared based on 16 articles on clinical presentation, 9 articles on diagnostic studies, and 30 articles on therapy. Subsequently, additional articles were identified and reviewed. When the pediatric literature was insufficient, the adult literature was also considered. Articles were evaluated using published criteria (13). The Committee based its recommendations on an integration of a review of the medical literature and expert opinion. Consensus was achieved by using the nominal group technique, a structured quantitative method, as described previously (14,15). By using the methods of the Canadian Preventive Services Task Force (16), the quality of evidence of each of the recommendations made by the committee was determined and is summarized (Table 1).

HOW RELIABLE ARE TESTS FOR *H. PYLORI* INFECTION?

Several invasive and noninvasive tests are available to detect *H. pylori* infection (Table 2). An ideal test for *H. pylori* is noninvasive or minimally invasive, highly accurate, inexpensive, and readily available and enables differentiation between active or past infection with the

TABLE 1. *Summary of recommendations and the quality of the supporting evidence*

Recommendations	Quality of evidence[a]
How reliable are tests for *H. pylori* infection?	
Currently, the diagnosis of *H. pylori*-mediated disease can be made reliably only through the use of endoscopy with biopsy.	II, III
Presently available commercial serologic tests are frequently unreliable for screening children for the presence of *H. pylori* infection.	II
Urea breath testing, although promising, has not been studied sufficiently in children.	II
When is testing indicated?	
It is recommended that testing be performed in children with endoscopically diagnosed, or radiographically definitive, duodenal or gastric ulcers.	I
It is recommended that children with recurrent abdominal pain, in the absence of documented ulcer disease, not be tested for *H. pylori* infection.	II
Testing for *H. pylori* infection is not recommended in asymptomatic children.	II
Routine screening of children with a family history of gastric cancer or recurrent peptic ulcer disease is not recommended.	II
Testing following treatment of documented *H. pylori* is recommended, especially with complicated peptic ulcer disease (i.e., bleeding, perforation, or obstruction). For patients who remain symptomatic after treatment, it is recommended that endoscopy and biopsy be performed to evaluate for the persistence of *H. pylori*-associated peptic ulcer disease.	I, II
If pathological evidence of MALT lymphoma is documented, then testing for *H. pylori* is recommended.	II
When is treatment of *H. pylori* infection indicated?	
Eradication treatment is recommended for children who have a duodenal ulcer or gastric ulcer identified at endoscopy and *H. pylori* detected on histology.	I
A prior history of documented duodenal or gastric ulcer disease is an indication for treatment if active *H. pylori* infection is documented.	I
There is no compelling evidence for treating children with *H. pylori* infection and non-ulcer dyspepsia or functional recurrent abdominal pain.	III
Treatment is not recommended for *H. pylori*-infected children residing in chronic care facilities; children with unexplained short stature; or children at increased risk for acquisition of infection, including asymptomatic children who have a family member with either peptic ulcer disease or gastric cancer.	III
What is the preferred treatment of *H. pylori* infections in children?	
It is recommended that treatment consist of three or four medications, given once or twice daily, for one to two weeks.	I

[a] Categories of the quallity of evidence: I Evidence obtained from at least one properly designed randomized controlled study. II-1 Evidence obtained from well-designed cohort or case-controlled trials without randomization. II-2 Evidence obtained from well-designed cohort or case-control analytic studies, preferably from more than one center or research group. II-3 Evidence obtained from multiple time series with or without the intervention. Dramatic results in uncontrolled experiments (such as the results of the introduction of penicillin treatment in the 1940's) could also be regarded as this type of evidence. III Opinions of respected authorities, based on clinical experience, descriptive studies, or reports of expert committees.

TABLE 2. *Tests for* Helicobacter pylori *and* Helicobacter-*related disorders*

Invasive tests requiring endoscopy
  Biopsies and histology
  Rapid urease testing
  Bacterial culture
  Polymerase chain reaction of bacterial DNA
Non-invasive tests
  Serum and whole blood antibody
  Saliva antibody
  Urine antibody
  Stool antigen
  Urea breath testing

organism. In addition, such a test enables discrimination between the presence of *H. pylori* infection and *H. pylori*–associated disease. Because no such ideal test currently exists, the advantages and drawbacks of tests that are available require critical appraisal and must be assessed for their suitability for use in children.

Failure to reach an accurate diagnosis carries considerable financial and social costs including the expense of more tests, repeated visits to health care providers, inappropriate treatment, and missed school or work. A definitive test, even if it is expensive, may result in overall cost savings (17).

It is important to emphasize that the accuracy of a diagnostic test is greatly impacted by the prevalence of *H. pylori* in the population tested. There is a need for studies to assess the accuracy and potential utility of various noninvasive diagnostic tests in populations in North America that differ in demographic factors that may influence the prevalence and natural history of *H. pylori* infection (18).

Invasive Testing Through Endoscopy

Biopsies and Histopathology

The definitive diagnosis of *H. pylori* and the evidence of the consequences of infection can be made reliably only by endoscopy with multiple biopsy specimens obtained in one or more regions of the stomach including antrum, body, and transition zones (i.e., cardia and incisura). Histology provides information regarding the presence of *H. pylori* and the severity and topographic distribution of gastritis including the presence of atrophic gastritis, intestinal metaplasia, and mucosa-associated lymphoid tissue (MALT) lymphoma (3). As in adults, biopsy specimens obtained in the prepyloric antrum have the highest yield in *H. pylori* infection. Tissue specimens often are also obtained from the body and the transition zones of the stomach, particularly if the patient has recently taken acid-suppressing medication (19). It is recommended that multiple biopsies be performed in children with endoscopically documented peptic ulcer disease or peptic ulcer suspected as a result of radiographic

study. The optimal staining of biopsy sections is best determined by local expert pathologists. Endoscopic examination of and specimens obtained in the esophagus, stomach, and duodenum also provide information about other upper gastrointestinal disorders that may be the cause of clinical symptoms including, for example, esophagitis and peptic ulcer disease that is not due to *H. pylori*.

There are drawbacks to diagnostic gastrointestinal endoscopy. It is a relatively invasive procedure requiring sedation or anesthesia. Furthermore, the test remains relatively expensive in many centers, and access to an endoscopist with specific pediatric expertise is limited in many geographic areas.

Rapid Urease Testing of Biopsy Tissues

Urease testing (CLO, TriMed, Kansas City, MO; Hp-Fast, GI Supply, Division of ChekMed Systems Inc., Camphill, PA; PyloriTek, Horizons International, Aguadilla, Puerto Rico) provides indirect identification of *H. pylori* infection within a few hours of endoscopy (20). However, these tests have a poor positive predictive value (as low as 50%) in children, even though the negative predictive value is high (97–98%) (20,21). The accuracy of the test is dependent on the number of tissue specimens tested, the location of biopsy sites, bacterial load, and previous usage of antibiotics and proton pump inhibitors, as well as the prevalence of *H. pylori* in the population tested.

Bacterial Culture

Culture of *H. pylori* from the gastric mucosa provides an opportunity to obtain a profile of antibiotic sensitivity that could identify potential treatment failure due to antibiotic resistance (22). Culture also provides a bacterial strain for use in epidemiologic studies to examine associations of virulence characteristics with disease outcome. However, bacterial culture for *H. pylori* is relatively expensive and success rates for recovery of the organism in many clinical laboratories are low (23). Currently, standardization of culture procedures has not been established, and bacterial cultures are only obtained routinely in research settings.

Polymerase Chain Reaction

Polymerase chain reaction (PCR) is a highly sensitive technique that can be used to detect the presence of *H. pylori* in body fluids (e.g., gastric juice and stool), tissues (e.g., gastric mucosa), and water (24). Testing of *H. pylori* genomic DNA by PCR can be used to advance knowledge at the molecular level—for example, by providing information about point mutations conferring resistance to antibiotics and about putative bacterial virulence factors. However, PCR is expensive, the assay is difficult to set up, specificity may be compromised by inadvertent contamination, and it is not widely available outside the research laboratory.

Noninvasive Testing

Immunoassay Tests to Detect H. pylori Antibodies

Enzyme-linked immunosorbent assays (ELISAs) to detect *H. pylori* antibodies are relatively inexpensive and easy to implement in the clinical setting. Many tests are available for use to test whole blood, plasma, or serum. However, compared with histology, the sensitivity and specificity of serologic assays are poor in both adults and children unless used in the populations in which they were initially developed (25). In general, the accuracy of serum-based immunoassays and whole-blood tests for use in the physician's office in symptomatic children in developed countries is poor, with a range of sensitivity of only 60% to 70% (26–28). Furthermore, age-related cutoff values for commercial immunologic tests have not been established for children. One immunoassay developed in a research center to detect *H. pylori*–specific immunoglobulin (Ig)G in children was 91% sensitive compared with sensitivity of less than 70% in three commercially available assays (28). In areas with low prevalence of *H. pylori* infection, such as in developed countries, testing of serum and whole blood is not sufficiently accurate to diagnose *H. pylori* infection in children. Accordingly, treatment regimens based on the results of these tests cannot be recommended. Serologic tests may not be used reliably to verify eradication of *H. pylori*, because antibody titers can remain positive for months, despite resolution of infection.

Saliva and Urine Tests for H. pylori Antibodies

Similar to serologic tests, saliva-based tests also detect the presence of *H. pylori*–specific IgG antibodies. The tests are easy to perform, painless, and inexpensive. Saliva tests are less sensitive than assays of serum or whole blood (29). The protein concentration of saliva appears to affect the accuracy of test results. Urine-based assays are easy to perform, require minimal labor for collection, and are painless (30). However, these assays are highly variable and are not yet commercially available. Therefore, saliva and urine assays for the detection of *H. pylori* antibodies cannot be recommended.

Stool Test for H. pylori Antigens

Testing of *H. pylori* antigens in stools has shown promising results in adults for the noninvasive diagnosis of gastric infection using a commercially available kit (31). Testing for *H. pylori* antigens in feces also appears to be accurate for use in monitoring the success of eradi-

cation therapy. However, patients may be reluctant to collect stool specimens. In addition, refrigerated stools are more difficult to test. Additional pediatric studies evaluating the accuracy of stool antigen testing for both initial diagnosis and posttreatment follow-up are required before specific recommendations can be considered (32).

Urea Breath Testing

Urea breath tests are noninvasive and have high sensitivity and specificity (>95%) both in adults (33) and children (34,35). The test requires the ingestion of either radiolabeled ^{14}C-urea or urea tagged with the stable isotope ^{13}C. Test results may be influenced by concurrent use of antibiotics and acid-suppressing medications and by the presence of other urease-producing organisms present in the oral cavity. Test parameters are currently laboratory-specific (e.g., dosages for differing ages of children, cutoff values, duration of fasting, use of a test meal, times of sampling, and timing of posttherapy testing) and have not been well standardized for children (36). In addition, urea breath testing is technically more difficult to perform in small children and infants, with failure rates in collection up to 10%, especially outside the clinical research setting (34).

In summary, the diagnosis of *H. pylori*–associated diseases currently can be made reliably only by endoscopy with biopsies. The most commonly used noninvasive test to screen adults for *H. pylori* infection is serology. Unfortunately, currently available commercial serologic tests are frequently unreliable for screening children for the presence of *H. pylori* infection. Current whole-blood, saliva, and urinary immunoassays are insufficiently sensitive or specific to be effective as diagnostic tools. Insufficient data are available in children to confirm the accuracy of the recently approved *H. pylori* stool antigen test. The urea breath test has the promise to provide noninvasive and accurate diagnosis of *H. pylori* infection; but currently, there is insufficient evidence that it can be used to reliably diagnose or exclude *H. pylori*–associated diseases.

WHEN IS TESTING INDICATED?

The primary goal of testing is to diagnose the cause of clinical symptoms and not simply to detect the presence of *H. pylori* infection. Testing is not helpful unless it will alter the management of the disease.

A variety of invasive and noninvasive tests exist for the detection of *H. pylori* infection, but their degree of sensitivity and specificity vary, as do their suitability for clinical use in children. Thus, there is potential for inappropriate testing or misuse of tests in children.

Endoscopically Diagnosed or Radiographically Definitive Peptic Ulcer

The causal relationship between *H. pylori* infection and primary duodenal ulcers is compelling (37). Therefore, it is recommended that testing for the presence of *H. pylori* infection be performed in children with endoscopically diagnosed or radiographically definitive duodenal ulcer. Although the data in children are less complete, evidence from studies in adults (38) supports the recommendation that testing for *H. pylori* also be performed in subjects with a documented gastric ulcer.

Abdominal Pain Unrelated to Peptic Ulcers

Several lines of evidence, including serologic surveys, endoscopic evaluations, and treatment trials indicate that *H. pylori* is not a frequent cause of recurrent abdominal pain in children. There have been six studies performed in North America, Europe, and Australia, with 2715 children evaluated by esophagogastroduodenoscopy and biopsy, serology, or urea breath test (39–44). Although 5% to 17% of children with abdominal pain had evidence of infection with *H. pylori*, 5% to 29% of children without abdominal pain were also infected with *H. pylori*. There are no convincing data to support routine testing of children with recurrent abdominal pain (39–45). Investigators have also looked for specific symptom patterns in *H. pylori*–infected children, but none so far has been detected (46–50). Future studies are needed to determine whether subsets of children with abdominal pain can be identified in whom signs and symptoms are caused by *H. pylori* infection. It is recommended that children with recurrent abdominal pain, in the absence of documented ulcer disease, not be tested for *H. pylori* infection.

Asymptomatic Children, Including Those at Increased Risk of Acquiring *H. pylori* Infection

There are no compelling data to support routine testing in asymptomatic children. Testing for *H. pylori* infection is not recommended in children without clinical symptoms, including those residing in long-term care facilities, children with short stature, and those at increased risk of acquiring *H. pylori* infection. In addition, purported extraintestinal manifestations of *H. pylori* infection have not been demonstrated in a convincing fashion (51). Accordingly, a test-and-treat approach is not recommended in these circumstances.

Family History of Gastric Cancer or Recurrent Peptic Ulcer Disease

No currently available data support routine testing in children with a positive family history of diseases related to *H. pylori* infection (52). Epidemiologic evidence in-dicates that there is a link between gastric cancers (both adenocarcinoma and lymphoma) and *H. pylori* infection. However, no studies have shown that *H. pylori* eradication during childhood prevents subsequent development of gastric malignancies. Until evidence is available to better define the role of *H. pylori* in a variety of gastric cancers and the role of *H. pylori* eradication in disease prevention, routine screening of children with a family history of gastric cancer or recurrent peptic ulcer disease is not recommended.

Histologic Evidence of Lymphoma

In the rare circumstance in which histopathologic evidence of MALT lymphoma is documented in a child, testing for *H. pylori* is recommended.

Follow-up of Therapy for *H. pylori* Infection

Testing to confirm eradication of infection and the resolution of associated symptoms and disease sequelae is advisable in selected children. Guidelines in adults recommend testing after treatment of complicated peptic ulcer (52), but studies in children are limited. As such, few data are available on the effectiveness of therapy in children, testing after treatment is recommended in those with complicated peptic ulcer disease (i.e., bleeding, perforation, or obstruction) or lymphoma. For patients who remain symptomatic, it is recommended that endoscopy and biopsy be performed to evaluate for the persistence of *H. pylori*-associated peptic ulcer disease. For patients with an uncomplicated ulcer who are asymptomatic after completion of eradication therapy, testing for persistence of infection is not necessary. However, some physicians advocate the use of urea breath testing in this clinical setting.

WHEN IS TREATMENT OF *H. PYLORI* INFECTION INDICATED?

Eradication therapy is recommended for children who have both known active *H. pylori* infection and symptomatic gastrointestinal disease. Known active *H. pylori* infection is defined as identification of the organisms by histopathologic examination or as a positive culture from endoscopic gastric biopsy. Serology is not a reliable test for active disease, because it may indicate past but not current infection with *H. pylori*.

There are no randomized controlled trials in children that determine the precise clinical settings in which eradication therapy is indicated. Although additional studies in children are needed (53), the available evidence supports the following recommendations.

Duodenal and Gastric Ulcers

Eradication treatment is recommended for children who have a duodenal ulcer or gastric ulcer identified at endoscopy and *H. pylori* documented by histopathology. A prior history of duodenal or gastric ulcer disease is also an indication for treatment if active *H. pylori* infection is documented. If a definitive ulcer is present on contrast radiography (e.g., an ulcer crater is present), eradication therapy is indicated if either a noninvasive or invasive test result is positive for *H. pylori*.

Lymphoma

The rare child with pathologic evidence of MALT lymphoma and *H. pylori* infection should be treated with eradication therapy. Further studies of pediatric patients with lymphoma should be performed to monitor the recurrence, progression, or remission of the tumor after therapy.

Atrophic Gastritis With Intestinal Metaplasia

Eradication treatment is recommended for the rare child who has pathologically proven atrophic gastritis with intestinal metaplasia, according to the updated Sydney classification of gastritis (54), plus coexisting *H. pylori* infection. Because of the preneoplastic nature of these pathologic changes, follow-up endoscopy is recommended to confirm that the *H. pylori* infection has been eradicated and to ensure that there is no subsequent progression of gastric mucosal disease.

Gastritis Without Peptic Ulcer Disease

The finding of *H. pylori*–associated gastritis in the absence of peptic ulcer disease during diagnostic endoscopy poses a dilemma for the endoscopist. The decision to treat *H. pylori*–associated gastritis without duodenal or gastric ulcer in this situation is subject to the judgment of the clinician and deliberations with the patient and family. Studies in adults on the effect of eradication treatment on abdominal symptoms have produced conflicting results (55–58). There are no randomized controlled trials in children. The long-term impact of the eradication of *H. pylori* and the healing of gastritis on the subsequent development of peptic ulcer disease, adenocarcinoma, or lymphoma is uncertain. Although there is a small lifetime risk of development of peptic ulcer disease associated with *H. pylori* gastritis, there are no randomized controlled trials demonstrating that eradication of *H. pylori* results in prevention of peptic ulcer disease. In addition, there are no data showing that eradication therapy influences the long-term risk for development of gastric cancers. Antibiotic treatment can result in adverse drug reactions, promote antibiotic resistance, and increase the

cost of care. Therefore, the *H. pylori* Infection Guideline Committee concludes that there is insufficient evidence to support either initiating or withholding eradication treatment in this situation.

Recurrent Abdominal Pain and Asymptomatic Children

There is no compelling evidence, at the present time, for treating children with *H. pylori* infection and either nonulcer dyspepsia or functional recurrent abdominal pain. There is also no convincing evidence currently available that asymptomatic children who have a family member with *H. pylori* infection, peptic ulcer, or gastric cancer need treatment.

WHAT IS THE PREFERRED TREATMENT OF *H. PYLORI* INFECTION IN CHILDREN?

The optimum treatment regimen for eradicating *H. pylori* in children has not been determined (59). Effective therapy in adults is defined as successful eradication of *H. pylori* infection in a minimum of 80% of treated subjects (60). Although it appears that treatment options that have been effective in adults will also be efficacious in children, controlled studies in pediatric populations are needed to confirm or refute this supposition. Unfortunately, the limited data currently available in children are open-label, case series and uncontrolled, anecdotal observations that do not meet the minimum criteria for determining efficacy. In vitro sensitivity of *H. pylori* to a specific drug does not guarantee that the bacterium will be effectively eradicated from the human stomach. Therefore, current treatment strategies to eradicate *H. pylori* have been developed primarily by trial-and-error methodology (61).

The single most important determinant of successful eradication therapy is compliance with the prescribed combination treatment regimen (62). There are well-described treatment failures due to suboptimal compliance. To enhance adherence to the treatment regimen, the number of medications prescribed, the frequency of administration, and the duration of therapy are best kept to the minimum required for successful treatment.

It is recommended that initial treatment consist of three medications, administered twice daily, for 1 to 2 weeks (63). Specifically, as shown in Table 3, three first-line therapy options are recommended for use in children and adolescents. For patients in whom initial treatment has failed, two other options are recommended, including one option with four medications. It is recommended that monotherapy and two-drug regimens be avoided, because they are ineffective and increase the likelihood

TABLE 3. *Recommended eradication therapies for* H. pylori *disease in children*

First-line options	Medications	Dosage
1	amoxicillin	50 mg/kg/day up to 1 g bid
	clarithromycin	15 mg/kg/day up to 500 mg bid
	proton pump inhibitor: omeprazole (or comparable acid inhibitory doses of another PPI)	1 mg/kg/day up to 20 mg bid
2	amoxicillin	50 mg/kg/day up to 1 g bid
	metronidazole	20 mg/kg/day–500 mg bid
	proton pump inhibitor: omeprazole (or comparable acid inhibitory doses of another PPI)	1 mg/kg/day up to 20 mg bid
3	clarithromycin	15 mg/kg/day up to 500 mg bid
	metronidazole	20 mg/kg/day up to 500 mg bid
	proton pump inhibitor: omeprazole (or comparable acid inhibitory doses of another PPI)	1 mg/kg/day up to 20 mg bid
Second-line options		
4	bismuth subsalicylate	1 tablet (262 mg) qid *or* 15 ml (17.6 mg/mL qid)
	metronidazole	20 mg/kg/day–500 mg bid
	proteon pump inhibitor: omeprazole (or comparable acid inhibitory doses of another PPI)	1 mg/kg/day up to 20 mg bid
	pus, an additional antibiotic: amoxicillin	50 mg/kg/day up to 1 g bid
	or tetracycline[a]	50 mg/kg/day up to 1 g bid
	or clarithromycin	15 mg/kg/day–500 mg bid
5	ranitidine bismuth-citrate	1 tablet qid
	clarithromycin	15 mg/kg/day–500 mg bid
	metronidazole	20 mg/kg/day–500 mg bid

Initial treatment should be provided in a twice daily regimen (to enhance compliance) for 7 to 14 days.

[a] Only for children 12 years of age or older.

bid, twice daily; qid, four times daily.

of acquired antibiotic resistance (64). Primary antimicrobial resistance also can result in treatment failure even when a three- or four-drug regimen is used. Resistance of *H. pylori* to nitroimidazoles causes an increase in the rate of treatment failures in regimens using metronidazole. An increasing prevalence of resistance to clarithromycin, documented in the past few years, particularly in Europe, could eventually impair the therapeutic effectiveness of this antibiotic in *H. pylori* treatment regimens. Results in some studies suggest that prior therapy with a proton pump inhibitor also reduces the effectiveness of eradication treatment protocols. Studies are needed to determine the relative importance of these risk factors in pediatric populations.

REFERENCES

1. Ernst PB, Gold BD. *Helicobacter pylori* in childhood: new insights into the immunopathogenesis of gastric disease and implications for managing infection in children. *J Pediatr Gastroenterol Nutr.* 1999;28:462–73.
2. Drumm B. *Helicobacter pylori* in the pediatric patient. *Gastroenterol Clin North Am.* 1993;22:169–82.
3. Dohil R, Hassall E, Jevon G, et al. Gastritis and gastropathy of childhood. *J Pediatr Gastroenterol Nutr.* 1999;29:378–94.
4. Huang J-Q, Sridhars CY, Hunt RH. Meta-analysis of the relationship between *Helicobacter pylori* seropositivity and gastric cancer. *Gastroenterology.* 1998;114:1169–79.
5. Watanabe T, Tada M, Nagai H, et al. *Helicobacter pylori* infection induces gastric cancer in Mongolian gerbils. *Gastroenterology.* 1998;115:642–8.
6. Webb PM, Knight T, Greaves S, et al. Relation between infection with *Helicobacter pylori* and living conditions in childhood: evidence for person to person transmission in early life. *BMJ.* 1994; 308:750–3.
7. Parsonnet J. The incidence of *Helicobacter pylori* infection. *Aliment Pharmacol Ther.* 1995;9:45–51.
8. Handt LK, Fox JG, Stalis IH, et al. Characterization of feline *Helicobacter pylori* strains and associated gastritis in a colony of domestic cats. *J Clin Microbiol.* 1995;33:2280–9.
9. Grubel P, Hoffman JS, Chong FK, et al. Vector potential of houseflies (Musca domestica) for *Helicobacter pylori*. *J Clin Microbiol.* 1997;35:1300–3.
10. Klein PD, Graham DY, Gaillour A, et al. Water source as a risk factor for *Helicobacter pylori* infection in Peruvian children. *Lancet.* 1991;337:1503–6.
11. Staat MA, Kruszon-Moran D, McQuillan GM, et al. A population-based serologic survey of *Helicobacter pylori* infection in children and adolescents in the United States. *J Infect Dis.* 1996;174: 1120–3.
12. Goodman KJ, Correa P. The transmission of *Helicobacter pylori*: a critical review of the evidence. *Int J Epidemiol.* 1995;24:875–87.
13. Sackett DL, Richardson WS, Rosenberg W, et al. *Evidence-based Medicine: How to Practice and Teach EBM.* Edinburgh: Churchill Livingston; 1998.
14. McMurray AR. Three decision-making aids: brainstorming, nominal group, and Delphi technique. *J Nurs Staff Dev.* 1994;10:62–5.
15. Cockeram AW. Clinical practice guidelines: help or hindrance? *J Pediatr Gastroenterol Nutr.* 1999;28:362–3.
16. Canadian Task Force on the Periodic Health Examination: the periodic health examination. *Can Med Assoc J.* 1979;121:1193–254.
17. Olson AD, Fendrick AM, Deutsch D, et al. Evaluation of initial noninvasive therapy in pediatric patients presenting with suspected ulcer disease. *Gastrointest Endosc.* 1996;44:554–1.
18. Rothman KJ, Greenland S. *Modern Epidemiology.* 2nd ed. Philadelphia: Lippincott–Raven; 1998.
19. Genta RM, Graham DY. Comparison of biopsy sites for the histopathologic diagnosis of *Helicobacter pylori*: a topographic study of *H. pylori* density and distribution. *Gastroenterology.* 1997;112: 2108–10.
20. Elitsur Y, Neace C. Detection of *Helicobacter pylori* organisms by Hp-fast in children. *Dig Dis Sci.* 1999;44:1169–72.
21. Elitsur Y, Hill I, Lichtman SN, et al. Prospective comparison of rapid urease tests (Pyloritek, CLO test) for the diagnosis of *Helicobacter pylori* infection in symptomatic children: a pediatric multicenter study. *Am J Gastroenterol.* 1998;93:217–9.

22. van der Hulst RW, van der Ende A, Homan A, et al. Influence of metronidazole resistance on efficacy of quadruple therapy for *Helicobacter pylori* eradication. *Gut.* 1998;42:166–9.

23. Holton J. Clinical relevance of culture: why, how, and when. *Helicobacter.* 1997;2(suppl 1):S25–33.

24. Westblom TU. Molecular diagnosis of *Helicobacter pylori*. *Immunol Invest.* 1997;26:163–74.

25. Breslin NP, O'Morain CA. Noninvasive diagnosis of *Helicobacter pylori*: a review. *Helicobacter.* 1997;2:111–7.

26. De Oliveira AMR, Rocha GA, Queiroz DMM, et al. Evaluation of enzyme-linked immunosorbent assay for the diagnosis of *Helicobacter pylori* infection in 157 children from different age groups with and without duodenal ulcer. *J Pediatr Gastroenterol Nutr.* 1999;28:157–61.

27. Czinn SJ. Serodiagnosis of *Helicobacter pylori* in pediatric patients. *J Pediatr Gastroenterol Nutr.* 1999;28:132–4.

28. Khanna B, Cutler A, Israel NR, et al. Use caution with serologic testing for *Helicobacter pylori* infection in children. *J Infect Dis.* 1998;178:460–5.

29. Fallone CA, Elizov M, Cleland P, et al. Detection of *Helicobacter pylori* infection by saliva IgG testing. *Am J Gastroenterol.* 1996; 91:1145–9.

30. Alemohammad MM, Foley TJ, Cohen H. Detection of immunoglobulin G antibodies to *Helicobacter pylori* in urine by an enzyme immunoassay method. *J Clin Microbiol.* 1993;31:2174–7.

31. Vaira D, Malfertheiner P, Megraud F, et al. Diagnosis of *Helicobacter pylori* with a new non-invasive antigen-based assay. *Lancet.* 1999;354:30–3.

32. Oderda G, Rapa A, Ronchi B, et al. Detection of *Helicobacter pylori* in stool specimens by non-invasive antigen enzyme immunoassay in children: multicentre Italian study. *BMJ.* 2000;320: 347–8.

33. Cutler AF, Havstad S, Ma CK, et al. Accuracy of invasive and noninvasive tests to diagnose *Helicobacter pylori* infection. *Gastroenterology.* 1995;109:136–41.

34. Rowland M, Lambert I, Gormally S, et al. Carbon 13-labeled urea breath test for the diagnosis of *Helicobacter pylori* infection in children. *J Pediatr.* 1997;131:815–20.

35. Bode G, Rothenbacher D, Brenner H, et al. Variation in the ^{13}C-urea breath test value by nationality in *Helicobacter pylori*-infected children. *Scand J Gastroenterol.* 1998;33:468–72.

36. Jones NL, Bourke B, Sherman PM. Breath testing for *Helicobacter pylori* infection in children: a breath of fresh air? *J Pediatr.* 1997; 131:791–3.

37. Sherman PM, Hassall E, Hunt RH, et al. Canadian *Helicobacter* study group consensus conference on the approach to *Helicobacter pylori* infection in children and adolescents. *Can J Gastroenterol.* 1999;13:553–9.

38. Hunt R, Thomson AB. Canadian *Helicobacter pylori* consensus conference. *Can J Gastroenterol.* 1998;12:31–41.

39. Van der Meer SB, Forget PP, et al. The prevalence of *Helicobacter pylori* serum antibodies in children with recurrent abdominal pain. *Eur J Pediatr.* 1992;151:799–801.

40. McCallion WA, Bailie AG, Ardill JE, et al. *Helicobacter pylori*, hypergastrinemia, and recurrent abdominal pain in children. *J Pediatr Surg.* 1995;30:427–9.

41. Chong SK, Lou Q, Asnicar MA, et al. *Helicobacter pylori* infection in recurrent abdominal pain in childhood: comparison of diagnostic tests and therapy. *Pediatrics.* 1995;96:211–5.

42. Bode G, Rothenbacher D, Brenner H, et al. *Helicobacter pylori* and abdominal symptoms: a population based study among preschool children in southern Germany. *Pediatrics.* 1998;101:634–7.

43. O'Donahoe JM, Sullivan PB, Scott R, et al. Recurrent abdominal pain and *Helicobacter pylori* in a community-based sample of London children. *Acta Paediatr.* 1996;85:961–4.

44. Hardikar W, Feekery C, Smith A, et al. *Helicobacter pylori* and recurrent abdominal pain in children. *J Pediatr Gastroenterol Nutr.* 1996;22:148–52.

45. Macarthur C, Saunder N, Feldman W. *Helicobacter pylori*, gastroduodenal disease, and recurrent abdominal pain in children. *JAMA.* 1995;273:729–34.

46. Gormally SM, Prakash N, Durnin MT, et al. Association of symptoms with *Helicobacter pylori* infection in children. *J Pediatr.* 1995;126:753–6.

47. Hardikar W, Davidson PM, Cameron DJ, et al. *Helicobacter pylori* infection in children. *J Gastroenterol Hepatol.* 1991;6:450–4.

48. Glassman MS, Schwarz Sm, Medow MS, et al. *Campylobacter pylori*-related gastrointestinal disease in children. Incidence and clinical findings. *Dig Dis Sci.* 1989;34:1501–4.

49. Reifen R, Rasooly I, Drumm B, et al. *Helicobacter pylori* infection in children: is there specific symptomatology. *Dig Dis Sci.* 1994; 39:1488–92.

50. Snyder JD, Hardy SC, Thorne GM, et al. Primary antral gastritis in young American children: low prevalence of *Helicobacter pylori*. *Dig Dis Sci.* 1994;39:1859–63.

51. Leontiadis GI, Sharma VK, Howden CW. Non-gastrointestinal tract associations of *Helicobacter pylori* infection. What is the evidence? *Arch Intern Med.* 1999;159:925–40.

52. Howden CW. For what conditions is there evidence-based justification for treatment of *Helicobacter pylori* infection? *Gastroenterology.* 1997;113:S107–112.

53. Sherman PM, Hunt RH. Why guidelines are required for treatment of *Helicobacter pylori* infection in children. *Clin Invest Med.* 1996; 19:362–7.

54. Dixon MF, Genta RM, Yardley JH, et al. Classification and grading of gastritis: the updated Sydney system. *Am J Surg Pathol.* 1994;20:1161–81.

55. Blum AL, Talley NJ, O'Morain C, et al. Lack of effect of treating *Helicobacter pylori* infection in patients with nonulcer dyspepsia: omeprazole plus clarithromycin and amoxicillin effect one year after treatment (OCAY) study group. *N Engl J Med.* 1998;339: 1875–81.

56. McColl K, Murray L, El-Omar E, et al. Symptomatic benefit from eradicating *Helicobacter pylori* infection in patients with nonulcer dyspepsia. *N Engl J Med.* 1998;339:1869–74.

57. Talley NJ, Janssens J, Lauritsen K, et al. Eradication of *Helicobacter pylori* in functional dyspepsia: randomized double blind placebo controlled trial with 12 months follow up. The Optimal Regimen Cures *Helicobacter* Induced Dyspepsia (ORCHID) study group. *BMJ.* 1999;318:833–7.

58. Talley NJ, Vakil N, Ballard D, et al. Absence of benefit from eradicating *Helicobacter pylori* in patients with nonulcer dyspepsia. *N Engl J Med.* 1999;3412:15:1106–11.

59. Blecker U, Gold BD. Treatment of *Helicobacter pylori* infection: a review. *Pediatr Infect Dis J.* 1997;16:391–9.

60. Harris A. Current regimens for treatment of *Helicobacter pylori* infection. *Br Med Bull.* 1998;54:195–205.

61. Peura D. *Helicobacter pylori*: rational management options. *Am J Med.* 1998;105:424–30.

62. Huang H-Q, Hunt RH. Treatment after failure: the problem of non-responders. *Gut.* 1999;45:140–5.

63. Rowland M, Imrie C, Bourke B, et al. How should *Helicobacter pylori* infected children be managed? *Gut.* 1999;45:1336–9.

64. Behrens R, Lang T, Keller KM, et al. Dual versus triple therapy of *Helicobacter pylori* infection: results of a multicentre trial. *Arch Dis Child.* 1999;81:68–70.

Guidelines for Preventing Opportunistic Infections Among Hematopoietic Stem Cell Transplant Recipients

The following guideline for preventing opportunistic infections among hematopoietic stem cell transplant recipients, developed by the Centers for Disease Control, the Infectious Disease Society of America, and the American Society of Blood and Marrow Transplantation, has been endorsed by the American Academy of Pediatrics.

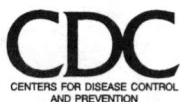

CENTERS FOR DISEASE CONTROL
AND PREVENTION

October 20, 2000 / Vol. 49 / No. RR-10

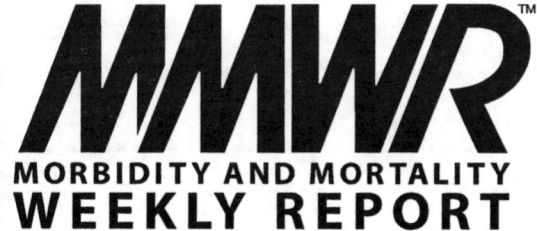

MORBIDITY AND MORTALITY
WEEKLY REPORT

Recommendations
and
Reports

Inside: **Continuing Education Examination**

Guidelines for Preventing Opportunistic Infections Among Hematopoietic Stem Cell Transplant Recipients

Recommendations of CDC, the Infectious Disease Society of America, and the American Society of Blood and Marrow Transplantation

U.S. DEPARTMENT OF HEALTH & HUMAN SERVICES
Centers for Disease Control and Prevention (CDC)
Atlanta, GA 30333

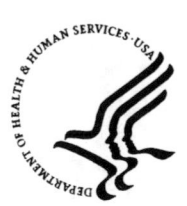

The *MMWR* series of publications is published by the Epidemiology Program Office, Centers for Disease Control and Prevention (CDC), U.S. Department of Health and Human Services, Atlanta, GA 30333.

SUGGESTED CITATION

Centers for Disease Control and Prevention. Guidelines for preventing opportunistic infections among hematopoietic stem cell transplant recipients: recommendations of CDC, the Infectious Disease Society of America, and the American Society of Blood and Marrow Transplantation.   MMWR 2000;49(No. RR-10):[inclusive page numbers].

Centers for Disease Control and Prevention .... Jeffrey P. Koplan, M.D., M.P.H.
Director

The material in this report was prepared for publication by
    National Center for Infectious Diseases .... James M. Hughes, M.D.
Director

        Division of AIDS, STD, and TB Laboratory Research .... Harold W. Jaffe, M.D.
Director

The production of this report as an *MMWR* serial publication was coordinated in
    Epidemiology Program Office .... Barbara R. Holloway, M.P.H.
Acting Director

    Office of Scientific and Health Communications .... John W. Ward, M.D.
Director
Editor, MMWR Series

        Recommendations and Reports .... Suzanne M. Hewitt, M.P.A.
Managing Editor

C. Kay Smith-Akin, M.Ed.
Project Editor

Lynda G. Cupell
Morie Higgins
Visual Information Specialists

Michele D. Renshaw
Erica R. Shaver
Technical Information Specialists

Abbreviations Used in This Publication

ANC	absolute neutrophil count
BAL	bronchoalveolar lavage
CDA	chlorodeoxyadenosine
CJD	Creutzfeldt-Jakob disease
CMV	cytomegalovirus
CRV	community-acquired respiratory virus
DNA	deoxyribonucleic acid
EBV	Epstein-Barr virus
EPA	Environmental Protection Agency
FDA	Food and Drug Administration
G-CSF	granulocyte colony-stimulating factor (filgastrim)
GM-CSF	granulocyte-macrophage colony-stimulating factor (sargramostim)
GVHD	graft-versus-host disease
HCW	health-care worker
HEPA filter	high-efficiency (>90%) particulate air filter
Hib	*Haemophilus influenzae* type b
HIV	human immunodeficiency virus
HLA	human lymphocyte antigen
HSCT	hematopoietic stem cell transplant; for this report, includes all blood- and marrow-derived hematopoietic stem cell transplants
HSV	herpes simplex virus
HTLV	human T-lymphotropic virus
IgA	immunoglobulin A
IgG	immunoglobulin G
IgM	immunoglobulin M
IVIG	intravenous immunoglobulin
LAF	laminar air flow
LD	Legionnaires' disease
LRI	lower respiratory infection
MIC	minimum inhibitory concentration
MRSA	methicillin-resistant *Staphylococcus aureus*
nvCJD	new variant Creutzfeldt-Jakob disease
OI	opportunistic infection
PCP	*Pneumocystis carinii* pneumonia
PCR	polymerase chain reaction
PZA/RIF	pyrazinamide/rifampin
RNA	ribonucleic acid
RSV	respiratory syncytial virus
TB	*Mycobacteria tuberculosis*
TMP-SMZ	trimethoprim-sulfamethasaxole
TST	tuberculin skin test
UCB	umbilical cord blood
URI	upper respiratory infection
VRE	vancomycin-resistant *Enterococcus*
VZIG	varicella-zoster immunoglobulin
VZV	varicella-zoster virus

The following CDC staff members prepared this report:

Clare A. Dykewicz, M.D., M.P.H.
Harold W. Jaffe, M.D., Director
Division of AIDS, STD, and TB Laboratory Research
National Center for Infectious Diseases

Jonathan E. Kaplan, M.D.
Division of AIDS, STD, and TB Laboratory Research
National Center for Infectious Diseases
Division of HIV/AIDS Prevention — Surveillance and Epidemiology
National Center for HIV, STD, and TB Prevention

in collaboration with
the Guidelines Working Group Members from CDC,
the Infectious Disease Society of America,
and the American Society of Blood and Marrow Transplantation

Clare A. Dykewicz, M.D., M.P.H., Chair
Harold W. Jaffe, M.D.
Thomas J. Spira, M.D.
Division of AIDS, STD, and TB Laboratory Research
William R. Jarvis, M.D.
Hospital Infections Program
National Center for Infectious Diseases, CDC

Jonathan E. Kaplan, M.D.
Division of AIDS, STD, and TB Laboratory Research
National Center for Infectious Diseases
Division of HIV/AIDS Prevention — Surveillance and Epidemiology
National Center for HIV, STD, and TB Prevention, CDC

Brian R. Edlin, M.D.
Division of HIV/AIDS Prevention—Surveillance and Epidemiology
National Center for HIV, STD, and TB Prevention, CDC

Robert T. Chen, M.D., M.A.
Beth Hibbs, R.N., M.P.H.
Epidemiology and Surveillance Division
National Immunization Program, CDC

Raleigh A. Bowden, M.D.
Keith Sullivan, M.D.
Fred Hutchinson Cancer Research Center
Seattle, Washington

David Emanuel, M.B.Ch.B.
Indiana University
Indianapolis, Indiana

David L. Longworth, M.D.
Cleveland Clinic Foundation
Cleveland, Ohio

Philip A. Rowlings, M.B.B.S., M.S.
International Bone Marrow Transplant Registry/
Autologous Blood and Marrow Transplant Registry
Milwaukee, Wisconsin

Robert H. Rubin, M.D.
Massachusetts General Hospital
Boston, Massachusetts
and
Massachusetts Institute of Technology
Cambridge, Massachusetts

Kent A. Sepkowitz, M.D.
Memorial-Sloan Kettering Cancer Center
New York, New York

John R. Wingard, M.D.
University of Florida
Gainesville, Florida

Additional Contributors

John F. Modlin, M.D.
Dartmouth Medical School
Hanover, New Hampshire

Donna M. Ambrosino, M.D.
Dana-Farber Cancer Institute
Boston, Massachusetts

Norman W. Baylor, Ph.D.
Food and Drug Administration
Rockville, Maryland

Albert D. Donnenberg, Ph.D.
University of Pittsburgh
Pittsburgh, Pennsylvania

Pierce Gardner, M.D.
State University of New York at Stony Brook
Stony Brook, New York

Roger H. Giller, M.D.
University of Colorado
Denver, Colorado

Neal A. Halsey, M.D.
Johns Hopkins University
Baltimore, Maryland

Chinh T. Le, M.D.
Kaiser-Permanente Medical Center
Santa Rosa, California

Deborah C. Molrine, M.D.
Dana-Farber Cancer Institute
Boston, Massachusetts

Keith M. Sullivan, M.D.
Fred Hutchinson Cancer Research Center
Seattle, Washington

Guidelines for Preventing Opportunistic Infections Among Hematopoietic Stem Cell Transplant Recipients

Recommendations of CDC, the Infectious Disease Society of America, and the American Society of Blood and Marrow Transplantation

Summary

CDC, the Infectious Disease Society of America, and the American Society of Blood and Marrow Transplantation have cosponsored these guidelines for preventing opportunistic infections (OIs) among hematopoietic stem cell transplant (HSCT) recipients. The guidelines were drafted with the assistance of a working group of experts in infectious diseases, transplantation, and public health. For the purposes of this report, HSCT is defined as any transplantation of blood- or marrow-derived hematopoietic stem cells, regardless of transplant type (i.e., allogeneic or autologous) or cell source (i.e., bone marrow, peripheral blood, or placental or umbilical cord blood). Such OIs as bacterial, viral, fungal, protozoal, and helminth infections occur with increased frequency or severity among HSCT recipients. These evidence-based guidelines contain information regarding preventing OIs, hospital infection control, strategies for safe living after transplantation, vaccinations, and hematopoietic stem cell safety. The disease-specific sections address preventing exposure and disease for pediatric and adult and autologous and allogeneic HSCT recipients. The goal of these guidelines is twofold: to summarize current data and provide evidence-based recommendations regarding preventing OIs among HSCT patients. The guidelines were developed for use by HSCT recipients, their household and close contacts, transplant and infectious diseases physicians, HSCT center personnel, and public health professionals. For all recommendations, prevention strategies are rated by the strength of the recommendation and the quality of the evidence supporting the recommendation. Adhering to these guidelines should reduce the number and severity of OIs among HSCT recipients.

INTRODUCTION

In 1992, the Institute of Medicine (*1*) recommended that CDC lead a global effort to detect and control emerging infectious agents. In response, CDC published a plan (*2*) that outlined national disease prevention priorities, including the development of guidelines for preventing opportunistic infections (OIs) among immunosuppressed persons. During 1995, CDC published guidelines for preventing OIs among persons infected with human immunodeficiency virus (HIV) and revised those guidelines during 1997 and 1999 (*3–5*). Because of the success of those guidelines, CDC sought to determine the need for expanding OI prevention activities to other immunosuppressed populations. An informal survey of hematology, oncology, and infectious disease specialists at transplant centers and a working group formed by CDC determined that guidelines were needed to help prevent OIs among hematopoietic stem cell transplant (HSCT)* recipients.

The working group defined OIs as infections that occur with increased frequency or severity among HSCT recipients, and they drafted evidence-based recommendations for preventing exposure to and disease caused by bacterial, fungal, viral, protozoal, or helminthic pathogens. During March 1997, the working group presented the first draft of these guidelines at a meeting of representatives from public and private health organizations. After review by that group and other experts, these guidelines were revised and made available during September 1999 for a 45-day public comment period after notification in the *Federal Register*. Public comments were added when feasible, and the report was approved by CDC, the Infectious Disease Society of America, and the American Society of Blood and Marrow Transplantation. The pediatric content of these guidelines has been endorsed also by the American Academy of Pediatrics. The hematopoietic stem cell safety section was endorsed by the International Society of Hematotherapy and Graft Engineering.

The first recommendations presented in this report are followed by recommendations for hospital infection control, strategies for safe living, vaccinations, and hematopoietic stem cell safety. Unless otherwise noted, these recommendations address allogeneic and autologous and pediatric and adult HSCT recipients. Additionally, these recommendations are intended for use by the recipients, their household and other close contacts, transplant and infectious diseases specialists, HSCT center personnel, and public health professionals.

Using These Guidelines

For all recommendations, prevention strategies are rated by the strength of the recommendation (Table 1) and the quality of the evidence (Table 2) supporting the recommendation. The principles of this rating system were developed by the Infectious Disease Society of America and the U.S. Public Health Service for use in the guidelines for preventing OIs among HIV-infected persons (*3–6*). This rating system allows assessments of recommendations to which adherence is critical.

BACKGROUND

HSCT is the infusion of hematopoietic stem cells from a donor into a patient who has received chemotherapy, which is usually marrow-ablative. Increasingly, HSCT has been used to treat neoplastic diseases, hematologic disorders, immunodeficiency syndromes, congenital enzyme deficiencies, and autoimmune disorders (e.g., systemic lupus erythematosus or multiple sclerosis) (*7–10*). Moreover, HSCT has become standard treatment for selected conditions (*7,11,12*). Data from the International Bone Marrow Transplant Registry and the Autologous Blood and Marrow Transplant Registry indicate that approximately 20,000 HSCTs were performed in North America during 1998 (Statistical

---

*For this report, HSCT is defined as any transplantation of blood- or marrow-derived hematopoietic stem cells, regardless of transplant type (e.g., allogeneic or autologous) or cell source (e.g., bone marrow, peripheral blood, or placental/umbilical cord blood). In addition, HSCT recipients are presumed immunocompetent at ≥24 months after HSCT if they are not on immunosuppressive therapy and do not have graft-versus-host disease (GVHD), a condition that occurs when the transplanted cells recognize that the recipient's cells are not the same cells and attack them.

Center of the International Bone Marrow Transplant Registry and Autologous Blood and Marrow Transplant Registry, unpublished data, 1998).

HSCTs are classified as either allogeneic or autologous on the basis of the source of the transplanted hematopoietic progenitor cells. Cells used in allogeneic HSCTs are harvested from a donor other than the transplant recipient. Such transplants are the most effective treatment for persons with severe aplastic anemia (13) and offer the only curative therapy for persons with chronic myelogenous leukemia (12). Allogeneic donors might be a blood relative or an unrelated donor. Allogeneic transplants are usually most successful when the donor is a human lymphocyte antigen (HLA)-identical twin or matched sibling. However, for allogeneic candidates who lack such a donor, registry organizations (e.g., the National Marrow Donor Program) maintain computerized databases that store information regarding HLA type from millions of volunteer donors (14–16). Another source of stem cells for allogeneic candidates without an HLA-matched sibling is a mismatched family member (17,18). However, persons who receive allogeneic grafts from donors who are not HLA-matched siblings are at a substantially greater risk for graft-versus-host disease (GVHD) (19). These persons are also at increased risk for suboptimal graft function and delayed immune system recovery (19). To reduce GVHD among allogeneic HSCTs, techniques have been developed to remove T-lymphocytes, the principal effectors of GVHD, from the donor graft. Although the recipients of T-lymphocyte–depleted marrow grafts generally have lower rates of GVHD, they also have greater rates of graft rejection, cytomegalovirus (CMV) infection, invasive fungal infection, and Epstein-Barr virus (EBV)-associated posttransplant lymphoproliferative disease (20).

The patient's own cells are used in an autologous HSCT. Similar to autologous transplants are syngeneic transplants, among whom the HLA-identical twin serves as the donor. Autologous HSCTs are preferred for patients who require high-level or marrow-ablative chemotherapy to eradicate an underlying malignancy but have healthy, undiseased bone marrows. Autologous HSCTs are also preferred when the immunologic antitumor effect of an allograft is not beneficial. Autologous HSCTs are used most frequently to treat breast cancer, non-Hodgkin's lymphoma, and Hodgkin's disease (21). Neither autologous nor syngeneic HSCTs confer a risk for chronic GVHD.

Recently, medical centers have begun to harvest hematopoietic stem cells from placental or umbilical cord blood (UCB) immediately after birth. These harvested cells are used primarily for allogeneic transplants among children. Early results demonstrate that greater degrees of histoincompatibility between donor and recipient might be tolerated without graft rejection or GVHD when UCB hematopoietic cells are used (22–24). However, immune system function after UCB transplants has not been well-studied.

HSCT is also evolving rapidly in other areas. For example, hematopoietic stem cells harvested from the patient's peripheral blood after treatment with hematopoietic colony-stimulating factors (e.g., granulocyte colony-stimulating factor [G-CSF or filgastrim] or granulocyte-macrophage colony-stimulating factor [GM-CSF or sargramostim]) are being used increasingly among autologous recipients (25) and are under investigation for use among allogeneic HSCT. Peripheral blood has largely replaced bone marrow as a source of stem cells for autologous recipients. A benefit of harvesting such cells from the donor's peripheral blood instead of bone marrow is that it eliminates the need for general anesthesia associated with bone marrow aspiration.

GVHD is a condition in which the donated cells recognize the recipient's cells as non-self and attack them. Although the use of intravenous immunoglobulin (IVIG) in the routine management of allogeneic patients was common in the past as a means of producing immune modulation among patients with GVHD, this practice has declined because of cost factors (26) and because of the development of other strategies for GVHD prophylaxis (27). For example, use of cyclosporine GVHD prophylaxis has become commonplace since its introduction during the early 1980s. Most frequently, cyclosporine or tacrolimus (FK506) is administered in combination with other immunosuppressive agents (e.g., methotrexate or corticosteroids) (27). Although cyclosporine is effective in preventing GVHD, its use entails greater hazards for infectious complications and relapse of the underlying neoplastic disease for which the transplant was performed.

Although survival rates for certain autologous recipients have improved (28,29), infection remains a leading cause of death among allogeneic transplants and is a major cause of morbidity among autologous HSCTs (29). Researchers from the National Marrow Donor Program reported that, of 462 persons receiving unrelated allogeneic HSCTs during December 1987–November 1990, a total of 66% had died by 1991 (15). Among primary and secondary causes of death, the most common cause was infection, which occurred among 37% of 307 patients (15).*

Despite high morbidity and mortality after HSCT, recipients who survive long-term are likely to enjoy good health. A survey of 798 persons who had received an HSCT before 1985 and who had survived for >5 years after HSCT, determined that 93% were in good health and that 89% had returned to work or school full time (30). In another survey of 125 adults who had survived a mean of 10 years after HSCT, 88% responded that the benefits of transplantation outweighed the side effects (31).

Immune System Recovery After HSCT

During the first year after an HSCT, recipients typically follow a predictable pattern of immune system deficiency and recovery, which begins with the chemotherapy or radiation therapy (i.e., the conditioning regimen) administered just before the HSCT to treat the underlying disease. Unfortunately, this conditioning regimen also destroys normal hematopoiesis for neutrophils, monocytes, and macrophages and damages mucosal progenitor cells, causing a temporary loss of mucosal barrier integrity. The gastrointestinal tract, which normally contains bacteria, commensal fungi, and other bacteria-carrying sources (e.g., skin or mucosa) becomes a reservoir of potential pathogens. Virtually all HSCT recipients rapidly lose all T- and B-lymphocytes after conditioning, losing immune memory accumulated through a lifetime of exposure to infectious agents, environmental antigens, and vaccines. Because transfer of donor immunity to HSCT recipients is variable and influenced by the timing of antigen exposure among donor and recipient, passively acquired donor immunity cannot be relied upon to provide long-term immunity against infectious diseases among HSCT recipients.

During the first month after HSCT, the major host-defense deficits include impaired phagocytosis and damaged mucocutaneous barriers. Additionally, indwelling intravenous catheters are frequently placed and left in situ for weeks to administer parenteral medications, blood products, and nutritional supplements. These catheters serve as another portal of entry for opportunistic pathogens from organisms colonizing the skin (e.g., coagulase-negative *Staphylococci*, *Staphylococcus aureus*, *Candida* species, and *Enterococci*) (32,33).

---

*Presently, no updated data have been published.

Engraftment for adults and children is defined as the point at which a patient can maintain a sustained absolute neutrophil count (ANC) of >500/mm³ and sustained platelet count of ≥20,000, lasting ≥3 consecutive days without transfusions. Among unrelated allogeneic recipients, engraftment occurs at a median of 22 days after HSCT (range: 6–84 days) (15). In the absence of corticosteroid use, engraftment is associated with the restoration of effective phagocytic function, which results in a decreased risk for bacterial and fungal infections. However, all HSCT recipients and particularly allogeneic recipients, experience an immune system dysfunction for months after engraftment. For example, although allogeneic recipients might have normal total lymphocyte counts within ≥2 months after HSCT, they have abnormal CD4/CD8 T-cell ratios, reflecting their decreased CD4 and increased CD8 T-cell counts (27). They might also have immunoglobulin G (IgG)$_2$, IgG$_4$, and immunoglobulin A (IgA) deficiencies for months after HSCT and have difficulty switching from immunoglobulin M (IgM) to IgG production after antigen exposure (32). Immune system recovery might be delayed further by CMV infection (34).

During the first ≥2 months after HSCT, recipients might experience acute GVHD that manifests as skin, gastrointestinal, and liver injury, and is graded on a scale of I–IV (32,35,36). Although autologous or syngeneic recipients might occasionally experience a mild, self-limited illness that is acute GVHD-like (19,37), GVHD occurs primarily among allogeneic recipients, particularly those receiving matched, unrelated donor transplants. GVHD is a substantial risk factor for infection among HSCT recipients because it is associated with a delayed immunologic recovery and prolonged immunodeficiency (19). Additionally, the immunosuppressive agents used for GVHD prophylaxis and treatment might make the HSCT recipient more vulnerable to opportunistic viral and fungal pathogens (38).

Certain patients, particularly adult allogeneic recipients, might also experience chronic GVHD, which is graded as either limited or extensive chronic GVHD (19,39). Chronic GVHD appears similar to autoimmune, connective-tissue disorders (e.g., scleroderma or systemic lupus erythematosus) (40) and is associated with cellular and humoral immunodeficiencies, including macrophage deficiency, impaired neutrophil chemotaxis (41), poor response to vaccination (42–44), and severe mucositis (19). Risk factors for chronic GVHD include increasing age, allogeneic HSCT (particularly those among whom the donor is unrelated or a non-HLA identical family member) (40), and a history of acute GVHD (24,45). Chronic GVHD was first described as occurring >100 days after HSCT but can occur 40 days after HSCT (19). Although allogeneic recipients with chronic GVHD have normal or high total serum immunoglobulin levels (41), they experience long-lasting IgA, IgG, and IgG subclass deficiencies (41,46,47) and poor opsonization and impaired reticuloendothelial function. Consequently, they are at even greater risk for infections (32,39), particularly life-threatening bacterial infections from encapsulated organisms (e.g., *Stre. pneumoniae*, *Ha. influenzae*, or *Ne. meningitidis*). After chronic GVHD resolves, which might take years, cell-mediated and humoral immunity function are gradually restored.

Opportunistic Pathogens After HSCT

HSCT recipients experience certain infections at different times posttransplant, reflecting the predominant host-defense defect(s) (Figure). Immune system recovery for HSCT recipients takes place in three phases beginning at day 0, the day of transplant.

FIGURE. Phases of opportunistic infections among allogeneic HSCT recipients

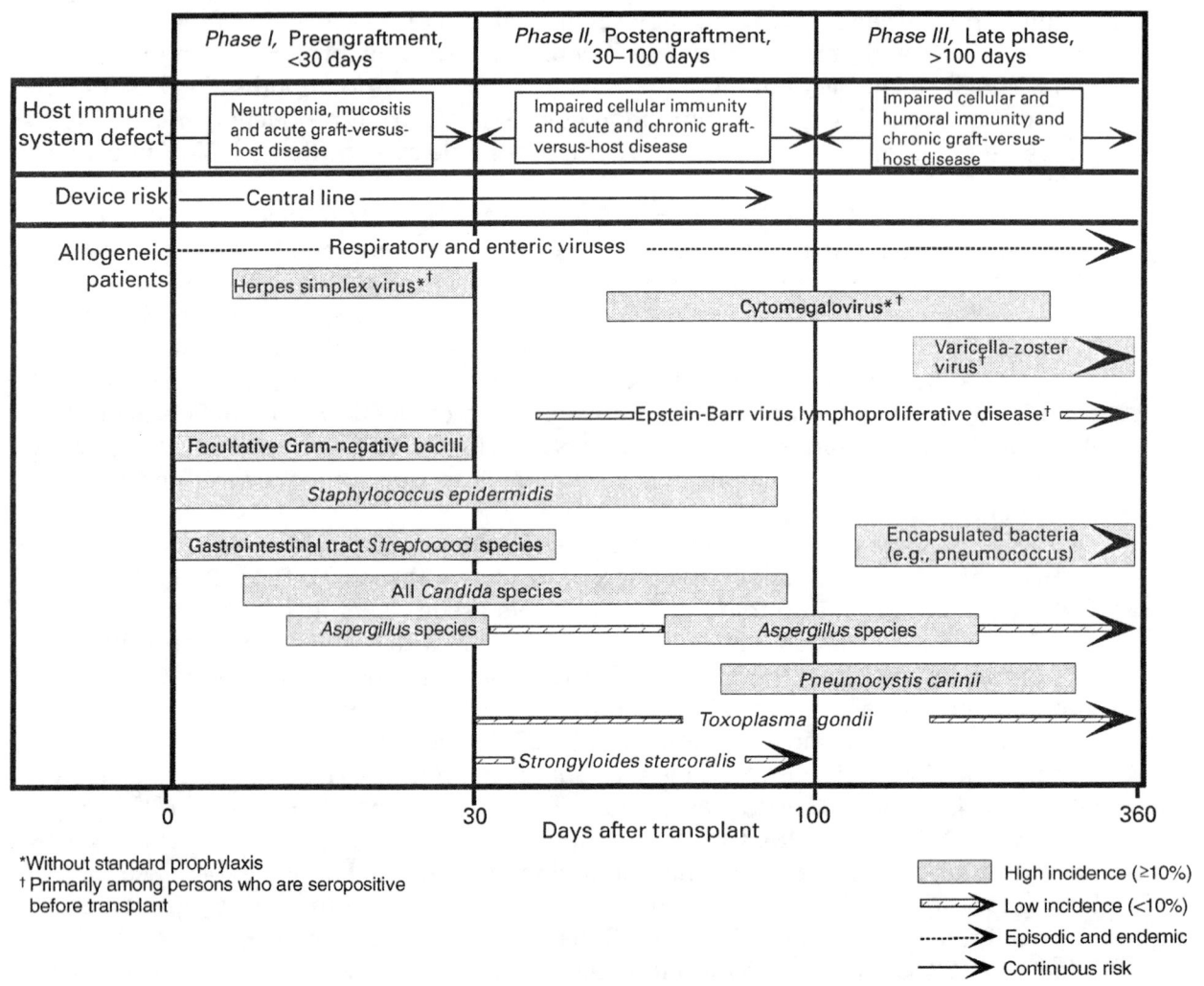

*Without standard prophylaxis
† Primarily among persons who are seropositive
  before transplant

Phase I is the preengraftment phase (<30 days after HSCT); phase II, the postengraftment phase (30–100 days after HSCT); and phase III, the late phase (>100 days after HSCT). Prevention strategies should be based on these three phases and the following information:

- **Phase I, preengraftment.** During the first month posttransplant, HSCT recipients have two critical risk factors for infection — prolonged neutropenia and breaks in the mucocutaneous barrier resulting from the HSCT preparative regimens and frequent vascular access required for patient care. Consequently, oral, gastro-intestinal, and skin flora are sources of infection. Prevalent pathogens include *Candida* species, and as neutropenia continues, *Aspergillus* species. Additionally, herpes simplex virus (HSV) reactivation can occur during this phase. During preengraftment, the risks for infection are the same for autologous or allogeneic patients, and OIs can appear as febrile neutropenia. Although a recipient's first fever during preengraftment is probably caused by a bacterial pathogen, rarely is an organism or site of infection identified. Instead, such infections are usually treated preemptively or empirically (*48*) until the neutropenia resolves (*49*). Growth factors can be administered during phase I to decrease neutropenia duration and complications (e.g., febrile neutropenia) (*50*).

- **Phase II, postengraftment.** Phase II is dominated by impaired cell-mediated immunity for allogeneic or autologous recipients. Scope and impact of this defect for allogeneic recipients are determined by the extent of GVHD and its immunosuppressive therapy. After engraftment, the herpes viruses, particularly CMV, are critical pathogens. At 30–100 days after HSCT, CMV causes pneumonia, hepatitis, and colitis and potentiates superinfection with opportunistic pathogens, particularly among patients with active GVHD. Other dominant pathogens during this phase include *Pneumocystis carinii* and *Aspergillus* species.

- **Phase III, late phase.** During phase III, autologous recipients usually have more rapid recovery of immune system function and, therefore, a lower risk for OIs than do allogeneic recipients. Because of cell-mediated and humoral immunity defects and impaired reticuloendothelial system function, allogeneic patients with chronic GVHD and recipients of alternate donor allogeneic transplants are at risk for certain infections during this phase. Alternate donors include matched unrelated, UCB, or mismatched family-related donors. These patients are at risk for infections that include CMV, varicella-zoster virus (VZV), EBV-related posttransplant lymphoproliferative disease, community-acquired respiratory viruses (CRV), and infections with encapsulated bacteria (e.g., *Ha. influenzae* and *Stre. pneumoniae*). Risk for these infections is approximately proportional to the severity of the patient's GVHD during phases II and III. Patients receiving mismatched allogeneic transplants have a higher attack rate and severity of GVHD and, therefore, a higher risk for OIs during phases II and III than do patients receiving matched allogeneic HSCTs. In contrast, patients undergoing autologous transplantation are primarily at risk for infection during phase I.

Preventing infections among HSCT recipients is preferable to treating infections. However, despite recent technologic advances, more research is needed to optimize health outcomes for HSCT recipients. Efforts to improve immune system reconstitution, particularly among allogeneic transplant recipients, and to prevent or resolve the immune dysregulation resulting from donor-recipient histoincompatibility and GVHD remain substantial challenges for preventing recurrent, persistent, or progressive infections among HSCT patients.

BACTERIAL INFECTIONS

General Recommendations

Preventing Exposure

Because bacteria are carried on the hands, health-care workers (HCWs) and others in contact with HSCT recipients should routinely follow appropriate hand-washing practices to avoid exposing recipients to bacterial pathogens (AIII).

Preventing Disease

Preventing Early Disease (0–100 Days After HSCT). Routine gut decontamination is not recommended for HSCT candidates (51–53) (DIII). Because of limited data, no recommendations can be made regarding the routine use of antibiotics for bacterial prophylaxis among afebrile, asymptomatic neutropenic recipients. Although studies have reported that using prophylactic antibiotics might reduce bacteremia rates after HSCT (51), infection-related fatality rates are not reduced (52). If physicians choose to use prophylactic antibiotics among asymptomatic, afebrile, neutropenic recipients, they should routinely review hospital and HSCT center antibiotic-susceptibility profiles, particularly when using a single antibiotic for antibacterial prophylaxis (BIII). The emergence of fluoquinolone-resistant coagulase-negative *Staphylococci* and *Es. coli* (51,52), vancomycin-intermediate *Sta. aureus* and vancomycin-resistant *Enterococcus* (VRE) are increasing concerns (54). Vancomycin should not be used as an agent for routine bacterial prophylaxis (DIII). Growth factors (e.g., GM-CSF and G-CSF) shorten the duration of neutropenia after HSCT (55); however, no data were found that indicate whether growth factors effectively reduce the attack rate of invasive bacterial disease.

Physicians should not routinely administer IVIG products to HSCT recipients for bacterial infection prophylaxis (DII), although IVIG has been recommended for use in producing immune system modulation for GVHD prevention. Researchers have recommended routine IVIG* use to prevent bacterial infections among the approximately 20%–25% of HSCT recipients with unrelated marrow grafts who experience severe

---

*Since November 1997, the United States has had a shortage of intravenous immunoglobulin (IVIG) (**Source:** CDC. Availability of immune globulin intravenous for treatment of immune deficient patients—United States, 1997–1998. MMWR 1999;48[8];159–162). Physicians who have difficulty obtaining IVIG should contact the following sources:

- American Red Cross Customer Service Center, (800) 261-5772;
- Alpha Therapeutic Corporation, (800) 421-0008;
- Baxter Healthcare Corporation, (847) 940-5955;
- Bayer Pharmaceutical Division, (800) 288-8370;
- Aventis Behring Customer Support, (800) 683-1288;
- Novartis Pharmaceuticals Corporation, (973) 781-8300, or the IVIG Emergency Hotline, (888) 234-2520; or
- Immune Deficiency Foundation, (800) 296-4433.

Physicians who are unable to obtain IVIG for a licensed indication from one of these sources should contact the Product Shortage Officer at the Food and Drug Administration's Center for Biologics Evaluation and Research, Office of Compliance, (301) 827-6220, for assistance.

hypogamma-globulinemia (e.g., IgG < 400 mg/dl) within the first 100 days after transplant (CIII). For example, recipients who are hypogammaglobulinemic might receive prophylactic IVIG to prevent bacterial sinopulmonary infections (e.g., from *Stre. pneumoniae*) (*8*) (CIII). For hypogammaglobulinemic allogeneic recipients, physicians can use a higher and more frequent dose of IVIG than is standard for non-HSCT recipients because the IVIG half-life among HSCT recipients (generally 1–10 days) is much shorter than the half-life among healthy adults (generally 18–23 days) (*56–58*). Additionally, infections might accelerate IgG catabolism; therefore, the IVIG dose for a hypogammaglobulinemic recipient should be individualized to maintain trough serum IgG concentrations >400–500 mg/dl (*58*) (BII). Consequently, physicians should monitor trough serum IgG concentrations among these patients approximately every 2 weeks and adjust IVIG doses as needed (BIII) (Appendix).

Preventing Late Disease (>100 Days After HSCT). Antibiotic prophylaxis is recommended for preventing infection with encapsulated organisms (e.g., *Stre. pneumoniae*, *Ha. influenzae*, or *Ne. meningitidis*) among allogeneic recipients with chronic GVHD for as long as active chronic GVHD treatment is administered (*59*) (BIII). Antibiotic selection should be guided by local antibiotic resistance patterns. In the absence of severe demonstrable hypogammaglobulinemia (e.g., IgG levels < 400 mg/dl, which might be associated with recurrent sinopulmonary infections), routine monthly IVIG administration to HSCT recipients >90 days after HSCT is not recommended (*60*) (DI) as a means of preventing bacterial infections.

Other Disease Prevention Recommendations. Routine use of IVIG among autologous recipients is not recommended (*61*) (DII). Recommendations for preventing bacterial infections are the same among pediatric or adult HSCT recipients.

Recommendations Regarding *Stre. pneumoniae*

Preventing Exposure

Appropriate care precautions should be taken with hospitalized patients infected with *Stre. pneumoniae* (*62,63*) (BIII) to prevent exposure among HSCT recipients.

Preventing Disease

Information regarding the currently available 23-valent pneumococcal polysaccharide vaccine indicates limited immunogenicity among HSCT recipients. However, because of its potential benefit to certain patients, it should be administered to HSCT recipients at 12 and 24 months after HSCT (*64–66*) (BIII). No data were found regarding safety and immunogenicity of the 7-valent conjugate pneumococcal vaccine among HSCT recipients; therefore, no recommendation regarding use of this vaccine can be made.

Antibiotic prophylaxis is recommended for preventing infection with encapsulated organisms (e.g., *Stre. pneumoniae*, *Ha. influenzae*, and *Ne. meningitidis*) among allogeneic recipients with chronic GVHD for as long as active chronic GVHD treatment is administered (*59*) (BIII). Trimethoprim-sulfamethasaxole (TMP-SMZ) administered for *Pneumocystis carinii* pneumonia (PCP) prophylaxis will also provide protection against pneumococcal infections. However, no data were found to support using TMP-SMZ prophylaxis among HSCT recipients solely for the purpose of preventing *Stre. pneumoniae* disease. Certain strains of *Stre. pneumoniae* are resistant to TMP-SMZ and penicillin. Recommendations for preventing pneumococcal infections are the same for allogeneic or autologous recipients.

As with adults, pediatric HSCT recipients aged ≥2 years should be administered the current 23-valent pneumococcal polysaccharide vaccine because the vaccine can be effective (BIII). However, this vaccine should not be administered to children aged <2 years because it is not effective among that age population (DI). No data were found regarding safety and immunogenicity of the 7-valent conjugate pneumococcal vaccine among pediatric HSCT recipients; therefore, no recommendation regarding use of this vaccine can be made.

Recommendations Regarding *Streptococci viridans*

Preventing Exposure

Because *Streptococci viridans* colonize the oropharynx and gut, no effective method of preventing exposure is known.

Preventing Disease

Chemotherapy-induced oral mucositis is a potential source of *Streptococci viridans* bacteremia. Consequently, before conditioning starts, dental consults should be obtained for all HSCT candidates to assess their state of oral health and to perform any needed dental procedures to decrease the risk for oral infections after transplant (67) (AIII).

Generally, HSCT physicians should not use prophylactic antibiotics to prevent *Streptococci viridans* infections (DIII). No data were found that demonstrate efficacy of prophylactic antibiotics for this infection. Furthermore, such use might select antibiotic-resistant bacteria, and in fact, penicillin- and vancomycin-resistant strains of *Streptococci viridans* have been reported (68). However, when *Streptococci viridans* infections among HSCT recipients are virulent and associated with overwhelming sepsis and shock in an institution, prophylaxis might be evaluated (CIII). Decisions regarding the use of *Streptococci viridans* prophylaxis should be made only after consultation with the hospital epidemiologists or infection-control practitioners who monitor rates of nosocomial bacteremia and bacterial susceptibility (BIII).

HSCT physicians should be familiar with current antibiotic susceptibilities for patient isolates from their HSCT centers, including *Streptococci viridans* (BIII). Physicians should maintain a high index of suspicion for this infection among HSCT recipients with symptomatic mucositis because early diagnosis and aggressive therapy are currently the only potential means of preventing shock when severely neutropenic HSCT recipients experience *Streptococci viridans* bacteremia (69).

Recommendations Regarding *Ha. influenzae* type b

Preventing Exposure

Adults with *Ha. influenzae* type b (Hib) pneumonia require standard precautions (62) to prevent exposing the HSCT recipient to Hib. Adults and children who are in contact with the HSCT recipient and who have known or suspected invasive Hib disease, including meningitis, bacteremia, or epiglottitis, should be placed in droplet precautions until 24 hours after they begin appropriate antibiotic therapy, after which they can be switched to standard precautions. Household contacts exposed to persons with Hib disease and who also have contact with HSCT recipients should be administered rifampin prophylaxis according to published recommendations (70,71); prophylaxis for household contacts of a patient with Hib disease are necessary if all contacts aged <4 years are not fully vaccinated (BIII) (Appendix). This recommendation is critical because the risk for invasive Hib disease among unvaccinated household contacts aged <4 years is increased, and rifampin can be effective in eliminating Hib carriage and preventing invasive Hib disease (*72–74*). Pediatric household contacts should be up-to-date with Hib vaccinations to prevent possible Hib exposure to the HSCT recipient (AII).

Preventing Disease

Although no data regarding vaccine efficacy among HSCT recipients were found, Hib conjugate vaccine should be administered to HSCT recipients at 12, 14, and 24 months after HSCT (BII). This vaccine is recommended because the majority of HSCT recipients have low levels of Hib capsular polysaccharide antibodies ≥4 months after HSCT (*75*), and allogeneic recipients with chronic GVHD are at increased risk for infection from encapsulated organisms (e.g., Hib) (*76,77*). HSCT recipients who are exposed to persons with Hib disease should be offered rifampin prophylaxis according to published recommendations (*70*) (BIII) (Appendix).

Antibiotic prophylaxis is recommended for preventing infection with encapsulated organisms (e.g., *Stre. pneumoniae*, *Ha. influenzae*, or *Ne. meningitidis*) among allogeneic recipients with chronic GVHD for as long as active chronic GVHD treatment is administered (*59*) (BIII). Antibiotic selection should be guided by local antibiotic-resistance patterns. Recommendations for preventing Hib infections are the same for allogeneic or autologous recipients. Recommendations for preventing Hib disease are the same for pediatric or adult HSCT recipients, except that any child infected with Hib pneumonia requires standard precautions with droplet precautions added for the first 24 hours after beginning appropriate antibiotic therapy (*62,70*) (BIII). Appropriate pediatric doses should be administered for Hib conjugate vaccine and for rifampin prophylaxis (*71*) (Appendix).

VIRAL INFECTIONS

Recommendations Regarding Cytomegalovirus

Preventing Exposure

HSCT candidates should be tested for the presence of serum anti-CMV IgG antibodies before transplantation to determine their risk for primary CMV infection and reactivation after HSCT (AIII). Only Food and Drug Administration (FDA) licensed or approved tests should be used. HSCT recipients and candidates should avoid sharing cups, glasses, and eating utensils with others, including family members, to decrease the risk for CMV exposure (BIII).

Sexually active patients who are not in long-term monogamous relationships should always use latex condoms during sexual contact to reduce their risk for exposure to CMV and other sexually transmitted pathogens (AII). However, even long-time monogamous pairs can be discordant for CMV infections. Therefore, during periods of immunocompromise, sexually active HSCT recipients in monogamous relationships should ask partners to be tested for serum CMV IgG antibody, and discordant couples should use latex condoms during sexual contact to reduce the risk for exposure to this sexually transmitted OI (CIII).

After handling or changing diapers or after wiping oral and nasal secretions, HSCT candidates and recipients should practice regular hand washing to reduce the risk for CMV exposure (AII). CMV-seronegative recipients of allogeneic stem cell transplants from CMV-seronegative donors (i.e., R-negative or D-negative) should receive only leukocyte-reduced or CMV-seronegative red cells or leukocyte-reduced platelets (<1 x 10^6 leukocytes/unit) to prevent transfusion-associated CMV infection (78) (AI). However, insufficient data were found to recommend use of leukocyte-reduced or CMV-seronegative red cells and platelets among CMV-seronegative recipients who have CMV-seropositive donors (i.e., R-negative or D-positive).

All HCWs should wear gloves when handling blood products or other potentially contaminated biologic materials (AII) to prevent transmission of CMV to HSCT recipients. HSCT patients who are known to excrete CMV should be placed under standard precautions (62) for the duration of CMV excretion to avoid possible transmission to CMV-seronegative HSCT recipients and candidates (AIII). Physicians are cautioned that CMV excretion can be episodic or prolonged.

Preventing Disease and Disease Recurrence

HSCT recipients at risk for CMV disease after HSCT (i.e., all CMV-seropositive HSCT recipients, and all CMV-seronegative recipients with a CMV-seropositive donor) should be placed on a CMV disease prevention program from the time of engraftment until 100 days after HSCT (i.e., phase II) (AI). Physicians should use either prophylaxis or preemptive treatment with ganciclovir for allogeneic recipients (AI). In selecting a CMV disease prevention strategy, physicians should assess the risks and benefits of each strategy, the needs and condition of the patient, and the hospital's virology laboratory support capability.

Prophylaxis strategy against early CMV (i.e., <100 days after HSCT) for allogeneic recipients involves administering ganciclovir prophylaxis to all allogeneic recipients at risk throughout phase II (i.e., from engraftment to 100 days after HSCT). The induction course is usually started at engraftment (AI), although physicians can add a brief prophylactic course during HSCT preconditioning (CIII) (Appendix).

Preemptive strategy against early CMV (i.e., <100 days after HSCT) for allogeneic recipients is preferred over prophylaxis for CMV-seronegative HSCT recipients of seropositive donor cells (i.e., D-positive or R-negative) because of the low attack rate of active CMV infection if screened or filtered blood product support is used (BII). Preemptive strategy restricts ganciclovir use for those patients who have evidence of CMV infection after HSCT. It requires the use of sensitive and specific laboratory tests to rapidly diagnose CMV infection after HSCT and to enable immediate administration of ganciclovir after CMV infection has been detected. Allogeneic recipients at risk should be screened ≥1 times/week from 10 days to 100 days after HSCT (i.e., phase II) for the presence of CMV viremia or antigenemia (AIII).

HSCT physicians should select one of two diagnostic tests to determine the need for preemptive treatment. Currently, the detection of CMV pp65 antigen in leukocytes (antigenemia) (79,80) is preferred for screening for preemptive treatment because it is more rapid and sensitive than culture and has good positive predictive value (79–81). Direct detection of CMV-DNA (deoxyribonucleic acid) by polymerase chain reaction (PCR) (82) is very sensitive but has a low positive predictive value (79). Although CMV-DNA PCR is less sensitive than whole blood or leukocyte PCR, plasma CMV-DNA PCR is useful during neutropenia, when the number of leukocytes/slide is too low to allow CMV pp65 antigenemia testing.

Virus culture of urine, saliva, blood, or bronchoalveolar washings by rapid shell-vial culture (*83*) or routine culture (*84,85*) can be used; however, viral culture techniques are less sensitive than CMV-DNA PCR or CMV pp65 antigenemia tests. Also, rapid shell-viral cultures require ≥48 hours and routine viral cultures can require weeks to obtain final results. Thus, viral culture techniques are less satisfactory than PCR or antigenemia tests. HSCT centers without access to PCR or antigenemia tests should use prophylaxis rather than preemptive therapy for CMV disease prevention (*86*) (BII). Physicians do use other diagnostic tests (e.g., hybrid capture CMV-DNA assay, Version 2.0 [*87*] or CMV pp67 viral RNA [ribonucleic acid] detection) (*88*); however, limited data were found regarding use among HSCT recipients, and therefore, no recommendation for use can be made.

Allogeneic recipients ≤100 days after HSCT (i.e., during phase II) should begin preemptive treatment with ganciclovir if CMV viremia or any antigenemia is detected or if the recipient has ≥2 consecutively positive CMV-DNA PCR tests (BIII). After preemptive treatment has been started, maintenance ganciclovir is usually continued until 100 days after HSCT or for a minimum of 3 weeks, whichever is longer (AI) (Appendix). Antigen or PCR tests should be negative when ganciclovir is stopped. Studies report that a shorter course of ganciclovir (e.g., for 3 weeks or until negative PCR or antigenemia occurs) (*89–91*) might provide adequate CMV prevention with less toxicity, but routine weekly screening by pp65 antigen or PCR test is necessary after stopping ganciclovir because CMV reactivation can occur (BIII).

Presently, only the intravenous formulation of ganciclovir has been approved for use in CMV prophylactic or preemptive strategies (BIII). No recommendation for oral ganciclovir use among HSCT recipients can be made because clinical trials evaluating its efficacy are still in progress. One group has used ganciclovir and foscarnet on alternate days for CMV prevention (*92*), but no recommendation can be made regarding this strategy because of limited data. Patients who are ganciclovir-intolerant should be administered foscarnet instead (*93*) (BII) (Appendix). HSCT recipients receiving ganciclovir should have ANCs checked ≥2 times/week (BIII). Researchers report managing ganciclovir-associated neutropenia by adding G-CSF (*94*) or temporarily stopping ganciclovir for ≥2 days if the patient's ANC is <1,000 (CIII). Ganciclovir can be restarted when the patient's ANC is ≥1,000 for 2 consecutive days. Alternatively, researchers report substituting foscarnet for ganciclovir if a) the HSCT recipient is still CMV viremic or antigenemic or b) the ANC remains <1,000 for >5 days after ganciclovir has been stopped (CIII) (Appendix). Because neutropenia accompanying ganciclovir administration is usually brief, such patients do not require antifungal or antibacterial prophylaxis (DIII).

Currently, no benefit has been reported from routinely administering ganciclovir prophylaxis to all HSCT recipients at >100 days after HSCT (i.e., during phase III). However, persons with high risk for late CMV disease should be routinely screened biweekly for evidence of CMV reactivation as long as substantial immunocompromise persists (BIII). Risk factors for late CMV disease include allogeneic HSCT accompanied by chronic GVHD, steroid use, low CD4 counts, delay in high avidity anti-CMV antibody, and recipients of matched unrelated or T-cell–depleted HSCTs who are at high risk (*95–99*). If CMV is still detectable by routine screening ≥100 days after HSCT, ganciclovir should be continued until CMV is no longer detectable (AI). If low-grade CMV antigenemia (<5 positive cells/slide) is detected on routine screening, the antigenemia test should be repeated in 3 days

(BIII). If CMV antigenemia indicates ≥5 cells/slide, PCR is positive, or the shell-vial culture detects CMV viremia, a 3-week course of preemptive ganciclovir treatment should be administered (BIII) (Appendix). Ganciclovir should also be started if the patient has had ≥2 consecutively positive viremia or PCR tests (e.g., in a person receiving steroids for GVHD or who received ganciclovir or foscarnet at <100 days after HSCT). Current investigational strategies for preventing late CMV disease include the use of targeted prophylaxis with antiviral drugs and cellular immunotherapy for those with deficient or absent CMV-specific immune system function.

If viremia persists after 4 weeks of ganciclovir preemptive therapy or if the level of antigenemia continues to rise after 3 weeks of therapy, ganciclovir-resistant CMV should be suspected. If CMV viremia recurs during continuous treatment with ganciclovir, researchers report restarting ganciclovir induction (*100*) or stopping ganciclovir and starting foscarnet (CIII). Limited data were found regarding the use of foscarnet among HSCT recipients for either CMV prophylaxis or preemptive therapy (*92,93*).

Infusion of donor-derived CMV-specific clones of CD8+ T-cells into the transplant recipient is being evaluated under FDA Investigational New Drug authorization; therefore, no recommendation can be made. Although, in a substantial cooperative study, high-dose acyclovir has had certain efficacy for preventing CMV disease (*101*), its utility is limited in a setting where more potent anti-CMV agents (e.g., ganciclovir) are used (*102*). Acyclovir is not effective in preventing CMV disease after autologous HSCT (*103*) and is, therefore, not recommended for CMV preemptive therapy (DII). Consequently, valacyclovir, although under study for use among HSCT recipients, is presumed to be less effective than ganciclovir against CMV and is currently not recommended for CMV disease prevention (DII).

Although HSCT physicians continue to use IVIG for immune system modulation, IVIG is not recommended for CMV disease prophylaxis among HSCT recipients (DI). Cidofovir, a nucleoside analog, is approved by FDA for the treatment of AIDS-associated CMV retinitis. The drug's major disadvantage is nephrotoxicity. Cidofovir is currently in FDA phase 1 trial for use among HSCT recipients; therefore, recommendations for its use cannot be made.

Use of CMV-negative or leukocyte-reduced blood products is not routinely required for all autologous recipients because most have a substantially lower risk for CMV disease. However, CMV-negative or leukocyte-reduced blood products can be used for CMV-seronegative autologous recipients (CIII). Researchers report that CMV-seropositive autologous recipients be evaluated for preemptive therapy if they have underlying hematologic malignancies (e.g., lymphoma or leukemia), are receiving intense conditioning regimens or graft manipulation, or have recently received fludarabine or 2-chlorodeoxyadenosine (CDA) (CIII). This subpopulation of autologous recipients should be monitored weekly from time of engraftment until 60 days after HSCT for CMV reactivation, preferably with quantitative CMV pp65 antigen (*80*) or quantitative PCR (BII).

Autologous recipients at high risk who experience CMV antigenemia (i.e., blood levels of ≥5 positive cells/slide) should receive 3 weeks of preemptive treatment with ganciclovir or foscarnet (*80*), but CD34+-selected patients should be treated at any level of antigenemia (BII) (Appendix). Prophylactic approach to CMV disease prevention is not appropriate for CMV-seropositive autologous recipients. Indications for the use of CMV prophylaxis or preemptive treatment are the same for children or adults.

Recommendations Regarding EBV

Preventing Exposure

All transplant candidates, particularly those who are EBV-seronegative, should be advised of behaviors that could decrease the likelihood of EBV exposure (AII). For example, HSCT recipients and candidates should follow safe hygiene practices (e.g., frequent hand washing [AIII] and avoiding the sharing of cups, glasses, and eating utensils with others) (104) (BIII), and they should avoid contact with potentially infected respiratory secretions and saliva (104) (AII).

Preventing Disease

Infusion of donor-derived, EBV-specific cytotoxic T-lymphocytes has demonstrated promise in the prophylaxis of EBV-lymphoma among recipients of T-cell–depleted unrelated or mismatched allogeneic recipients (105,106). However, insufficient data were found to recommend its use. Prophylaxis or preemptive therapy with acyclovir is not recommended because of lack of efficacy (107,108) (DII).

Recommendations Regarding HSV

Preventing Exposure

HSCT candidates should be tested for serum anti-HSV IgG before transplant (AIII); however, type-specific anti-HSV IgG serology testing is not necessary. Only FDA-licensed or -approved tests should be used. All HSCT candidates, particularly those who are HSV-seronegative, should be informed of the importance of avoiding HSV infection while immunocompromised and should be advised of behaviors that will decrease the likelihood of HSV exposure (AII). HSCT recipients and candidates should avoid sharing cups, glasses, and eating utensils with others (BIII). Sexually active patients who are not in a long-term monogamous relationship should always use latex condoms during sexual contact to reduce the risk for exposure to HSV as well as other sexually transmitted pathogens (AII). However, even long-time monogamous pairs can be discordant for HSV infections. Therefore, during periods of immunocompromise, sexually active HSCT recipients in such relationships should ask partners to be tested for serum HSV IgG antibody. If the partners are discordant, they should consider using latex condoms during sexual contact to reduce the risk for exposure to this sexually transmitted OI (CIII). Any person with disseminated, primary, or severe mucocutaneous HSV disease should be placed under contact precautions for the duration of the illness (62) (AI) to prevent transmission of HSV to HSCT recipients.

Preventing Disease and Disease Recurrence

Acyclovir. Acyclovir prophylaxis should be offered to all HSV-seropositive allogeneic recipients to prevent HSV reactivation during the early posttransplant period (109–113) (AI). Standard approach is to begin acyclovir prophylaxis at the start of the conditioning therapy and continue until engraftment occurs or until mucositis resolves, whichever is longer, or approximately 30 days after HSCT (BIII) (Appendix). Without supportive data from controlled studies, routine use of antiviral prophylaxis for >30 days after HSCT to prevent HSV is not recommended (DIII). Routine acyclovir prophylaxis is not indicated for

HSV-seronegative HSCT recipients, even if the donors are HSV-seropositive (DIII). Researchers have proposed administration of ganciclovir prophylaxis alone (*86*) to HSCT recipients who required simultaneous prophylaxis for CMV and HSV after HSCT (CIII) because ganciclovir has in vitro activity against CMV and HSV 1 and 2 (*114*), although ganciclovir has not been approved for use against HSV.

Valacyclovir. Researchers have reported valacyclovir use for preventing HSV among HSCT recipients (CIII); however, preliminary data demonstrate that very high doses of valacyclovir (8 g/day) were associated with thrombotic thrombocytopenic purpura/ hemolytic uremic syndrome among HSCT recipients (*115*). Controlled trial data among HSCT recipients are limited (*115*), and the FDA has not approved valacyclovir for use among recipients. Physicians wishing to use valacyclovir among recipients with renal impairment should exercise caution and decrease doses as needed (BIII) (Appendix).

Foscarnet. Because of its substantial renal and infusion-related toxicity, foscarnet is not recommended for routine HSV prophylaxis among HSCT recipients (DIII).

Famciclovir. Presently, data regarding safety and efficacy of famciclovir among HSCT recipients are limited; therefore, no recommendations for HSV prophylaxis with famciclovir can be made.

Other Recommendations

HSV prophylaxis lasting >30 days after HSCT might be considered for persons with frequent recurrent HSV (CIII) (Appendix). Acyclovir can be used during phase I for administration to HSV-seropositive autologous recipients who are likely to experience substantial mucositis from the conditioning regimen (CIII). Antiviral prophylaxis doses should be modified for use among children (Appendix), but no published data were found regarding valacyclovir safety and efficacy among children.

Recommendations Regarding VZV

Preventing Exposure

HSCT candidates should be tested for the presence of serum anti-VZV IgG antibodies (AIII). However, these tests are not 100% reliable, particularly among severely immuno-suppressed patients. Researchers recommend that a past history of varicella accompanied by a positive titer is more likely to indicate the presence of immunity to VZV than a low positive titer alone. All HSCT candidates and recipients, particularly those who are VZV-seronegative, should be informed of the potential seriousness of VZV disease among immunocompromised persons and advised of strategies to decrease their risk for VZV exposure (*116–122*) (AII).

Although researchers report that the majority of VZV disease after HSCT is caused by reactivation of endogenous VZV, HSCT candidates and recipients who are VZV-seronegative, or VZV-seropositive and immunocompromised, should avoid exposure to persons with active VZV infections (*123*) (AII). HCWs, family members, household contacts, and visitors who are healthy and do not have a reported history of varicella infection or who are VZV-seronegative should receive VZV vaccination before being allowed to visit or have direct contact with an HSCT recipient (AIII). Ideally, VZV-susceptible family members, household contacts, and potential visitors of immunocompromised HSCT recipients should be vaccinated as soon as the decision is made to perform HSCT. The vaccination dose or doses should be completed ≥4 weeks before the conditioning regimen begins or ≥6 weeks (42 days) before the HSCT is performed (BIII).

HSCT recipients and candidates undergoing conditioning therapy should avoid contact with any VZV vaccine recipient who experiences a rash after vaccination (BIII). When this rash occurs, it usually appears 14–21 days after VZV vaccination (median: 22 days; range: 5–35 days) (personal communication from Robert G. Sharrar, M.D., Merck & Co., Inc.). However, to date, no serious disease has been reported among immunocompromised patients from transmission of VZV vaccine virus, and the VZV vaccine strain is susceptible to acyclovir.

All HSCT recipients with VZV disease should be placed under airborne and contact precautions (62) (AII) to prevent transmission to other HSCT recipients. Contact precautions should be continued until all skin lesions are crusted. Airborne precautions should be instituted 10 days after exposure to VZV and continued until 21 days after last exposure or 28 days postexposure if the patient received varicella-zoster immunoglobulin (VZIG)* (62) (AI) because a person infected with VZV can be infectious before the rash appears.

Preventing Disease

VZIG. VZV-seronegative HSCT recipients should be administered VZIG as soon as possible but ideally within 96 hours after close or household contact with a person having either chickenpox or shingles if the HSCT recipient is not immunocompetent (i.e., allogeneic patient <24 months after HSCT, ≥24 months after HSCT and on immunosuppressive therapy, or having chronic GVHD) (AII). Researchers report VZIG administration for VZV exposure as described for HSCT recipients who were VZV-seropositive before HSCT (CIII).

Because of the high morbidity of VZV-associated disease among severely immunocompromised HSCT recipients and until further data are published, HSCT physicians should administer VZIG to all VZV-seronegative HSCT recipients or candidates undergoing conditioning therapy who are exposed to a VZV vaccinee having a varicella-like rash (BIII). Researchers also report VZIG administration for this situation for VZV-seropositive HSCT recipients and candidates undergoing conditioning therapy (CIII). These recommendations are made because the vaccinee might be unknowingly incubating wild-type varicella, particularly during the first 14 days after varicella vaccination, and because vaccine-strain VZV has been rarely transmitted by VZV vaccinees with vesicular rashes postvaccination (121).

If VZV-seronegative HSCT recipients or candidates undergoing conditioning therapy are closely exposed to varicella >3 weeks after receiving VZIG, they should be administered another dose of VZIG (120) (BIII). Researchers also recommend VZIG administration for this condition for VZV-seropositive HSCT recipients and candidates undergoing conditioning therapy (CIII).

---

*VZIG is distributed by FFF Enterprises, Inc., under contract with the American Red Cross, except in Massachusetts where it is distributed by the Massachusetts Public Health Biologic Laboratories (now a unit of the University of Massachusetts) (19). FFF Enterprises, Inc., can be contacted at
   FFF Enterprises, Inc.
   41093 County Center Drive
   Temecula, CA 92591
   Phone: (800) 522-4448

Antiviral Drugs. Any HSCT recipient or candidate undergoing conditioning therapy who experiences a VZV-like rash (particularly after exposure to a person with wild-type varicella or shingles) should receive preemptive intravenous acyclovir until ≥2 days after all lesions have crusted (BIII) (Appendix). Any HSCT recipient or candidate undergoing conditioning therapy who experiences a VZV-like rash after exposure to a VZV vaccinee with a rash should be administered intravenous acyclovir preemptively to prevent severe, disseminated VZV disease (BII). Acyclovir should be administered until 2 days after all lesions have crusted.

Long-term acyclovir prophylaxis to prevent recurrent VZV infection (e.g., during the first 6 months after HSCT) is not routinely recommended (*124–126*) (DIII); however, this therapy could be considered for use among HSCT recipients with severe, long-term immunodeficiency (CIII). When acyclovir resistance occurs among patients, HSCT physicians should use foscarnet for preemptive treatment of VZV disease (*127*) (BIII). Researchers report valacyclovir use for preventing HSV among HSCT recipients (CIII). However, preliminary data demonstrate that very high doses of valacyclovir (8 g/day) were associated with thrombotic thrombocytopenic purpura/hemolytic uremic syndrome among HSCT recipients (*115*). Controlled trial data regarding HSCT recipients are limited (*115*), and the FDA has not approved valacyclovir for use among HSCT recipients. Physicians wishing to use valacyclovir among HSCT recipients with renal impairment should exercise caution and decrease doses as needed (BIII) (Appendix). No data were found demonstrating safety and efficacy of preemptive treatment of famciclovir against herpes zoster among HSCT recipients. Consequently, no recommendation for its use can be made.

Live-Attenuated VZV Vaccine. VZV vaccine use is contraindicated among HSCT recipients <24 months after HSCT (*128*) (EIII). Use of VZV vaccine among HSCT recipients is restricted to research protocols for recipients ≥24 months after HSCT who are presumed immunocompetent. Further research is needed to determine the safety, immunogenicity, and efficacy of VZV vaccine among HSCT recipients.

Other Recommendations

An inactivated VZV vaccine has been used investigationally among HSCT recipients (*129*); however, more studies are needed before a recommendation regarding its use can be made. Recommendations for VZV prevention are the same for allogeneic or autologous recipients. Recommendations for preventing VZV disease among pediatric or adult HSCT recipients are the same, except that appropriate dose adjustments for VZIG should be made for pediatric HSCT recipients (AIII) (Appendix).

Recommendations Regarding CRV Infections: Influenza, Respiratory Syncytial Virus, Parainfluenza Virus, and Adenovirus

Preventing Exposure

Preventing CRV exposure is critical in preventing CRV disease (*130,131*). To prevent nosocomial CRV transmission, HSCT recipients and their HCWs should always follow HSCT infection control guidelines (AIII). To minimize the risk for CRV transmission, HCWs and visitors with upper respiratory infection (URI) symptoms should be restricted from contact with HSCT recipients and HSCT candidates undergoing conditioning therapy (AIII). At a minimum, active clinical surveillance for CRV disease should be conducted on all hospitalized HSCT recipients and candidates undergoing conditioning therapy; this clinical surveillance should include daily screening for signs and symptoms of CRV (e.g., URI or lower respiratory infection [LRI]) (AIII). Viral cultures of asymptomatic HSCT candidates are unlikely to be useful. HSCT recipients with URI or LRI symptoms should be placed under contact precautions to avoid transmitting infection to other HSCT candidates and recipients, HCWs, and visitors until the etiology of illness is identified (62) (BIII). Optimal isolation precautions should be modified as needed after the etiology is identified (AIII). HSCT recipients and candidates, their family members and visitors, and all HCWs should be informed regarding CRV infection control measures and the potential severity of CRV infections among HSCT recipients (130–140) (BIII). Physicians have routinely conducted culture-based CRV surveillance among HSCT recipients; however, the cost effectiveness of this approach has not been evaluated.

Influenza vaccination of family members and close or household contacts is strongly recommended during each influenza season (i.e., October–May) starting the season before HSCT and continuing ≥24 months after HSCT (141) (AI) to prevent influenza exposure among the recipients or candidates. All family members and close or household contacts of HSCT recipients who remain immunocompromised ≥24 months after HSCT should continue to be vaccinated annually as long as the HSCT recipient's immunocompromise persists (141) (AI). Seasonal influenza vaccination is strongly recommended for all HCWs of HSCT recipients (142,143) (AI).

If HCWs, family members, or other close contacts of HSCT recipients receive influenza vaccination during an influenza A outbreak, they should receive amantadine or rimantadine chemoprophylaxis for 2 weeks after influenza vaccination (BI) while the vaccinee experiences an immunologic response to the vaccine. Such a strategy is likely to prevent transmission of influenza A to HCWs and other close contacts of HSCT recipients, which could prevent influenza A transmission to HSCT recipients themselves. However, if a nosocomial outbreak occurs with an influenza A strain that is not contained in the available influenza vaccine, all healthy family members, close and household contacts, and HCWs of HSCT recipients and candidates should be administered influenza A chemoprophylaxis with amantadine or rimantadine until the end of the outbreak (141) (BIII).

In 1999, two neuroaminidase inhibitors (zanamivir and oseltamivir) were approved for treatment of influenza, but are not currently approved for prophylaxis. To date, experience is limited regarding use of zanamivir or oseltamivir in the treatment or prophylaxis of influenza among HSCT settings. However, HCWs, family members, or other close contacts can be offered a neuroaminidase inhibitor (e.g., zanamivir or oseltamivir) using the same strategies outlined previously, if a) rimantadine or amantadine cannot be tolerated, b) the outbreak strain of influenza A is amantadine or rimantadine-resistant, or c) the outbreak strain is influenza B (144–147) (BI). Zanamivir can be administered to persons aged ≥12 years, and oseltamivir can be administered to persons aged ≥18 years. Patients with influenza should be placed under droplet and standard precautions (AIII) to prevent transmission of influenza to HSCT recipients. HCWs with influenza should be excused from patient care until they are no longer infectious (AIII).

Preventing Disease

HSCT physicians should determine the etiology of a URI in an HSCT recipient or candidate undergoing conditioning therapy, if possible, because respiratory syncytial virus (RSV), influenza, parainfluenza, and adenovirus URIs can progress to more serious LRI, and certain CRVs can be treated (BIII). Appropriate diagnostic samples include nasopharyngeal washes, swabs or aspirates, throat swabs, and bronchoalveolar lavage (BAL) fluid. HSCT candidates with URI symptoms at the time conditioning therapy is scheduled to start should postpone their conditioning regimen until the URIs resolve, if possible, because certain URIs might progress to LRI during immunosuppression (*131,133,137,138*) (BIII).

Recommendations Regarding Influenza. Life-long seasonal influenza vaccination is recommended for all HSCT candidates and recipients, beginning during the influenza season before HSCT and resuming ≥6 months after HSCT (*142*) (BIII). Influenza vaccinations administered to HSCT recipients <6 months after HSCT are unlikely to be beneficial and are not recommended (*142*) (DII). HSCT recipients <6 months after HSCT should receive chemoprophylaxis with amantadine or rimantadine during community or nosocomial influenza A outbreaks (BIII). These drugs are not effective against influenza B. Additionally, antiviral-resistant strains of influenza can emerge during treatment with amantadine or rimantadine and transmission of resistant strains can occur (*148,149*). During such outbreaks, HSCT recipients 6–24 months after HSCT, or >24 months after HSCT and still substantially immunocompromised (i.e., receiving immunosuppressive therapy, have had a relapse of their underlying disease, or have GVHD) and who have not yet received a current influenza vaccination, should be vaccinated against influenza immediately (BIII). Additionally, to allow sufficient time for the patient to experience an immunologic response to influenza vaccine, chemoprophylaxis with amantadine or rimantadine can be used for these HSCT recipients for 2 weeks after vaccination during a nosocomial or community influenza A outbreak (CIII). Influenza A chemoprophylaxis with amantadine or rimantadine has been recommended for all influenza A-exposed HSCT recipients <24 months after HSCT or ≥24 months after HSCT and substantially immunocompromised regardless of vaccination history, because of their likely suboptimal immunologic response to influenza vaccine (*142,143*). However, no recommendation regarding such chemoprophylaxis can be made because of lack of data.

To prevent severe disease, early preemptive therapy with amantadine or rimantadine has been reported for HSCT recipients with unexplained acute URI or LRI symptoms during a community or nosocomial outbreak of influenza A (*141*). However, the effectiveness in preventing influenza-related complications and the safety of this strategy have not been evaluated among HSCT recipients. Therefore, data are insufficient to make a recommendation.

Neuroaminidase inhibitors (zanimivir and oseltamivir), intravenous and aerosol ribavirin, and combination drug therapy (e.g., rimantadine or amantadine with ribavirin or interferon) (*143,150–153*) have been proposed for investigational, preemptive treatment to prevent severe influenza disease among HSCT recipients. However, because of lack of data, no recommendation for use of these strategies among HSCT recipients can be made.

Recommendations Regarding RSV. Respiratory secretions of any hospitalized HSCT candidate or recipient who experiences signs or symptoms of CRV infection should be tested promptly by viral culture and rapid diagnostic tests for RSV (BIII). If two diagnostic samples taken ≥2 days apart do not identify a respiratory pathogen despite persistence of respiratory symptoms, BAL and further testing are advised (BIII). This testing is critical because of the high morbidity and case fatality of RSV disease among HSCT recipients (*154,155*). HSCT recipients, particularly those who are preengraftment and at highest risk for severe RSV pneumonia, should have their illness diagnosed early (i.e., during RSV URI), and their illness should be treated aggressively to prevent fatal RSV disease (BIII).

Although a definitive, uniformly effective preemptive therapy for RSV infection among HSCT recipients has not been identified, certain strategies have been proposed, including use of aerosolized ribavirin (*155,156*), RSV antibodies (i.e., passive immunization with high RSV-titered IVIG or RSV immunoglobulin) in combination with aerosolized ribavirin (*137,157*), and RSV monoclonal antibody (*158*). Clinical trials are currently underway to evaluate the efficacy of these strategies. No recommendation regarding the optimal method for RSV prevention and preemptive therapy can be made because of limited data. Further, current data do not support use of intravenous ribavirin for preemptive therapy for RSV pneumonia among HSCT recipients (*60*) (DIII), and no commercially licensed vaccines against RSV are currently available.

Recommendations Regarding Parainfluenza Virus and Adenovirus. Immunoprophylaxis, chemoprophylaxis, and preemptive treatment for parainfluenza virus and adenovirus infections among HSCT recipients have been proposed (*159,160*). However, no recommendation can be made in these guidelines because of insufficient data. No commercially licensed vaccines against parainfluenza or adenovirus are currently available.

Other Disease Prevention Recommendations

The recommendations for preventing CRV infections and their recurrence are the same for allogeneic or autologous recipients. Generally, these recommendations apply to children or adults (*161–164*), but with appropriate adjustments in antiviral drug and influenza vaccine doses for children (Appendix).

For pediatric HSCT recipients and candidates aged >6 months, annual seasonal influenza vaccination is recommended HSCT (BIII). Children aged <9 years who are receiving influenza vaccination for the first time require two doses administered ≥1 months apart (AI). Healthy children who receive influenza vaccination for the first time might not generate protective antibodies until 2 weeks after receipt of the second dose of influenza vaccine. Therefore, during an influenza A outbreak, pediatric recipients aged <9 years, ≥6 months after HSCT, and receiving their first influenza vaccination, should be administered ≥6 weeks of influenza A chemoprophylaxis after the first dose of influenza vaccine (*141*) (BIII) (Appendix). Amantadine and rimantadine are not FDA-approved for children aged <1 year (*141,161*) (DIII).

To prevent RSV disease, researchers report substituting RSV-IVIG for IVIG during RSV season (i.e., November–April) for pediatric recipients (i.e., children aged <18 years) who receive routine IVIG therapy (*164*) (i.e., those with hypogammaglobulinemia) (CIII) (Appendix). Other researchers report that pediatric recipients with RSV can be considered for preemptive therapy (e.g., during URI or early LRI) with aerosolized ribavirin (CIII), although this therapy remains controversial (*164*) (Appendix). Droplet and contact precautions for the duration of illness are required for pediatric recipients for the duration of adenovirus (*62*) (AIII).

HEALTH SCIENCES BROOKFIELD LIBRARY CORK

FUNGAL INFECTIONS

General Recommendations

Preventing Exposure

Limited data were found that demonstrate to what extent preventing fungal exposures is effective in preventing infection and disease. However, HSCT recipients and candidates undergoing conditioning therapy have been advised to avoid contact with certain areas and substances, including foods, that might increase a patient's risk for fungal exposures (CII). Specific precautions have included avoiding areas of high dust exposure (e.g., excavation sites, areas of building construction or renovation, chicken coops, and caves), occupations involving soil, and foods that contain molds (e.g., blue cheese).

Preventing Disease

Growth factors (e.g., GM-CSF and G-CSF) shorten the duration of neutropenia after HSCT (*165*); however, no data were found that indicate which growth factors effectively reduce the attack rate of invasive fungal disease. Therefore, no recommendation for use of growth factors solely for prophylaxis against invasive fungal disease can be made.

Topical antifungal drugs, which are applied to the skin or mucosa (e.g., nystatin or clotrimazole), might reduce fungal colonization in the area of application. However, these agents have not been proven to prevent generation of locally invasive or disseminated yeast infections (e.g., candidiasis) or mold infections (e.g., aspergillosis) and are not recommended for their prophylaxis (DII). Performing fungal surveillance cultures is not indicated for asymptomatic HSCT recipients (*166,167*) (DII), but cultures should be obtained from symptomatic HSCT recipients (BIII).

Recommendations Regarding Yeast Infections

Preventing Exposure

Invasive candidiasis is usually caused by dissemination of endogenous *Candida* species that have colonized a patient's gastrointestinal tract (*168*). Consequently, methods of preventing exogenous yeast exposure usually do not prevent invasive yeast infections after HSCT. However, because *Candida* species can be carried on the hands, HCWs and others in contact with HSCT recipients should follow appropriate hand-washing practices to safeguard patients from exposure (AIII).

Preventing Disease

Allogeneic recipients should be administered fluconazole prophylaxis to prevent invasive disease with fluconazole-susceptible *Candida* species during neutropenia, particularly among centers where *Can. albicans* is the predominant cause of invasive fungal disease preengraftment (AI) (Appendix). Because candidiasis occurs during phase I (*169*), fluconazole (400 mg/day by mouth or intravenously) should be administered (*169,170*) from the day of HSCT until engraftment (AII). However, fluconazole is not effective against certain *Candida* species, including *Can. krusei* (*171*) and *Can. glabrata* and is, therefore, not recommended for their prevention (DI). Further studies are needed to determine the optimal duration of fluconazole prophylaxis. Preliminary studies have reported that low-dose fluconazole prophylaxis (100–200 mg/day by mouth) among neutropenic patients has variable efficacy in preventing candidiasis (*172*). Therefore, this therapy is not recommended for HSCT recipients (DII). Oral, nonabsorbable antifungal drugs, including oral amphotericin B (500 mg suspension every 6 hours), nystatin, and clotrimazole troches, might reduce superficial colonization and control local mucosal candidiasis, but have not been demonstrated to reduce invasive candidiasis (CIII).

Other Recommendations

HSCT candidates with candidemia or invasive candidiasis can safely receive transplants (*173*) if a) their infection was diagnosed early and treated immediately and aggressively with amphotericin B or alternatively with appropriate doses of fluconazole if the organism is susceptible; and b) evidence of disease control is reported (e.g., by serial computed tomography scans) before the transplant (BIII). Such patients should continue receiving therapeutic doses of an appropriate antifungal drug throughout phase I (BII) and until a careful review of clinical, laboratory, and serial computed tomography scans verifies resolution of candidiasis (BII).

Because autologous recipients generally have an overall lower risk for invasive fungal infection than allogeneic recipients, certain autologous recipients do not require routine antiyeast prophylaxis (DIII). However, researchers recommend administering antiyeast prophylaxis to a subpopulation of autologous recipients with underlying hematologic malignancies (e.g., lymphoma or leukemia) and who have or will have prolonged neutropenia and mucosal damage from intense conditioning regimens or graft manipulation, or have received fludarabine or 2-CDA recently (BIII). Recommendations regarding preventing invasive yeast infections among pediatric or adult HSCT recipients are the same, except that appropriate dose adjustments for prophylactic drugs should be made for pediatric recipients (Appendix).

Recommendations Regarding Mold Infections

Preventing Exposure

Nosocomial mold infections among HSCT recipients result primarily from respiratory exposure to and direct contact with fungal spores (*174*). Ongoing hospital construction and renovation have been associated with an increased risk for nosocomial mold infection, particularly aspergillosis, among severely immunocompromised patients (*175–177*). Therefore, whenever possible, HSCT recipients who remain immunocompromised should avoid hospital construction or renovation areas (AIII). When constructing new HSCT centers or renovating old ones, hospital planners should ensure that rooms for HSCT patients have an adequate capacity to minimize fungal spore counts through use of

- high-efficiency (>90%) particulate air (HEPA) filtration (*140,178,179*) (BIII);

- directed room airflow (i.e., positive air pressure in patient rooms in relation to corridor air pressure) so that air from patient rooms flows into the corridor (*180*) (BIII);

- correctly sealed rooms, including correctly sealed windows and electrical outlets (*140*) (BIII);

- high rates of room air exchange (i.e., >12 air changes/hour) (*140,178*) (BIII); and

- barriers between patient care and renovation or construction areas (e.g., sealed plastic) that prevent dust from entering patient care areas and that are impermeable to *Aspergillus* species (*175,179*) (BIII).

Additionally, HSCT centers should be cleaned with care, particularly after hospital renovation or construction, to avoid exposing HSCT recipients and candidates to mold spores (*174,176*) (BIII).

Preventing Disease

No regimen has been reported to be clearly effective or superior in preventing aspergillosis, and therefore, no recommendation can be made. Further studies are needed to determine the optimal strategy for aspergillosis prevention. Moderate-dose (0.5 mg/kg/day) amphotericin B (*181–184*), low-dose (0.1–0.25 mg/kg/day) amphotericin B (*185–187*), intranasal amphotericin B spray (*188*), lipid formulations of amphotericin B (*182,189*), and aerosolized amphotericin B (*190*) have been administered for aspergillosis prophylaxis, but data are limited regarding the safety and efficacy of these formulations among HSCT recipients. Additionally, itraconazole capsules are not recommended for fungal prophylaxis among HSCT recipients (*191*) (DII) for three reasons. First, itraconazole capsules are poorly absorbed gastrointestinally, particularly among patients who are fasting (*192*) or receiving cytotoxic agents (*193*). Second, persons taking itraconazole capsules do not achieve steady-state serum levels for 2 weeks (*188,194*), and when achieved, these levels are lower than the average *Aspergillus* species minimum inhibitory concentration (MIC) among HSCT recipients (*195*). Third, itraconazole has adverse interactions with other drugs (e.g., antiepileptics, rifampin, oral hypoglycemics, protease inhibitors, vinca alkaloids, cyclosporine, methylprednisolone, and warfarin-like anticoagulants) (*196*). Trials assessing the efficacy of the recently licensed cyclodextrin oral solution and intravenous formulations of itraconazole in preventing invasive fungal disease among HSCT recipients are in progress; however, no recommendations regarding its use for *Aspergillus* species infection prophylaxis can be made. For HSCT recipients whose respiratory specimens are culture positive for *Aspergillus* species, acute invasive aspergillosis should be diagnosed presumptively (*197*) and treated preemptively and aggressively (e.g., with intravenous amphotericin) (AIII).

The risk for aspergillosis recurrence has been high among allogeneic recipients with preexisting invasive aspergillosis. Previously, allogeneic HSCTs were avoided among persons with uncontrolled, proven aspergillosis. However, HSCT center personnel have recently reported successful allogeneic or autologous HSCT among a limited number of persons who have had successfully treated, prior invasive pulmonary aspergillosis (*198–200*). Because of limited data, no recommendations regarding strategies for preventing aspergillosis recurrence can be made.

PROTOZOAL AND HELMINTHIC INFECTIONS

Recommendations Regarding PCP

Preventing Exposure

Although a possible cause of PCP is reactivation of latent infection among immunocompromised persons, cases of person-to-person transmission of PCP have been reported (201–206). Generally, standard precautions should be used for patients with PCP (62) (BIII), but researchers have reported patients with PCP being isolated (201,204) and contact precautions being used if evidence existed of person-to-person transmission in the institution (CIII). This subject remains controversial, and until further data are published, HSCT recipients should avoid exposure to persons with PCP (62) (CIII).

Preventing Disease and Disease Recurrence

Physicians should prescribe PCP prophylaxis for allogeneic recipients throughout all periods of immunocompromise (207) after engraftment. Prophylaxis should be administered from engraftment until 6 months after HSCT (AII) for all patients, and >6 months after HSCT for the duration of immunosuppression for those who a) are receiving immunosuppressive therapy (e.g. prednisone or cyclosporine) (AI), or b) have chronic GVHD (BII). However, PCP prophylaxis can be initiated before engraftment if engraftment is delayed (CIII). Researchers report an additional 1- to 2-week course of PCP prophylaxis before HSCT (i.e., day –14 to day –2) (CIII).

Preferred PCP prophylaxis is TMP-SMZ (AII); however, if TMP-SMZ is administered before engraftment, the associated myelosuppression could delay engraftment, and patients might experience sensitivity to the drug. Every effort should be made to keep such patients on the drug, including assessment of desensitization therapy, although data regarding this technique among HSCT recipients are limited. For patients who cannot tolerate TMP-SMZ, physicians can choose to use alternative PCP prophylaxis regimens (e.g., dapsone) (208) (BIII). Use of aerosolized pentamidine (209) is associated with the lowest PCP prevention rates and should only be used if other agents cannot be tolerated. Atovaquone is a possible alternative drug for PCP prophylaxis among dapsone-intolerant persons with HIV infection (210); however, no recommendation regarding use of atovaquone among HSCT recipients can be made because of lack of data. Although data are limited, concomitant use of leucovorin (folinic acid) and TMP-SMZ is not recommended (211,212) (DIII). A patient's history of PCP should not be regarded as a contraindication to HSCT (213) (DIII).

Recurrent PCP among HSCT recipients is rare; however, patients with continued immunosuppression should remain on PCP prophylaxis until their immunosuppression is resolved (AI). The regimen recommended for preventing toxoplasmosis recurrence among HSCT recipients (i.e., TMP-SMZ) will also prevent PCP recurrence.

Other Recommendations

PCP prophylaxis should be considered for autologous recipients who have underlying hematologic malignancies (i.e., lymphoma or leukemia), are receiving intense conditioning regimens or graft manipulation, or have recently received fludarabine or 2-CDA

(*207,214*) (BIII). PCP prophylaxis should be administered ≥6 months after HSCT if substantial immunosuppression or immunosuppressive therapy (e.g., steroids) persists (CIII). Use of PCP prophylaxis among other autologous recipients is controversial (CIII). Generally, indications for PCP prophylaxis are the same among children or adults, but pediatric doses should be used (Appendix).

Recommendations Regarding *Toxoplasma gondii*

Preventing Exposure

All HSCT recipients should be provided information regarding strategies to reduce their risk for *Toxoplasma* species exposure. Researchers report that potential donors for allogeneic HSCT be tested for *To. gondii* antibodies (*215,216*) by using FDA-licensed or -approved screening tests that include IgG antibody testing because *To. gondii* has been reported to be transmitted by leukocyte transfusion (*217*) and HSCT (*218,219*) (CIII).

Preventing Disease and Disease Recurrence

Because most toxoplasmosis among HSCT recipients is caused by disease reactivation, researchers report that candidates for allogeneic HSCT can be tested for IgG antibody to determine whether they are at risk for disease reactivation after HSCT (*215,216,218*) (CIII). However, the value of such testing is controversial because a limited number of patients who were seronegative for *To. gondii* pretransplant experienced the infection posttransplant (*220*). If testing is performed, only FDA-licensed or -approved screening tests should be used.

Researchers recommend toxoplasmosis prophylaxis for seropositive allogeneic recipients with active GVHD or a prior history of toxoplasmic chorioretinitis (*221,222*), but data demonstrating efficacy are limited (CIII). The optimal prophylactic regimen for toxoplasmosis among HSCT recipients has not been determined, but a proposed drug is TMP-SMZ (BII), although allogeneic recipients have experienced break-through clinical disease despite TMP-SMZ prophylaxis (*218*). For patients who are TMP-SMZ–intolerant, a combination of clindamycin, pyramethamine, and leucovorin can be substituted for *To. gondii* prophylaxis (Appendix). After therapy for toxoplasmosis, HSCT recipients should continue receiving suppressive doses of TMP-SMZ or an alternate regimen for the duration of their immunosuppression (BIII) (Appendix).

Other Recommendations

Recipients of autologous transplants are at negligible risk for toxoplasmosis reactivation (*218*). No prophylaxis or screening for toxoplasmosis infection is recommended for such patients (DIII). Indications for toxoplasmosis prophylaxis are the same among children or adults, but pediatric doses should be used among children (Appendix).

Recommendations Regarding *Strongyloides stercoralis*

Preventing Exposure

Allogeneic recipients should avoid contact with outhouses and cutaneous exposure to soil or other surfaces that might be contaminated with human feces (*223*) (AIII). Allogeneic recipients who work in settings (e.g., hospitals or institutions) where they could be exposed to fecal matter should wear gloves when working with patients or in areas with potential fecal contamination (AIII).

Preventing Disease and Disease Recurrence

Travel and residence histories should be obtained for all patients before HSCT to determine any exposures to high-risk areas (e.g., such moist temperate areas as the tropics, subtropics, or the southeastern United States and Europe) (223) (BIII). HSCT candidates who have unexplained peripheral eosinophilia or who have resided in or traveled to areas endemic for strongyloidiasis, even during the distant past, should be screened for asymptomatic strongyloidiasis before HSCT (BIII). Serologic testing with an enzyme-linked immunosorbent assay is the preferred screening method and has a sensitivity and specificity of >90% (223,224) (BIII). FDA-licensed or -approved screening tests should be used. Although stool examinations for strongyloidiasis are specific, the sensitivity obtained from ≥3 stool examinations is 60%–70%; the sensitivity obtained from concentrated stool exams is, at best, 80% (223). A total of ≥3 stool examinations should be performed if serologic tests are unavailable or if strongyloidiasis is clinically suspected in a seronegative patient (BIII).

HSCT candidates whose screening tests before HSCT are positive for *Strongyloides* species, and those with an unexplained eosinophilia and a travel or residence history indicative of exposure to *Strongyloides stercoralis* should be empirically treated before transplantation (225,226), preferably with ivermectin (BIII), even if seronegative or stool-negative (Appendix).

To prevent recurrence among HSCT candidates with parasitologically confirmed strongyloidiasis, cure after therapy should be verified with ≥3 consecutive negative stool examinations before proceeding with HSCT (AIII). Data are insufficient to recommend a drug prophylaxis regimen after HSCT to prevent recurrence of strongyloidiasis. HSCT recipients who had strongyloidiasis before or after HSCT should be monitored carefully for signs and symptoms of recurrent infection for 6 months after treatment (BIII).

Other Recommendations

Hyperinfection strongyloidiasis has not been reported after autologous HSCT; however, the same screening precautions should be used among autologous recipients (BIII). Indications for empiric treatment for strongyloidiasis before HSCT are the same among children or adults except for children weighing <15 kg, for whom the preferred drug is thiabendazole (BIII) (Appendix).

Recommendations Regarding *Trypanosoma cruzi*

Preventing Exposure

HSCT physicians should be aware that *Trypanosoma cruzi*, the etiologic agent of Chagas' disease, can be transmitted congenitally, through blood transfusion (227), and possibly through HSCT. Additionally, treatment for persons infected with *Tr. cruzi* is not always effective, even during the acute stage of infection (227). Therefore, potential donors who were born, received a blood transfusion, or ever lived for ≥6 months in a Chagas' disease endemic area (e.g., parts of South and Central America and Mexico) should be screened serologically for anti-*Tr. cruzi* serum IgG antibody (228) (BIII). Persons who lived <6 months in a Chagas'-endemic area but who had high-risk living conditions (e.g., having had extensive exposure to the Chagas' disease vector — the reduviid bug — or having lived in dwellings with mud walls, unmilled logs and sticks, or a thatched roof) should also be screened for evidence of *Tr. cruzi* infection (BIII). Because Chagas' disease can be transmitted congenitally, researchers report that any person with extensive multigenerational maternal family histories of cardiac disease (e.g., cardiomegaly and arrhythmias) should be screened serologically for serum IgG anti-*Tr. cruzi* antibodies (*227*) (CIII). To decrease the risk for misdiagnosis by false-positive or false-negative serologic tests, *Tr. cruzi* screening should consist of ≥2 conventional serologic tests (e.g., enzyme immunoassay, indirect hemagglutination, indirect fluorescent antibody) or ≥1 conventional serologic tests, followed by a confirmatory serologic test (e.g., radioimmunoprecipitation assay) (*229*) (BIII). Persons with active Chagas' disease should not serve as HSCT donors (DIII). Researchers also recommend deferral of HSCT donation for a past history of Chagas' disease (CIII).

Preventing Disease

HSCT candidates who are at risk for being infected with *Tr. cruzi* should be screened for serum IgG anti-*Tr. cruzi* antibody (*228*) (BIII). *Tr. cruzi* seropositivity is not a contraindication to HSCT (*228,230*). However, if an acute illness occurs in a *Tr. cruzi*-seropositive HSCT recipient, particularly during neutropenia, *Tr. cruzi* reactivation should be included in the differential diagnosis (*230*) (BIII). Researchers have proposed use of beznidazole or nifurtimox for preemptive therapy or prophylaxis of recurrent *Tr. cruzi* among seropositive HSCT recipients (*230,231*), but insufficient data were found to make a recommendation.*

Other Recommendations

Recommendations are the same for autologous or allogeneic recipients. However, recurrence of Chagas' disease is probably less likely to occur among autologous recipients because of the shorter duration of immunosuppression. Recommendations are the same among children or adults.

HOSPITAL INFECTION CONTROL

Room Ventilation

HSCT center personnel should follow published guidelines for hospital room design and ventilation (*140,180*) (BIII). HSCT centers should also prevent birds from gaining access to hospital air-intake ducts (*140,174*) (AII). All allogeneic recipients should be placed in rooms with >12 air exchanges/hour (*232,233*) and point-of-use HEPA filters that are capable of removing particles ≥0.3 μm in diameter (*140,178,180,233*) (AIII). Correct filtration is critical in HSCT centers with ongoing construction and renovation (*179*). When portable HEPA filters are used as adjuncts to the primary ventilation system, they must be placed centrally in patient rooms so that space is available around all surfaces to allow free air circulation (BIII). The need for environmental HEPA filtration for autologous recipients has not been established. However, HEPA-filtered rooms should

---

*For additional information regarding the epidemiology of Chagas' disease, contact CDC/ National Center for Infectious Diseases/Division of Parasitic Diseases, (770) 488-7760.

be evaluated for autologous recipients if they experience prolonged neutropenia, a substantial risk factor for nosocomial aspergillosis (CIII).

A laminar air flow (LAF) room contains filtered air that moves in parallel, unidirectional flow — the air enters the room from one wall and exits the room on the opposite wall (232). Although LAF has been demonstrated to protect patients from infection during aspergillosis outbreaks related to hospital construction (234,235), the value of routine LAF room use for all HSCT recipients is doubtful because substantial overall survival benefit has not been reported (236). During 1983, LAF rooms were preferred for allogeneic recipients with aplastic anemia and HLA-identical sibling donors because use of regular rooms was associated with a mortality rate that was approximately four times higher than for those recipients treated in LAF rooms (237). However, the survival of aplastic anemia HSCT recipients during the late 1990s exceeds that reported during the early 1980s, and no studies have been done to determine whether HSCT recipients with aplastic anemia still have an improved survival rate when treated in an LAF room. Therefore, HSCT centers need not construct LAF rooms for each HSCT recipient. Use of LAF rooms, if available, is optional (CII).

Hospital rooms should have directed airflow so that air intake occurs at one side of the room and air exhaust occurs at the opposite side (140) (BIII). Each hospital room should also be well-sealed (e.g, around windows and electrical outlets) (140) (BIII). To provide consistent positive pressure in the recipient's room, HSCT centers should maintain consistent pressure differentials between the patient's room and the hallway or anteroom at >2.5 Pa (i.e., 0.01 inches by water gauge) (232,233) (BIII). Generally, hospital rooms for HSCT recipients should have positive room air pressure when compared with any adjoining hallways, toilets, and anterooms, if present.

Anterooms should have positive air pressure compared with hallways (180). An exception is the HSCT recipient with an active disease that has airborne transmission (e.g., pulmonary or laryngeal *Mycobacteria tuberculosis* [TB] or measles). These HSCT patients should be placed in negative isolation rooms (62) (BIII), and a room with an anteroom is recommended for such patients (180) (BIII).

Whenever possible, HSCT centers should have self-closing doors to maintain constant pressure differentials among the HSCT recipients' room and anterooms, if available, and hallways (233) (BIII). To enable the nursing staff to observe the HSCT recipient even when the doors are closed, windows can be installed in either the door or the wall of the HSCT recipient's room (233) (CIII).

HSCT centers should provide backup emergency power and redundant air-handling and pressurization systems to maintain a constant number of air exchanges and room pressurization in the center when the central ventilation system is shut off for maintenance and repair (238) (BIII). Additionally, infection control personnel should work with maintenance personnel to develop protocols to protect HSCT centers at all times from bursts of mold spores that might occur when air-handling systems are restarted after routine maintenance shut-downs (BIII).

Construction, Renovation, and Building Cleaning

Construction and Renovation

Hospital construction and renovation have been associated with an increased risk for nosocomial fungal infection, particularly aspergillosis, among severely immunocompromised patients (175,176). Therefore, persons responsible for HSCT center construction or renovation should consult published recommendations regarding environmental controls during construction (*239,240*) (AIII).

Whenever possible, HSCT recipients, HCWs, and visitors should avoid construction or renovation areas (*240*) (AIII). Also, equipment and supplies used by HSCT recipients or their HCWs should not be exposed to construction or renovation areas (*240*). When planning for construction or renovation, the HSCT center should include plans for intensified aspergillosis-control measures (AIII). Construction and renovation infection control planning committees should include engineers, architects, housekeeping staff, infection control personnel, the director of the HSCT center, the administration, and safety officers (*241*) (BIII).

When constructing new HSCT centers, planners should ensure that patient rooms will have adequate capacity to minimize fungal spore counts by following room ventilation recommendations. During outdoor construction and demolition, the intake air should be sealed (BIII), if possible; if not, filters should be checked frequently. Additionally, to protect HSCT patient care areas during fire drills and emergencies, weather stripping should be placed around stairwell doors, or alternatively, the stairwell air should be filtered to the level of safety of the adjacent hospital air (BIII). False ceilings should be avoided whenever possible (*174*) (BII). If use of false ceilings cannot be avoided, the area above false ceilings should be vacuumed routinely to minimize dust and, therefore, fungal exposure to patients (*174*) (BIII).

During hospital construction or renovation, hospitals should construct rigid, dust-proof barriers with airtight seals (*242*) between patient care and construction or renovation areas to prevent dust from entering patient care areas; these barriers (i.e., sealed drywall) should be impermeable to *Aspergillus* species (*140,175,176,179,240*) (BIII). If impervious barriers cannot be created around the construction or renovation area, patients should be moved from the area until renovation or construction is complete and the area has been cleaned appropriately (*176*) (BIII). HSCT centers should direct pedestrian traffic occurring near construction or renovation areas away from patient care areas to limit the opening and closing of doors or other barriers that might cause dust dispersion, entry of contaminated air, or tracking of dust into patient areas (*140*), particularly those in the HSCT center (*176*) (BIII). If possible, specific corridors, entrances, and exits should be dedicated to construction use only (*240*). An elevator to which patients do not have access also should be dedicated to construction use only (*240*). Construction workers, whose clothing might be contaminated with *Aspergillus* species spores, should use the construction elevator and avoid contact with patients, patient care areas, other elevators, and nonconstruction areas (BIII).

Hospital construction or renovation areas should have negative air pressure relative to that in adjacent patient care areas, if no contraindications exist for such pressure differential (*140,176,179,240,242*) (BIII). Ideally, air from the construction or renovation areas should be exhausted to the outside of the hospital (*176*) (BIII) or if recirculated, it should be HEPA-filtered first (BIII).

Researchers have proposed that HSCT recipients wear the N95 respirator to prevent mold exposure during transportation near hospital construction or renovation areas (CIII) because the N95 respirators are regarded as effective against any aerosol. However, to be maximally effective, N95 respirators must be fit-tested and all users must be trained. With correct personnel fit-testing and training, N95 respirators reliably reduce aerosol exposure by 90%. Without fit-testing and training, aerosol exposure would be reduced but not necessarily by 90% (*243*). For patients who cannot use or tolerate an

N95 respirator, researchers have proposed using the powered air purifying respirator (*244,245*), which can be used by patients in wheelchairs. Limitations of the powered air purifying respirator include its cost and that it is not appropriate for young children and infants. General limitations of using respirators are that no commercially available respirator, including N95, has been tested specifically for its efficacy in reducing exposure to *Aspergillus* species in hospital construction or renovation areas, and no studies have been done that assess the usefulness and acceptability of using respirators among HSCT recipients. Standard surgical masks provide negligible protection against mold spores and are not recommended for this indication (DIII).

Newly constructed or renovated areas should be cleaned before patients are allowed to enter them (*140,176*) (AIII). Decontamination of fungal-contaminated areas that cannot be extracted and replaced should be done using copper-8-quinolate (*179*) (BIII). Also, areas above false ceilings located under or adjacent to construction areas should be vacuumed (*174*) (BIII). Additionally, the ventilation, direction of airflow, and room pressurization should be tested and correctly adjusted before patients are allowed to enter (BIII).

Cleaning

HSCT centers should be cleaned ≥1 times/day with special attention to dust control (BIII). Exhaust vents, window sills, and all horizontal surfaces should be cleaned with cloths and mop heads that have been premoistened with an FDA- or Environmental Protection Agency (EPA)-registered hospital disinfectant (BIII). Thorough cleaning during and after any construction activity, including minor renovation projects, is critical (BIII).

HSCT center personnel should prohibit exposures of patients to such activities as vacuuming or other floor or carpet vacuuming that could cause aerosolization of fungal spores (e.g., *Aspergillus* species) (*140*) (AIII). Accordingly, doors to patient rooms should be closed when vacuuming HSCT center corridors. All vacuum cleaners used in the HSCT center should be fitted with HEPA filters. An FDA- or EPA-registered disinfectant (*246,247*) should be used daily for environmental disinfection and when wet vacuuming is performed in the HSCT center (BIII). If an HSCT center provides care for infants, phenolic disinfectants can be used to clean the floors only if the compound is diluted according to the product label; but phenolic compounds should not be used to clean basinets or incubators (*246*) (DIII).

Water leaks should be cleaned up and repaired as soon as possible but within 72 hours to prevent mold proliferation in floor and wall coverings, ceiling tiles, and cabinetry in and around all HSCT patients care areas (BIII). If cleanup and repair are delayed ≥72 hours after the water leak, the involved materials should be assumed to contain fungi and handled accordingly. Use of a moisture meter to detect water penetration of walls should be used whenever possible to guide decision-making (*238*) (BIII). For example, if the wall does not have <20% moisture content ≥72 hours after water penetration, it should be removed (BIII). Design and selection of furnishings should focus on creating and maintaining a dust-free environment. Flooring and finishes (i.e., wall coverings, window shades, and countertops) used in HSCT centers should be scrubbable, nonporous, easily disinfected, and they should collect minimal dust (BIII).

Isolation and Barrier Precautions

HSCT center personnel should follow published guidelines for hospital isolation practices, including CDC guidelines for preventing nosocomial infections (*62,140,248*) (AIII).

However, the efficacy of specific isolation and barrier precautions in preventing nosocomial infections among HSCT recipients has not been evaluated.

HSCT recipients should be placed in private (i.e., single-patient) rooms (BIII). If contact with body fluids is anticipated, standard precautions should be followed (AIII). These precautions include hand washing and wearing appropriate gloves, surgical masks or eye and face protection, and gowns during procedures and activities that are likely to generate splashes or sprays of blood, body fluids, secretions or excretions, or cause soiling of clothing (62). When indicated, HSCT recipients should also be placed on airborne, droplet, or contact precautions in addition to standard precautions (62) (AIII). Careful observation of isolation precautions is critical in preventing transmission of infectious agents among HSCT recipients, HCWs, visitors, and other HSCT recipients. Physicians are cautioned that HSCT recipients might have a prolonged or episodic excretion of organisms (e.g., CMV).

Researchers have proposed that HSCT recipients wear surgical mask and gloves when exiting their hospital rooms before engraftment (CIII). All HSCT recipients who are immunocompromised (phases I–III of immune system recovery) and candidates undergoing conditioning therapy should minimize the time spent in crowded areas of the hospital (e.g., waiting areas and elevators) (BIII) to minimize potential exposure to persons with CRV infections.

Hand Hygiene

Hand washing is the single-most critical and effective procedure for preventing nosocomial infection (62). All persons, but particularly HCWs, should wash their hands before entering and after leaving the rooms of HSCT recipients and candidates undergoing conditioning therapy (62,249) or before and after any direct contact with patients regardless of whether they were soiled from the patient, environment, or objects (AI). HSCT recipients should be encouraged to practice safe hand hygiene (e.g., washing hands before eating, after using the toilet, and before and after touching a wound) (BIII). Hand washing should be done with an antimicrobial soap and water (AIII); alternatively, use of hygienic hand rubs is another acceptable means of maintaining hand hygiene (250,251). If gloves are worn, HCWs should put them on in the patient's room after hand washing and then discard them in the same patient's room before washing hands again after exiting the room. When worn, gloves should always be changed between patients or when soiled before touching a clean area (e.g., change gloves after touching the perineum and before going to a "clean" area) (AIII). Appropriate gloves should be used by all persons when handling potentially contaminated biological materials (AII). Items worn on the hands and fingers (e.g., rings or artificial nails [248,252]) and adhesive bandage strips, can create a nidus for pathogenic organisms that is difficult to clean. Thus, HCWs should avoid wearing such items whenever possible (BII).

Equipment

All HSCT center personnel should sterilize or disinfect and maintain equipment and devices using only EPA-registered compounds as directed by established guidelines (140,180,246,247,253–256) (AIII). HSCT center personnel should monitor opened and unopened wound-dressing supplies (e.g., adhesive bandages [257,258] and surgical and elastic adhesive tape [259]) to detect mold contamination and prevent subsequent cutaneous transmission to patients (BII).

Monitoring should consist of discarding all bandages and wound dressings that are out of date, have damaged packaging, or are visually contaminated by construction debris or moisture (BIII). When arm boards are used to provide support for intravenous lines, only sterile dressing materials should be used (*260*), and arm boards should be changed frequently (e.g., daily) (BIII). Additionally, unsterile tongue depressors inserted into a piece of foam tubing should not be used as splints for intravenous and arterial catheter sites because these have been associated with an outbreak of fatal invasive nosocomial *Rhizopus microsporus* among preterm (i.e., very low-birth–weight) infants (*261*) (DII). HSCT centers should not install carpeting in hallways outside (DII) or in patient rooms (DIII) because contaminated carpeting has been associated with outbreaks of aspergillosis among HSCT recipients (*262,263*).

Plants, Play Areas, and Toys

Although to date, exposure to plants and flowers has not been conclusively reported to cause fungal infections among HSCT recipients, most researchers strongly recommend that plants and dried or fresh flowers should not be allowed in the rooms of hospitalized HSCT candidates undergoing conditioning therapy and HSCT recipients (phases I–III of immune system recovery) because *Aspergillus* species have been isolated from the soil of potted ornamental plants (e.g., cacti), the surface of dried flower arrangements, and fresh flowers (*140,174,178,264*) (BIII).

Play areas for pediatric HSCT recipients and candidates undergoing conditioning therapy should be cleaned and disinfected ≥1 times/week and as needed (BIII). Only toys, games, and videos that can be kept clean and disinfected should be allowed in the HSCT center (BIII). HSCT centers should follow published recommendations for washing and disinfecting toys (*265*) (BIII). All HSCT center toys, games, and videos should be routinely and thoroughly washed or wiped down when brought into the HSCT center and thereafter ≥1 times/week and as needed by using a nontoxic FDA- or EPA-registered disinfectant (*246,247,265*) followed by a water rinse (BIII). Cloth or plush toys should be washed in a hot cycle of a washing machine or dry-cleaned ≥1 times/week and as needed (BIII). Alternatively, machine washing in a cold cycle is acceptable if laundry chemicals for cold water washing are used in proper concentration (*265*). Hard plastic toys should be scrubbed with warm soapy water using a brush to clean crevices, rinsed in clean water, immersed in a mild bleach solution, which should be made fresh daily, for 10–20 minutes, rinsed again, and allowed to air dry (*246*). Alternatively, hard plastic toys can be washed in a dishwasher or hot cycle of a washing machine (BIII). Broviac dolls* should be disassembled upon completion of play and washed with a nontoxic FDA- or EPA-registered disinfectant (*246,247*), rinsed with tap water, and allowed to air dry before other children are allowed to play with them (BIII). Toys that cannot be washed, disinfected, or dry-cleaned after use should be avoided (BIII). Infants, toddlers, and children who put toys in their mouths should not share toys (*265*) (DIII). For children in isolation, researchers recommend the following:

- Disposable play items should be offered whenever possible (BIII).

- Before returning a washable toy used in an isolation room to the pediatric play room for use by another child, it should be cleaned again as previously described (BIII).

---

*Broviac dolls are used to demonstrate medical procedures (e.g., insertion of catheters) to children to lessen their fears.

- When a child is taken out of isolation, toys, games, and videos used during the period of isolation and that might serve as fomites for infection should be thoroughly disinfected with a nontoxic FDA- or EPA-registered disinfectant (*246,247,265*) (BIII). After use in isolation rooms, cloth or plush toys should be placed in a plastic bag and separated from unused toys. All cloth or plush toys used in isolation rooms should be washed in a washing machine or dry-cleaned before being used in a nonisolation room (BIII). Toys that cannot be disinfected or dry-cleaned after use in an isolation room should be discarded (BIII).

Water-retaining bath toys have been associated with an outbreak of *Pseudomonas aeruginosa* in a pediatric oncology ward (*266*); therefore, these toys should not be used by immunocompromised HSCT recipients and candidates (DII). Occupational and physical therapy items should be cleaned and disinfected as previously described (BIII). Soil-based materials (e.g., clay or potting soil) should be avoided (BIII).

HCWs

HSCT center personnel should have a written comprehensive policy regarding their immunizations and vaccinations, and that policy should meet current CDC, Advisory Committee on Immunization Practices, and Healthcare Infection Control Practices Advisory Committee recommendations (*267*) (BIII). Immunizations are needed to prevent transmission of vaccine-preventable diseases to HSCT recipients and candidates undergoing conditioning therapy. All HCWs with diseases transmissible by air, droplet, and direct contact (e.g., VZV, infectious gastroenteritis, HSV lesions of lips or fingers, and URIs) should be restricted from patient contact and temporarily reassigned to other duties (AI). HSCT center personnel should follow published recommendations regarding the duration of work restrictions for HCWs with infectious diseases (*268,269*) (BIII). HSCT center HCWs with bloodborne viruses (e.g., HIV or hepatitis B or C viruses) should not be restricted from patient contact (DIII) as long as they do not perform procedures that pose a high risk for injury that could result in patient exposure to the HCW's blood or body fluids. Work exclusion policies should be designed to encourage HCWs to report their illnesses or exposures (AII).

HSCT Center Visitors

Hospitals should have written policies for screening HSCT center visitors, particularly children, for potentially infectious conditions. Such screening should be performed by clinically trained HCWs (BII). Visitors who might have communicable infectious diseases (e.g., URIs, flu-like illnesses, recent exposure to communicable diseases, an active shingles rash whether covered or not, a VZV-like rash within 6 weeks of receiving a live-attenuated VZV vaccine, or a history of receiving an oral polio vaccine within the previous 3–6 weeks) should not be allowed in the HSCT center or allowed to have direct contact with HSCT recipients or candidates undergoing conditioning therapy (AII). No absolute minimum age requirement for HSCT center visitors exists; however, all visitors must be able to understand and follow appropriate hand washing and isolation precautions (AIII). The number of HSCT center visitors at any one time should be restricted to a number that permits the nursing staff to perform appropriate screening for contagious diseases and adequate instruction and supervision of hand washing, glove and mask use, and biosafety precautions (BIII).

Patient Skin and Oral Care

To optimize skin care, HSCT recipients should take daily showers or baths during and after transplantation (BIII), using a mild soap (BIII). Skin care during neutropenia should also include daily inspection of skin sites likely to be portals of infection (e.g., the perineum and intravascular access sites) (BIII). HSCT recipients and candidates undergoing conditioning therapy should maintain good perineal hygiene to minimize loss of skin integrity and risk for infection (BIII). To facilitate this precaution, HSCT center personnel should develop protocols for patient perineal care, including recommendations for gentle but thorough perineal cleaning after each bowel movement and thorough drying of the perineum after each urination (BIII). Females should always wipe the perineum from front to back after using the toilet to prevent fecal contamination of the urethra and urinary tract infections (AIII). Moreover, to prevent vaginal irritation, menstruating immunocompromised HSCT recipients should not use tampons (DIII) to avoid the risk for cervical and vaginal abrasions. Additionally, the use of rectal thermometers, enemas, suppositories, and rectal exams are contraindicated among HSCT recipients to avoid skin or mucosal breakdown (DIII).

All HSCT candidates and their caregivers should be educated regarding the importance of maintaining good oral and dental hygiene for at least the first year after HSCT to reduce the risk for oral and dental infections (AIII). For example, HSCT candidates should be informed that establishment of the best possible periodontal health before HSCT is a substantial step in avoiding short- and long-term oral infections and that maintenance of safe oral hygiene after HSCT can minimize the severity of infections and facilitate healing of mucositis, particularly before engraftment (BIII).

All HSCT candidates should receive a dental evaluation and relevant treatment before conditioning therapy begins (270,271) (AIII). Likely sources of dental infection should be vigorously eliminated (271) (AIII). For example, teeth with moderate to severe caries should be restored; ill-fitting dental prostheses should be repaired; and teeth compromised by moderate to severe periodontal disease should be extracted (271). Ideally, 10–14 days should elapse between the completion of tissue-invasive oral procedures and onset of conditioning therapy to allow for adequate healing and monitoring for postsurgical complications (AIII).

HSCT recipients with mucositis and HSCT candidates undergoing conditioning therapy should maintain safe oral hygiene by performing oral rinses 4–6 times/day with sterile water, normal saline, or sodium bicarbonate solutions (270) (AIII). HSCT recipients and candidates should brush their teeth ≥2 times/day with a soft regular toothbrush (270) (BIII). If the recipient cannot tolerate these brushings, use of an ultrasoft toothbrush or toothette (i.e., foam swab on a stick), can be used (CIII), but physicians should be aware that using the latter products are less desirable than using soft regular or ultrasoft toothbrushes because the toothettes remove less dental debris (270). Using toothpaste is optional, depending on the recipient's tolerance (270) (CIII). HSCT recipients and candidates undergoing conditioning therapy who are skilled at dental flossing should floss daily if this can be done without trauma (BIII). Routine dental supervision is advised to monitor and guide the patient's maintenance of oral and dental hygiene (BIII). To decrease the risk for mechanical trauma and infection of oral mucosa, fixed orthodontic appliances and space maintainers should not be worn from the start of conditioning therapy until preengraftment mucositis resolves, and these devices should not be worn during any subsequent periods of mucositis (270) (DIII). Dental and transplant teams and the patient's community dentist should coordinate removal of these appliances and long-term rehabilitation of any oral lesions (BIII). However, patients who normally wear removable dental prostheses might be able to wear them during conditioning therapy before HSCT and during mucositis after HSCT, depending on the degree of tissue integrity at the denture-bearing sites and the ability of the patient to maintain denture hygiene on a daily basis (CIII).

Preventing Bacterial Intravascular Catheter-Related Infections

HSCT center personnel are advised to implement published guidelines for preventing intravascular device-related infections (33) (AIII). Contact with tap water at the central venous catheter site should be avoided (BIII). For long-term central venous access among children, HSCT physicians can use a totally implantable device among children aged <4 years if the anticipated duration of vascular access is >30 days (CII). However, such a device among children aged <4 years is not generally used as the actual HSCT infusion site because a) problems with skin fragility contraindicate repeated punctures over the port site and b) the port device might have an insufficient number of lumens for optimal patient management immediately after HSCT.

To prevent bloodstream infections associated with needleless intravenous access devices, HSCT recipients should a) cover and protect the catheter tip or end cap during bathing or showering to protect it from tap water contamination, b) change the device in accordance with manufacturers' recommendations, if available, and c) have a caregiver perform intravenous infusions whenever possible (272,273) (BII). Also, HSCT recipients and their caregivers should be educated regarding proper care of needleless intravenous access devices (272) (BII). No recommendation regarding the use of antibiotic-impregnated central venous catheters among HSCT recipients can be made because of lack of data.

Control of Specific Nosocomial Infections

Recommendations Regarding Legionella Species

HSCT physicians should always include Legionnaires' disease (LD) in the differential diagnosis of pneumonia among HSCT recipients (140) (AIII). Appropriate tests to confirm LD include a) culturing sputum, BAL, and tissue specimens; b) testing BAL specimens for Legionellae by direct fluorescent antibody; and c) testing for Legionella pneumophila serogroup 1 antigen in urine. The incubation period for LD is usually 2–10 days; thus, laboratory-confirmed legionellosis that occurs in a patient who has been hospitalized continuously for ≥10 days before the onset of illness is regarded as a definite case of nosocomial LD, and a laboratory-confirmed infection that occurs 2–9 days after hospital admission is a possible case of nosocomial LD (140). When a case of laboratory-confirmed nosocomial LD (274,275) is identified in a person who was in the inpatient HSCT center during all or part of the 2–10 days before illness onset, or if two or more cases of laboratory-confirmed LD occur among patients who had visited an outpatient HSCT center, hospital personnel should

- report the case(s) to the local or state health department if the disease is reportable in that state or if assistance is needed (140) (AIII); and

- in consultation with the hospital infection control team, conduct a thorough epidemiologic and environmental investigation to determine the likely environmental source(s) of *Legionella* species (e.g., showers, tap water faucets, cooling towers, and hot water tanks) (*274,276*) (AI).

The source of *Legionella* infection should be identified and decontaminated or removed (AIII). Extensive hospital investigations of an isolated case of possible nosocomial LD might not be indicated if the patient has had limited contact with the inpatient center during most of the incubation period (CIII). Because HSCT recipients are at much higher risk for disease and death from legionellosis compared with other hospitalized persons (*274*), periodic routine culturing for *Legionellae* in water samples from the center's potable water supply could be regarded as part of an overall strategy for preventing LD in HSCT centers (CIII). However, the optimal methodology (i.e., frequency or number of sites) for environmental surveillance cultures in HSCT centers has not been determined, and the cost-effectiveness of this strategy has not been evaluated. Because HSCT recipients are at high risk for LD and no data were found to determine a safe concentration of *Legionellae* organisms in potable water, the goal, if environmental surveillance for *Legionellae* is undertaken, should be to maintain water systems with no detectable organisms (AIII). Physicians should suspect legionellosis among HSCT recipients with nosocomial pneumonia even when environmental surveillance cultures do not yield *Legionellae* (AIII). If *Legionella* species are detected in the water supplying an HSCT center, the following should be done until *Legionella* species are no longer detected by culture:

- The water supply should be decontaminated (*140*) (AII).

- HSCT recipients should be given sponge baths with water that is not contaminated with *Legionella* species (e.g., not with the HSCT center's *Legionella* species-contaminated potable water system) (BIII).

- Patients should not take showers in LD-contaminated water (DIII).

- Water from faucets containing LD-contaminated water should not be used in patient rooms or the HSCT center and outpatient clinic to avoid creating infectious aerosols (CIII).

- HSCT recipients should be given sterile water instead of tap water for drinking, brushing teeth, or flushing nasogastric tubes during Legionellosis outbreaks (BIII).

HSCT center personnel should use only sterile water (i.e., not distilled unsterile water) for rinsing nebulization devices and other semicritical respiratory-care equipment after cleaning or disinfecting and for filling reservoirs of nebulization devices (*140*) (BII). HSCT centers should not use large-volume room air humidifiers that create aerosols (e.g., by Venturi principle, ultrasound, or spinning disk) and, thus, are actually nebulizers (*140*) (DI) unless these humidifier or nebulizers are sterilized or subjected to daily high-level disinfection and filled with sterile water only (*140*) (CIII).

When a new hospital with an HSCT center is constructed, the cooling towers should be placed so that the tower drift is directed away from the hospital's air-intake system, and the cooling towers should be designed so that the volume of aerosol drift is minimized (*140*) (BII). For operational hospital cooling towers, hospitals should

- install drift eliminators,

- regularly use an effective biocide,

- maintain cooling towers according to the manufacturer's recommendations, and

- keep adequate maintenance records (*140*) (BII).

HSCT physicians are encouraged to consult published recommendations regarding preventing nosocomial Legionellosis (*140,277*) (BIII). No data were found to determine whether drinking tap water poses a risk for *Legionella* exposure among HSCT recipients in the absence of an outbreak.

Recommendations Regarding Methicillin-Resistant Sta. aureus

HSCT center HCWs should follow basic infection control practices (e.g., hand washing between patients and use of barrier precautions, including wearing gloves whenever entering the methicillin-resistant *Sta. aureus* [MRSA] infected or colonized patient's room); these practices are essential for MRSA control (*62*) (AII). If MRSA is a substantial problem in the HSCT center and evidence exists of ongoing MRSA transmission, MRSA infected or colonized patients should be treated as a cohort (e.g., cared for exclusively by a limited number of HCWs) (BIII). HSCT transplant recipients with recurrent *Sta. aureus* infections should undergo extensive evaluation for persistent colonization, including cultures of nares, groin, axilla, and ostomy sites (e.g., tracheostomy or gastrointestinal tube) (BIII). For patients with recurrent MRSA infection, elimination of the carrier state should be attempted by applying a 2% mupirocin calcium ointment to the nares (BIII), although this strategy has been only marginally effective in certain institutions (*278*) (Appendix). High-level mupirocin-resistant MRSA has been reported in Europe, the Middle East, and South America (*279–283*) but is uncommon in the United States. As with any antibiotic, incorrect or overuse of mupirocin can result in mupirocin-resistant *Staphylococci*; therefore, mupirocin use should be reserved for infection control strategies only (*279,280*). For patients who fail mupirocin, physicians have used bacitracin, TMP-SMZ, or rifampin administered with another antibiotic, but no standardized protocol using these drugs for this indication has been evaluated and no recommendations can be made because of lack of data. Selection of a systemic antibiotic should be guided by susceptibility patterns.

Intravascular cannulas or other implantable devices that are infected or colonized with MRSA should be removed (AIII). Patients with MRSA should be placed under contact precautions until all antibiotics are discontinued and until three consecutive cultures, taken ≥1 weeks apart, are negative (*62*) (BIII). Screening cultures for MRSA include the anterior nares, any body site previously positive for MRSA, and any wounds or surgical sites.

Recommendations Regarding Staphylococcus Species with Reduced Susceptibility to Vancomycin

All HSCT centers should have sufficient laboratory capability to identify all *Staphylococci* isolates and their susceptibility patterns to antibiotics, including vancomycin (*284,285*) (AIII). Additionally, all HSCT center personnel should conduct routine surveillance for the emergence of *Staphylococcus* species strains with reduced susceptibility to vancomycin (*285,286*) (AIII). Reduced susceptibility should be considered for all *Sta. aureus* strains that have a vancomycin MIC of ≥4 µg/mL and all coagulase-negative

Staphylococci that have a vancomycin MIC of ≥8 µg/mL. If repeat testing of the organism in pure culture confirms the genus, species, and elevated vancomycin MICs, the following steps should be taken (*287*):

- The laboratory should immediately contact hospital infection control personnel, the patient's clinical center, and the patient's attending physician, as well as the local or state health department, and CDC's Hospital Infections Program Help Desk ([404] 639-6106 or [800] 893-0485) (*284,285,287,288*) (AIII).

- The HSCT center's infection control personnel, in collaboration with appropriate authorities (i.e., state and local health departments and CDC) should promptly initiate an epidemiologic and laboratory investigation (*287,288*) (AIII) and follow published guidelines for the control of such species (*285,287,288*) (BIII).

- Medical and nursing staff should

  — institute contact precautions (e.g., wearing of gown and gloves, using antibacterial soap for hand washing, and wearing masks when contamination of the HCW with secretions is likely) as recommended for multidrug-resistant organisms (*62,284,287*);

  — minimize the number of persons with access to colonized or infected patients (*287*); and

  — treat as a cohort colonized or infected patients (e.g., care for them exclusively with a limited number of HCWs) (*286,287*) (AIII).

- If a patient in an HSCT center is colonized or infected with *Staphylococci* that have reduced susceptibility to vancomycin, the infection control personnel should follow published guidelines for the control of such species (*285,287,288*) (BIII).

Avoiding overuse and misuse of antibiotics will decrease the emergence of *Staphylococcus* species with reduced susceptibility to vancomycin (*286,287*). Therefore, medical and ancillary staff members who are responsible for monitoring antimicrobial use patterns in the facility should routinely review vancomycin-use patterns (*284,285,287*) (AIII). Additionally, HSCT center personnel should institute prudent use of all antibiotics, particularly vancomycin, to prevent the emergence of *Staphylococcus* with reduced susceptibility to vancomycin (*284,285,287–289*) (AII). Intravascular cannulas or other implantable devices that are infected or colonized with *Staphylococcus* species strains with reduced susceptibility to vancomycin should be removed (AIII).

Recommendations Regarding VRE

Use of intravenous vancomycin is associated with VRE emergence. Vancomycin and all other antibiotics, particularly antianaerobic agents (e.g., metronidazole and third-generation cephalosporins) must be used judiciously (*284,290–292*) (AII). Oral vancomycin use can be limited by treating recurrences of *Cl. difficile* diarrhea with oral metronidazole instead of vancomycin (BIII). Physicians have placed patients with a history of VRE or VRE colonization into continuous isolation during clinic visits and hospitalizations; however, this practice is controversial because certain non-HSCT recipients might clear VRE from their stools. No recommendation regarding use of continuous isolation among HSCT recipients can be made because of lack of data. To control VRE exposure, strict adherence to the following standard infection control measures is necessary (292) (AI):

- Wash hands with antibacterial soap before entering and after leaving HSCT recipients' rooms, particularly those who have VRE colonization or infection; alternatively, wash hands with a waterless antiseptic agent (e.g., an alcohol-based rinse or gel) (250).

- Whenever possible, treat as a cohort patients who are known to be colonized or infected with VRE (290).

- Disinfect patient rooms and equipment (291,293), including surfaces of the hospital ward environment (e.g., floors, walls, bed frames, doors, bathroom surfaces) with an FDA- or EPA-registered disinfectant (246,247). A nontoxic disinfectant should be used for pediatric areas (BIII).

- Place patients with VRE under contact precautions until all antibiotics are discontinued (CIII) and repeated cultures are negative (62) (BIII). HCWs should always wear gloves when in the VRE patient or carrier's room and discard gloves in the patient's room before exiting.

No evidence exists that treating VRE carriers is beneficial; therefore, chronic antibiotic treatment of carriers is not recommended (DIII). HSCT recipients and candidates should be screened for VRE colonization at the time of interfacility transfer to allow for immediate institution of appropriate infection control practices and to minimize transmission of VRE between and within facilities (294) (BII). However, the role of outpatient surveillance in VRE control is unknown; such surveillance is costly and should not be undertaken in nonoutbreak settings (DIII). A history of having resolved VRE bacteremia or being a VRE carrier are not contraindications to HSCT (BIII).

Recommendations Regarding Cl. difficile

HSCT physicians should follow published recommendations for preventing and controlling Cl. difficile disease, including minimizing the duration of antibiotic therapy and number of antibiotics used for any indication (295,296) (AIII). All patients with Cl. difficile disease should be placed under contact precautions for the duration of illness (62) (AII). All HCWs who anticipate contact with a Cl. difficile-infected patient or the patient's environment or possessions should put on gloves before entering the patient's room (62,295–298) and before handling the patient's secretions and excretions (AI). During Cl. difficile outbreaks, HSCT center personnel should restrict use of antibiotics (e.g., clindamycin) (299) (BII). To prevent transmission of Cl. difficile to patients during nosocomial Cl. difficile outbreaks, HSCT center HCWs should a) use disposable rectal thermometers or tympanic thermometers; b) disinfect gastrointestinal endoscopes with 2% glutaraldehyde immersion for 10 minutes or use an equivalent disinfectant strategy (255,256); and c) perform surface sterilization of the hospital ward environment (e.g., floors, walls, bed frames, doors, bathroom surfaces) with an FDA- or EPA-registered sterilant (e.g., phosphate-buffered sodium hypochlorite solution [1,660 ppm available chloride]; unbuffered hypochlorite solution [500 ppm available chloride]; 0.04% formaldehyde and 0.03% glutaraldehyde [255,295,300]; or ethylene oxide [247,296]) (BII). Additionally, physicians should treat patients with Cl. difficile disease with antibiotics as recommended in published reports (62,295) (BII).

Certain researchers also recommend antibiotic treatment of *Cl. difficile* carriers (*301*). However, other researchers have reported that treatment of asymptomatic *Cl. difficile* carriers with metronidazole is not effective and that treatment with vancomycin is only effective temporarily (i.e., <2 months after treatment) (*302*). Consequently, no recommendation regarding treatment of asymptomatic *Cl. difficile* carriers can be made. Similarly, although symptomatic *Cl. difficile* disease recurrence or relapse occurs among 7%–20% of patients (*295*), data are insufficient to make a recommendation for preventing multiple *Cl. difficile* relapses.

The following practices are not recommended for *Cl. difficile* control:

- routine stool surveillance cultures for *Cl. difficile* for asymptomatic patients or HCWs, even during outbreaks (DIII);

- culturing HCWs' hands for *Cl. difficile* (DIII); or

- treating patients presumptively for *Cl. difficile* disease pending toxin results (DIII), unless the patient is very sick with a compatible syndrome or the hospital has a high prevalence of *Cl. difficile* (CIII).

Prophylactic use of lyophilized *Saccharomyces boulardii* to reduce diarrhea among antibiotic recipients is not recommended because this therapy is not associated with a substantial reduction in diarrhea associated with *Cl. difficile* disease (*303*) and has been associated with *Saccharomyces boulardii* fungemia (*304*) (DII).

Recommendations Regarding CRV Infections

Physicians should institute appropriate precautions and infection control measures for preventing nosocomial pneumonia among hospitalized HSCT recipients and candidates undergoing conditioning therapy, particularly during community or nosocomial CRV outbreaks (*140*) (AIII). Patients with URI or LRI symptoms should be placed under a) contact precautions for most viral respiratory infections including varicella; b) droplet precautions for influenza or adenovirus; or c) airborne precautions for measles or varicella to avoid transmitting infection to other HSCT candidates and recipients as well as to HCWs and visitors (BIII). Identifying HSCT recipients with RSV infection and placing them under contact precautions immediately (AIII) to prevent nosocomial transmission is critical. When suctioning the respiratory tract of patients with URI or LRI symptoms, HCWs should wear gowns, surgical masks, and eye protection to avoid contamination from the patient's respiratory secretions. All protective clothing (e.g., gown, gloves, surgical mask, and eye protection) should be put on when entering a patient's room and discarded in the same room before exiting; protective clothing should always be changed between patient rooms (*140*) (AIII). When caring for an HSCT recipient or candidate undergoing conditioning therapy with URI or LRI, HCWs and visitors should change gloves and wash hands a) after contact with a patient; b) after handling respiratory secretions or objects contaminated with secretions from one patient and before contact with another patient, object, or environmental surface; and c) between contacts with a contaminated body site and the respiratory tract of or respiratory device used on the same patient (*140*) (AII). This practice is critical because most respiratory infections are usually transmitted by contact, particularly by hand to nose and eye. Therefore just wearing a mask, without appropriate hand washing, glove-wearing, or use of eye protection is insufficient to prevent transmission of CRV infections.

Researchers have proposed that HSCT recipients or candidates undergoing conditioning therapy be placed under contact precautions during nosocomial outbreaks (*131*) (CIII). Even when no nosocomial or community outbreak of CRV infections exists, all persons who enter the HSCT center should be screened daily for URI symptoms, including visitors and HCWs (BIII). Researchers also describe systems where HCWs provide daily verification (e.g., using sign-in sheets) that they are free of URI symptoms before being allowed to provide HSCT patient care. HCWs and visitors with URI symptoms should be restricted from contact with HSCT recipients and candidates undergoing conditioning therapy to minimize the risk for CRV transmission (*131*) (AIII). All HCWs with URI symptoms should be restricted from patient contact and reassigned to nonpatient care duties until the HCW's symptoms resolve (BIII). Visitors with URI symptoms should be asked to defer their visit to the HSCT center (*131*) until their URI symptoms resolve (BIII).

Respiratory secretions of any hospitalized HSCT candidate or recipient with signs or symptoms of CRV infection should be tested promptly by viral culture and rapid diagnostic tests for CRV (BIII). Appropriate samples include nasopharyngeal washes, swabs, aspirates, throat swabs, and BAL fluid. This practice is critical because preemptive treatment of certain CRVs (e.g., influenza and RSV) (*133*) might prevent severe disease and death among HSCT recipients. Viral shedding among HSCT recipients with CRV infection has been reported to last ≤4 months for influenza (*143*), ≤2 years for adenovirus (*305,306*), and ≤22 days for RSV (*136*); however, RSV viral shedding has been reported to last 112 days in a child with severe combined immunodeficiency (*307*). Therefore, to prevent nosocomial transmission of CRV (*136*), HSCT center HCWs should recognize that prolonged CRV shedding can occur when determining the duration of appropriate precautions for CRV-infected HSCT recipients or candidates undergoing conditioning therapy (CIII). HSCT centers should use serial testing by using cultures from nasopharyngeal swabs, throat swabs or aspirates, or rapid antigen tests to help determine whether patients have stopped shedding influenza virus (BIII). Researchers have proposed that HSCT physicians conduct routine CRV surveillance among HSCT recipients to detect outbreaks and implement infection control measures as early as possible (CIII). During RSV season, HSCT recipients and candidates with signs or symptoms should be tested for RSV infection (i.e., the presence of RSV antigen in respiratory secretions tested by enzyme-linked immunosorbent assay and viral culture) starting with admission to the HSCT center. All patients who are RSV-antigen positive should be treated as a cohort during nosocomial RSV outbreaks because this practice reduces nosocomial RSV transmission (*130,131*) (BII). Symptomatic HCWs should be excluded from patient contact until symptoms resolve. HCWs and visitors with infectious conjunctivitis should be restricted from direct patient contact until the drainage resolves (i.e., usually, 5–7 days for adenovirus) and the ophthalmology consultant concurs that the infection and inflammation have resolved (*268*) (AII) to avoid possible transmission of adenovirus to HSCT recipients.

Preventing CRV exposure among HSCT recipients after hospital discharge is more challenging because of high CRV prevalence. Preventive measures should be individualized in accordance with the immunologic status and tolerance of the patient. In outpatient waiting rooms, patients with CRV infections should be separated to the extent possible from other patients (BIII).

Recommendations Regarding TB

HSCT candidates should be screened for TB by careful medical history and chart review to ascertain any history of prior TB exposure (AIII) because immunocompromised persons have higher risk for progression from latent TB infection to active disease (*244*). Also, physicians can administer a tuberculin skin test (TST) using the Mantoux method with five tuberculin units of purified protein derivative (CIII); but because of a patient's immunocompromise, this test might not be reliable. If a TST is administered, either the Tubersol® or Aplisol® formulation of purified protein derivative can be used (*244,308*). Persons with a recently positive TST or a history of a positive TST and no prior preventive therapy should be administered a chest radiograph and evaluated for active TB (*309*) (AI). For immunocompromised persons, a positive TST is defined as ≥5 mm of induration (*309,310*) because of their decreased ability to mount a delayed hypersensitivity response (CIII). Because immunosuppressive therapy decreases the sensitivity of the TST, HSCT physicians should not rely solely on the TST to determine whether latent TB infection is present and whether preventive therapy should be administered to HSCT recipients or candidates (DIII). Instead, a full 9-month course of isonicotinic acid hydrazide preventive therapy should be administered to immunocompromised HSCT recipients or candidates who have been substantially exposed to someone with active, infectious (i.e., sputum-smear positive) pulmonary or laryngeal TB, regardless of the HSCT recipient's or candidate's TST status (*309*) (BIII). A full 9-month course of isonicotinic acid hydrazide preventive therapy should also be administered to HSCT recipients or candidates with a positive TST who were not previously treated and have no evidence of active TB disease (*309*) (AIII) (Appendix). Routine anergy screening might not be reliable among HSCT recipients and candidates undergoing conditioning therapy and, therefore, is not recommended (DIII). An HSCT should not be canceled or delayed because of a positive TST (DIII).

Use of a 2-month course of a daily pyrazinamide/rifampin (PZA/RIF) regimen has been recommended as an alternate preventive therapy for persons with TB (*309*). However, limited data were found regarding safety and efficacy of this regimen among non-HIV–infected persons. Furthermore, rifampin has substantial drug interactions with certain medications, including cyclosporine, tacrolimus (FK506), corticosteroids, fluconazole, and pain medications. Therefore, routine use of the 2-month PZA/RIF prophylactic regimen among HSCT recipients is not recommended (DIII). However, this regimen can be used for HSCT candidates who are not at risk for serious rifampin drug interactions and whose HSCT is not scheduled until ≥2 weeks after completion of the 2-month PZA/RIF course (CIII). This delay will diminish the possibility of adverse effects of rifampin on drugs used for routine HSCT OI prophylaxis (e.g., fluconazole) (*311*). An HSCT candidate or recipient who has been exposed to an active case of extrapulmonary, and therefore, noninfectious TB does not require preventive therapy (DIII).

HSCT center personnel should follow guidelines regarding the control of TB in healthcare facilities (*244,245*), including instituting airborne precautions and negative-pressure rooms for patients with suspected or confirmed pulmonary or laryngeal TB (*62,244*) (AII). HCWs should wear N95 respirators, even in isolation rooms, to protect themselves from possible TB transmission from patients with active pulmonary or laryngeal TB, particularly during cough-inducing procedures (*62,244,245,312*) (AIII). To be maximally effective, respirators (e.g., N95) must be fit-tested, and all respirator users must be trained to use them correctly (*243*) (AIII). Unless they become soiled or damaged, changing N95 respirators between patient rooms is not necessary (DIII). Bacillus of Calmette and Guérin vaccination is contraindicated among HSCT candidates and recipients because it might cause disseminated or fatal disease among immunocompromised persons (*313,314*) (EII). No role has been identified for chronic suppressive therapy or follow-up surveillance cultures among HSCT recipients who have a history of successfully treated TB (DIII).

Infection Control Surveillance

HSCT center personnel are advised to follow standard guidelines for surveillance of antimicrobial use and nosocomial pathogens and their susceptibility patterns (*315*) (BIII). HSCT center personnel should not perform routine fungal or bacterial cultures of asymptomatic HSCT recipients (*166,167*) (DII). In the absence of epidemiologic clusters of infections, HSCT center personnel should not perform routine periodic bacterial surveillance cultures of the HSCT center environment or of equipment or devices used for respiratory therapy, pulmonary-function testing, or delivery of inhalation anesthesia (*140*) (DIII). Researchers recommend that hospitals perform routine sampling of air, ceiling tiles, ventilation ducts, and filters to test for molds, particularly when construction or renovation occurs near or around the rooms of immunocompromised patients (*167,174*) or when clinical surveillance demonstrates a possible increase in mold (i.e., aspergillosis) cases (CIII). Strategies that might decrease fungal spores in the ventilation system include eliminating access of birds (i.e., primarily pigeons) to air-intake systems, removing bird droppings from the air-intake ducts, and eliminating moss from the hospital roof (*174*). Furthermore, in the absence of a nosocomial fungal outbreak, HSCT centers need not perform routine fungal cultures of devices and dust in the rooms of HSCT recipients and candidates undergoing conditioning therapy (DIII). HSCT center personnel should routinely perform surveillance for the number of aspergillosis cases occurring among HSCT recipients, particularly during hospital construction or renovation (BIII). A two-fold or greater increase in the attack rate of aspergillosis during any 6-month period indicates that the HSCT center environment should be evaluated for breaks in infection control techniques and procedures and that the ventilation system should be investigated carefully (*174*) (BIII).

STRATEGIES FOR SAFE LIVING AFTER HSCT — PREVENTING EXPOSURE AND DISEASE

Avoiding Environmental Exposures

HSCT recipients and candidates undergoing conditioning therapy, particularly allogeneic recipients, and parents of pediatric HSCT recipients and candidates should be educated regarding strategies to avoid environmental exposures to opportunistic pathogens (AIII).

Preventing Infections Transmitted by Direct Contact

HSCT recipients and candidates should wash their hands thoroughly (i.e., with soap and water) and often. For example, hands should be washed

- before eating or preparing food;

- after changing diapers;

- after gardening or touching plants or dirt;

- after touching pets or animals;

- after touching secretions or excretions or items that might have had contact with human or animal stool (e.g., clothing, bedding, toilets, or bedpans);

- after going outdoors; and

- before and after touching wounds (*249*) (AIII).

Conscientious hand washing is critical during the first 6 months after HSCT and during other periods of substantial immunosuppression (e.g., GVHD, systemic steroid use, or relapse of the underlying disease for which the transplant was performed) (AIII). Pediatric HSCT recipients and candidates should be supervised by adults during hand washing to ensure thorough cleaning (*316*) (BIII). Hand washing should be performed with an antimicrobial soap and water (AIII); alternatively, use of hygienic hand rubs is an acceptable means of maintaining hand hygiene (*250,251*). HSCT recipients who visit or live on farms should follow published recommendations for preventing cryptosporidiosis (*5,316,317–319*) (BIII).

Preventing Respiratory Infections

To prevent respiratory infections after hospital discharge, HSCT recipients should observe the following precautions:

- Frequent and thorough hand washing is critical (BIII), but HSCT recipients should also avoid touching their mucus membranes, unless they have washed their hands first, to avoid inoculating themselves with CRV.

- HSCT recipients should avoid close contact with persons with respiratory illnesses (BIII). When close contact is unavoidable, those persons with respiratory illnesses should be encouraged to wash their hands frequently and to wear surgical masks or, at a minimum, smother their sneezes and coughs in disposable tissues. Alternatively, the HSCT recipient can wear a surgical mask (CIII).

- HSCT recipients should avoid crowded areas (e.g., shopping malls or public elevators) where close contact with persons with respiratory illnesses is likely (BIII).

- HSCT candidates or recipients should be advised that certain activities and occupations (e.g., work in health-care settings, prisons, jails, or homeless shelters) can increase their risk for TB exposure (BIII). In deciding whether a patient should continue activities in these settings, physicians should evaluate the patient's specific duties, the precautions used to prevent TB exposure in the workplace, and the prevalence of TB in the community. The decision to continue or terminate such activities should be made jointly between patient and physician (BIII). HSCT recipients should avoid exposure to persons with active tuberculosis, particularly during the first 6 months after HSCT and during other periods of substantial immunosuppression (e.g., GVHD, systemic steroid use, or relapse of the underlying disease for which the transplant was performed) (BIII).

Researchers report that allogeneic recipients should avoid construction or excavation sites or other dust-laden environments for the first 6 months after HSCT and during other periods of substantial immunosuppression (e.g., GVHD, systemic steroid use, or relapse of the underlying disease for which the transplant was performed) to avoid exposures to molds (CIII). Researchers also report that outpatient HSCT recipients should be advised of travel routes to the HSCT center that will avoid or minimize exposure to construction sites (CIII).

Coccidioidomycosis is uncommon after allogeneic HSCT; however, researchers report that HSCT recipients traveling to or residing in coccidioidomycosis-endemic areas (e.g., the American southwest, Mexico, and Central and South America) should avoid or minimize exposure to disturbed soil, including construction or excavation sites, areas with recent earthquakes, farms, or other rural areas (CIII). Histoplasmosis (*Histoplasma capsulatum*) after allogeneic HSCT is also rare; however, researchers report that HSCT recipients in histoplasmosis-endemic areas should avoid exposure to chicken coops and other bird-roosting sites and caves for the first 6 months after HSCT and during periods of substantial immunosuppression (e.g., GVHD, systemic steroid use, or relapse of the underlying disease for which the transplant was performed) (CIII).

Smoking tobacco and exposure to environmental tobacco smoke are risk factors for bacterial and CRV infections among healthy adults and children (*320–325*); consequently, logic dictates that physicians advise HSCT recipients not to smoke and to avoid exposure to environmental tobacco smoke (CIII). However, no data were found that specifically assess whether smoking or environmental smoke exposure are risk factors for OIs among HSCT recipients. Researchers have reported that marijuana smoking might be associated with generation of invasive pulmonary aspergillosis among immunocompromised persons, including HSCT recipients (*326–329*). Therefore, HSCT recipients should refrain from smoking marijuana to avoid *Aspergillus* species exposure (*326,330–334*) (BIII).

Preventing Infections Transmitted Through Direct Contact and Respiratory Transmission

Researchers have proposed that immunocompromised HSCT recipients and candidates who are undergoing conditioning therapy avoid gardening or direct contact with soil, plants, or their aerosols to reduce exposure to potential pathogens (e.g., *To. gondii*, *Hi. capsulatum*, *Cryptococcus neoformans*, *Nocardia* species, and *Aspergillus* species) (CIII). HSCT recipients, particularly allogeneic recipients, could wear gloves while gardening or touching plants or soil (*335*) (CIII), and they should avoid creating plant or soil aerosols (BIII). Additionally, they should always wash their hands afterwards (*335*) and care for skin abrasions or cuts sustained during soil or plant contact (AIII).

Persons whose occupations involve animal contact (e.g., veterinarians, pet store employees, farmers, or slaughterhouse workers) could be at increased risk for toxoplasmosis and other zoonotic diseases. Although data are insufficient to justify a general recommendation against HSCT recipients working in such settings, these exposures should be avoided during the first 6 months after HSCT and during other periods of substantial immunosuppression (e.g., GVHD, systemic steroid use, or relapse of the underlying disease for which the transplant was performed) (BIII).

Safe Sex

Sexually active HSCT recipients should avoid sexual practices that could result in oral exposure to feces (*5,316*) (AIII). Sexually active patients who are not in long-term monogamous relationships should always use latex condoms during sexual contact to reduce their risk for exposure to CMV, HSV, HIV, hepatitis B and C, and other sexually transmitted pathogens (AII). However, even long-time monogamous partners can be discordant for these infections. Therefore, during periods of immunocompromise, sexually active HSCT recipients in such relationships should consider using latex condoms during sexual contact to reduce the risk for exposure to these sexually transmitted infections (CIII).

Pet Safety

Preventing Pet-Transmitted Zoonotic Infections

HSCT physicians should advise recipients and candidates undergoing conditioning therapy of the potential infection risks posed by pet ownership; however, they should not routinely advise HSCT recipients to part with their pets, with limited exceptions. Generally, immunocompromised HSCT recipients and candidates undergoing conditioning therapy should minimize direct contact with animals (*336,337*), particularly those animals that are ill (e.g., with diarrhea) (*335*) (BIII). Immunocompromised persons who choose to own pets should be more vigilant regarding maintenance of their pet's health than immunocompetent pet owners (BIII). This recommendation means seeking veterinary care for their pet early in the pet's illness to minimize the possible transmission of the pet's illness to the owner (*335*) (BIII). Feeding pets only high-quality commercial pet foods reduces the possibility of illness caused by spoiled or contaminated foods, thus reducing the possibility of transmitting illness from the pet to the HSCT recipient. If eggs, poultry, or meat products are given to the pet as supplements, they should be well-cooked. Any dairy products given to pets should be pasteurized (*335*) (BIII). Pets should be prevented from drinking toilet bowl water and from having access to garbage; pets should not scavenge, hunt, or eat other animals' feces (*335*) (BIII).

If HSCT recipients have contact with pets or animals, they should wash their hands after handling them (particularly before eating) and after cleaning cages; HSCT recipients should avoid contact with animal feces to reduce the risk for toxoplasmosis, cryptosporidiosis, salmonellosis, and campylobacteriosis (*335*) (BIII). Adults should supervise hand washing of pediatric HSCT recipients (BIII). Immunocompromised HSCT recipients and candidates should not clean pet litter boxes or cages or dispose of animal waste (DIII). If this cannot be avoided, patients should wear disposable gloves during such activities and wash their hands thoroughly afterwards (BIII). Immunocompromised HSCT recipients and candidates should avoid adopting ill or juvenile pets (e.g., aged <6 months for cats) (*335*) and any stray animals (*5,316*) (BIII). Any pet that experiences diarrhea should be checked by a veterinarian for infection with *Cryptosporidium* (*5,316*), *Giardia* species (*335*), *Salmonella*, and *Campylobacter* (*5,335,337*) (BIII).

Immunocompromised HSCT recipients and candidates should not have contact with reptiles (e.g., snakes, lizards, turtles, or iguanas) (DII) to reduce their risk for acquiring salmonellosis (*335,338–341*). Additionally, patients should be informed that salmonellosis can occur from fomite contact alone (*342*). Therefore, HSCT recipients and candidates should avoid contact with a reptile, its food, or anything that it has touched, and if such contact occurs, recipients and candidates should wash their hands thoroughly afterwards (AIII). Immunocompromised HSCT recipients and candidates should avoid contact with ducklings and chicks because of the risk for acquiring *Salmonella* or

Campylobacter species infections (*338,343*) (BIII). Immunocompromised HSCT recipients and candidates should avoid contact with exotic pets (e.g., nonhuman primates) (BIII). Bird cage linings should be cleaned regularly (e.g., daily) (*337*). All persons, but particularly immunocompromised HSCT candidates and recipients, should wear gloves whenever handling items contaminated with bird droppings (*337*) (BIII) because droppings can be a source of *Cryptococcus neoformans*, *Mycobacterium avium*, or *Hi. capsulatum*. However, routine screening of healthy birds for these diseases is not recommended (*335*) (DIII). To minimize potential exposure to *Mycobacterium marinum*, immunocompromised HSCT recipients and candidates should not clean fish tanks (DIII). If this task cannot be avoided, patients should wear disposable gloves during such activities and wash their hands thoroughly afterwards (*335,337*) (BIII).

Preventing Toxoplasmosis

The majority of toxoplasmosis cases in the United States is acquired through eating undercooked meat (*335,337*). However, all HSCT recipients and candidates, particularly those who are *To. gondii* seronegative, should be informed of the risks for contracting toxoplasmosis from cat feces (BIII), but need not be advised to give away their cats (DII). For households with cats, litter boxes should not be placed in kitchens, dining rooms, or other areas where food preparation and eating occur (*335*). Additionally, litter boxes should be cleaned daily by someone other than the HSCT recipient during the first 6 months after HSCT and during periods of substantial immunosuppression (e.g., GVHD, steroid use, or relapse of the underlying disease for which the transplant was performed) to reduce the risk for transmitting toxoplasmosis to the HSCT recipient (BIII). Daily litter box changes will minimize the risk for fecal transmission of *To. gondii* oocysts, because fecal oocysts require ≥2 days of incubation to become infectious. If HSCT recipients perform this task during the first 6 months after HSCT and during subsequent periods of substantial immunocompromise (e.g., during GVHD, systemic steroid use, or relapse of the underlying neoplastic disease for which the transplant was performed), they should wear disposable gloves (*335*). Gloves should be discarded after a single use (BIII). Soiled, dried litter should be disposed of carefully to prevent aerosolizing the *To. gondii* oocysts (BIII). Cat feces (but not litter) can be flushed down the toilet (BIII). Also, persons who clean cat litter, particularly HSCT recipients, should wash their hands thoroughly with soap and water afterwards to reduce their risk for acquiring toxoplasmosis (BIII).

HSCT recipients and candidates with cats should keep their cats inside (BIII) and should not adopt or handle stray cats (DIII). Cats should be fed only canned or dried commercial food or well-cooked table food, not raw or undercooked meats, to eliminate the possibility of causing an illness that could be transmitted from the cat to the HSCT recipient (BIII). Pet cats of HSCT recipients do not need to be tested for toxoplasmosis (EII). Playground sandboxes should be kept covered when not in use to prevent cats from soiling them (BIII). HSCT recipients and candidates undergoing conditioning therapy should avoid drinking raw goat's milk to decrease the risk for acquiring toxoplasmosis (BIII).

Water and Other Beverage Safety

Although limited data were found regarding the risks for and epidemiology of *Cryptosporidium* disease among HSCT recipients, HSCT recipients are prudent to avoid possible exposures to *Cryptosporidium* (BIII) because it has been reported to cause severe, chronic diarrhea, malnutrition, and death among other immunocompromised persons (*5,318,319*). HSCT recipients should avoid walking, wading, swimming, or playing in recreational water (e.g., ponds or lakes) that is likely to be contaminated with *Cryptosporidium, Es. coli* O157:H7 (*344–346*), sewage, or animal or human waste (BII). HSCT recipients should also avoid swallowing such water (e.g., while swimming) (*5,344,346*) as well as any water taken directly from rivers and lakes (*5,316*) (AIII).

HSCT recipients should not use well water from private wells or from public wells in communities with limited populations (DIII) because tests for microbial contamination are performed too infrequently (e.g., in certain locations, tests are performed ≤1 times/ month) to detect sporadic bacterial contamination. However, drinking well water from municipal wells serving highly populated areas is regarded as safe from bacterial contamination because the water is tested ≥2 times/day for bacterial contamination. If HSCT recipients consume tap water, they should routinely monitor mass media (e.g., radio, television, or newspapers) in their area to immediately implement any boil-water advisories that might be issued for immunocompromised persons by state or local governments (BIII). A boil-water advisory means that all tap water should be boiled for ≥1 minutes before it is consumed. Tap water might not be completely free of *Cryptosporidium*. To eliminate the risk for *Cryptosporidium* exposure from tap water, HSCT recipients can boil tap water for ≥1 minutes before consuming it (e.g., drinking or brushing teeth) (*5*) (CIII). Alternately, they can use certain types of water filters (*316*) or a home distiller (*317*) to reduce their risk for *Cryptosporidium* (*5*) and other waterborne pathogens (CIII). If a home water filter* is used, it should be capable of removing particles ≥1 μm in diameter, or filter by reverse osmosis. However, the majority of these filters are not capable of removing smaller microbes (e.g., bacteria or viruses), and therefore, should only be used on properly treated municipal water. Further, the majority of these devices would not be appropriate for use on an unchlorinated private well to control viral or bacterial pathogens. Bottled water can be consumed if it has been processed to remove *Cryptosporidium* by one of three processes — reverse osmosis, distillation, or 1-μm particulate absolute filtration. To confirm that a specific bottled water has undergone one of these processes, HSCT recipients should contact the bottler directly.[†]

Patients can take other precautions in the absence of boil-water advisories to further reduce their risk for cryptosporidiosis. These extra precautions include avoiding fountain beverages and ice made from tap water at restaurants, bars, and theaters (*5*), fruit drinks made from frozen concentrate mixed with tap water, and iced tea or coffee made with tap water (*317*). Drinks that are likely to be *Cryptosporidium* safe for HSCT recipients include nationally distributed brands of bottled or canned carbonated soft drinks and beers (*5*); commercially packaged noncarbonated drinks that contain fruit juice; fruit juices that do not require refrigeration until after opening (e.g., those that are stored unrefrigerated on grocery shelves) (*5*); canned or bottled soda, seltzer or fruit drinks; steaming hot (≥175 F) tea or coffee (*317*); juices labeled as pasteurized; and nationally distributed brands of frozen fruit juice concentrate that are reconstituted with water from

---

*For a list of filters certified under NSF Standard 053 for cyst (i.e., *Cryptosporidium*) removal, contact the NSF International consumer line at (800) 673-8010 or <http://www.nsf.org/notice/ crypto.html>.

[†] The International Bottled Water Association can be contacted at (703) 683-5213 from 9 a.m. to 5 p.m. EST or anytime at their Internet site (<http://www.bottledwater.org>) to obtain contact information regarding water bottlers.

a safe source (5). HSCT recipients should not drink unpasteurized milk or fruit or vegetable juices (e.g., apple cider or orange juice) to avoid infection with *Brucella* species, *Es. coli* O157:H7, *Salmonella* species, *Cryptosporidium*, and others (*319,347–351*) (DII).

Food Safety

HSCT candidates and household or family members who prepare food for them after HSCT should review food safety practices that are appropriate for all persons (*352*) (AIII), and food preparers should be educated regarding additional food safety practices appropriate for HSCT recipients. This review and education should be done before the conditioning regimen (i.e., chemotherapy and radiation) begins (BIII). Adherence to these guidelines will decrease the risk for foodborne disease among HSCT recipients.

Food Safety Practices Appropriate for All Persons

Raw poultry, meats, fish, and seafood should be handled on separate surfaces (e.g., cutting board or counter top) from other food items. Food preparers should always use separate cutting boards (i.e., one for poultry and other meats and one for vegetables and remaining cutting or carving tasks) (AIII), or the board(s) should be washed with warm water and soap between cutting different food items (AIII). To prevent foodborne illnesses caused by *Campylobacter jejuni* and *Salmonella enteritidis*, which can cause severe and invasive infections among immunocompromised persons (*353,354*), uncooked meats should not come in contact with other foods (BIII).

After preparing raw poultry, meats, fish, and seafood and before preparing other foods, food handlers should wash their hands thoroughly in warm, soapy water. Any cutting boards, counters, knives, and other utensils used should be washed thoroughly in warm, soapy water also (AIII). Food preparers should keep shelves, counter tops, refrigerators, freezers, utensils, sponges, towels, and other kitchen items clean (AIII). All fresh produce should be washed thoroughly under running water before serving (*355*) (AIII). Persons preparing food should follow published U.S. Department of Agriculture recommendations regarding safe food thawing (*356*) (BIII).

Persons cooking food for HSCT recipients should follow established guidelines for monitoring internal cooking temperatures for meats (*357*) (AII). The only method for determining whether the meat has been adequately cooked is to measure its internal temperature with a thermometer because the color of the meat after cooking does not reliably reflect the internal temperature. Different kinds of meat should be cooked to varying internal temperatures, all ≥150 F (AII). Specifically, the U.S. Department of Agriculture recommends that poultry be cooked to an internal temperature of 180 F; other meats and egg-containing casseroles and souffles should be cooked to an internal temperature of ≥160 F. Cold foods should be stored at <40 F; hot foods should be kept at >140 F (BIII). Food preparers should

- wash their hands before and after handling leftovers (AIII);

- use clean utensils and food-preparation surfaces (AIII);

- divide leftovers into small units and store in shallow containers for quick cooling (AII);

- refrigerate leftovers within 2 hours of cooking (AII).

- discard leftovers that were kept at room temperature for >2 hours (AIII);

- reheat leftovers or heat partially cooked foods to ≥165 F throughout before serving (AII);

- bring leftover soups, sauces, and gravies to a rolling boil before serving (AIII); and

- follow published guidelines for cold storage of food (352) (AII).

Additional Food Safety Practices Appropriate for HSCT Recipients

HSCT recipients' diets should be restricted to decrease the risk for exposure to foodborne infections from bacteria, yeasts, molds, viruses, and parasites (BIII). Currently, a low microbial diet is recommended for HSCT recipients (358,359) (BIII). This diet should be continued for 3 months after HSCT for autologous recipients. Allogeneic recipients should remain on the diet until all immunosuppressive drugs (e.g., cyclosporine, steroids, and tacrolimus) are discontinued. However, the HSCT physician should have final responsibility for determining when the diet can be discontinued safely. Only one study has reported that dietary changes (e.g., consuming yogurt) have decreased the risk for mycotic infections (e.g., candidal vaginitis) (360) (Table 3). HSCT recipients should not eat any raw or undercooked meat, including beef, poultry, pork, lamb, venison or other wild game, or combination dishes containing raw or undercooked meats or sweetbreads from these animals (e.g., sausages or casseroles) (AII). Also, HSCT recipients should not consume raw or undercooked eggs or foods that might contain them (e.g., certain preparations of hollandaise sauce, Caesar and other salad dressings, homemade mayonnaise, and homemade eggnog) because of the risk for infection with *Salmonella enteritidis* (354) (AII). HSCT recipients should not consume raw or undercooked seafood (e.g., oysters or clams) to prevent exposure to *Vibrio* species, viral gastroenteritis, and *Cryptosporidium parvum* (361–364) (AII).

HSCT recipients and candidates should only consume meat that is well-done when they or their caretakers do not have direct control over food preparation (e.g., when eating in a restaurant) (AI). To date, no evidence exists in the United States that eating food at a fast food restaurant is riskier than eating at a conventional sit-down restaurant. Generally, HSCT candidates undergoing conditioning therapy and HSCT recipients with neutropenia (i.e., ANC < 1,000/ml^3), GVHD, or immunosuppression should avoid exposures to naturopathic medicines that might contain molds (365) (DIII). HSCT recipients wishing to take naturopathic medications are advised to use them only as prescribed by a licensed naturopathic physician working in consultation with the recipient's transplant and infectious disease physicians (CIII).

Travel Safety

Travel to developing countries can pose substantial risks for exposure to opportunistic pathogens for HSCT recipients, particularly allogeneic recipients chronically immunosuppressed. HSCT recipients should not plan travel to developing countries without consulting their physicians (AIII), and travel should not occur until the period of severe immunosuppression has resolved. Generally, allogeneic recipients should not plan travel to developing countries for 6–12 months after HSCT, particularly if GVHD has occurred. Autologous recipients can travel to developing countries 3–6 months after HSCT if their physicians agree.

HSCT recipients should be informed regarding strategies to minimize the risk for acquiring foodborne and waterborne infections while traveling. They should obtain updated, detailed health information for international travelers from health organizations (*366,367*) (AIII). Generally, while traveling in developing countries, HSCT recipients should avoid consuming the following (BIII):

- raw fruits and vegetables,

- tap water or any potentially untreated or contaminated water,

- ice made from tap water or any potentially contaminated water,

- unpasteurized milk or any unpasteurized dairy products,

- fresh fruit juices,

- food and drinks from street vendors, and

- raw or undercooked eggs.

Steaming hot foods, fruits peeled by oneself, bottled and canned processed drinks, and hot coffee or tea are probably safe (*367,368*). Travelers should plan for treating their drinking water while in developing countries. If bottled water is not available, boiling is the best method of making water safe. However, if boiling water is not feasible, the traveler should carry supplies for disinfecting water (e.g., commercially available iodine disinfection tablets or a portable water filter) (*366,368*).

Antimicrobial prophylaxis for traveler's diarrhea is not recommended routinely for HSCT recipients traveling to developing countries (DIII) because traveler's diarrhea is not known to be more frequent or more severe among immunocompromised hosts. However, HSCT physicians who wish to provide prophylaxis to HSCT recipients who are traveling can prescribe a fluoroquinolone (e.g., ciprofloxacin hydrochloride) or TMP-SMZ (CIII), although resistance to TMP-SMZ is now common and resistance to fluoroquinolones is increasing in tropical areas (Appendix). Researchers recommend using bismuth subsalicylate to prevent traveler's diarrhea among adults (*366*). However, no data were found regarding safety and efficacy among HSCT recipients, and salicylates are not recommended for use among persons aged <18 years because salicylates are associated with Reye's syndrome (*369*).

HSCT recipients' immunization status should be assessed and their vaccinations updated as needed before travel (*366*). Influenza chemoprophylaxis with rimantadine or amantadine can be used for immunocompromised HSCT recipients who are traveling outside the continental United States and who could be exposed to influenza A (CIII).

HSCT RECIPIENT VACCINATIONS

Antibody titers to vaccine-preventable diseases (e.g., tetanus, polio, measles, mumps, rubella, and encapsulated organisms) decline during the 1–4 years after allogeneic or autologous HSCT (*66,370–373*) if the recipient is not revaccinated. Clinical relevance of decreased antibodies to vaccine-preventable diseases among HSCT recipients is not immediately apparent because a limited number of cases of vaccine-preventable diseases are reported among U.S. recipients. However, vaccine-preventable diseases still pose risks to the U.S. population. Additionally, evidence exists that certain vaccine-preventable diseases (e.g., encapsulated organisms) can pose increased risk for HSCT recipients (*66*); therefore, HSCT recipients should be routinely revaccinated after HSCT so that they can experience immunity to the same vaccine-preventable diseases as others (Table 4).

HSCT center personnel have developed vaccination schedules for HSCT recipients (*374*). One study determined that HSCT center personnel used 3–11 different vaccination schedules per vaccine (*374*); consequently, the study authors requested national guidelines for doses and timing of vaccines after HSCT to eliminate confusion among HSCT center personnel regarding how to vaccinate their patients. To address this need, an interim vaccination schedule for HSCT recipients was drafted in collaboration with partner organizations, including CDC's Advisory Committee on Immunization Practices. The purpose of the vaccination schedule in these guidelines is to provide guidance for HSCT centers (Table 4). Although limited data were found regarding safety and immunogenicity (e.g., serologic studies of antibody titers after vaccination) among HSCT recipients, no data were found regarding vaccine efficacy among HSCT recipients (e.g., which determine whether vaccinated HSCT recipients have decreased attack rates of disease compared with unvaccinated HSCT recipients). Because certain HSCT recipients have faster immune system recovery after HSCT than others, researchers have proposed that different vaccination schedules be recommended for recipients of different types of HSCT. However, to date, data are too limited to do so. Therefore, the same vaccination schedule is recommended for all HSCT recipients (e.g., allogeneic, autologous, and bone marrow, peripheral, or UCB grafts) until additional data are published. In the tables, vaccines have only been recommended for use among HSCT recipients if evidence exists of safety and immunogenicity for those recipients. Vaccination of family members, household contacts, and HCWs are also recommended to minimize exposure of vaccine-preventable diseases among HSCT recipients (Tables 5–8).

HEMATOPOIETIC STEM CELL SAFETY

With allogeneic HSCT, the life of the recipient might depend on the timely selection of an acceptable HLA-matched donor. Only a limited number of HLA-matched donors might be identified; hence, the transplant physician often has to accept a higher risk for transmission of an infectious agent through HSCT than would be permitted for routine blood transfusion. This section provides strategies for the HSCT physician to minimize transmission of infectious diseases, whenever possible, from donors to recipients.*† Whether to select a donor who is at risk for or who has an infectious disease transmissible by HSCT, should be determined on a case-by-case basis (AIII) and is the final responsibility of the HSCT physician (AIII). If the only possible donor is at risk for or known to be infected with a bloodborne pathogen and the patient is likely to succumb rapidly from his or her disease if an HSCT is not received, the physician must carefully weigh the risks and benefits of using potentially infected donor cells. No person should be denied a potentially life-saving HSCT procedure solely on the basis of the risk for an infectious disease. However, HSCT physicians should avoid transplanting any infected or infectious donor hematopoietic stem cell product unless no other stem cell product can be obtained and

---

*The U.S. Public Health Service is reexamining the current donor deferral recommendations regarding risk behaviors for donors of organs, cells, tissues, xenotransplantation, and reproductive cells and tissue, including semen, and revisions to these guidelines could become necessary as the research evolves.

† Guidelines for screening UCB donors and their mothers are evolving and will not be addressed in this document.

the risk for death from not undergoing transplantation is deemed to be greater than the risk for morbidity or death from the infection that could potentially be transmitted (DII). If such a product is selected for use, it should be done on a case-by-case basis (*375*) and the following should be noted in the recipient's chart:

- knowledge and authorization of the recipient's HSCT physician regarding the potential for transmission of an infectious agent during HSCT, and

- advance informed consent from the recipient or recipient's legal guardian acknowledging the possible transmission of an infectious agent during the transplantation (AIII).

Subsequently, the HSCT physician should include the infectious agent in the differential diagnosis of any illness that the HSCT recipient experiences so that the infection, if transmitted, can be diagnosed early and treated preemptively, if possible. Infectious products (except those in which CMV seropositivity is the only evidence of infectiousness) should be labeled as being a biohazard or as untested for biohazards, as applicable. Tissue intended for autologous use should be labeled "For Autologous Use Only — Use Only for (Patient's Name)."

Preventing Transmission of Infections from HSCT Donors to Recipients

All prospective HSCT donors should be evaluated through a physical history and examination to determine their general state of health and whether they pose a risk for transmitting infectious diseases to the recipient (*376*). To detect transmissible infections, all HSCT donor collection site personnel should follow up-to-date published guidelines and standards for donor screening (e.g., medical history), physical exam, and serologic testing (*377–383*) (AIII). Initial donor screening and physical exam should be performed ≤8 weeks before the planned donation (BIII). Donor serologic testing should be done ≤30 days before donation to detect potentially transmissible infections (BII); additionally, researchers recommend that donors be retested ≤7 days before collection. If testing is done >7 days before donation, donor screening should be repeated to ensure that no new risk behaviors have occurred during the interval between the original screening and the time of donation (BIII). This practice is critical because if new behavioral risk factors have occurred, the potential donor might need to be deferred. Screening and testing should be done on all allogeneic or syngeneic donors (AIII). Screening and testing of autologous donors is recommended to ensure the safety of laboratory personnel and to prevent cross contamination (BIII). If autologous donors are not tested, their autologous units should be specially labeled and handled as if potentially infected (BIII). For donors screened in the United States, FDA-licensed or -approved tests should be used in accordance with the manufacturers' instructions (AIII), and the donor samples should be tested in laboratories certified by the Clinical Laboratory Improvement Amendments of 1988 (AIII).

All HSCT donors should be in good general health (*376*) (BIII). Acute or chronic illness in the prospective donor should be investigated to determine the etiology. Generally, persons who are ill should not be HSCT donors (DIII). A flu-like illness in a prospective donor at the time of evaluation or between the time of evaluation and donation should prompt evaluation of and serologic testing for infections that might pose a risk to the recipient (e.g., EBV, CMV, *To. gondii*) (BIII). Persons with a positive serum EBV-viral capsid antigen IgM but negative serum EBV-viral capsid antigen IgG should not serve as donors for allogeneic T-cell–depleted HSCT, particularly for unrelated or mismatched transplants, until their serum EBV-viral capsid antigen IgG becomes positive (DIII). Persons with acute toxoplasmosis should not donate until the acute illness has resolved (DII); however, physicians should be aware that persons who are asymptomatically seropositive for *To. gondii* might transmit this infection through HSCT (*218*).

Prospective donors with symptoms of active TB should be evaluated for that disease (*383*) (BIII). Prospective donors with active TB should not donate (EIII) until the TB is well-controlled (e.g., no longer contagious as determined by the donor's primary physician) after appropriate medical therapy. However, no known risk exists from transplanting marrow from an untreated, tuberculin-positive donor who has no evidence of active disease. Screening potential donors for TB with Mantoux skin tests (DIII) is not necessary. Prospective HSCT donors who reside in or have traveled to areas endemic for rickettsia or other tickborne pathogens and who are suspected of having an acute tickborne infection should be temporarily deferred as donors until infection with these pathogens is excluded (DIII). Relevant pathogens include *Rickettsia rickettsii*, *Babesia microti* and other *Babesia* species, *Coxiella burnetii*, and the Colorado tick fever virus, which are the etiologic agents of Rocky Mountain spotted fever, babesiosis, Q fever, and Colorado tick fever, respectively; these pathogens have been reported to be transmitted by blood transfusion (*384–388*). Researchers recommend deferral for a past history of Q fever or babesiosis because these infections can be chronic and the babesiosis parasite might persist despite appropriate therapy (*389*) (CIII). Additionally, researchers have recommended deferring persons with acute human ehrlichiosis (e.g., human active human granulocytic ehrlichiosis [*390*], human monocytic ehrlichiosis, as well as any infections from *Ehrlichia ewingii*) from HSCT donation (CIII).

The medical history of the prospective HSCT donor should include the following:

- History of vaccinations (*377*) during the 4 weeks before donation (AII). If the potential donor is unsure of vaccinations received, his or her records should be reviewed. HSCT donation should be deferred for 4 weeks after the donor receives any live-attenuated vaccine (e.g., rubeola [measles], mumps, rubella [German measles], oral polio, varicella, yellow fever, and oral typhoid vaccines) (EIII). This deferral will avoid the possibility of infusing a live infectious agent into an HSCT recipient. HSCT donation need not be deferred for persons who have recently received toxoid or killed (i.e., inactivated), recombinant viral, bacterial, or rickettsial vaccines as long as the donor is asymptomatic and afebrile (*389*) (BIII). Such vaccines include tetanus toxoid, diphtheria toxoid, hepatitis A and B, cholera, influenza (i.e., killed intramuscular vaccine), meningococcal, paratyphoid, pertussis, plague, polio (i.e., inactivated polio vaccine), rabies, typhoid (i.e., inactivated intramuscular vaccine), or typhus vaccines (*389*).

- Travel history (BIII) to determine whether the donor has ever resided in or traveled to countries with endemic diseases that might be transmitted through HSCT (e.g., malaria). Permanent residents of nonendemic countries who have traveled to an area that CDC regards as endemic for malaria can be accepted as HSCT donors if 1 year has elapsed since the donor's departure from the endemic area and if the donor has been free of malaria symptoms, regardless of whether he or she received antimalarial chemoprophylaxis. Because cases of

HSCT-transmitted malaria have been reported (*391,392*), persons who have had malaria and received appropriate treatment should be deferred from HSCT donation for 3 years after becoming asymptomatic. Immigrants, refugees, citizens, or residents for ≥5 years of endemic countries can be accepted as HSCT donors if 3 years have elapsed since they departed the malarious area and if they have been free of malaria symptoms.

- History of Chagas' disease and leishmaniasis. Persons with active Chagas' disease or leishmaniasis should not serve as HSCT donors (DIII) because these diseases can be transmitted by transfusion (*227,229,231,393–395*). Researchers also recommend deferral of HSCT donation if a past history exists of either of these diseases because the parasite can persist despite therapy (*227–229,231, 389,393–395*) (CIII).

- History of any deferral from plasma or blood donation. The reason for such a deferral (*376*) and whether it was based on a reported infectious disease or behavioral or other risk factor should be investigated (BIII).

- History of viral hepatitis. A person with a history of viral hepatitis after his or her eleventh birthday should be excluded from HSCT donation (BIII).

- History of blood product transfusion, solid organ transplantation, or transplantation of tissue within the last 12 months (BIII). Such persons should be excluded from HSCT donation (DIII). Xenotransplant product recipients and their close contacts should be indefinitely deferred from donating any blood products, including hematopoietic stem cells, whole blood, or other blood components including plasma, leukocytes, and tissues (*396*) (AIII). Close contacts to be deferred from donations include persons who have engaged repeatedly in activities that could result in an intimate exchange of body fluids with a xenotransplantation product recipient. Such close contacts could include sexual partners, household members who share razors or toothbrushes, and HCWs or laboratory personnel with repeated percutaneous, mucosal, or other direct exposures.

- History of risk factors for classic Creutzfeldt-Jakob disease (CJD), including any blood relative with Creutzfeldt-Jakob disease, receipt of a human pituitary-derived growth hormone or receipt of a corneal or dura mater graft (*383,397–399*) (BIII). Potential HSCT donors should also be screened for new variant Creutzfeldt-Jakob Disease (nvCJD) risk factors, including a history of cumulative travel or residence in the United Kingdom for ≥6 months during 1980–1996 or receipt of injectable bovine insulin since 1980, unless the product was not manufactured since 1980 from cattle in the United Kingdom (*398*) (BIII). The clinical latency period for iatrogenic, classic CJD can be >30 years (*398*), and transmission of classic CJD by blood products is highly unlikely (*398*). Although no classic or nvCJD has ever been reported among HSCT recipients, persons with a history of classic or nvCJD risk factors should be excluded from donation for unrelated HSCT (DIII) if a choice exists between two otherwise equally suitable donors. The risk for transmitting classic or nvCJD from an HSCT donor to a recipient is unknown, but researchers believe that persons with nvCJD risk factors could be at higher risk for transmitting nvCJD to HSCT recipients than persons with classic CJD risk factors.

- Past medical history that indicates the donor has clinical evidence of or is at high risk for acquiring a bloodborne infection (e.g., HIV-1 or -2, human T-lymphotropic virus [HTLV]-I or -II, hepatitis C, or hepatitis B) (*381,383*), including

  — men who have had sex with another man during the preceding 5 years (*381,383*) (BIII);

  — persons who report nonmedical intravenous, intramuscular, or subcutaneous injection of drugs during the preceding 5 years (*381*) (BIII);

  — persons with hemophilia or related clotting disorders who have received human-derived clotting factor concentrates (*381*) (BIII);

  — persons who have engaged in sex in exchange for money or drugs during the preceding 5 years (*381*) (BIII);

  — persons who have had sex during the preceding 12 months with any person described previously (*381*) or with a person known or suspected to have HIV (*381*) or hepatitis B infections (BIII);

  — persons who have been exposed during the preceding 12 months to known or suspected HIV, hepatitis B- or C-infected blood through percutaneous inoculation or through contact with an open wound, nonintact skin, or mucous membrane (*381*) (BIII);

  — inmates of correctional systems (*379–381*) and persons who have been incarcerated for >72 consecutive hours during the previous 12 months (BIII);

  — persons who have had or have been treated for syphilis or gonorrhea during the preceding 12 months (*376,379,380*) (BIII); and

  — persons who within 12 months have undergone tattooing, acupuncture, ear or body piercing (*380,400,401*) in which shared instruments are known to have been used (BIII) or other nonsterile conditions existed.

Persons reporting any of these past medical histories should be excluded from donation (DIII).

The following serologic tests should be performed for each prospective donor:

- HIV-1 antigen, anti-HIV-1 and -2, anti-HTLV-I and -II, hepatitis B surface antigen, total antihepatitis B core antigen, antihepatitis C, anti-CMV, and a serologic test for syphilis (*376,379,380,383*) (AIII). Potential donors who have repeatedly reactive screening tests for HIV-1 antigen, anti-HIV-1 or -2, anti-HTLV-I or -II, antihepatitis C, hepatitis B surface antigen, or antihepatitis B core antigen should be excluded as HSCT donors (*381*) (EII). Persons who refuse infectious disease testing should also be excluded as HSCT donors (*381*) (EIII).

- Investigational nucleic acid tests to detect hepatitis C virus RNA and HIV RNA are currently being used in the United States to screen blood donors and could be used for screening HSCT donors. If nucleic acid tests are approved by FDA, these tests should be incorporated into routine screening regimens for HSCT donors. When nucleic acid testing is done for HIV and hepatitis C investigationally, a positive result should exclude the potential donor.

All infectious disease testing and results should be reported to the HSCT physician before the candidate's conditioning regimen begins (*381*) (AIII). Bone marrow should be collected using sterile technique in a medically acceptable setting and according to standard operating procedures (AIII).

HSCT transplant center personnel should keep accurate records of all HSCT received and the disposition of each sample obtained (*381*). These tracking records must be separate from patients' medical records (e.g., in a log book) so that this information is easily obtainable. Recorded information should include the donor identification number, name of procurement of distribution center supplying the HSCT, recipient-identifying information, name of recipient's physician, and dates of a) receipt by the HSCT center and b) either transplantation to the recipient or further distribution (*381*) (AIII). All centers for donation, transplantation, or collection of hematopoietic stem cells should keep records of donor screening and testing, and HSCT harvesting, processing, testing, cryopreservation, storage, and infusion or disposal of each aliquot of donated hematopoietic progenitor cells for ≥10 years after the date of implantation, transplantation, infusion, or transfer of the product (*378*) (AIII). However, if that date is not known, records should be retained ≥10 years after the product's distribution, disposition, or expiration, whichever is latest.

Pediatric Donors

Children aged >18 months who are born to mothers with or at risk for HIV infection, who have not been breast-fed during the past 12 months, and whose HIV antibody tests, physical examination, and medical records do not indicate evidence of HIV infection can be accepted as donors (*381*) (BIII). Children aged <18 months who are born to mothers with or at risk for HIV infection and who have not been breast-fed by an HIV-infected woman during the past 12 months can be accepted as donors only if HIV infection has been excluded according to established criteria (*402*) (BIII). Children who have been breast-fed by an HIV-infected woman during the past 12 months should be excluded as stem cell donors regardless of HIV infection status (AIII). The mother and, if possible, the father of all pediatric stem-cell donors who are at risk for perinatal transmission of HIV and other bloodborne infections, should be interviewed by a health-care professional competent to elicit information regarding risk factors for possible bloodborne infection in the potential pediatric donor (AIII). Children who meet any of the adult donor exclusion criteria should not become HSCT donors (*381*) (EIII).

Preventing Infection from Extraneous Contamination of Donated Units

Personnel of donation, collection, or transplantation centers, cell-processing laboratories, and courier services should follow current standards for detecting and preventing extrinsic bacterial and fungal contamination of collected stem cell units at the collection site, during processing and transportation, and at the transplant center (*376*) (AIII). Quality improvement programs and procedure manuals of collection centers, cell-processing laboratories, and transplant programs should include strategies for preventing transplant-associated infections. For example, collection centers should use aseptic techniques when collecting marrow, peripheral blood, and UCB hematopoietic stem cells (*376,378*) (AIII). Whenever possible, closed systems should be used for pooling hematopoietic stem cells during a collection procedure (BIII) because higher rates of microbial contamination seen in marrow harvests versus blood stem cell collections can be caused by use of open collecting systems (*375,403,404*). The highest risk for extraneous microbial contamination of hematopoietic stem cells occurs during extensive manipulation and processing in the laboratory (*404,405*). Potential sources include unprotected hands and laboratory equipment and freezers (*406*), particularly the liquid phases of liquid nitrogen freezers (*407*). Therefore, stem cell processing should be performed according to current standards (*378*) using approved manufacturing practices (AIII). Hematopoietic stem cell units thawed in a water bath should be enclosed in a second bag (i.e., double-bagged technique) to prevent contamination of the ports or caps from unsterile bath water (*407*) (BIII). Additionally, water baths should be cleaned routinely (BIII) and certain researchers have proposed that the bath contain sterile water (*407*) (CIII). Researchers also report sterilizing liquid nitrogen freezers before initial use for hematopoietic stem cell storage (*407*) until fungal and bacterial cultures are negative (CIII).

Cell-processing laboratory personnel should implement programs to detect extrinsic bacterial or fungal contamination of collected stem cell units, ideally before transplantation (AIII). Although repeated cultures are costly (*408*), donated hematopoietic stem cells should be cultured for aerobic bacteria and fungi ≥1 times during initial processing and freezing (BIII). Researchers also have proposed adding anaerobic bacterial cultures and culturing twice, once at the end of processing, and once after thawing just before use (*407*) (CIII). If bacterial culture results are positive, antibiotic-susceptibility tests should be performed (BIII). Results of cultures and antibiotic-susceptibility tests should be provided to the transplant physician before release of a cryopreserved marrow or blood stem cell unit, and as soon as feasible for transplants infused before completion of culture incubation (BIII).

Collection center, cell-processing laboratory, and transplant program personnel should maintain active surveillance of infections among persons who have received hematopoietic stem cells from those facilities to collect data regarding the number of infections after HSCT that might have been caused by exogenous contamination of donor stem cells (BIII) because this type of infection has been reported (*405*).

In Utero or Fetal HSCT

No national standards exist for in utero or fetal HSCT, and the overall risks for transmitting infections to a fetus through HSCT (*409,410*) have not been determined. However, in addition to precautions appropriate for adult recipients, physicians performing in utero or fetal HSCT are advised to evaluate potential donors for evidence of active infectious diseases that could cause serious congenital infections (e.g., rubella, varicella, CMV, syphilis, or *To. gondii*) in the fetus (CIII).

Acknowledgments

The authors gratefully acknowledge the assistance of the following persons in the preparation of this report: Jon S. Abramson, M.D.; Saundra N. Aker, R.D.; George J. Alangaden, M.D.; Ann Arvin, M.D.; Carol Baker, M.D.; Michael Boeckh, M.D.; Brian J. Bolwell, M.D.; John M. Boyce, M.D.; C. Dean Buckner, M.D.; Pranatharthi H. Chandrasekar, M.D.; D.W. Chen, M.D., M.P.H.; Joan Chesney, M.D.; Raymond Chinn, M.D.; Christina Cicogna, M.D.; Dennis Confer, M.D.; Stella M. Davies, M.D., Ph.D.; Alfred DeMaria, Jr., M.D.; David W. Denning, M.B.B.S.; Joseph Fay, M.D.; Stephen Forman, M.D.; Michael Gerber, M.D.; Anne A. Gershon, M.D.; Stuart L. Goldberg, M.D.; Marie Gourdeau, M.D.; Christine J. Hager, Ph.D.; Rebecca Haley, M.D.; Liana Harvath, Ph.D.; Kelly Henning, M.D.; Steve Heyse; Elizabeth Higgs; Kevin High, M.D.; Mary M. Horowitz, M.D.; Craig W.S. Howe, M.D., Ph.D.; David D. Hurd, M.D.; Hakan Kuyu, M.D.; Amelia A. Langston, M.D.; Catherine Laughlin, Ph.D.; Hillard M. Lazarus, M.D.; Joseph H. Laver, M.D.; Helen Leather, Phar.D.; Paul R. McCurdy, M.D.; Carole Miller, M.D.; I. George Miller, M.D.; Per Ljungman, M.D., Ph.D.; Paul R. McCurdy, M.D.; Richard J. O'Reilly, M.D.; Gary Overturf, M.D.; Jan E. Patterson, M.D.; Lauren Patton, D.D.S.; Doug Peterson, D.D.S., Ph.D.; Donna Przepiorka, M.D., Ph.D.; Philip A. Pizzo, M.D.; Charles G. Prober, M.D.; Issam Raad, M.D.; Elizabeth C. Reed, M.D.; Frank Rhame, M.D.; Olle Ringdén, M.D.; Stephen M. Rose, Ph.D.; Scott D. Rowley, M.D.; Pablo Rubinstein, M.D.; Martin Ruta; Joel Ruskin, M.D.; Thomas N. Saari, M.D.; Stephen Schoenbaum, M.D.; Mark Schubert, D.D.S., M.S.D.; Jane D. Siegel, M.D.; Jacqueline Sheridan; Alicia Siston, M.D.; Trudy N. Small, M.D.; Frank O. Smith, M.D.; Ruth Solomon, M.D.; Cladd Stevens, M.D.; Patrick J. Stiff, M.D.; Andrew J. Streifel, M.P.H.; Donna A. Wall, M.D.; Thomas Walsh, M.D.; Phyllis Warkentin, M.D.; Robert A. Weinstein, M.D.; Estella Whimbey, M.D.; Richard Whitley, M.D.; Catherine Wilfert, M.D.; Drew J. Winston, M.D.; Jeffrey Wolf, M.D.; Andrew Yeager, M.D.; John A. Zaia, M.D.; and Carol Zukerman.

Contributions from the following CDC staff are also gratefully acknowledged: Larry J. Anderson, M.D.; Fred Angulo, D.V.M.; Richard Besser, M.D.; Jay C. Butler, M.D.; Donald Campbell; Mary E. Chamberland, M.D.; James Childs, Sc.D.; Nancy J. Cox, Ph.D.; Robert B. Craven, M.D.; Jackie Curlew; Vance J. Dietz, M.D., M.P.H.T.M.; Richard Facklam, Ph.D.; Cindy R. Friedman, M.D.; Keiji Fukuda, M.D., M.P.H.; Rana A. Hajjeh, M.D.; Barbara Herwaldt, M.D., M.P.H.; AnnMarie Jenkins; Dennis D. Juranek, D.V.M., M.Sc.; Paul Kilgore, M.D.; William Kohn, D.D.S.; Jacobus Kool, M.D., D.T.M.H.; John R. Livengood, M.D., M.Phil.; Eric Mast, M.D., M.P.H.; Michael McNeil, M.D., M.P.H.; Robin R. Moseley, M.A.T.; Thomas R. Navin, M.D.; Adelisa Panlilio, M.D., M.P.H.; Monica Parise, M.D.; Michele Pearson, M.D.; Bradford A. Perkins, M.D.; Renee Ridzon, M.D.; Martha Rogers, M.D.; Nancy Rosenstein, M.D.; Charles Rupprecht, Ph.D., V.M.D.; Peter Schantz, Ph.D.; Lawrence B. Schonberger, M.D., M.P.H.; Jane Seward, M.B.B.S., M.P.H.; John A. Stewart, M.D.; Raymond Strikas, M.D.; Robert V. Tauxe, M.D., M.P.H.; Theodore Tsai, M.D.; Rodrigo Villar, M.D.; David Wallace; and Sherilyn Wainwright, D.V.M., M.D.

The contributions of staff from other federal and nongovernmental agencies are also gratefully acknowledged: Agency for Healthcare Research and Quality; Food and Drug Administration; Health Resources and Services Administration; National Institutes of Health; National Cancer Institute; National Heart, Lung, and Blood Institute; National Institute for Allergy and Infectious Diseases; CDC's Advisory Committee on Immunization Practices; American Academy of Pediatrics' Committee on Infectious Diseases; American Association of Blood Banks; Hospital Infection Control Advisory Committee; International Society of Hematotherapy and Graft Engineering; National Marrow Donor Program; Southwest Oncology Group; Foundation for the Accreditation of Hematopoietic Cell Therapy; and Society for Healthcare Epidemiology of America.

References

Introduction

1. Institute of Medicine/Committee on Emerging Microbial Threats to Health. Emerging infections: microbial threats to health in the United States. Lederberg J, Shope RE, and Oaks SC Jr., eds. Washington, DC: National Academy Press, 1992. Available at <http://books.nap.edu/books/0309047412/html/index.html>. Accessed June 28, 2000.
2. CDC. Addressing emerging infectious disease threats: a prevention strategy for the United States. Atlanta, GA: US Department of Health and Human Services, Public Health Service, CDC, 1994. Available at <http://www.cdc.gov/ncidod/publications/eid_plan>. Accessed May 17, 2000.
3. CDC. USPHS/IDSA guidelines for the prevention of opportunistic infections in persons infected with human immunodeficiency virus: a summary. MMWR 1995;44(No. RR-8): 1–34.
4. CDC. 1997 USPHS/IDSA guidelines for the prevention of opportunistic infections in persons infected with human immunodeficiency virus. MMWR 1997;46(No. RR-12):1–46.
5. CDC. 1999 USPHS/IDSA guidelines for the prevention of opportunistic infections in persons infected with human immunodeficiency virus. MMWR 1999;48(No. RR-10):1–66.
6. Gross PA, Barrett TL, Dellinger EP, et al. Purpose of quality standards for infectious diseases. Clin Infect Dis 1994;18(3):421.

Background

7. Appelbaum FR. Use of bone marrow and peripheral blood stem cell transplantation in the treatment of cancer. CA Cancer J Clin 1996;46(3):142–64.
8. Kessinger A, Armitage JO. Use of peripheral stem cell support of high-dose chemotherapy. In: DeVita VT Jr., Hellman S, Rosenberg SA, eds. Important advances in oncology 1993. Philadelphia, PA: J.B.Lippincott Co. 1993.
9. Bortin MM, Horowitz MM, Gale RP, et al. Changing trends in allogeneic bone marrow transplantation for leukemia in the 1980s. JAMA 1992;268(5):607–12.
10. Sobocinski KA, Horowitz MM, Rowlings PA, et al. Bone marrow transplantation—1994: a report from the International Bone Marrow Transplant Registry and the North American Autologous Bone Marrow Transplant Registry. J Hematother 1994;3:95–102.
11. Zittoun RA, Mandelli F, Willemze R, et al. Autologous or allogeneic bone marrow transplantation compared with intensive chemotherapy in acute myelogenous leukemia. New Engl J Med 1995;332(4):217–23.
12. Thomas ED, Clift RA, Fefer A, et al. Marrow transplantation for the treatment of chronic myelogenous leukemia. Ann Intern Med 1986;104(2):155–63.
13. Storb R, Longton G, Anasetti C, et al. Changing trends in marrow transplantation for aplastic anemia [Review]. Bone Marrow Transplant 1992;10(suppl 1):45–52.
14. Mackinnon S, Hows JM, Goldman JM, et al. Bone marrow transplantation for chronic myeloid leukemia: the use of histocompatible unrelated volunteer donors. Exp Hematol 1990;18(5):421–5.
15. Kernan NA, Bartsch G, Ash RC, et al. Analysis of 462 transplantations from unrelated donors facilitated by the National Marrow Donor Program. N Engl J Med 1993;328(9): 593–602.
16. Nademanee AP, Schmidt GM, Parker P, et al. Outcome of matched unrelated donor bone marrow transplantation in patients with hematologic malignancies using molecular typing for donor selection and graft-versus-host disease prophylaxis regimen of cyclosporine, methotrexate, and prednisone. Blood 1995;86:1228–34.
17. Clift RA, Hansen JA, Thomas ED, et al. Marrow transplantation from donors other than HLA-identical siblings. Transplant 1979;28(3):235–42.
18. Beatty PG, Clift RA, Mickelson EM, et al. Marrow transplantation from related donors other than HLA-identical siblings. N Engl J Med 1985;313(13):765–71.
19. Ferrara JL, Deeg HJ. Graft-versus-host disease [Review]. N Engl J Med 1991;324(10): 667–74.

20. Marmont AM, Horowitz MM, Gale RP, et al. T-cell depletion of HLA-identical transplants in leukemia. Blood 1991;78(8):2120–30.
21. Rowlings PA. 1996 summary slides show current use and outcome of blood and marrow transplantation. Autologous Blood & Marrow Transplant Registry—North America: ABMTR Newsletter 1996;3(1):6–12.
22. Rubinstein P, Rosenfield RE, Adamson JW, Stevens CE. Stored placental blood for unrelated bone marrow reconstitution [Review]. Blood 1993;81(7):1679–90.
23. Kurtzberg J, Laughlin M, Graham ML, et al. Placental blood as a source of hematopoietic stem cells for transplantation into unrelated recipients. N Engl J Med 1996;335(3): 157–66.
24. Wagner JE, Rosenthal J, Sweetman R, et al. Successful transplantation of HLA-matched and HLA-mismatched umbilical cord blood from unrelated donors: analysis of engraftment and acute graft-versus-host disease. Blood 1996;88(3):795–802.
25. Meropol NJ, Overmoyer BA, Stadtmauer EA. High-dose chemotherapy with autologous stem cell support for breast cancer. Oncology (Huntingt) 1992;6(12):53–60, 63; discussion, 63–4, 69; published erratum, Oncology (Huntingt) 1993;7(3):105.
26. Sullivan KM, Storek J, Kopecky KJ, et al. Controlled trial of long-term administration of intravenous immunoglobulin to prevent late infection and chronic graft-vs.-host disease after marrow transplantation: clinical outcome and effect on subsequent immune recovery. Biol Blood Marrow Transplant 1996;2(1):44–53.
27. Lazarus HM, Vogelsang GB, Rowe JM. Prevention and treatment of acute graft-versus-host disease: the old and the new; a report from The Eastern Cooperative Oncology Group (ECOG) [Review]. Bone Marrow Transplant 1997;19(6):577–600.
28. Antman KH, Rowlings PA, Vaughn WP, et al. High-dose chemotherapy with autologous hematopoietic stem cell support for breast cancer in North America. J Clin Oncol 1997;15(5):1870–9.
29. Nevill TJ, Shepherd JD, Nantel SH, et al. Stem cell transplant-related mortality (TRM) 1985–1996: the Vancouver experience [Abstract 4426]. Blood 1997;90(10)(suppl 1 [part 2 of 2]):373b.
30. Duell T, van Lint MT, Ljungman P, et al. Health and functional status of long-term survivors of bone marrow transplantation. Ann Intern Med 1997;126(3):184–92.
31. Bush NE, Haberman M, Donaldson G, Sullivan KM. Quality of life of 125 adults surviving 6–18 years after bone marrow transplantation. Soc Sci Med 1995;40(4):479–90.
32. Ochs L, Shu XO, Miller J, et al. Late infections after allogeneic bone marrow transplantation: comparison of incidence in related and unrelated donor transplant recipients. Blood 1995;86(10):3979–86.
33. Pearson ML. Guideline for prevention of intravascular device-related infections. Part I. Intravascular device-related infections: an overview. Am J Infect Control 1996;24:262–93.
34. Paulin T, Ringdén O, Lönnqvist B. Faster immunological recovery after bone marrow transplantation in patients without cytomegalovirus infection. Transplant 1985;39(4): 377–84.
35. Armitage JO. Bone marrow transplantation. N Engl J Med 1994;330(12):827–38.
36. Thomas ED, Storb R, Clift RA, et al. Bone marrow transplantation (second of two parts) [Review]. N Engl J Med 1975;292(17):895–902.
37. Yeager AM, Vogelsang GB, Jones RJ, et al. Induction of cutaneous graft-versus-host disease by administration of cyclosporine to patients undergoing autologous bone marrow transplantation for acute myeloid leukemia. Blood 1992;79(11):3031–5.
38. Rinehart JJ, Balcerzak SP, Sagone AL, LoBuglio AF. Effects of corticosteroids on human monocyte function. J Clin Invest 1974;54(6):1337–43.
39. Atkinson K, Horowitz MM, Gale RP, et al. Consensus among bone marrow transplanters for diagnosis, grading and treatment of chronic graft-versus-host disease. Bone Marrow Transplant 1989;4(3):247–54.

40. Sullivan KM, Agura E, Anasetti C, et al. Chronic graft-versus-host disease and other late complications of bone marrow transplantation. Semin Hematol 1991;28(3):250–9.

41. Witherspoon RP, Storb R, Ochs HD, et al. Recovery of antibody production in human allogeneic marrow graft recipients: influence of time posttransplantation, the presence or absence of chronic graft-versus-host disease, and antithymocyte globulin treatment. Blood 1981;58(2):360–8.

42. Lum LG, Munn NA, Schanfield MS, Storb R. Detection of specific antibody formation to recall antigens after human bone marrow transplantation. Blood 1986;67(3):582–7.

43. Ambrosino DM, Molrine DC. Critical appraisal of immunization strategies for the prevention of infection in the compromised host. Hematol Oncol Clin North Am 1993;7(5):1027–50.

44. Lum LG. Kinetics of immune reconstitution after human marrow transplantation. Blood 1987;69(2):369–80.

45. Shulman HM, Sullivan KM, Weiden PL, et al. Chronic graft-versus-host syndrome in man: a long-term clinicopathologic study of 20 Seattle patients. Am J Med 1980;69(2):204–17.

46. Izutsu KT, Sullivan KM, Schubert MM, et al. Disordered salivary immunoglobulin secretion and sodium transport in human chronic graft-versus-host disease. Transplant 1983;35(5): 441–6.

47. Aucouturier P, Barra A, Intrator L, et al. Long lasting IgG subclass and antibacterial polysaccharide antibody deficiency after allogeneic bone marrow transplantation. Blood 1987;70(3):779–85.

48. Hughes WT, Armstrong D, Bodey GP, et al. 1997 guidelines for the use of antimicrobial agents in neutropenic patients with unexplained fever [Review]. Clin Infect Dis 1997;25(3): 551–73.

49. Pizzo PA, Hathorn JW, Hiemenz J, et al. Randomized trial comparing ceftazidime alone with combination antibiotic therapy in cancer patients with fever and neutropenia. N Engl J Med 1986;315(9):552–8.

50. Amgen, Inc. Filgrastim. In: Physician's desk reference. 54th edition. Montvale, NJ: Medical Economics Company, Inc., 2000:528–33.

Bacterial Infections

51. Cruciani M, Rampazzo R, Malena M, et al. Prophylaxis with fluoroquinolones for bacterial infections in neutropenic patients: a meta-analysis. Clin Infect Dis 1996(4);23:795–805.

52. Murphy M, Brown AE, Sepkowitz KA, et al. Fluoroquinolone prophylaxis for the prevention of bacterial infections in patients with cancer—is it justified [Letter]? Clin Infect Dis 1997;25(2):346–8.

53. Cometta A, Calandra T, Bille J, Glauser MP. *Escherichia coli* resistant to fluoroquinolones in patients with cancer and neutropenia. N Engl J Med 1994;330(17):1240–1.

54. Kirkpatrick BD, Harrington SM, Smith D, et al. Outbreak of vancomycin-dependent *Enterococcus faecium* in a bone marrow transplant unit. Clin Infect Dis 1999;29(5): 1268–73.

55. Vose JM, Armitage JO. Clinical applications of hematopoietic growth factors. J Clin Oncol 1995;13(4):1023–35.

56. Rand KJ, Houck H, Ganju A, Babington RG, Elfenbein GJ. Pharmacokinetics of cytomegalovirus specific IgG antibody following intravenous immunoglobulin in bone marrow transplant patients. Bone Marrow Transplant 1989;4(6):679–83.

57. Bosi A, De Majo E, Guidi S, et al. Kinetics of anti-CMV antibodies after administration of intravenous immunoglobulins to bone marrow transplant recipients. Haematologica 1990;75(2):109–12.

58. Buckley RH, Schiff RI. Use of intravenous immune globulin in immunodeficiency diseases. N Engl J Med 1991;325(2):110–7.

59. Bowden RA, Myers JD. Infection complicating bone marrow transplantation. In: Rubin RH, Young LS, eds. Clinical approach to infection in the compromised host. 3rd edition. New York, NY: Plenum Medical Book Co., 1994:601–28.

60. Sullivan KM, Storek J, Kopecky KJ, et al. Controlled trial of long-term administration of intravenous immunoglobulin to prevent late infection and chronic graft-versus-host disease following marrow transplantation: clinical outcome and effect on subsequent immune recovery. Biol Blood Marrow Transplant 1996;2:44–53.

61. Wolff SN, Fay JW, Herzig RH, et al. High-dose weekly intravenous immunoglobulin to prevent infections in patients undergoing autologous bone marrow transplantation or severe myelosuppressive therapy. Ann Intern Med 1993;118(12):937–42.

62. Garner JS. Guideline for isolation precautions in hospitals. Hospital Infection Control Practices Advisory Committee. Infect Control Hosp Epidemiol 1996;17(1):53–80; published erratum, Infect Control Hosp Epidemiol 1996;17(4):214.

63. CDC. Prevention of pneumococcal disease: recommendations of the Advisory Committee on Immunization Practices (ACIP). MMWR 1997;46(No. RR-8):1–24.

64. Winston DJ, Schiffman G, Wang DC, et al. Pneumococcal infections after human bone-marrow transplantation. Ann Intern Med 1979;91(6):835–41.

65. Hammarström V, Pauksen K, Azinge J, et al. Pneumococcal immunity and response to immunization with pneumococcal vaccine in bone marrow transplant patients: the influence of graft versus host reaction. Support Care Cancer 1993;1:195–9.

66. Guinan EC, Molrine DC, Antin JH, et al. Polysaccharide conjugate vaccine responses in bone marrow transplant patients. Transplant 1994;57(5):677–84.

67. Schubert MM, Peterson DE, Lloid ME. Oral complications. In: Thomas ED, Blume KG, Forman SJ, eds. Hematopoietic cell transplantation. 2nd ed. Oxford, England: Blackwell Science, Inc., 1999;751–63.

68. Alcaide F, Linares JA, Pallares R, et al. In vitro activities of 22 ß-lactam antibiotics against penicillin-resistant and penicillin-susceptible viridans group Streptococci isolated from blood. Antimicrob Agents Chemother 1995;39(10):2243–7.

69. Steiner M, Villablanca J, Kersey J, et al. Viridans streptococcal shock in bone marrow transplant patients. Am J Hematol 1993;42(4):354–8.

70. American Academy of Pediatrics/Committee on Infectious Diseases. Haemophilus influenzae infections. In: Pickering LK, ed. 2000 red book: report of the Committee on Infectious Diseases. 25th ed. Elk Grove Village, IL: American Academy of Pediatrics; 2000:262–72.

71. CDC. Recommendations for use of Haemophilus b conjugate vaccines and a combined diphtheria, tetanus, pertussis, and Haemophilus b vaccine: recommendations of the Advisory Committee on Immunization Practices (ACIP). MMWR 1993;42(No. RR-13):1–15.

72. Granoff DM, Basden M. Haemophilus influenzae infections in Fresno County, California: a prospective study of the effects of age, race, and contact with a case on incidence of disease. J Infect Dis 1980;141(1):40–6.

73. Band JD, Fraser DW, Ajello G. Prevention of Haemophilus influenzae type b disease. JAMA 1984;251(18):2381–6.

74. Band JD, Fraser DW, Hightower AW, Broome CV. Prophylaxis of Haemophilus influenzae type b disease [Letter]. JAMA 1984;252(23):3249–50.

75. Barra A, Cordonnier C, Prezilosi MP, et al. Immunogenicity of Haemophilus influenzae type b conjugate vaccine in allogeneic bone marrow transplant recipients. J Infect Dis 1992;166(5):1021–8.

76. Sable CA, Donowitz GA. Infections in bone marrow transplant recipients. Clin Infect Dis 1994;18(3):273–84; quiz 282–4.

77. Roy V, Ochs L, Weisdorf D. Late infections following allogeneic bone marrow transplantation: suggested strategies for prophylaxis [Review]. Leuk Lymphoma 1997;26(1–2):1–15.

Viral Infections
78. Bowden RA, Slichter SJ, Sayers M, et al. Comparison of filtered leukocyte-reduced and cytomegalovirus (CMV) seronegative blood products for the prevention of transfusion-associated CMV infection after marrow transplantation. Blood 1995;86(9):3598–603.

79. Boeckh M, Gooley TA, Myerson D, Cunningham T, Schoch G, Bowden RA. Cytomegalovirus pp65 antigenemia-guided early treatment with ganciclovir versus ganciclovir at engraftment after allogeneic marrow transplantation: a randomized double blind study. Blood 1996;88(10):4063–71.

80. Boeckh M, Stevens-Ayers T, Bowden R. Cytomegalovirus pp65 antigenemia after autologous marrow and peripheral blood stem cell transplantation. J Infect Dis 1996;174(5):907–12.

81. Boeckh M, Bowden R. Cytomegalovirus infection in marrow transplantation. In: Buckner CD, Clift RA, ed. Technical and biological components of marrow transplantation. Boston, MA: Kluwer Academic Publishers, 1995:97–136.

82. Einsele H, Ehninger G, Hebart H, et al. Polymerase chain reaction monitoring reduces the incidence of cytomegalovirus disease and the duration and side effect of antiviral therapy after bone marrow transplantation. Blood 1995;86(7):2815–20.

83. Mendez JC, Sia IG, Paya CV. Human cytomegalovirus. In: Lennette EH, Smith TF, eds. Laboratory diagnosis of viral infections. 3rd ed., revised and expanded. New York, NY: Marcel Decker, Inc., 1999: 361–72.

84. Goodrich JM, Mori M, Gleaves CA, et al. Early treatment with ganciclovir to prevent cytomegalovirus disease after allogeneic bone marrow transplant. N Engl J Med 1991;325(23):1601–7.

85. Schmidt GM, Horak DA, Niland JC, Duncan SR, Forman SJ, Zaia JA. Randomized controlled trial of prophylactic ganciclovir for cytomegalovirus pulmonary infection in recipients of allogeneic bone marrow transplants. New Engl J Med 1991;324(15):1005–11.

86. Goodrich JM, Bowden RA, Fisher L, Keller C, Schoch G. Meyers JD. Ganciclovir prophylaxis to prevent cytomegalovirus disease after allogeneic marrow transplant. Ann Intern Med 1993;118(3):173–8.

87. Mazzulli T, Drew LW, Yen-Lieberman B, et al. Multicenter comparison of the Digene Hybrid Capture CMV DNA Assay (Version 2.0), the pp65 antigenemia assay, and cell culture for the detection of cytomegalovirus viremia. J Clin Microbiol 1999;37(4):958–63.

88. Gerna G, Baldanti F, Middeldorp JM, et al. Clinical significance of expression of human cytomegalovirus pp67 late transcript in heart, lung, and bone marrow transplant recipients as determined by nucleic acid sequence-based amplification. J Clin Microbiol 1999;37(4):902–11.

89. Singhal S, Mehta J, Powles R, et al. Three weeks of ganciclovir for cytomegalovirus after allogeneic bone marrow transplantation. Bone Marrow Transplant 1995;15(5):777–81.

90. Verdonck LF, Dekker AW, Rozenberg-Arska M, van den Hoek MR. Risk-adapted approach with a short course of ganciclovir to prevent cytomegalovirus (CMV) pneumonia in CMV-seropositive recipients of allogeneic bone marrow transplants. Clin Infect Dis 1997;24(5): 901–7.

91. Zaia J, Gallez-Hawkins GM, Longmate J, et al. Late bacterial and fungal sepsis and mortality after BMT are increased by duration of early ganciclovir preemptive therapy for CMV infection [Abstract 2128]. Blood 1998;92(10)(suppl 1 [part 1 of 2]):518a.

92. Bacigalupo A, Bregante S, Tedone E, et al. Combined foscarnet-ganciclovir treatment for cytomegalovirus infections after allogeneic hematopoietic stem cell transplantation. Transplant 1996;62(3);376–80.

93. Moretti S, Zikos P, Van Lint MT, et al. Foscarnet vs ganciclovir for cytomegalovirus (CMV) antigenemia after allogeneic hematopoietic stem cell transplantation (HSCT): a randomized study. Bone Marrow Transplant 1998;22(2):175–80.

94. Boeckh M, Hoy C, Torok-Storb B. Occult cytomegalovirus infection of marrow stroma. Clin Infect Dis 1998;26(1):209–10.

95. Krause H, Hebart H, Jahn G, Muller CA, Einsele H. Screening for CMV-specific T-cell proliferation to identify patients at risk of developing late onset CMV disease. Bone Marrow Transplant 1997;19(11):1111–16.

96. Gor D, Sabin C, Prentice HG, et al. Longitudinal fluctuations in cytomegalovirus load in bone marrow transplant patients: relationship between peak virus load, donor/recipient serostatus, acute GVHD and CMV disease. Bone Marrow Transplant 1998;21(6):597–605.

97. Zaia JA, Gallez-Hawkins GM, Teftmeier BR, et al. Late cytomegalovirus disease in marrow transplantation is predicted by virus load in plasma. J Infect Dis 1997;176(3):782–5.

98. Ljungman P, Aschan J, Azinge JN, et al. Cytomegalovirus viremia and specific T-helper cell responses as predictors of disease after allogeneic marrow transplantation. Br J Haematol 1993;83(1):118–24.

99. Lazzarotto T, Varani S, Spezzacatena P, et al. Delayed acquisition of high-avidity anti-cytomegalovirus antibody is correlated with prolonged antigenemia in solid organ transplant recipients. J Infect Dis 1998;178(4):1145–9.

100. Boeckh M, Gallez-Hawkins GM, Myerson D, Zaia JA, Bowden RA. Plasma polymerase chain reaction for cytomegalovirus DNA after allogeneic marrow transplantation: comparison with polymerase chain reaction using peripheral blood leukocytes, pp65 antigenemia, and viral culture. Transplant 1997;64(1):108–13.

101. Prentice HG, Gluckman E, Powles RL, et al. Impact of long-term acyclovir on cytomegalovirus infection and survival after allogeneic bone marrow transplantation. Lancet 1994;343(8900):749–53.

102. Boeckh M, Gooley TA, Bowden RA. Effect of high-dose acyclovir on survival in allogeneic marrow transplant recipients who received ganciclovir at engraftment or for cytomegalovirus pp65 antigenemia. J Infect Dis 1998;178(4):1153–7.

103. Boeckh M, Gooley TA, Reusser P, Buckner CD, Bowden RA. Failure of high-dose acyclovir to prevent cytomegalovirus disease after autologous marrow transplantation. J Infect Dis 1995;172(4):939–43.

104. American Public Health Association. Mononucleosis, infectious. In: Chin J, ed. Control of communicable diseases manual. 17th ed. Washington, DC: American Public Health Association, 2000:350–2.

105. Papadopoulos E, Ladanyi M, Emanuel D, et al. Infusions of donor leukocytes to treat Epstein-Barr virus-associated lymphoproliferative disorders after allogeneic bone marrow transplantation. New Engl J Med 1994;330(17):1185–91.

106. Rooney CM, Smith CA, Ng CY, et al. Infusion of cytotoxic T cells for the prevention and treatment of Epstein-Barr virus-induced lymphoma in allogeneic transplant recipients. Blood 1998;92(5):1549–55.

107. Shapiro RS, McClain K, Frizzera G, et al. Epstein-Barr virus associated B cell lymphoproliferative disorders following bone marrow transplantation. Blood 1988;71(5): 1234–43.

108. Zutter MM, Martin PJ, Sale GE, et al. Epstein-Barr virus lymphoproliferation after bone marrow transplantation. Blood 1988;72(2):520–9.

109. Saral R, Burns WH, Laskin OL, Santos GW, Lietman PS. Acyclovir prophylaxis of herpes-simplex-virus infections. N Engl J Med 1981;305(2):63–7.

110. Gluckman E, Lotsberg J, Devergie A, et al. Prophylaxis of herpes infections after bone marrow transplantation by oral acyclovir. Lancet 1983;2(8352):706–8.

111. Wade JC, Newton B, McLaren C, Flournoy N, Keeney RE, Meyers JD. Intravenous acyclovir to treat mucocutaneous herpes simplex virus infection after marrow transplantation: a double-blind trial. Ann Intern Med 1982;96(3):265–9.

112. Wade JC, Newton B, Flournoy N, Meyers JD. Oral acyclovir for prevention of herpes simplex reactivation after marrow transplantation. Ann Intern Med 1984;100(6):823–8.

113. Johnson JR, Egaas S, Gleaves CA, Hackman R, Bowden RA. Hepatitis due to herpes simplex virus in marrow-transplant recipients. Clin Infect Dis 1992;14(1):38–45.

114. Crumpacker CS. Ganciclovir [Review]. New Engl J Med 1996;335(10):721–9.

115. Chulay JD, Bell AR, Miller GB, and the International Valaciclovir HSV Study Group. Long-term safety of valaciclovir for suppression of herpes simplex virus infections [Abstract 105]. In: Infectious Diseases Society of America (IDSA) Program and Abstracts, 34th annual meeting, September 18–20, 1996, New Orleans, Louisiana;55.

116. Han CS, Miller W, Haake R, Weisdorf D. Varicella zoster infection after bone marrow transplantation: incidence, risk factors, and complications. Bone Marrow Transplant 1994;13(3):277–83.

117. Lawrence R, Gershon AA, Holzman R, Steinberg SP. Risk of zoster after varicella vaccination in children with leukemia. New Engl J Med 1988;318(9):543–8.

118. Locksley RM, Fluornoy N, Sullivan KM, Meyers JD. Infection with varicella-zoster virus after marrow transplantation. J Infect Dis 1985;152(6):1172–81.

119. Schuchter LM, Wingard J, Piantadose S, Burns WH, Santos GW, Saral R. Herpes zoster infection after autologous bone marrow transplantation. Blood 1989;74(4):1424–27.

120. CDC. Prevention of varicella: recommendations of the Advisory Committee on Immunization Practices (ACIP). MMWR 1996;45(No. RR-11):1–36.

121. CDC. Prevention of varicella: updated recommendations of the Advisory Committee on Immunization Practices (ACIP). MMWR 1999;48(No. RR-06):1–5.

122. Wacker P, Hartmann O, Benhamou E, Salloum E, Lamerle J. Varicella-zoster virus infections after autologous bone marrow transplantation in children. Bone Marrow Transplant 1989;4(2):191–4.

123. Josephson A, Gombert ME. Airborne transmission of nosocomial varicella from localized zoster. J Infect Dis 1988;158(1):238–41.

124. Sempere A, Sanz GF, Senent L, et al. Long-term acyclovir prophylaxis for prevention of varicella zoster virus infection after autologous bone stem cell transplantation in patients with acute leukemia. Bone Marrow Transplant 1992;10(6):495–8.

125. Selby PJ, Powles RL, Easton D, et al. Prophylactic role of intravenous and long-term oral acyclovir after allogeneic bone marrow transplantation. Br J Cancer 1989;59(3):434–8.

126. Ljungman P, Wilczek H, Gahrton G, et al. Long-term acyclovir prophylaxis in bone marrow transplant recipients and lymphocyte proliferation to herpes antigens in vitro. Bone Marrow Transplant 1986;1(2):185–92.

127. Cirrelli R, Herne K, McCrary M, Lee P, Tyrine, SK. Famciclovir: review of clinical efficacy and safety [Review]. Antiviral Res 1996;29(2–3):141–51.

128. Cat LK, Yamauchi NK. Varicella vaccine in immunocompromised patients [Review]. Annuals of Pharmacology 1996;30(2):181–4.

129. Redman RL, Nader S, Zerboni L, et al. Early reconstitution of immunity and decreased severity of herpes zoster in bone marrow transplant recipients immunized with inactivated varicella vaccine. J Infect Dis 1997;176(3):578–85.

130. Garcia R, Raad I, Abi-Said D, et al. Nosocomial respiratory syncytial virus infections: prevention and control in bone marrow transplant patients. Infect Control Hosp Epidemiol 1997;18(6):412–6.

131. Raad I, Abbas J, Whimbey E. Infection control of nosocomial respiratory viral disease in the immunocompromised host. Am J Med 1997;102(3A):48–52.

132. Sable CA, Hayden FG. Orthomyxoviral and paramyxoviral infections in transplant patients [Review]. Infect Dis Clin North Am 1995;9(4):987–1003.

133. Whimbey E, Champlin R, Couch RB, et al. Community respiratory virus infections among hospitalized adult bone marrow transplant recipients. Clin Infect Dis 1996;22(5):778–82.

134. Whimbey E, Englund JA, Couch RB. Community respiratory virus infections in immunocompromised patients with cancer. Am J Med 1997;102(3A):10–8.

135. Bowden RA. Respiratory virus infections in bone marrow transplant: the Fred Hutchinson Cancer Research Center experience. Am J Med 1997;102(3A):27–30.

136. Harrington RD, Hooton RD, Hackman RC, et al. Outbreak of respiratory syncytial virus in a bone marrow transplant center. J Infect Dis 1992;165(6):987–93.

137. Whimbey E, Champlin R, Englund JA, et al. Combination therapy with aerosolized ribavirin and intravenous immunoglobulin for respiratory syncytial virus disease in adult bone marrow transplant recipients. Bone Marrow Transplant 1995;16(3):393–9.

138. Folz RJ, Elkordy MA. Coronavirus pneumonia following autologous bone marrow transplantation for breast cancer. Chest 1999;115(3):901–5.

139. Whimbey E, Elting LS, Couch RB, et al. Influenza A virus infection among hospitalized adult bone marrow transplant recipients. Bone Marrow Transplant 1994;13(4):437–40.

140. CDC. Guideline for prevention of nosocomial pneumonia. Respiratory Care 1994;39(12): 1191–236.

141. CDC. Prevention and control of influenza: recommendations of the Advisory Committee on Immunization Practices (ACIP). MMWR 2000;49(No. RR-3):1–38.

142. Engelhard D, Nagler A, Hardan I, et al. Antibody response to a two-dose regimen of influenza vaccine in allogeneic T cell-depleted and autologous BMT recipients. Bone Marrow Transplant 1993;11(1):1–5.

143. Hayden FG. Prevention and treatment of influenza in immunocompromised patients. Am J Med 1997;102(3A):55–60.

144. Monto AS, Robinson DP, Herlocher ML, Hinson JM Jr, Elliott MJ, Crisp A. Zanamivir in the prevention of influenza among healthy adults: a randomized controlled trial. JAMA 1999;282(1):31–5.

145. Hayden FG, Atmar RL, Schilling M, et al. Use of the selective oral neuraminidase inhibitor oseltamivir to prevent influenza. New Engl J Med 1999;341(18):1336–43.

146. Hayden FG, Gubareva L, Klein T, et al. Inhaled zanamivir for preventing transmission of influenza in families [Abstract LB-2]. In: Final program, abstracts and exhibits addendum, 38th Interscience Conference on Antimicrobial Agents and Chemotherapy. Washington, DC: American Society for Microbiology, 1991:1.

147. CDC. Neuraminidase inhibitors for treatment of influenza A and B infections. MMWR 1999;48(No. RR-14):1–10.

148. Englund JA, Champlin RE, Wyde PR, et al. Common emergence of amantadine- and rimantadine-resistant influenza A viruses in symptomatic immunocompromised adults. Clin Infect Dis 1998;26(6):1418–24.

149. Klimov AI, Rocha E, Hayden FG, et al. Prolonged shedding of amantadine-resistant influenzae A viruses by immunodeficient patients: detection by polymerase chain reaction-restriction analysis. J Infect Dis 1995;172(5):1352–55.

150. Knight V, Gilbert BE. Ribavirin aerosol treatment of influenza [Review]. Infect Dis Clin North Am 1987;1(2):441–57.

151. Hayden FG, Sabie CA, Connor JD, Lane J. Intravenous ribavirin by constant infusion for serious influenza and parainfluenza virus infection. Antiviral Therapy 1996;1:51–6.

152. Hayden FG, Treanor JJ, Betts RF, Lobo M, Esinhart JD, Hussey EK. Safety and efficacy of the neuraminidase inhibitor GG167 in experimental human influenza. JAMA 1996;275(4): 295–9.

153. Hayden FG. Combination antiviral therapy for respiratory virus infections. Antiviral Res 1996;29(1):45–8.

154. Martin MA, Bock MJ, Pfaller MA, Wenzel RP. Respiratory syncytial virus infections in adult bone marrow transplant recipients [Letter]. Lancet 1988;1(8599):1396–7.

155. Hertz MI, Englund JA, Snover D, Bitterman PB, McGlave PB. Respiratory syncytial virus-induced acute lung injury in adult patients with bone marrow transplants: a clinical approach and review of the literature [Review]. Medicine 1989;68(5):269–81.

156. Win N, Mitchell D, Pugh S, Russell NH. Successful therapy with ribavirin of late onset respiratory syncytial virus pneumonitis complicating allogeneic bone transplantation. Clin Lab Haematol 1992;14(1):29–32.

157. DeVincenzo JP, Leombuno D, Soiffer RJ, Siber GR. Immunotherapy of respiratory syncytial virus pneumonia following bone marrow transplantation. Bone Marrow Transplant 1996;17(6):1051–6.

158. Boeckh M, Bowden RA, Berrey MM, et al. Phase I evaluation of a RSV-specific humanized monoclonal antibody (MEDI-493) after hematopoietic stem cell transplantation (HSCT) [Abstract MN-20]. 38th Interscience Conference on Antimicrobial Agents and Chemotherapy, September 24–27, 1998, San Diego, CA;593.

159. Flomenberg P, Babbitt J, Drobyski WR, et al. Increasing incidence of adenovirus disease in bone marrow transplant recipients. J Infect Dis 1994;169(4):775–81.

160. Englund JA, Piedra PA, Whimbey EA. Prevention and treatment of respiratory syncytial virus and parainfluenza viruses in immunocompromised patients. Am J Med 1997;102(3A):61–70.

161. American Academy of Pediatrics. Influenza. In: Pickering LK, ed. 2000 red book: report of the Committee on Infectious Diseases. 25th ed. Elk Grove Village, IL: American Academy of Pediatrics, 2000:351–9.

162. American Academy of Pediatrics. Parainfluenza viral infections. In: Pickering LK, ed. 2000 red book: report of the Committee on Infectious Diseases. 25th ed. Elk Grove Village, IL: American Academy of Pediatrics, 2000:419–20.

163. American Academy of Pediatrics. Adenovirus infections. In: Pickering LK, ed. 2000 red book: report of the Committee on Infectious Diseases. 25th ed. Elk Grove Village, IL: American Academy of Pediatrics, 2000:162–3.

164. American Academy of Pediatrics. Respiratory syncytial virus. In: Pickering LK, ed. 2000 red book: report of the Committee on Infectious Diseases. 25th ed. Elk Grove Village, IL: American Academy of Pediatrics, 2000:483–7.

Fungal Infections

165. Vose JM, Armitage JO. Clinical applications of hematopoietic growth factors. J Clin Oncol 1995;13(4):1023–35.

166. Riley DK, Pavia AT, Beatty PG, Denton D, Carroll KC. Surveillance cultures in bone marrow transplant recipients: worthwhile or wasteful? Bone Marrow Transplant 1995;15(3):469–73.

167. Walsh TJ. Role of surveillance cultures in prevention and treatment of fungal infections. National Cancer Institute Monograph No. 9;1990:43–5.

168. Crawford SW. Bone-marrow transplantation and related infections. Semin Respir Infect 1993;8(3):183–90.

169. Goodman JL, Winston DJ, Greenfield RA, et al. Controlled trial of fluconazole to prevent fungal infections in patients undergoing bone marrow transplantation. N Engl J Med 1992;326(13):845–51.

170. Slavin MA, Osborne B, Adams R, et al. Efficacy and safety of fluconazole prophylaxis for fungal infections after marrow transplantation—a prospective, randomized, double-blind study. J Infect Dis 1995;171(6):1545–52.

171. Reed EC. Infectious complications during autotransplantation [Review]. Hematol Oncol Clin North Am 1993;7:717–35.

172. Donowitz G, Harman C. Low dose fluconazole prophylaxis in neutropenia [Abstract 024]. 9th International Symposium on Infections in the Immunocompromised Host, Assisi, Italy, June 23–26, 1996.

173. Bjerke JW, Meyers JD, Bowden RA. Hepatosplenic candidiasis—a contraindication to marrow transplantation? Blood 1994;84(8):2811–4.

174. Walsh TJ, Dixon DM. Nosocomial aspergillosis: environmental microbiology, hospital epidemiology, diagnosis and treatment. Eur J Epidemiol 1989;5(2):131–42.

175. Weems JJ Jr, Davis BJ, Tablan OC, Kaufman L, Martone WJ. Construction activity: an independent risk factor for invasive aspergillosis and zygomycosis in patients with hematologic malignancy. Infect Control 1987;8(2):71–5.

176. Krasinski K, Holzman RS, Hanna B, Greco MA, Graff M, Bhogal M. Nosocomial fungal infection during hospital renovation. Infection Control 1985;6(7):278–82.

177. Thio CL, Smith D, Merz WG, et al. Refinements of environmental assessment during an outbreak investigation of invasive aspergillosis in a leukemia and bone marrow transplant unit. Infect Control Hosp Epidemiol 2000;21(1):18–23.

178. Rhame FS, Streifel AJ, Kersey JH Jr, McGlave PB. Extrinsic risk factors for pneumonia in the patient at high risk of infection [Review]. Am J Med 1984;76(5A):42–52.

179. Opal SM, Asp AA, Cannady, PB Jr, Morse PL, Burton LJ, Hammer PG 2nd. Efficacy of infection control measures during a nosocomial outbreak of disseminated aspergillosis associated with hospital construction. J Infect Dis 1986;153(3):634–7.

180. American Institute of Architects Academy of Architecture for Health, with assistance from the US Department of Health and Human Services. Guidelines for design and construction of hospital and medical facilities. Washington, DC: American Institute of Architects Press, 1996–67:58.

181. Bowden RA, Cays M, Gooley T, Mamelok RD, van Burik JA. Phase I study of amphotericin B colloidal dispersion for the treatment of invasive fungal infections after marrow transplant. J Infect Dis 1996;173(5):1208–15.

182. Kruger W, Stockschlader M, Russman B, et al. Experience with liposomal amphotericin-B in 60 patients undergoing high-dose therapy and bone marrow or peripheral blood stem cell transplantation. Br J Haematol 1995;91(3):684–90.

183. Ringdén O, Tollemar J, Dahllof G, Tyden G. High cure rate of invasive fungal infections in immunocompromised children using AmBisome. Transplant Proc 1994;26(1):175–7.

184. Andstrom EE, Ringdén O, Remberger M, Svahn BM, Tollemar J. Safety and efficacy of liposomal amphotericin B in allogeneic bone marrow transplant recipients. Mycoses 1996;39(5–6):185–93.

185. O'Donnell MR, Schmidt GM, Tegtmeier BR, et al. Prediction of systemic fungal infection in allogeneic marrow recipients: impact of amphotericin prophylaxis in high-risk patients. J Clin Oncol 1994;12(4):827–34.

186. Rousey SR, Russler S, Gottlieb M, Ash RC. Low-dose amphotericin B prophylaxis against invasive *Aspergillus* infections in allogeneic marrow transplantation. Am J Med 1991;91(5):484–92.

187. Perfect JR, Klotman ME, Gilbert CC, et al. Prophylactic intravenous amphotericin B in neutropenic autologous bone marrow transplant recipients. J Infect Dis 1992;165(5):891–7.

188. Wade JC. Chapter 5: epidemiology of *Candida* infections. In: Bodey GP, ed. Candidiasis: pathogenesis, diagnosis and treatment. New York, NY: Raven Press, Ltd., 1993:85–107.

189. Tollemar J, Ringdén O, Andersson S, et al. Prophylactic use of liposomal amphotericin B (AmBisome) against fungal infections: a randomized trial in bone marrow transplant recipients. Transplant Proc 1993;25(1 part 2):1495–7.

190. Conneally E, Cafferkey MT, Daly PA, Keane CT, McCann SR. Nebulized amphotericin B as prophylaxis against invasive aspergillosis in granulocytopenic patients. Bone Marrow Transplant 1990;5(6):403–6.

191. Cleary JD, Taylor JW, Chapman SW. Itraconazole in antifungal therapy. Ann of Pharmacother 1992;26(4):502–9.

192. Jennings TS, Hardin TC. Treatment of aspergillosis with itraconazole [Review]. Annals of Pharmacother 1993;27(10):1206–11.

193. Poirier JM, Berlioz F, Isnard F, Chrymol G. Marked intra- and inter-patient variability of itraconazole steady state plasma concentrations. Thérapie 1996;51(2):163–7.

194. Prentice AG, Warnock DW, Johnson SA, Phillips MJ, Oliver DA. Multiple dose pharmacokinetics of an oral solution of itraconazole in autologous bone marrow transplant recipients. J Antimicrob Chemother 1994;34(2):247–52.

195. Tam JY, Hamed KA, Blume K, Prober CG. Use of itraconazole in treatment of prevention of invasive aspergillosis in bone marrow transplant recipients [Abstract 813]. 33rd Interscience Conference on Antimicrobial Agents and Chemotherapy (ICAAC), New Orleans, LA, 1993;268.

196. Ortho Biotech, Inc. Itraconazole. In: Physician's desk reference (PDR), Montvale, NJ: Medical Economics Company, 2000:2131–4.

197. Denning DW. Invasive aspergillosis [Review]. Clin Infect Dis 1998;26(4):781–803; quiz 804–5.

198. McWhinney PHM, Kibbler CC, Hamon MD, et al. Progress in the diagnosis and management of aspergillosis in bone marrow transplantation: 13 years' experience. Clin Infect Dis 1993;17(3):397–404.

199. Lupinetti FM, Behrendt DM, Giller RH, Trigg ME, de Alarcon P. Pulmonary resection for fungal infection in children undergoing bone marrow transplantation. J Thorac Cardiovasc Surg 1992;104(3):684–7.

200. Richard C, Romon I, Baro J, et al. Invasive pulmonary aspergillosis prior to BMT in acute leukemia patients does not predict a poor outcome. Bone Marrow Transplant 1993;12(3):237–41.

Protozoal and Helminthic Infections

201. Brazinsky JH, Phillips JE. Pneumocystis pneumonia transmission between patients with lymphoma. JAMA 1969;209(10):1527.

202. Chave JP, David S, Wauters JP, Van Meller G, Francioli P. Transmission of *Pneumocystic carinii* from AIDS patients to other immunosuppressed patients: a cluster of *Pneumocystis carinii* pneumonia in renal transplant patients. AIDS 1991;5(8):927–32.

203. Goesch TR, Götz G, Stellbrinck KH, Albrecht H. Weh HJ, Hossfeld DK. Possible transfer of *Pneumocystis carinii* between immunodeficient patients [Letter]. Lancet 1990;336(8715):627.

204. Bensousan T, Garo B, Islam S, Bourbigot B, Cledes J, Garre M. Possible transfer of *Pneumocystic carinii* between kidney transplant recipients [Letter]. Lancet 1990;336(8722):1066–7.

205. Ruskin J, Remington JS. Compromised host and infection. I: *Pneumocystic carinii* pneumonia. JAMA 1967;202(12):1070–4.

206. Watanabe JM, Chinchinian H, Weitz C, McIlvanie SK. *Pneumocystis carinii* pneumonia in a family. JAMA 1965;193(8):685–6.

207. Tuan IZ, Dennison D, Weisdorf DJ. *Pneumocystis carinii* pneumonitis following bone marrow transplantation. Bone Marrow Transplant 1992;10(3):267–72.

208. Maltezou HC, Petropoulos D, Choroszy M, et al. Dapsone for *Pneumocystic carinii* prophylaxis in children undergoing bone marrow transplantation [Review]. Bone Marrow Transplant 1997;20(10):879–81.

209. Link H, Vöhringer H-F, Wingen F, Bragas B, Schwardt A, Ehninger G. Pentamidine aerosol prophylaxis of *Pneumocystis carinii* pneumonia after BMT. Bone Marrow Transplant 1993;11(5):403–6.

210. Chan C, Montaner J, Lefebvre EA, et al. Atovaquone suspension compared with aerosolized pentamidine for prevention of *Pneumocystis carinii* pneumonia in human immunodeficiency virus-infected subjects intolerant of trimethoprim or sulfonamides. J Infect Dis 1999;180(2):369–76.

211. Nunn PP, Allistone JC. Resistance to trimethoprim-sulfamethoxazole in the treatment of *Pneumocystis carinii* pneumonia: implication of folinic acid. Chest 1984;86(1):149–50.

212. Safrin S, Lee BL, Sande MA. Adjunctive folinic acid with trimethoprim-sulfamethoxazole for *Pneumocystic carinii* pneumonia in AIDS patients is associated with an increased risk of therapeutic failure and death. J Infect Dis 1994;170(4):912–7.

213. Martino R, Martínez, Brunet S, Sureda A. Successful bone marrow transplantation in patients with recent *Pneumocystis carinii* pneumonia: report of two cases [Letter]. Bone Marrow Transplant 1995;16(3):491.

214. Castagnola E, Dini G, Lanino E, et al. Low CD4 lymphocyte count in a patient with *P. carinii* pneumonia after autologous bone marrow transplantation. Bone Marrow Transplant 1995;15(16):977–8.

215. Derouin F, Devergie A, Auber P, et al. Toxoplasmosis in bone marrow transplant recipients: report of seven cases and review [Review]. Clin Infect Dis 1992;15(2):267–70.

216. Koneru B, Anaissie E, Tricot G, et al. High incidence of and mortality from *Toxoplasma gondii* infections in T-cell depleted allogeneic bone marrow transplant recipients

[Abstract 987]. 39th Annual American Society of Hematology Meeting, San Diego, CA, December 5–9, 1997;224A.

217. Siegel SE, Lunde MN, Gelderman AH, et al. Transmission of toxoplasmosis by leukocyte transfusion. Blood 1971;37(4):388–94.

218. Slavin MA, Meyers JD, Remington JS, Hackman RC. *Toxoplasma gondii* infection in marrow transplant recipients: a 20 year experience. Bone Marrow Transplant 1994;13(5): 549–57.

219. Jurges E, Young Y, Eltumi M, et al. Transmission of toxoplasmosis by bone marrow transplant associated with Campath-1G. Bone Marrow Transplant 1992;9(1):65–6.

220. Chandrasekar PH, Momin F, Bone Marrow Transplant Team. Disseminated toxoplasmosis in marrow recipients: a report of three cases and a review of the literature. Bone Marrow Transplant 1997;19(7):685–9.

221. Foot ABM, Garin YJF, Ribaud P, Devergie A, Derouin F, Gluckman E. Prophylaxis of toxoplasmosis with pyrimethamine/sulfadoxine (Fansidar) in bone marrow transplant recipients. Bone Marrow Transplant 1994;14(2):241–5.

222. Peacock JE Jr, Greven CM, Cruz JM, Hurd DD. Fansidar: reactivation toxoplasmic retinochoroiditis in patients undergoing bone marrow transplantation: is there a role for chemoprophylaxis [Review]? Bone Marrow Transplant 1995;15(6):983–7.

223. Liu LX, Weller PF. Strongyloidiasis and other intestinal nematode infections [Review]. Infect Dis Clin North Am 1993;7(3):655–82.

224. Conway DJ, Atkins NS, Lillywhite JE, et al. Immunodiagnosis of *Strongyloides stercoralis* infection: a method for increasing the specificity of the indirect ELISA. Trans R Soc Trop Med Hyg 1993;87(2):173–6.

225. Fishman JA. *Pneumocystis carinii* and parasitic infections in the immunocompromised host. In: Rubin RH, Young LS, eds. Clinical approach to infection in the compromised host 3rd edition. New York, NY: Plenum Medical Book Company, 1994;275–334.

226. Fishman JA. *Pneumocystis carinii* and parasitic infections in transplantation. Infect Dis Clin North Am 1995;9(4):1005–44.

227. Leiby DA, Fucci MH, Stumpf RJ. *Trypanosoma cruzi* in a low- to moderate-risk blood donor population: seroprevalence and possible congenital transmission. Transfusion 1999;39(3):310–5.

228. Dictar M, Sinagra A, Verón MT, et al. Recipients and donors of bone marrow transplants suffering from Chagas' disease: management and preemptive therapy of parasitemia. Bone Marrow Transplant 1998;21(4):391–3.

229. Moraes-Souza H, Bordin JO. Strategies for prevention of transfusion-associated Chagas' disease. Transfus Med Rev 1996;10(3):161–70.

230. Altclas J, Sinagra A, Jaimovich G, et al. Reactivation of chronic Chagas' disease following allogeneic bone marrow transplantation and successful pre-emptive therapy with benznidazole. Transplant Infectious Disease 1999;1:135–7.

231. Altclas J, Jaimovich G, Milovic V, Klein F, Feldman L. Chagas' disease after bone marrow transplantation. Bone Marrow Transplant 1996;18(2):447–8.

Hospital Infection Control
232. Streifel AJ. Chapter 80: design and maintenance of hospital ventilation systems and the prevention of airborne nosocomial infections. In: Mayhall CG, ed. Hospital epidemiology and infection control. 2nd ed. Philadelphia, PA: Lippincott Williams & Wilkins 1999; 1211–21.

233. Streifel AJ, Marshall JW. Parameters for ventilation controlled environments in hospitals. In: Moschandreas DJ, ed. Design, construction, and operation of healthy buildings; solutions to global and regional concerns. Atlanta, GA: American Society of Heating, Refrigerating and Air-Conditioning Engineers Press, 1998;305–9.

234. Barnes RA, Rogers TR. Control of an outbreak of nosocomial aspergillosis by laminar airflow isolation. J Hosp Infect 1989;14(2):89–94.

235. Sheretz FJ, Belani A, Kramer BS, et al. Impact of air filtration on nosocomial *Aspergillus* infections: unique risk to bone marrow transplant recipients. Am J Med 1987;83(4):709–18.

236. Walter EA, Bowden RA. Infection in the bone marrow transplant recipient [Review]. Infect Dis Clin North Am 1995;9(4):823–47.

237. Storb R, Prentice RL, Buckner CD, et al. Graft-versus-host disease and survival in patients with aplastic anemia treated by marrow grafts from HLA-identical siblings. N Engl J Med 1983;308(6):302–7.

238. Streifel AJ. Maintenance and engineering; biomedical engineering; support services and facilities management. In: Association for Professionals in Infection Control and Epidemiology, Inc. Principles and practice. 2nd ed. St. Louis, MO: Mosby, 2000 (in press).

239. Vesley D, Streifel AJ. Chapter 69: environmental services. In: Mayhall CG, ed. Hospital epidemiology and infection control. 2nd ed. Philadelphia, PA: Lippincott Williams & Wilkins, 1999;1047–53.

240. Carter CD, Barr BA. Infection control issues in construction and renovation. Infect Control Hosp Epidemiol 1997;18(8):587–96.

241. Loo VG, Bertrand C, Dixon C, et al. Control of construction-associated nosocomial aspergillosis in an antiquated hematology unit. Infect Control Hospital Epidemiol 1996;17(6):360–4.

242. Rask DR, Dziekan B, Swincicki WC, et al. Air quality control during renovation in health care facilities. In: Moschandreas DJ, ed. Design, construction, and operation of healthy buildings; solutions to global and regional concerns. Atlanta, GA: American Society of Heating, Refrigerating, and Air-Conditioning Engineers Press, 1998:291–304.

243. CDC. Laboratory performance evaluation of N95 filtering facepiece respirators, 1996. MMWR 1998;47(48):1045–9.

244. CDC. Guidelines for preventing the transmission *Mycobacterium tuberculosis* in health-care facilities, 1994. MMWR 1994;43(No. RR-13):1–132.

245. CDC/National Institute of Occupational Safety and Health. Protect yourself against tuberculosis—a respiratory protection guide for health care workers. Cincinnati, OH: US Department of Health and Human Services, US Public Health Service, CDC, National Institute for Occupational Health and Safety, 1995; DHHS publication no. (NIOSH) 96-102:1–132. Available at <http://www.cdc.gov/niosh>. Accessed May 15, 2000.

246. Rutala WA. APIC guideline for selection and use of disinfectants. Am J Infect Control 1996;24(4):313–42.

247. National Antimicrobial Information Network. List of EPA registered products. Available at <http://ace.orst.edu/info/nain/lists.htm>. Accessed May 15, 2000.

248. Mangram AJ, Horan TC, Pearson ML, Silver LC, Jarvis WR, Hospital Infection Control Practices Advisory Committee. Guideline for prevention of surgical site infection, 1999. Infect Control Hosp Epidemiol 1999;20(4):247–80 or Am J Infect Control 1999;27(2):97–134.

249. Garner JS, Favero MS. Guideline for handwashing and hospital environmental control, 1985; supersedes guideline for hospital environmental control published in 1981. Available at <http://www.cdc.gov/ncidod/hip/Guide/handwash.htm>. Accessed May 15, 2000.

250. Rotter ML. Chapter 87: hand washing and hand disinfection. In: Mayhall CG, ed. Hospital epidemiology and infection control. 2nd ed. Baltimore, MD: Lippincott Williams and Wilkins, 1999:1339–55.

251. Larson EL. APIC guideline for handwashing and hand antisepsis in health care settings. Am J Infect Control 1995;23(4):251–69.

252. McNeil SA, Foster CL, Kauffman CA. Effect of hand cleansing with antimicrobial soap gel on microbial colonization of artificial nails (AN) [Abstract 1696]. 39th Interscience Conference on Antimicrobial Agents and Chemotherapy Abstracts, San Francisco, CA, 1999;635.

253. CDC/National Center for Infectious Diseases/Hospital Infections Program. Sterilization or disinfection of medical devices: general principles. Atlanta, GA: US Department of Health and Human Services, CDC, 2000. Available at <http://www.cdc.gov/ncidod/hip/sterile/sterilgp.htm>. Accessed May 15, 2000.

254. Favero MS, Bond WW. Chapter 24: sterilization, disinfection, and antisepsis in the hospital. In: Hauser WJ Jr, Herrmann KL, Isenberg HD, Shadomy HJ, eds. Manual of clinical microbiology. Washington DC: American Society for Microbiology, 1991:183–200.

255. Johnson S, Gerding DN. Chapter 29: *Clostridium difficile*. In: Mayhall CG, ed. Hospital epidemiology and infection control. 2nd ed., Philadelphia, PA: Lippincott Williams & Wilkins, 1999:467–76.

256. Rutala WA, Weber DJ. Disinfection of endoscopes: review of new chemical sterilants used for high-level disinfection. Infect Control and Hospital Epidemiol 1999;20(1):69–75; published erratum, Infect Control Hosp Epidemiol 1999;20(5):302.

257. CDC. Nosocomial outbreak of *Rhizopus* infections associated with Elastoplast® wound dressings—Minnesota. MMWR 1978;27(5):33–4.

258. CDC. Follow-up on *Rhizopus* infections associated with Elastoplast® bandages—United States. MMWR 1978;27(28):243–4.

259. Bryce EA, Walker M, Scharf S, et al. Outbreak of cutaneous aspergillosis in a tertiary-care hospital. Infect Control Hosp Epidemiol 1996;17(3):170–2.

260. McCarty JM, Flam MS, Pullen G, Jones R, Kassel SH. Outbreak of primary cutaneous aspergillosis related to intravenous arm boards. J Pediatr 1986;108(5 Pt 1):721–4.

261. Mitchell SJ, Gray J, Morgan MEI, Hocking MC, Durbin GM. Nosocomial infection with *Rhizopus microsporus* in preterm infants: association with wooden tongue depressors. Lancet 1996;348(9025):441–3.

262. Gerson SL, Parker P, Jacobs MR, Creger R, Lazarus HM. Aspergillosis due to carpet contamination [Letter]. Infect Control Hosp Epidemiol 1994;15(4 Pt 1):221–3.

263. Richet H, McNeil M, Pewters W, et al. *Aspergillus flavus* in a bone marrow transplant unit (BMTU): pseudofungemia traced to hallway carpeting [Abstract F-23]. 89th Annual Meeting of the American Society for Microbiology, New Orleans, Louisiana, May 14–18, 1989:462.

264. Staib F. Ecological and epidemiological aspects of *Aspergilli* pathogenic for man and animal in Berlin (West). Zentrablatt fur Bakteriologie, Mikrobiologie, und Hygiene—Series A 1984;257(2):240–5.

265. CDC. ABCs of safe and healthy child care: an on-line handbook for child care providers. Atlanta, GA: US Department of Health and Human Services, CDC, 2000. Available at <http://www.cdc.gov/ncidod/hip/ABC/abc.htm>. Accessed May 15, 2000.

266. Buttery JP, Alabaster SJ, Heine RG, et al. Multiresistant *Pseudomonas aeruginosa* outbreak in a pediatric oncology ward related to bath toys. Pediatr Infect Dis J 1998;17(6):509–13.

267. CDC. Immunization of health care workers: recommendations of the Advisory Committee on Immunization Practices (ACIP) and the Hospital Infection Control Practices Advisory Committee. MMWR 1997;46(No. RR-18):1–42.

268. Bolyard EA, Tablan OC, Williams WW, et al. Guideline for infection control in health care personnel. Infect Control Hospital Epidemiol 1998;19(6):407–63.

269. Stover BH, Bratcher DF. Varicella-zoster virus: infection, control, and prevention [Review]. Am J Infect Control 1998;26(3):369–83; quiz 382–4.

270. Schubert MM, Peterson DE, Lloid ME. Oral complications. In: Thomas ED, Blume KG, Forman SJ, eds. Hematopoietic cell transplantation. 2nd ed. Oxford, England: Blackwell Science, Inc., 1999;751–63.

271. Wilkes JD. Prevention and treatment of oral mucositis following cancer chemotherapy [Review]. Semin Oncol 1998;25(5):538–51.

272. Toscano CM, Bell M, Zukerman C, et al. Bloodstream infections (BSI) associated with needleless device use, bathing practices and home infusion [Poster abstract P3]. 48th Annual Epidemic Intelligence Service Conference, April 19–23, 1999, Atlanta, GA;47.

273. Do AN, Ray BJ, Banerjee SN, et al. Bloodstream infection associated with needleless device use and the importance of infection-control practices in the home health care setting. J Infect Dis 1999;179(2):442–8.

274. Kool JL, Fiore AE, Kioski CM, et al. More than 10 years of unrecognized nosocomial transmission of Legionnaires' disease among transplant patients. Infect Control Hosp Epidemiol 1998;19(12):898–904.

275. CDC. Sustained transmission of nosocomial Legionnaires' disease—Arizona and Ohio. MMWR 1997;46(19):416–21.

276. Lepine LA, Jernigan DB, Butler JC, et al. Recurrent outbreak of nosocomial Legionnaires' disease detected by urinary antigen testing: evidence for long-term colonization of a hospital plumbing system. Infect Control Hosp Epidemiol 1998;19(12):905–10.

277. Muraca PW, Yu VL, Goetz A. Disinfection of water distribution systems for *Legionella*: a review of application procedures and methodologies [Review]. Infect Control Hosp Epidemiol 1990;11(2):79–88.

278. Harbarth S, Dharan S, Liassine N, Herrault P, Auckenthaler R, Pittet D. Randomized, placebo-controlled, double-blind trial to evaluate the efficacy of mupirocin for eradicating carriage of methicillin-resistant *Staphylococcus aureus*. Antimicrob Agents Chemother 1999;43(6):1412–6.

279. Leski TA, Gniadkowski M, Skoczynska A, Stefaniuk E, Trzcinski K, Hryniewicz W. Outbreak of mupirocin-resistant *Staphylococci* in a hospital in Warsaw, Poland, due to plasmid transmission and clonal spread of several strains. J Clin Microbiol 1999;37(9):2781–8.

280. Schmitz FJ, Lindenlauf E, Hofmann B, et al. Prevalence of low- and high-level mupirocin resistance in *Staphylococci* from 19 European hospitals. J Antimicrob Chemother 1998;42(4):489–95.

281. Irish D, Eltringham I, Teall A, et al. Control of an outbreak of an epidemic methicillin-resistant *Staphylococcus aureus* also resistant to mupirocin. J Hosp Infect 1998;39(1):19–26.

282. Udo EE, Farook VS, Mokadas EM, Jacob LE, Sanyal SC. Molecular fingerprinting of mupirocin-resistant methicillin-resistant *Staphylococcus aureus* from a burn unit. Int J Infect Dis 1998–99;3(2):82–7.

283. Bastos MC, Mondino PJ, Azevedo ML, Santos KR, Giambiagi-deMarval M. Molecular characterization and transfer among *Staphylococcus* strains of a plasmid conferring high-level resistance to mupirocin. Eur J Clin Microbiol Infect Dis 1999;18(6):393–8.

284. CDC. Recommendations for preventing the spread of vancomycin resistance: recommendations of the Hospital Infection Control Practices Advisory Committee (HICPAC). MMWR 1995;44(No. RR-12):1–13.

285. CDC. Update: *Staphylococcus aureus* with reduced susceptibility to vancomycin—United States, 1997. MMWR 1997;46(35):813–5.

286. Smith TL, Pearson ML, Wilcox KR, et al. Emergence of vancomycin resistance in *Staphylococcus aureus*. N Engl J Med 1999;340(7):493–501.

287. CDC. Interim guidelines for prevention and control of staphylococcal infection associated with reduced susceptibility to vancomycin. MMWR 1997;46(27):626–35.

288. CDC. Reduced susceptibility of *Staphylococcus aureus* to vancomycin—Japan, 1996. MMWR 1997;46(27):624–35.

289. Waldvogel FA. New resistance in *Staphylococcus aureus*. N Engl J Med 1999;340(7):556–7.

290. Montecalvo MA, Shay DK, Patel P, et al. Bloodstream infections with vancomycin-resistant *Enterococci*. Arch Intern Med 1996;156:1458–62.

291. Hospital Infection Control Practices Advisory Committee (HICPAC). Recommendations for preventing the spread of vancomycin resistance. Infect Control Hosp Epidemiol 1995;16:105–13.

292. Kirkpatrick BD, Harrington SM, Smith D, et al. Outbreak of vancomycin-dependent *Enterococcus faecium* in a bone marrow transplant unit. Clin Infect Dis 1999;29(5):1268–73.

293. Byers KE, Durbin LJ, Simonton BM, Anglim AM, Adel KA, Farr BM. Disinfection of hospital rooms contaminated with vancomycin-resistant *Enterococcus faecium*. Infect Control Hosp Epidemiol 1998;19(4):261–4.

294. Trick WE, Kuehnert MJ, Quirk SB, et al. Regional dissemination of vancomycin-resistant *Enterococci* resulting from interfacility transfer of colonized patients. J Infect Dis 1999;180(2):391–6.

295. Gerding DN, Johnson S, Peterson LR, Mulligan ME, Silva J Jr. *Clostridium difficile*-associated diarrhea and colitis [Review]. Infect Control Hosp Epidemiol 1995;16(8): 459–77.

296. Johnson S, Gerding DN. *Clostridium difficile*-associated diarrhea. Clin Infect Dis 1998;26:1027–36; quiz 1035–6.

297. McFarland LV, Mulligan M, Kwok RY, Stamm WE. Nosocomial acquisition of *Clostridium difficile* infection. N Engl J Med 1989;321(3):204–10.

298. Johnson S, Gerding DN, Olson MM, et al. Prospective, controlled study of vinyl glove use to interrupt *Clostridium difficile* nosocomial transmission. Am J Med 1990;88(2): 137–40.

299. Pear SM, Williamson T, Bettin K, Gerding DN, Galgiami JN. Decrease in nosocomial *Clostridium difficile*-associated diarrhea by restricting clindamycin use. Ann Intern Med 1994;120(4):272–7.

300. Kaatz GW, Gitlin SD, Schaberg DR et al. Acquisition of *Clostridium difficile* from the hospital environment. Am J Epidemiol 1988;127(6):1289–94.

301. Delmee M, Vandercam B, Avesani V, Michaux JL. Epidemiology and prevention of *Clostridium difficile* infections in a leukemia unit. Eur J Clin Microbiol 1987;6(6):623–7.

302. Johnson S, Homann SR, Bettin KM, et al. Treatment of asymptomatic *Clostridium difficile* carriers (fecal excretors) with vancomycin or metronidazole. Ann Intern Med 1992;117(4):297–302.

303. Surawicz CM, Elmer GW, Speelman P, McFarland LV, Chinn J, Van Belle G. Prevention of antibiotic associated diarrhea by *Saccharomyces boulardii*: a prospective study. Gastroenterology 1989;96(4):981–8.

304. Niault M, Thomas F, Prost J, Ansai FH, Kalfon P. Fungemia due to *Saccharomyces* species in a patient treated with enteral *Saccharomyces boulardii*. Clin Infect Dis 1999;28:930.

305. Fox JP, Brandt CD, Wasserman FE, et al. Virus watch program: a continuing surveillance of viral infections in metropolitan New York families. VI: observations of adenovirus infections: virus excretion patterns, antibody response, efficacy of surveillance, patterns of infections, and relation to illness. Am J Epidemiol 1969;89(1):25–50.

306. Hillis WO, Cooper MR, Bang FB. Adenovirus infection in West Bengal. I: persistence of viruses in infants and young children. Indian J Med Res 1973;61(7):980–8.

307. Hall CB, Powell KR, MacDonald DE, et al. Respiratory syncytial virus infection in children with compromised immune function. New Engl J Med 1986;315(2):77–81.

308. Villarino ME, Burman W, Wang YC, et al. Comparable specificity of 2 commercial tuberculin reagents in persons at low risk for tuberculous infection. JAMA 1999;281(2):169–71.

309. American Thoracic Society/CDC. Targeted tuberculin testing and treatment of latent tuberculosis infection. Am J Respir Crit Care Med 2000;161(4, part 2):S221–47.

310. American Academy of Pediatrics. Tuberculosis. In: Pickering LK, ed. 2000 red book: report of the Committee on Infectious Diseases. 25th ed. Elk Grove Village, IL: American Academy of Pediatrics;2000:593–613.

311. CDC. Notice to readers: use of short-course tuberculosis preventive therapy regimens in HIV-seronegative persons. MMWR 1998;47(42):911–2.

312. Fennelly KP. Transmission of tuberculosis during medical procedures [Letter]. Clin Infect Dis 1997;25:1273–5.

313. Talbot EA, Perkins MD, Silva SFM, Frothingham R. Disseminated Bacille Calmette-Guérin disease after vaccination: case report and review. Clin Infect Dis 1997;24(6):1139–46.

314. CDC. Role of BCG vaccine in the prevention and control of tuberculosis in the United States: a joint statement by the Advisory Council for the Elimination of Tuberculosis and the Advisory Committee on Immunization Practices. MMWR 1996;45(No. RR-4):13.

315. Gaynes RP, Horan TC. Chapter 85: surveillance of nosocomial infections. In: Mayhall CG, ed. Hospital epidemiology and infection control. 2nd ed. Philadelphia, PA: Lippincott Williams & Wilkins, 1999:1285–317.

Strategies for Safe Living After HSCT — Prevention of Exposure and Disease

316. CDC/National Center for Infectious Diseases/Working Group on Waterborne Cryptosporidiosis. Cryptosporidium and water: a public health handbook. Atlanta, GA: US Department of Health and Human Services, CDC, 1997. Available at <http://www.cdc.gov/ncidod/diseases/crypto/crypto.pdf>. Accessed May 15, 2000.

317. CDC/National Center for Infectious Diseases. Cryptosporidiosis [Fact sheet]. Atlanta, GA: US Department of Health and Human Services, CDC, 1999. Available at <http://www.cdc.gov/ncidod/dpd/parasites/cryptosporidiosis/factsht_cryptosporidiosis.htm>. Accessed May 15, 2000.

318. American Academy of Pediatrics. Cryptosporidiosis. In: Pickering LK, ed. 2000 red book: report of the Committee on Infectious Diseases. 25th ed. Elk Grove Village, IL: American Academy of Pediatrics 2000:223–4.

319. American Public Health Association. Cryptosporidiosis. In: Chin J, ed. Control of communicable diseases manual. 17th ed. Washington, DC: American Public Health Association, 2000:134–7.

320. DiFranza JR, Lew RA. Morbidity and mortality in children associated with the use of tobacco products by other people. Pediatrics 1996;97(4):560–8.

321. Cohen S, Tyrrell DA, Russell MA, Jarvis MJ, Smith AP. Smoking, alcohol consumption, and susceptibility to the common cold. Am J Pub Health 1993;83(9):1277–83.

322. Fischer M, Hedberg K, Cardosi P, et al. Tobacco smoke as a risk factor for meningococcal disease. Pediatr Infect Dis J 1997;16:979–83.

323. Lipsky BA, Boyko EJ, Inui TS, Koepsell TD. Risk factors for acquiring pneumococcal infections. Arch Intern Med 1986;146:2179–85.

324. Hall CB, Hall WJ, Gala CL, MaGill FB, Leddy JP. Long-term prospective study in children after respiratory syncytial virus infection. J Pediatr 1984;105(3):358–64.

325. Nuorti JP, Butler JC, Farley MM, et al. Cigarette smoking and invasive pneumococcal disease. New Engl J Med 2000;342(10):681–9.

326. Levitz SM, Diamond RD. Aspergillosis and marijuana [Letter]. Ann Intern Med 1991;115(7):578–9.

327. Marks WH, Florence L, Lieberman J, et al. Successfully treated invasive pulmonary aspergillosis associated with smoking marijuana in a renal transplant recipient [Review]. Transplant 1996;61(12):1771–4.

328. Chusid MJ, Gelfand JA, Nutter C, Fauci AS. Letter: pulmonary aspergillosis, inhalation of contaminated marijuana smoke, chronic granulomatous disease. Ann Intern Med 1975;82(5):682–3.

329. Hamadeh R, Ardehali A, Locksley RM, York MK. Fatal aspergillosis associated with smoking contaminated marijuana in a marrow transplant recipient. Chest 1988;94(2):432–3.

330. Kurup VP, Resnick A, Kagen SL, Cohen SH, Fink JN. Allergenic fungi and actinomycetes in smoking materials and their health implications. Mycopathologia 1983;82(1):61–4.

331. Kagen SL. *Aspergillus*: an inhalable contaminant of marihuana. N Engl J Med 1981;304(8):483–4.

332. Schwartz IS. Marijuana and fungal infection [Letter]. Am J Clin Pathol 1985;84(2):256.

333. Schwartz IS. Non-*Aspergillus* sinusitis and marijuana use [Letter]. Am J Clin Pathol 1992;97(4):601–2.

334. Llamas R, Hart R, Schneider NS. Allergic bronchopulmonary aspergillosis associated with smoking moldy marihuana. Chest 1978;73(6):871–2.

335. Angulo FJ, Glaser CA, Juranek DD, Lappin MR, Regnery RL. Caring for pets of immunocompromised persons. J Am Vet Med Assoc 1994;205(12):1711–8.

336. Elliott DL, Tolle SW, Goldberg L, Miller JB. Pet-associated illness. New Engl J Med 1985;313(16):985–94.

337. Glaser CA, Angulo FJ, Rooney JA. Animal-associated opportunistic infections among persons infected with the human immunodeficiency virus. Clin Infect Dis 1994;18:14–24.

338. Adams RM. Animals in schools: a zoonosis threat? Pediatr Infect Dis J 1998;17(2):174–6.

339. Dalton C, Hoffman R, Pape J. Iguana-associated salmonellosis in children. Pediatr Infect Dis J 1995;14(4):319–20.

340. CDC. Reptile-associated salmonellosis—selected states, 1996–1998. MMWR 1999;48(44):1009–13.

341. CDC. Errata: Reptile-associated salmonellosis—selected states, 1996–1998. MMWR 1999;48(45):1051.

342. Mermin J, Hoar B, Angulo FJ. Iguanas and *Salmonella marina* infection in children: a reflection of the increasing incidence of reptile-associated salmonellosis in the United States. Pediatr 1997;99(3):399–402.

343. CDC. Salmonellosis associated with chicks and ducklings—Michigan and Missouri, Spring 1999. MMWR 2000;49(14):297–9.

344. CDC. Lake-associated outbreak of *Escherichia coli* O157:H7—Illinois, 1995. MMWR 1996;45(21):437–9.

345. CDC. Outbreak of cryptosporidiosis associated with a water sprinkler foundation— Minnesota, 1997. MMWR 1998;47(40):856–60.

346. Kramer MH, Sorhage FE, Goldstein ST, Dalley E, Wahlquist SP, Herwaldt BL. First reported outbreak in the United States of cryptosporidiosis associated with a recreational lake. Clin Infect Dis 1998;26(1):27–33.

347. al-Eissa YA, Kambal AM, al-Nasser MN, al-Habib SA, al-Fawaz IM, al-Zamil FA. Childhood brucellosis: a study of 102 cases. Pediatr Infect Dis J 1990;9(2):74–9.

348. Keene WE, Hedberg K, Herriott DE, et al. Prolonged outbreak of *Escherichia coli* O157:H7 infections caused by commercially distributed raw milk. J Infect Dis 1997;176(3):815–8.

349. CDC. Outbreak of *Escherichia coli* O157:H7 infections associated with drinking unpasteurized commercial apple juice—British Columbia, California, Colorado, and Washington, October 1996. MMWR 1996;45(44):975.

350. CDC. Outbreaks of *Escherichia coli* O157:H7 infection and cryptosporidiosis associated with drinking unpasteurized apple cider—Connecticut and New York, October 1996. MMWR 1997;46(1):4–8.

351. CDC. Outbreak of *Salmonella* serotype Muenchen infections associated with unpasteurized orange juice—United States and Canada, June 1999. MMWR 1999;48(27): 582–5.

352. CDC/National Center for Infectious Diseases. Handle and prepare food safely. Atlanta, GA: US Department of Health and Human Services, CDC, 2000. Available at <http:// www.cdc.gov/ncidod/op/food.htm>. Accessed May 15, 2000.

353. CDC. Outbreak of *Campylobacter* enteritis associated with cross-contamination of food— Oklahoma, 1996. MMWR 1998;47(7):129–31.

354. CDC. Outbreaks of *Salmonella* serotype enteritidis infection associated with consumption of raw shell eggs—United States, 1994–1995. MMWR 1996;45(34):737–42.

355. CDC. Foodborne outbreak of cryptosporidiosis—Spokane, Washington, 1997. MMWR 1998;47(27):565–7.

356. US Department of Agriculture/Food Safety and Inspection Service. Big thaw—safe defrosting methods. Washington, DC: US Department of Agriculture, Food Safety and Inspection Service, Consumer Education and Information, 1996;1–2. Available at <http://www.fsis.usda.gov/OA/news/bigthaw.htm>. Accessed May 15, 2000.

357. US Department of Agriculture/Food Safety and Inspection Service. Kitchen thermometers. Washington, DC: US Department of Agriculture Consumer, Food Safety and Inspection Service, Education and Information, 2000 (in press).

358. Moe GL. Chapter 12: low-microbial diets for patients with granulocytopenia. In: Bloch AS, ed. Nutrition management of the cancer patient. Rockville, MD: Aspen Publishing, Inc., 1990:125–34.

359. Aker SN, Lenssen P. Chapter 80: nutritional support of patients with hematologic malignancies. In: Benz EJ Jr, Cohen HJ, Burie B, et al., eds. Hematology: basic principles and practice, 3rd ed. New York, NY: Churchill Livingstone, 2000:1501–14.

360. Hilton E, Isenberg HD, Alperstein P, France K, Borenstein MT. Ingestion of yogurt containing *Lactobacillus acidophilus* as prophylaxis for candidal vaginitis. Ann Intern Med 1992;116(5):353–7.

361. CDC. *Vibrio vulnificus* infections associated with eating raw oysters—Los Angeles, 1996. MMWR 1996;45(29):621–4.

362. CDC. Outbreak of *Vibrio parahaemolyticus* infection associated with eating raw oysters and clams harvested from Long Island Sound—Connecticut, New Jersey, and New York, 1998. MMWR 1999;48(03):48–51.

363. CDC. Viral gastroenteritis associated with eating oysters—Louisiana, December 1996–January 1997. MMWR 1997;46(47):1109–12.

364. Fayer R, Lewis EJ, Trout JM, et al. *Cryptosporidium parvum* in oysters from commercial harvesting sites in Chesapeake Bay. Emerg Infect Dis 1999;5(5):706–10.

365. Oliver MR, van Voorhis WC, Boeckh M, Mattson D, Bowden RA. Hepatic mucormycosis in a bone marrow transplant recipient who ingested naturopathic medicine. Clin Infect Dis 1996;22:521–4.

366. CDC. Health Information for international travel 1999–2000. Atlanta, GA: US Department of Health and Human Services, CDC, 1999. Available at <http://www.cdc.gov/travel/yellowbk99.pdf>. Accessed May 16, 2000.

367. World Health Organization. Guide on safe food for travelers. Geneva, Switzerland: World Health Organization, 1997:1–4. Available at <http://www.who.int/dsa/cat98/trav8.htm>. Accessed May 15, 2000.

368. CDC/National Center for Infectious Diseases. Food and water precautions and traveler's diarrhea prevention. Atlanta, GA: US Department of Health and Human Services, CDC, 2000;1–2. Available at <http://www.cdc.gov/travel/foodwatr.htm>. Accessed May 15, 2000.

369. Belay E, Bresee JS, Holman RC, Khan AS, Shahriari A, Schonberger LB. Reye's syndrome in the United States from 1981 through 1997. New Engl J Med 1999;340(18):1377–82.

HSCT Recipient Vaccinations

370. Pauksen K, Hammarström V, Ljungman P, et al. Immunity to poliovirus and immunization with inactivated poliovirus vaccine after autologous bone marrow transplantation. Clin Infect Dis 1994;18(4):547–52.

371. Pauksen K, Duraj V, Ljungman P, et al. Immunity to and immunization against measles, rubella and mumps in patients after autologous bone marrow transplantation. Bone Marrow Transplant 1992;9(6):427–32.

372. Ljungman P, Wiklund-Hammarsten M, Duraj V, et al. Responses to tetanus toxoid immunization after allogeneic bone marrow transplantation. J Infect Dis 1990;162(2):496–500.

373. Ljungman P, Fridell E, Lonnqvist B, et al. Efficacy and safety of vaccination of marrow transplant recipients with a live attenuated measles, mumps, and rubella vaccine. J Infect Dis 1989;159(4):610–5.

374. Henning KJ, White MH, Sepkowitz KA, Armstrong D. National survey of immunization practices following allogeneic bone marrow transplantation. JAMA 1997;277(14): 1148–51.

Hematopoietic Stem Cell Safety

375. Padley D, Koontz F, Trigg ME, Gingrich R, Strauss RG. Bacterial contamination rates following processing of bone marrow and peripheral blood progenitor cell preparations. Transfusion 1996;36(1):53–6.

376. National Marrow Donor Program.® Standards: effective September 1, 1999. 17th ed. Minneapolis, MN: National Marrow Donor Program, 1999:1–35.

377. Progenitor Cell Standards Task Force. Standards for hematopoietic progenitor cells. Bethesda, MD: American Association of Blood Banks, 1996:1–36.

378. Foundation for the Accreditation of Hematopoietic Cell Therapy. Standards for hematopoietic progenitor cell collection, processing and transplantation. 1st ed.-North America. Omaha, NE: FAHCT Accreditation Office, 1996:1–58.

379. Food and Drug Administration. Memorandum, June 8, 1995: recommendations for the deferral of current and recent inmates of correctional institutions as donors of whole blood, blood components, source leukocytes, and source plasma. Rockville, MD: US Department of Health and Human Services, Food and Drug Administration, 1995. Available at <http://www.fda.gov/cber/bldmem/6_8_95.txt>. Accessed May 16, 2000.

380. American Association of Blood Banks. New uniform donor history questionnaire issued [Association bulletin 99-10]. American Association of Blood Banks News 1999;(Nov/Dec):13–21.

381. CDC. Guidelines for preventing transmission of human immunodeficiency virus through transplantation of human tissue and organs. MMWR 1994;43(No. RR-8):1–17.

382. CDC. Public health service inter-agency guidelines for screening donors of blood, plasma, organs, tissues, and semen for evidence of hepatitis B and hepatitis C. MMWR 1991;40(No. RR-4):1–17.

383. Food and Drug Administration. Suitability determination for donors of human cellular and tissue-based products [Proposed rule]. Federal Register 1999;64:52696–723. Available at <http://www.fda.gov/cber/rules/suitdonor.pdf>. Accessed May 16, 2000.

384. Wells GM, Woodward TE, Fiset P, Hornick RB. Rocky Mountain spotted fever caused by blood transfusion. JAMA 1978;239(26):2763–65.

385. Herwaldt BL, Kjemtrup AM, Conrad PA, et al. Transfusion-transmitted babesiosis in Washington State: first reported case caused by a WA1-type parasite. J Infect Dis 1997;175(5):1259–62.

386. Dobroszycki J, Herwaldt BL, Boctor F, et al. Cluster of transfusion-associated babesiosis cases traced to a single asymptomatic donor. JAMA 1999;281(10):927–30.

387. CDC. Q fever—California. MMWR 1977;26(10):86, 91.

388. CDC. Transmission of Colorado tick fever virus by blood transfusion—Montana. MMWR 1975;24:422–7.

389. American Association of Blood Banks. Standards for blood banks and transfusion services. 19th ed. Bethesda, MD: American Association of Blood Banks, 1999:1–98.

390. Klein MB, Miller JS, Nelson CM, Goodman JL. Primary bone marrow progenitors of both granulocytic and monocytic lineages are susceptible to infection with the agent of human granulocytic ehrlichiosis. J Infect Dis 1997;176(5):1405–9.

391. Dharmasena F, Gordon-Smith EC. Transmission of malaria by bone marrow transplantation [Letter]. Transplant 1986;42(2):228.

392. Villeneuve L, Cassaing S, Magnaval JF, et al. *Plasmodium falciparum* infection following allogeneic bone-marrow transplantation. Ann Trop Med Parasitol 1999;93(5):533–5.

393. Leiby DA, Lenes BA, Tibbals MA, Tames-Olmedo MT. Prospective evaluation of a patient with *Trypanosoma cruzi* infection transmitted by transfusion. New Engl J Med 1999; 341(16):1237–9.

394. Leiby DA, Read EJ, Lenes BA, et al. Seroepidemiology of *Trypanosoma cruzi*, etiologic agent of Chagas' disease, in US blood donors. J Infect Dis 1997;176:1047–52.

395. Dodd RY. Transmission of parasites by blood transfusion [Review]. Vox Sang 1998;74(suppl 2):161–3.

396. Food and Drug Administration. Guidance for industry: precautionary measures to reduce the possible risk of transmission of zoonoses by blood and blood products from xenotransplantation products recipients and their contacts—12/23/99 [Draft guidance]. Rockville, MD: US Department of Health and Human Services, Food and Drug Administration, 1999;1–11. Available at <http://www.fda.gov/cber/guidelines.htm>. Accessed May 16, 2000.

397. CDC. Creutzfeldt-Jakob disease associated with cadaveric dura mater grafts—Japan, January 1979–May 1996. MMWR 1997;46(45):1066–9.

398. Food and Drug Administration. Guidance for industry: revised precautionary measures to reduce the possible risk of transmission of Creutzfeldt-Jakob Disease (CJD) and new variant Creutzfeldt-Jakob disease (nvCJD) by blood and blood products—11/23/99. Rockville, MD: US Department of Health and Human Services, Food and Drug Administration, 1999;1–16. Available at <http://www.fda.gov/cber/guidelines.htm>. Accessed May 16, 2000.

399. Will RG, Alpers MP, Dormont D, Schonberger LB, Tateishi J. Infectious and sporadic prion diseases. In: Prusiner SB, ed. Prion biology and diseases. Cold Spring Harbor, NY: Cold Spring Harbor Laboratory Press, 1999:465–507.

400. Food and Drug Administration. Memorandum, April 23, 1992: revised recommendations for the prevention of Human Immunodeficiency Virus (HIV) transmission by blood and blood products. Rockville, MD: US Department of Health and Human Services, Food and Drug Administration, 1992:1–24. Available at <http://www.fda.gov/cber/memo.htm>. Accessed May 16, 2000.

401. Pugatch D, Mileno M, Rich JD. Possible transmission of human immunodeficiency virus type 1 from body piercing. Clin Infect Dis 1998;26(3):767–8.

402. CDC. 1995 revised guidelines for prophylaxis against *Pneumocystic carinii* pneumonia for children infected with or perinatally exposed to human immunodeficiency virus. MMWR 1995;44(No. RR-4):1–11.

403. Attarian H, Bensinger WI, Buckner CD, McDonald DL, Rowley SD. Microbial contamination of peripheral blood stem cell collections. Bone Marrow Transplant 1996;17(5):699–702.

404. Rowley SD, Davis J, Dick J, et al. Bacterial contamination of bone marrow grafts intended for autologous and allogeneic bone marrow transplantation: incidence and clinical significance. Transfusion 1988;28(2):109–12.

405. Webb IJ, Coral FS, Andersen JW, et al. Sources and sequelae of bacterial contamination of hematopoietic cell components: implications for the safety of hematotherapy and graft engineering. Transfusion 1996;36(9):782–8.

406. Meyers JD, Huff JC, Holmes KK, Thomas ED, Bryan JA. Parenterally transmitted hepatitis A associated with platelet transfusions: epidemiologic study of an outbreak in a marrow transplantation center. Ann Intern Med 1974;81(2):145–51.

407. Fountain D, Ralston M, Higgins N, et al. Liquid nitrogen freezers: a potential source of microbial contamination of hematopoietic stem cell components. Transfusion 1997;37(6):585–91.

408. Nasser RM, Hajjar I, Sandhaus LM, et al. Routine cultures of bone marrow and peripheral stem cell harvests: clinical impact, cost analysis, and review. Clin Infect Dis 1998;27(4):886–8.

409. Flake AW, Roncarolo MG, Puck JM, et al. Treatment of x-linked severe combined immunodeficiency by in utero transplantation of paternal bone marrow. N Engl J Med 1996;335(24):1806–10.

410. Flake AW, Zanjani ED. In utero hematopoietic stem cell transplantation: a status report. JAMA 1997;278(11):932–7.

TABLE 1. Evidence-based rating system used to determine strength of recommendations

Category	Definition	Recommendation
A	Strong evidence for efficacy and substantial clinical benefit	Strongly recommended
B	Strong or moderate evidence for efficacy, but only limited clinical benefit	Generally recommended
C	Insufficient evidence for efficacy; or efficacy does not outweigh possible adverse consequences (e.g., drug toxicity or interactions) or cost of chemoprophylaxis or alternative approaches	Optional
D	Moderate evidence against efficacy or for adverse outcome	Generally not recommended
E	Strong evidence against efficacy or of adverse outcome	Never recommended

Source: Adapted from CDC. 1999 USPHS/IDSA guidelines for the prevention of opportunistic infections in persons infected with human immunodeficiency virus. MMWR 1999;48(RR-10):1–66.

TABLE 2. Evidence-based rating system used to determine quality of evidence supporting recommendation

Category	Definition
I	Evidence from at least one well-executed randomized, controlled trial
II	Evidence from at least one well-designed clinical trial without randomization; cohort or case-controlled analytic studies (preferably from more than one center); multiple time-series studies; or dramatic results from uncontrolled experiments
III	Evidence from opinions of respected authorities based on clinical experience, descriptive studies, or reports of expert committees

Source: Adapted from CDC. 1999 USPHS/IDSA guidelines for the prevention of opportunistic infections in persons infected with human immunodeficiency virus. MMWR 1999;48(RR-10):1–66.

TABLE 3. Foods that pose a high risk for hematopoietic stem cell transplant (HSCT) recipients and safer substitutions

Foods That Pose a High Risk	Safer Substitutions
Raw and undercooked eggs* and foods containing them (e.g., french toast, omelettes, salad dressings, egg nog, and puddings)	Pasteurized or hard boiled eggs
Unpasteurized dairy products (e.g., milk, cheese, cream, butter, and yogurt)	Pasteurized dairy products
Fresh-squeezed, unpasteurized fruit and vegetable juices	Pasteurized juices
Unpasteurized cheeses or cheeses containing molds	Pasteurized cheeses
Undercooked or raw poultry, meats, fish, and seafood	Cooked poultry, well-done meats, cooked fish, and seafood
Vegetable sprouts (e.g., alfalfa, bean, and other seed sprouts)[†]	Should be avoided
Raw fruits with a rough texture (e.g., raspberries)[§]	Should be avoided
Smooth raw fruits	Should be washed under running water, peeled, or cooked
Unwashed raw vegetables[¶]	Should be washed under running water, peeled, or cooked
Undercooked or raw tofu	Cooked tofu (i.e., cut into ≤1-inch cubes and boiled for ≥5 minutes in water or broth before eating or using in recipes)
Raw or unpasteurized honey	Should be avoided
Deli meats, hot dogs, and processed meats**	Should be avoided unless further cooked
Raw, uncooked grain products	Cooked grain products including bread, cooked, and ready-to-eat cold cereal, pretzels, popcorn, potato chips, corn chips, tortilla chips, cooked pasta, and rice
Maté tea[††]	Should be avoided
All moldy and outdated food products	Should be avoided
Unpasteurized beer (e.g., home-brewed and certain microbrewery beer)	Pasteurized beer (i.e., retail bottled or canned, or draft beer that has been pasteurized after fermentation)
Raw, uncooked brewers yeast	Should be avoided; HSCT recipients should avoid any contact with raw yeast (e.g., they should not make bread products themselves)
Unroasted raw nuts	Cooked nuts
Roasted nuts in the shell	Canned or bottled roasted nuts or nuts in baked products

* **Source:** CDC. Outbreaks of *Salmonella* serotype enteritidis infection associated with consumption of raw shell eggs—United States, 1994–1995. MMWR 1996; 45(34):737–42.
† **Source:** Taormina PJ, Beuchat LR, Slutsker L. Infections associated with eating seed sprouts: an international concern. Emerg Infect Dis 1999;5(5):626–34.
§ **Source:** Herwaldt BL, Ackers ML. Outbreak in 1996 of cyclosporiasis associated with imported raspberries. New Engl J Med 1997;336(22):1548–56.
¶ **Source:** CDC. Foodborne outbreak of cryptosporidiosis—Spokane, Washington, 1997. MMWR 1998;47(27):565–7.
** **Source:** CDC. Update: multistate outbreak of listeriosis—United States, 1998–1999. MMWR 1999;47(51):1117–8.
†† **Source:** Kusminsky G, Dictar M, Arduino S, Zylberman M, Sanchez Avalos JC. Do not drink Maté: an additional source of infection in South American neutropenic patients. Bone Marrow Transplant 1996;17(1):127.

TABLE 4. Recommended vaccinations for hematopoietic stem cell transplant* (HSCT) recipients, including both allogeneic and autologous recipients

For these guidelines, HSCT recipients are presumed immunocompetent at ≥24 months after HSCT if they are not on immunosuppressive therapy and do not have graft-versus-host disease (GVHD).

Vaccine or toxoid	Time after HSCT			Rating
	12 months	14 months	24 months	
Inactivated vaccine or toxoid				
Diphtheria, tetanus, pertussis				
Children aged <7 years*	Diphtheria toxoid-tetanus toxoid-pertussis vaccine (DTP) or diphtheria toxoid-tetanus toxoid (DT)†	DTP or DT	DTP or DT	BIII
Children aged ≥7 years§	Tetanus-diphtheria toxoid (Td)	Td	Td	BII
Haemophilus influenzae type b (Hib) conjugate¶	Hib conjugate	Hib conjugate	Hib conjugate	BII
Hepatitis (HepB)**	HepB	HepB	HepB	BIII
23-valent pneumococcal polysaccharide (PPV23)††	PPV23	—	PPV23	BIII
Hepatitis A§§	Routine administration not indicated			Not rated because of limited data
Influenza¶¶	Lifelong, seasonal administration, beginning before HSCT and resuming at ≥6 months after HSCT			BII
Meningococcal***	Routine administration not indicated			Not rated because of limited data
Inactivated polio (IPV)†††	IPV	IPV	IPV	BII
Rabies§§§	Routine administration not indicated			Not rated because of limited data
Lyme disease	Routine administration not indicated; limited data regarding safety, efficacy, or immunogenicity among HSCT recipients			Not rated because of limited data
Live-attenuated vaccine				
Measles-mumps-rubella (MMR)¶¶¶ *****††††	—	—	MMR	BIII
Varicella vaccine§§§§	Contraindicated for HSCT recipients			EIII
Rotavirus vaccine	Not recommended for any person in the United States¶¶¶¶			EII

TABLE 4. (Continued) Recommended vaccinations for hematopoietic stem cell transplant* (HSCT) recipients, including both allogeneic and autologous recipients

* Studies report that an HSCT recipient can be primed if the donor has had primary vaccination series. Studies also report that a recipient's antibody titer before HSCT might affect the titer 1 year after HSCT (**Source:** Lum LG. Kinetics of immune reconstitution after human marrow transplantation. Blood 1987;69[2]:369–80). No data were found regarding safety and immunogenicity of pertussis vaccination among HSCT recipients.

† DT should be used whenever a contraindication exists to pertussis vaccination.

§ HSCT recipients should be revaccinated with tetanus–diphtheria toxoids every 10 years, as routinely recommended for all adolescents and adults (**Sources:** CDC. Diphtheria, tetanus, and pertussis: recommendations of vaccine use and other prevention measures; recommendations of the Advisory Committee on Immunization Practices [ACIP]. MMWR 1991;40[No. RR-10]:1–28; and CDC. Use of vaccines and immunoglobulin in persons with altered immunocompetence: recommendations of the Advisory Committee on Immunization Practices [ACIP]. MMWR 1993;42[No. RR-4]:1–18).

¶ Hib conjugate vaccine is recommended for HSCT recipients of any age (**Sources:** CDC. Recommendations for use of *Haemophilus* b conjugate vaccines and a combined diphtheria, tetanus, pertussis, and *Haemophilus* b vaccine: recommendations of the Advisory Committee on Immunization Practices [ACIP]. MMWR 1993;42[No. RR-13]:1–15; and CDC. Use of vaccines and immunoglobulin in persons with altered immunocompetence: recommendations of the Advisory Committee on Immunization Practices [ACIP]. MMWR 1993;42[No. RR-4]:1–18).

** Hepatitis B vaccination is recommended for all susceptible persons aged ≤18 years and for adults who have risk factors for hepatitis B virus infection (**Sources:** CDC. Hepatitis B virus: a comprehensive strategy for eliminating transmission in the United States through universal childhood vaccination; recommendations of the Immunization Practices Advisory Committee [ACIP]. MMWR 1991;40[No. RR-13]:1–25; and CDC. Notice to readers: update; recommendations to prevent hepatitis B virus transmission—United States. MMWR 1995;44[30]:574–5). ACIP hepatitis B vaccination recommendations indicate that high doses (40 μg/dose) are recommended for adult dialysis patients and other immunocompromised adults (**Source:** CDC. Notice to readers: update; recommendations to prevent hepatitis B virus transmission—United States. MMWR 1995;44[30]:574–5). No data were found regarding immunocompromised children and their response to higher doses of vaccine. Postvaccination testing for antibody to hepatitis B surface antigen is recommended 1–2 months after the third vaccine dose to ensure protection among immunocompromised persons (**Source:** CDC. Notice to readers: update; recommendations to prevent hepatitis B virus transmission—United States. MMWR 1995;44[30]:574–5). Persons who do not respond to the primary vaccine series should complete a second 3-dose series.

†† The 23-valent pneumococcal polysaccharide vaccine might not be protective against pneumococcal infection among HSCT recipients. The second dose of vaccine is not a booster dose, but provides a second chance for immunologic response among persons who failed to respond to the first dose (**Source:** Guinan EC, Molrine DC, Antin JH, et al. Polysaccharide conjugate vaccine responses in bone marrow transplant patients. Transplant 1994;57[5]:677–84). Adjunctive antibiotic prophylaxis against encapsulated organisms, including pneumococcal disease, is recommended for allogeneic recipients with chronic GVHD (**Source:** Bortin MM, Horowitz MM, Gale RP, et al. Changing trends in allogeneic bone marrow transplantation for leukemia in the 1980s. JAMA 1992;268[5]:607–12). No data were found regarding safety and immunogenicity of the 7-valent conjugate pneumococcal vaccine among HSCT recipients; therefore, no recommendation regarding use of this vaccine can be made.

§§ No data were found regarding immunogenicity, safety, and efficacy of hepatitis A vaccine among HSCT recipients. Researchers report that hepatitis A vaccination can be used for investigational use among HSCT recipients aged ≥24 months at ≥12 months after HSCT and who are at increased risk for hepatitis A or its adverse consequences (e.g., persons with chronic liver disease, including chronic GVHD, and children living in areas with consistently elevated hepatitis A incidence) (**Source:** CDC. Prevention of hepatitis A through active or passive immunization: recommendations of the Advisory Committee on Immunization Practices [ACIP]. MMWR 1999;48[No. RR-12]:1–37).

¶¶ Children aged <9 years receiving influenza vaccination for the first time require two doses. Children aged ≤12 years should receive only split-virus influenza vaccine. Persons aged >12 years can receive whole- or split-virus vaccine. ACIP's and the American Academy of Pediatrics' dosing schedule should be used (**Sources:** American Academy of Pediatrics. Influenza. In: Pickering LK, ed. 2000 red book: report of the Committee on Infectious Diseases. 25th ed. Elk Grove Village, IL: American Academy of Pediatrics, 2000:351–9; and CDC. Prevention and control of influenza: recommendations of the Advisory Committee on Immunization Practices [ACIP]. MMWR 2000;49[No. RR-3]:1–38). For optimal influenza prevention, both vaccination and influenza chemoprophylaxis should be used among HSCT recipients.

*** Administration of meningococcal vaccine should be evaluated for HSCT recipients who live in endemic areas or areas experiencing outbreaks (**Source:** CDC. Control and prevention of meningococcal disease and control and prevention of serogroup C meningococcal disease: evaluation and management of suspected outbreaks. MMWR 1997;46[No. RR-5]:1–21). However, meningococcal vaccine immunogenicity and efficacy among HSCT recipients have not been studied.

††† Inactivated polio virus vaccine is immunogenic among HSCT recipients, although no data were found regarding efficacy and more data are needed regarding optimal methods and timing of immunization (**Sources:** Henning KJ, White MH, Sepkowitz KA, Armstrong D. National survey of immunization practices following allogeneic bone marrow transplantation. JAMA 1997;277[14]:1148–51; and CDC. Poliomyelitis prevention in the United States: introduction of a sequential vaccination schedule of inactivated poliovirus vaccine followed by oral poliovirus vaccine; recommendations of the Advisory Committee on Immunization Practices [ACIP]. MMWR 1997;46[No. RR-3]:1–25).

TABLE 4. (*Continued*) Recommended vaccinations for hematopoietic stem cell transplant* (HSCT) recipients, including both allogeneic and autologous recipients

§§§   Clinicians can administer preexposure rabies vaccine to HSCT recipients with potential occupational exposures to rabies (**Source:** CDC. Human rabies prevention—United States, 1999: recommendations of the Advisory Committee on Immunization Practices [ACIP] MMWR 1999;48[No. RR-1]:1–21; and published erratum, MMWR 1999;48[1]:16). However, the safety and immunogenicity of rabies vaccination among HSCT recipients has not been studied. Preexposure rabies vaccination should probably be delayed until 12–24 months after HSCT. Administration of rabies vaccine with human rabies immunoglobulin postexposure can be administered anytime after HSCT as indicated. Existing ACIP and American Academy of Pediatrics guidelines for postexposure human rabies immunoglobulin and vaccine administration should be followed, which include administering 5 doses of rabies vaccine administered on days 0, 3, 7, 14, and 28 postexposure (**Sources:** American Academy of Pediatrics. Rabies. In: Pickering LK, ed. 2000 red book: report of the Committee on Infectious Diseases. 25th ed. Elk Grove Village, IL: American Academy of Pediatrics;2000:475–82; and CDC. Human rabies prevention—United States, 1999: recommendations of the Advisory Committee on Immunization Practices [ACIP] MMWR 1999;48[No. RR-1]:1–21; published erratum, MMWR 1999;48[1]:16).

¶¶¶   The first dose of measles-mumps-rubella vaccine should be administered ≥24 months after HSCT if the HSCT recipient is presumed immunocompetent. The second measles-mumps-rubella dose is recommended 6–12 months later (BIII); however, the benefit of a second dose among HSCT recipients has not been evaluated. During outbreaks, the second dose can be administered 4 weeks after the first dose (**Source:** CDC. Use of vaccines and immunoglobulin in persons with altered immunocompetence: recommendations of the Advisory Committee on Immunization Practices [ACIP]. MMWR 1993;42[No. RR-4]:1–18).

*****   The half-life of intravenous immunoglobulin is decreased among HSCT recipients, but its effect on vaccine immunogenicity has not been evaluated. ACIP's and the American Academy of Pediatrics' recommendations regarding intervals between administration of immunoglobulin preparations for various indications and vaccines containing live measles virus should be used (**Sources:** American Academy of Pediatrics. Measles. In: Pickering LK, ed. 2000 red book: report of the Committee on Infectious Diseases. 25th ed. Elk Grove Village, IL: American Academy of Pediatrics. 2000:385–96; CDC. Measles, mumps, and rubella—vaccine use and strategies for elimination of measles, rubella, and congenital rubella syndrome and control of mumps: recommendations of the Advisory Committee on Immunization Practices [ACIP]. MMWR 1998;47[No. RR-8]:1–48; and CDC. General recommendations on immunization: recommendations of the Advisory Committee on Immunization Practices [ACIP]. MMWR 1994;43[No. RR-1]:1–38).

†††††   Use of live vaccines (e.g., measles-mumps-rubella) is indicated only among immunocompetent persons and is contraindicated for recipients after HSCT who are not presumed immunocompetent (**Sources:** CDC. Prevention of varicella: recommendations of the Advisory Committee on Immunization Practices [ACIP]. MMWR 1996;45[No. RR-11]:1–36; and CDC. General recommendations on immunization: recommendations of the Advisory Committee on Immunization Practices [ACIP]. MMWR 1994;43[No. RR-1]:1–38). Further research is needed to determine the safety, immunogenicity, and efficacy of varicella vaccine among HSCT recipients.

§§§§§   To protect HSCT recipients from varicella exposure, all varicella-susceptible health-care workers, family members, and close contacts of the recipient should be vaccinated against varicella (**Source:** American Academy of Pediatrics. Varicella-zoster infections. In: Pickering LK, ed. 2000 red book: report of the committee on Infectious diseases. 25th ed. Elk Grove Village, IL: American Academy of Pediatrics;2000:624–38).

¶¶¶¶¶   **Source:** CDC. Withdrawal of rotavirus vaccine recommendation. MMWR 1999;48[43]:1007.

Additional Notes: All indicated nonlive vaccines should be administered to HSCT recipients regardless of HSCT type or presence of GVHD. Live-attenuated vaccines, (e.g., measles-mumps-rubella, varicella, Bacillus Calmette-Guérin, yellow fever, and oral typhoid vaccines) should not be administered to any HSCT recipient with active GVHD or immunosuppression (**Source:** CDC. Role of BCG [Bacillus of Calmette and Guérin] vaccine in the prevention and control of tuberculosis in the United States: a joint statement by the Advisory Council for the Elimination of Tuberculosis and the Advisory Committee on Immunization Practices. MMWR 1996;45[No. RR-4]:1–18). To date, no adverse events have been reported (e.g., exacerbation of GVHD) among vaccinated HSCT recipients. However, data regarding immunization among HSCT recipients are limited and further studies are needed to evaluate safety, efficacy, and immunogenicity of the proposed HSCT immunization schedule. Use of combination vaccines is encouraged (**Source:** CDC. Combination vaccines for childhood immunization: recommendations of the Advisory Committee on Immunization Practices [ACIP], the American Academy of Pediatrics [AAP], and the American Academy of Family Physicians [AAFP]. MMWR 1999;48[No. RR-5]:1–15). No contraindications to simultaneous administration of any vaccines exist, except cholera and yellow fever. Adverse events after vaccination should be reported promptly to the Vaccine Adverse Event Reporting System (VAERS), P.O. Box 1100, Rockville, MD 20849-1100. Forms and information can be obtained from VAERS ([800] 822-7967). If the HSCT recipient has lapsed immunizations after HSCT (i.e., has missed one or more vaccine doses), the immunization schedule does not have to be restarted. Instead, the missing vaccine dose should be administered as soon as possible or during the next scheduled clinic appointment.

Table 5. Vaccinations for family, close contacts, and health-care workers (HCWs) of hematopoietic stem cell transplantation (HSCT) recipients*

Vaccine	Recommendations for use	Rating
Hepatitis A[†]	Routine vaccination is recommended for persons at increased risk for hepatitis A or its adverse consequences (e.g., persons with chronic liver disease or persons traveling to hepatitis A-endemic countries) and for children aged ≥24 months living in areas with consistently elevated hepatitis A incidence.[†]	BII
Influenza[§][¶]	Household contacts — Vaccination is strongly recommended during each influenza season (i.e., October–May) beginning in the season before the transplant and continuing to ≥24 months after HSCT. All household contacts of immunocompromised HSCT recipients should be vaccinated annually as long as these conditions persist.	AI
	HCWs and home caregivers — Annual vaccination is strongly recommended during each influenza season.	AI
Polio**	Vaccination is not routinely recommended for adults but should be administered when polio vaccination is indicated according to published Advisory Committee on Immunization Practices guidelines; when polio vaccine is administered, inactivated polio vaccine should be used.	AI
Measles-mumps-rubella[††]	Vaccination is recommended for all persons who are aged ≥12 months and who are not pregnant or immunocompromised.	AI
Rotavirus[§§]	Contraindicated because intussusception has been reported among infants during the first 1–2 weeks after rotavirus vaccination with substantially increased frequency.	EII
Varicella[¶¶]	Vaccination should be administered to all susceptible HCWs, household contacts, and family members who are aged ≥12 months and who are not pregnant or immunocompromised. When varicella vaccination is administered to persons aged ≥13 years, 2 doses are required, administered 4–8 weeks apart.	AIII

* This vaccination schedule refers only to vaccine-preventable diseases that are spread person-to-person.

† **Source:** CDC. Prevention of hepatitis A through active or passive immunization: recommendations of the Advisory Committee on Immunization Practices (ACIP). MMWR 1999;48(No. RR-12):1–37.

§ Children aged <9 years receiving influenza vaccination for the first time require 2 doses. Children aged ≤12 years should receive only split-virus influenza vaccine. Persons aged >12 years can receive whole- or split-virus vaccine (**Sources:** CDC. Prevention and control of influenza: recommendations of the Advisory Committee on Immunization Practices [ACIP]. MMWR 2000;49[No. RR-3]:1–38; and CDC. Immunization of health care workers: recommendations of the Advisory Committee on Immunization Practices [ACIP] and the Hospital Infection Control Practices Advisory Committee. MMWR 1997;46[No. RR-18]:1–42).

¶ If HCWs, family members, or other close contacts of HSCT recipients receive influenza vaccination during an influenza A outbreak, they should also receive amantadine or rimantadine chemoprophylaxis for 2 weeks after the influenza vaccination (BI) while the vaccinee develops an immunologic response to the vaccine. However, if a nosocomial outbreak occurs with an influenza A strain that is not contained in the available influenza vaccine, HCWs, family members, and other close contacts of HSCT recipients and candidates should be administered influenza A chemoprophylaxis with amantadine or rimantadine until the end of the outbreak (**Source:** CDC. Prevention and control of influenza: recommendations of the Advisory Committee on Immunization Practices [ACIP]. MMWR 2000;49[No. RR-3]:1–38) (BIII). HCWs, family members, or other close contacts can be offered a neuroaminidase inhibitor (e.g., zanamivir or oseltamivir) using the same strategies outlined previously, if one or more of the following exists: a) rimantadine or amantadine cannot be tolerated; b) the outbreak strain of influenza A is amantadine- or rimantadine-resistant; or c) the outbreak strain is influenza B (**Sources:** Monto AS, Robinson DP, Herlocher ML, Hinson JM Jr, Elliott MJ, Crisp A. Zanamivir in the prevention of influenza among healthy adults: a randomized controlled trial. JAMA 1999;282[1]:31–5; Hayden FG, Atmar RL, Schilling M, et al. Use of the selective oral neuraminidase inhibitor oseltamivir to prevent influenza. New Engl J Med 1999;341[18]:1336–43; Hayden FG, Gubareva L, Klein T, et al. Inhaled zanamivir for preventing transmission of influenza in families [Abstract LB-2]. In: Final program, abstracts and exhibits addendum, 38th Interscience Conference on Antimicrobial Agents and Chemotherapy. Washington, DC: American Society for Microbiology, 1991:1; and CDC. Neuraminidase inhibitors for treatment of influenza A and B infections. MMWR 1999;48[No. RR-14]:1–10) (BI). Zanamivir can be administered to persons aged ≥12 years, and oseltamivir can be administered to persons aged ≥18 years.

** **Caution:** Vaccine-strain polio virus in oral polio vaccine can be transmitted person-to-person; therefore, oral polio vaccine administration is contraindicated among household contacts of immunocompromised persons. If oral polio vaccine is inadvertently administered to a household contact of an HSCT recipient, ACIP's and the American Academy of Pediatrics' recommendations should be followed to minimize close contact with the immunocompromised person for 4–6 weeks after vaccination (**Sources:** American Academy of Pediatrics. Poliovirus infections. In: Pickering LK, ed. 2000 red book: report of the Committee on Infectious Diseases. 25th ed. Elk Grove Village, IL: American Academy of Pediatrics, 2000:465–70; CDC. Immunization of health care workers: recommendations of the Advisory Committee on Immunization Practices (ACIP) and the Hospital Infection Control

Table 5. (*Continued*) **Vaccinations for family, close contacts, and health-care workers (HCWs) of hematopoietic stem cell transplantation (HSCT) recipients***

Practices Advisory Committee. MMWR 1997;46[No. RR-18]:1–42; and CDC. Poliomyelitis prevention in the United States: introduction of a sequential vaccination schedule of inactivated poliovirus vaccine followed by oral poliovirus vaccine; recommendations of the Advisory Committee on Immunization Practices [ACIP]. MMWR 1997;46[No. RR-3]:1–25). Although vaccine-associated paralytic poliomyelitis has not been reported among HSCT recipients after exposure to household contacts inadvertently vaccinated with oral polio vaccine, inactivated polio vaccine should be used among family members, close contacts, and HCWs to avoid person-to-person transmission of vaccine-strain polio virus (**Source**: CDC. Poliomyelitis prevention in the United States: introduction of a sequential vaccination schedule of inactivated poliovirus vaccine followed by oral poliovirus vaccine; recommendations of the Advisory Committee on Immunization Practices [ACIP]. MMWR 1997;46[No. RR-3]:1–25).

†† No evidence exists that live-attenuated vaccine-strain viruses in measles-mumps-rubella vaccine have ever been transmitted from person-to-person, except rubella vaccine virus from a nursing mother to her infant (**Source**: CDC. Measles, mumps, and rubella—vaccine use and strategies for elimination of measles, rubella, and congenital rubella syndrome and control of mumps: recommendations of the Advisory Committee on Immunization Practices [ACIP]. MMWR 1998;47[No. RR-8]:1–48).

** HCWs, family members, close contacts and visitors who do not have a documented history of varicella-zoster infection or who are seronegative should receive this vaccination before being allowed to visit or have direct contact with an HSCT recipient (AIII). Ideally, varicella-zoster–susceptible HCWs, family members, household contacts, and potential visitors of immunocompromised HSCT recipients should be vaccinated as soon as the decision to perform an HSCT is made. The vaccination dose or doses should be completed ≥4 weeks before the conditioning regimen begins or ≥6 weeks (42 days) before contact with the HSCT recipient is planned (BIII). If a varicella vaccinee develops a postvaccination rash within 42 days of vaccination, the vaccinee should avoid contact with HSCT recipients until all rash lesions are crusted or the rash has resolved (**Sources**: CDC. Prevention of varicella: recommendations of the Advisory Committee on Immunization Practices [ACIP]. MMWR 1996;45[No. RR-11]:1–36; and CDC. Immunization of health care workers: recommendations of the Advisory Committee on Immunization Practices [ACIP] and the Hospital Infection Control Practices Advisory Committee. MMWR 1997;46[No. RR-18]:1–42).

TABLE 6. Vaccinations for hematopoietic stem cell transplant (HSCT) recipients traveling to areas endemic for selected vaccine-preventable diseases

Vaccine	Recommendations for use	Rating
Bacillus of Calmette and Guérin (live-attenuated vaccine)	Use of live-attenuated vaccine is contraindicated among HSCT recipients at <24 months after HSCT and among all persons who are immunocompromised.* No data were found regarding use among HSCT recipients.	EIII
Cholera	Vaccination is not indicated. No data were found regarding safety and immunogenicity among HSCT recipients.[†]	DIII
Hepatitis A	No data were found regarding immunogenicity, safety, or efficacy of hepatitis A vaccine among HSCT recipients; therefore, intramuscular immunoglobulin use is preferred for hepatitis A prophylaxis among HSCT recipients. However, administration of intramuscular immunoglobulin does not replace avoidance behaviors (e.g., careful selection of food and water).[§] Researchers recommend that hepatitis A vaccination be evaluated for investigational use among HSCT recipients aged ≥24 months; however, no recommendation can be made because of limited data.	Not rated because of limited data
Japanese B encephalitis	No data were found regarding safety, immunogenicity, or efficacy among HSCT recipients.[¶]	Not rated because of limited data
Lyme disease	No data were found regarding safety, immunogenicity, or efficacy among HSCT recipients.	Not rated because of limited data
Meningococcal vaccine	Vaccine should be administered to HSCT recipients traveling to endemic areas or to areas experiencing outbreaks.** However, meningococcal vaccine immunogenicity and efficacy have not been studied among HSCT recipients.	Not rated because of limited data
Plague	No data were found regarding safety, immunogenicity, or efficacy among HSCT recipients.[††]	Not rated because of limited data
Polio (inactivated polio vaccine only)	Booster dose can be administered as indicated.[§§]	CIII
Rabies	Researchers recommend that administration of a preexposure series be evaluated for persons at ≥12 months after HSCT if they anticipate travel to endemic areas.[¶¶] However, no data were found regarding safety, immunogenicity, or efficacy among HSCT recipients.	Not rated because of limited data
Typhoid, oral (live-attenuated vaccine)	Use of oral typhoid vaccine (live-attenuated strain) is contraindicated among HSCT recipients at <24 months after HSCT and among those who are immunocompromised.*** No data were found regarding safety, immunogenicity, or efficacy among HSCT recipients.	EIII
Typhoid (intramuscular)	No data were found regarding safety, immunogenicity, or efficacy among HSCT recipients.	Not rated because of limited data
Yellow fever (live-attenuated vaccine)	Use of live-attenuated vaccine is contraindicated among HSCT recipients at <24 months after HSCT and among all immunocompromised persons.[†††] No data were found regarding safety, immunogenicity, or efficacy among HSCT recipients.	EIII

* **Source:** CDC. Role of BCG [Bacillus of Calmette and Guérin] vaccine in the prevention and control of tuberculosis in the United States: a joint statement by the Advisory Council for the Elimination of Tuberculosis and the Advisory Committee on Immunization Practices. MMWR 1996;45(No. RR-4):1–18.

[†] **Source:** CDC. Recommendations of the Immunization Practices Advisory Committee: cholera vaccine. MMWR 1988;37(40):617–8; 623–4.

[§] **Source:** CDC. Prevention of hepatitis A through active or passive immunization: recommendations of the Advisory Committee on Immunization Practices (ACIP). MMWR 1999;48(No. RR-12):1–37.

[¶] **Source:** CDC. Inactivated Japanese encephalitis virus vaccine: recommendations of the Advisory Committee on Immunization Practices (ACIP). MMWR 1993;42(No. RR-1):1–15.

** **Source:** CDC. Control and prevention of meningococcal disease and control and prevention of serogroup C meningococcal disease: evaluation and management of suspected outbreaks. MMWR 1997;46(No. RR-5):1–21.

TABLE 6. (*Continued*) **Vaccinations for hematopoietic stem cell transplant (HSCT) recipients traveling to areas endemic for selected vaccine-preventable diseases**

†† **Source**: CDC. Prevention of plague: recommendations of the Advisory Committee on Immunization Practices (ACIP). MMWR 1996;45(No. RR-14):1–15.

§§ **Source**: CDC. Poliomyelitis prevention in the United States: introduction of a sequential vaccination schedule of inactivated poliovirus vaccine followed by oral poliovirus vaccine; recommendations of the Advisory Committee on Immunization Practices (ACIP). MMWR 1997;46(No. RR-3):1–25.

¶¶ **Source**: CDC. Human rabies prevention—United States, 1999: recommendations of the Advisory Committee on Immunization Practices (ACIP) MMWR 1999;48(No. RR-1):1–21; published erratum, MMWR 1999;48(1):16.

*** **Source**: CDC. Typhoid immunization: recommendations of the Advisory Committee on Immunization Practices (ACIP). MMWR 1994;43(No. RR-14):1–7.

††† **Source**: CDC. Yellow fever vaccine: recommendations of the Immunization Practices Advisory Committee (ACIP). MMWR 90;39(No. RR-6):1–6.

Additional Note: Specific advice for international travelers, including information regarding endemic diseases by country, is available through CDC's automated travelers' hotline at (404) 332-4559; by facsimile at (404) 335-4565; on the Internet at <http://www.cdc.gov>; and by file transfer protocol at <ftp.cdc.gov>.

TABLE 7. Use of passive immunization for hematopoietic stem cell transplant (HSCT) recipients exposed to vaccine-preventable diseases

Preparation	Recommendations for Use	Rating
Cytomegalovirus immunoglobulin	Not recommended for prophylaxis among HSCT recipients because of its lack of efficacy.*	DI
Hepatitis B immunoglobulin	Immunocompromised persons who have percutaneous or permucosal exposure to hepatitis B virus should receive 2 doses administered 1 month apart. For immunocompetent persons, the need for postexposure prophylaxis depends on the vaccination history and antibody to hepatitis B surface antigen response status of the exposed person.[†]	CIII
Human rabies immunoglobulin	Should be administered with rabies vaccine at anytime after HSCT as indicated for postexposure rabies prophylaxis. Existing Advisory Committee on Immunization Practices guidelines for postexposure should be followed, with 5 doses of rabies vaccine administered on days 0, 3, 7, 14, and 28 postexposure.[§]	CIII
Respiratory syncytial virus immunoglobulin[¶]	Because of high rates of case fatality from respiratory syncytial virus pneumonia among HSCT recipients, HSCT physicians can administer HSCT recipients with upper or lower respiratory infection preemptive therapy with a high titer of neutralizing antibodies to prevent severe disease and death until controlled trials can be performed.**	CIII
Respiratory syncytial virus monoclonal antibody	Physicians can use respiratory syncytial virus monoclonal antibody[††] investigationally as preemptive therapy (Appendix).	Not rated because of limited data
Tetanus immunoglobulin	Postexposure vaccination should be administered with or without tetanus immunoglobulin as indicated for tetanus exposure[§§] that occurs anytime after HSCT.	CIII
Varicella-zoster immunoglobulin[¶¶]	Ideally, should be administered to HSCT recipients ≤96 hours after close contact with a person with varicella or shingles if the HSCT recipient is at a) <24 months after HSCT or b) ≥24 months after HSCT and still immunocompromised. Administration can extend the varicella incubation period from 10–21 days to 10–28 days. If the HSCT recipient experiences a varicella-zoster virus-like rash after contact with or exposure to a person with varicella or herpes zoster, antiviral drug therapy should be administered until ≥2 days after all lesions have crusted.***	AII
Intramuscular immunoglobulin	Should be administered to hepatitis A-susceptible HSCT recipients who anticipate hepatitis A exposure, (e.g., during travel to endemic areas) and for postexposure prophylaxis as indicated.[†††] Should also be administered after measles exposure among HSCT recipients who were not vaccinated against measles after HSCT.[§§§]	BIII
Intravenous immunoglobulin[¶¶¶]	Can be administered to HSCT recipients with severe hypogammaglobulinemia (immunoglobulin G < 400 mg/dl) ≤100 days after HSCT to prevent bacterial infections**** (Appendix).	CIII

* **Source:** Boeckh M, Bowden R. Cytomegalovirus infection in marrow transplantation. In: Buckner CD, ed. Technical and biological components of marrow transplantation. Boston, MA: Kluwer Academic Publishers, 1995:97–136.

† **Source:** CDC. Immunization of health care workers: recommendations of the Advisory Committee on Immunization Practices (ACIP) and the Hospital Infection Control Practices Advisory Committee. MMWR 1997;46(No. RR-18):1–42.

§ **Sources:** American Academy of Pediatrics. Rabies. In: Pickering LK, ed. 2000 red book: report of the Committee on Infectious Diseases. 25th ed. Elk Grove Village, IL: American Academy of Pediatrics;2000:475–82; and CDC. Human rabies prevention—United States, 1999: recommendations of the Advisory Committee on Immunization Practices (ACIP) MMWR 1999;48(No. RR-1):1–21; published erratum, MMWR 1999;48(1):16.

TABLE 7. (*Continued*) **Use of passive immunization for hematopoietic stem cell transplant (HSCT) recipients exposed to vaccine-preventable diseases**

¶ Researchers recommend substituting respiratory syncytial virus immunoglobulin for intravenous immunoglobulin for HSCT recipients on replacement intravenous immunoglobulin therapy during respiratory syncytial virus season (i.e., November–April) (**Source**: American Academy of Pediatrics. Respiratory syncytial virus. In: Pickering LK, ed. 2000 red book: report of the Committee on Infectious Diseases. 25th ed. Elk Grove Village, IL: American Academy of Pediatrics;2000:483–7) (CIII). However, no data were found demonstrating safety and efficacy of respiratory syncytial virus immunoglobulin use among HSCT recipients.

§§ **Source**: CDC. Diphtheria, tetanus, and pertussis: recommendations of vaccine use and other prevention measures; recommendations of the Advisory Committee on Immunization Practices (ACIP). MMWR 1991;40(No. RR-10):1–28.

¶¶ If intravenous immunoglobulin replacement therapy (>250 mg/kg) has been administered <2 weeks before varicella or zoster rash exposure, varicella-zoster immunoglobulin administration is probably not required. Varicella-zoster immunoglobulin is distributed by the American Red Cross, except in Massachusetts, where it is distributed by the Massachusetts Public Health Biologic Laboratories (now a unit of the University of Massachusetts) (**Source**: CDC. Prevention of varicella: recommendations of the Advisory Committee on Immunization Practices [ACIP]. MMWR 1996;45[No. RR-11]:1–36).

*** **Source**: CDC. Prevention of varicella: recommendations of the Advisory Committee on Immunization Practices (ACIP). MMWR 1996;45(No. RR-11):1–36.

††† **Source**: CDC. Prevention of hepatitis A through active or passive immunization: recommendations of the Advisory Committee on Immunization Practices (ACIP). MMWR 1999;48(No. RR-12):1–37.

§§§ **Sources**: CDC. Measles, mumps, and rubella—vaccine use and strategies for elimination of measles, rubella, and congenital rubella syndrome and control of mumps: recommendations of the Advisory Committee on Immunization Practices (ACIP). MMWR 1998;47(No. RR-8):1–48; and Eibl MM, Wedgwood RJ. Intravenous immunoglobulin: a review. Immunodeficiency Reviews 1989;1:1–42.

¶¶¶ When administered, serum immunoglobulin G levels should be monitored regularly (e.g., every 2 weeks).

**** **Sources**: Antman KH, Rowlings PA, Vaughn WP, et al. High-dose chemotherapy with autologous hematopoietic stem cell support for breast cancer in North America. J Clin Oncol 1997;15(5):1870–9; and Wolff SN, Fay JW, Herzig RH, et al. High-dose weekly intravenous immunoglobulin to prevent infections in patients undergoing autologous bone marrow transplantation or severe myelosuppressive therapy. Ann Intern Med 1993;118(12):937–42.

Additional Notes: Intravenous immunoglobulin can be obtained from the American Red Cross Blood Services, although shortages occasionally occur. Physicians who have difficulty obtaining urgently needed intravenous immunoglobulin and other immunoglobulin products are advised to contact any of the following:

- American Red Cross Customer Service Center, (800) 261-5772;
- Alpha Therapeutic Corporation, (800) 421-0008;
- Baxter Healthcare Corporation, (847) 940-5955;
- Bayer Pharmaceutical Division, (800) 288-8370;
- Aventis Behring Customer Support, (800) 683-1288;
- Novartis Pharmaceuticals Corporation, (973) 781-8300, or the Intravenous Immunoglobulin Emergency Hotline, (888) 234-2520; or
- Immune Deficiency Foundation, (800) 296-4433.

Physicians who are unable to obtain intravenous immunoglobulin for a licensed indication from one of these sources should contact the Product Shortage Officer at the Food and Drug Administration's Center for Biologics Evaluation and Research, Office of Compliance, (301) 827-6220, for assistance. Patients with immunoglobulin E anti-immunoglobulin A antibodies are at high risk for experiencing anaphylaxis from immunoglobulin administration (**Source**: Burks AW, Sampson HA, Buckley RH. Anaphylactic reactions after gamma globulin administration in patients with hypogammaglobulinemia. New Engl J Med 1986;314[9]:560–4). Therefore, persons with immunoglobulin A deficiency should not be administered standard immunoglobulin preparations (DIII; BIII). However, researchers report that use of immunoglobulin A-depleted immunoglobulin preparations can be used with caution in these persons (**Sources**: Burks AW, Sampson HA, Buckley RH. Anaphylactic reactions after gamma globulin administration in patients with hypogammaglobulinemia. New Engl J Med 1986;314[9]:560–4; Siberry GK, Iannone R, eds. Harriet Lane handbook: a manual for pediatric house officers. 15th ed.; St. Louis, MO: Mosby, Inc., 2000:339;739; and Stiehm ER. Human intravenous immunoglobulin in primary and secondary antibody deficiencies [Review]. Pediatr Infect Dis J 1997;16[7]:696–707).

TABLE 8. Vaccine information

Vaccine or toxoid	Trade name	Manufacturer/ telephone number	Storage recommendation
Diphtheria toxoid-tetanus toxoid-pertussis vaccine	Tripedia®	Aventis Pasteur, Inc. (800) Vaccine	Store at 2–8 C (36–46 F); do not freeze
	Infanrix®	SmithKline Beecham (800) 877-1158	
	Acel-Imune®	Wyeth-Lederle (800) 572-8221	
	Certiva®	North American Vaccine (888) 628-2829	
Diphtheria toxoid-tetanus toxoid-pertussis vaccine–*Haemophilus influenzae* type b	Tetramune®	Wyeth-Lederle (800) 572-8221	Store at 2–8 C (36–46 F); do not freeze
	DTP/ACTHib®	Aventis Pasteur, Inc. (800) Vaccine	
	TriHibit®		
Tetanus-diphtheria toxoid (adult) and Diphtheria-tetanus toxoid (pediatric)	Generic	Aventis Pasteur, Inc. (800) Vaccine Wyeth-Lederle (800) 572-8221	Store at 2–8 C (36–46 F); do not freeze
Haemophilus influenzae type b	ACTHib®	Aventis Pasteur, Inc. (800) Vaccine	Store at 2–8 C (36–46 F); do not freeze
	HibTiter®	Wyeth-Lederle (800) 572-8221	
	PedvaxHIB®	Merck Human Health Division (800) MerckRX (ordering) (800) NSCmerc (questions)	
	OmniHIB®	SmithKline Beecham (800) 877-1158	
Haemophilus influenzae type b-Hepatitis B	COMVAX®	Merck Human Health Division (800) MerckRX (ordering) (800) NSCmerc (questions)	Store at 2–8 C (36–46 F); do not freeze
Inactivated polio vaccine	IPOL®	Aventis Pasteur, Inc. (800) Vaccine	
Measles-mumps-rubella Measles-rubella Mumps-rubella Measles Mumps Rubella	M-M-R II® M-R-Vax II® Biavax II® Attenuvax® Mumpsvax® Meruvax II®	Merck Human Health Division (800) MerckRX (ordering) (800) NSCmerc (questions)	Store at 2–8 C (36–46 F); freezing is permissible
Varicella	Varivax®		Maintain in a frozen state of –15 C (5 F) or colder
Hepatitis A	Vaqta® Havix®	SmithKline Beecham (800) 877-1158	Store at 2–8 C (36–46 F); do not freeze
Hepatitis B	Engerix-B® Recombivax B®	Merck Human Health Division (800) MerckRX (ordering) (800) NSCmerc (questions)	Store at 2–8 C (36–46 F); do not freeze
Influenza	Fluzone®	Aventis Pasteur, Inc. (800) Vaccine	Store at 2–8 C (36–46 F); do not freeze
	Fluvirin®	Celltech Medeva Pharmaceutical (800) 234-5535	
	Flu-Shield®	Wyeth-Ayerst Laboratories (800) 358-7443	
	Fluogen®	Monarch Pharmaceuticals (888) 358-6436	
Japanese encephalitis	JE-VAX	Research Foundation for Microbial Diseases of Osaka University, Japan; Distributed by Aventis Pasteur, Inc. (800) Vaccine SmithKline Beecham	Store at 2–8 C (36–46 F); do not freeze

TABLE 8. (*Continued*) Vaccine information

Vaccine or toxoid	Trade name	Manufacturer/ telephone number	Storage recommendation
Lyme disease	LYMErix™	(800) 877-1158	Store at 2–8 C 36–46 F); do not freeze
Pneumococcal 23-valent	Pru-Immune-23®	Wyeth-Lederle (800) 572-8221	Store at 2–8 C (36–46 F); do not freeze
	Pneumovax 23®	Merck Human Health Division (800) MerckRX (ordering) (800) NSCmerc (questions)	
Meningococcal	Menomune-A/C/Y/W-135®	Aventis Pasteur, Inc. (800) Vaccine	Store at 2–8 C (36–46 F); do not freeze
Rabies	Generic	BioPort Corporation (517) 327-1500; distributed by SmithKline Beecham (800) 877-1158	Store at 2–8 C (36–46 F); do not freeze
	Imovax Rabies® and Imovax Rabies ID® RabAvert™	Aventis Pasteur, Inc. (800) Vaccine Chiron Corporation (800) 244-7668	
Typhoid	Typhoid Vaccine U.S. P.	Wyeth-Lederle (800) 572-8221	
Typhoid Vi polysaccharide	Typhim Vi™	Aventis Pasteur, Inc. (800) Vaccine	

Notes: Persons needing additional vaccine information or CDC's Advisory Committee on Immunization Practices guidelines can contact the CDC Immunization Hotline at (800) CDC-SHOT ([800] 232-7468) or at <http:// www.cdc.gov/ nip>. Adverse events after vaccination should be reported promptly to the Vaccine Adverse Event Reporting System (VAERS), P.O. Box 1100, Rockville, MD 20849-1100. Forms and information can be obtained from VAERS at (800) 822-7967.

Appendix

Dosing Charts for Preventing Opportunistic Infections Among Hematopoietic Stem Cell Transplant Recipients

I. Preventive regimens for adult or adolescent hematopoietic stem cell transplant (HSCT) recipients

Pathogen: Cytomegalovirus

Indication	First choice	Alternatives
Universal prophylaxis for cytomegalovirus disease among all allogeneic adult or adolescent HSCT recipients at risk throughout phase II (i.e., from engraftment to day 100 after HSCT)	Ganciclovir, 5 mg/kg/dose intravenously every 12 hours for 5–7 days, followed by 5–6 mg/kg intravenously daily for 5 days/ week from engraftment until day 100 after HSCT (AI)	Foscarnet, 60 mg/kg intravenously every 12 hours for 7 days, followed by 90–120 mg/kg intravenously daily until day 100 after HSCT (CIII)
Or preemptive cytomegalovirus treatment administered <100 days after HSCT to all allogeneic adult or adolescent HSCT recipients at risk: Start ganciclovir when the patient experiences any level of cytomegalovirus antigenemia or viremia or has ≥2 consecutively positive cytomegalovirus-DNA polymerase chain reaction tests	Ganciclovir, 5 mg/kg/dose intravenously every 12 hours for 7–14 days, followed by 5 mg/kg/day for 5 days/week until day 100 after HSCT or for a minimum of 3 weeks, whichever is longer (AI); or administer ganciclovir for a total of 3–6 weeks; antigen or polymerase chain reaction tests should be negative when ganciclovir is stopped; reinstitute ganciclovir if subsequent weekly cytomegalovirus antigenemia screening tests become positive (BI)	
Preemptive treatment for cytomegalovirus seropositive autologous adult or adolescent HSCT recipients at <100 days after HSCT: Start ganciclovir when antigenemia is ≥5 cells/slide, but CD34+-selected patients should be treated at any level of antigenemia*	Ganciclovir, 5 mg/kg/dose intravenously every 12 hours for 7 days, followed by 5 mg/kg/day intravenously for 5 days/week for 2 weeks (BII)	
Preemptive treatment of allogeneic adult or adolescent HSCT recipients >100 days after HSCT: Start ganciclovir when a) antigenemia is ≥5 cells/slide or b) the patient has had ≥2 consecutively positive viremia or polymerase chain reaction tests (e.g., in a person receiving steroids for graft-versus-host disease or who received ganciclovir or foscarnet at <100 days after HSCT)	Ganciclovir, 5 mg/kg/dose intravenously every 12 hours for 7 days, followed by 5 mg/kg/day intravenously for 5 days/week for 2 weeks (BIII)	

* **Source**: Holmberg LA, Boeckh M, Hooper H, et al. Increased incidence of cytomegalovirus disease after autologous CD34-selected peripheral blood stem cell transplantation [Clinical observations, interventions, and therapeutic trials]. Blood 1999;94(12):4029–35.

Notes: Patients who do not tolerate standard doses of ganciclovir should be administered foscarnet. Ganciclovir and foscarnet doses should be modified for renal impairment. Prehydration is required for foscarnet administration.

Pathogen: Herpes simplex virus

Indication	First choice	Alternatives
Prevention of herpes simplex virus reactivation among seropositive adult or adolescent HSCT recipients: Start acyclovir at the beginning of conditioning therapy and continue until engraftment or until mucositis resolves (i.e., approximately 30 days after HSCT for allogeneic HSCT recipients)	Acyclovir, 200 mg by mouth 3 times/day or 250 mg/m^2/dose infused over 1 hour intravenously every 12 hours (BIII)	Valacyclovir, 500 mg by mouth daily (CIII)

Note: For patients requiring prophylaxis for cytomegalovirus and herpes simplex virus after engraftment, ganciclovir alone provides effective prophylaxis for both pathogens.

Pathogen: Varicella-zoster virus

Indication	First choice	Alternatives
Prevention of varicella-zoster virus disease after exposure among adult or adolescent HSCT recipients who are at <24 months after HSCT or who are at ≥24 months after HSCT and on immunosuppressive therapy or have chronic graft-versus-host disease: Ideally, administer prophylaxis within 96 hours (preferably, within 48 hours) after close contact with a person who has chickenpox or shingles	Varicella-zoster immunoglobulin, 5 vials (1.25 ml each or 625 units total) intramuscularly (All)	None

Pathogen: Influenza

Indication	First choice	Alternatives
Prevention of influenza A or B among adult or adolescent HSCT recipients	Lifelong annual seasonal (i.e., October–May) influenza vaccination starting before HSCT and restarting 6 months after HSCT (BIII); whole- or split-virus influenza vaccine, 0.5 ml/dose intramuscularly	None
Prophylaxis and preemptive treatment among all HSCT recipients during community and nosocomial outbreaks of influenza A	Rimantadine, 100 mg by mouth 2 times/day (CIII)	Amantadine, 100 mg by mouth 2 times/day (CIII)

Notes: Rimantadine dose should be reduced for patients with impaired renal function or for severely impaired hepatic function. Amantadine dose should be reduced for renal impairment.

Pathogen: Bacterial infections, general prophylaxis

Indication	First choice	Alternatives
Prevention of bacterial infections among allogeneic adult or adolescent HSCT recipients with severe hypogammaglobulinemia (i.e., serum immunoglobulin G level < 400 mg/dl) at <100 days after HSCT	Intravenous immunoglobulin, 500 mg/kg/week (CIII)	None

Notes: Patients with immunoglobulin E anti-immunoglobulin A antibodies are at high risk for experiencing anaphylaxis from immunoglobulin administration (**Source:** Burks AW, Sampson HA, Buckley RH. Anaphylactic reactions after gamma globulin administration in patients with hypogammaglobulinemia. New Engl J Med 1986;314[9]:560–4). Therefore, persons with immunoglobulin A deficiency should not receive standard immunoglobulin products (**Source:** Siberry GK, Iannone R, eds. Harriet Lane handbook: a manual for pediatric house officers. 15th ed.; St. Louis, MO: Mosby, Inc., 2000:339;739) (DIII). However, researchers have reported that use of immunoglobulin A-depleted immunoglobulin preparations can be used with caution among these persons (**Sources:** Burks AW, Sampson HA, Buckley RH. Anaphylactic reactions after gamma globulin administration in patients with hypogammaglobulinemia. New Engl J Med 1986;314[9]:560–4; Stiehm ER. Human intravenous immunoglobulin in primary and secondary antibody deficiencies [Review]. Pediatr Infect Dis J 1997;16[7]:696–707; and American Academy of Pediatrics. Passive immunization. In: Pickering LK, ed. 2000 red book: report of the Committee on Infectious Diseases. 25th ed. Elk Grove Village, IL: American Academy of Pediatrics;2000:41–53). Researchers also propose checking serum immunoglobulin G levels every 2 weeks among patients receiving intravenous immunoglobulin replacement therapy.

Pathogen: *Streptococcus pneumoniae*

Indication	First choice	Alternatives
Prevention of pneumococcal disease among adult or adolescent HSCT recipients	23-valent pneumococcal polysaccharide vaccine at 12 and 24 months after HSCT (BIII)	None

Note: Penicillin-resistant *Streptococcus pneumoniae* is increasing in the United States.

Pathogen: *Haemophilus influenzae* type b

Indication	First choice	Alternatives
Prevention of invasive *Haemophilus influenzae* type b (Hib) disease among adult or adolescent HSCT recipients	Hib conjugate vaccine administered at 12, 14, and 24 months after HSCT (BII)	None
Generally, HSCT recipients who are household contacts of a person with Hib disease should be administered rifampin prophylaxis* (BIII); however, prophylaxis is not needed for adult or adolescent HSCT recipients who are household contacts of a person with Hib disease if all household contacts aged <4 years are fully vaccinated	Rifampin 600 mg by mouth daily for 4 days (BIII)	

* **Source**: American Academy of Pediatrics. *Haemophilus influenzae* infections. In: Pickering LK, ed. 2000 red book: report of the Committee on Infectious Diseases. 25th ed. Elk Grove Village, IL: American Academy of Pediatrics;2000:262–72.

Pathogen: Methicillin-resistant *Staphylococcus aureus*

Indication	First choice	Alternatives
Elimination of methicillin-resistant *Staphylococcus aureus* carrier state among adults or adolescents to prevent this disease among chronic carriers	Mupirocin calcium ointment 2%; use a cotton-tipped applicator or equivalent to apply to nares 2 times/day for 5 days or to wounds daily for 2 weeks	None

Pathogen: *Candida* **species**

Indication	First choice	Alternatives
Prophylaxis for disease from fluconazole-susceptible *Candida* species among a) allogeneic adult or adolescent HSCT recipients or b) autologous adult or adolescent HSCT recipients with lymphoma or leukemia and who have or will have prolonged neutropenia and mucosal damage from intense conditioning regimens or graft manipulation or who have recently received fludarabine or 2-chlorodeoxyadenosine: Administer prophylaxis from the day of transplantation (i.e., day 0) until engraftment (i.e., approximately 30 days after HSCT) or until 7 days after the absolute neutrophil count > 1,000 cells/mm³	Fluconazole, 400 mg by mouth or intravenously daily (AI)	None

Pathogen: *Pneumocystis carinii*

Indication	First choice	Alternatives
Prophylaxis for *Pneumocystis carinii* pneumonia among a) all allogeneic adult or adolescent HSCT recipients or b) autologous adult or adolescent HSCT recipients with underlying hematologic malignancies (e.g., lymphoma or leukemia) or for those receiving intense conditioning regimens or graft manipulation or for those who have recently received fludarabine or 2-chlorodeoxyadenosine:* Administer prophylaxis from time of engraftment for ≥6 months after HSCT; continue >6 months after HSCT for the duration of immunosuppression for all persons who a) are receiving immunosuppressive therapy (e.g., prednisone or cyclosporine) or who b) have chronic graft-versus-host disease	Trimethoprim-sulfamethoxazole, 1 double-strength tablet by mouth daily or 1 single-strength tablet by mouth daily or 1 double-strength tablet by mouth 3 times/week (AII); researchers also recommend administering prophylaxis for 1–2 weeks before HSCT (i.e., day –14 to –2) (CIII)	Dapsone, 50 mg by mouth 2 times/day or 100 mg by mouth daily (BIII) or pentamidine, 300 mg every 3–4 weeks by Respirgard II™ nebulizer (CIII)

* **Source**: Tuan IZ, Dennison D, Weisdorf DJ. *Pneumocystis carinii* pneumonitis after bone marrow transplantation. Bone Marrow Transplant 1992;10(3):267–72.

Note: Patients who are receiving sulfadiazine-pyrimethamine for toxoplasmosis therapy are protected against *Pneumocystis carinii* and do not need additional prophylaxis.

Pathogen: *Toxoplasma gondii*

Indication	First choice	Alternatives
Prophylaxis of *Toxoplasma gondii* disease among seropositive allogeneic adult or adolescent HSCT recipients: Start after engraftment and administer as long as patients remain on immunosuppressive therapy (i.e., generally, until 6 months after HSCT)	Trimethoprim-sulfamethoxazole, 1 double-strength tablet by mouth daily or 1 single-strength tablet by mouth daily or 1 double-strength table by mouth 3 times/week (AII)	For those persons who are intolerant of trimethoprim-sulfamethoxazole, the following drugs can be substituted: Clindamycin, 300–450 mg by mouth every 6–8 hours; plus pyrimethamine, 25–75 mg by mouth daily; plus leucovorin, 10–25 mg by mouth 4 times/day (CIII)

Note: Among allogeneic HSCT recipients, clinical toxoplasmosis has occurred despite the use of trimethoprim-sulfamethoxazole for *Pneumocystis carinii* prophylaxis (**Source**: Slavin MA, Meyers JD, Remington JS, Hackman RC. *Toxoplasma gondii* infection in marrow transplant recipients: a 20 year experience. Bone Marrow Transplant 1994;13[5]:549–57).

Pathogen: _Strongyloides_ species

Indication	First choice	Alternatives
Prevention of strongyloidiasis hyperinfection among adult or adolescent HSCT candidates whose HSCT screening tests are positive for _Strongyloides_ species or who have an unexplained eosinophilia and a travel or residence history suggestive of exposure to _Strongyloides stercoralis_: Administer prophylaxis before HSCT	Ivermectin, 200 µg/kg by mouth daily for 2 consecutive days* (BIII); 1 tablet = 6 mg; doses administered as follows: Body weight (kg) / Oral dose <15 / Not recommended ≥15–24 / ½ tablet 25–35 / 1 tablet 36–50 / 1½ tablets 51–65 / 2 tablets 66–79 / 2½ tablets ≥80 / 200 µg/kg	Albendazole, 400 mg by mouth daily for 3 days or thiabendazole, 25 mg/kg by mouth 2 times/day for 2 days (BIII); maximum dose, 3 g/ 24 hours

*__Sources__: Liu LX, Weller PF. Strongyloidiasis and other intestinal nematode infections [Review]. Infect Dis Clin North Am 1993;7(3):655–82; and Naquira C, Jimenez G, Guerra JG, et al. Ivermectin for human strongyloidiasis and other intestinal helminths. Am J Trop Med Hyg 1989;40:304–9.

Notes: Among immunocompromised patients, multiple courses at 2-week intervals might be required; however, cure might not be achievable. Safety and efficacy of ivermectin has not been established during pregnancy. Albendazole and thiabendazole are contraindicated during pregnancy.

Pathogen: Traveler's diarrhea

Indication	First choice	Alternatives
Prophylaxis among adult or adolescent HSCT recipients who are immunocompromised and who plan to travel in developing countries	Ciprofloxacin, 500 mg by mouth daily for the duration of stay in developing countries (BIII) or bismuth subsalicylate, 2 oz by mouth 4 times/day or 2 tablets by mouth 4 times/day; can be administered for ≤3 weeks to prevent travelers' diarrhea in adults aged >18 years only	Trimethoprim-sulfamethoxazole, 1 double-strength tablet by mouth daily for the duration of stay in developing country (CIII)

Notes: Use of aspirin-containing products including bismuth subsalicylate is contraindicated in persons aged <18 years unless prescribed by a physician because these products have been associated with Reye's syndrome (**Source**: Belay E, Bresee JS, Holman RC, Khan AS, Shahriari A, Schonberger LB. Reye's syndrome in the United States from 1981 through 1997. New Engl J Med 1999;340[18]:1377–82). Ciprofloxacin, norfloxacin, and ofloxacin are not approved for use among children aged <18 years.

Pathogen: *Mycobacteria tuberculosis*

Indication	First choice	Alternatives
Prevention of *Mycobacteria tuberculosis* among a) highly immunocompromised adult or adolescent HSCT recipients or candidates who have been substantially exposed to someone with active, infectious (e.g., sputum smear positive) pulmonary or laryngeal tuberculosis, regardless of the HSCT recipient's or candidate's tuberculin skin test status, or b) adult or adolescent HSCT recipients or candidates with a positive tuberculin skin test and who were not previously treated and have no evidence of active tuberculosis disease	Isoniazid, 5 mg/kg/day by mouth or intramuscularly for 9 months (i.e., for ≥270 doses);* maximum dose, 300 mg/day, and pyridoxine (vitamin B₆), 25–50 mg by mouth daily for 9 months; administer to nutritionally deficient HSCT recipients and candidates while on isoniazid preventive therapy to reduce the occurrence of isoniazid-induced neuropathy* (BIII)	None

*Source: CDC. Prevention and treatment of tuberculosis among patients infected with human immunodeficiency virus: principles of therapy and revised recommendations. MMWR 1998;47(No. RR-20):1–58.

Notes: A twice-weekly schedule of isoniazid and pyridoxine can be administered (CIII). The twice-weekly isoniazid dose is 15 mg/kg by mouth or intramuscularly (maximum dose, 900 mg). The twice-weekly pyridoxine dose is 50–100 mg by mouth. A 2-month pyrazinamide/rifampin preventive therapy regimen can be used for HSCT candidates who are not at risk for serious rifampin drug interactions and whose HSCT is not scheduled until ≥2 weeks after the 2-month course is completed (**Sources**: CDC. Notice to readers: use of short-course tuberculosis preventive therapy regimens in HIV-seronegative persons. MMWR 1998;47[42]:911–2; and CDC. Prevention and treatment of tuberculosis among patients infected with human immunodeficiency virus: principles of therapy and revised recommendations. MMWR 1998;47[No. RR-20]:1–58) (CIII). The usual pyrazinamide dose is 15–30 mg/kg/day by mouth or 50–70 mg/kg/dose by mouth 2 times/week (maximum daily pyrazinamide dose, 2.0 gm; maximum twice-weekly dose, 3.5 gm). Rifampin dose is 10 mg/kg/day by mouth or intravenously or 10 mg/kg/dose administered 2 times/week by mouth or intravenously (maximum rifampin dose, 600 mg). Routine use of a 2-month pyrazinamide/rifampin preventive therapy regimen is not recommended after HSCT because of the risk for serious rifampin drug interactions (DIII). Persons who have been exposed to rifampin- and isoniazid-resistant tuberculosis should be placed on preventive therapy regimens that involve ≥2 antituberculosis drugs to which the infecting strain is susceptible, and a tuberculosis specialist should be consulted (**Source**: CDC. Prevention and treatment of tuberculosis among patients infected with human immunodeficiency virus: principles of therapy and revised recommendations. MMWR 1998;47[No. RR-20]:1–58) (BIII). A tuberculosis specialist should also be consulted for patients who are intolerant to isoniazid (AIII). All intermittent dosing strategies should be administered as directly observed therapy (AIII).

II. Preventive regimens for pediatric hematopoietic stem cell transplant (HSCT) recipients

Pathogen: Cytomegalovirus

Indication	First choice	Alternatives
Universal prophylaxis for cytomegalovirus disease among all allogeneic pediatric HSCT recipients at risk throughout phase II (i.e., from engraftment to day 100 after HSCT)	Ganciclovir, 5 mg/kg/dose intravenously every 12 hours for 5–7 days, followed by 5 mg/kg/dose intravenously daily for 5 days/week from engraftment until day 100 after HSCT (AI)	Foscarnet, 60 mg/kg intravenously every 12 hours for 14 days, followed by 90–120 mg/kg/day until day 100 after HSCT (CIII)
Or preemptive cytomegalovirus treatment administered <100 days after HSCT to all allogeneic pediatric HSCT recipients at risk: Start ganciclovir when the patient experiences any level of cytomegalovirus antigenemia or viremia or has ≥2 consecutively positive cytomegalovirus-DNA polymerase chain reaction tests	Ganciclovir, 5 mg/kg/dose intravenously every 12 hours for 7–14 days, followed by 5 mg/kg/day for 5 days/week until day 100 after HSCT or for a minimum of 3 weeks, whichever is longer (AI); or administer ganciclovir for a total of 3–6 weeks; antigen or polymerase chain reaction tests should be negative when ganciclovir is stopped; reinstitute ganciclovir if subsequent weekly cytomegalovirus antigenemia screening tests become positive (BI)	
Preemptive treatment for cytomegalovirus seropositive autologous pediatric HSCT recipients at <100 days after HSCT: Start ganciclovir when antigenemia is ≥5 cells/slide, but CD34+-selected patients should be treated at any level of antigenemia*	Ganciclovir, 5 mg/kg/dose intravenously every 12 hours for 7 days, followed by 5 mg/kg/day intravenously for 5 days/week for 2 weeks (BII)	
Preemptive treatment of allogeneic pediatric HSCT recipients >100 days after HSCT: Start ganciclovir when a) antigenemia is ≥5 cells/slide or b) the patient has had ≥2 consecutively positive viremia or polymerase chain reaction tests (e.g., in a person receiving steroids for graft-versus-host disease or who received ganciclovir or foscarnet at <100 days after HSCT)	Ganciclovir, 5 mg/kg/dose intravenously every 12 hours for 7 days, followed by 5 mg/kg/day intravenously for 5 days/week for 2 weeks (BIII)	

* **Source:** Holmberg LA, Boeckh M, Hooper H, et al. Increased incidence of cytomegalovirus disease after autologous CD34-selected peripheral blood stem cell transplantation [Clinical observations, interventions, and therapeutic trials]. Blood 1999;94(12):4029–35.

Notes: Patients who do not tolerate standard doses of ganciclovir should be administered foscarnet. Ganciclovir and foscarnet doses should be modified for renal impairment. Prehydration is required for foscarnet administration.

Pathogen: Herpes simplex virus

Indication	First choice	Alternatives
Prevention of herpes simplex virus reactivation among seropositive pediatric HSCT recipients: Start acyclovir at the beginning of conditioning therapy and continue until engraftment or until mucositis resolves (i.e., approximately 30 days after HSCT for allogeneic HSCT recipients)	Acyclovir, 250 mg/m^2/dose intravenously every 8 hours (BIII) or 125 mg/m^2/dose intravenously every 6 hours (CIII)	Acyclovir 600–1,000 mg/24 hours by mouth, divided in 3–5 doses/day

Note: For patients requiring prophylaxis for cytomegalovirus and herpes simplex virus after engraftment, ganciclovir alone provides effective prophylaxis for both pathogens. Valacyclovir is not approved for use among children.

Pathogen: Varicella-zoster virus

Indication	First choice	Alternatives
Prevention of varicella-zoster virus disease after exposure among pediatric HSCT recipients who are at <24 months after HSCT or who are at ≥24 months after HSCT and on immunosuppressive therapy or have chronic graft-versus-host disease: Ideally, administer prophylaxis within 96 hours (preferably, within 48 hours) after close contact with a person who has chickenpox or shingles	Varicella-zoster immunoglobulin, 125 units (1.25 ml)/10 kg (22 lbs) of body weight administered intramuscularly; maximum dose, 625 units or 5 vials (AII); doses administered as follows: Body weight (kg) Dose Number of vials 0–10 125 units 1 10.1–20 250 units 2 20.1–30 375 units 3 30.1–40 500 units 4 >40 kg 625 units 5	Limited data demonstrate that a 1-week course of high-dose acyclovir might prevent varicella

Pathogen: Influenza

Indication	First choice	Alternatives
Prevention of influenza A and B among pediatric HSCT recipients	Lifelong annual seasonal (i.e., October–May) influenza vaccination before HSCT and resuming ≥6 months after HSCT (BIII); doses administered as follows:	None

Age	Number of doses	Type of influenza vaccine
6–35 mo	0.25 ml	Split-virus*
3–8 years	0.5 ml	Split-virus*
9–12 years	0.5 ml	Split-virus
>12 years	0.5 ml	Whole- or split-virus

Indication	First choice	Alternatives
Prophylaxis and preemptive treatment of influenza A among pediatric HSCT recipients during nosocomial or community influenza A outbreaks	Rimantadine, for children aged 1–9 years, 5 mg/kg/day once daily or divided in 2 doses (CIII); maximum daily dose, 150 mg; for children aged ≥10 years (weight, <40 kg), 5 mg/kg/day by mouth, divided in 2 doses; for children aged ≥10 years (weight, ≥40 kg), 100 mg by mouth 2 times/day	Amantadine, for children aged 1–9 years, 5 mg/kg/day; maximum daily dose, 150 mg; for children aged ≥10 years (weight, <40 kg), 5 mg/kg/day by mouth, divided in 2 doses; for children aged ≥10 years (weight, ≥40 kg), 100 mg by mouth 2 times/day; maximum daily dose, 200 mg

* Children aged <9 years receiving influenza vaccination for the first time require 2 doses of vaccine spaced ≥1 months apart.

Notes: Neither rimantadine nor amantadine are Federal Drug Administration-approved for children aged <1 year. Rimantadine and amantadine doses should be reduced for patients with impaired renal function.

Pathogen: Respiratory syncytial virus

Indication	First choice	Alternatives
Prophylaxis for respiratory syncytial virus (RSV) lower respiratory infection among hypogammaglobulinemic pediatric HSCT recipients	RSV intravenous immunoglobulin can be administered in place of intravenous immunoglobulin during RSV season (i.e., November–April in the United States) for pediatric HSCT recipients who are on routine intravenous immunoglobulin therapy* (e.g., those with hypogammaglobulinemia) (CIII); usual RSV intravenous immunoglobulin dose is 750 mg/kg/month or a 1-mg/1-mg dosing substitution of RSV intravenous immunoglobulin for intravenous immunoglobulin can be used for patients who normally require high intravenous immunoglobulin doses to maintain serum immunoglobulin G > 400 mg/dl; can administer more frequently than monthly as needed to keep serum immunoglobulin G > 400 mg/dl	None
Preemptive treatment of RSV upper respiratory infection or early lower respiratory infection among pediatric HSCT recipients	Aerosolized ribavirin,* 6 g/300 ml sterile water to make a concentration of 20 mg/ml; administer 18 hours/day for 10 days in a tent (CIII); for HSCT recipients with lower respiratory infections who cannot tolerate a tent or who have RSV upper respiratory infection, administer ribavirin as 2 g for 2 hours every 8 hours by face mask for 10 days; use small particle aerosol generator model SPAG-2	

*__Source__: American Academy of Pediatrics. Respiratory syncytial virus. In: Pickering LK, ed. 2000 red book: report of the Committee on Infectious Disease. 25th ed. Elk Grove Village, IL: American Academy of Pediatrics;2000: 483–7.

Notes: RSV intravenous immunoglobulin is contraindicated among patients with immunoglobulin A deficiency or who might have allergic reactions or anaphylaxis when receiving blood products containing immunoglobulin A (DIII). RSV monoclonal antibody is under investigational use among HSCT recipients for treatment with ribavirin but not for prophylaxis.

Pathogen: Bacterial infections, general prophylaxis

Indication	First choice	Alternatives
Prevention of bacterial infections among allogeneic pediatric HSCT recipients with severe hypogammaglobulinemia (i.e., serum immunoglobulin G level < 400 mg/dl) at <100 days after HSCT	Intravenous immunoglobulin 400 mg/kg/month; increase dose or frequency as needed to keep serum immunoglobulin G levels > 400 mg/dl (CIII)	None

Notes: Patients with immunoglobulin E anti-immunoglobulin A antibodies are at high risk for experiencing anaphylaxis from immunoglobulin administration (**Source**: Burks AW, Sampson HA, Buckley RH. Anaphylactic reactions after gamma globulin administration in patients with hypogammaglobulinemia. New Engl J Med 1986;314[9]:560–4). Therefore, persons with immunoglobulin A deficiency should not receive standard immunoglobulin products (**Source**: Siberry GK, Iannone R, eds. Harriet Lane handbook: a manual for pediatric house officers. 15th ed.; St. Louis, MO: Mosby, Inc., 2000:339;739) (DIII). However, researchers report that use of immunoglobulin A-depleted immunoglobulin preparations can be used with caution in these persons (**Sources**: Burks AW, Sampson HA, Buckley RH. Anaphylactic reactions after gamma globulin administration in patients with hypogammaglobulinemia. New Engl J Med 1986;314[9]:560–4; Siberry GK, Iannone R, eds. Harriet Lane handbook: a manual for pediatric house officers. 15th ed.; St. Louis, MO: Mosby, Inc., 2000:339;739; Stiehm ER. Human intravenous immunoglobulin in primary and secondary antibody deficiencies [Review]. Pediatr Infect Dis J 1997;16[7]:696–707; American Academy of Pediatrics. Passive immunization. In: Pickering LK, ed. 2000 red book: report of the Committee on Infectious Diseases. 25th ed. Elk Grove Village, IL: American Academy of Pediatrics;2000:41–53). Researchers also propose checking serum immunoglobulin G levels every 2 weeks for patients receiving intravenous immunoglobulin replacement therapy.

Pathogen: *Streptococcus pneumoniae*

Indication	First choice	Alternatives
Prevention of pneumococcal disease among pediatric HSCT recipients	23-valent pneumococcal polysaccharide vaccine at 12 and 24 months after HSCT (BIII)	None

Notes: The 23-valent pneumococcal polysaccharide vaccine should not be administered to children aged <2 years because of lack of efficacy (DI). Penicillin-resistant *Streptococcus pneumoniae* is increasing in the United States.

Pathogen: *Haemophilus influenzae* type b

Indication	First choice	Alternatives
Prevention of invasive *Haemophilus influenzae* type b (Hib) disease among pediatric HSCT recipients	Hib conjugate vaccine administered at 12, 14, and 24 months after HSCT (BII)	None
Generally, pediatric HSCT recipients who are household contacts of a person with Hib disease should be administered rifampin prophylaxis* (BIII); however, prophylaxis is not needed for pediatric HSCT recipients who are household contacts of a person with Hib disease if all household contacts aged <4 years are fully vaccinated	Rifampin, administered as follows: Age Dose 0–1 mo 10 mg/kg by mouth daily for 4 days >1 mo 20mg/kg by mouth daily for 4 days Maximum dose, 600 mg/day (BIII)	None

* **Source:** American Academy of Pediatrics. *Haemophilus influenzae* infections. In: Pickering LK, ed. 2000 red book: report of the Committee on Infectious Diseases. 25th ed. Elk Grove Village, IL: American Academy of Pediatrics;2000:262–72.

Pathogen: Methicillin-resistant *Staphylococcus aureus*

Indication	First choice	Alternatives
Elimination of methicillin-resistant *Staphylococcus aureus* carrier state among pediatric patients to prevent this disease among chronic carriers	Mupirocin calcium ointment 2%; use a cotton-tipped applicator or equivalent to apply to nares 2 times/day for 5 days or to wounds daily for 2 weeks*	Bacitracin is regarded safe for use among children, and the dose is the same as for mupirocin; however, no standardized protocol has been evaluated

* Safety of mupirocin calcium ointment 2% use among children aged <12 years has not be established.

Pathogen: *Candida* species

Indication	First choice	Alternatives
Prophylaxis for disease from fluconazole-susceptible *Candida* species among a) allogeneic pediatric HSCT recipients or b) autologous pediatric HSCT recipients with lymphoma or leukemia and who have or will have prolonged neutropenia and mucosal damage from intense conditioning regimens or graft manipulation or who have recently received fludarabine or 2-chlorodeoxyadenosine: Administer prophylaxis from the day of transplantation (i.e., day 0) until engraftment (i.e., approximately 30 days after HSCT) or until 7 days after the absolute neutrophil count > 1,000 cells/mm^3	Fluconazole, for children aged 6 months–13 years, administer 3–6 mg/kg/day by mouth or intravenously (AI); maximum dose, 600 mg/day; for children aged >13 years, administer 400 mg by mouth or intravenously daily (AI)	None

Pathogen: *Pneumocystis carinii*

Indication	First choice	Alternatives
Prophylaxis for *Pneumocystis carinii* pneumonia among a) all allogeneic pediatric HSCT recipients or b) autologous pediatric HSCT recipients with underlying hematologic malignancies (e.g., lymphoma or leukemia) or for those receiving intense conditioning regimens or graft manipulation or for those who have recently received fludarabine or 2-chlorodeoxyadenosine:* Administer prophylaxis from time of engraftment for ≥6 months after HSCT; continue >6 months after HSCT for the duration of immunosuppression for all persons who a) are receiving immunosuppressive therapy (e.g., prednisone or cyclosporine) or who b) have chronic graft-versus-host disease	Trimethoprim-sulfamethoxazole, 150 mg trimethoprim/750 mg sulfamethoxazole/m²/day by mouth in 2 divided doses 3 times/week on consecutive days (AII); or a single dose by mouth 3 times/week on consecutive days; or by mouth in 2 divided doses daily for 7 days; or by mouth in 2 divided doses 3 times/week on alternate days; researchers also report administering prophylaxis for 1–2 weeks before HSCT (i.e., day –14 to –2) (CIII)	Dapsone, for HSCT recipients aged ≥1 months, 2 mg/kg (maximum dose, 100 mg) by mouth daily (BIII); or intravenous pentamidine, 4 mg/kg every 2–4 weeks; or aerosolized pentamidine, for HSCT recipients aged ≤5 years, 9 mg/kg/dose; or for HSCT recipients aged >5 years, 300 mg; should be administered every month by Respirgard II™ nebulizer (CIII)

* **Source:** Tuan IZ, Dennison D, Weisdorf DJ. *Pneumocystis carinii* pneumonitis after bone marrow transplantation. Bone Marrow Transplant 1992;10(3):267–72.

Notes: Trimethoprim-sulfamethoxazole is not recommended for patients aged <2 months because of risk for kernicterus. Patients who are receiving sulfadiazine-pyrimethamine for toxoplasmosis therapy are protected against *Pneumocystis carinii* and do not need additional prophylaxis.

Pathogen: *Toxoplasma gondii*

Indication	First choice	Alternatives
Prophylaxis of *Toxoplasma gondii* disease among seropositive allogeneic pediatric HSCT recipients: Start after engraftment and administer as long as patients remain on immunosuppressive therapy (i.e., generally, until 6 months after HSCT)	Trimethoprim-sulfamethoxazole, 150 mg trimethoprim/750 mg sulfamethoxazole/m²/day by mouth in 2 divided doses 3 times/week on consecutive days (AII); or a single dose by mouth 3 times/ week on consecutive days; or by mouth in 2 divided doses daily for 7 days; or by mouth in 2 divided doses 3 times/weekly on alternate days	For those persons who are intolerant of trimethoprim-sulfamethoxazole, the following drugs can be substituted: Clindamycin, 20–30 mg/kg/day by mouth, divided in 4 divided doses daily; plus pyrimethamine, 1 mg/ kg by mouth daily; plus leucov- orin, 5 mg by mouth every 3 days (CIII)

Note: Trimethoprim-sulfamethoxazole is not recommended for patients aged <2 months because of risk for kernict- erus. Among allogeneic HSCT recipients, clinical toxoplasmosis has occurred despite the use of trimethoprim- sulfamethoxazole for *Pneumocystis carinii* prophylaxis (**Source**: Slavin MA, Meyers JD, Remington JS, Hackman RC. *Toxoplasma gondii* infection in marrow transplant recipients: a 20 year experience. Bone Marrow Transplant 1994;13[5]:549–57).

Pathogen: *Strongyloides* species

Indication	First choice	Alternatives
Prevention of strongyloidiasis hyperinfection among pediatric HSCT candidates whose HSCT screening tests are positive for *Strongyloides* species or who have an unexplained eosinophilia and a travel or residence history suggestive of exposure to *Strongyloides stercoralis*: Administer prophylaxis before HSCT	Ivermectin, 200 µg/kg by mouth daily for 2 consecutive days* (BIII); 1 tablet = 6 mg; doses administered as follows: Body weight (kg) / Oral dose <15 — Not recommended ≥15–24 — ½ tablet 25–35 — 1 tablet 36–50 — 1½ tablets 51–65 — 2 tablets 66–79 — 2½ tablets ≥80 — 200 µg/kg	Thiabendazole, 25 mg/kg 2 times daily for 2 days; maximum dose, 3 g/24 hours

* **Sources**: Liu LX, Weller PF. Strongyloidiasis and other intestinal nematode infections [Review]. Infect Dis Clin North Am 1993;7(3):655–82; and Naquira C, Jimenez G, Guerra JG, et al. Ivermectin for human strongyloidiasis and other intestinal helminths. Am J Trop Med Hyg 1989;40:304–9.

Notes: Ivermectin safety among children weighing <15 kg has not been established. Among immunocompromised patients, multiple courses of ivermectin at 2-week intervals might be required; however, cure might not be achievable. Safety and efficacy of ivermectin has not been established during pregnancy. Thiabendazole is contraindicated during pregnancy.

Pathogen: Traveler's diarrhea

Indication	First choice	Alternatives
Prophylaxis among pediatric HSCT recipients who are immunocompromised and who plan to travel in developing countries	Trimethoprim-sulfamethoxazole, 150 mg trimethoprim/750 mg sulfamethoxazole/m²/day by mouth, divided in 2 doses 3 times/week on consecutive days (CIII); can be administered for duration of stay in developing country	Trimethoprim-sulfamethoxazole, single dose by mouth 3 times/week on consecutive days

Notes: Use of aspirin-containing products including bismuth subsalicylate is contraindicated in persons aged <18 years unless prescribed by a physician because these products have been associated with Reye's syndrome (**Source:** Belay E, Bresee JS, Holman RC, Khan AS, Shahriari A, Schonberger LB. Reye's syndrome in the United States from 1981 through 1997. New Engl J Med 1999;340[18]:1377–82). Trimethoprim-sulfamethoxazole is not recommended for patients aged <2 months because of risk for kernicterus. Resistance to trimethoprim-sulfamethoxazole is common in tropical areas. Usual doses of trimethoprim-sulfamethoxazole for *Pneumocystis carinii* pneumonia prophylaxis should provide limited protection against traveler's diarrhea.

Pathogen: *Mycobacteria tuberculosis*

Indication	First choice	Alternatives
Prevention of *Mycobacteria tuberculosis* among a) highly immunocompromised pediatric HSCT recipients or candidates who have been exposed to someone with active, infectious (e.g., sputum smear positive) pulmonary or laryngeal tuberculosis, regardless of the HSCT recipient's or candidate's tuberculin skin test status, or b) pediatric HSCT recipients or candidates with a positive tuberculin skin test and who were not previously treated and have no evidence of active tuberculosis disease	Isoniazid, 10–20 mg/kg/day by mouth or intramuscularly for 9 months (i.e., for ≥270 doses);* maximum dose, 300 mg/day, and pyridoxine (vitamin B$_6$), 1–2 mg/kg/day by mouth daily for 9 months; dose required might vary by age and condition;† administer to nutritionally deficient HSCT recipients and candidates while on isoniazid preventive therapy to reduce the occurrence of isoniazid-induced neuropathy* (BIII)	None

* **Sources:** American Academy of Pediatrics. Tuberculosis. In: Pickering LK, ed. 2000 red book: report of the Committee on Infectious Diseases. 25th ed. Elk Grove Village, IL: American Academy of Pediatrics;2000:593–613; CDC. Prevention and treatment of tuberculosis among patients infected with human immunodeficiency virus: principles of therapy and revised recommendations. MMWR 1998;47(No. RR-20):1–58; and CDC. Notice to readers: use of short-course tuberculosis preventive therapy regimens in HIV-seronegative persons. MMWR 1998;47(42):911–2.

† **Source:** Siberry GK, Iannone R, eds. Harriet Lane handbook: a manual for pediatric house officers. 15th ed.; St. Louis, MO: Mosby, Inc., 2000:834–5.

Notes: A twice-weekly schedule of isoniazid and pyridoxine can be administered (CIII). The twice-weekly isoniazid dose is 20–40 mg/kg by mouth or intramuscularly (maximum dose, 900 mg). A 2-month pyrazinamide/rifampin preventive therapy regimen can be used for HSCT candidates who are not at risk for serious rifampin drug interactions and whose HSCT is not scheduled until ≥2 weeks after the 2-month course is completed. Rifampin dose is 10–20 mg/kg/day by mouth or intravenously or 10–20 mk/kg/dose by mouth or intravenously, administered 2 times/week (maximum pyrazinamide dose, 3.5 g; maximum rifampin dose, 600 mg) (**Sources:** CDC. Notice to readers: use of short-course tuberculosis preventive therapy regimens in HIV-seronegative persons. MMWR 1998;47[42]:911–2; and CDC. Prevention and treatment of tuberculosis among patients infected with human immunodeficiency virus: principles of therapy and revised recommendations. MMWR 1998;47[No. RR-20]:1–58.) (CIII). The usual pyrazinamide dose is 15–30 mg/kg/day by mouth or 50–70 mg/kg/dose by mouth 2 times/week (maximum) (maximum daily pyrazinamide dose, 2 g). Routine use of a 2-month pyrazinamide/rifampin preventive therapy regimen is not recommended after HSCT because of the risk for serious rifampin drug interactions (DIII). Persons who have been exposed to rifampin- and isoniazid-resistant tuberculosis should be placed on preventive therapy regimens that involve ≥2 antituberculosis drugs to which the infecting strain is susceptible (**Source:** CDC. Prevention and treatment of tuberculosis among patients infected with human immunodeficiency virus: principles of therapy and revised recommendations. MMWR 1998;47[No. RR-20]:1–58), and a tuberculosis specialist should be consulted (BIII). A tuberculosis specialist should also be consulted for patients who are intolerant to isoniazid (AIII). All intermittent dosing strategies should be administered as directly observed therapy (AIII).

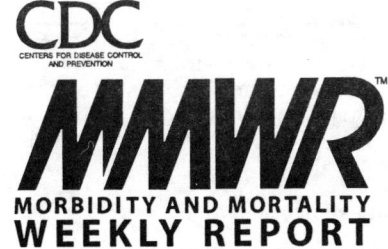

October 20, 2000 / Vol. 49 / No. RR-10

Recommendations
and
Reports

Continuing Education Activity
Sponsored by CDC

Guidelines for Preventing Opportunistic Infections Among Hematopoietic Stem Cell Transplant Recipients: Recommendations of CDC, the Infectious Disease Society of America, and the American Society of Blood and Marrow Transplantation

EXPIRATION — OCTOBER 20, 2001

You must complete and return the response form electronically or by mail by **October 20, 2001,** to receive continuing education credit. If you answer all of the questions, you will receive an award letter for 4.5 hours Continuing Medical Education (CME) credit, 0.45 hour Continuing Education Units (CEUs), or 5.3 hours Continuing Nursing Education (CNE) credit. If you return the form electronically, you will receive educational credit immediately. If you mail the form, you will receive educational credit in approximately 30 days. No fees are charged for participating in this continuing education activity.

INSTRUCTIONS
By Internet
1. Read this *MMWR* (Vol. 49, RR-10), which contains the correct answers to the questions beginning on the next page.
2. Go to the *MMWR* Continuing Education Internet site at <http://www.cdc.gov/mmwr/cme/conted.html>.
3. Select which exam you want to take and select whether you want to register for CME, CEU, or CNE credit.
4. Fill out and submit the registration form.
5. Select exam questions. To receive continuing education credit, you must answer all of the questions. Questions with more than one correct answer will instruct you to "Indicate all that apply."
6. Submit your answers no later than **October 20, 2001.**
7. Immediately print your Certificate of Completion for your records.

By Mail
1. Read this *MMWR* (Vol. 49, RR-10), which contains the correct answers to the questions beginning on the next page.
2. Complete all registration information on the response form, including your name, mailing address, phone number, and e-mail address, if available.
3. Indicate whether you are registering for CME, CEU, or CNE credit.
4. Select your answers to the questions, and mark the corresponding letters on the response form. To receive continuing education credit, you must answer all of the questions. Questions with more than one correct answer will instruct you to "Indicate all that apply."
5. Sign and date the response form or a photocopy of the form and send no later than **October 20, 2001,** to
    Fax: 404-639-4198   Mail: MMWR CE Credit
                                                 Office of Scientific and Health Communications
                                                 Epidemiology Program Office, MS C-08
                                                 Centers for Disease Control and Prevention
                                                 1600 Clifton Rd, N.E.
                                                 Atlanta, GA 30333
6. Your Certificate of Completion will be mailed to you within 30 days.

ACCREDITATION

Continuing Medical Education (CME). This activity has been planned and implemented in accordance with the Essential Areas and Policies of the Accreditation Council for Continuing Medical Education through the joint sponsorship of CDC, the Infectious Disease Society of America, and the American Society of Blood and Marrow Transplantation. CDC is accredited by the Accreditation Council for Continuing Medical Education (ACCME) to provide continuing medical education for physicians. CDC designates this educational activity for a maximum of 4.5 hours in category 1 credit towards the AMA Physician's Recognition Award. Each physician should claim only those hours of credit that he/she actually spent in the educational activity.

Continuing Education Unit (CEU). CDC has been approved as an authorized provider of continuing education and training programs by the International Association for Continuing Education and Training and awards 0.45 hour Continuing Education Units (CEUs).

Continuing Nursing Education (CNE). This activity for 5.3 contact hours is provided by CDC, which is accredited as a provider of continuing education in nursing by the American Nurses Credentialing Center's Commission on Accreditation.

Goals and Objectives

This *MMWR* provides guidelines for preventing opportunistic infections (OIs) among hematopoietic stem cell transplant (HSCT) recipients. The goals of these guidelines are to summarize current data regarding preventing opportunistic infections among HSCT recipients and provide evidence-based recommended strategies for preventing these OIs. Upon completion of this educational activity, the reader should be able to identify strategies for a) preventing exposure and disease from bacterial, viral, fungal, protozoa, and helminth infections and b) hospital infection control, safe living, vaccinations, and hematopoietic stem cell safety.

To receive continuing education credit, please answer all of the following questions.

1. **What are the three phases of immune system recovery after HSCT?**

    A. Phase I, –45–21 days; phase II, 30–100 days; and phase III, >100 days.

    B. Phase I, 0–21 days; phase II, 30–90 days; and phase III, >90 days.

    C. Phase I, 0–30 days; phase II, 30–120 days; and phase III, >120–365 days.

    D. Phase I, <30 days; phase II, 30–100 days; and phase III, >100 days.

    E. None of the above.

2. **Which opportunistic infections commonly occur during phase I?**

    A. Cytomegalovirus, *Pneumocystis carinii* pneumonia, and aspergillosis.

    B. Cytomegalovirus, *Pneumocystis carinii* pneumonia, and varicella-zoster virus.

    C. Herpes simplex virus, cytomegalovirus, and *Candida* species.

    D. Herpes simplex virus, *Candida* species, and aspergillosis.

    E. Herpes simplex virus, aspergillosis, and varicella-zoster virus.

3. **HSCT recipients should avoid eating which of the following foods?**

    A. Raw or undercooked meat.

    B. Unpasteurized dairy products.

    C. Vegetable sprouts.

    D. Soft cheese.

    E. All of the above.

4. **Which of the following statements is true regarding vaccinations that HSCT recipients should receive?**

    A. Diphtheria and tetanus toxoids at 12, 14, and 24 months after HSCT.

    B. Measles, mumps, rubella vaccinations at 12 and 24 months after HSCT.

    C. Pneumococcal vaccinations at 12, 14, and 24 months after HSCT.

    D. Varicella-zoster immunoglobulin at 24 months after HSCT.

    E. Oral polio vaccine at 12, 14, and 24 months after HSCT.

5. **Recommended aspergillosis prophylaxis is . . .**

    A. Fluconazole, 400 mg by mouth or intravenously daily.

    B. Fluconazole, 200 mg by mouth or intravenously daily.

    C. Amphotericin B, 1 mg/kg/day intravenously.

    D. Itraconazole capsules, 200 mg by mouth daily.

    E. None of the above.

6. **Which of the following statements is not true regarding use of laminar air flow rooms in HSCT centers?**

    A. Substantial survival benefit has been reported for all HSCT recipients.

    B. Substantial survival benefit has been reported for allogeneic HSCT recipients with aplastic anemia and human lymphocyte antigen-identical sibling donors.

    C. Patients are protected from infection during aspergillosis outbreaks related to hospital construction.

    D. Use of laminar air flow rooms for HSCT recipients is optional.

7. The number of recommended air exchanges per hour in an HSCT recipient's hospital room is . . .

    A. <6.

    B. <8.

    C. <10.

    D. >12.

    E. ≥15.

8. Patient rooms in HSCT centers should have negative air pressure when compared with hallways and anterooms.

    A. True.

    B. False.

9. HSCT recipients should be cared for routinely by using . . .

    A. standard precautions.

    B. airborne precautions.

    C. droplet precautions.

    D. contact precautions.

    E. all of the above.

10. The single-most critical and effective procedure for preventing nosocomial infection is . . .

    A. following isolation precautions.

    B. following ventilation precautions.

    C. hand washing.

    D. environmental disinfection.

    E. excluding visitors experiencing illness from the HSCT center.

11. An HSCT recipient can be exposed safely to visitors with . . .

    A. an upper respiratory infection.

    B. a covered shingles rash.

    C. a varicella-zoster virus-like rash occurring ≤4 weeks after the person has received a varicella-zoster virus vaccination.

    D. a history of oral polio vaccination within the previous 3–6 weeks.

    E. a history of vaccination with inactivated polio vaccine within the previous 3–6 weeks.

12. When constructing cooling towers for a new hospital with an HSCT center, all of the following should be done to prevent legionellosis except . . .

    A. installing drift eliminators.

    B. regularly using an effective biocide.

    C. maintaining the cooling towers according to the manufacturer's directions.

    D. locating the cooling towers so that drift is directed towards the hospital's air-intake system.

    E. keeping adequate maintenance records.

13. Which of the following animals is a safe pet for HSCT recipients?

    A. Reptile.

    B. Duckling.

    C. Nonhuman primate.

    D. Cat aged ≥6 months.

    E. Stray dog.

In questions 14–17, match the recommended prophylaxis drug with the pathogen it protects against.

14. Acyclovir.   A. *Candida* species.

15. Foscarnet.   B. *Aspergillus* species.

16. Dapsone.   C. Herpes simplex virus.

17. Fluconazole.   D. Cytomegalovirus.

                                          E. *Pneumocystis carinii.*

Correct answers for questions 1–17.

1. D; 2. D; 3. E; 4. A; 5. E; 6. A; 7. D; 8. B; 9. A; 10. C; 11. E; 12. D; 13. D; 14. C; 15. D; 16. E; 17. A.

18. **Indicate your work setting.**

  A. State/local health department.

  B. Other public health setting.

  C. Hospital clinic/private practice.

  D. Managed care organization.

  E. Academic institution.

  F. Other.

19. **Which best describes your professional activities?**

  A. Patient care — emergency/urgent care department.

  B. Patient care — inpatient.

  C. Patient care — primary-care clinic or office.

  D. Laboratory/pharmacy.

  E. Public health.

  F. Other.

20. **I plan to use these recommendations as the basis for . . .** (*Indicate all that apply.*)

  A. health education materials.

  B. insurance reimbursement policies.

  C. local practice guidelines.

  D. public policy.

  E. other.

21. **Each month, approximately how many patients do you see?**

  A. None.

  B. 1–5.

  C. 6–20.

  D. 21–50.

  E. 51–100.

  F. >100.

22. **How much time did you spend reading this report and completing the exam?**

  A. 2–2.5 hours.

  B. More than 2.5 hours but fewer than 3 hours.

  C. 3–3.5 hours.

  D. More than 3.5 hours but fewer than 4 hours.

  E. More than 4.5 hours.

23. After reading this report, I am confident I can identify strategies for preventing exposure and disease from bacterial infections among HSCT recipients.

   A. Strongly agree.
   B. Agree.
   C. Neither agree nor disagree.
   D. Disagree.
   E. Strongly disagree.

24. After reading this report, I am confident I can identify strategies for preventing exposure and disease from viral infections among HSCT recipients.

   A. Strongly agree.
   B. Agree.
   C. Neither agree nor disagree.
   D. Disagree.
   E. Strongly disagree.

25. After reading this report, I am confident I can identify strategies for preventing exposure and disease from fungal infections among HSCT recipients.

   A. Strongly agree.
   B. Agree.
   C. Neither agree nor disagree.
   D. Disagree.
   E. Strongly disagree.

26. After reading this report, I am confident I can identify strategies for preventing exposure and disease from protozoa infections among HSCT recipients.

   A. Strongly agree.
   B. Agree.
   C. Neither agree nor disagree.
   D. Disagree.
   E. Strongly disagree.

27. After reading this report, I am confident I can identify strategies for preventing exposure and disease from helminth infections among HSCT recipients.

   A. Strongly agree.
   B. Agree.
   C. Neither agree nor disagree.
   D. Disagree.
   E. Strongly disagree.

28. After reading this report, I am confident I can identify strategies for hospital infection control for HSCT recipients.

   A. Strongly agree.
   B. Agree.
   C. Neither agree nor disagree.
   D. Disagree.
   E. Strongly disagree.

29. **After reading this report, I am confident I can identify strategies for safe living for HSCT recipients.**

    A. Strongly agree.

    B. Agree.

    C. Neither agree nor disagree.

    D. Disagree.

    E. Strongly disagree.

30. **After reading this report, I am confident I can identify strategies for vaccinations for HSCT recipients.**

    A. Strongly agree.

    B. Agree.

    C. Neither agree nor disagree.

    D. Disagree.

    E. Strongly disagree.

31. **After reading this report, I am confident I can identify strategies for hematopoietic stem cell safety for HSCT recipients.**

    A. Strongly agree.

    B. Agree.

    C. Neither agree nor disagree.

    D. Disagree.

    E. Strongly disagree.

32. **The objectives are relevant to the goal of this report.**

    A. Strongly agree.

    B. Agree.

    C. Neither agree nor disagree.

    D. Disagree.

    E. Strongly disagree.

33. **The figure, tables, and appendix are useful.**

    A. Strongly agree.

    B. Agree.

    C. Neither agree nor disagree.

    D. Disagree.

    E. Strongly disagree.

34. **Overall, the presentation of the report enhanced my ability to understand the material.**

    A. Strongly agree.

    B. Agree.

    C. Neither agree nor disagree.

    D. Disagree.

    E. Strongly disagree.

35. **These recommendations will affect my practice.**

    A. Strongly agree.

    B. Agree.

    C. Neither agree nor disagree.

    D. Disagree.

    E. Strongly disagree.

MMWR Response Form for Continuing Education Credit
October 20, 2000/Vol. 49/No. RR-10

Guidelines for Preventing Opportunistic Infections Among Hematopoietic Stem Cell
Transplant Recipients: Recommendations of CDC, the Infectious Disease Society of
America, and the American Society of Blood and Marrow Transplantation

To receive continuing education credit, you must
1. *provide your contact information;*
2. *indicate your choice of CME, CEU, or CNE credit;*
3. *answer all of the test questions;*
4. *sign and date this form or a photocopy;*
5. *submit your answer form by October 20, 2001.*
*Failure to complete these items can result in a delay or rejection of
your application for continuing education credit.*

_____

Last Name   First Name

Street/Address or P.O. Box

Apartment or Suite

City   State   Zip Code

Check One
- [ ] CME Credit
- [ ] CEU Credit
- [ ] CNE Credit

*Fill in the appropriate blocks to indicate your answers. Remember, you must answer all of the questions to receive
continuing education credit!*

1. [ ] A [ ] B [ ] C [ ] D [ ] E
2. [ ] A [ ] B [ ] C [ ] D [ ] E
3. [ ] A [ ] B [ ] C [ ] D [ ] E
4. [ ] A [ ] B [ ] C [ ] D [ ] E
5. [ ] A [ ] B [ ] C [ ] D [ ] E
6. [ ] A [ ] B [ ] C [ ] D
7. [ ] A [ ] B [ ] C [ ] D [ ] E
8. [ ] A [ ] B
9. [ ] A [ ] B [ ] C [ ] D [ ] E
10. [ ] A [ ] B [ ] C [ ] D [ ] E
11. [ ] A [ ] B [ ] C [ ] D [ ] E
12. [ ] A [ ] B [ ] C [ ] D [ ] E
13. [ ] A [ ] B [ ] C [ ] D [ ] E
14. [ ] A [ ] B [ ] C [ ] D [ ] E
15. [ ] A [ ] B [ ] C [ ] D [ ] E
16. [ ] A [ ] B [ ] C [ ] D [ ] E
17. [ ] A [ ] B [ ] C [ ] D [ ] E
18. [ ] A [ ] B [ ] C [ ] D [ ] E [ ] F

19. [ ] A [ ] B [ ] C [ ] D [ ] E [ ] F
20. [ ] A [ ] B [ ] C [ ] D [ ] E
21. [ ] A [ ] B [ ] C [ ] D [ ] E [ ] F
22. [ ] A [ ] B [ ] C [ ] D [ ] E
23. [ ] A [ ] B [ ] C [ ] D [ ] E
24. [ ] A [ ] B [ ] C [ ] D [ ] E
25. [ ] A [ ] B [ ] C [ ] D [ ] E
26. [ ] A [ ] B [ ] C [ ] D [ ] E
27. [ ] A [ ] B [ ] C [ ] D [ ] E
28. [ ] A [ ] B [ ] C [ ] D [ ] E
29. [ ] A [ ] B [ ] C [ ] D [ ] E
30. [ ] A [ ] B [ ] C [ ] D [ ] E
31. [ ] A [ ] B [ ] C [ ] D [ ] E
32. [ ] A [ ] B [ ] C [ ] D [ ] E
33. [ ] A [ ] B [ ] C [ ] D [ ] E
34. [ ] A [ ] B [ ] C [ ] D [ ] E
35. [ ] A [ ] B [ ] C [ ] D [ ] E

Detach or Photocopy

_____ _____
Signature   **Date I Completed Exam**

In this report, Clare A. Dykewicz, M.D., M.P.H., and Harold W. Jaffe, M.D., have included a discussion regarding products that are not labeled for use or are still investigational.

Use of trade names and commercial sources is for identification only and does not imply endorsement by the U.S. Department of Health and Human Services.

References to non-CDC sites on the Internet are provided as a service to *MMWR* readers and do not constitute or imply endorsement of these organizations or their programs by CDC or the U.S. Department of Health and Human Services. CDC is not responsible for the content of pages found at these sites.

MMWR

The *Morbidity and Mortality Weekly Report (MMWR)* Series is prepared by the Centers for Disease Control and Prevention (CDC) and is available free of charge in electronic format and on a paid subscription basis for paper copy. To receive an electronic copy on Friday of each week, send an e-mail message to *listserv@listserv.cdc.gov*. The body content should read *SUBscribe mmwr-toc*. Electronic copy also is available from CDC's World-Wide Web server at *http://www.cdc.gov/mmwr* or from CDC's file transfer protocol server at *ftp://ftp.cdc.gov/pub/ Publications/mmwr/*. To subscribe for paper copy, contact Superintendent of Documents, U.S. Government Printing Office, Washington, DC 20402; telephone (202) 512-1800.

Data in the weekly *MMWR* are provisional, based on weekly reports to CDC by state health departments. The reporting week concludes at close of business on Friday; compiled data on a national basis are officially released to the public on the following Friday. Address inquiries about the *MMWR* Series, including material to be considered for publication, to: Editor, *MMWR* Series, Mailstop C-08, CDC, 1600 Clifton Rd., N.E., Atlanta, GA 30333; telephone (888) 232-3228.

All material in the *MMWR* Series is in the public domain and may be used and reprinted without permission; citation as to source, however, is appreciated.

☆U.S. Government Printing Office: 2000-533-206/28042 Region IV

Guidelines for the Prevention of Intravascular Catheter-Related Infections

- *Clinical Practice Guideline*

Guidelines for the Prevention of Intravascular Catheter-Related Infections

Naomi P. O'Grady, MD*; Mary Alexander, BS‡; E. Patchen Dellinger, MD§;
Julie L. Gerberding, MD, MPH‖; Stephen O. Heard, MD¶; Dennis G. Maki, MD#; Henry Masur, MD*;
Rita D. McCormick, RN**; Leonard A. Mermel, DO‡‡; Michele L. Pearson, MD§§; Issam I. Raad, MD‖‖;
Adrienne Randolph, MD, MSc¶¶; and Robert A. Weinstein, MD##

ABSTRACT. These guidelines have been developed for practitioners who insert catheters and for persons responsible for surveillance and control of infections in hospital, outpatient, and home health-care settings. This report was prepared by a working group comprising members from professional organizations representing the disciplines of critical care medicine, infectious diseases, health-care infection control, surgery, anesthesiology, interventional radiology, pulmonary medicine, pediatric medicine, and nursing. The working group was led by the Society of Critical Care Medicine (SCCM), in collaboration with the Infectious Disease Society of America (IDSA), Society for Healthcare Epidemiology of America (SHEA), Surgical Infection Society (SIS), American College of Chest Physicians (ACCP), American Thoracic Society (ATS), American Society of Critical Care Anesthesiologists (ASCCA), Association for Professionals in Infection Control and Epidemiology (APIC), Infusion Nurses Society (INS), Oncology Nursing Society (ONS), Society of Cardiovascular and Interventional Radiology (SCVIR), American Academy of Pediatrics (AAP), and the Healthcare Infection Control Practices Advisory Committee (HICPAC) of the Centers for Disease Control and Prevention (CDC) and is intended to replace the *Guideline for Prevention of Intravascular Device-Related Infections* published in 1996. These guidelines are intended to provide evidence-based recommendations for preventing catheter-related infections. Major areas of emphasis include 1) educating and training health-care providers who insert and maintain catheters; 2) using maximal sterile barrier precautions during central venous catheter insertion; 3) using a 2% chlorhexidine preparation for skin antisepsis; 4) avoiding routine replacement of central venous catheters as a strategy to prevent infection; and 5) using antiseptic/antibiotic impregnated short-term central venous catheters if the rate of infection is high despite adherence to other strategies (ie, education and training, maximal sterile barrier precautions, and 2% chlorhexidine for skin antisepsis). These guidelines also identify performance indicators that can be used locally by health-care institutions or organizations to monitor their success in implementing these evidence-based recommendations. *Pediatrics* 2002; 110(5). URL: http://www.pediatrics.org/cgi/content/full/110/5/e51; *catheter-related bloodstream infections, intensive care unit, central venous catheter, peripherally inserted central catheter, guidelines.*

ABBREVIATIONS. CRBSI, catheter-related bloodstream infections; HICPAC, Healthcare Infection Control Practices Advisory Committee; CDC, Centers for Disease Control and Prevention; ICU, intensive care unit; BSI, bloodstream infection; CVC, central venous catheter; PICC, peripherally inserted central catheter; NNIS, National Nosocomial Infection Surveillance; RR, relative risk; CI, confidence interval; IV, intravenous; FDA, US Food and Drug Administration; VRE, vancomycin-resistant enterococcus; VCH, vancomycin/ciprofloxacin/heparin; VH, vancomycin/heparin.

INTRODUCTION

This report provides health-care practitioners with background information and specific recommendations to reduce the incidence of intravascular catheter-related bloodstream infections (CRBSI). These guidelines replace the *Guideline for Prevention of Intravascular Device-Related Infections*, which was published in 1996.[1]

The *Guidelines for the Prevention of Intravascular Catheter-Related Infections* have been developed for practitioners who insert catheters and for persons who are responsible for surveillance and control of infections in hospital, outpatient, and home health-care settings. This report was prepared by a working group composed of professionals representing the disciplines of critical care medicine, infectious diseases, health-care infection control, surgery, anesthesiology, interventional radiology, pulmonary medicine, pediatrics, and nursing. The working group was led by the Society of Critical Care Medicine (SCCM), in collaboration with Infectious Disease Society of America (IDSA), Society for Healthcare Epidemiology of America (SHEA), Surgical Infection Society (SIS), American College of Chest Physicians (ACCP), American Thoracic Society (ATS), American Society of Critical Care Anesthesiologists (ASCCA), Association for Professionals in Infection Control and Epidemiology (APIC), Infusion Nurses Society (INS), Oncology Nursing Society (ONS), Society of Cardiovascular and Interventional Radiology

From the *National Institutes of Health, Bethesda, Maryland; ‡Infusion Nurses Society, Cambridge, Massachusetts; §University of Washington, Seattle, Washington; ‖Office of the Director, CDC, Atlanta, Georgia; ¶University of Massachusetts Medical School, Worcester, Massachusetts; #University of Wisconsin Medical School, Madison, Wisconsin; **University of Wisconsin Hospital and Clinics, Madison, Wisconsin; ‡‡Rhode Island Hospital and Brown University School of Medicine, Providence, Rhode Island; §§Division of Healthcare Quality Promotion, National Center for Infectious Diseases Centers for Disease Control and Prevention, Atlanta, Georgia; ‖‖M. D. Anderson Cancer Center, Houston, Texas; ¶¶The Children's Hospital, Boston, Massachusetts; and ##Cook County Hospital and Rush Medical College, Chicago, Illinois.
Received for publication; Mar 8 2002; accepted Mar 8, 2002.
Address correspondence to Naomi P. O'Grady, MD, National Institutes of Health, Department of Critical Care Medicine, 9000 Rockville Pike, Bldg 10, Rm 7D43, Bethesda, MD 20892.
PEDIATRICS (ISSN 0031 4005). Copyright © 2002 by the American Academy of Pediatrics.

APPENDIX A

Examples of Clinical Definitions for Catheter-Related Infections Localized Catheter Colonization

Significant growth of a microorganism (>15 CFU) from the catheter tip, subcutaneous segment of the catheter, or catheter hub

Exit Site Infection

Erythema or induration within 2 cm of the catheter exit site, in the absence of concomitant BSI and without concomitant purulence

Clinical Exit Site Infection (or Tunnel Infection)

Tenderness, erythema, or site induration >2 cm from the catheter site along the subcutaneous tract of a tunneled (eg, Hickman, Broviac) catheter, in the absence of concomitant BSI

Pocket Infection

Purulent fluid in the subcutaneous pocket of a totally implanted intravascular catheter that might or might not be associated with spontaneous rupture and drainage or necrosis of the overlaying skin, in the absence of concomitant BSI

Infusate-Related BSI

Concordant growth of the same organism from the infusate and blood cultures (preferably percutaneously drawn) with no other identifiable source of infection

CRBSI

Bacteremia/fungemia in a patient with an intravascular catheter with at least 1 positive blood culture obtained from a peripheral vein, clinical manifestations of infections (ie, fever, chills, and/or hypotension), and no apparent source for the BSI except the catheter. One of the following should be present: a positive semiquantitative (>15 CFU/catheter segment) or quantitative (>103 CFU/catheter segment catheter) culture whereby the same organism (species and antibiogram) is isolated from the catheter segment and peripheral blood; simultaneous quantitative blood cultures with a >5:1 ratio CVC versus peripheral; differential period of CVC culture versus peripheral blood culture positivity of >2 hours.

Surveillance Definitions for Primary BSIs, NNIS System

Laboratory-Confirmed BSI

Should meet at least 1 of the following criteria:
Criterion 1: Patient has a recognized pathogen cultured from 1 or more blood cultures, and the pathogen cultured from the blood is not related to an infection at another site.
Criterion 2: Patient has at least 1 of the following signs or symptoms: fever (>100.4°F [>38°C]), chills, or hypotension, and at least 1 of the following:

1. Common skin contaminant (eg, diphtheroids, *Bacillus* species, *Propionibacterium* species, coagulase-negative staphylococci, micrococci) cultured from 2 or more blood cultures drawn on separate occasions
2. Common skin contaminant (eg, diphtheroids, *Bacillus* species, *Propionibacterium* species, coagulase-negative staphylococci, micrococci) cultured from at least 1 blood culture from a patient with an intravenous line, and the physician institutes appropriate antimicrobial therapy
3. Positive antigen test on blood (eg, *Hemophilus influenzae*, *Streptococcus pneumoniae*, *Neisseria meningitides*, group B streptococcus)
and signs and symptoms with positive laboratory results are not related to an infection at another site.

Criterion 3: Patient aged <1 year has at least 1 of the following signs or symptoms: fever (>100.4°F [>38°C]), hypo-

thermia (<98.6°F [<37°C]), apnea, or bradycardia, and at least 1 of the following:

1. Common skin contaminant (eg, diphtheroids, *Bacillus* species, *Propionibacterium* species, coagulase-negative staphylococci, micrococci) cultured from 2 or more blood cultures drawn on separate occasions
2. Common skin contaminant (eg, diphtheroids, *Bacillus* species, *Propionibacterium* species, coagulase-negative staphylococci, micrococci) cultured from at least 1 blood culture from a patient with an intravenous line, and the physician institutes appropriate antimicrobial therapy
3. Positive antigen test on blood (eg, *H influenzae*, *S pneumoniae*, *N meningitides*, group B streptococcus)
and signs and symptoms with positive laboratory results are not related to an infection at another site.

Clinical Sepsis

Should meet at least 1 of the following criteria:
Criterion 1: Patient has at least 1 of the following clinical signs with no other recognized cause: fever (>100.4°F [>38°C]), hypotension (systolic pressure <90 mmHg), or oliguria (<20 mL/h), and blood culture not done or no organisms or antigen detected in blood and no apparent infection at another site, and physician institutes treatment for sepsis.
Criterion 2: Patient aged <1 year has at least 1 of the following clinical signs or symptoms with no other recognized cause: fever (>100.4°F [>38°C]), hypothermia (<98.6°F [<37°C]), apnea, or bradycardia, and blood culture not done or no organisms or antigen detected in blood and no apparent infection at another site, and physician institutes treatment for sepsis.

Catheter-Associated BSI

Defined by the following:
• Vascular access device that terminates at or close to the heart or 1 of the great vessels. An umbilical artery or vein catheter is considered a central line.
• BSI is considered to be associated with a central line if the line was in use during the 48-hour period before development of the BSI. If the time interval between onset of infection and device use is >48 hours, then there should be compelling evidence that the infection is related to the central line.

Arterial or Venous Infection

Included are arteriovenous graft, shunt, fistula, or intravenous cannulation. Should meet at least 1 of the following criteria:
Criterion 1: Patient has organisms cultured from arteries or veins removed during a surgical operation and blood culture not done or no organisms cultured from blood.
Criterion 2: Patient has evidence of arterial or venous infection seen during a surgical operation or histopathologic examination.
Criterion 3: Patient has at least 1 of the following signs or symptoms with no other recognized cause: fever (>100.4°F [>38°C]), pain, erythema, or heat at involved vascular site and >15 CFUs cultured from an intravascular cannula tip using a semiquantitative culture method and blood culture not done or no organisms cultured from blood.
Criterion 4: Patient has purulent drainage at the involved vascular site and blood culture not done or no organisms cultured from blood.
Criterion 5: Patient aged <1 year has at least 1 of the following signs or symptoms with no other recognized cause: fever (>100.4°F [>38°C]), hypothermia (<98.6°F [<37°C]), apnea, bradycardia, lethargy, or pain, erythema or heat at involved vascular site and >15 colonies cultured from intravascular cannula tip using semiquantitative method and blood culture not done or no organisms cultured from blood.

(SCVIR), American Academy of Pediatrics (AAP), and the Healthcare Infection Control Practices Advisory Committee (HICPAC) of the Centers for Disease Control and Prevention (CDC). The recommendations presented in this report reflect consensus of HICPAC and other professional organizations.

INTRAVASCULAR CATHETER-RELATED INFECTIONS IN ADULT AND PEDIATRIC PATIENTS: AN OVERVIEW

Background

Intravascular catheters are indispensable in modern-day medical practice, particularly in intensive care units (ICUs). Although such catheters provide necessary vascular access, their use puts patients at risk for local and systemic infectious complications, including local site infection, CRBSI, septic thrombophlebitis, endocarditis, and other metastatic infections (eg, lung abscess, brain abscess, osteomyelitis, and endophthalmitis).

Health-care institutions purchase millions of intravascular catheters each year. The incidence of CRBSI varies considerably by type of catheter, frequency of catheter manipulation, and patient-related factors (eg, underlying disease and acuity of illness). Peripheral venous catheters are the devices most frequently used for vascular access. Although the incidence of local or bloodstream infections (BSIs) associated with peripheral venous catheters is usually low, serious infectious complications produce considerable annual morbidity because of the frequency with which such catheters are used. However, the majority of serious catheter-related infections are associated with central venous catheters (CVCs), especially those that are placed in patients in ICUs. In the ICU setting, the incidence of infection is often higher than in the less acute in-patient or ambulatory setting. In the ICU, central venous access might be needed for extended periods of time; patients can be colonized with hospital-acquired organisms; and the catheter can be manipulated multiple times per day for the administration of fluids, drugs, and blood products. Moreover, some catheters can be inserted in urgent situations, during which optimal attention to aseptic technique might not be feasible. Certain catheters (eg, pulmonary artery catheters and peripheral arterial catheters) can be accessed multiple times per day for hemodynamic measurements or to obtain samples for laboratory analysis, augmenting the potential for contamination and subsequent clinical infection.

The magnitude of the potential for CVCs to cause morbidity and mortality resulting from infectious complications has been estimated in several studies.[2] In the United States, 15 million CVC days (ie, the total number of days of exposure to CVCs by all patients in the selected population during the selected time period) occur in ICUs each year.[2] If the average rate of CVC-associated BSIs is 5.3 per 1,000 catheter days in the ICU,[3] approximately 80,000 CVC-associated BSIs occur in ICUs each year in the United States. The attributable mortality for these BSIs has ranged from no increase in mortality in studies that controlled for severity of illness,[4–6] to 35% increase in mortality in prospective studies that did not use this control.[7,8] Thus, the attributable mortality remains unclear. The attributable cost per infection is an estimated $34,508–$56,000,[5,9] and the annual cost of caring for patients with CVC-associated BSIs ranges from $296 million to $2.3 billion.[10]

A total of 250,000 cases of CVC-associated BSIs have been estimated to occur annually if entire hospitals are assessed rather than ICUs exclusively.[11] In this case, attributable mortality is an estimated 12%–25% for each infection, and the marginal cost to the health-care system is $25,000 per episode.[11]

Therefore, by several analyses, the cost of CVC-associated BSI is substantial, both in terms of morbidity and in terms of financial resources expended. To improve patient outcome and reduce health-care costs, strategies should be implemented to reduce the incidence of these infections. This effort should be multidisciplinary, involving health-care professionals who insert and maintain intravascular catheters, health-care managers who allocate resources, and patients who are capable of assisting in the care of their catheters. Although several individual strategies have been studied and shown to be effective in reducing CRBSI, studies using multiple strategies have not been conducted. Thus, it is not known whether implementing multiple strategies will have an additive effect in reducing CRBSI, but it is logical to use multiple strategies concomitantly.

Terminology and Estimates of Risk

The terminology used to identify different types of catheters is confusing, because many clinicians and researchers use different aspects of the catheter for informal reference. A catheter can be designated by the type of vessel it occupies (eg, peripheral venous, central venous, or arterial); its intended life span (eg, temporary or short-term versus permanent or long-term); its site of insertion (eg, subclavian, femoral, internal jugular, peripheral, and peripherally inserted central catheter [PICC]); its pathway from skin to vessel (eg, tunneled versus nontunneled); its physical length (eg, long versus short); or some special characteristic of the catheter (eg, presence or absence of a cuff, impregnation with heparin, antibiotics or antiseptics, and the number of lumens). To accurately define a specific type of catheter, all of these aspects should be described (Table 1).

The rate of all catheter-related infections (including local infections and systemic infections) is difficult to determine. Although CRBSI is an ideal parameter because it represents the most serious form of catheter-related infection, the rate of such infection depends on how CRBSI is defined.

Health-care professionals should recognize the difference between surveillance definitions and clinical definitions. The surveillance definitions for catheter-associated BSI includes all BSIs that occur in patients with CVCs, when other sites of infection have been excluded (Appendix A). That is, the surveillance definition overestimates the true incidence of CRBSI because not all BSIs originate from a catheter. Some bacteremias are secondary BSIs from undocumented

TABLE 1.   Catheters Used for Venous and Arterial Access

Catheter Type	Entry Site	Length	Comments
Peripheral venous catheters (short)	Usually inserted in veins of forearm or hand	<3 in	Phlebitis with prolonged use; rarely associated with bloodstream infection
Peripheral arterial catheters	Usually inserted in radial artery; can be placed in femoral, axillary, brachial, posterior tibial arteries	<3 in	Low infection risk; rarely associated with bloodstream infection
Midline catheters	Inserted via the antecubital fossa into the proximal basilic or cephalic veins; does not enter central veins	3–8 in	Anaphylactoid reactions have been reported with catheters made of elastomeric hydrogel; lower rates of phlebitis than short peripheral catheters
Nontunneled CVCs	Percutaneously inserted into central veins (subclavian, internal jugular, or femoral)	8 cm or longer, depending on patient size	Account for majority of CRBSI
Pulmonary artery catheters	Inserted through a Teflon introducer in a central vein (subclavian, internal jugular, or femoral)	30 cm or longer, depending on patient size	Usually heparin bonded; similar rates of bloodstream infection as CVC; subclavian site preferred to reduce infection risk
PICCs	Inserted into basilic, cephalic, or brachial veins and enter the superior vena cava	20 cm or longer, depending on patient size	Lower rate of infection than nontunneled CVCs
Tunneled CVCs	Implanted into subclavian, internal jugular, or femoral veins	8 cm or longer, depending on patient size	Cuff inhibits migration of organisms into catheter tract, lower rate of infection than nontunneled CVC
Totally implantable	Tunneled beneath skin and have devices subcutaneous port accessed with a needle; implanted in subclavian or internal jugular vein	8 cm or longer, depending on patient size	Lowest risk for CRBSI; improved patient self-image; no need for local catheter site care; surgery required for catheter removal
Umbilical catheters	Inserted into either umbilical vein or umbilical artery	6 cm or less, depending on patient size	Risk for CRBSI similar to catheters placed in umbilical vein versus artery

sources (eg, postoperative surgical sites, intra-abdominal infections, and hospital-associated pneumonia or urinary tract infections). Thus, surveillance definitions are really definitions for catheter-associated BSIs. A more rigorous definition might include only those BSIs for which other sources were excluded by careful examination of the patient record, and where a culture of the catheter tip demonstrated substantial colonies of an organism identical to those found in the bloodstream. Such a clinical definition would focus on catheter-related BSIs. Therefore, to accurately compare a health-care facility's infection rate to published data, comparable definitions also should be used.

CDC and the Joint Commission on Accreditation of Healthcare Organizations (JCAHO) recommend that the rate of catheter-associated BSIs be expressed as the number of catheter associated BSIs per 1,000 CVC days.[12,13] This parameter is more useful than the rate expressed as the number of catheter-associated infections per 100 catheters (or percentage of catheters studied), because it accounts for BSIs over time and therefore adjusts risk for the number of days the catheter is in use.

Epidemiology and Microbiology

Since 1970, CDC's National Nosocomial Infection Surveillance System (NNIS) has been collecting data on the incidence and etiologies of hospital-acquired infections, including CVC-associated BSIs in a group of nearly 300 US hospitals. The majority of hospital-acquired BSIs are associated with the use of a CVC, with BSI rates being substantially higher among patients with CVCs than among those without CVCs. Rates of CVC-associated BSI vary considerably by

hospital size, hospital service/unit, and type of CVC. During 1992–2001, NNIS hospitals reported ICU rates of CVC-associated BSI ranging from 2.9 (in a cardiothoracic ICU) to 11.3 (in a neonatal nursery for infants weighing <1,000 g) BSIs per 1,000 CVC days (Table 2).[14]

The relative risk (RR) of catheter-associated BSI also has been assessed in a meta-analysis of 223 prospective studies of adult patients.[11] RR of infection was best determined by analyzing rates of infection both by BSIs per 100 catheters and BSIs per 1,000 catheter days. These rates, and the NNIS-derived data, can be used as benchmarks by individual hos-

TABLE 2.   Pooled Means of the Distribution of CVC-Associated Bloodstream Infection Rates in Hospitals That Report to the NNIS System, January 1992 to June 2001

Type of ICU	Number of ICUs	Catheter Days	Pooled Mean/ 1000 Catheter Days
Coronary	102	252 325	4.5
Cardiothoracic	64	419 674	2.9
Medical	135	671 632	5.9
Medical/surgical			
Major teaching	123	579 704	5.3
All others	180	863 757	3.8
Neurosurgical	47	123 780	4.7
Nursery, high risk			
≤1000 g	138	438 261	11.3
1001–1500 g	136	213 351	6.9
1501–2500 g	132	163 697	4.0
>2500 g	133	231 573	3.8
Pediatric	74	291 831	7.6
Surgical	153	900 948	5.3
Trauma	25	116 709	7.9
Respiratory	7	21 265	3.4

Issued August 2001.[290,291]

pitals to estimate how their rates compare with other institutions. Rates are influenced by patient-related parameters, such as severity of illness and type of illness (eg, third-degree burns versus postcardiac surgery), and by catheter-related parameters, such as the condition under which the catheter was placed (eg, elective versus urgent) and catheter type (eg, tunneled versus nontunneled or subclavian versus jugular).

Types of organisms that most commonly cause hospital-acquired BSIs change over time. During 1986–1989, coagulase-negative staphylococci, followed by *Staphylococcus aureus*, were the most frequently reported causes of BSIs, accounting for 27% and 16% of BSIs, respectively (Table 3).[15] Pooled data from 1992 through 1999 indicate that coagulase-negative staphylococci, followed by enterococci, are now the most frequently isolated causes of hospital-acquired BSIs.[12] Coagulase-negative staphylococci account for 37%[12] and *S aureus* account for 12.6% of reported hospital-acquired BSIs.[12] Also notable was the susceptibility pattern of *S aureus* isolates. In 1999, for the first time since NNIS has been reporting susceptibilities, >50% of all *S aureus* isolates from ICUs were resistant to oxacillin.[12]

In 1999, enterococci accounted for 13.5% of BSIs, an increase from 8% reported to NNIS during 1986–1989. The percentage of enterococcal ICU isolates resistant to vancomycin also is increasing, escalating from 0.5% in 1989 to 25.9% in 1999.[12]

Candida spp caused 8% of hospital-acquired BSIs reported to NNIS during 1986–1989,[15,16] and during 1992–1999.[12,17,18] Resistance of *Candida* spp to commonly used antifungal agents is increasing. Although NNIS has not reported the percentage of BSIs caused by non-*albicans* species or fluconazole susceptibility data, other epidemiologic and clinical data document that fluconazole resistance is an increasingly relevant consideration when designing empiric therapeutic regimens for CRBSIs caused by yeast. Data from the Surveillance and Control of Pathogens of Epidemiologic Importance (SCOPE) Program documented that 10% of *C albicans* bloodstream isolates from hospitalized patients were resistant to fluconazole.[17] Additionally, 48% of *Candida* BSIs were caused by non-*albicans* species, including *C glabrata* and *C krusei*, which are more likely than *C albicans* to demonstrate resistance to fluconazole and itraconazole.[18,19]

Gram-negative bacilli accounted for 19% of catheter-associated BSIs during 1986–1989[15] compared with 14% of catheter-associated BSIs during 1992–1999.[12] An increasing percentage of ICU-related isolates are caused by *Enterobacteriaceae* that produce extended-spectrum β-lactamases (ESBLs), particularly *Klebsiella pneumoniae*.[20] Such organisms not only are resistant to extended-spectrum cephalosporins, but also to frequently used, broad spectrum antimicrobial agents.

Pathogenesis

Migration of skin organisms at the insertion site into the cutaneous catheter tract with colonization of the catheter tip is the most common route of infection for peripherally inserted, short-term catheters.[21,22] Contamination of the catheter hub contributes substantially to intraluminal colonization of long-term catheters.[23–25] Occasionally, catheters might become hematogenously seeded from another focus of infection. Rarely, infusate contamination leads to CRBSI.[26]

Important pathogenic determinants of catheter-related infection are 1) the material of which the device is made and 2) the intrinsic virulence factors of the infecting organism. In vitro studies demonstrate that catheters made of polyvinyl chloride or polyethylene are likely less resistant to the adherence of microorganisms than are catheters made of Teflon, silicone elastomer, or polyurethane.[27,28] Therefore, the majority of catheters sold in the United States are no longer made of polyvinyl chloride or polyethylene. Some catheter materials also have surface irregularities that enhance the microbial adherence of certain species (eg, coagulase-negative staphylococci, *Acinetobacter calcoaceticus*, and *Pseudomonas aeruginosa*[29–31]); catheters made of these materials are especially vulnerable to microbial colonization and subsequent infection. Additionally, certain catheter materials are more thrombogenic than others, a characteristic that also might predispose to catheter colonization and catheter-related infection.[31,32] This association has led to emphasis on preventing catheter-related thrombus as an additional mechanism for reducing CRBSI.

The adherence properties of a given microorganism also are important in the pathogenesis of catheter-related infection. For example, *S aureus* can adhere to host proteins (eg, fibronectin) commonly present on catheters.[33,34] Also, coagulase-negative staphylococci adhere to polymer surfaces more readily than do other pathogens (eg, *Escherichia coli* or *S aureus*). Additionally, certain strains of coagulase-negative staphylococci produce an extracellular polysaccharide often referred to as "slime."[35,36] In the presence of catheters, this slime potentiates the pathogenicity of coagulase-negative staphylococci by allowing them to withstand host defense mechanisms (eg, acting as a barrier to engulfment and killing by polymorphonuclear leukocytes) or by making them less susceptible to antimicrobial agents (eg, forming a matrix that binds antimicrobials before their contact with the organism cell wall).[37] Certain *Candida* spp, in the presence of glucose-containing fluids, might produce slime similar to that of their bacterial counterparts, potentially explaining

TABLE 3. Most Common Pathogens Isolated From Bloodstream Infections [12,15]

Pathogen	1986–1989 (%)	1992–1999 (%)
Coagulase-negative staphylococci	27	37
S aureus	16	13
Enterococcus	8	13
Gram-negative rods	19	14
E coli	6	2
Enterobacter	5	5
P aeruginosa	4	4
K pneumoniae	4	3
Candida species	8	8

the increased proportion of BSIs caused by fungal pathogens among patients receiving parenteral nutrition fluids.[38]

STRATEGIES FOR PREVENTION OF CATHETER-RELATED INFECTIONS IN ADULT AND PEDIATRIC PATIENTS

Quality Assurance and Continuing Education

Measures to minimize the risk for infection associated with intravascular therapy should strike a balance between patient safety and cost effectiveness. As knowledge, technology, and health-care settings change, infection control and prevention measures also should change. Well-organized programs that enable health-care providers to provide, monitor, and evaluate care and to become educated are critical to the success of this effort. Reports spanning the past two decades have consistently demonstrated that risk for infection declines following standardization of aseptic care,[39–43] and that insertion and maintenance of intravascular catheters by inexperienced staff might increase the risk for catheter colonization and CRBSI.[43,44] Specialized "IV teams" have shown unequivocal effectiveness in reducing the incidence of catheter-related infections and associated complications and costs.[45–45] Additionally, infection risk increases with nursing staff reductions below a critical level.[48]

Site of Catheter Insertion

The site at which a catheter is placed influences the subsequent risk for catheter-related infection and phlebitis. The influence of site on the risk for catheter infections is related in part to the risk for thrombophlebitis and density of local skin flora.

Phlebitis has long been recognized as a risk for infection. For adults, lower extremity insertion sites are associated with a higher risk for infection than are upper extremity sites.[49–51] In addition, hand veins have a lower risk for phlebitis than do veins on the wrist or upper arm.[52]

The density of skin flora at the catheter insertion site is a major risk factor for CRBSI. Authorities recommend that CVCs be placed in a subclavian site instead of a jugular or femoral site to reduce the risk for infection. No randomized trial satisfactorily has compared infection rates for catheters placed in jugular, subclavian, and femoral sites. Catheters inserted into an internal jugular vein have been associated with higher risk for infection than those inserted into a subclavian or femoral vein.[22,53,54] Femoral catheters have been demonstrated to have relatively high colonization rates when used in adults.[55] Femoral catheters should be avoided, when possible, because they are associated with a higher risk for deep venous thrombosis than are internal jugular or subclavian catheters[56–60] and because of a presumption that such catheters are more likely to become infected. However, studies in pediatric patients have demonstrated that femoral catheters have a low incidence of mechanical complications and might have an equivalent infection rate to that of nonfemoral catheters.[61–63] Thus, in adult patients, a

subclavian site is preferred for infection control purposes, although other factors (eg, the potential for mechanical complications, risk for subclavian vein stenosis, and catheter-operator skill) should be considered when deciding where to place the catheter. In a meta-analysis of eight studies, the use of bedside ultrasound for the placement of CVCs substantially reduced mechanical complications compared with the standard landmark placement technique (RR = 0.22; 95% confidence interval [CI] = 0.10–0.45).[64] Consideration of comfort, security, and maintenance of asepsis as well as patient-specific factors (eg, preexisting catheters, anatomic deformity, and bleeding diathesis), RR of mechanical complications (eg, bleeding and pneumothorax), the availability of bedside ultrasound, and the risk for infection should guide site selection.

Type of Catheter Material

Teflon or polyurethane catheters have been associated with fewer infectious complications than catheters made of polyvinyl chloride or polyethylene.[27,65,66] Steel needles used as an alternative to catheters for peripheral venous access have the same rate of infectious complications as do Teflon catheters.[67,68] However, the use of steel needles frequently is complicated by infiltration of intravenous (IV) fluids into the subcutaneous tissues, a potentially serious complication if the infused fluid is a vesicant.[68]

Hand Hygiene and Aseptic Technique

For short peripheral catheters, good hand hygiene before catheter insertion or maintenance, combined with proper aseptic technique during catheter manipulation, provides protection against infection. Good hand hygiene can be achieved through the use of either a waterless, alcohol-based product[69] or an antibacterial soap and water with adequate rinsing.[70] Appropriate aseptic technique does not necessarily require sterile gloves; a new pair of disposable nonsterile gloves can be used in conjunction with a "no-touch" technique for the insertion of peripheral venous catheters. However, gloves are required by the Occupational Safety and Health Administration as standard precautions for the prevention of bloodborne pathogen exposure.

Compared with peripheral venous catheters, CVCs carry a substantially greater risk for infection; therefore, the level of barrier precautions needed to prevent infection during insertion of CVCs should be more stringent. Maximal sterile barrier precautions (eg, cap, mask, sterile gown, sterile gloves, and large sterile drape) during the insertion of CVCs substantially reduces the incidence of CRBSI compared with standard precautions (eg, sterile gloves and small drapes).[22,71] Although the efficacy of such precautions for insertion of PICCs and midline catheters has not been studied, the use of maximal barrier precautions also is probably applicable to PICCs.

Skin Antisepsis

In the United States, povidone iodine has been the most widely used antiseptic for cleansing arterial catheter and CVC-insertion sites.[72] However, in one study, preparation of central venous and arterial sites with a 2% aqueous chlorhexidine gluconate lowered BSI rates compared with site preparation with 10% povidone-iodine or 70% alcohol.[73] Commercially available products containing chlorhexidine have not been available until recently; in July 2000, the US Food and Drug Administration (FDA) approved a 2% tincture of chlorhexidine preparation for skin antisepsis. Other preparations of chlorhexidine might not be as effective. Tincture of chlorhexidine gluconate 0.5% is no more effective in preventing CRBSI or CVC colonization than 10% povidone iodine, as demonstrated by a prospective, randomized study of adults.[74] However, in a study involving neonates, 0.5% chlorhexidine reduced peripheral IV colonization compared with povidone iodine (20/418 versus 38/408 catheters; p = 0.01).[75] This study, which did not include CVCs, had an insufficient number of participants to assess differences in BSI rates. A 1% tincture of chlorhexidine preparation is available in Canada and Australia, but not yet in the United States. No published trials have compared a 1% chlorhexidine preparation to povidone-iodine.

Catheter Site Dressing Regimens

Transparent, semipermeable polyurethane dressings have become a popular means of dressing catheter insertion sites. Transparent dressings reliably secure the device, permit continuous visual inspection of the catheter site, permit patients to bathe and shower without saturating the dressing, and require less frequent changes than do standard gauze and tape dressings; the use of these dressings saves personnel time.

In the largest controlled trial of dressing regimens on peripheral catheters, the infectious morbidity associated with the use of transparent dressings on approximately 2,000 peripheral catheters was examined.[65] Data from this study suggest that the rate of colonization among catheters dressed with transparent dressings (5.7%) is comparable to that of those dressed with gauze (4.6%) and that no clinically substantial differences exist in either the incidences of catheter-site colonization or phlebitis. Furthermore, these data suggest that transparent dressings can be safely left on peripheral venous catheters for the duration of catheter insertion without increasing the risk for thrombophlebitis.[65]

A meta-analysis has assessed studies that compared the risk for catheter-related BSIs for groups using transparent dressings versus groups using gauze dressing.[76] The risk for CRBSIs did not differ between the groups. The choice of dressing can be a matter of preference. If blood is oozing from the catheter insertion site, gauze dressing might be preferred.

In a multi-center study, a chlorhexidine-impregnated sponge (Biopatch) placed over the site of short-term arterial and CVCs reduced the risk for catheter colonization and CRBSI.[77] No adverse systemic effects resulted from use of this device.

Catheter Securement Devices

Sutureless securement devices can be advantageous over suture in preventing catheter-related BSIs. One study, which involved only a limited number of patients and was underpowered, compared a sutureless device with suture for the securement of PICCS; in this study, CRBSI was reduced in the group of patients that received the sutureless device.[78]

In-Line Filters

In-line filters reduce the incidence of infusion-related phlebitis.[79,80] No data support their efficacy in preventing infections associated with intravascular catheters and infusion systems. Proponents of filters cite several potential benefits to using these filters, including 1) reducing the risk for infection from contaminated infusate or proximal contamination (ie, introduced proximal to the filter); 2) reducing the risk for phlebitis in patients who require high doses of medication or in those in whom infusion-related phlebitis already has occurred; 3) removing particulate matter that might contaminate IV fluids[81]; and 4) filtering endotoxin produced by gram-negative organisms in contaminated infusate[82] These theoretical advantages should be tempered by the knowledge that infusate-related BSI is rare and that filtration of medications or infusates in the pharmacy is a more practical and less costly way to remove the majority of particulates. Furthermore, in-line filters might become blocked, especially with certain solutions (eg, dextran, lipids, and mannitol), thereby increasing the number of line manipulations and decreasing the availability of administered drugs.[83] Thus, for reducing the risk for CRBSI, no strong recommendation can be made in favor of using in-line filters.

Antimicrobial/Antiseptic Impregnated Catheters and Cuffs

Certain catheters and cuffs that are coated or impregnated with antimicrobial or antiseptic agents can decrease the risk for CRBSI and potentially decrease hospital costs associated with treating CRBSIs, despite the additional acquisition cost of an antimicrobial/antiseptic impregnated catheter.[84] All of the studies involving antimicrobial/antiseptic impregnated catheters have been conducted using triple-lumen, noncuffed catheters in adult patients whose catheters remained in place <30 days. Although all of the studies have been conducted in adults, these catheters have been approved by FDA for use in patients weighing >3 kg. No antiseptic or antimicrobial impregnated catheters currently are available for use in weighing <3 kg.

Chlorhexidine/Silver Sulfadiazine

Catheters coated with chlorhexidine/silver sulfadiazine only on the external luminal surface have been studied as a means to reduce CRBSI. Two meta-analyses[2,85] demonstrated that such catheters reduced the risk for CRBSI compared with standard noncoated catheters. The mean duration of catheter placement in one meta-analysis ranged from 5.1 to

11.2 days.[86] The half-life of antimicrobial activity against *S epidermidis* is 3 days in vitro for catheters coated with chlorhexidine/silver sulfadiazine; this antimicrobial activity decreases over time.[87] The benefit for the patients who receive these catheters will be realized within the first 14 days.[86] A second-generation catheter is now available with chlorhexidine coating both the internal and external luminal surfaces. The external surface has three times the amount of chlorhexidine and extended release of the surface bound antiseptics than that in the first generation catheters. The external surface coating of chlorhexidine is combined with silver-sulfadiazine, and the internal surface is coated with chlorhexidine alone. Preliminary studies indicate that prolonged anti-infective activity provides improved efficacy in preventing infections.[88] Although rare, anaphylaxis has been reported with the use of these chlorhexidine/silver sulfadiazine catheters in Japan.[89] Whether patients will become colonized or infected with organisms resistant to chlorhexidine/silver sulfadiazine has not been determined.[86]

Chlorhexidine/silver sulfadiazine catheters are more expensive than standard catheters. However, one analysis has suggested that the use of chlorhexidine/silver sulfadiazine catheters should lead to a cost savings of $68 to $391 per catheter[90] in settings in which the risk for CRBSI is high despite adherence to other preventive strategies (eg, maximal barrier precautions and aseptic techniques). Use of these catheters might be cost effective in ICU patients, burn patients, neutropenic patients, and other patient populations in which the rate of infection exceeds 3.3 per 1,000 catheter days.[86]

Minocycline/Rifampin

In a multicenter randomized trial, CVCs impregnated on both the external and internal surfaces with minocycline/rifampin were associated with lower rates of CRBSI when compared with the first-generation chlorhexidine-silver sulfadiazine impregnated catheters.[91] The beneficial effect began after day 6 of catheterization. None of the catheters were evaluated beyond 30 days. No minocycline/rifampin-resistant organisms were reported. However, in vitro data indicate that these impregnated catheters could increase the incidence of minocycline and rifampin resistance among pathogens, especially staphylococci. The half-life of antimicrobial activity against *S epidermidis* is 25 days with catheters coated with minocycline/rifampin, compared with 3 days for the first-generation catheters coated with chlorhexidine/silver sulfadiazine in vitro.[87] In vivo, the duration of antimicrobial activity of the minocycline/rifampin catheter is longer than that of the first-generation chlorhexidine/silver sulfadiazine catheter.[91] No comparative studies have been published using the second-generation chlorhexidine/silver sulfadiazine catheter. Studies are needed to evaluated whether the improved performance of the minocyline/rifampin catheters results from the antimicrobial agents used or from the coating of both the internal and external surfaces. As with chlorhexidine/silver sulfadiazine catheters, some clinicians have recom-

mended that the minocycline/rifampin catheters be considered in patient populations when the rate of CRBSI exceeds 3.3 per 1,000 catheter days.[86] Others suggest that reducing all rates of CRBSI should be the goal.[92] The decision to use chlorhexidine/silver sulfadiazine or minocycline/rifampin impregnated catheters should be based on the need to enhance prevention of CRBSI after standard procedures have been implemented (eg, educating personnel, using maximal sterile barrier precautions, and using 2% chlorhexidine skin antisepsis) and then balanced against the concern for emergence of resistant pathogens and the cost of implementing this strategy.

Platinum/Silver

Ionic metals have broad antimicrobial activity and are being used in catheters and cuffs to prevent CRBSI. A combination platinum/silver impregnated catheter is available in Europe and has recently been approved by FDA for use in the United States. Although these catheters are being marketed for their antimicrobial properties, no published studies have been presented to support an antimicrobial effect.

Silver Cuffs

Ionic silver has been used in subcutaneous collagen cuffs attached to CVCs.[93] The ionic silver provides antimicrobial activity and the cuff provides a mechanical barrier to the migration of microorganisms along the external surface of the catheter. In studies of catheters left in place ≥20 days, the cuff failed to reduce the incidence of CRBSI.[94,95] Two other studies of short-term catheters could not demonstrate efficacy because of the minimal number of CRBSIs observed.[93,96]

Systemic Antibiotic Prophylaxis

No studies have demonstrated that oral or parenteral antibacterial or antifungal drugs might reduce the incidence of CRBSI among adults.[97–99] However, among low birth weight infants, two studies have assessed vancomycin prophylaxis; both demonstrated a reduction in CRBSI but no reduction in mortality.[100,101] Because the prophylactic use of vancomycin is an independent risk factor for the acquisition of vancomycin-resistant enterococcus (VRE),[102] the risk for acquiring VRE likely outweighs the benefit of using prophylactic vancomycin.

Antibiotic/Antiseptic Ointments

Povidone-iodine ointment applied at the insertion site of hemodialysis catheters has been studied as a prophylactic intervention to reduce the incidence of catheter-related infections. One randomized study of 129 hemodialysis catheters demonstrated a reduction in the incidence of exit-site infections, catheter-tip colonization, and BSIs with the routine use of povidone-iodine ointment at the catheter insertion site compared with no ointment at the insertion site.[103]

Several studies have evaluated the effectiveness of mupirocin ointment applied at the insertion sites of CVCs as a means to prevent CRBSI.[104–106] Although mupirocin reduced the risk for CRBSI,[106] mupirocin ointment also has been associated with mupirocin resistance,[107,108] and might adversely affect the integrity of polyurethane catheters.[109,110]

Nasal carriers of *S aureus* have a higher risk for acquiring CRBSI than do noncarriers.[103,111] Mupirocin ointment has been used intranasally to decrease nasal carriage of *S aureus* and lessen the risk for CRBSI. However, resistance to mupirocin develops in both *S aureus* and coagulase-negative staphylococci soon after routine use of mupirocin is instituted.[107,108]

Other antibiotic ointments applied to the catheter insertion site also have been studied and have yielded conflicting results.[112–114] In addition, rates of catheter colonization with *Candida* spp might be increased with the use of antibiotic ointments that have no fungicidal activity.[112,114] To avoid compromising the integrity of the catheter, any ointment that is applied to the catheter insertion site should be checked against the catheter and ointment manufacturers' recommendations regarding compatibility.

Antibiotic Lock Prophylaxis

To prevent CRBSI, antibiotic lock prophylaxis has been attempted by flushing and filling the lumen of the catheter with an antibiotic solution and leaving the solution to dwell in the lumen of the catheter. Three studies have demonstrated the usefulness of such prophylaxis in neutropenic patients with long-term catheters.[115–117] In two of the studies, patients received either heparin alone (10 U/ml) or heparin plus 25 micrograms/ml of vancomycin. The third study compared vancomycin/ciprofloxacin/heparin (VCH) to vancomycin/heparin (VH) and then to heparin alone. The rate of CRBSI with vancomycin-susceptible organisms was significantly lower (VCH, p = 0.022; VH, p = 0.028) and the time to the first episode of bacteremia with vancomycin-susceptible organisms was substantially longer (VCH, p = 0.036; VH, p = 0.011) in patients receiving either vancomycin/ciprofloxacin/heparin or vancomycin/heparin compared with heparin alone.[115–117] One study involving a limited number of children revealed no difference in rates of CRBSI between children receiving a heparin flush compared with those receiving heparin and vancomycin.[118] However, because the use of vancomycin is an independent risk factor for the acquisition of VRE,[102] this practice is not recommended routinely.

An anticoagulant/antimicrobial combination comprising minocycline and ethylenediaminetetraacetic acid (EDTA) has been proposed as a lock solution because it has antibiofilm and antimicrobial activity against gram-positive, gram-negative, and *Candida* organisms,[119] as well as anticoagulant properties. However, no controlled or randomized trials have demonstrated its efficacy.

Anticoagulants

Anticoagulant flush solutions are used widely to prevent catheter thrombosis. Because thrombi and fibrin deposits on catheters might serve as a nidus for microbial colonization of intravascular catheters,[120,121] the use of anticoagulants might have a role in the prevention of CRBSI.

In a meta-analysis evaluating the benefit of heparin prophylaxis (3 U/ml in TPN, 5,000 U every 6 or 12 hours flush, or 2,500 U low molecular weight heparin subcutaneously) in patients with short-term CVCs, the risk for catheter-related central venous thrombosis was reduced with the use of prophylactic heparin.[122] However, no substantial difference in the rate for CRBSI was observed. Because the majority of heparin solutions contain preservatives with antimicrobial activity, whether any decrease in the rate of CRBSI is a result of the reduced thrombus formation, the preservative, or both is unclear.

The majority of pulmonary artery, umbilical, and central venous catheters are available with a heparin-bonded coating. The majority are heparin-bonded with benzalkonium chloride, which provides the catheters with antimicrobial activity[123] and provides an anti-thrombotic effect.[124]

Warfarin also has been evaluated as a means for reducing CRBSI by reducing thrombus formation on catheters.[125,126] In patients with long-term CVCs, low-dose warfarin (ie, 1 mg/day) reduced the incidence of catheter thrombus. No data demonstrate that warfarin reduces the incidence of CRBSI.

Replacement of Catheters

Peripheral Venous Catheters

Scheduled replacement of intravascular catheters has been proposed as a method to prevent phlebitis and catheter-related infections. Studies of short peripheral venous catheters indicate that the incidence of thrombophlebitis and bacterial colonization of catheters increases when catheters are left in place >72 hours.[66,67,127] However, rates of phlebitis are not substantially different in peripheral catheters left in place 72 hours compared with 96 hours.[128] Because phlebitis and catheter colonization have been associated with an increased risk for catheter-related infection, short peripheral catheter sites commonly are rotated at 72–96-hour intervals to reduce both the risk for infection and patient discomfort associated with phlebitis.

Midline Catheters

Midline catheters have been associated with lower rates of phlebitis than short peripheral catheters and with lower rates of infection than CVCs.[129–131] In one prospective study of 140 midline catheters, their use was associated with a BSI rate of 0.8 per 1,000 catheter-days.[131] No specific risk factors, including duration of catheterization, were associated with infection. Midline catheters were in place a median of 7 days, but for as long as 49 days. Although the findings of this study suggested that midline catheters can be changed only when there is a specific indication, no prospective, randomized studies have assessed the benefit of routine replacement as a strategy to prevent CRBSI associated with midline catheters.

CVCs, Including PICCs and Hemodialysis Catheters

Catheter replacement at scheduled time intervals as a method to reduce CRBSI has not lowered rates.

Two trials have assessed a strategy of changing the catheter every 7 days compared with a strategy of changing catheters as needed.[132,133] One of these studies involved 112 surgical ICU patients needing CVCs, pulmonary artery catheters, or peripheral arterial catheters,[132] whereas the other study involved only subclavian hemodialysis catheters.[133] In both studies, no difference in CRBSI was observed in patients undergoing scheduled catheter replacement every 7 days compared with patients whose catheters were replaced as needed.

Scheduled guidewire exchanges of CVCs is another proposed strategy for preventing CRBSI. The results of a meta-analysis of 12 randomized controlled trials assessing CVC management failed to prove any reduction of CRBSI rates through routine replacement of CVCs by guidewire exchange compared with catheter replacement on an as-needed basis.[134] Thus, routine replacement of CVCs is not necessary for catheters that are functioning and have no evidence of causing local or systemic complications.

Catheter replacement over a guidewire has become an accepted technique for replacing a malfunctioning catheter or exchanging a pulmonary artery catheter for a CVC when invasive monitoring no longer is needed. Catheter insertion over a guidewire is associated with less discomfort and a significantly lower rate of mechanical complications than are those percutaneously inserted at a new site[135]; in addition, this technique provides a means of preserving limited venous access in some patients. Replacement of temporary catheters over a guidewire in the presence of bacteremia is not an acceptable replacement strategy, because the source of infection is usually colonization of the skin tract from the insertion site to the vein.[22,135] However, in selected patients with tunneled hemodialysis catheters and bacteremia, catheter exchange over a guidewire, in combination with antibiotic therapy, might be an alternative as a salvage strategy in patients with limited venous access.[136–139]

Hemodialysis Catheters

The use of catheters for hemodialysis is the most common factor contributing to bacteremia in dialysis patients.[140,141] The RR for bacteremia in patients with dialysis catheters is sevenfold the risk for patients with primary arteriovenous fistulas.[142] Despite the National Kidney Foundation's effort to reduce the number of hemodialysis patients maintained with catheter access, catheter use increased from 12.7% in 1995 to 22.2% in 1999.[143] Rates for bacteremia per 100 patient months were 0.2 for arteriovenous fistulas, 0.5 for grafts, 5.0 for cuffed catheters, and 8.5 for noncuffed catheters (CDC, unpublished data, 1999).

To reduce the rate of infection, hemodialysis catheters should be avoided in favor of arteriovenous fistulas and grafts. If temporary access is needed for dialysis, a cuffed catheter is preferable to a noncuffed catheter, even in the ICU setting, if the catheter is expected to stay in place for >3 weeks.[11,144]

Pulmonary Artery Catheters

Pulmonary artery catheters are inserted through a Teflon introducer and typically remain in place an average of 3 days. The majority of pulmonary artery catheters are heparin bonded, which reduces not only catheter thrombosis but also microbial adherence to the catheter.[145] Meta-analysis indicates that standard nonheparin-bonded pulmonary artery catheter rates of CRBSI are 5.5 per 1,000 catheter days; for heparin-bonded pulmonary artery catheters, this rate is 2.6 per 1,000 catheter days.[11] Because the majority of pulmonary artery catheters are heparin-bonded, the RR of infection with these catheters is similar to that of CVC (2.6 versus 2.3 per 1,000 catheter days).[11]

A prospective study of 442 pulmonary artery catheters demonstrated an increased risk for CRBSI after 5 days (0/442 CRBSI before 5 days versus 5/442 CSBSI after 5 days; $P < 0.001$).[146] A prospective observational study of 71 pulmonary artery catheters demonstrated higher infection rates in catheters left in place longer than 7 days (2% before 7 days versus 16% after 7 days; $P = 0.056$).[147] However, no studies indicate that catheter replacement at scheduled time intervals is an effective method to reduce CRBSI.[132,135] In patients who continue to require hemodynamic monitoring, pulmonary artery catheters do not need to be changed more frequently than every 7 days. No specific recommendation can be made regarding routine replacement of catheters that need to be in place for >7 days.

Pulmonary artery catheters are usually packaged with a thin plastic sleeve that prevents touch contamination when placed over the catheter. In a study of 166 catheters, patients who were randomly assigned to have their catheters self-contained within this sleeve had a reduced risk for CRBSI compared with those who had a pulmonary artery catheter placed without the sleeve ($P = 0.002$).[148]

Peripheral Arterial Catheters

Peripheral arterial catheters are usually inserted into the radial or femoral artery and permit continuous blood pressure monitoring and blood gas measurements. The rate of CRBSI is comparable to that of temporary CVCs (2.9 versus 2.3 per 1,000 catheter days).[11] One study of peripheral arterial catheters demonstrated no difference in infection rates between changing catheters at scheduled times and changing arterial catheters on an as-needed basis.[132] One observational study of 71 arterial catheters revealed that 10 local infections and four CRBSIs occurred in patients who had peripheral arterial catheters in place for >4 days compared with one local infection and no CRBSIs in patients whose catheters were in place <4 days ($P < 0.05$).[147] Because the risk for CRBSI is likely similar to that of short-term CVCs, arterial catheters can be approached in a similar way. No specific recommendation can be made regarding replacement of catheters that need to be in place for >5 days.

APPENDIX B. Summary of Recommended Frequency of Replacements for Catheters, Dressings, Administration Sets, and Fluids

Catheter	Replacement and Relocation of Device	Replacement of Catheter Site Dressing	Replacement of Administration Sets	Hang Time for Parenteral Fluids
Peripheral venous catheters	In adults, replace catheter and rotate site no more frequently than every 72–96 h. Replace catheters inserted under emergency basis and insert a new catheter at a different site within 48 h. In pediatric patients, do not replace peripheral catheters unless clinically indicated.	Replace dressing when the catheter is removed or replaced or when the dressing becomes damp, loosened, or soiled. Replace dressings more frequently in diaphoretic patients. In patients who have large bulky dressings that prevent palpation or direct visualization of the catheter insertion site, remove the dressing and visually inspect the catheter at least daily and apply a new dressing.	Replace IV tubing, including add-on devices, no more frequently than at 72-h intervals unless clinically indicated. Replace tubing used to administer blood, blood products, or lipid emulsions within 24 h of initiating the infusion. No recommendation for replacement of tubing used for intermittent infusions. Consider short extension tubing connected to the catheter to be a portion of the device. Replace such short extension tubing when the catheter is changed.	No recommendation for the hang time of IV fluids, including non–lipid-containing parenteral nutrition fluids. Complete infusion of lipid-containing parenteral nutrition fluids (eg, 3-in-1 solutions) within 24 h of hanging the fluid. Complete infusion of lipid emulsions alone within 12 h of hanging the fluid. Complete infusions of blood products within 4 h of hanging the product.
Midline catheters	No recommendation for the frequency of the catheter replacement	As above.	As above.	As above.
Peripheral arterial catheters	In adults, do not replace catheters routinely to prevent catheter-related infection. In pediatric patients, no recommendation for the frequency of catheter replacement. Replace disposable or reusable transducers at 96-hour intervals. Replace continuous flush device at the time the transducer is replaced.	Replace dressing when the catheter is replaced; when the dressing becomes damp, loosened, or soiled; or when inspection of the site is necessary.	Replace the IV tubing at the time the transducer is replaced (ie, 96-h intervals).	Replace the flush solution at the time the transducer is replaced (ie, 96-h intervals).
CVCs including peripherally inserted central catheters and hemodialysis catheters*	Do not routinely replace catheters.	Replace gauze dressings every 2 d and transparent dressings every 7 d on short-term catheters. Replace the dressing when the catheter is replaced; when the dressing becomes damp, loosened, or soiled; or when inspection of the site is necessary.	Replace IV tubing and add-on devices no more frequently than at 72-h intervals. Replace tubing used to administer blood products or lipid emulsions within 24 h of initiating the infusion.	No recommendation for the hang time of IV fluids, including non–lipid-containing parenteral nutrition fluids. Complete infusions of lipid-containing fluids within 24 h of hanging the fluid.
Pulmonary artery catheters	Do not replace catheter to prevent catheter-related infection.	As above.	As above.	As above.
Umbilical catheters	Do not routinely replace catheters.	Not applicable.	Replace IV tubing and add-on devices no more frequently than at 72-h intervals. Replace tubing used to administer blood products or lipid emulsions within 24 h of initiating the infusion.	No recommendations for the hang time of IV fluids, including non–lipid-containing parenteral nutrition fluids. Complete infusion of lipid-containing fluids within 24 h of hanging the fluid.

* Includes nontunneled catheters, tunneled catheters, and totally implanted devices.

Replacement of Administration Sets

The optimal interval for routine replacement of IV administration sets has been examined in three well-controlled studies. Data from each of these studies reveal that replacing administration sets no more frequently than 72 hours after initiation of use is safe and cost-effective.[149–151] Data from a more recent study demonstrated that rates of phlebitis were not substantially different if administration sets were left in place 96 hours compared with 72 hours.[128] When a fluid that enhances microbial growth is infused (eg, lipid emulsions and blood products), more frequent changes of administration sets are indicated, because these products have been identified as independent risk factors for CRBSI.[152–158]

Stopcocks (used for injection of medications, administration of IV infusions, and collection of blood samples) represent a potential portal of entry for microorganisms into vascular access catheters and IV fluids. Stopcock contamination is common, occurring in 45% and 50% in the majority of series. Whether such contamination is a substantial entry point of CRBSI has been difficult to prove.

"Piggyback" systems are used as an alternative to stopcocks. However, they also pose a risk for contamination of the intravascular fluid if the device entering the rubber membrane of an injection port is exposed to air or comes into direct contact with nonsterile tape used to fix the needle to the port. Modified piggyback systems have the potential to prevent contamination at these sites.[159]

Needleless Intravascular Catheter Systems

Attempts to reduce the incidence of sharp injuries and the resultant risk for transmission of bloodborne infections to health-care workers have led to the design and introduction of needleless infusion systems. When the devices are used according to manufacturers' recommendations, they do not substantially affect the incidence of CRBSI.[160–167]

Multidose Parenteral Medication Vials

Parenteral medications commonly are dispensed in multidose, parenteral medication vials that might be used for prolonged periods for one or more patients. Although the overall risk for extrinsic contamination of multidose vials is likely minimal,[168] the consequences of contamination might result in life-threatening infection.[169,170] Single-use vials are frequently preservative-free and might pose a risk for contamination if they are punctured several times.

SPECIAL CONSIDERATIONS FOR INTRAVASCULAR CATHETER-RELATED INFECTIONS IN PEDIATRIC PATIENTS

Prevention of CRBSI in children requires additional considerations, although only certain studies have been performed specifically in children. Pediatric data have been derived largely from studies in neonatal or pediatric ICUs and pediatric oncology patients.

Epidemiology

As in adults, the majority of BSIs in children are associated with the use of an intravascular catheter. From 1995 through 2000, the pooled mean catheter-associated BSI rate for all pediatric ICUs reporting data to NNIS was 7.7 per 1,000 catheter days.[171,172] Umbilical catheter and CVC-associated BSI rates for neonatal ICUs ranged from 11.3 per 1,000 catheter days in children with birth weight <1,000 g to 4.0 per 1,000 catheter days in children whose birth weight was >2,500 g.[171] Catheter utilization rates were comparable in adult and pediatric ICUs.[172,173]

Microbiology

As in adults, the majority of CRBSIs in children are caused by coagulase-negative staphylococci. During 1992–1999, these bacteria accounted for 37.7% of BSIs in pediatric ICUs reporting to NNIS.[12] Exposure to lipids has been identified as an independent risk factor for development of coagulase-negative staphylococcal bacteremia in very low birth weight infants (ie, those weighing <1,000 g) (odds ratio [OR] = 9.4; 95% CI = 1.2–74.2),[155] as well as candidemia in the neonatal ICU (OR = 5.33; 95% CI = 1.23–48.4).[154] Gram-negative bacteria accounted for 25% of BSIs reported in pediatric ICUs,[172] whereas enterococci and *Candida* spp accounted for 10% and 9%, respectively.[172]

Peripheral Venous Catheters

As in adults, the use of peripheral venous catheters in pediatric patients might be complicated by phlebitis, infusion extravasation, and catheter infection.[174] Catheter location, infusion of parenteral nutritional fluids with continuous IV lipid emulsions, and length of ICU stay before catheter insertion have all increased pediatric patients' risk for phlebitis. However, contrary to the risk in adults, the risk for phlebitis in children has not increased with the duration of catheterization.[174,175]

Peripheral Arterial Catheters

In a prospective study of 340 peripheral arterial catheters in children, the following two risk factors for catheter-related infection were identified: 1) use of an arterial system that permitted backflow of blood into the pressure tubing and 2) duration of catheterization.[176] Although a correlation was found between duration of arterial catheterization and risk for catheter colonization, the risk remained constant for 2–20 days at 6.2%.[176]

Umbilical Catheters

Although the umbilical stump becomes heavily colonized soon after birth, umbilical-vessel catheterization often is used for vascular access in newborn infants. Umbilical vessels can be cannulated easily and permit both collection of blood samples and measurement of hemodynamic status. The incidences of catheter colonization and BSI are similar for umbilical vein catheters and umbilical artery catheters. In several studies, an estimated 40%–55% of umbilical artery catheters were colonized and 5%

resulted in CRBSI; umbilical vein catheters were associated with colonization in 22%–59% of cases[177-179] and with CRBSI in 3%–8% of cases.[178] Although CRBSI rates are similar for umbilical catheters in the high position (ie, above the diaphragm) compared with the low position (ie, below the diaphragm and above the aortic bifurcation), catheters placed in the high position result in a lower incidence of vascular complications without an increase in adverse sequelae.[178]

Risk factors for infection differ for umbilical artery and umbilical vein catheters. In one study, neonates with very low birth weight who also received antibiotics for >10 days were at increased risk for umbilical artery CRBSIs.[178] In comparison, those with higher birth weight and receipt of parenteral nutrition fluids were at increased risk for umbilical vein CRBSI. Duration of catheterization was not an independent risk factor for infection of either type of umbilical catheter.

CVCs

Because of the limited vascular sites in children, attention should be given to the frequency with which catheters are replaced in these patients. In a study in which survival analysis techniques were used to examine the relation between the duration of central venous catheterization and complications in pediatric ICU patients, all of the patients studied (n = 397) remained uninfected for a median of 23.7 days.[180] In addition, no relation was found between duration of catheterization and the daily probability of infection ($r = 0.21$; $P > 0.1$), suggesting that routine replacement of CVCs likely does not reduce the incidence of catheter-related infection.[180]

Catheter Site Care

Although data regarding the use of the chlorhexidine-impregnated sponge (Biopatch in children are limited, one randomized, controlled study involving 705 neonates reported a substantial decrease in colonized catheter tips in infants in the Biopatch group compared with the group that had standard dressings (15% versus 24%; RR = 0.6; 95% CI = 0.5–0.9), but no difference in the rates of CRBSI or BSI without a source. Biopatch was associated with localized contact dermatitis in infants of very low birth weight. Of 98 neonates with very low birth weight, 15 (15%) developed localized contact dermatitis; four (1.5%) of 237 neonates weighing >1,000 g developed this reaction ($P < 0.0001$). Infants with gestational age <26 weeks who had CVCs placed at age <8 days were at increased risk for having localized contact dermatitis, whereas no infants in the control group developed this local reaction.[181]

Performance Indicators

Performance indicators for reducing CRBSI are 1) implementation of educational programs that include didactic and interactive components for those who insert and maintain catheters; 2) use of maximal sterile barrier precautions during catheter placement; 3) use of chlorhexidine for skin antisepsis; and 4) rates of catheter discontinuation when the catheter is no longer essential for medical management. The impact these recommendations will have on individual institutions should be evaluated using specific performance indicators.

RECOMMENDATIONS FOR PLACEMENT OF INTRAVASCULAR CATHETERS IN ADULTS AND CHILDREN

These recommendations are designed to reduce the infectious complications associated with intravascular catheter use. Recommendations should be considered in the context of the institution's experience with catheter-related infections, experience with other adverse catheter-related complications (eg, thrombosis, hemorrhage, and pneumothorax), and availability of personnel skilled in the placement of intravascular devices. Recommendations are provided for 1) intravascular-catheter use in general; 2) specific devices; and 3) special circumstances (ie, intravascular-device use in pediatric patients and CVC use for parenteral nutrition and hemodialysis access). Recommendations regarding the frequency of replacing catheters, dressings, administration sets, and fluids also are provided (Appendix B).

As in previous guidelines issued by CDC and HICPAC, each recommendation is categorized on the basis of existing scientific data, theoretical rationale, applicability, and economic impact. The CDC/HICPAC system for categorizing recommendations is as follows:

Category IA. Strongly recommended for implementation and strongly supported by well-designed experimental, clinical, or epidemiologic studies.

Category IB. Strongly recommended for implementation and supported by some experimental, clinical, or epidemiologic studies, and a strong theoretical rationale.

Category IC. Required by state or federal regulations, rules, or standards.

Category II. Suggested for implementation and supported by suggestive clinical or epidemiologic studies or a theoretical rationale.

Unresolved issue. Represents an unresolved issue for which evidence is insufficient or no consensus regarding efficacy exists.

  I. Health-care worker education and training
    A. Educate health-care workers regarding the indications for intravascular catheter use, proper procedures for the insertion and maintenance of intravascular catheters, and appropriate infection-control measures to prevent intravascular catheter-related infections.[39,43,45-47,182-187] **Category IA**
    B. Assess knowledge of and adherence to guidelines periodically for all persons who insert and manage intravascular catheters.[39,43,46,182,188] **Category IA**
    C. Ensure appropriate nursing staff levels in ICUs to minimize the incidence of CRBSIs.[48,189,190] **Category IB**
  II. Surveillance
    A. Monitor the catheter sites visually or by palpation through the intact dressing on a reg-

ular basis, depending on the clinical situation of individual patients. If patients have tenderness at the insertion site, fever without obvious source, or other manifestations suggesting local or BSI, the dressing should be removed to allow thorough examination of the site[1,191–193] **Category IB**

B. Encourage patients to report to their healthcare provider any changes in their catheter site or any new discomfort. **Category II**

C. Record the operator, date, and time of catheter insertion and removal, and dressing changes on a standardized form. **Category II**

D. Do not routinely culture catheter tips.[8,194,195] **Category IA**

III. Hand hygiene

A. Observe proper hand-hygiene procedures either by washing hands with conventional antiseptic-containing soap and water or with waterless alcohol-based gels or foams. Observe hand hygiene before and after palpating catheter insertion sites, as well as before and after inserting, replacing, accessing, repairing, or dressing an intravascular catheter. Palpation of the insertion site should not be performed after the application of antiseptic, unless aseptic technique is maintained[43,70,196–200] **Category IA**

B. Use of gloves does not obviate the need for hand hygiene.[43,198,199] **Category IA**

IV. Aseptic technique during catheter insertion and care

A. Maintain aseptic technique for the insertion and care of intravascular catheters.[22,71,201,202] **Category IA**

B. Wear clean or sterile gloves when inserting an intravascular catheter as required by the Occupational Safety and Health Administration Bloodborne Pathogens Standard. **Category IC.** Wearing clean gloves rather than sterile gloves is acceptable for the insertion of peripheral intravascular catheters if the access site is not touched after the application of skin antiseptics. Sterile gloves should be worn for the insertion of arterial and central catheters.[201,203] **Category IA**

C. Wear clean or sterile gloves when changing the dressing on intravascular catheters. **Category IC**

V. Catheter insertion

Do not routinely use arterial or venous cutdown procedures as a method to insert catheters.[204–206] **Category IA**

VI. Catheter site care

A. Cutaneous antisepsis

1. Disinfect clean skin with an appropriate antiseptic before catheter insertion and during dressing changes. Although a 2% chlorhexidine-based preparation is preferred, tincture of iodine, an iodophor, or 70% alcohol can be used.[73,75,207,208] **Category IA**

2. No recommendation can be made for the use of chlorhexidine in infants aged <2 months. **Unresolved issue**

3. Allow the antiseptic to remain on the insertion site and to air dry before catheter insertion. Allow povidone iodine to remain on the skin for at least 2 minutes, or longer if it is not yet dry before insertion.[73,75,207,208] **Category IB**

4. Do not apply organic solvents (eg, acetone and ether) to the skin before insertion of catheters or during dressing changes.[209] **Category IA**

VII. Catheter-site dressing regimens

A. Use either sterile gauze or sterile, transparent, semipermeable dressing to cover the catheter site.[146,210–212] **Category IA**

B. Tunneled CVC sites that are well healed might not require dressings. **Category II**

C. If the patient is diaphoretic, or if the site is bleeding or oozing, a gauze dressing is preferable to a transparent, semi-permeable dressing.[146,210–212] **Category II**

D. Replace catheter-site dressing if the dressing becomes damp, loosened, or visibly soiled.[146,210] **Category IB**

E. Change dressings at least weekly for adult and adolescent patients depending on the circumstances of the individual patient.[211] **Category II**

F. Do not use topical antibiotic ointment or creams on insertion sites (except when using dialysis catheters) because of their potential to promote fungal infections and antimicrobial resistance.[107,213] **Category IA** (See Central Venous Catheters, Including PICCs, Hemodialysis, and Pulmonary Artery Catheters, in Adult and Pediatric Patients, Section II.I.)

G. Do not submerge the catheter under water. Showering should be permitted if precautions can be taken to reduce the likelihood of introducing organisms into the catheter (eg, if the catheter and connecting device are protected with an impermeable cover during the shower.[214,215] **Category II**

VIII. Selection and replacement of intravascular catheters

A. Select the catheter, insertion technique, and insertion site with the lowest risk for complications (infectious and noninfectious) for the anticipated type and duration of IV therapy.[22,55,59,216–218] **Category IA**

B. Promptly remove any intravascular catheter that is no longer essential.[219,220] **Category IA**

C. Do not routinely replace central venous or arterial catheters solely for the purposes of reducing the incidence of infection.[134,135,221] **Category IB**

D. Replace peripheral venous catheters at least every 72–96 hours in adults to prevent phlebitis.[128] Leave peripheral venous catheters in place in children until IV therapy is completed, unless complications (eg, phlebitis and infiltration) occur.[174,175,222,223] **Category IB**

E. When adherence to aseptic technique cannot be ensured (ie, when catheters are inserted during a medical emergency), replace all catheters as soon as possible and after no longer than 48 hours.[22,71,201,202] **Category II**

F. Use clinical judgment to determine when to replace a catheter that could be a source of infection (eg, do not routinely replace catheters in patients whose only indication of infection is fever). Do not routinely replace venous catheters in patients who are bacteremic or fungemic if the source of infection is unlikely to be the catheter.[224] **Category II**

G. Replace any short-term CVC if purulence is observed at the insertion site, which indicates infection.[224,225] **Category IB**

H. Replace all CVCs if the patient is hemodynamically unstable and CRBSI is suspected.[224,225] **Category II**

I. Do not use guidewire techniques to replace catheters in patients suspected of having catheter-related infection.[134,135] **Category IB**

IX. Replacement of administration sets[a], needleless systems, and parenteral fluids

A. Administration sets

1. Replace administration sets, including secondary sets and add-on devices, no more frequently than at 72-hour intervals, unless catheter-related infection is suspected or documented.[23,149–151] **Category IA**

2. Replace tubing used to administer blood, blood products, or lipid emulsions (those combined with amino acids and glucose in a 3-in-1 admixture or infused separately) within 24 hours of initiating the infusion.[158,226–229] **Category IB**. If the solution contains only dextrose and amino acids, the administration set does not need to be replaced more frequently than every 72 hours.[226] **Category II**

3. Replace tubing used to administer propofol infusions every 6 or 12 hours, depending on its use, per the manufacturer's recommendation.[230] **Category IA**

B. Needleless intravascular devices

1. Change the needleless components at least as frequently as the administration set.[160–162,164–167] **Category II**

2. Change caps no more frequently than every 72 hours or according to manufacturers' recommendations.[160,162,165,166] **Category II**

3. Ensure that all components of the system are compatible to minimize leaks and breaks in the system.[163] **Category II**

4. Minimize contamination risk by wiping the access port with an appropriate antiseptic and accessing the port only with sterile devices.[162,163,165] **Category IB**

C. Parenteral fluids

1. Complete the infusion of lipid-containing solutions (eg, 3-in-1 solutions) within 24 hours of hanging the solution.[156–158,226,229] **Category IB**

2. Complete the infusion of lipid emulsions alone within 12 hours of hanging the emulsion. If volume considerations require more time, the infusion should be completed within 24 hours.[156–158] **Category IB**

3. Complete infusions of blood or other blood products within 4 hours of hanging the blood.[231–234] **Category II**

4. No recommendation can be made for the hang time of other parenteral fluids. **Unresolved issue**

X. IV-injection ports

A. Clean injection ports with 70% alcohol or an iodophor before accessing the system[164,235,236] **Category IA**

B. Cap all stopcocks when not in use.[235] **Category IB**

XI. Preparation and quality control of IV admixtures

A. Admix all routine parenteral fluids in the pharmacy in a laminar-flow hood using aseptic technique.[237,238] **Category IB**

B. Do not use any container of parenteral fluid that has visible turbidity, leaks, cracks, or particulate matter or if the manufacturer's expiration date has passed.[237] **Category IB**

C. Use single-dose vials for parenteral additives or medications when possible.[237,239] **Category II**

D. Do not combine the leftover content of single-use vials for later use.[237,239] **Category IA**

E. If multidose vials are used

1. Refrigerate multidose vials after they are opened if recommended by the manufacturer. **Category II**

2. Cleanse the access diaphragm of multidose vials with 70% alcohol before inserting a device into the vial.[236] **Category IA**

3. Use a sterile device to access a multidose vial and avoid touch contamination of the device before penetrating the access diaphragm.[235,240] **Category IA**

4. Discard multidose vial if sterility is compromised.[235,240] **Category IA**

XII. In-line filters
Do not use filters routinely for infection-control purposes.[80,241] **Category IA**

XIII. IV-therapy personnel
Designate trained personnel for the insertion

---

[a]Administration sets include the area from the spike of tubing entering the fluid container to the hub of the vascular access device. However, a short extension tube might be connected to the catheter and might be considered a portion of the catheter to facilitate aseptic technique when changing administration sets.

and maintenance of intravascular catheters.[46,47,210,242] **Category IA**

XIV. Prophylactic antimicrobials
Do not administer intranasal or systemic antimicrobial prophylaxis routinely before insertion or during use of an intravascular catheter
to prevent catheter colonization or
BSI.[97,98,108,243] **Category IA**

PERIPHERAL VENOUS CATHETERS, INCLUDING MIDLINE CATHETERS, IN ADULT AND PEDIATRIC PATIENTS

I. Selection of peripheral catheter
  A. Select catheters on the basis of the intended
     purpose and duration of use, known com-
     plications (eg, phlebitis and infiltration),
     and experience of individual catheter oper-
     ators.[67,68,244] **Category IB**
  B. Avoid the use of steel needles for the ad-
     ministration of fluids and medication that
     might cause tissue necrosis if extravasation
     occurs.[67,68] **Category IA**
  C. Use a midline catheter or PICC when the
     duration of IV therapy will likely exceed 6
     days.[244] **Category IB**
II. Selection of peripheral-catheter insertion site
  A. In adults, use an upper- instead of a lower-
     extremity site for catheter insertion. Replace
     a catheter inserted in a lower-extremity site
     to an upper-extremity site as soon as possi-
     ble.[67,245] **Category IA**
  B. In pediatric patients, the hand, the dorsum
     of the foot, or the scalp can be used as the
     catheter insertion site. **Category II**
  C. Replacement of catheter
     1. Evaluate the catheter insertion site daily,
        by palpation through the dressing to dis-
        cern tenderness and by inspection if a
        transparent dressing is in use. Gauze and
        opaque dressings should not be removed
        if the patient has no clinical signs of in-
        fection. If the patient has local tenderness
        or other signs of possible CRBSI, an
        opaque dressing should be removed and
        the site inspected visually. **Category II**
     2. Remove peripheral venous catheters if
        the patient develops signs of phlebitis
        (eg, warmth, tenderness, erythema, and
        palpable venous cord), infection, or a
        malfunctioning catheter.[66] **Category IB**
     3. In adults, replace short, peripheral ve-
        nous catheters at least 72–96 hours to
        reduce the risk for phlebitis. If sites for
        venous access are limited and no evi-
        dence of phlebitis or infection is present,
        peripheral venous catheters can be left in
        place for longer periods, although the
        patient and the insertion sites should be
        closely monitored.[66,128,247] **Category IB**
     4. Do not routinely replace midline cathe-
        ters to reduce the risk for infection.[131]
        Category IB

     5. In pediatric patients, leave peripheral
        venous catheters in place until IV ther-
        apy is completed, unless a complication
        (eg, phlebitis and infiltration) oc-
        curs.[174,175,222,223] **Category IB**
III. Catheter and catheter-site care
    Do not routinely apply prophylactic topical an-
    timicrobial or antiseptic ointment or cream to
    the insertion site of peripheral venous cathe-
    ters.[107,213] **Category IA**

CVCs, INCLUDING PICCs, HEMODIALYSIS, AND PULMONARY ARTERY CATHETERS, IN ADULT AND PEDIATRIC PATIENTS

I. Surveillance
  A. Conduct surveillance in ICUs and other pa-
     tient populations to determine CRBSI rates,
     monitor trends in those rates, and assist in
     identifying lapses in infection-control prac-
     tices.[3,12,16,247–250] **Category IA**
  B. Express ICU data as the number of catheter-
     associated BSIs per 1,000 catheter-days for
     both adults and children and stratify by
     birth weight categories for neonatal ICUs to
     facilitate comparisons with national data in
     comparable patient populations and health-
     care settings.[3,12,16,247–250] **Category IB**
  C. Investigate events leading to unexpected
     life-threatening or fatal outcomes. This in-
     cludes any process variation for which a
     recurrence would likely present an adverse
     outcome.[13] **Category IC**
II. General principles
  A. Use a CVC with the minimum number of
     ports or lumens essential for the manage-
     ment of the patient.[251–254] **Category IB**
  B. Use an antimicrobial or antiseptic-impreg-
     nated CVC in adults whose catheter is ex-
     pected to remain in place >5 days if, after
     implementing a comprehensive strategy to
     reduce rates of CRBSI, the CRBSI rate re-
     mains above the goal set by the individual
     institution based on benchmark rates (Table
     2) and local factors. The comprehensive
     strategy should include the following three
     components: educating persons who insert
     and maintain catheters, use of maximal ster-
     ile barrier precautions, and a 2% chlorhexi-
     dine preparation for skin antisepsis during
     CVC insertion.[84–86,90,91,255] **Category IB**
  C. No recommendation can be made for the
     use of impregnated catheters in children.
     Unresolved issue
  D. Designate personnel who have been trained
     and exhibit competency in the insertion of
     catheters to supervise trainees who perform
     catheter insertion.[39,43,46,182,187,188] **Category
     IA**
  E. Use totally implantable access devices for
     patients who require long-term, intermit-
     tent vascular access. For patients requiring
     frequent or continuous access, a PICC or

tunneled CVC is preferable.[256,257] **Category II**

F. Use a cuffed CVC for dialysis if the period of temporary access is anticipated to be prolonged (eg, >3 weeks).[144,258] **Category IB**

G. Use a fistula or graft instead of a CVC for permanent access for dialysis.[142] **Category IB**

H. Do not use hemodialysis catheters for blood drawing or applications other than hemodialysis except during dialysis or under emergency circumstances. **Category II**

I. Use povidone-iodine antiseptic ointment at the hemodialysis catheter exit site after catheter insertion and at the end of each dialysis session only if this ointment does not interact with the material of the hemodialysis catheter per manufacturer's recommendation.[103,114,144] **Category II**

III. Selection of catheter insertion site

A. Weigh the risk and benefits of placing a device at a recommended site to reduce infectious complications against the risk for mechanical complications (eg, pneumothorax, subclavian artery puncture, subclavian vein laceration, subclavian vein stenosis, hemothorax, thrombosis, air embolism, and catheter misplacement).[22,55,59,218] **Category IA**

B. Use a subclavian site (rather than a jugular or a femoral site) in adult patients to minimize infection risk for nontunneled CVC placement.[22,55,59,60] **Category IA**

C. No recommendation can be made for a preferred site of insertion to minimize infection risk for a tunneled CVC.[61–63] **Unresolved issue**

D. Place catheters used for hemodialysis and pheresis in a jugular or femoral vein rather than a subclavian vein to avoid venous stenosis if catheter access is needed.[259–263] **Category IA**

IV. Maximal sterile barrier precautions during catheter insertion

A. Use aseptic technique including the use of a cap, mask, sterile gown, sterile gloves, and a large sterile sheet, for the insertion of CVCs (including PICCS) or guidewire exchange.[22,71] **Category IA**

B. Use a sterile sleeve to protect pulmonary artery catheters during insertion.[148] **Category IB**

V. Replacement of catheter

A. Do not routinely replace CVCs, PICCs, hemodialysis catheters, or pulmonary artery catheters to prevent catheter-related infections.[132,134,135] **Category IB**

B. Do not remove CVCs or PICCs on the basis of fever alone. Use clinical judgment regarding the appropriateness of removing the catheter if infection is evidenced elsewhere or if a noninfectious cause of fever is suspected.[224,264] **Category II**

C. Guidewire exchange

1. Do not use guidewire exchanges routinely for nontunneled catheters to prevent infection.[135,265] **Category IB**

2. Use a guidewire exchange to replace a malfunctioning nontunneled catheter if no evidence of infection is present.[135,265] **Category IB**

3. Use a new set of sterile gloves before handling the new catheter when guidewire exchanges are performed.[22,71] **Category II**

VI. Catheter and catheter-site care

A. General measures
Designate one port exclusively for hyperalimentation if a multilumen catheter is used to administer parenteral nutrition.[266] **Category II**

B. Antibiotic lock solutions
Do not routinely use antibiotic lock solutions to prevent CRBSI. Use prophylactic antibiotic lock solution only in special circumstances (eg, in treating a patient with a long-term cuffed or tunneled catheter or port who has a history of multiple CRBSIs despite optimal maximal adherence to aseptic technique).[115,116,267,268] **Category II**

C. Catheter-site dressing regimens

1. Replace the catheter-site dressing when it becomes damp, loosened, or soiled or when inspection of the site is necessary.[65,146,211] **Category IA**

2. Replace dressings used on short-term CVC sites every 2 days for gauze dressings and at least every 7 days for transparent dressings, except in those pediatric patients in which the risk for dislodging the catheter outweighs the benefit of changing the dressing.[211] **Category IB**

3. Replace dressings used on tunneled or implanted CVC sites no more than once per week, until the insertion site has healed.[211] **Category IB**

4. No recommendation can be made regarding the necessity for any dressing on well-healed exit sites of long-term cuffed and tunneled CVCs. **Unresolved issue**

D. No recommendation can be made for the use of chlorhexidine sponge dressings to reduce the incidence of infection. **Unresolved issue**

E. Do not use chlorhexidine sponge dressings in neonates aged <7 days or of gestational age <26 weeks.[181] **Category II**

F. No recommendation can be made for the use of sutureless securement devices. **Unresolved issue**

G. Ensure that catheter-site care is compatible with the catheter material.[109,110] **Category IB**

H. Use a sterile sleeve for all pulmonary artery catheters.[148] **Category IB**

ADDITIONAL RECOMMENDATIONS FOR PERIPHERAL ARTERIAL CATHETERS AND PRESSURE MONITORING DEVICES FOR ADULT AND PEDIATRIC PATIENTS

I. Selection of pressure monitoring system
Use disposable, rather than reusable, transducer assemblies when possible.[269–273] **Category IB**

II. Replacement of catheter and pressure monitoring system
A. Do not routinely replace peripheral arterial catheters to prevent catheter-related infections.[132,147,221,274] **Category II**
B. Replace disposable or reusable transducers at 96-hour intervals. Replace other components of the system (including the tubing, continuous-flush device, and flush solution) at the time the transducer is replaced.[22,270] **Category IB**

III. Care of pressure monitoring systems
A. General measures
  1. Keep all components of the pressure monitoring system (including calibration devices and flush solution) sterile.[269,275–277] **Category IA**
  2. Minimize the number of manipulations of and entries into the pressure monitoring system. Use a closed-flush system (ie, continuous flush), rather than an open system (ie, one that requires a syringe and stopcock), to maintain the patency of the pressure monitoring catheters.[272,278] **Category II**
  3. When the pressure monitoring system is accessed through a diaphragm rather than a stopcock, wipe the diaphragm with an appropriate antiseptic before accessing the system.[272] **Category IA**
  4. Do not administer dextrose-containing solutions or parenteral nutrition fluids through the pressure monitoring circuit.[272,279,280] **Category IA**
B. Sterilization or disinfection of pressure monitoring systems
  1. Use disposable transducers.[272,279–282] **Category IB**
  2. Sterilize reusable transducers according to the manufacturers' instructions if the use of disposable transducers is not feasible.[272,279–282] **Category IA**

RECOMMENDATIONS FOR UMBILICAL CATHETERS

I. Replacement of catheters
A. Remove and do not replace umbilical artery catheters if any signs of CRBSI, vascular insufficiency, or thrombosis are present.[283] **Category II**
B. Remove and do not replace umbilical venous catheters if any signs of CRBSI or thrombosis are present.[283] **Category II**
C. No recommendation can be made for treating through an umbilical venous catheter

suspected of being infected. **Unresolved issue**
D. Replace umbilical venous catheters only if the catheter malfunctions. **Category II**

II. Catheter-site care
A. Cleanse the umbilical insertion site with an antiseptic before catheter insertion. Avoid tincture of iodine because of the potential effect on the neonatal thyroid. Other iodine-containing products (eg, povidone-iodine) can be used.[75,177,178,284,285] **Category IB**
B. Do not use topical antibiotic ointment or creams on umbilical catheter insertion sites because of the potential to promote fungal infections and antimicrobial resistance.[107,213] **Category IA**
C. Add low doses of heparin (0.25–1.0 F/ml) to the fluid infused through umbilical arterial catheters.[286–288] **Category IB**
D. Remove umbilical catheters as soon as possible when no longer needed or when any sign of vascular insufficiency to the lower extremities is observed. Optimally, umbilical artery catheters should not be left in place >5 days.[283,289] **Category II**
E. Umbilical venous catheters should be removed as soon as possible when no longer needed but can be used up to 14 days if managed aseptically.[290,291] **Category II**

REFERENCES

1. Pearson ML. Guideline for prevention of intravascular device-related infections. Part I. Intravascular device-related infections: an overview. The Hospital Infection Control Practices Advisory Committee. *Am J Infect Control.* 1996;24:262-277
2. Mermel LA. Prevention of intravascular catheter-related infections. *Ann Intern Med.* 2000;132:391–402
3. CDC. National Nosocomial Infections Surveillance (NNIS) System report, data summary from October 1986–April 1998, issued June 1998. *Am J Infect Control.* 1998;26:522–533
4. Digiovine B, Chenoweth C, Watts C, Higgins M. The attributable mortality and costs of primary nosocomial bloodstream infections in the intensive care unit. *Am J Respir Crit Care Med.* 1999;160:976–981
5. Rello J, Ochagavia A, Sabanes E, et al. Evaluation of outcome of intravenous catheter-related infections in critically ill patients. *Am J Respir Crit Care Med.* 2000;162:1027–1030
6. Soufir L, Timsit JF, Mahe C, Carlet J, Regnier B, Chevret S. Attributable morbidity and mortality of catheter-related septicemia in critically ill patients: a matched, risk-adjusted, cohort study. *Infect Control Hosp Epidemiol.* 1999;20:396–401
7. Collignon PJ. Intravascular catheter associated sepsis: a common problem. The Australian Study on Intravascular Catheter Associated Sepsis. *Med J Aust.* 1994;161:374–378
8. Pittet D, Tarara D, Wenzel RP. Nosocomial bloodstream infection in critically ill patients. Excess length of stay, extra costs, and attributable mortality. *JAMA.* 1994;271:1598–1601
9. Dimick JB, Pelz RK, Consunji R, Swoboda SM, Hendrix CW, Lipsett PA. Increased resource use associated with catheter-related bloodstream infection in the surgical intensive care unit. *Arch Surg.* 2001; 136:229–234
10. Mermel LA. Correction: catheter related bloodstream-infections. *Ann Intern Med.* 2000;133:395
11. Kluger DM, Maki DG. The relative risk of intravascular device related bloodstream infections in adults [abstract]. In: *Abstracts of the 39th Interscience Conference on Antimicrobial Agents and Chemotherapy.* San Francisco, CA: American Society for Microbiology; 1999:514
12. CDC. National Nosocomial Infections Surveillance (NNIS) System report, data summary from January 1990–May 1999, issued June 1999. *Am J Infect Control.* 1999;27:520–532
13. Joint Commission on the Accreditation of Healthcare Organizations. Accreditation manual for hospitals. In: Joint Commission on the Ac-

creditation of Healthcare Organizations, ed. Chicago, IL: Joint Commission on the Accreditation of Healthcare Organizations; 1994: 121–140

14. CDC. National Nosocomial Infections Surveillance (NNIS) System report, data summary from January 1992–June 2001, issued August 2001. *Am J Infect Control.* 2001;6:404–421

15. Schaberg DR, Culver DH, Gaynes RP. Major trends in the microbial etiology of nosocomial infection. *Am J Med.* 1991;91(suppl):S72–S75

16. Banerjee SN, Emori TG, Culver DH, et al. Secular trends in nosocomial primary bloodstream infections in the United States, 1980–1989. National Nosocomial Infections Surveillance System. *Am J Med.* 1991; 91(suppl):S86–S89

17. Pfaller MA, Jones RN, Messer SA, Edmond MB, Wenzel RP. National surveillance of nosocomial blood stream infection due to *Candida albicans:* frequency of occurrence and antifungal susceptibility in the SCOPE Program. *Diagn Microbiol Infect Dis.* 1998;31:327–332

18. Pfaller MA, Jones RN, Messer SA, Edmond MB, Wenzel RP. National surveillance of nosocomial blood stream infection due to species of *Candida* other than *Candida albicans:* frequency of occurrence and antifungal susceptibility in the SCOPE Program. *Diagn Microbiol Infect Dis.* 1998;30:121–129

19. Nguyen MH, Peacock JE Jr, Morris AJ, et al. The changing face of candidemia: emergence of non-*Candida albicans* species and antifungal resistance. *Am J Med.* 1996;100:617–623

20. Fridkin SK, Gaynes RP. Antimicrobial resistance in intensive care units. *Clin Chest Med.* 1999;20:303–316

21. Maki DG, Weise CE, Sarafin HW. A semiquantitative culture method for identifying intravenous-catheter-related infection. *N Engl J Med.* 1977;296:1305–1309

22. Mermel LA, McCormick RD, Springman SR, Maki DG. The pathogenesis and epidemiology of catheter-related infection with pulmonary artery Swan-Ganz catheters: a prospective study utilizing molecular subtyping. *Am J Med.* 1991;91(suppl):S197–S205

23. Sitges-Serra A, Linares J, Perez JL, Jaurrieta E, Lorente L. A randomized trial on the effect of tubing changes on hub contamination and catheter sepsis during parenteral nutrition. *Parenter Enteral Nutr.* 1985; 9:322–325

24. Linares J, Sitges-Serra A, Garau J, Perez JL, Martin R. Pathogenesis of catheter sepsis: a prospective study with quantitative and semiquantitative cultures of catheter hub and segments. *J Clin Microbiol.* 1985; 21:357–360

25. Raad II, Costerton W, Sabharwal U, Sacilowski M, Anaissie E, Bodey GP. Ultrastructural analysis of indwelling vascular catheters: a quantitative relationship between luminal colonization and duration of placement. *J Infect Dis.* 1993;168:400–407

26. Maki DG. Infections associated with intravascular lines. In: Remington JS, ed. *Current Clinical Topics in Infectious Diseases.* New York, NY: McGraw-Hill; 1982:309–363

27. Sheth NK, Franson TR, Rose HD, Buckmire FL, Cooper JA, Sohnle PG. Colonization of bacteria on polyvinyl chloride and Teflon intravascular catheters in hospitalized patients. *J Clin Microbiol.* 1983;18: 1061–1063

28. Ashkenazi S, Weiss E, Drucker MM, Bodey GP. Bacterial adherence to intravenous catheters and needles and its influence by cannula type and bacterial surface hydrophobicity. *J Lab Clin Med.* 1986;107:136–140

29. Locci R, Peters G, Pulverer G. Microbial colonization of prosthetic devices. IV. Scanning electron microscopy of intravenous catheters invaded by yeasts. *Zentralbl Bakteriol Mikrobiol Hyg [B].* 1981;173: 419–424

30. Locci R, Peters G, Pulverer G. Microbial colonization of prosthetic devices. I. Microtopographical characteristics of intravenous catheters as detected by scanning electron microscopy. *Zentralbl Bakteriol Mikrobiol Hyg [B].* 1981;173:285–292

31. Nachnani GH, Lessin LS, Motomiya T, Jensen WN, Bodey GP. Scanning electron microscopy of thrombogenesis on vascular catheter surfaces. *N Engl J Med.* 1972;286:139–140

32. Stillman RM, Soliman F, Garcia L, Sawyer PN. Etiology of catheter-associated sepsis. Correlation with thrombogenicity. *Arch Surg.* 1977; 112:1497–1499

33. Herrmann M, Lai QJ, Albrecht RM, Mosher DF, Proctor RA. Adhesion of *Staphylococcus aureus* to surface-bound platelets: role of fibrinogen/fibrin and platelet integrins. *J Infect Dis.* 1993;167:312–322

34. Herrmann M, Suchard SJ, Boxer LA, Waldvogel FA, Lew PD. Thrombospondin binds to *Staphylococcus aureus* and promotes staphylococcal adherence to surfaces. *Infect Immun.* 1991;59:279–288

35. Ludwicka A, Uhlenbruck G, Peters G, et al. Investigation on extracellular slime substance produced by *Staphylococcus epidermidis. Zentralbl Bakteriol Mikrobiol Hyg.* 1984;258:256–267

36. Gray ED, Peters G, Verstegen M, Regelmann WE. Effect of extracellular slime substance from *Staphylococcus epidermidis* on the human cellular immune response. *Lancet.* 1984;1:365–367

37. Farber BF, Kaplan MH, Clogston AG. *Staphylococcus epidermidis* extracted slime inhibits the antimicrobial action of glycopeptide antibiotics. *J Infect Dis.* 1990;161:37–40

38. Branchini ML, Pfaller MA, Rhine-Chalberg J, Frempong T, Isenberg HD. Genotypic variation and slime production among blood and catheter isolates of *Candida parapsilosis. J Clin Microbiol.* 1994;32: 452–456

39. Sherertz RJ, Ely EW, Westbrook DM, et al. Education of physicians-in-training can decrease the risk for vascular catheter infection. *Ann Intern Med.* 2000;132:641–648

40. Ryan JA Jr, Abel RM, Abbott WM, et al. Catheter complications in total parenteral nutrition: a prospective study of 200 consecutive patients. *N Engl J Med.* 1974;290:757–761

41. Sanders RA, Sheldon GF. Septic complications of total parenteral nutrition: a five year experience. *Am J Surg.* 1976;132:214–220

42. Murphy LM, Lipman TO. Central venous catheter care in parenteral nutrition: a review. *Parenter Enteral Nutr.* 1987;11:190–201

43. Eggimann P, Harbarth S, Constantin MN, Touveneau S, Chevrolet JC, Pittet D. Impact of a prevention strategy targeted at vascular-access care on incidence of infections acquired in intensive care. *Lancet.* 2000;355:1864–1868

44. Armstrong CW, Mayhall CG, Miller KB, et al. Prospective study of catheter replacement and other risk factors for infection of hyperalimentation catheters. *J Infect Dis.* 1986;154:808–816

45. Nehme AE. Nutritional support of the hospitalized patient: the team concept. *JAMA.* 1980;243:1906–1908

46. Soifer NE, Borzak S, Edlin BR, Weinstein RA. Prevention of peripheral venous catheter complications with an intravenous therapy team: a randomized controlled trial. *Arch Intern Med.* 1998;158:473–477

47. Tomford JW, Hershey CO. The IV therapy team: impact on patient care and costs of hospitalization. *NITA.* 1985;8:387–389

48. Fridkin SK, Pear SM, Williamson TH, Galgiani JN, Jarvis WR. The role of understaffing in central venous catheter-associated bloodstream infections. *Infect Control Hosp Epidemiol.* 1996;17:150–158

49. Bansmer G, Keith D, Tesluk H. Complications following use of indwelling catheters of inferior vena cava. *JAMA.* 1958;167:1606–1611

50. Crane C. Venous interruption of septic thrombophlebitis. *N Engl J Med.* 1960;262:947–951

51. Indar R. The dangers of indwelling polyethelene cannulae in deep veins. *Lancet.* 1959;1:284–286

52. Maki DG, Mermel LA. Infections due to infusion therapy. In: Bennett JV, Brachman PS, eds. *Hospital Infections.* 4th ed. Philadelphia, PA: Lippencott-Raven; 1998:689–724

53. Heard SO, Wagle M, Vijayakumar E, et al. Influence of triple-lumen central venous catheters coated with chlorhexidine and silver sulfadiazine on the incidence of catheter-related bacteremia. *Arch Intern Med.* 1998;158:81–87

54. Richet H, Hubert B, Nitemberg G, et al. Prospective multicenter study of vascular-catheter-related complications and risk factors for positive central-catheter cultures in intensive care unit patients. *J Clin Microbiol.* 1990;28:2520–2525

55. Goetz AM, Wagener MM, Miller JM, Muder RR. Risk of infection due to central venous catheters: effect of site of placement and catheter type. *Infect Control Hosp Epidemiol.* 1998;19:842–845

56. Joynt GM, Kew J, Gomersall CD, Leung VY, Liu EK. Deep venous thrombosis caused by femoral venous catheters in critically ill adult patients. *Chest.* 2000;117:178–183

57. Mian NZ, Bayly R, Schreck DM, Besserman EB, Richmand D. Incidence of deep venous thrombosis associated with femoral venous catheterization. *Acad Emerg Med.* 1997;4:1118–1121

58. Durbec O, Viviand X, Potie F, Vialet R, Albanese J, Martin C. A prospective evaluation of the use of femoral venous catheters in critically ill adults. *Crit Care Med.* 1997;25:1986–1989

59. Trottier SJ, Veremakis C, O'Brien J, Auer AI. Femoral deep vein thrombosis associated with central venous catheterization: results from a prospective, randomized trial. *Crit Care Med.* 1995;23:52–59

60. Merrer J, De Jonghe B, Golliot F, et al. Complications of femoral and subclavian venous catheterization in critically ill patients: a randomized controlled trial. *JAMA.* 2001;286:700–707

61. Venkataraman ST, Thompson AE, Orr RA. Femoral vascular catheterization in critically ill infants and children. *Clin Pediatr.* 1997;36: 311–319

62. Stenzel JP, Green TP, Fuhrman BP, Carlson PE, Marchessault RP. Percutaneous femoral venous catheterizations: a prospective study of complications. *J Pediatr.* 1989;114:411–415

63. Goldstein AM, Weber JM, Sheridan RL. Femoral venous access is safe in burned children: an analysis of 224 catheters. *J Pediatr.* 1997;130: 442–446

64. Randolph AG, Cook DJ, Gonzales CA, Pribble CG. Ultrasound guidance for placement of central venous catheters: a meta-analysis of the literature. *Crit Care Med.* 1996;24:2053–2058

65. Maki DG, Ringer M. Evaluation of dressing regimens for prevention of infection with peripheral intravenous catheters: gauze, a transparent polyurethane dressing, and an iodophor-transparent dressing. *JAMA.* 1987;258:2396–2403

66. Maki DG, Ringer M. Risk factors for infusion-related phlebitis with small peripheral venous catheters: a randomized controlled trial. *Ann Intern Med.* 1991;114:845–854

67. Band JD, Maki DG. Steel needles used for intravenous therapy: morbidity in patients with hematologic malignancy. *Arch Intern Med.* 1980; 140:31–34

68. Tully JL, Friedland GH, Baldini LM, Goldmann DA. Complications of intravenous therapy with steel needles and Teflon catheters: a comparative study. *Am J Med.* 1981;70:702–706

69. Pittet D, Hugonnet S, Harbath S, et al. Effectiveness of a hospital-wide programme to improve compliance with hand hygiene. *Lancet.* 2000; 356:1307–1309

70. Larson EL, Rackoff WR, Weiman M, et al. APIC guideline for handwashing and hand antisepsis in health care settings. *Am J Infect Control.* 1995;23:251–269

71. Raad II, Hohn DC, Gilbreath BJ, et al. Prevention of central venous catheter-related infections by using maximal sterile barrier precautions during insertion. *Infect Control Hosp Epidemiol.* 1994;15:231–238

72. Clemence MA, Walker D, Farr BM. Central venous catheter practices: results of a survey. *Am J Infect Control.* 1995;23:5–12

73. Maki DG, Ringer M, Alvarado CJ. Prospective randomised trial of povidone-iodine, alcohol, and chlorhexidine for prevention of infection associated with central venous and arterial catheters. *Lancet.* 1991; 338:339–343

74. Humar A, Ostromecki A, Direnfeld J, et al. Prospective randomized trial of 10% povidone-iodine versus 0.5% tincture of chlorhexidine as cutaneous antisepsis for prevention of central venous catheter infection. *Clin Infect Dis.* 2000;31:1001–1007

75. Garland JS, Buck RK, Maloney P, et al. Comparison of 10% povidone-iodine and 0.5% chlorhexidine gluconate for the prevention of peripheral intravenous catheter colonization in neonates: a prospective trial. *Pediatr Infect Dis J.* 1995;14:510–516

76. Hoffmann KK, Weber DJ, Samsa GP, Rutala WA. Transparent polyurethane film as an intravenous catheter dressing: a meta-analysis of the infection risks. *JAMA.* 1992;267:2072–2076

77. Maki DG, Mermel LA, Klugar D, et al. The efficacy of a chlorhexidine impregnated sponge (Biopatch) for the prevention of intravascular catheter-related infection- a prospective randomized controlled multicenter study [abstract]. Presented at the Interscience Conference on Antimicrobial Agents and Chemotherapy. Toronto, Ontario, Canada: American Society for Microbiology, 2000

78. Yamamoto AJ, Solomon JA, Soulen MC, et al. Sutureless securement device reduces complications of peripherally inserted central venous catheters. *J Vasc Interv Radiol.* 2002;13:77–81

79. Rusho WJ, Bair JN. Effect of filtration on complications of postoperative intravenous therapy. *Am J Hosp Pharm.* 1979;36:1355–1356

80. Maddox RR, John JF Jr, Brown LL, Smith CE. Effect of inline filtration on postinfusion phlebitis. *Clin Pharm.* 1983;2:58–61

81. Turco SJ, Davis NM. Particulate matter in intravenous infusion fluids—phase 3. *Am J Hosp Pharm.* 1973;30:611–613

82. Baumgartner TG, Schmidt GL, Thakker KM, et al. Bacterial endotoxin retention by inline intravenous filters. *Am J Hosp Pharm.* 1986;43: 681–684

83. Butler DL, Munson JM, DeLuca PP. Effect of inline filtration on the potency of low-dose drugs. *Am J Hosp Pharm.* 1980;37:935–941

84. Raad II, Darouiche R, Dupuis J, et al. Central venous catheters coated with minocycline and rifampin for the prevention of catheter-related colonization and bloodstream infections: a randomized, double-blind trial. The Texas Medical Center Catheter Study Group. *Ann Intern Med.* 1997;127:267–274

85. Veenstra DL, Saint S, Saha S, Lumley T, Sullivan SD. Efficacy of antiseptic-impregnated central venous catheters in preventing catheter-related bloodstream infection: a meta-analysis. *JAMA.* 1999;281: 261–267

86. Maki DG, Stolz SM, Wheeler S, Mermel LA. Prevention of central venous catheter-related bloodstream infection by use of an antiseptic-impregnated catheter: a randomized, controlled trial. *Ann Intern Med.* 1997;127:257–266

87. Raad II, Darouiche R, Hachem R, Mansouri M, Bodey GP. The broad-spectrum activity and efficacy of catheters coated with minocycline and rifampin. *J Infect Dis.* 1996;173:418–424

88. Bassetti S, Hu J, D'Agostino RB Jr, Sherertz RJ. Prolonged antimicrobial activity of a catheter containing chlorhexidine-silver sulfadiazine extends protection against catheter infections in vivo. *Antimicrob Agents Chemother.* 2001;45:1535–1538

89. Oda T, Hamasaki J, Kanda N, Mikami K. Anaphylactic shock induced by an antiseptic-coated central venous catheter. *Anesthesiology.* 1997; 87:1242–1244

90. Veenstra DL, Saint S, Sullivan SD. Cost-effectiveness of antiseptic-impregnated central venous catheters for the prevention of catheter-related bloodstream infection. *JAMA.* 1999;282:554–560

91. Darouiche RO, Raad II, Heard SO, et al. A comparison of two antimicrobial-impregnated central venous catheters. Catheter Study Group. *N Engl J Med.* 1999;340:1–8

92. Institute of Medicine. *To Err Is Human: Building a Safer Health System.* Washington, DC: National Academy Press; 2000

93. Maki DG, Cobb L, Garman JK, Shapiro JM, Ringer M, Helgerson RB. An attachable silver-impregnated cuff for prevention of infection with central venous catheters: a prospective randomized multicenter trial. *Am J Med.* 1988;85:307–314

94. Dahlberg PJ, Agger WA, Singer JR, et al. Subclavian hemodialysis catheter infections: a prospective, randomized trial of an attachable silver-impregnated cuff for prevention of catheter-related infections. *Infect Control Hosp Epidemiol.* 1995;16:506–511

95. Groeger JS, Lucas AB, Coit D, et al. A prospective, randomized evaluation of the effect of silver impregnated subcutaneous cuffs for preventing tunneled chronic venous access catheter infections in cancer patients. *Ann Surg.* 1993;218:206–210

96. Bonawitz SC, Hammell EJ, Kirkpatrick JR. Prevention of central venous catheter sepsis: a prospective randomized trial. *Am Surg.* 1991; 57:618–623

97. McKee R, Dunsmuir R, Whitby M, Garden OJ. Does antibiotic prophylaxis at the time of catheter insertion reduce the incidence of catheter-related sepsis in intravenous nutrition? *J Hosp Infect.* 1985;6:419–425

98. Ranson MR, Oppenheim BA, Jackson A, Kamthan AG, Scarffe JH. Double-blind placebo controlled study of vancomycin prophylaxis for central venous catheter insertion in cancer patients. *J Hosp Infect.* 1990;15:95–102

99. Ljungman P, Hagglund H, Bjorkstrand B, Lonnqvist B, Ringden O. Peroperative teicoplanin for prevention of gram-positive infections in neutropenic patients with indwelling central venous catheters: a randomized, controlled study. *Support Care Cancer.* 1997;5:485–458

100. Kacica MA, Horgan MJ, Ochoa L, Sandler R, Lepow ML, Venezia RA. Prevention of gram-positive sepsis in neonates weighing less than 1500 g. *J Pediatr.* 1994;125:253–258

101. Spafford PS, Sinkin RA, Cox C, Reubens L, Powell KR. Prevention of central venous catheter-related coagulase-negative staphylococcal sepsis in neonates. *J Pediatr.* 1994;125:259–263

102. CDC. Recommendations for preventing the spread of vancomycin resistance. Recommendations of the Hospital Infection Control Practices Advisory Committee (HICPAC). *MMWR Recomm Rep.* 1995; 44(No. RR-12):1–13

103. Levin A, Mason AJ, Jindal KK, Fong IW, Goldstein MB. Prevention of hemodialysis subclavian vein catheter infections by topical povidone-iodine. *Kidney Int.* 1991;40:934–938

104. Casewell MW. The nose: an underestimated source of *Staphylococcus aureus* causing wound infection. *J Hosp Infect.* 1998;40(suppl):S3–S11

105. Hill RL, Fisher AP, Ware RJ, Wilson S, Casewell MW. Mupirocin for the reduction of colonization of internal jugular cannulae—a randomized controlled trial. *J Hosp Infect.* 1990;15:311–321

106. Sesso R, Barbosa D, Leme IL, et al. *Staphylococcus aureus* prophylaxis in hemodialysis patients using central venous catheter: effect of mupirocin ointment. *J Am Soc Nephrol.* 1998;9:1085–1092

107. Zakrzewska-Bode A, Muytjens HL, Liem KD, Hoogkamp-Korstanje JA. Mupirocin resistance in coagulase-negative staphylococci, after topical prophylaxis for the reduction of colonization of central venous catheters. *J Hosp Infect.* 1995;31:189–193

108. Miller MA, Dascal A, Portnoy J, Mendelson J. Development of mupirocin resistance among methicillin-resistant *Staphylococcus aureus* after widespread use of nasal mupirocin ointment. *Infect Control Hosp Epidemiol.* 1996;17:811–813

109. Rao SP, Oreopoulos DG. Unusual complications of a polyurethane PD catheter. *Perit Dial Int.* 1997;17:410–412

110. Riu S, Ruiz CG, Martinez-Vea A, Peralta C, Oliver JA. Spontaneous rupture of polyurethane peritoneal catheter: a possible deleterious

effect of mupirocin ointment. *Nephrol Dial Transplant.* 1998;13: 1870–1871

111. von Eiff C, Becker K, Machka K, Stammer H, Peters G. Nasal carriage as a source of *Staphylococcus aureus* bacteremia. *N Engl J Med.* 2001;344: 11–16

112. Zinner SH, Denny-Brown BC, Braun P, Burke JP, Toala P, Kass EH. Risk of infection with intravenous indwelling catheters: effect of application of antibiotic ointment. *J Infect Dis.* 1969;120:616–619

113. Norden CW. Application of antibiotic ointment to the site of venous catheterization—a controlled trial. *J Infect Dis.* 1969;120:611–615

114. Maki DG, Band JD. A comparative study of polyantibiotic and iodophor ointments in prevention of vascular catheter-related infection. *Am J Med.* 1981;70:739–744

115. Henrickson KJ, Axtell RA, Hoover SM, et al. Prevention of central venous catheter-related infections and thrombotic events in immunocompromised children by the use of vancomycin/ciprofloxacin/heparin flush solution: a randomized, multicenter, double-blind trial. *J Clin Oncol.* 2000;18:1269–1278

116. Carratala J, Niubo J, Fernandez-Sevilla A, et al. Randomized, double-blind trial of an antibiotic-lock technique for prevention of gram-positive central venous catheter-related infection in neutropenic patients with cancer. *Antimicrob Agents Chemother.* 1999;43:2200–2204

117. Schwartz C, Henrickson KJ, Roghmann K, Powell K. Prevention of bacteremia attributed to luminal colonization of tunneled central venous catheters with vancomycin-susceptible organisms. *J Clin Oncol.* 1990;8:1591–1597

118. Rackoff WR, Weiman M, Jakobowski D, et al. A randomized, controlled trial of the efficacy of a heparin and vancomycin solution in preventing central venous catheter infections in children. *J Pediatr.* 1995;127:147–151

119. Raad II, Buzaid A, Rhyne J, et al. Minocycline and ethylenediaminetetraacetate for the prevention of recurrent vascular catheter infections. *Clin Infect Dis.* 1997;25:149–151

120. Raad II, Luna M, Khalil SA, Costerton JW, Lam C, Bodey GP. The relationship between the thrombotic and infectious complications of central venous catheters. *JAMA.* 1994;271:1014–1016

121. Timsit JF, Farkas JC, Boyer JM, et al. Central vein catheter-related thrombosis in intensive care patients: incidence, risk factors, and relationship with catheter-related sepsis. *Chest.* 1998;114:207–213

122. Randolph AG, Cook DJ, Gonzales CA, Andrew M. Benefit of heparin in central venous and pulmonary artery catheters: a meta-analysis of randomized controlled trials. *Chest.* 1998;113:165–171

123. Mermel LA, Stolz SM, Maki DG. Surface antimicrobial activity of heparin-bonded and antiseptic-impregnated vascular catheters. *J Infect Dis.* 1993;167:920–924

124. Pierce CM, Wade A, Mok Q. Heparin-bonded central venous lines reduce thrombotic and infective complications in critically ill children. *Intensive Care Med.* 2000;26:967–972

125. Bern MM, Lokich JJ, Wallach SR, et al. Very low doses of warfarin can prevent thrombosis in central venous catheters: a randomized prospective trial. *Ann Intern Med.* 1990;112:423–428

126. Boraks P, Seale J, Price J, et al. Prevention of central venous catheter associated thrombosis using minidose warfarin in patients with haematological malignancies. *Br J Haematol.* 1998;101:483–486

127. Collin J, Collin C. Infusion thrombophlebitis. *Lancet.* 1975;2:458

128. Lai KK. Safety of prolonging peripheral cannula and i.v. tubing use from 72 hours to 96 hours. *Am J Infect Control.* 1998;26:66–70

129. Fontaine PJ. Performance of a new softening expanding midline catheter in home intravenous therapy patients. *J Intraven Nurs.* 1991;14: 91–99

130. Harwood IR, Greene LM, Kozakowski-Koch JA, Rasor JS. New peripherally inserted midline catheter: a better alternative for intravenous antibiotic therapy in patients with cystic fibrosis. *Pediatr Pulmonol.* 1992;12:233–239

131. Mermel LA, Parenteau S, Tow SM. The risk of midline catheterization in hospitalized patients. A prospective study. *Ann Intern Med.* 1995; 123:841–844

132. Eyer S, Brummitt C, Crossley K, Siegel R, Cerra F. Catheter-related sepsis: prospective, randomized study of three methods of long-term catheter maintenance. *Crit Care Med.* 1990;18:1073–1079

133. Uldall PR, Merchant N, Woods F, Yarworski U, Vas S. Changing subclavian haemodialysis cannulas to reduce infection. *Lancet.* 1981;1: 1373

134. Cook D, Randolph A, Kernerman P, et al. Central venous catheter replacement strategies: a systematic review of the literature. *Crit Care Med.* 1997;25:1417–1424

135. Cobb DK, High KP, Sawyer RG, et al. A controlled trial of scheduled replacement of central venous and pulmonary-artery catheters. *N Engl J Med.* 1992;327:1062–1068

136. Robinson D, Suhocki P, Schwab SJ. Treatment of infected tunneled venous access hemodialysis catheters with guidewire exchange. *Kidney Int.* 1998;53:1792–1794

137. Beathard GA. Management of bacteremia associated with tunneled-cuffed hemodialysis catheters. *J Am Soc Nephrol.* 1999;10:1045–1049

138. Saad TF. Bacteremia associated with tunneled, cuffed hemodialysis catheters. *Am J Kidney Dis.* 1999;34:1114–1124

139. Duszak R Jr, Haskal ZJ, Thomas-Hawkins C, et al. Replacement of failing tunneled hemodialysis catheters through pre-existing subcutaneous tunnels: a comparison of catheter function and infection rates for de novo placements and over-the-wire exchanges. *J Vasc Interv Radiol.* 1998;9:321–327

140. Jaar BG, Hermann JA, Furth SL, Briggs W, Powe NR. Septicemia in diabetic hemodialysis patients: comparison of incidence, risk factors, and mortality with nondiabetic hemodialysis patients. *Am J Kidney Dis.* 2000;35:282–292

141. Powe NR, Jaar B, Furth SL, Hermann J, Briggs W. Septicemia in dialysis patients: incidence, risk factors, and prognosis. *Kidney Int.* 1999;55:1081–1090

142. Hoen B, Paul-Dauphin A, Hestin D, Kessler M. EPIBACDIAL: a multicenter prospective study of risk factors for bacteremia in chronic hemodialysis patients. *J Am Soc Nephrol.* 1998;9:869–976

143. Tokars JI, Miller ER, Alter MJ, et al. National surveillance of dialysis-associated diseases in the United States, 1997. *Semin Dial.* 2000;13: 75–85

144. Foundation NK. III. NKF-K/DOQI Clinical practice guidelines for vascular access: update 2000. *Am J Kidney Dis.* 2001;37(suppl): S137–S181

145. Mermel LA. Intravascular catheters impregnated with benzalkonium chloride. *J Antimicrob Chemother.* 1993;32:905–906

146. Maki DG, Stolz SS, Wheeler S, Mermel LA. A prospective, randomized trial of gauze and two polyurethane dressings for site care of pulmonary artery catheters: implications for catheter management. *Crit Care Med.* 1994;22:1729–1737

147. Raad II, Umphrey J, Khan A, Truett LJ, Bodey GP. The duration of placement as a predictor of peripheral and pulmonary arterial catheter infections. *J Hosp Infect.* 1993;23:17–26

148. Cohen Y, Fosse JP, Karoubi P, et al. The "hands-off" catheter and the prevention of systemic infections associated with pulmonary artery catheter: a prospective study. *Am J Respir Crit Care Med.* 1998;157: 284–287

149. Josephson A, Gombert ME, Sierra MF, Karanfil LV, Tansino GF. The relationship between intravenous fluid contamination and the frequency of tubing replacement. *Infect Control.* 1985;6:367–370

150. Maki DG, Botticelli JT, LeRoy ML, Thielke TS. Prospective study of replacing administration sets for intravenous therapy at 48- vs 72-hour intervals: 72 hours is safe and cost-effective. *JAMA.* 1987;258: 1777–1781

151. Snydman DR, Donnelly-Reidy M, Perry LK, Martin WJ. Intravenous tubing containing burettes can be safely changed at 72 hour intervals. *Infect Control.* 1987;8:113–116

152. Hanna HA, Raad II. Blood products: a significant risk factor for long-term catheter-related bloodstream infections in cancer patients. *Infect Control Hosp Epidemiol.* 2001;22:165–166

153. Raad II, Hanna HA, Awad A, et al. Optimal frequency of changing intravenous administration sets: is it safe to prolong use beyond 72 hours? *Infect Control Hosp Epidemiol.* 2001;22:136–139

154. Saiman L, Ludington E, Dawson JD, et al. Risk factors for *Candida* species colonization of neonatal intensive care unit patients. *Pediatr Infect Dis J.* 2001;20:1119–1124

155. Avila-Figueroa C, Goldmann DA, Richardson DK, Gray JE, Ferrari A, Freeman J. Intravenous lipid emulsions are the major determinant of coagulase-negative staphylococcal bacteremia in very low birth weight newborns. *Pediatr Infect Dis J.* 1998;17:10–17

156. Crocker KS, Noga R, Filibeck DJ, Krey SH, Markovic M, Steffee WP. Microbial growth comparisons of five commercial parenteral lipid emulsions. *J Parenter Enteral Nutr.* 1984;8:391–395

157. Jarvis WR, Highsmith AK. Bacterial growth and endotoxin production in lipid emulsion. *J Clin Microbiol.* 1984;19:17–20

158. Melly MA, Meng HC, Schaffner W. Microbiol growth in lipid emulsions used in parenteral nutrition. *Arch Surg.* 1975;110:1479–1481

159. Inoue Y, Nezu R, Matsuda H, et al. Prevention of catheter-related sepsis during parenteral nutrition: effect of a new connection device. *J Parenter Enteral Nutr.* 1992;16:581–585

160. Arduino MJ, Bland LA, Danzig LE, McAllister SK, Aguero SM. Micro-

biologic evaluation of needleless and needle-access devices. *Am J Infect Control.* 1997;25:377–380

161. Brown JD, Moss HA, Elliott TS. The potential for catheter microbial contamination from a needleless connector. *J Hosp Infect.* 1997;36:181–189

162. Cookson ST, Ihrig M, O'Mara EM, et al. Increased bloodstream infection rates in surgical patients associated with variation from recommended use and care following implementation of a needleless device. *Infect Control Hosp Epidemiol.* 1998;19:23–27

163. Do AN, Ray BJ, Banerjee SN, et al. Bloodstream infection associated with needleless device use and the importance of infection-control practices in the home health care setting. *J Infect Dis.* 1999;179:442–448

164. Luebke MA, Arduino MJ, Duda DL, et al. Comparison of the microbial barrier properties of a needleless and a conventional needle-based intravenous access system. *Am J Infect Control.* 1998;26:437–441

165. McDonald LC, Banerjee SN, Jarvis WR. Line-associated bloodstream infections in pediatric intensive-care-unit patients associated with a needleless device and intermittent intravenous therapy. *Infect Control Hosp Epidemiol.* 1998;19:772–777

166. Mendelson MH, Short LJ, Schechter CB, et al. Study of a needleless intermittent intravenous-access system for peripheral infusions: analysis of staff, patient, and institutional outcomes. *Infect Control Hosp Epidemiol.* 1998;19:401–406

167. Seymour VM, Dhallu TS, Moss HA, Tebbs SE, Elliot TS. A prospective clinical study to investigate the microbial contamination of a needleless connector. *J Hosp Infect.* 2000;45:165–168

168. Longfield RN, Smith LP, Longfield JN, Coberly J, Cruess D. Multiple-dose vials: persistence of bacterial contaminants and infection control implications. *Infect Control.* 1985;6:194–199

169. Henry B, Plante-Jenkins C, Ostrowska K. An outbreak of *Serratia marcescens* associated with the anesthetic agent propofol. *Am J Infect Control.* 2001;29:312–315

170. Grohskopf LA, Roth VR, Feikin DR, et al. *Serratia liquefaciens* bloodstream infections from contamination of epoetin alfa at a hemodialysis center. *N Engl J Med.* 2001;344:1491–1497

171. CDC. National Nosocomial Infections Surveillance (NNIS) System report, data summary from April 1995–April 2000, issued June 2000. *Am J Infect Control.* 2000;28:429–435

172. Richards MJ, Edwards JR, Culver DH, Gaynes RP. Nosocomial infections in pediatric intensive care units in the United States: National Nosocomial Infections Surveillance System. *Pediatrics.* 1999;103:103–109

173. Richards MJ, Edwards JR, Culver DH, Gaynes RP. Nosocomial infections in medical intensive care units in the United States: National Nosocomial Infections Surveillance System. *Crit Care Med.* 1999;27:887–892

174. Garland JS, Dunne WM Jr, Havens P, et al. Peripheral intravenous catheter complications in critically ill children: a prospective study. *Pediatrics.* 1992;89:1145–1150

175. Garland JS, Nelson DB, Cheah TE, Hennes HH, Johnson TM. Infectious complications during peripheral intravenous therapy with Teflon catheters: a prospective study. *Pediatr Infect Dis J.* 1987;6:918–921

176. Furfaro S, Gauthier M, Lacroix J, Nadeau D, Lafleur L, Mathews S. Arterial catheter-related infections in children: a 1-year cohort analysis. *Am J Dis Child.* 1991;145:1037–1043

177. Krauss AN, Albert RF, Kannan MM. Contamination of umbilical catheters in the newborn infant. *J Pediatr.* 1970;77:965–969

178. Landers S, Moise AA, Fraley JK, Smith EO, Baker CJ. Factors associated with umbilical catheter-related sepsis in neonates. *Am J Dis Child.* 1991;145:675–680

179. Balagtas RC, Bell CE, Edwards LD, Levin S. Risk of local and systemic infections associated with umbilical vein catheterization: a prospective study in 86 newborn patients. *Pediatrics.* 1971;48:359–367

180. Stenzel JP, Green TP, Fuhrman BP, Carlson PE, Marchessault RP. Percutaneous central venous catheterization in a pediatric intensive care unit: a survival analysis of complications. *Crit Care Med.* 1989;17:984–988

181. Garland JS, Alex CP, Mueller CD, et al. A randomized trial comparing povidone-iodine to a chlorhexidine gluconate-impregnated dressing for prevention of central venous catheter infections in neonates. *Pediatrics.* 2001;107:1431–1436

182. Davis D, O'Brien MA, Freemantle N, Wolf FM, Mazmanian P, Taylor-Vaisey A. Impact of formal continuing medical education: do conferences, workshops, rounds, and other traditional continuing education activities change physician behavior or health care outcomes? *JAMA.* 1999;282:867–874

183. Conly JM, Hill S, Ross J, Lertzman J, Louie TJ. Handwashing practices in an intensive care unit: the effects of an educational program and its relationship to infection rates. *Am J Infect Control.* 1989;17:330–339

184. East SA. Planning, implementation, and evaluation of a successful hospital-based peripherally inserted central catheter program. *J Intraven Nurs.* 1994;17:189–192

185. Kyle KS, Myers JS. Peripherally inserted central catheters. Development of a hospital-based program. *J Intraven Nurs.* 1990;13:287–290

186. BeVier PA, Rice CE. Initiating a pediatric peripherally inserted central catheter and midline catheter program. *J Intraven Nurs.* 1994;17:201–205

187. Tomford JW, Hershey CO, McLaren CE, Porter DK, Cohen DI. Intravenous therapy team and peripheral venous catheter-associated complications: a prospective controlled study. *Arch Intern Med.* 1984;144:1191–1194

188. Wenzel RP, Wentzel RP. The development of academic programs for quality assessment. *Arch Intern Med.* 1991;151:653–654

189. Robert J, Fridkin SK, Blumberg HM, et al. The influence of the composition of the nursing staff on primary bloodstream infection rates in a surgical intensive care unit. *Infect Control Hosp Epidemiol.* 2000;21:12–17

190. Vicca AF. Nursing staff workload as a determinant of methicillin-resistant *Staphylococcus aureus* spread in an adult intensive therapy unit. *J Hosp Infect.* 1999;43:109–113

191. White MC, Ragland KE. Surveillance of intravenous catheter-related infections among home care clients. *Am J Infect Control.* 1994;22:231–235

192. Lorenzen AN, Itkin DJ. Surveillance of infection in home care. *Am J Infect Control.* 1992;20:326–329

193. White MC. Infections and infection risks in home care settings. *Infect Control Hosp Epidemiol.* 1992;13:535–539

194. Raad II, Baba M, Bodey GP. Diagnosis of catheter-related infections: the role of surveillance and targeted quantitative skin cultures. *Clin Infect Dis.* 1995;20:593–597

195. Widmer AF, Nettleman M, Flint K, Wenzel RP. The clinical impact of culturing central venous catheters: a prospective study. *Arch Intern Med.* 1992;152:1299–1302

196. Boyce JM, Farr BM, Jarvis WR, et al. Guideline for hand hygiene in the healthcare setting. *Am J Infect Control.* 2002. In press

197. Bischoff WE, Reynolds TM, Sessler CN, Edmond MB, Wenzel RP. Handwashing compliance by health care workers: the impact of introducing an accessible, alcohol-based hand antiseptic. *Arch Intern Med.* 2000;160:1017–1021

198. Pittet D, Dharan S, Touveneau S, Sauvan V, Perneger TV. Bacterial contamination of the hands of hospital staff during routine patient care. *Arch Intern Med.* 1999;159:821–826

199. Simmons B, Bryant J, Neiman K, Spencer L, Arheart K. The role of handwashing in prevention of endemic intensive care unit infections. *Infect Control Hosp Epidemiol.* 1990;11:589–594

200. Boyce JM, Kelliher S, Vallande N. Skin irritation and dryness associated with two hand-hygiene regimens: soap-and-water hand washing versus hand antisepsis with an alcoholic hand gel. *Infect Control Hosp Epidemiol.* 2000;21:442–448

201. Capdevila JA. Catheter-related infection: an update on diagnosis, treatment, and prevention. *Int J Infect Dis.* 1998;2:230–236

202. Abi-Said D, Raad II, Umphrey J, Gonzalez V, Richardson D, Marts K, Hohn D. Infusion therapy team and dressing changes of central venous catheters. *Infect Control Hosp Epidemiol.* 1999;20:101–105

203. CDC. Update: universal precautions for prevention of transmission of human immunodeficiency virus, hepatitis B virus, and other blood-borne pathogens in health-care settings. *MMWR Morb Mortal Wkly Rep.* 1988;37:377–382, 388

204. Povoski SP. A prospective analysis of the cephalic vein cutdown approach for chronic indwelling central venous access in 100 consecutive cancer patients. *Ann Surg Oncol.* 2000;7:496–502

205. Arrighi DA, Farnell MB, Mucha P Jr, Ilstrup DM, Anderson DL. Prospective, randomized trial of rapid venous access for patients in hypovolemic shock. *Ann Emerg Med.* 1989;18:927–930

206. Ahmed Z, Mohyuddin Z. Complications associated with different insertion techniques for Hickman catheters. *Postgrad Med J.* 1998;74:104–107

207. Little JR, Murray PR, Traynor PS, Spitznagel E. A randomized trial of povidone-iodine compared with iodine tincture for venipuncture site disinfection: effects on rates of blood culture contamination. *Am J Med.* 1999;107:119–125

208. Mimoz O, Pieroni L, Lawrence C, et al. Prospective, randomized trial of two antiseptic solutions for prevention of central venous or arterial catheter colonization and infection in intensive care unit patients. *Crit Care Med.* 1996;24:1818–1823

209. Maki DG, McCormack KN. Defatting catheter insertion sites in total parenteral nutrition is of no value as an infection control measure. Controlled clinical trial. *Am J Med.* 1987;83:833–840

210. Bijma R, Girbes AR, Kleijer DJ, Zwaveling JH. Preventing central venous catheter-related infection in a surgical intensive-care unit. *Infect Control Hosp Epidemiol.* 1999;20:618–620

211. Rasero L, Degl'Innocenti M, Mocali M, et al. Comparison of two different time interval protocols for central venous catheter dressing in bone marrow transplant patients: results of a randomized, multicenter study. *Haematologica.* 2000;85:275–279

212. Madeo M, Martin CR, Turner C, Kirkby V, Thompson DR. A randomized trial comparing Arglaes (a transparent dressing containing silver ions) to Tegaderm (a transparent polyurethane dressing) for dressing peripheral arterial catheters and central vascular catheters. *Intensive Crit Care Nurs.* 1998;14:187–191

213. Flowers RH, Schwenzer KJ, Kopel RF, Fisch MJ, Tucker SI, Farr BM. Efficacy of an attachable subcutaneous cuff for the prevention of intravascular catheter-related infection: a randomized, controlled trial. *JAMA.* 1989;261:878–883

214. Robbins J, Cromwell P, Korones DN. Swimming and central venous catheter-related infections in the child with cancer. *J Pediatr Oncol Nurs.* 1999;16:51–56

215. Howell PB, Walters PE, Donowitz GR, Farr BM. Risk factors for infection of adult patients with cancer who have tunneled central venous catheters. *Cancer.* 1995;75:1367–1375

216. Goetz AM, Miller J, Wagener MM, Muder RR. Complications related to intravenous midline catheter usage: a 2-year study. *J Intraven Nurs.* 1998;21:76–80

217. Martin C, Viviand X, Saux P, Gouin F. Upper-extremity deep vein thrombosis after central venous catheterization via the axillary vein. *Crit Care Med.* 1999;27:2626–2629

218. Robinson JF, Robinson WA, Cohn A, Garg K, Armstrong JD. Perforation of the great vessels during central venous line placement. *Arch Intern Med.* 1995;155:1225–1228

219. Lederle FA, Parenti CM, Berskow LC, Ellingson KJ. The idle intravenous catheter. *Ann Intern Med.* 1992;116:737–738

220. Parenti CM, Lederle FA, Impola CL, Peterson LR. Reduction of unnecessary intravenous catheter use: internal medicine house staff participate in a successful quality improvement project. *Arch Intern Med.* 1994;154:1829–1832

221. Thomas F, Burke JP, Parker J, et al. The risk of infection related to radial vs femoral sites for arterial catheterization. *Crit Care Med.* 1983; 11:807–812

222. Nelson DB, Garland JS. The natural history of Teflon catheter-associated phlebitis in children. *Am J Dis Child.* 1987;141:1090–1092

223. Shimandle RB, Johnson D, Baker M, Stotland N, Karrison T, Arnow PM. Safety of peripheral intravenous catheters in children. *Infect Control Hosp Epidemiol.* 1999;20:736–740

224. O'Grady NP, Barie PS, Bartlett J, et al. Practice parameters for evaluating new fever in critically ill adult patients. Task Force of the American College of Critical Care Medicine of the Society of Critical Care Medicine in collaboration with the Infectious Disease Society of America. *Crit Care Med.* 1998;26:392–408

225. Mermel LA, Farr BM, Sherertz RJ, et al. Guidelines for the management of intravascular catheter-related infections. *Clin Infect Dis.* 2001; 32:1249–1272

226. Mershon J, Nogami W, Williams JM, Yoder C, Eitzen HE, Lemons JA. Bacterial/fungal growth in a combined parenteral nutrition solution. *J Parenter Enteral Nutr.* 1986;10:498–502

227. Gilbert M, Gallagher SC, Eads M, Elmore MF. Microbial growth patterns in a total parenteral nutrition formulation containing lipid emulsion. *J Parenter Enteral Nutr.* 1986;10:494–497

228. Maki DG, Martin WT. Nationwide epidemic of septicemia caused by contaminated infusion products. IV. Growth of microbial pathogens in fluids for intravenous infusions. *J Infect Dis.* 1975;131:267–272

229. Didier ME, Fischer S, Maki DG. Total nutrient admixtures appear safer than lipid emulsion alone as regards microbial contamination: growth properties of microbial pathogens at room temperature. *J Parenter Enteral Nutr.* 1998;22:291–296

230. Bennett SN, McNeil MM, Bland LA, et al. Postoperative infections traced to contamination of an intravenous anesthetic, propofol. *N Engl J Med.* 1995;333:147–154

231. Roth VR, Arduino MJ, Nobiletti J, et al. Transfusion-related sepsis due to *Serratia liquefaciens* in the United States. *Transfusion.* 2000;40:931–935

232. Blajchman MA. Reducing the risk of bacterial contamination of cellular blood components. *Dev Biol Stand.* 2000;102:183–193

233. Barrett BB, Andersen JW, Anderson KC. Strategies for the avoidance of

234. Wagner SJ, Friedman LI, Dodd RY. Transfusion-associated bacterial sepsis. *Clin Microbiol Rev.* 1994;7:290–302

235. Plott RT, Wagner RF Jr, Tyring SK. Iatrogenic contamination of multidose vials in simulated use. A reassessment of current patient injection technique. *Arch Dermatol.* 1990;126:1441–1444

236. Salzman MB, Isenberg HD, Rubin LG. Use of disinfectants to reduce microbial contamination of hubs of vascular catheters. *J Clin Microbiol.* 1993;31:475–479

237. ASHP Council on Professional Affairs. ASHP guidelines on quality assurance for pharmacy-prepared sterile products. *Am J Health Syst Pharm.* 2000;57:1150–1169

238. Herruzo-Cabrera R, Garcia-Caballero J, Vera-Cortes ML, et al. Growth of microorganisms in parenteral nutrient solutions. *Am J Hosp Pharm.* 1984;41:1178–1180

239. Green KA, Shouldachi B, Schoer K, Moro D, Blend R, McGeer A. Gadolinium-based MR contrast media: potential for growth of microbial contaminants when single vials are used for multiple patients. *AJR Am J Roentgenol.* 1995;165:669–671

240. Arrington ME, Gabbert KC, Mazgaj PW, Wolf MT. Multidose vial contamination in anesthesia. *AANA J.* 1990;58:462–466

241. Falchuk KH, Peterson L, McNeil BJ. Microparticulate-induced phlebitis: its prevention by in-line filtration. *N Engl J Med.* 1985;312: 78–82

242. Cohran J, Larson E, Roach H, Blane C, Pierce P. Effect of intravascular surveillance and education program on rates of nosocomial bloodstream infections. *Heart Lung.* 1996;25:161–164

243. Netto dos Santos KR, de Souza Fonseca L, Gontijo Filho PP. Emergence of high-level mupirocin resistance in methicillin-resistant *Staphylococcus aureus* isolated from Brazilian university hospitals. *Infect Control Hosp Epidemiol.* 1996;17:813–816

244. Ryder MA. Peripheral access options. *Surg Oncol Clin North Am.* 1995; 4:395–427

245. Maki DG, Goldman DA, Rhame FS. Infection control in intravenous therapy. *Ann Intern Med.* 1973;79:867–887

246. Tager IB, Ginsberg MB, Ellis SE, et al. An epidemiologic study of the risks associated with peripheral intravenous catheters. *Am J Epidemiol.* 1983;118:839–851

247. Horan TC, Emori TG. Definitions of key terms used in the NNIS System. *Am J Infect Control.* 1997;25:112–116

248. Khuri-Bulos NA, Shennak M, Agabi S, et al. Nosocomial infections in the intensive care units at a university hospital in a developing country: comparison with National Nosocomial Infections Surveillance intensive care unit rates. *Am J Infect Control.* 1999;27:547–552

249. Pittet D, Wenzel RP. Nosocomial bloodstream infections. Secular trends in rates, mortality, and contribution to total hospital deaths. *Arch Intern Med.* 1995;155:1177–1184

250. CDC. Monitoring hospital-acquired infections to promote patient safety—United States, 1990–1999. *MMWR Morb Mortal Wkly Rep.* 2000;49: 149–153

251. Clark-Christoff N, Watters VA, Sparks W, Snyder P, Grant JP. Use of triple-lumen subclavian catheters for administration of total parenteral nutrition. *J Parenter Enteral Nutr.* 1992;16:403–407

252. Early TF, Gregory RT, Wheeler JR, Snyder SO Jr, Gayle RG. Increased infection rate in double-lumen versus single-lumen Hickman catheters in cancer patients. *South Med J.* 1990;83:34–36

253. Hilton E, Haslett TM, Borenstein MT, Tucci V, Isenberg HD, Singer C. Central catheter infections: single- versus triple-lumen catheters: influence of guide wires on infection rates when used for replacement of catheters. *Am J Med.* 1988;84:667–672

254. Yeung C, May J, Hughes R. Infection rate for single lumen v triple lumen subclavian catheters. *Infect Control Hosp Epidemiol.* 1988;9: 154–158

255. Collin GR. Decreasing catheter colonization through the use of an antiseptic-impregnated catheter: a continuous quality improvement project. *Chest.* 1999;115:1632–1640

256. Groeger JS, Lucas AB, Thaler HT, et al. Infectious morbidity associated with long-term use of venous access devices in patients with cancer. *Ann Intern Med.* 1993;119:1168–1174

257. Pegues D, Axelrod P, McClarren C, et al. Comparison of infections in Hickman and implanted port catheters in adult solid tumor patients. *J Surg Oncol.* 1992;49:156–162

258. Moss AH, Vasilakis C, Holley JL, Foulks CJ, Pillai K, McDowell DE. Use of a silicone dual-lumen catheter with a Dacron cuff as a long-term vascular access for hemodialysis patients. *Am J Kidney Dis.* 1990;16: 211–215

259. Schillinger F, Schillinger D, Montagnac R, Milcent T. Post catheteriza-

tion vein stenosis in haemodialysis: comparative angiographic study of 50 subclavian and 50 internal jugular accesses. *Nephrol Dial Transplant.* 1991;6:722–724

260. Cimochowski GE, Worley E, Rutherford WE, Sartain J, Blondin J, Harter H. Superiority of the internal jugular over the subclavian access for temporary dialysis. *Nephron.* 1990;54:154–161

261. Barrett N, Spencer S, McIvor J, Brown EA. Subclavian stenosis: a major complication of subclavian dialysis catheters. *Nephrol Dial Transplant.* 1988;3:423–425

262. Trerotola SO, Kuhn-Fulton J, Johnson MS, Shah H, Ambrosius WT, Kneebone PH. Tunneled infusion catheters: increased incidence of symptomatic venous thrombosis after subclavian versus internal jugular venous access. *Radiology.* 2000;217:89–93

263. Macdonald S, Watt AJ, McNally D, Edwards RD, Moss JG. Comparison of technical success and outcome of tunneled catheters inserted via the jugular and subclavian approaches. *J Vasc Interv Radiol.* 2000;11:225–231

264. Widmer AF. Management of catheter-related bacteremia and fungemia in patients on total parenteral nutrition. *Nutrition.* 1997;13(suppl):S18–S25

265. Powell C, Kudsk KA, Kulich PA, Mandelbaum JA, Fabri PJ. Effect of frequent guidewire changes on triple-lumen catheter sepsis. *J Parenter Enteral Nutr.* 1988;12:462–464

266. Snydman DR, Murray SA, Kornfeld SJ, Majka JA, Ellis CA. Total parenteral nutrition-related infections: prospective epidemiologic study using semiquantitative methods. *Am J Med.* 1982;73:695–699

267. Easom A. Prophylactic antibiotic lock therapy for hemodialysis catheters. *Nephrol Nurs J.* 2000;27:75

268. Vercaigne LM, Sitar DS, Penner SB, Bernstein K, Wang GQ, Burczynski FJ. Antibiotic-heparin lock: in vitro antibiotic stability combined with heparin in a central venous catheter. *Pharmacotherapy.* 2000;20:394–399

269. Donowitz LG, Marsik FJ, Hoyt JW, Wenzel RP. *Serratia marcescens* bacteremia from contaminated pressure transducers. *JAMA.* 1979;242:1749–1751

270. Luskin RL, Weinstein RA, Nathan C, Chamberlin WH, Kabins SA. Extended use of disposable pressure transducers: a bacteriologic evaluation. *JAMA.* 1986;255:916–920

271. Maki DG, Hassemer CA. Endemic rate of fluid contamination and related septicemia in arterial pressure monitoring. *Am J Med.* 1981;70:733–738

272. Mermel LA, Maki DG. Epidemic bloodstream infections from hemodynamic pressure monitoring: signs of the times. *Infect Control Hosp Epidemiol.* 1989;10:47–53

273. Tenold R, Priano L, Kim K, Rourke B, Marrone T. Infection potential of nondisposable pressure transducers prepared prior to use. *Crit Care Med.* 1987;15:582–583

274. Leroy O, Billiau V, Beuscart C, et al. Nosocomial infections associated with long-term radial artery cannulation. *Intensive Care Med.* 1989;15:241–246

275. Fisher MC, Long SS, Roberts EM, Dunn JM, Balsara RK. *Pseudomonas maltophilia* bacteremia in children undergoing open heart surgery. *JAMA.* 1981;246:1571–1574

276. Stamm WE, Colella JJ, Anderson RL, Dixon RE. Indwelling arterial catheters as a source of nosocomial bacteremia: an outbreak caused by *Flavobacterium* species. *N Engl J Med.* 1975;292:1099–1102

277. Weinstein RA, Emori TG, Anderson RL, Stamm WE. Pressure transducers as a source of bacteremia after open heart surgery: report of an outbreak and guidelines for prevention. *Chest.* 1976;69:338–344

278. Shinozaki T, Deane RS, Mazuzan JE Jr, Hamel AJ, Hazelton D. Bacterial contamination of arterial lines: a prospective study. *JAMA.* 1983;249:223–225

279. Solomon SL, Alexander H, Eley JW, et al. Nosocomial fungemia in neonates associated with intravascular pressure-monitoring devices. *Pediatr Infect Dis.* 1986;5:680–685

280. Weems JJ Jr, Chamberland ME, Ward J, Willy M, Padhye AA, Solomon SL. *Candida parapsilosis* fungemia associated with parenteral nutrition and contaminated blood pressure transducers. *J Clin Microbiol.* 1987;25:1029–1032

281. Beck-Sague CM, Jarvis WR, Brook JH, et al. Epidemic bacteremia due to *Acinetobacter baumannii* in five intensive care units. *Am J Epidemiol.* 1990;132:723–733

282. Villarino ME, Jarvis WR, O'Hara C, Bresnahan J, Clark N. Epidemic of *Serratia marcescens* bacteremia in a cardiac intensive care unit. *J Clin Microbiol.* 1989;27:2433–2436

283. Boo NY, Wong NC, Zulkifli SS, Lye MS. Risk factors associated with umbilical vascular catheter-associated thrombosis in newborn infants. *J Paediatr Child Health.* 1999;35:460–465

284. Cronin WA, Germanson TP, Donowitz LG. Intravascular catheter colonization and related bloodstream infection in critically ill neonates. *Infect Control Hosp Epidemiol.* 1990;11:301–308

285. Miller KL, Coen PE, White WJ, Hurst WJ, Achey BE, Lang CM. Effectiveness of skin absorption of tincture of I in blocking radioiodine from the human thyroid gland. *Health Phys.* 1989;56:911–914

286. Ankola PA, Atakent YS. Effect of adding heparin in very low concentration to the infusate to prolong the patency of umbilical artery catheters. *Am J Perinatol.* 1993;10:229–232

287. Horgan MJ, Bartoletti A, Polansky S, Peters JC, Manning TJ, Lamont BM. Effect of heparin infusates in umbilical arterial catheters on frequency of thrombotic complications. *J Pediatr.* 1987;111:774–778

288. David RJ, Merten DF, Anderson JC, Gross S. Prevention of umbilical artery catheter clots with heparinized infusates. *Dev Pharmacol Ther.* 1981;2:117–126

289. Fletcher MA, Brown DR, Landers S, Seguin J. Umbilical arterial catheter use: report of an audit conducted by the Study Group for Complications of Perinatal Care. *Am J Perinatol.* 1994;11:94–99

290. Seguin J, Fletcher MA, Landers S, Brown D, Macpherson T. Umbilical venous catheterizations: audit by the Study Group for Complications of Perinatal Care. *Am J Perinatol.* 1994;11:67–70

291. Loisel DB, Smith MM, MacDonald MG, Martin GR. Intravenous access in newborn infants: impact of extended umbilical venous catheter use on requirement for peripheral venous lines. *J Perinatol.* 1996;16:461–466

292. Garner JS, Jarvis WR, Emori TG, Horan TC, Hughes JM. CDC definitions for nosocomial infections, 1988. *Am J Infect Control.* 1988;16:128–140

293. Garner JS, Jarvis WR, Emori TG, Horan TC, Hughes JM. CDC definitions for nosocomial infections, 1988 [erratum]. *Am J Infect Control.* 1988;16:177

Practice Guidelines for the Treatment of Lyme Disease

• •

The following guideline for the treatment of lyme disease, developed by the Infectious Diseases Society of America, has been endorsed by the American Academy of Pediatrics.

GUIDELINES FROM THE INFECTIOUS DISEASES SOCIETY OF AMERICA

Practice Guidelines for the Treatment of Lyme Disease

Gary P. Wormser,[1] Robert B. Nadelman,[1]
Raymond J. Dattwyler,[2] David T. Dennis,[6]
Eugene D. Shapiro,[7] Allen C. Steere,[9]
Thomas J. Rush,[5] Daniel W. Rahn,[10]
Patricia K. Coyle,[3] David H. Persing,[11]
Durland Fish,[8] and Benjamin J. Luft[4]

[1]*Division of Infectious Diseases, Department of Medicine, New York Medical College, Valhalla,* [2]*Division of Allergy, Immunology and Lyme Disease, Department of Medicine,* [3]*Department of Neurology, and* [4]*Department of Medicine, Health Sciences Center, State University of New York at Stony Brook, and* [5]*private practice, Briarcliff Manor, New York;* [6]*Division of Vector-Borne Infectious Diseases, National Center for Infectious Diseases, Centers for Disease Control and Prevention, Fort Collins, Colorado; Departments of* [7]*Pediatrics and* [8]*Epidemiology and Public Health, Yale University School of Medicine, New Haven, Connecticut;* [9]*Tufts University School of Medicine, New England Medical Center, Boston, Massachusetts;* [10]*Office of Medical Management, Medical College of Georgia, Augusta; and* [11]*Diagnostics Development, Corixa Corporation, and Infectious Disease Research Institute, Seattle Life Sciences Center, Seattle, Washington*

Executive Summary

Tick bites and prophylaxis. The best currently available method for preventing infection with *Borrelia burgdorferi* is to avoid vector tick exposure. If exposure to *Ixodes scapularis* or *Ixodes pacificus* ticks is unavoidable, measures recommended to reduce the risk of infection include using both protective clothing and tick repellents, checking the entire body for ticks daily, and promptly removing attached ticks, before transmission of *B. burgdorferi* can occur (A-III [see tables 1 and 2 for recommendation categories, indicated in parentheses throughout this text]).

Routine use of either antimicrobial prophylaxis (E-I) or serological tests (D-III) after a tick bite is not recommended. Some experts recommend antibiotic therapy for patients bitten by *I. scapularis* ticks that are estimated to have been attached for >48 h (on the basis of the degree of engorgement of the tick with blood), in conjunction with epidemiological information regarding the prevalence of tick-transmitted infection (C-III). However, accurate determinations of species of tick and degree of engorgement are not routinely possible, and data are insufficient to demonstrate efficacy of antimicrobial therapy in this setting.

Persons who remove attached ticks should be monitored closely for signs and symptoms of tick-borne diseases for up to 30 days and specifically for the occurrence of a skin lesion at the site of the tick bite (which may suggest Lyme disease) or a temperature >38°C (which may suggest human granulo-

cytic ehrlichiosis [HGE] or babesiosis). Persons who develop a skin lesion or other illness within 1 month after removing an attached tick should promptly seek medical attention for assessment of the possibility of having acquired a tick-borne disease (A-II).

Health care practitioners, particularly those in areas where Lyme disease is endemic, should become familiar with its clinical manifestations, recommended practices for testing for it, and therapy for the disease, as well as for HGE and babesiosis (A-III).

Testing of ticks for tick-borne infectious organisms is not recommended, except in research studies (D-III).

Prior vaccination with the recently licensed recombinant outer-surface protein A (OspA) vaccine preparation reduces the risk of developing Lyme disease associated with tick bites but should not alter the above recommendations (A-I).

Early Lyme disease. Administration of doxycycline (100 mg twice daily) or amoxicillin (500 mg 3 times daily) for 14–21 days is recommended for treatment of early localized or early disseminated Lyme disease associated with erythema migrans, in the absence of neurological involvement or third-degree atrioventricular heart block (A-I). In prospective studies, these agents have been shown to be effective in treating erythema migrans and associated symptoms. Doxycycline has the advantage of being efficacious for treatment of HGE, which may occur simultaneously with early Lyme disease. Doxycycline is relatively contraindicated during pregnancy or lactation and for children aged <8 years.

Because of its higher cost, cefuroxime axetil (500 mg orally twice daily), which is as effective as doxycycline in the treatment of erythema migrans (A-I), should be reserved as an alternative agent for those patients who can take neither doxycycline nor amoxicillin. For children, we recommend amoxicillin at a dos-

---

Reprints or correspondence: Dr. Gary P. Wormser, Room 209 SE, Macy Pavilion, Westchester Medical Center, Valhalla, NY 10595.

Clinical Infectious Diseases 2000; 31(Suppl 1):S1–14
© 2000 by the Infectious Diseases Society of America. All rights reserved.
1058-4838/2000/310S1-0001$03.00

Table 1. Categories indicating the strength of each recommendation for or against use.

Category	Definition
A	Good evidence to support a recommendation for use
B	Moderate evidence to support a recommendation for use
C	Poor evidence to support a recommendation for or against use
D	Moderate evidence to support a recommendation against use
E	Good evidence to support a recommendation against use

NOTE.   Table is adapted from [1].

age of 50 mg/kg/d, divided into 3 doses per day (maximum, 500 mg/dose), or doxycycline (for those aged ≥8 years) at a dosage of 1–2 mg/kg twice per day (maximum, 100 mg/dose) (B-II). Cefuroxime axetil, at a dosage of 30 mg/kg/d, divided into 2 doses daily (maximum, 500 mg/dose), is an acceptable alternative agent (B-III).

Macrolide antibiotics are not recommended as first-line therapy for early Lyme disease (E-I). When used, they should be reserved for patients who are intolerant of amoxicillin, doxycycline, and cefuroxime axetil. Possible regimens for adults are as follows: azithromycin, 500 mg orally daily for 7–10 days; erythromycin, 500 mg orally 4 times daily for 14–21 days; and clarithromycin, 500 mg orally twice daily for 14–21 days. Possible dosages for children are the following: azithromycin, 10 mg/kg/d (maximum, 500 mg/d); erythromycin, 12.5 mg/kg 4 times daily (maximum, 500 mg/dose); and clarithromycin, 7.5 mg/kg twice daily (maximum, 500 mg/dose). Patients treated with macrolides should be closely followed.

Ceftriaxone (2 g iv daily), although effective, is not superior to oral agents and is not recommended as a first-line agent for treatment of Lyme disease in the absence of neurological involvement or third-degree atrioventricular heart block (E-I).

The use of ceftriaxone (2 g once daily iv for 14–28 days) in early Lyme disease is recommended for acute neurological disease manifested by meningitis or radiculopathy (B-II). Intravenous penicillin G at a dosage of 18–24 million units daily, divided into doses given every 4 h (for patients with normal renal function), may be a satisfactory alternative (B-II). Cefotaxime (2 g iv every 8 h) may also be a satisfactory alternative (B-II). For adult patients who are intolerant of both penicillin and cephalosporins, doxycycline (200–400 mg/d) in 2 divided doses given orally (or iv if the patient is unable to take oral medications) for 14–28 days may be adequate (B-II).

For children, we recommend ceftriaxone (75–100 mg/kg/d) in a single daily iv dose (maximum, 2 g) (B-II) or cefotaxime (150–200 mg/kg/d) divided into 3 or 4 iv doses (maximum, 6 g/d) (B-III) for 14–28 days. An alternative is iv penicillin G (200,000–400,000 units/kg/d; maximum, 18–24 million units/d) divided into doses given every 4 h for those with normal renal function (B-II).

Patients with first- or second-degree atrioventricular heart block associated with early Lyme disease should be treated with the same antimicrobial regimens as patients with erythema migrans without carditis (see paragraphs 1 and 2 of the recom-

mendations in this section, above) (B-III). We recommend that patients with third-degree atrioventricular heart block be treated with parenteral antibiotics such as ceftriaxone (see paragraphs 5 and 6 of the recommendations in this section, above) in the hospital, although there are no clinical trials to support this recommendation (B-III). A temporary pacemaker may also be required.

Although antibiotic treatment does not hasten the resolution of seventh-cranial-nerve palsy associated with *B. burgdorferi* infection, antibiotics should be given to prevent further sequelae (B-II). There was disagreement among panel members on the neurological evaluation of patients with seventh-cranial-nerve palsy. Some members perform a CSF examination on all patients with seventh-cranial-nerve palsy, whereas others reserve lumbar puncture for patients for whom there is strong clinical suspicion of CNS involvement (e.g., severe headache or nuchal rigidity). Patients whose CSF examinations yield normal findings may be treated with the same regimens used for patients with erythema migrans (B-III), whereas patients for whom there is clinical and laboratory evidence of CNS involvement should be treated with regimens effective against meningitis (see paragraphs 5 and 6 of the recommendations in this section, above) (B-II).

Treatment for pregnant patients can be identical to that for nonpregnant patients with the same disease manifestation, except that tetracyclines should be avoided (B-III).

Lyme arthritis.   Lyme arthritis usually can be treated successfully with antimicrobial agents administered orally or intravenously. Administration of doxycycline (100 mg twice daily orally) or amoxicillin (500 mg 3 times daily), in each instance for 28 days, is recommended for patients without clinically evident neurological disease (B-II). For children, we recommend administration of doxycycline (1–2 mg/kg twice per day; maximum, 100 mg/dose), which can be given to patients aged ≥8 years, or amoxicillin (50 mg/kg/d, divided into 3 doses per day; maximum, 500 mg/dose) for 28 days (B-II).

Oral therapy is easier to administer than iv antibiotics, is associated with fewer serious complications, and is considerably less expensive. Its disadvantage is that some patients treated with oral agents have subsequently manifested overt neuroborreliosis, which may require iv therapy for successful treat-

Table 2. Grades indicating the quality of evidence on which recommendations are based.

Grade	Definition
I	Evidence from at least 1 properly randomized, controlled trial
II	Evidence from at least 1 well-designed clinical trial without randomization, from cohort or case-controlled analytic studies (preferably from >1 center), from multiple time-series studies, or from dramatic results of uncontrolled experiments
III	Evidence from opinions of respected authorities that is based on clinical experience, descriptive studies, or reports of expert committees

ment. Further controlled trials are needed to compare oral with iv therapy.

Neurological evaluation, including lumbar puncture, should be done for patients if there is a strong clinical suspicion of neurological involvement. Patients with both arthritis and objective evidence of neurological disease should receive iv ceftriaxone (2 g once daily for 14–28 days) (A-II). Alternative therapies include iv cefotaxime (2 g iv every 8 h) (B-III) or iv penicillin G (18–24 million units daily, divided into doses given every 4 h for patients with normal renal function) (B-II). Because of low blood levels, the long-acting benzathine preparation of penicillin is not recommended (D-III). For children, we recommend administration of ceftriaxone (75–100 mg/kg/d in a single daily iv dose; maximum, 2 g) (B-III) or cefotaxime (150–200 mg/kg/d divided into 3 or 4 iv doses; maximum, 6 g/d) (B-III) for 14–28 days. An alternative is iv penicillin G (200,000–400,000 units/kg/d; maximum, 18–24 million units/d), divided into doses given every 4 h for those with normal renal function (B-III).

For patients who have persistent or recurrent joint swelling after recommended courses of antibiotic therapy, we recommend repeat treatment with another 4-week course of oral antibiotics or with a 2- to 4-week course of iv ceftriaxone (B-III). Clinicians should consider waiting several months before initiating repeat treatment with antimicrobial agents because of the anticipated slow resolution of inflammation after treatment. If patients have persistent arthritis despite 2 courses of oral therapy or one course of iv therapy, symptomatic treatment with nonsteroidal anti-inflammatory agents is recommended; intra-articular steroids may also be of benefit (B-III). If persistent synovitis is associated with significant pain or if it limits function, arthroscopic synovectomy can reduce the period of joint inflammation (B-II).

Late neuroborreliosis affecting the CNS or peripheral nervous system. For patients with late neurological disease affecting the CNS or peripheral nervous system, treatment with ceftriaxone (2 g once a day iv for 2–4 weeks) is recommended (B-II). Alternative parenteral therapy may include administration of cefotaxime (2 g iv every 8 h) (B-II) or iv penicillin G (18–24 million units daily, divided into doses given every 4 h for patients with normal renal function) (B-II). Response to treatment is usually slow and may be incomplete. However, unless relapse is shown by reliable objective measures, repeat treatment is not recommended. For children, a 14–28-day course of treatment with ceftriaxone (75–100 mg/kg/d in a single daily iv dose; maximum, 2 g) is recommended (B-II). An alternative is cefotaxime (150–200 mg/kg/d iv, divided into 3 or 4 doses; maximum, 6 g/d) (B-II). Another alternative is iv penicillin G (200,000–400,000 units/kg/d, divided into doses given every 4 h for those with normal renal function; maximum, 18–24 million units/d) (B-II).

Chronic Lyme disease or post–Lyme disease syndrome. After an episode of Lyme disease that is treated appropriately, some persons have a variety of subjective complaints (such as myalgia,

arthralgia, or fatigue). Some of these patients have been classified as having "chronic Lyme disease" or "post–Lyme disease syndrome," which are poorly defined entities. These patients appear to be a heterogeneous group. Although European patients rarely have been reported to have residual infection with *B. burgdorferi*, this has yet to be convincingly demonstrated either in a large series of appropriately treated European patients or in a study of North American patients.

Randomized controlled studies of treatment of patients who remain unwell after standard courses of antibiotic therapy for Lyme disease are in progress. To date, there are no convincing published data that repeated or prolonged courses of either oral or iv antimicrobial therapy are effective for such patients. The consensus of the Infectious Diseases Society of America (IDSA) expert-panel members is that there is insufficient evidence to regard "chronic Lyme disease" as a separate diagnostic entity.

Objective

The objective of these practice guidelines is to provide clinicians and other health care practitioners with recommendations for management of cases in which either Lyme disease has been diagnosed or the patient was bitten by an *Ixodes* tick in North America (tables 1 and 2) [1]. Lyme disease is endemic in several regions of the United States, particularly areas of the Northeast, Upper Midwest, and Northwest [2]. It is the most frequent vector-borne disease in the United States. Adults and children of both sexes can be affected. These patients are evaluated and treated by general practitioners, pediatricians, and internists, as well as by infectious disease specialists, dermatologists, rheumatologists, neurologists, orthopedists, obstetricians, and ophthalmologists. Because the genospecies of *B. burgdorferi* that cause Lyme disease in North America are different from those that cause Lyme borreliosis in Eurasia, recommendations were based, whenever possible, on studies conducted in the United States.

In the treatment of this disease, as in all infectious diseases, basic medical and scientific principles should be considered. In selecting an antibiotic, there should be evidence of activity in vitro, evidence of penetration into the infected sites, and clinical studies to support the treatment regimen. The reader is referred to other sources for information on diagnostic aspects of Lyme disease [3–9].

Prevention of Tick Bites

The best currently available method for preventing infection with *B. burgdorferi* and other *Ixodes*-transmitted infections is to avoid tick-infested areas [10]. If exposure to *I. scapularis* or *I. pacificus* ticks is unavoidable, a number of measures may help to decrease the risk that ticks will attach and subsequently transmit infection. The use of protective clothing (shirt tucked into pants and pants tucked into socks) may interfere with attachment by ticks by increasing the time required for ticks to find exposed skin, thus facilitating their recognition and removal. By wearing light-colored clothing (to provide a background with which the tick contrasts), persons in areas of endemicity may also be more likely to see (and remove) ticks before they have attached.

Daily inspections of the entire body to locate (and remove) ticks also provide an opportunity to prevent transmission of tick-borne infections [11, 12]. Attached ticks should be removed promptly with fine-toothed forceps, if possible [13]. Tick and insect repellents applied to the skin and clothing provide additional protection [10, 14, 15].

Tick Bites and Prophylaxis

Primary Management Options

For patients who remove attached ticks, we considered the following management options: (1) treating all such persons; (2) treating only persons believed to be at high risk (e.g., those removing a nymphal or adult vector tick [*I. scapularis* or *I. pacificus*] after 48 h of attachment); (3) treating only persons who develop erythema migrans or other clinical signs and symptoms of tick-borne infection; and (4) treating all persons who seroconvert from negativity to positivity (optimally with a 4-fold increase in titer) for serum antibodies to *B. burgdorferi* (acute and follow-up blood specimens from all persons who are bitten would need to be collected and tested for antibodies in paired specimens).

Outcome

The panel weighed both the risks and the consequences of developing Lyme disease (including the risk of late complications) for persons bitten by vector ticks *(I. scapularis* or *I. pacificus)* against the cost and adverse effects of prophylactic antimicrobials. The effect of the different strategies on quality of life was considered. In addition, we considered the effect of the recent licensing of a recombinant OspA vaccine for prevention of Lyme disease [16]. The principal desired outcome is prevention of Lyme disease. Another desired outcome is the prevention of other *Ixodes*-borne illnesses, including babesiosis and HGE. Concurrent infection and disease with these organisms have been described [17–19].

Evidence

Option 1: treating with antimicrobials all persons who remove vector ticks (I. scapularis *or* I. pacificus) *that have become attached.* Although some practitioners routinely treat patients that have been bitten by *I. scapularis* [20], several prospective, randomized double-blind clinical trials involving persons who were bitten by *I. scapularis* ticks and then were treated with placebo, penicillin, tetracycline, or amoxicillin each led to con-

clusions that routine antimicrobial prophylaxis is not warranted [21–23]. A meta-analysis of these studies (in which >600 persons were enrolled) did not indicate that antimicrobial prophylaxis is effective (pooled OR, 0.0; 95% CI, 0.0–1.5; $P = .12$) [24]. The authors of the meta-analysis estimated that if amoxicillin rather than doxycycline were used (to enable small children and pregnant or lactating women to receive prophylaxis), 8 cases of drug-associated rash, including 1 severe life-threatening reaction, would occur for every 10 cases of early Lyme disease that were prevented [24].

In addition, 3 cases of minor amoxicillin-related adverse effects (e.g., diarrhea) would occur for every case of Lyme disease that was prevented. In 2 studies of prophylaxis for tick bites in which adverse effects of the antimicrobials used for prophylaxis were reported, the risk of acquiring Lyme disease after a tick bite was no different than the risk of developing adverse effects from the prophylactic antibiotics [21, 22].

One cost-effectiveness analysis concluded that a 2-week course of doxycycline is indicated when the probability of infection with *B. burgdorferi* after a tick bite is ≥.036 and should be considered when the theoretical probability ranges from .01 to .035 [25]. Many experts, however, disagree with key assumptions in the model. Furthermore, doxycycline is relatively contraindicated for women who are either pregnant or breastfeeding, as well as for children aged <8 years.

Some practitioners prescribe a 10-to-14-day course of amoxicillin for pregnant women who have been bitten by *I. scapularis*, because case reports have suggested that adverse outcomes for the fetus may be associated with pregnancies complicated by Lyme borreliosis [26]. Increasing data from clinical and epidemiological studies, however, suggest that favorable outcomes can be expected when pregnant women with Lyme borreliosis are treated with standard antibiotic regimens [27–29].

In addition to *B. burgdorferi*, other potential pathogens may be present in *I. scapularis* ticks [30, 31]. Babesiosis and HGE can occur independently or together with Lyme disease [17, 18, 32]. Administration of doxycycline is effective in the treatment of patients with HGE [33] but is not recommended as therapy for babesiosis. There are no published clinical data regarding the efficacy of prophylaxis with doxycycline against either of these infections.

Option 2: treating with antimicrobials only persons believed to be at high risk (e.g., those who have removed a nymphal or adult vector tick [I. scapularis *or* I. pacificus] *after 48 h of attachment).* Entomological studies have shown that *B. burgdorferi* is rarely transmitted by *I. scapularis* within the first 48 h of attachment to laboratory animals [11, 12]. This "grace period" is required for spirochetes to migrate from the gut into the salivary glands of infected ticks once feeding commences [34]. Thus, ticks that have been attached for <48 h theoretically cannot transmit *B. burgdorferi* infection. However, this is not true for HGE or babesiosis, since the organisms that cause these diseases are already present in the salivary glands before feeding (D. Fish, unpublished data, and [35]).

The option of treating selectively persons with "high-risk" tick bites to prevent Lyme disease assumes that the species, stage, degree of engorgement, and infection status of the tick, as well as the probability of transmission of infection, can be readily ascertained. This is rarely true. Many different tick species bite humans, and some "ticks" removed from humans are actually spiders, scabs, lice, or dirt and thus pose no risk of Lyme disease [36, 37]. Methods for determining the infection status of ticks removed from patients are experimental and are not standardized. One study found that patients who removed partially engorged ticks that were calculated to have been attached for ≥72 h were significantly more likely to develop *B. burgdorferi* infection than were patients who removed ticks that had been attached for an estimated duration of <72 h (*P* = .008) [37]. However, even if the risk of Lyme disease is increased with partially engorged ticks, no study has demonstrated that antimicrobials are effective in reducing the risk of infection after a tick bite.

Option 3: treating with antimicrobials only persons who develop erythema migrans or other clinical manifestations of Lyme disease or other tick-transmitted diseases. The great majority of persons with *B. burgdorferi* infection present with erythema migrans [16, 38–40]. Since primary erythema migrans lesions occur at the site of a tick bite [41–44], a person who removes a tick would be likely to detect and to seek care for a rash that subsequently develops at that location. Patients who develop fever in the absence of erythema migrans after an *Ixodes* tick bite should be evaluated for HGE and/or babesiosis in areas where these infections are endemic [33, 45, 46].

In a placebo-treated population observed prospectively in a large, multicenter vaccine trial, some volunteers developed serological evidence of asymptomatic *B. burgdorferi* infection [16]. Whether antibiotic therapy is beneficial for such patients is unknown, a question in need of further study. (See next paragraph [option 4] for caveats concerning serological diagnosis.)

Option 4: treating with antimicrobials all persons who seroconvert from negativity to positivity for serum antibodies to B. burgdorferi when acute and follow-up serum samples are tested simultaneously. Although assessment of acute- and convalescent-phase serologies is a standard means of identifying individuals with a variety of infectious diseases, the utility of this approach for identifying infection with *B. burgdorferi* following a tick bite is unknown. Present serological assays for Lyme disease have substantial limitations [3–7], and their use is not recommended for screening of persons lacking objective manifestations of Lyme disease [3, 4, 6, 7].

Recommendations

The best currently available method for preventing infection with *B. burgdorferi* and other *Ixodes*-transmitted infections is to avoid vector tick exposure. If exposure to *I. scapularis* or *I. pacificus* ticks is unavoidable, measures recommended to reduce the risk of infection include using both protective clothing and tick repellents, checking the entire body for ticks daily, and promptly removing attached ticks before transmission of *B. burgdorferi* can occur (A-III).

Routine use of either antimicrobial prophylaxis (E-I) or serological tests (D-III) after a tick bite is not recommended. Some experts recommend antibiotic therapy for patients bitten by *I. scapularis* ticks that are estimated to have been attached for >48 h (on the basis of the degree of engorgement of the tick with blood), in conjunction with epidemiological information regarding the prevalence of tick-transmitted diseases (C-III). However, accurate determinations of tick species and degree of engorgement are not routinely possible, and data are insufficient to demonstrate efficacy of antimicrobials in this setting.

Persons who remove attached ticks should be monitored closely for signs and symptoms of tick-borne diseases for up to 30 days and specifically for the occurrence of a skin lesion at the site of the tick bite (which may suggest Lyme disease) or a temperature >38°C (which may suggest HGE or babesiosis). Persons who develop a skin lesion or other illness within 1 month after removing an attached tick should promptly seek medical attention for assessment of the possibility of having acquired a tick-borne disease (A-II).

Health care practitioners, particularly those in areas where Lyme disease is endemic, should become familiar with the clinical manifestations of and recommended practices for testing and therapy for Lyme disease, as well as for HGE and babesiosis (A-III).

Testing of ticks for tick-borne infectious organisms is not recommended, except in research studies (D-III).

Prior vaccination with the recently licensed recombinant OspA vaccine preparation reduces the risk of developing Lyme disease associated with tick bites but should not alter the above recommendations (A-I).

Early Lyme Disease

Primary Management Options

We considered the following management options for early Lyme disease: oral antimicrobial therapy for early localized infection (i.e., solitary erythema migrans) and oral versus iv therapy for cases of early disseminated infection (i.e., patients presenting with multiple erythema migrans lesions, carditis, cranial-nerve palsy, meningitis, or acute radiculopathy). Borrelial lymphocytoma was not addressed because of its rarity in North America (its primary causative organism, *Borrelia afzelii,* is an exclusively Eurasian genospecies).

Outcome

The panel weighed both the risks and the consequences of developing late complications of Lyme disease and the possible adverse effects of antimicrobial therapy. The desired outcome is to resolve the symptoms and signs of early Lyme disease and to prevent late complications.

Evidence

At least 7 randomized prospective trials have addressed the treatment of early Lyme disease in the United States [47–53]. All studies used erythema migrans as the disease-defining criterion. Six studies recruited patients with either localized or disseminated early Lyme disease [47–52], whereas 1 study required disseminated early disease for enrollment [53]. Differing criteria were used to define treatment success and failure in the various studies. Most studies defined "failure" by the occurrence of objective clinical manifestations, but subjective symptoms were considered evidence of treatment failure in some studies.

The etiology of residual patient complaints after treatment may include an inflammatory response, unrelated to active infection, or alternative disease processes. Failure rates were not considered in the context of background complaints in an otherwise "healthy" population. For example, in a recent random telephone survey collecting self-reported health information, the prevalence of chronic joint symptoms in adults ranged from 12.3% to 22.7% [54]. In a study of adult members in a health maintenance organization in Seattle, ~20% reported fatigue of at least 6 months' duration that interfered with normal activities [55]. Twelve percent of a control group of children without Lyme disease in another study mentioned fatigue as a symptom [56]. In rheumatology practice, a prevalence of 15%–20% for fibromyalgia is common [57]. Nearly 85% of the general population may experience at least 1 somatic symptom in a 6-week period, and 81% of healthy university students and hospital staff members described at least 1 such symptom over a 3-day interval [58, 59]. Thus, the occurrence of arthralgia, myalgia, and fatigue after treatment for early Lyme disease must be evaluated in the context of background complaints for a significant proportion of patients.

In addition, the possibility of coinfection with other pathogens such as *Babesia microti* and the *Ehrlichia* species that causes HGE was not considered in any of the treatment studies of early Lyme disease. In a separate study in an area in which babesiosis is endemic, most patients who had residual complaints after treatment for early Lyme disease had evidence of coinfection with *B. microti* [17]. Specific treatment with antiparasitic agents directed against this microorganism was effective in diminishing symptoms in 1 study [60].

The first randomized clinical trial of treatment of erythema migrans compared erythromycin, tetracycline, and penicillin at dosages of 250 mg 4 times daily for 10 days and included 112 adult patients [47]. Signs and symptoms after treatment were considered to be either "minor" (headache, fatigue, supraventricular tachycardia, arthralgias, brief arthritis of <2 weeks' duration, or isolated facial palsy) or "major" (meningitis, meningoencephalitis, carditis, or recurrent attacks of arthritis). Approximately 15% of patients had transient intensification of symptoms during the first 24 h of therapy, consistent with a Jarisch-Herxheimer reaction. Erythema migrans and its associated symptoms resolved significantly faster in patients treated with penicillin or tetracycline than in patients treated with erythromycin ($P < .05$). In addition, treatment with tetracycline or penicillin was associated with a lower rate of occurrence of "major" manifestations by these criteria, compared with the occurrence rate associated with erythromycin.

Overall, "minor" posttreatment signs and symptoms occurred in ~45% of patients. Extending therapy to 20 days with tetracycline in a subsequent study by the same investigators had no effect on the frequency of posttreatment symptoms [47]. The results of these studies supported the findings of an earlier open trial of oral penicillin therapy [61]. It could be concluded that erythema migrans was responsive to antibiotic treatment but optimal therapy was not defined.

Subsequent small studies found that doxycycline and amoxicillin (plus probenecid), which are the tetracycline and β-lactam preparations most commonly prescribed in current clinical practice for patients with erythema migrans, were effective therapies, and that the efficacies of each drug regimen were similar [48, 49].

A multicenter study that compared cefuroxime axetil (500 mg twice daily for 20 days) with doxycycline (100 mg 3 times daily for 20 days) in 123 patients with erythema migrans demonstrated satisfactory outcomes for ~90% of patients followed for 1 year after treatment [50]. Seventy-one percent of patients in the cefuroxime group and 76% in the doxycycline group were completely cured, whereas 19% and 16% of patients, respectively, had persistent subjective complaints but their conditions improved. Although treatment was considered to have failed for 10% of patients, most of these patients did not have objective evidence of continuing active infection.

A second multicenter study, in which 232 patients with erythema migrans were randomized to receive either cefuroxime or doxycycline for 20 days, confirmed that the 2 drugs had comparable efficacy [51]. Consistent with earlier reports, a Jarisch-Herxheimer–like reaction occurred during the first 24 h of therapy in 12% of patients in each treatment group.

A multicenter, double-blind, randomized prospective trial compared azithromycin (500 mg once daily for 7 days) with amoxicillin (500 mg 3 times daily for 20 days) in the treatment of patients with erythema migrans [52]. Amoxicillin was found to be significantly more effective than azithromycin in resolving the acute manifestations of erythema migrans completely and in preventing relapse within a 6-month period. Of 217 evaluable patients, only 4% of those treated with amoxicillin relapsed,

Table 3. Recommended antimicrobial regimens for treatment of patients with Lyme disease.

Recommendation, drug	Dosage for adults	Dosage for children
Preferred oral		
Amoxicillin	500 mg t.i.d.	50 mg/kg/d divided into 3 doses (maximum, 500 mg/dose)
Doxycycline	100 mg b.i.d.[a]	Age <8 y: not recommended; age ≥8 y: 1–2 mg/kg b.i.d. (maximum, 100 mg/dose)
Alternative oral		
Cefuroxime axetil	500 mg b.i.d.	30 mg/kg/d divided into 2 doses (maximum, 500 mg/dose)
Preferred parenteral		
Ceftriaxone	2 g iv once daily	75–100 mg/kg iv per day in a single dose (maximum, 2 g)
Alternative parenteral		
Cefotaxime	2 g iv t.i.d.	150–200 mg/kg/d iv divided into 3 or 4 doses (maximum, 6 g/d)
Penicillin G	18–24 million units iv/d divided into doses given q4h[b]	200,000–400,000 units/kg/d, divided into doses given q4h[b] (maximum, 18–24 million units/d)

[a] Tetracyclines are relatively contraindicated for pregnant or lactating women.
[b] The penicillin dosage should be reduced for patients with impaired renal function.

compared with 16% of those treated with azithromycin ($P = .005$). A higher symptom score before treatment correlated with persistent symptoms after treatment.

Only 1 study has specifically addressed the treatment of acute disseminated nonneurological Lyme disease. This prospective, randomized multicenter trial revealed that in the absence of clinically apparent CNS involvement, oral doxycycline (100 mg twice daily for 3 weeks) was similar in efficacy to iv ceftriaxone (2 g daily for 2 weeks) [53].

In most of the controlled trials, patients assigned to be treated with either doxycycline or amoxicillin received therapy for ~3 weeks. However, similar success rates have been reported in studies in which 14-day treatment courses with these antibiotics were used [62, 63]. Although none of the prospective studies included pregnant patients, there are no data to suggest that these patients should be treated differently from other patients with Lyme disease, except that tetracycline therapy should be avoided [64].

Several conclusions can be drawn from these trials. Doxycycline, amoxicillin, and cefuroxime axetil are efficacious in the treatment of early Lyme disease. Most patients respond promptly and completely. Some individuals have persistent subjective complaints despite therapy that otherwise appears curative. Less than 10% of infected individuals fail to respond to antibiotic therapy, as evidenced by objective manifestations of persistent infection, and repeat treatment is rarely required. In general, patients who are more systemically ill (e.g., febrile with significant constitutional complaints) at the time of diagnosis take longer to have a complete response to therapy. Coinfection with other tick-borne infections or inadequately recognized CNS infection at the time of institution of antibiotic therapy may be the explanation for antibiotic failures in some circumstances.

Despite excellent activity against B. burgdorferi in vitro [65], the macrolides that have been studied systematically, namely, erythromycin [47] and azithromycin [52] in the United States and roxithromycin [66] in Europe, are less effective than other therapeutic agents (reviewed in [67]). Clarithromycin has not been studied in a controlled trial [68].

All antimicrobials effective in early Lyme disease are associated with a low frequency of serious adverse effects. Drug-induced rashes occur with both amoxicillin [52] and cefuroxime [50, 51]. Doxycycline may cause photosensitivity [50, 51], which may be problematic since early Lyme disease occurs most commonly during the summer months. Individuals treated with doxycycline are advised to avoid exposure to the sun while receiving therapy. In addition, doxycycline is relatively contraindicated for children aged <8 years and for women who are pregnant or breast-feeding.

Cefuroxime axetil is much more expensive than doxycycline or amoxicillin; therefore, its administration is not recommended as first-line therapy (table 3).

In contrast to the second-generation cephalosporin cefuroxime and certain third-generation cephalosporins (e.g., ceftriaxone), first-generation cephalosporins such as cephalexin are inactive in vitro against B. burgdorferi and are ineffective clinically [69, 70].

Available evidence regarding treatment of acute neurological Lyme disease in the United States is based on small case series. Patients with Lyme meningitis or acute radiculopathy respond to iv penicillin [71], although ceftriaxone is more widely used for this indication because of its convenient once-daily dosing [72]. European trials have found iv penicillin to be as effective as cefotaxime or ceftriaxone [73, 74] and cefotaxime to be as effective as ceftriaxone [75]. Doxycycline administered orally or iv has also been used successfully in Europe [76–79], but

Table 4. Recommended therapy for patients with Lyme disease.

Indication	Treatment	Duration, d
Tick bite	None recommended; observe	
Erythema migrans	Oral regimen[a,b]	14–21
Acute neurological disease		
Meningitis or radiculopathy	Parenteral regimen[a,c]	14–28
Cranial-nerve palsy	Oral regimen[a]	14–21
Cardiac disease		
1st or 2d degree heart block	Oral regimen[a]	14–21
3d degree heart block	Parenteral regimen[a,d]	14–21
Late disease		
Arthritis without neurological disease	Oral regimen[a]	28
Recurrent arthritis after oral regimen	Oral regimen[a] or	28
	parenteral regimen[a]	14–28
Persistent arthritis after 2 courses of antibiotics	Symptomatic therapy	
CNS or peripheral nervous system disease	Parenteral regimen[a]	14–28
Chronic Lyme disease or post–Lyme disease syndrome	Symptomatic therapy[e]	

  [a] See table 3.

  [b] For adult patients who are intolerant of amoxicillin, doxycycline, and cefuroxime axetil, alternatives are azithromycin (500 mg orally daily for 7–10 days), erythromycin (500 mg orally 4 times per day for 14–21 days), or clarithromycin (500 mg orally twice daily for 14–21 days [except during pregnancy]). The recommended dosages of these agents for children are as follows: azithromycin, 10 mg/kg daily (maximum, 500 mg/d); erythromycin, 12.5 mg/kg 4 times daily (maximum, 500 mg/dose); clarithromycin, 7.5 mg/kg twice daily (maximum, 500 mg/dose). Patients treated with macrolides should be closely followed.

  [c] For nonpregnant adult patients intolerant of both penicillin and cephalosporins, doxycycline (200–400 mg/d orally [or iv if oral medications cannot be taken], divided into 2 doses) may be adequate.

  [d] A temporary pacemaker may be required.

  [e] See the discussion of Chronic Lyme Disease or Post–Lyme Disease Syndrome in the text.

experience with this agent for the treatment of patients with meningitis due to Lyme disease in the United States is limited.

Cranial-nerve palsy has been treated satisfactorily with oral antibiotics [38, 80]. There was disagreement among panel members, however, on the neurological evaluation of patients with seventh-cranial-nerve palsy. Some members perform a lumbar puncture for all individuals with Lyme disease–associated seventh-cranial-nerve palsy. Others reserve lumbar puncture for those patients for whom there is strong clinical evidence of CNS involvement (e.g., severe headache or nuchal rigidity).

Patients whose CSF examinations yield normal findings may be treated with the same regimens used for patients with erythema migrans, whereas those with clinical and laboratory evidence of CNS involvement should be treated with regimens effective against meningitis. Since the frequency and rate of recovery of seventh-cranial-nerve palsy in patients treated with antibiotics appear to be the same as in untreated patients, the principal goal of therapy is to prevent the development of later clinical manifestations [80].

No studies have specifically addressed the treatment of carditis. Cardiac involvement in North American Lyme disease primarily manifests as atrioventricular heart block and usually occurs within the first several weeks of infection, often in conjunction with erythema migrans [81]. First- and second-degree atrioventricular heart blocks resolve during therapy with oral antibiotics. Because of the potential for life-threatening complications, patients with third-degree atrioventricular heart block should be closely monitored in the hospital. Most panel members treat such patients with iv ceftriaxone, although there is no evidence that parenteral therapy is more effective than

oral therapy. Insertion of a temporary pacemaker may be necessary for patients with third-degree heart block in some circumstances.

Recommendations

Administration of doxycycline (100 mg twice daily) or amoxicillin (500 mg 3 times daily) for 14–21 days is recommended for treatment of early localized or early disseminated Lyme disease associated with erythema migrans, in the absence of neurological involvement or third-degree atrioventricular heart block (tables 3 and 4) (A-I). In prospective studies, these agents have been shown to be effective in the treatment of erythema migrans and associated symptoms.

Doxycycline has the advantage of being efficacious for treatment of HGE, which may occur simultaneously with early Lyme disease. Doxycycline is relatively contraindicated during pregnancy or lactation and for children aged <8 years. Because of its higher cost, cefuroxime axetil, which is as effective as doxycycline in the treatment of erythema migrans (A-I), should be reserved as an alternative agent for those patients who can take neither doxycycline nor amoxicillin. For children, amoxicillin or doxycycline (for those aged ≥8 years) is recommended (tables 3 and 4) (B-II). Cefuroxime axetil is an acceptable alternative agent (B-III).

Administration of macrolide antibiotics is not recommended as first-line therapy for early Lyme disease (E-I). When used, they should be reserved for patients who are intolerant of amoxicillin, doxycycline, and cefuroxime axetil (table 4). Patients treated with macrolides should be closely followed.

Ceftriaxone (2 g iv daily), although effective, is not superior to oral agents and is therefore not recommended for treatment of Lyme disease in the absence of neurological involvement or third-degree atrioventricular heart block (E-I).

The use of ceftriaxone (2 g once daily iv for 14–28 days) in early Lyme disease is recommended for acute neurological disease manifested by meningitis or radiculopathy (tables 3 and 4) (B-II). Parenteral therapy with penicillin G or cefotaxime may be a satisfactory alternative (B-II). For adult patients who are intolerant of both penicillin and cephalosporins, doxycycline (200–400 mg/d in 2 divided doses orally [or iv if the patient is unable to take oral medications]) for 14–28 days may be adequate (B-II).

For children, iv ceftriaxone (B-II) or cefotaxime (B-III) is recommended (tables 3 and 4); penicillin G given iv is an alternative (B-II).

Patients with first- or second-degree atrioventricular heart block associated with early Lyme disease should be treated in the same manner as patients with erythema migrans without carditis (tables 3 and 4) (B-III). We recommend that patients with third-degree atrioventricular heart block be treated with parenteral antibiotics such as ceftriaxone (table 3) in the hospital, although there are no clinical trial data to support this recommendation (B-III). A temporary pacemaker may also be required.

Although antibiotic treatment does not hasten the resolution of seventh-cranial-nerve palsy associated with *B. burgdorferi* infection, antibiotics should be given to prevent further sequelae (B-II). There was disagreement among panel members on the neurological evaluation of patients with seventh-cranial-nerve palsy. Some members perform a CSF examination of all patients with seventh-cranial-nerve palsy, whereas others reserve lumbar puncture for those in whom there is strong clinical evidence of CNS involvement (e.g., severe headache or nuchal rigidity).

Patients whose CSF examinations yield normal findings may be treated with the same regimens used for patients with erythema migrans (B-III). Those with clinical and laboratory evidence of CNS involvement should be treated with regimens effective against meningitis (tables 3 and 4) (B-II).

Treatment for pregnant patients can be identical to that for nonpregnant patients with the same disease manifestation, except that tetracyclines should be avoided (B-III).

Late Lyme Disease

Options

The panel considered various oral and parenteral antimicrobial regimens for treatment of the late manifestations of Lyme disease. Late manifestations include arthritis (oligoarticular), encephalopathy (characterized primarily by memory deficit, irritability, and somnolence), and neuropathy (manifested primarily by distal paresthesias or radicular pain). Acrodermatitis

chronica atrophicans was not addressed because of its rarity in North America (its primary causative organism, *B. afzelii,* is an exclusively Eurasian genospecies). Because of the lack of evaluable data on ophthalmologic complications, which are very rare, the panel was unable to make recommendations concerning keratitis and other possible ocular manifestations of Lyme disease.

The response to treatment of late manifestations is typically slow, and improvement or resolution of symptoms may take weeks or months. However, appropriate antibiotic treatment results in eventual recovery in most patients.

Outcome

The panel compared the risks and consequences of ineffective treatment of late Lyme disease with the problems resulting from adverse effects of antimicrobial therapies. The desired outcome is to treat effectively the late complications of Lyme disease while minimizing the adverse effects of antibiotic therapy. It has not been shown nor is it anticipated that *B. burgdorferi* will develop resistance to antibiotics, but the indiscriminate use of antibiotics exacerbates the problem of antibiotic-resistant community-acquired infections with other bacteria.

Evidence

The first study of antibiotic treatment in patients with Lyme arthritis was initiated in 1980 [82]. The regimens tested were those used for the treatment of tertiary syphilis, and the study design was a double-blind, placebo-controlled trial. The patients had intermittent or chronic Lyme arthritis primarily affecting the knees, and all patients were subsequently shown to be seropositive for antibodies to *B. burgdorferi*. In the first phase of the study, 40 patients were randomized to receive im benzathine penicillin G (7.2 million units) or placebo. In the second phase, 20 patients were treated with iv penicillin G (20 million units per day for 10 days). Of the 20 patients who received im benzathine penicillin, 7 (35%) had complete resolution of joint involvement soon after treatment, compared with none of 20 patients who were given placebo ($P < 0.02$). Of the 20 patients treated the following year with iv penicillin G, 11 (55%) had complete resolution of the arthritis soon after treatment. It was concluded that parenteral penicillin was often effective in the treatment of Lyme arthritis, but a number of patients failed to respond.

Subsequently, a series of studies was begun to test the efficacy of iv ceftriaxone in the treatment of late Lyme disease. In comparison with penicillin, the advantages of ceftriaxone are its excellent CSF penetration and long serum half-life, which permits once-a-day dosing for outpatient management. In 1987, a case series of 7 patients with Lyme arthritis or chronic neuroborreliosis, who were refractory to oral or iv penicillin therapy, were then treated with iv ceftriaxone (2 or 4 g/d for 2 weeks) [83]. All 5 patients who had arthritis responded to ceftriaxone therapy, and for 5 of the 6 patients with limb paresthesias, a reduction in symptoms and improvement of nerve-conduction study findings were noted.

In a follow-up study, 23 patients with Lyme arthritis or late neuroborreliosis were randomly assigned to receive penicillin (20 million units per day iv for 10 days) or ceftriaxone (4 g/d iv for 14 days) [84]. Of the 13 patients who received ceftriaxone, none had objective evidence of persistent disease after treatment, although 3 had mild arthralgias and 1 complained of fatigue and memory difficulty. In contrast, 5 of the 10 patients who received iv penicillin continued to have fatigue, memory deficit, or recurrent oligoarthritis. For 4 of these 5 patients, symptoms resolved after repeat treatment with ceftriaxone.

In a subsequent study, 31 patients with Lyme arthritis or chronic neuroborreliosis were randomly assigned to receive 2 or 4 g/d of ceftriaxone for 2 weeks [84]. After treatment, 3 of the 31 patients had persistent encephalopathy, 2 had persistent neuropathy, and 3 had no diminishment of their arthritis. The overall frequency of persistent symptoms among patients was 13%, which was similar in both treatment groups. In an open-label, randomized, multicenter study, 143 evaluable patients with manifestations of late Lyme disease, primarily Lyme arthritis, were treated with iv ceftriaxone (2 g/d for either 2 or 4 weeks) [85]. In 76% of those treated for 2 weeks and 70% of those treated for 4 weeks, symptoms resolved after treatment (the *P* value was not significant). The most common persistent symptoms were arthralgia, pain, weakness, malaise, and fatigue.

The principal conclusions of these 2 studies were that the efficacy of iv ceftriaxone at a dosage of 2 g/d was equivalent to that at a dosage of 4 g/d, and a 2-week course was as efficacious as a 4-week course for the treatment of late Lyme disease. However, some patients had persistent symptoms despite ceftriaxone treatment.

At the same time that studies were being carried out to assess parenteral antibiotic regimens, oral therapy was also found to be effective in the treatment of patients with Lyme arthritis. In 1983 and 1984, 14 children with Lyme arthritis were treated orally with either phenoxymethyl penicillin or tetracycline for 10–30 days [86]. Thirteen experienced no further attacks of arthritis at follow-up at 4–24 months after treatment, whereas 1 patient's symptoms did not resolve until after a 10-day course of iv penicillin.

From 1986 through 1991, 48 adult and pediatric patients with Lyme arthritis were randomly assigned to receive either doxycycline (100 mg orally twice a day) or amoxicillin and probenecid (500 mg of each 4 times a day), in each instance for 30 days [87]. Eighteen of the 20 evaluable patients treated with doxycycline and 16 of the 18 evaluable patients who completed the amoxicillin regimen had resolution of arthritis within 13 months after enrollment in the study. However, neuroborreliosis later developed in 5 patients, 4 of whom were treated with the amoxicillin/probenecid regimen. The concomitant use of pro-benecid with amoxicillin may be inadvisable, because probenecid may impair penetration of β-lactam antibiotics into brain parenchyma [72, 88].

In retrospect, it was noted that all 5 patients reported subtle distal paresthesias or memory impairment at the time of enrollment. It was concluded that patients with Lyme arthritis can usually be treated successfully with oral antibiotics, but practitioners must be aware of subtle neurological symptoms that may require treatment with iv antibiotics.

In a cost-effectiveness analysis, iv therapy was found to be no more cost-effective than oral therapy for patients with Lyme arthritis; iv therapy was more likely to result in serious complications and was substantially more expensive [89]. Therefore, the authors concluded that oral antibiotics are to be preferred in the initial treatment of Lyme arthritis in the absence of concomitant neurological involvement.

Not all patients with Lyme arthritis respond to antibiotic therapy. In 1 treatment trial, none of the 16 patients with Lyme arthritis who were treated with iv ceftriaxone (2 g daily for 2 weeks) had resolution of arthritis within 3 months after completion of therapy [87]. That study's enrollment requirement of continuous joint swelling for at least 3 months despite treatment with other recommended parenteral or oral antibiotic regimens differed from requirements in previous studies.

These 16 patients were also found to have distinctive immunogenetic and immune markers, including a high frequency of human leukocyte antigen–DR4 specificity and of antibody reactivity with OspA of the spirochete. More recent data based on PCR testing of serial joint fluid samples suggest that arthritis may persist in a small number of patients despite eradication of the spirochete [90]. The observation that there are epitopes of OspA that cross-react with human leukocyte function–associated antigen-1 [91] suggests that immune phenomena might explain the persistent joint inflammation in these cases.

Arthroscopic synovectomy has been used successfully in the treatment of patients whose arthritis persists despite antibiotic therapy. Of 20 patients who underwent this procedure for refractory chronic Lyme arthritis of the knee, 16 (80%) had resolution of joint inflammation during the first month following surgery or soon thereafter [92]. The remaining 4 patients (20%) had persistent or recurrent synovitis.

Patients with late Lyme disease associated with prominent neurological features also respond to antibiotic therapy. In trials conducted from 1987 through 1989, 27 adult patients with Lyme encephalopathy, polyneuropathy, or both were treated with iv ceftriaxone (2 g/d for 2 weeks) [93]. In addition to clinical signs and symptoms, outcome measures included CSF analyses and neuropsychological tests of memory. Response to therapy was usually gradual and did not begin until several months after treatment. When response was measured 6 months after treatment, 17 patients (63%) had uncomplicated improvement, 6 (22%) had improvement but then relapsed, and 4 (15%) had no change in their condition.

In a subsequent study, the same investigators treated 18 adult patients with Lyme encephalopathy with iv ceftriaxone (2 g/d for 30 days) [94]. Of the 18 patients, 16 had abnormal verbal or visual memory scores on neuropsychological tests and 16 had CSF abnormalities, most commonly production of intrathecal antibody to *B. burgdorferi* or an elevated total protein level. As determined 6 months after treatment, 14 (93%) of the 15 patients examined had diminished symptoms, and verbal memory scores for the 15 patients were significantly improved (*P* < .01). The total CSF protein values were significantly less for the 10 patients who had follow-up analyses (*P* < .05). At 12–24 months, all patients' conditions were back to normal or improved (1 of the 18 patients was given repeat treatment after 8 months).

It was concluded that Lyme encephalopathy may be associated with active infection of the nervous system and that the infection in most patients can be treated successfully with a 30-day course of iv ceftriaxone. Whether a 30-day course is superior to 14 days of treatment is unclear. Although the data are much more limited, the conditions of children with neurocognitive abnormalities attributed to Lyme disease also appear to improve after 2–4 weeks of iv ceftriaxone [95].

The third-generation cephalosporin cefotaxime has been tested in Europe and has been found to be effective in the treatment of late Lyme disease [96]. Although cefotaxime has to be administered 3–4 times daily (compared with once daily administration of ceftriaxone), it does not cause the biliary complications that have been associated with ceftriaxone therapy [97].

Recommendations

Lyme arthritis. Lyme arthritis can usually be treated successfully with antimicrobial agents administered orally or iv (tables 3 and 4). Administration of doxycycline or amoxicillin, in each instance for 28 days, is recommended for patients without clinical evidence of neurological disease (B-II). For children, doxycycline (for those aged ≥8 years) or amoxicillin is recommended (tables 3 and 4) (B-II). Oral therapy is easier to administer than iv antibiotics, is associated with fewer serious complications, and is considerably less expensive. Its disadvantage is that some patients treated with oral agents have subsequently manifested overt neuroborreliosis, which may require iv therapy for successful treatment. Further controlled trials are needed to compare oral with iv therapy.

Neurological evaluation, including lumbar puncture, should be done for patients for whom there is a strong clinical suspicion of neurological involvement. Patients with arthritis and objective evidence of neurological disease should receive parenteral therapy with ceftriaxone (tables 3 and 4) (A-II). Alternative parenteral agents include cefotaxime (B-III) and penicillin G (B-II). The long-acting benzathine preparation of penicillin achieves only low levels in the blood and therefore is not recommended (D-III). For children, ceftriaxone iv (B-III) or cefotaxime (B-III) is recommended (tables 3 and 4); penicillin G administered iv is an alternative (B-III).

For patients who have persistent or recurrent joint swelling after recommended courses of antibiotic therapy, we recommend repeat treatment with another 4-week course of oral antibiotics or with a 2- to 4-week course of ceftriaxone iv (tables 3 and 4) (B-III). Clinicians should consider waiting several months before initiating repeat treatment with antimicrobial agents, because of the anticipated slow resolution of inflammation after treatment. If patients have persistent arthritis despite 2 courses of oral therapy or 1 course of iv therapy, symptomatic treatment with nonsteroidal anti-inflammatory agents is recommended; intra-articular steroids may also be of benefit (B-III). If persistent synovitis is associated with significant pain or if it limits function, arthroscopic synovectomy can reduce the period of joint inflammation (B-II).

Late neuroborreliosis affecting the CNS or the peripheral nervous system. For patients with late neurological disease affecting the CNS or peripheral nervous system, treatment with ceftriaxone (2 g once a day iv for 2–4 weeks) is recommended (tables 3 and 4) (B-II). Alternative parenteral therapy may include administration of cefotaxime (B-II) or penicillin G (B-II). Response to treatment is usually slow and may be incomplete. However, unless relapse is shown by reliable objective measures, repeat treatment is not recommended. For children, treatment with ceftriaxone is recommended (tables 3 and 4) (B-II). Cefotaxime or penicillin G administered iv are alternatives (B-II).

Chronic Lyme Disease or Post–Lyme Disease Syndrome

Following an episode of Lyme disease that is treated appropriately, some persons have a variety of subjective complaints (such as myalgia, arthralgia, or fatigue). Some of these patients have been classified as having "chronic Lyme disease" or "post–Lyme disease syndrome," which are poorly defined entities. These patients appear to be a heterogeneous group. Although European patients rarely have been reported to have residual infection (or perhaps reinfection) with *B. burgdorferi* [98], this has yet to be substantiated either in a large series of appropriately treated European patients or in a study of North American patients. Residual subjective symptoms that last weeks or months also may persist after other medical diseases (both infectious and noninfectious). It has also been recognized that the prevalence of fatigue and/or arthralgias in the general population is >10% [52–56, 58, 59, 99].

In areas of endemicity, coinfection with *B. microti* or the *Ehrlichia* species that causes HGE may explain persistent symptoms for a small number of these patients [17, 19]. Randomized controlled studies of treatment of patients who remain unwell after standard courses of antibiotic therapy for Lyme disease are in progress. To date, there are no convincing published data showing that repeated or prolonged courses of oral or iv antimicrobial therapy are effective for such patients. The consensus of the IDSA expert-panel members is that there is insufficient evidence to regard "chronic Lyme disease" as a separate diagnostic entity.

Acknowledgments

We thank Drs. Peter Gross, John Nowakowski, Karl Li, and José Munoz for helpful comments, as well as Betty Bosler, Eleanor Bramesco, and Lisa Giarratano for assistance.

References

1. Gross PA, Barrett TL, Dellinger EP, et al. Purpose of quality standards for infectious diseases. Clin Infect Dis 1994;18:421.
2. Centers for Disease Control and Prevention. Recommendations for the use of Lyme disease vaccine: recommendations of the Advisory Committee on Immunization Practices (ACIP). MMWR Morb Mortal Wkly Rep 1999;48:1–25.
3. Brown SL, Hansen SL, Langone JJ. Role of serology in the diagnosis of Lyme disease. JAMA 1999;282:62–6.
4. Wormser GP, Aguero-Rosenfeld ME, Nadelman RB. Lyme disease serology: problems and opportunities. JAMA 1999;282:79–80.
5. Aguero-Rosenfeld ME, Roberge J, Carbonaro CA, Nowakowski J, Nadelman RB, Wormser GP. Effects of Osp A vaccination on Lyme disease serologic testing. J Clin Microbiol 1999;37:3718–21.
6. American College of Physicians. Guidelines for laboratory evaluation in the diagnosis of Lyme disease. Ann Intern Med 1997;127:1106–8.
7. Tugwell P, Dennis DT, Weinstein A. et al. Clinical guideline. II. Laboratory evaluation in the diagnosis of Lyme disease. Ann Intern Med 1997;127:1109–23.
8. Halperin JJ. Logigian EL, Finkel MF, Pearl RA. Practice parameters for the diagnosis of patients with nervous system Lyme borreliosis (Lyme disease). Neurology 1996;46:619–27.
9. Nadelman RB, Wormser GP. Erythema migrans and early Lyme disease. Am J Med 1995;98(Suppl 4A):15S–24S.
10. Fishbein DB, Dennis DT. Tick-borne diseases—a growing risk. N Engl J Med 1995;333:452–3.
11. Piesman J, Mather TN, Sinsky RJ, Spielman A. Duration of tick attachment and Borrelia burgdorferi transmission. J Clin Microbiol 1987;25:557–8.
12. Piesman J, Maupin GO, Campos EG, Happ CM. Duration of adult female Ixodes dammini attachment and transmission of Borrelia burgdorferi with description of a needle aspiration isolation method. J Infect Dis 1991;163:895–7.
13. Needham GR. Evaluation of 5 popular methods for tick removal. Pediatrics 1985;75:997–1002.
14. Fradin MS. Mosquitoes and mosquito repellents: a clinician's guide. Ann Intern Med 1998;128:931–40.
15. US Environmental Protection Agency, Office of Pesticide Programs. Using insect repellents safely. Publication EPA-735/F-93-052R. Washington, DC: US Environmental Protection Agency, 1996.
16. Steere AC, Sikand VK, Meurice F, et al. Vaccination against Lyme disease with recombinant Borrelia burgdorferi outer-surface lipoprotein A with adjuvant. N Engl J Med 1998;339:209–15.
17. Krause PJ, Telford SR III, Spielman A, et al. Concurrent Lyme disease and babesiosis: evidence for increased severity and duration of illness. JAMA 1996;275:1657–60.
18. Nadelman RB, Horowitz HW, Hsieh T-C, et al. Simultaneous human ehrlichiosis and Lyme borreliosis. N Engl J Med 1997;337:27–30.
19. Duffy J, Pittlekow MR, Kolbert CP, Ruttledge BJ, Persing DH. Coinfection with Borrelia burgdorferi and the agent of human granulocytic ehrlichiosis. Lancet 1997;349:399.
20. Fix AD, Strickland GT, Grant J. Tick bites and Lyme disease in an endemic setting: problematic use of serologic testing and prophylactic antibiotic therapy. JAMA 1998;279:206–10.
21. Costello CM, Steere AC, Pinkerton RE, Feder HM Jr. A prospective study of tick bites in an endemic area for Lyme disease. J Infect Dis 1989;159:136–9.
22. Shapiro ED, Gerber MA, Holabird ND, et al. A controlled trial of antimicrobial prophylaxis for Lyme disease after deer-tick bites. N Engl J Med 1992;327:1769–73.
23. Agre F, Schwartz R. The value of early treatment of deer tick bite for the prevention of Lyme disease. Am J Dis Child 1993;147:945–7.
24. Warshafsky S, Nowakowski J, Nadelman RB, Kamer RS, Peterson SJ, Wormser GP. Efficacy of antibiotic prophylaxis for prevention of Lyme disease. J Gen Intern Med 1996;11:329–33.
25. Magid D, Schwartz B, Craft J, Schwartz JS. Prevention of Lyme disease after tick bites: a cost effectiveness analysis. N Engl J Med 1992;327:534–41.
26. Schlesinger PA, Duray PH, Burke SA, Steere AC, Stillman MT. Maternal-fetal transmission of the Lyme disease spirochete, Borrelia burgdorferi. Ann Intern Med 1985;103:67–8.
27. Maraspin V. Cimperman J, Lotric-Furlan S, Pleterski-Rigler D, Strle F. Treatment of erythema migrans in pregnancy. Clin Infect Dis 1996;22:788–93.
28. Williams CL, Strobino B, Weinstein A, Spierling P, Medici F. Maternal Lyme disease and congenital malformation: a cord blood serosurvey in endemic and control areas. Paediatr Perinat Epidemiol 1995;9:320–30.
29. Strobino BA, Williams CL, Abid S, Chalson R, Spierling P. Lyme disease and pregnancy outcome: a prospective study of 2000 prenatal patients. Am J Obstet Gynecol 1993;169:367–74.
30. Spielman A, Wilson ML, Levine JF. Piesman J. Ecology of Ixodes dammini–borne human babesiosis and Lyme disease. Annu Rev Entomol 1985;30:439–60.
31. Telford SR III. Dawson JE, Katavalos P, Warner CK, Kolbert CP, Persing DH. Perpetuation of the agent of human granulocytic ehrlichiosis in a deer tick-rodent cycle. Proc Natl Acad Sci USA 1996;93:6209–14.
32. Piesman J, Hicks TC, Sinsky RJ. Obin G. Simultaneous transmission of Borrelia burgdorferi and Babesia microti by individual nymphal Ixodes dammini ticks. J Clin Microbiol 1987;25:2012–3.
33. Bakken JS, Krueth J, Wilson-Nordskog C, Tilden RL, Asanovich K, Dumler JS. Clinical and laboratory characteristics of human granulocytic ehrlichiosis. JAMA 1996;275:199–205.
34. Ribeiro JM, Mather TN, Piesman J, Spielman A. Dissemination and salivary delivery of Lyme disease spirochetes in vector ticks (Acari: Ixodidae). J Med Entomol 1987;24:201–5.
35. Piesman J, Lewengrub S, Rudzinska MA, Spielman A. Babesia microti: prolonged survival of salavarian piroplasms in nymphal Ixodes dammini. Exp Parasitol 1987;64:292–9.
36. Saltzman MB, Rubin LG, Sood SK. Prevention of Lyme disease after tick bites [letter]. N Engl J Med 1993;328:137.
37. Sood SK, Salzman MB, Johnson BJB, et al. Duration of tick attachment as a predictor of the risk of Lyme disease in an area in which Lyme disease is endemic. J Infect Dis 1997;175:996–9.
38. Steere AC. Lyme disease. N Engl J Med 1989;321:586–96.
39. Gerber MA, Shapiro ED, Burke GS, et al. Lyme disease in children in southeastern Connecticut. N Engl J Med 1996;335:1270–4.
40. Wormser GP, McKenna D, Nadelman RB, Nowakowski J, Weinstein A. Lyme disease in children [letter]. N Engl J Med 1997;336:1107.
41. Berger BW. Dermatologic manifestations of Lyme disease. Rev Infect Dis 1989;11:S1475–81.
42. Nadelman RB, Nowakowski J, Forseter G, et al. The clinical spectrum of early Lyme borreliosis in patients with culture positive erythema migrans. Am J Med 1996;100:502–8.

43. Melski JW, Reed KD, Mitchell PD, Barth GD. Primary and secondary erythema migrans in central Wisconsin. Arch Dermatol 1993;129:709–16.

44. Steere AC, Bartenhagen NH, Craft JE, et al. The early clinical manifestations of Lyme disease. Ann Intern Med 1983;99:76–82.

45. Aguero-Rosenfeld ME, Horowitz HW, Wormser GP, et al. Human granulocytic ehrlichiosis: a case series from a single medical center in New York State. Ann Intern Med 1996;125:904–8.

46. White DJ, Talarico J, Chang H-G, Birkhead GS, Heimberger T, Morse DL. Human babesiosis in New York State: review of 139 hospitalized cases and analysis of prognostic factors. Arch Intern Med 1998;158:2149–54.

47. Steere AC, Hutchinson GJ, Rahn DW, et al. Treatment of early manifestations of Lyme disease. Ann Intern Med 1983;99:22–6.

48. Dattwyler RJ, Volkman DJ, Conaty SM, Platkin SP, Luft BJ. Amoxicillin plus probenecid versus doxycycline for treatment of erythema migrans borreliosis. Lancet 1990;336:1404–6.

49. Massarotti EM, Luger SW, Rahn DW, et al. Treatment of early Lyme disease. Am J Med 1992;92:396–403.

50. Nadelman RB, Luger SW, Frank E, et al. Comparison of cefuroxime axetil and doxycycline in the treatment of early Lyme disease. Ann Intern Med 1992;117:273–80.

51. Luger SW, Paparone P, Wormser GP, et al. Comparison of cefuroxime axetil and doxycycline in treatment of patients with early Lyme disease associated with erythema migrans. Antimicrob Agents Chemother 1995:39:661–7.

52. Luft BJ, Dattwyler RJ, Johnson RC, et al. Azithromycin compared with amoxicillin in the treatment of erythema migrans: a double-blind, randomized, controlled trial. Ann Intern Med 1996;124:785–91.

53. Dattwyler RJ, Luft BJ, Kunkel M, et al. Ceftriaxone compared with doxycycline for the treatment of acute disseminated Lyme disease. N Engl J Med 1997;337:289–94.

54. Centers for Disease Control and Prevention. Prevalence and impact of chronic joint symptoms: 7 states, 1996. MMWR Morb Mortal Wkly Rep 1998;47:345–51.

55. Buchwald D, Umali P, Umali J, Kith P, Pearlman T, Komaroff AL. Chronic fatigue and the chronic fatigue syndrome: prevalence in a Pacific Northwest Health Care System. Ann Intern Med 1995;123:81–8.

56. Wang TJ, Sangha O, Phillips CB, et al. Outcomes of children treated for Lyme disease. J Rheumatol 1998;25:2249–53.

57. Wolfe F, Cathey MA. Prevalence of primary and secondary fibrositis. J Rheum 1983;10:965–8.

58. Reidenberg MM, Lowenthal DT. Adverse nondrug reactions. N Engl J Med 1968;279:678–9.

59. Verbrugge LM, Ascione FJ. Exploring the iceberg. Common symptoms and how people care for them. Med Care 1987:25:539–69.

60. Krause PJ, Spielman A, Telford SR III, et al. Persistent parasitemia after acute babesiosis. N Engl J Med 1998;339:160–5.

61. Steere AC, Malawista SE, Newman JH, Spieler PN, Bartenhagen NH. Antibiotic therapy in Lyme disease. Ann Intern Med 1980;93:1–8.

62. Nowakowski J, McKenna D, Nadelman RB, et al. Two weeks' therapy with doxycycline or amoxicillin to treat patients with culture-proven erythema migrans [abstract 383]. In: Program and abstracts of the 8th International Conference on Lyme Borreliosis and Other Emerging Tick-borne Diseases (Munich), 20–24 June 1999.

63. Nowakowski J, Nadelman RB, Forseter G, McKenna D, Wormser GP. Doxycycline versus tetracycline therapy for Lyme disease associated with erythema migrans. J Am Acad Dermatol 1995;32:223–7.

64. Treatment of Lyme disease. Med Lett Drugs Ther1992;34:95–7.

65. Dever LL, Jorgensen JH, Barbour AG. Comparative in vitro activities of clarithromycin, azithromycin, and erythromycin against Borrelia burgdorferi. Antimicrob Agents Chemother 1993;37:1704–6.

66. Hansen K, Hovmark A, Lebech A-M, et al. Roxithromycin in Lyme borreliosis: discrepant results of an in vitro and in vivo animal susceptibility study and a clinical trial in patients with erythema migrans. Acta Derm Venereol 1992;72:297–300.

67. Wormser GP. Lyme disease: insights into the use of antimicrobials for prevention and treatment in the context of experience with other spirochetal infections. Mt Sinai J Med 1995;62:188–95.

68. Dattwyler RJ, Grunwaldt E, Luft BJ. Clarithromycin in treatment of early Lyme disease: a pilot study. Antimicrob Agents Chemother 1996;40:468–9.

69. Nowakowski J, McKenna D, Nadelman RB, Cooper D, Bittker S, Holmgren D, Pavia C, Johnson RC, Wormser GP. Failure of treatment with cephalexin for Lyme disease. Arch Fam Med 2000;9:563–7.

70. Agger WA, Callister SM, Jobe DA. In vitro susceptibilities of Borrelia burgdorferi to 5 oral cephalosporins and ceftriaxone. Antimicrob Agents Chemother 1992;36:1788–90.

71. Steere AC, Pachner AR, Malawista SE. Neurologic abnormalities of Lyme disease: successful treatment with high-dose intravenous penicillin. Ann Intern Med 1983;99:767–72.

72. Wormser GP. Treatment and prevention of Lyme disease, with emphasis on antimicrobial therapy for neuroborreliosis and vaccination. Semin Neurol 1997;17:45–52.

73. Pfister HW, PreacMursic V, Wilske B, Einhaupl KM. Cefotaxime vs penicillin G for acute neurologic manifestations in Lyme borreliosis: a prospective randomized study. Arch Neurol 1989;46:1190–4.

74. Mullegger RR, Millner MM, Stanek G, Spork KD. Penicillin G sodium and ceftriaxone in the treatment of neuroborreliosis in children: a prospective study. Infection 1991;19:279–83.

75. Pfister H-W, Preac-Mursic V, Wilske B, Schielke E, Sorgel F, Einhaupl KM. Randomized comparison of ceftriaxone and cefotaxime in Lyme neuroborreliosis. J Infect Dis 1991;163:311–8.

76. Dotevall L, Alestig K, Hanner P, Norkrans G, Hagberg L. The use of doxycycline in nervous system Borrelia burgdorferi infection. Scand J Infect Dis Suppl 1988;53:74–9.

77. Dotevall L, Hagberg L. Successful oral doxycycline treatment of Lyme disease–associated facial palsy and meningitis. Clin Infect Dis 1999;28:569–74.

78. Karlsson M, Hammers-Berggren S, Lindquist L, Stiernstedt G, Svenungsson B. Comparison of intravenous penicillin G and oral doxycycline for treatment of Lyme neuroborreliosis. Neurology 1994;44:1203–7.

79. Kohlhepp W, Oschmann P, Mertens H-G. Treatment of Lyme borreliosis: randomized comparison of doxycycline and penicillin G. J Neurol 1989;236:464–9.

80. Clark JR, Carlson RD, Sasaki CT, Pachies AR, Steere AC. Facial paralysis in Lyme disease. Laryngoscope 1985;95:1341–5.

81. Steere AC, Batsford WP, Weinberg M, et al. Lyme carditis: cardiac abnormalities of Lyme disease. Ann Intern Med 1980;93:8–16.

82. Steere AC, Green J, Schoen RT, et al. Successful parenteral penicillin therapy of established Lyme arthritis. N Engl J Med 1985;312:869–74.

83. Dattwyler RJ, Halperin JJ, Pass H, Luft BJ. Ceftriaxone as effective therapy for refractory Lyme disease. J Infect Dis 1987;155:1322–5.

84. Dattwyler RJ, Halperin JJ, Volkman DJ, Luft BJ. Treatment of late Lyme borreliosis: randomized comparison of ceftriaxone and penicillin. Lancet 1988;1:1191–4.

85. Dattwyler RJ, Luft BJ, Maladorno D, et al. Treatment of late Lyme disease—a comparison of 2 weeks vs. 4 weeks of ceftriaxone [abstract 662]. In: Proceedings of the 7th International Congress on Lyme Borreliosis (San Francisco), 16–21 June 1996.

86. Eichenfield AH, Goldsmith DP, Benach JL, et al. Childhood Lyme arthritis: experience in an endemic area. J Pediatr 1986;109:753–8.

87. Steere AC, Levin RE, Molloy PJ, et al. Treatment of Lyme arthritis. Arthritis Rheum 1994;37:878–88.

88. Fishman RA. Blood-brain and CSF barriers to penicillin and related organic acids. Arch Neurol 1966;15:113–24.

89. Eckman MH, Steere AC, Kalish RA, Pauker SG. Cost effectiveness of oral as compared with intravenous antibiotic treatment for patients with early Lyme disease or Lyme arthritis. N Engl J Med 1997;337:357–63.

90. Nocton JJ, Dressler F, Rutledge BJ, Rys PN, Persing DH, Steere AC. De-

tection of *Borrelia burgdorferi* by polymerase chain reaction in synovial fluid from patients with Lyme arthritis. N Engl J Med **1994**;330:229–34.

91. Gross DM, Forsthuber T, Tary-Lehmann M, et al. Identification of LFA-1 as a candidate autoantigen in treatment resistant Lyme arthritis. Science **1998**;281:703–6.

92. Schoen RT, Aversa JM, Rahn DW, Steere AC. Treatment of refractory chronic Lyme arthritis with arthroscopic synovectomy. Arthritis Rheum **1991**;34: 1056–60.

93. Logigian EL, Kaplan RF, Steere AC. Chronic neurologic manifestations of Lyme disease. N Engl J Med **1990**;323:1438–44.

94. Logigian EL, Kaplan RF, Steere AC. Successful treatment of Lyme encephalopathy with intravenous ceftriaxone. J Infect Dis **1999**;180:377–83.

95. Bloom BJ, Wyckoff PM, Meissner HC, Steere AC. Neurocognitive abnor-

malities in children after classic manifestations of Lyme disease. Pediatr Infect Dis J **1998**;17:189–96.

96. Hassler D, Zoller L, Haude A, Hufnagel HD, Heinrich F, Sonntag HG. Cefotaxime versus penicillin in the late stage of Lyme disease: prospective, randomized therapeutic approach. Infection **1990**;18:16–20.

97. Ettestad PJ, Campbell GL, Welbel SF, et al. Biliary complications in the treatment of unsubstantiated Lyme disease. J Infect Dis **1995**;171:356–61.

98. Preac-Mursic V, Weber K, Pfister HW, et al. Survival of *Borrelia burgdorferi* in antibiotically treated patients with Lyme borreliosis. Infection **1989**; 17:355–9.

99. Chen MK. The epidemiology of self-perceived fatigue among adults. Prev Med **1986**;15:74–81.

The Management of Minor Closed Head Injury in Children

• *Clinical Practice Guideline*
• *Technical Report Summary*

Readers of this clinical practice guideline are urged to review the technical report to enhance the evidence-based decision-making process. The full technical report is available on the enclosed CD-ROM.

AMERICAN ACADEMY OF PEDIATRICS

The Management of Minor Closed Head Injury in Children

Committee on Quality Improvement, American Academy of Pediatrics

Commission on Clinical Policies and Research, American Academy of Family Physicians

ABSTRACT. The American Academy of Pediatrics (AAP) and its Committee on Quality Improvement in collaboration with the American Academy of Family Physicians (AAFP) and its Commission on Clinical Policies and Research, and in conjunction with experts in neurology, emergency medicine and critical care, research methodologists, and practicing physicians have developed this practice parameter. This parameter provides recommendations for the management of a previously neurologically healthy child with a minor closed head injury who, at the time of injury, may have experienced temporary loss of consciousness, experienced an impact seizure, vomited, or experienced other signs and symptoms. These recommendations derive from a thorough review of the literature and expert consensus. The methods and results of the literature review and data analyses including evidence tables can be found in the technical report. This practice parameter is not intended as a sole source of guidance for the management of children with minor closed head injuries. Rather, it is designed to assist physicians by providing an analytic framework for the evaluation and management of this condition. It is not intended to replace clinical judgment or establish a protocol for all patients with a minor head injury, and rarely will provide the only appropriate approach to the problem.

The practice parameter, "The Management of Minor Closed Head Injury in Children," was reviewed by the AAFP Commission on Clinical Policies and Research and individuals appointed by the AAFP and appropriate committees and sections of the AAP including the Chapter Review Group, a focus group of office-based pediatricians representing each AAP District: Gene R. Adams, MD; Robert M. Corwin, MD; Diane Fuquay, MD; Barbara M. Harley, MD; Thomas J. Herr, MD, Chair; Kenneth E. Matthews, MD; Robert D. Mines, MD; Lawrence C. Pakula, MD; Howard B. Weinblatt, MD; and Delosa A. Young, MD.

The supporting data are contained in a technical report available at http://www.pediatrics.org/cgi/content/full/104/6/e78.

ABBREVIATIONS. AAP, American Academy of Pediatrics; AAFP, American Academy of Family Physicians; CT, cranial computed tomography; MRI, magnetic resonance imaging.

The recommendations in this statement do not indicate an exclusive course of treatment or serve as a standard of medical care. Variations, taking into account individual circumstances, may be appropriate.
PEDIATRICS (ISSN 0031 4005). Copyright © 1999 by the American Academy of Pediatrics.

Minor closed head injury is one of the most frequent reasons for visits to a physician.[1] Although >95 000 children experience a traumatic brain injury each year in the United States,[2] consensus is lacking about the acute care of children with minor closed head injury. The evaluation and management of injured children may be influenced by local practice customs, settings where children are evaluated, the type and extent of financial coverage, and the availability of technology and medical staffing.

Because of the magnitude of the problem and the potential seriousness of closed head injury among children, the AAP and the American Academy of Family Physicians (AAFP) undertook the development of an evidence-based parameter for health care professionals who care for children with minor closed head injury. In this document, the term Subcommittee is used to denote the Subcommittee on Minor Closed Head Injury, which reports to the AAP Committee on Quality Improvement, and the AAFP Commission on Clinical Policies, Research, and Scientific Affairs.

While developing this practice parameter, the Subcommittee attempted to find evidence of benefits resulting from 1 or more patient management options. However, at many points, adequate data were not available from the medical literature to provide guidance for the management of children with mild head injury. When such data were unavailable, we did not make specific recommendations for physicians and other professionals but instead we presented a range of practice options deemed acceptable by the Subcommittee.

An algorithm at the end of this parameter presents recommendations and options in the context of direct patient care. Management is discussed for the initial evaluation of a child with minor closed head injury, and the disposition after evaluation. These recommendations and options may be modified to fit the needs of individual patients.

PURPOSE AND SCOPE

This practice parameter is specifically intended for previously neurologically healthy children of either sex 2 through 20 years of age, with isolated minor closed head injury.

The parameter defines children with minor closed head injury as those who have normal mental status at the initial examination, who have no abnormal or focal findings on neurologic (including fundoscopic) examination, and who have no physical evidence of skull fracture (such as hemotympanum, Battle's sign, or palpable bone depression).

This parameter also is intended to address children who may have experienced temporary loss of consciousness (duration <1 minute) with injury, may have had a seizure immediately after injury, may have vomited after injury, or may have exhibited signs and symptoms such as headache and lethargy. The treatment of these children is addressed by this parameter, provided that they seem to be normal as described in the preceding paragraph at the time of evaluation.

This parameter is not intended for victims of multiple trauma, for children with unobserved loss of consciousness, or for patients with known or suspected cervical spine injury. Children who may otherwise fulfill the criteria for minor closed head injury, but for whom this parameter is not intended include patients with a history of bleeding diatheses or neurologic disorders potentially aggravated by trauma (such as arteriovenous malformations or shunts), patients with suspected intentional head trauma (eg, suspected child abuse), or patients with a language barrier.

The term brief loss of consciousness in this parameter refers to a duration of loss of consciousness of 1 minute or less. This parameter does not make any inference that the risk for intracranial injury changes with any specific length of unconsciousness lasting <1 minute. The treatment of children with loss of consciousness of longer duration is not addressed by this parameter.

Finally, this parameter refers only to the management of children evaluated by a health care professional immediately or shortly after (within 24 hours) injury. This parameter is not intended for the management of children who are initially evaluated >24 hours after injury.

METHODS FOR PARAMETER DEVELOPMENT

The literature review encompassed original research on minor closed head trauma in children, including studies on the prevalence of intracranial injury, the sensitivity and specificity of different imaging modalities, the utility of early diagnosis of intracranial injury, the effectiveness of various patient management strategies, and the impact of minor closed head injury on subsequent child health. Research was included if it had data exclusively on children or identifiable child-specific data, if cases were comparable with the case definition in the parameter, and if the data were published in a peer-reviewed journal. Review articles and articles based solely on expert opinion were excluded.

An initial search was performed on several computerized databases including Medline (1966–1993) using the terms head trauma and head injury. The search was restricted to infants, children, and adolescents, and to English-language articles published after 1966. A total of 422 articles were identified. Titles and abstracts were reviewed by the Subcommittee and articles were reviewed if any reviewer considered the title relevant. This process identified 168 articles that were sent to Subcommittee members with a literature review form to categorize study design, identify study questions, and abstract pertinent data. In addition, reference lists in the articles were reviewed for additional sources, and 125 additional articles were identified. After excluding review articles and other studies not meeting entry criteria, a total of 64 articles were included for review. All articles were reabstracted by the methodologists and the data summarized on evidence tables. Differences in case definition, outcome definition, and study samples precluded pooling of data among studies.

The published data proved extremely limited for a number of study questions, and direct queries were placed to several authors for child-specific data. Because these data have not been formally published, the Subcommittee does not rest strong conclusions on them; however, they are included in the Technical Report. The Technical Report produced along with this practice parameter contains supporting scientific data and analysis including evidence tables and is available at http://www.pediatrics.org/cgi/content/full/104/6/e78.

SUMMARY

Initial Evaluation and Management of the Child With Minor Closed Head Injury and No Loss of Consciousness

Observation

For children with minor closed head injury and no loss of consciousness, a thorough history and appropriate physical and neurologic examination should be performed. Observation in the clinic, office, emergency department, or at home, under the care of a competent caregiver is recommended for children with minor closed head injury and no loss of consciousness. Observation implies regular monitoring by a competent adult who would be able to recognize abnormalities and to seek appropriate assistance. The use of cranial computed tomography (CT) scan, skull radiograph, or magnetic resonance imaging (MRI) is not recommended for the initial evaluation and management of the child with minor closed head injury and no loss of consciousness.

Initial Evaluation of the Child With Minor Closed Head Injury With Brief Loss of Consciousness

Observation or Cranial CT Scan

For children with minor closed head injury and brief loss of consciousness (<1 minute), a thorough history and an appropriate physical and neurologic examination should be performed. Observation, in the office, clinic, emergency department, hospital, or home under the care of a competent caregiver, may be used to evaluate children with minor closed head injury with brief loss of consciousness. Cranial CT scanning may also be used, in addition to observation, in the initial evaluation and management of children with minor closed head injury with loss of consciousness.

The use of skull radiographs or MRI in the initial management of children with minor closed head injury and loss of consciousness is not recommended. However, there are limited situations in which MRI and skull radiography are options (see sections on skull radiographs and on MRI).

Patient Management Considerations

Many factors may influence how management strategies influence outcomes for children with minor closed head injury. These factors include: 1) the prevalence of intracranial injury, 2) the percentage of intracranial injuries that need medical or neurosurgical intervention (ie, the percentage of these injuries that, if left undiagnosed or untreated, leads to disability or death), 3) the relative accuracy of clinical examination, skull radiographs, and CT scans as diagnostic tools to detect such intracranial injuries that benefit from medical or neurosurgical intervention, 4) the efficacy of treatment for intracranial injuries, and 5) the detrimental effect on outcome, if any, of delay from the time of injury to the time of diagnosis and intervention.

This last factor, delay of diagnosis and intervention, is particularly relevant when trying to decide between a clinical strategy of immediate CT scanning of all patients as opposed to a strategy that relies primarily on patient observation, with CT scanning reserved for rare patients whose conditions change. To our knowledge, no published studies were available for review that compared clinically meaningful outcomes (ie, morbidity or mortality) between children receiving different management regimens such as immediate neuroimaging, or observation. Although some studies were able to demonstrate the presence of intracranial abnormalities on CT scans or MRIs among children with minor head injury, no known evidence suggested that immediate neuroimaging of asymptomatic children improved outcomes for these children, compared with the outcomes for children managed primarily with examination and observation.

Initial Management of the Child With Minor Closed Head Injury and No Loss of Consciousness

Minor closed head injury without loss of consciousness is a common occurrence in childhood. Available data suggest that the risk of intracranial injury is negligible in this situation. Population-based studies have found that fewer than 1 in 5000 patients with minor closed head injury and no loss of consciousness have intracranial injuries that require medical or neurosurgical intervention. In 1 study of 5252 low-risk patients, mostly adults, none were found to have an intracranial injury after minor head injury.[3] Comparably sized studies do not exist for children. In 2 much smaller studies of children with minor head injury, among those with normal neurologic examination findings and no loss of consciousness, amnesia, vomiting, headache, or mental status abnormalities, no children had abnormal CT scan findings.[4,5]

Observation

Among children with minor closed head injury and no loss of consciousness, a thorough history and appropriate physical and neurologic examination

should be performed. Subcommittee consensus was that observation, in the clinic, office, emergency department, or home under the care of a competent observer, be used as the primary management strategy. If on examination the patient's condition appears normal (as outlined earlier), no additional tests are needed and the child can be safely discharged to the care of a responsible caregiver. The recommended duration of observation is discussed in the section titled "Disposition of the Child With Minor Head Injury."

CT Scan/MRI

With such a low prevalence of intracranial injury, the Subcommittee believed that the marginal benefits of early detection of intracranial injury afforded by routine brain imaging studies such as CT or MRI were outweighed by considerations of cost, inconvenience, resource allocation, and possible side effects attributable to sedation or inappropriate interventions (eg, medical, surgical, or other interventions based on incidental CT findings in asymptomatic children).

Skull Radiographs

Skull radiographs have only a very limited role in the evaluation of children with minor closed head injury, no loss of consciousness, and no signs of skull fracture (ie, no palpable depression, hemotympanum, or Battle's sign). The substantial rate of false-positive results provided by skull radiographs (ie, a skull fracture detected on skull radiographs in the absence of intracranial injury) along with the low prevalence of intracranial injury among this specific subset of patients, leads to a low predictive value of skull radiographs. Most children with abnormal skull radiographs will not harbor significant intracranial lesions and conversely intracranial injury occurs in the absence of a skull fracture detected on skull radiographs.

There may be some clinical scenarios in which a practitioner desires imaging such as the case of a child with a scalp hematoma over the course of the meningeal artery. In situations such as these, the Subcommittee believes that clinical judgment should prevail. However, given the relatively low predictive value of skull radiographs, the Subcommittee believes that, if imaging is desired, cranial CT scan is the more satisfactory imaging modality.

Initial Management of the Child With Minor Closed Head Injury and Brief Loss of Consciousness

Among children with minor closed head injury, loss of consciousness is uncommon but is associated with an increased risk for intracranial injury. Studies performed since the advent of CT scanning suggest that children with loss of consciousness, or who demonstrate amnesia at the time of evaluation, or who have headache or vomiting at the time of evaluation, have a prevalence of intracranial injury detectable on CT that ranges from 0% to 7%.[5-8] Although most of these intracranial lesions will remain clinically insignificant, a substantial proportion of children, between 2% and 5% of those with minor head injury and loss of consciousness, may require neurosurgical intervention.[6-8] The differences in findings among studies are likely attributable to differences in selection criteria, along with random variation among studies with limited sample size. Although these findings might have been biased somewhat if more seriously injured patients were preferentially selected for CT scans, even studies in which patients were explicitly stated to be neurologically normal and asymptomatic found children with clinically significant injuries that required intervention.[6]

In past studies of children with minor head injury, patient selection may have led to overestimates of the prevalence of intracranial injury. Many of these studies looked at patients referred to emergency departments or trauma centers, patients brought to emergency departments after examination in the field by emergency personnel, or patients for whom the reason for obtaining CT scans was not clearly stated. These factors may have led to the selection of a patient population at higher risk for intracranial injury than the patients specifically addressed in this practice parameter.

As evidence of this, population-based studies before the widespread availability of CT scanning found the prevalence of clinically significant intracranial injury after minor closed head injury to be far less than estimated by the aforementioned studies. One study found a prevalence of intracranial injury that required neurosurgery to be as low as .02%.[9] This discrepancy is consistent also with the fact that many lesions currently identified with cranial CT were not recognized before the availability of this technology. Because most of these lesions do not progress or require neurosurgical intervention, most would not have been diagnosed in studies before the availability of CT scan.

Observation

As discussed earlier, the Subcommittee did not find evidence to show that immediate neuroimaging of asymptomatic children produced demonstrable benefits compared with a management strategy of initial observation alone. In light of these considerations, there was Subcommittee consensus based on limited evidence that for children who are neurologically normal after minor closed head injury with loss of consciousness, patient observation was an acceptable management option.

If the health care practitioner chooses observation alone, it may be performed in the clinic, office, emergency department, hospital, or at home under the care of a competent observer, typically a parent or suitable guardian. If the observer seems unable to follow or comply with the instructions for home observation, observation under the supervision of a health care practitioner is to be considered.

CT Scan

Data that support the routine use of CT scanning of children with minor head injury and loss of consciousness indicate that children with intracranial lesions after minor closed head injury are not easily distinguishable clinically from the large majority with no intracranial injury.[10,11] Children with nonspecific signs such as headache, vomiting, or lethargy after minor closed head injury may be more likely to have intracranial injury than children without such signs. However, these clinical signs are of limited predictive value, and most children with headache, lethargy, or vomiting after minor closed head injury do not have demonstrable intracranial injury. In addition, some children with intracranial injury do not have any signs or symptoms. Because of these findings, many investigators have concluded that the physical and neurologic examination are inadequate predictors of intracranial injury, and that cranial CT is more sensitive than physical and neurologic examinations for the diagnosis of intracranial injury.

The most accurate and rapid means of detecting intracranial injury would be with a clinical protocol that routinely obtained intracranial imaging for all children after head injury. Rapid diagnosis and treatment of subdural hematomas was found in 1 study to significantly reduce morbidity and mortality among severely injured adults.[12] However, this result was not replicated in other studies of subdural or epidural hematomas[13-15] and similar studies have not addressed less severely head injured children, or children with minor closed head injury.

CT itself is a safe procedure. However, some healthy children require sedation or anesthesia, and the benefits gained from cranial CT should be carefully weighed against the possible harm of sedating and/or anesthetizing a large number of children. In addition, CT scans obtained for asymptomatic children may show incidental findings that lead to subsequent unnecessary medical or surgical interventions. To our knowledge, no data are available that demonstrate that children who undergo CT scanning early after minor closed head injury with loss of consciousness have different outcomes compared with children who receive observation alone after injury. A clinical trial comparing the risks and benefits of immediate CT scanning with simple monitored observation for children with minor closed head injury has not been performed, primarily because intracranial injury after minor closed head injury is so rare that the cost and logistics of such a study would be prohibitive. As a result, the risk–benefit ratio for the evaluation and management modalities of CT scanning or observation is unknown.

Simple observation by a reliable parent or guardian is the management option with the least initial costs, while CT scans typically cost less than observation performed in the hospital. A study that compares costs of CT and observation strategies would need data on the cost of following up children with positive CT scans, as well as the potential costs associated with late detection and emergency therapy among those managed by observation alone.

Because of these considerations, there was Subcommittee consensus based on limited evidence that for children who are neurologically normal after minor closed head injury with loss of consciousness, cranial CT scanning along with observation was also an acceptable management option.

Skull Radiographs

Before the availability of CT imaging, skull radiographs were a common means to evaluate children with head injury. Skull radiographs may identify skull fractures, but they do not directly show brain injury or other intracranial trauma. Although intracranial injury is more common in the presence of a skull fracture, many studies have demonstrated that intracranial lesions are not always associated with skull fractures and that skull fractures do not always indicate an underlying intracranial lesion.[7,8,16]

Large studies of children and adults have shown that the sensitivity of skull radiographs for identifying intracranial injury in children is quite low (~25% in some studies). More recent studies limited to children have reported sensitivities between 50% and 100%, with the latter higher figure reported from studies of adolescent patients.[7,8,15,16] The specificity of skull radiographs for intracranial injury (the proportion of patients without intracranial injury who have normal radiographs) has been reported as between 53% and 97% in these same studies. Given the limited specificity of skull radiographs and the low prevalence of intracranial injury, the skull radiographs would likely be interpreted as abnormal for a substantial proportion of patients without intracranial injury. Furthermore, the low sensitivity of the radiographs will result in the interpretation of skull radiographs as normal for some patients with intracranial injury.

The Subcommittee consensus was that skull radiographs have only a limited role in the management of the child with loss of consciousness. If imaging is desired by the health care practitioner and if CT and skull radiographs are available, the Subcommittee believes that CT scanning is the imaging modality of choice, based on the increased sensitivity and specificity of CT scans. When CT scanning is not readily available, skull radiographs may assist the practitioner to define the extent of injury and risk for intracranial injury. In this situation, there was Subcommittee consensus that, for a child who has suffered minor closed head injury with loss of consciousness, skull radiographs are an acceptable management option. However, as noted, skull fractures may be detected on skull radiographs in the absence of intracranial injury, and intracranial injury may be present when no skull fracture is detected on skull radiographs. These limitations should be considered carefully by physicians who elect to use skull radiographs. Regardless of findings on skull films (should the physician elect to obtain them) close observation, as described previously, remains a cornerstone of patient management.

MRI

MRI is another available modality for neuroimaging. Although MRI has been shown to be more sensitive than cranial CT in detecting certain types of intracranial abnormalities, CT is more sensitive for hyperacute and acute intracranial hemorrhage (especially subarachnoid hemorrhage). CT is more quickly and easily performed than MRI, and costs for CT scans generally are less than those for MRI. The consensus of the Subcommittee was that cranial CT offered substantial advantages over MRI in the acute care of children with minor closed head injury.

As is the case with skull radiographs, there may be situations in which CT scanning is not readily available and the health care professional desires to obtain imaging studies. There was Subcommittee consensus that, for a child who has experienced minor closed head injury with loss of consciousness, MRI to evaluate the intracranial status of the child was an acceptable management option.

Disposition of Children With Minor Closed Head Injury

Children Managed by Observation Alone

Children who appear neurologically normal after minor closed head injury are at very low risk for subsequent deterioration in their condition and are unlikely to require medical intervention. Therefore, although observation is recommended for patients after the initial evaluation is completed, such observation may take place in many different settings. The strategy chosen by the health care practitioner may depend on the resources available for observation. Other factors, such as the distance and time it would take to reach appropriate care if the patient's clinical status worsened, may influence where observation occurs.

Historically, when hospitalization has been used to observe children after head injury, the length of stay averaged 12 to 48 hours. This practice was based on the reasoning that most life-threatening complications occur within 24 hours after head injury. The Subcommittee believes that a prudent duration of observation would extend at least 24 hours, and could be accomplished in any combination of locations, including the emergency department, hospital, clinic, office, or home. However, it is important for physicians, parents, and other guardians to have a high index of suspicion about any change in the patient's clinical status for several days after the injury. Parents or guardians require careful instruction to seek medical attention if the patient's condition worsens at any time during the first several days after injury.

In all cases, the health care professional is to make a careful assessment of the parent or guardian's anticipated compliance with the instructions to monitor the patient. If the caregiver is incompetent, unavailable, intoxicated, or otherwise incapacitated, other provisions must be made to ensure adequate observation of the child. These provisions may differ based on the characteristics of each case.

The physician has an important role in educating the parents or guardians of children with minor closed head injury. Understandable, printed instructions should be given to the parent or guardian detailing how to monitor the patient and including information on how and when to seek medical attention if necessary. All children discharged should be released to the care of a reliable parent or guardian who has adequate transportation and who has the capability to seek medical attention if the child's condition worsens.

Children Evaluated by Cranial CT

Neurologically normal patients with normal cranial CT scans are at extremely low risk for subsequent problems. Although there are many reports of patients with head injuries in whom extradural or intracerebral bleeding developed after an initial stable clinical period,[18-22] there are only a few reports of patients in whom extradural or intracerebral bleeding developed after a postinjury CT scan was interpreted as normal.[23-25] Most often when such cases have been described, the patients had sustained a more severe initial head injury than the patient for whom this parameter is intended, and the neurologic status of the patients was not intact at the initial examination following the injury. A number of studies have demonstrated the safety of using cranial CT as a triage instrument for neurologically normal and clinically stable patients after minor closed head injury.[26-31]

Patients may be discharged from the hospital for observation by a reliable observer if the postinjury CT scan is interpreted as normal. The length of observation should be similar to that described in the preceding section. If the cranial CT reveals abnormalities, proper disposition depends on a thorough consideration of the abnormalities and, when warranted, consultations with appropriate subspecialists.

Research Issues

Classification of Head Injury in Children and Prognostic Features

Much remains to be learned about minor closed head injury in children. The implications of clinical events such as loss of consciousness and signs or symptoms such as seizures, nausea, vomiting, and headache remain unclear. Data on patients with low-risk head injuries but with loss of consciousness, such as the data provided on a primarily adult population, are not available for children. Moreover, this practice parameter deals with clinically normal patients who did not lose consciousness at the time of injury and with patients who did lose consciousness with injury. Children with minor head injury, who have experienced loss of consciousness, vomiting or seizures have been found to have a prevalence of intracranial injury ranging from 2% to 5%. Questions remain about the selection of patients for many of these studies, and there is considerable uncertainty about the generalizability of these results to patients within this parameter.

Future studies on minor closed head injury should assess the relationship between characteristics such as these and the risk for intracranial injury among children who are clinically asymptomatic. Specifically, studies should address the question of whether such a history of loss of consciousness is associated with an increased risk for clinically significant intracranial abnormalities. Such studies should not be limited to patients seen in referral settings, but instead should cover patients from a wide range of settings, including those managed in clinics and offices, and if possible, those managed over the phone.

These studies should also address the independent prognostic value of other signs and symptoms for which the clinical significance in children is uncertain. In particular, practitioners are often faced with managing patients who are asymptomatic except for episodes of repeated vomiting or moderate to severe headache. The Subcommittee did not find evidence in the literature that helped differentiate the risk status of children with such symptoms from children without such symptoms. If studies are performed on this population, information should be collected on the presence of signs or symptoms including posttraumatic seizures, nausea with or without vomiting, posttraumatic amnesia, scalp lacerations and hematomas, headache, and dizziness, and their relationship to intracranial injury.

The Benefit of Early Detection of, and Intervention for, Intracranial Lesions in Asymptomatic Children

The outcome for asymptomatic patients found to have intracranial hematomas is of particular interest. Additional studies are needed to determine whether a strategy of immediate CT scan provides measurably improved outcomes for children with minor closed head injury compared with a strategy of observation followed by CT scan for children whose clinical status changes. Although rapid detection and neurosurgical intervention for intracranial injuries such as subdural hematomas has been shown to improve outcome in some studies of patients with more serious head injuries, it is unclear whether the same benefit would accrue to asymptomatic neurologically normal children.

A randomized, controlled trial would provide the most direct information on the risks and benefits of each management strategy. However, such a study would be extremely difficult and expensive to perform because of the rarity of adverse outcomes. Retrospective observational studies among children with minor head injury could be performed more easily and at less cost. However, correct characterization of the patient's clinical status before any treatment strategy or diagnostic procedure would be essential to eliminate bias in the evaluation of the comparison groups.

Finally, if such studies are performed to compare different diagnostic and management strategies, the outcomes should include not only mortality and short-term morbidity, but also long-term outcomes such as persistent psychological problems or learning disorders.

The Management of the Asymptomatic Patient With Intracranial Hemorrhage

The optimal management and prognosis for asymptomatic patients with intracranial hemorrhage is unknown. Because surgery is not always indicated or beneficial, some neurosurgeons and neurologists now advocate an expectant approach of close observation for small intracranial and extradural hemato-

Evaluation and Triage of Children and Adolescents With Minor Head Trauma

Algorithm

1 Patient older than 2–20 years with head injury presents to clinician for evaluation

2 Clinician stabilizes patient's condition if necessary, obtains history, and performs physical examination

3 Does the patient have any of the following:
(1) multiple trauma; OR
(2) known or suspected cervical spine injury; OR
(3) preexisting neurologic disorder; OR
(4) bleeding diathesis; OR
(5) suspected intentional head trauma; OR
(6) language barrier between patient or parents and provider; OR
(7) presence of drugs or alcohol?

— Yes →

4 Exit clinical algorithm to appropriate individualized patient management

No ↓

5 Does child have abnormal results of skull or eye examination and/or abnormal results of neurologic examination? (A) (See text for definition of abnormal results.)

— Yes →

No ↓

6 Is there a history of brief loss of consciousness with this injury?

— No (B) →

7 Does physician believe home observation is appropriate AND parent(s) is competent to observe?

— Yes →

8 Observe at home. (B, C)

No ↓

10 Observe in hospital or other facility. (B, C)

Yes ↓

9 Physician and patient or parents discuss clinical options:
(1) Observation (C); or
(2) Imaging (D, E, F).

11 Do signs and/ or symptoms of intracranial problems develop?

— Yes →

12
(1) Arrange emergency consultation with appropriate specialist; AND
(2) Consider emergency CT scan; AND/OR
(3) Arrange for transfer to a facility with definitive neurosurgical care facilities.
(I)

No ↓

14 Arrange appropriate follow-up

13 Does physician in consultation with patient or parents, choose observation? (C)

— Yes →

No ↓

15 Is CT scan available? (C)

— Yes →

16 Perform CT scan of head

→

17 Does CT scan reveal lesion that requires surgery or does it reveal other abnormality?

— Yes →

18 Arrange consultation with appropriate specialist (H)

No ↓

20 Return to Box 7 (G)

No ↓

19 Arrange appropriate referral or transfer for imaging or reconsider observation

mas, considering hematoma size, shift of intracranial structures, and other factors.

If all asymptomatic children with minor head injury undergo cranial CT scanning, a substantial number of patients with an abnormal result on CT may undergo surgery that is unnecessary or even harmful. Additional research is needed to determine the proper management of asymptomatic children with intracranial hemorrhage. Outcome measures should include mortality and morbidity outcomes such as seizures, learning disabilities, and behavioral disabilities.

Research Into Other Imaging Modalities

As newer modalities for neuroimaging are developed and disseminated, careful evaluation of their relative utility is necessary before they are used for patients with minor closed head injury. Although such new modalities frequently provide new and different types of information to the health care professional, it is important that they be submitted to scientific study to assess their effect on patient outcome.

Algorithm

The notes below are integral to the algorithm. The letters in parentheses correspond to the algorithm.

A. This parameter addresses the management of previously neurologically healthy children with minor closed head injury who have normal mental status on presentation, no abnormal or focal findings on neurologic (including fundoscopic) examination, and no physical evidence of skull fracture (such as hemotympanum, Battle's sign, or palpable depression).

B. Observation in the clinic, office, emergency department, or home, under the care of a competent caregiver is recommended for children with minor closed head injury and no loss of consciousness.

C. Observation in the office, clinic, emergency department, hospital, or home under the care of a competent caregiver may be used to manage children with minor closed head injury with loss of consciousness.

D. Cranial CT scanning along with observation may also be used in the initial evaluation and management of children with minor closed head injury with brief loss of consciousness.

E. If imaging is desired by the health care practitioner and if both CT and skull radiography are available, CT scanning is the imaging modality of choice, because of its increased sensitivity and specificity. When CT scanning is not readily available, skull radiographs may assist the practitioner to define the risk for intracranial injury. However skull fractures may be detected on skull radiographs in the absence of intracranial injury, and occasionally intracranial injury is present despite the absence of a skull fracture detected on skull radiographs. These limitations should be considered by physicians who elect to use skull radiographs. Whether the changed probabilities for harboring an intracranial injury based on the results of the skull radiographs is sufficient to alter the management strategy may depend on the preferences of the family and physician.

F. In some studies MRI has been shown to be more sensitive than CT in diagnosing certain intracranial lesions. However, there is currently no appreciable difference between CT and MRI in the diagnosis of clinically significant acute intracranial injury and bleeding that requires neurosurgical intervention. CT is more quickly and easily performed than MRI, and the costs for CT scans generally are less than those for MRI. Because of this, the consensus among the Subcommittee was that cranial CT offered advantages over MRI in the acute care of children with minor closed head injury.

G. Neurologically normal patients with a normal cranial CT scan are at very low risk for subsequent deterioration. Patients may be discharged from the hospital for observation by a reliable observer if the postinjury CT scan is normal. The decision to observe at home takes into consideration the delay that would ensue if the child had to return to the hospital as well as the reliability of the parents or other caregivers. Otherwise, depending on the preferences of the patient and physician, observation also may take place in the office, clinic, emergency department, or hospital.

H. If the cranial CT reveals abnormalities, proper disposition depends on a thorough consideration of the abnormalities and, when warranted, consultation with appropriate subspecialists.

I. If the child's neurologic condition worsens during observation, a thorough neurologic examination is to be performed, along with immediate cranial CT after the patient's condition is stabilized. If a repeat CT scan shows new intracranial pathologic abnormalities, consultation with the appropriate subspecialist is warranted.

AAP COMMITTEE ON QUALITY IMPROVEMENT, 1992–1997
David A. Bergman, MD, Chairperson
Richard D. Baltz, MD
James R. Cooley, MD
John B. Coombs, MD
Michael J. Goldberg, MD, Sections Liaison
Charles J. Homer, MD, MPH, Section on Epidemiology Liaison
Paul V. Miles, MD
Lawrence F. Nazarian, MD, 1992–1994
Thomas A. Riemenschneider, MD, 1992–1995
Kenneth B. Roberts, MD
Daniel W. Shea, MD, 1992–1995
William M. Zurhellen, MD

SUBCOMMITTEE ON MANAGEMENT OF MINOR HEAD INJURY
John B. Coombs, MD, Chairperson
Hanan Bell, PhD, AAFP, Methodologic Consultant
Robert L. Davis, MD, MPH, AAP, Consultant
Theodore G. Ganiats, MD, AAFP
Michael D. Hagen, MD, AAFP, 1992–1993
Jack Haller, MD, AAP, Consultant
Charles J. Homer, MD, MPH, AAP, Subcommittee Methodologist
David M. Jaffee, MD, AAP Section on Emergency Medicine Liaison
Hector James, MD, AAP
Larry Kleinman, MD, AAP, Consultant 1992–1994
Jane Knapp, MD, AAP
J. Michael Dean, MD, AAP
Patricia Nobel, MD, AAP
Sanford Schneider, MD, AAP

AAFP COMMISSION ON CLINICAL POLICIES AND RESEARCH, 1996–1997
Joseph E. Scherger, MD, MPH, Chairperson, 1997
Richard G. Roberts, MD, JD, Chairperson, 1996
Roman M. Hendrickson, MD
William J. Hueston, MD, 1996
Stephen J. Spann, MD
Thomas Gilbert, MD, MPH, 1997
Theodore G. Ganiats, MD
William R. Phillips, MD, MPH

Richard K. Zimmerman, MD, MPH
Lee A. Green, MD, MPH
Jonathan E. Rodnick, MD
Barbara P. Yawn, MD, MSc
Linda L. Barrett, MD, Resident Representative,
  1997
Enrico G. Jones, MD, Resident Representative,
  1996
Theresa-Ann Clark, Student Representative
Ross R. Black, MD, Liaison, Commission on
  Quality and Scope of Practice
Leah Raye Mabry, MD, Liaison, Commision on
  Public Health
Herbert F. Young, MD, MA, Staff Executive
Hanan S. Bell, PhD, Assistant Staff Executive

REFERENCES

1. Levin HS, Mattis S, Ruff RM, et al. Neurobehavioral outcome following minor head injury: a three-center study. *J Neurosurg.* 1987;66:234–243
2. Krauss JF, Black MA, Hessol N, et al. The incidence of acute brain injury and serious impairment in a defined population. *Am J Epidemiol.* 1984;119:186–201
3. Masters SJ, McClean PM, Arcarese JS, et al. Skull radiograph examinations after head trauma: recommendations by a multidisciplinary panel and validation study. *N Engl J Med.* 1987;316:84–91
4. Hennes H, Lee M, Smith D, Sty JR, Losek J. Clinical predictors of severe head trauma in children. *Am J Dis Child.* 1988;142:1045–1047
5. Dietrich AM, Bowman MJ, Ginn-Pease ME, Kusnick E, King DR. Pediatric head injuries: can clinical factors reliably predict an abnormality on computed tomography? *Ann Emerg Med.* 1993;22:1535–1540
6. Dacey RG Jr, Alves WM, Rimel RW, Winn HR, Jane JA. Neurosurgical complications after apparently minor head injury: assessment of risk in a series of 610 patients. *J Neurosurg.* 1986;65:203–210
7. Hahn YS, McLone DG. Risk factors in the outcome of children with minor head injury. *Pediatr Neurosurg.* 1993;19:135–142
8. Rosenthal BW, Bergman I. Intracranial injury after moderate head trauma in children. *J Pediatr.* 1989;115:346–350
9. Teasdale GM, Murray G, Anderson E, et al. Risks of acute traumatic intracranial complications in hematoma in children and adults: implications for head injuries. *Br Med J.* 1990;300:363–367
10. Rivara F, Taniguchi D, Parish RA, et al. Poor prediction of positive computed tomographic scans by clinical criteria in symptomatic pediatric head trauma. *Pediatrics.* 1987;80:579–584
11. Davis RL, Mullen N, Makela M, Taylor JA, Cohen W, Rivara FP. Cranial computed tomography scans in children after minimal head injury with loss of consciousness. *Ann Emerg Med.* 1994;24:640–645
12. Seelig JM, Becker DP, Miller JD, Greenberg RP, Ward JD, Choi SC. Traumatic acute subdural hematoma: major mortality reduction in comatose patients treated within four hours. *N Engl J Med.* 1981;304:1511–1518
13. Chen TY, Wong CW, Chang CN, et al. The expectant treatment of asymptomatic supratentorial epidural hematomas. *Neurosurgery.* 1993;32:176–179
14. Hatashita S, Koga N, Hosaka Y, Takagi S. Acute subdural hematoma: severity of injury, surgical intervention, and mortality. *Neurol Med Chir (Tokyo).* 1993;33:13–18
15. Lobato RD, Rivas JJ, Gomez PA, et al. Head injured patients who talk and deteriorate into coma. *J Neurosurg.* 1991;75:256–261
16. Zimmerman RA, Bilaniuk LT, Gennarelli T, Bruce D, Dolinskas C, Uzzell B. Cranial computed tomography in diagnosis and management of acute head trauma. *AJR Am J Roentgenol.* 1978;131:27–34
17. Borovich B, Braun J, Guilburd JN, et al. Delayed onset of traumatic extradural hematoma. *J Neurosurg.* 1985;63:30–34
18. Miller JD, Murray LS, Teasdale GM. Development of a traumatic intracranial hematoma after a ''minor'' head injury. *Neurosurgery.* 1990;27:669–673
19. Rosenthal BW, Bergman I. Intracranial injury after moderate head trauma in children. *J Pediatr.* 1989;115:346–350
20. Dacey RG, Alves WM, Rimel RW, Winn HR, Jane JA. Neurosurgical complications after apparently minor head injury. *J Neurosurg.* 1986;65:203–210
21. Deitch D, Kirshner HS. Subdural hematoma after normal CT. *Neurology.* 1989;39:985–987
22. Poon WS, Rehman SU, Poon CY, Li AK. Traumatic extradural hematoma of delayed onset is not a rarity. *Neurosurgery.* 1992;30:681–686
23. Brown FD, Mullan S, Duda EE. Delayed traumatic intracerebral hematomas. *J Neurosurg.* 1978;48:1019–1022
24. Lipper MH, Kishore PR, Girevendulis AK, Miller JD, Becker DP. Delayed intracranial hematoma in patients with severe head injury. *Radiology.* 1979;133:645–649
25. Diaz FG, Yock DH Jr, Larson D, Rockswold GL. Early diagnosis of delayed posttraumatic intracerebral hematomas. *J Neurosurg.* 1979;50:217–223
26. Stein SC, Ross SE. The value of computed tomographic scans in patients with low-risk head injuries. *Neurosurgery.* 1990;29:638–640
27. Stein SC, Ross SE. Mild head injury: a plea for routine early CT scanning. *J Trauma.* 1992;33:11–13
28. Harad FT, Kerstein MD. Inadequacy of bedside clinical indicators in identifying significant intracranial injury in trauma patients. *J Trauma.* 1992;32:359–363
29. Livingston DH, Loder PA, Koziol J, Hunt CD. The use of CT scanning to triage patients requiring admission following minimal head injury. *J Trauma.* 1991;31:483–489
30. Feurman T, Wackym PA, Gade GF, Becker DP. Value of skull radiography, head computed tomographic scanning, and admission for observation in cases of minor head injury. *Neurosurgery.* 1988;22:449–453
31. Livingston DH, Loder PA, Hunt CD. Minimal head injury: is admission necessary? *Am Surg.* 1991;57:14–17

Technical Report Summary:
Minor Head Injury in Children

Charles J. Homer, MD, MPH, and Lawrence Kleinman, MD, MPH

ABSTRACT

Minor head trauma affecting children is a common reason for medical consultation and evaluation. In order to provide evidence on which to base a clinical practice guideline for the American Academy of Pediatrics, we undertook a systematic review of the literature on minor head trauma in children.

Methods. **Medline and Health databases were searched for articles published between 1966 and 1993 on head trauma or head injury, limited to infants, children, and adolescents. Abstracts were reviewed for relevance to mild head trauma consistent with the index case defined by the AAP subcommittee. Relevant articles were identified, reviewed, and abstracted. Additional citations were identified by review of references and expert suggestions. Unpublished data were also identified through contact with authors highlighting child-specific information. Abstracted data were summarized in evidence tables. The process was repeated in 1998, updating the review for articles published between 1993 and 1997.**

Results. **A total of 108 articles were abstracted from 1033 abstracts and articles identified through the various search strategies. Variation in definitions precluded any pooling of data from different studies. Prevalence of intracranial injury in children with mild head trauma varied from 0% to 7%. Children with no clinical risk characteristics are at lower risk than are children with such characteristics; the magnitude of increased risk was inconsistent across studies. Computed tomography scan is most sensitive and specific for detection of intracranial abnormalities; sensitivity and specificity of skull radiographs ranged from 21% to 100% and 53% to 97%, respectively. No high quality studies tested alternative strategies for management of such children. Outcome studies are inconclusive as to the impact of minor head trauma on long-term cognitive function.**

Conclusions. **The literature on mild head trauma does not provide a sufficient scientific basis for evidence-based recommendations about most of the key issues in clinical management. More consistent definitions and multisite assessments are needed to clarify this field. Pediatrics 1999;104(6). URL:http://www.pediatrics.org/ cgi/content/full/104/6/e78.** *Keywords: head trauma, imaging, literature review.*

Minor head trauma affecting a child is a common reason for medical consultation and evaluation. No consensus exists concerning the appropriate diagnostic assessment of such children. Previous surveys of physicians indicated significant variation in practice, and examination of hospitalization rates shows substantial regional variation for this condition. The American Academy of Pediatrics, in coordination with the American Academy of Family Physicians, launched an initiative to develop a clinical practice guideline to reduce variation and improve the quality of care of children with minor head trauma.

This report provides the technical information on the literature concerning minor head trauma in children that was used by the American Academy of Pediatrics/American Academy of Family Physicians' subcommittee in formulating this guideline.

METHODS

The literature review included the following salient aspects of minor head trauma in children:

- Prevalence of intracranial injury
- Sensitivity and specificity of different imaging modalities in detecting intracranial injury, including skull radiography, computed tomography (CT), and magnetic resonance imaging (MRI)
- Utility of early diagnosis of intracranial injury
- Effectiveness of alternative management strategies, and
- Impact of minor head injury on subsequent child health.

The data included for review met the following criteria:

1. publication in a peer-reviewed journal,
2. data related exclusively to children or was identifiable as being specifically related to children, and
3. assurance that cases described in the article were comparable with the case described in the practice guideline. Review articles and expert opinion were excluded.

A medical librarian undertook an initial search of several computerized databases, including Medline (1966–1993) and Health, searching terms of head trauma and head injury, restricted to infancy, children, and adolescents. Four hundred twenty-two articles were identified. Titles and abstracts were reviewed by 4 initial reviewers, including the subcommittee chairperson, American Academy of Pediatrics staff, and methodologic consultants, and articles were obtained when reviewers considered the title to be relevant. Through this process, 168 articles were identified.

Articles were sent to subcommittee members with an article review form, which asked reviewers to categorize the study design, identify the study question, and abstract the data to enable data pooling and meta-analysis. In addition, reviewers were asked to check the article references to see whether additional sources could be found.

Of the initial 168 articles sent out, reviewers excluded 134 papers and included 34 papers in their reviews.

An additional 125 references were identified through bibliography tracing, of which 30 were included for review by the epidemiologist/pediatrician consultants.

All articles included were then abstracted again by the epidemiologist/pediatrician consultants, and the data were compiled using summary tables and evidence tables. Differences in case definition, outcome definition, and study samples precluded pooling of data to arrive at common estimates.

Because the published data proved extremely limited for a number of study questions, direct queries were given to several authors for child-specific data. Because these data have not been formally published, we did not rest strong conclusions on them; when available, however, they are presented with this report.

Because of the lengthy period between the initial review of the literature and final approval of the guideline, a second literature review was performed to assure that the literature review was current. This literature review used the same search headings and targeted the period between January 1, 1993, and July 1, 1997. For this review, only an electronic search was performed. The review identified an additional 486 abstracts, of which 44 were selected for detailed review by the epidemiologist and 11 included in the evidence tables.

RESULTS

In general, interpretation of clinical studies of head trauma was complicated by several characteristics of the literature. Specifically, the head trauma literature suffers by the non-standardized ways of categorizing head injury, clinical examinations, radiologic outcomes, and clinical outcomes, and by the inconsistent reporting of the subjects included in a study population.

The results of the literature review are presented by each area for which evidence was sought.

Risk of Intracranial Injury

Ten published articles were identified that provided estimates of the prevalence of intracranial injury in children with mild head injury, with CT scans used as the "gold standard". Among these articles, however, 3 included patients with more severe symptoms or findings than specified by the guideline case description (including Glasgow coma scale [GCS] scores as low as 13), and 1 included trivial abnormalities on CT as the principal outcome measure. Among those studies restricting their subjects to GCS scores of 15, and considering abnormal findings to be subdural, extradural, or intracerebral hematomas, ranges of the prevalence of intracranial injury ranged from 0% to 7%. The high estimate of 7% comes from a study in which both initial and delayed (24-hour) CT scans were obtained for most patients; how many patients were referred for care at this institution because of clinical deterioration was not noted.

Three unpublished studies provided prevalence estimates of intracranial injuries ranging from 4% to 10% among patients with a GCS score of 15, without focal neurologic findings, but with either a history of (brief) loss of consciousness or amnesia (J. Finkelstein, 1994; S. C. Stein, 1994; S. C. Stein, 1994).

We sought to determine within these articles whether any clinical characteristics were associated with the presence or absence of significant CT scan abnormalities. Two studies indicated that among patients with a GCS score of 15, normal neurologic examinations, no history of loss of consciousness or amnesia, no vomiting, headache, or subtle changes in mental status, there were no abnormal CT scan findings. One additional case series (49 children) found that no child with a GCS of 15, a completely normal neurologic examination, and no trauma aside from the head injury experienced an intracranial lesion, even with a history of loss of consciousness or amnesia. The upper limits for the 95% confidene interval for this estimate is 6%, and the

analysis that identified this group of predictors is exploratory; no confirmatory analyses were undertaken in a second dataset.

One pediatric study used surgery for intracranial bleeding as an indicator of intracranial injury. This study found that .017% of cases with a GCS score of 15 required surgery.

We conclude from these data that:

- the true prevalence of intracranial injury following mild head injury is not clearly known;

- the population as defined by the head trauma task force is likely heterogeneous in its risk;

- children with clinically trivial head injury—no loss of consciousness or amnesia, normal examinations, no vomiting, headache, and a GCS score of 15—are at substantially <1% risk of having an intracranial abnormality of immediate clinical significance;

- children with mild head injury but who have experienced loss of consciousness, amnesia, vomiting, or seizures are at higher risk of having an intracranial injury detected using CT, likely in the 1% to 5% range, with a significantly lower amount requiring any intervention (see below).

We extended this section of the literature review to examine the significance of the abnormalities detected by CT scanning in such patients. No studies randomly assigned patients with abnormal CT scans to receive or not receive surgery. Rather, several reports on the management decisions among those children found to have abnormal CT scans. These studies, and the unpublished data provided to us, indicated that between 20% and 80% of children with abnormal CT scans underwent a neurosurgical procedure, a proportion of which was intracranial pressure monitoring only.

Imaging Modalities

Through the 1970s and early 1980s, controversy raged concerning the role of skull radiography in the assessment of acute head trauma. Although fewer articles are now being written on this topic, the lack of access to CT scanners in some practice settings prompted review of this literature.

We identified 5 studies that examined the sensitivity and specificity of skull radiographs for the detection of intracranial injury, using intracranial abnormality or bleeding as determined by CT scanning as the gold standard. These studies found that the sensitivity of skull films varied from 50% to 100%; 1 of the studies showing 100% sensitivity was restricted to adolescents. The specificity of skull films for intracranial injury (ie, the proportion of patients without intracranial injury who have normal films) has been reported to be between 53% and 97%. Thus, a substantial proportion of patients without intracranial injury will have abnormal skull films.

A few studies have examined the role of MRI in head trauma. These studies indicate that although subtle forms of neural injury can be better detected by MRI, and that isodense subdural collections (as may be found in chronic subdural injuries in adults) also may be more readily identified, in acute settings with children MRI offers no advantage in detecting lesions of clinical concern.

We conclude from this literature that 1) although an abnormal skull film increases the likelihood of a significant intracranial lesion, the test is not of sufficient sensitivity or specificity to be clinically useful in most settings, and 2) CT is sufficiently sensitive and specific as the imaging modality of choice at this time; in most cases, a normal CT scan in a child who meets the case definition provides assurance that subsequent adverse outcomes are very unlikely. A cohort of 399 such children (GCS .12 and normal CT scan) found 3 patients who were readmitted within 1 month, 1 of whom had an intercranial contusion, but none required neurosurgical intervention. Rarely, cases are reported in the literature of children with normal CT scans who subsequently develop "flash edema," or, even more rarely, intracranial (especially epidural) hematomas.

Utility of Early Diagnosis

In the course of the literature review, because the reviewers identified several papers and unpublished reports that noted a higher frequency of intracranial abnormalities than the subcommittee members had anticipated, the subcommittee requested that literature examining the utility of the early diagnosis of these abnormalities be examined. Little child-specific data are available that relate to this question, ie, "Are children with apparently mild head trauma who are discovered to have an intracranial injury better off if the discovery is made sooner rather than later?" Although a classic and often cited study of comatose adults with subdural hematoma showed a dramatic benefit associated with rapid diagnosis and treatment, subsequent study has not replicated that report for either subdural or epidural bleeding. Small case series have similarly not found a correlation between delay in diagnosis of intracranial bleeding and outcome in children. The extreme limitations of these reports in their sample size, and the appropriately nonrandom allocation of time to diagnosis and treatment make any inferences from this work extremely limited.

Effectiveness of Alternative Management Strategies

An ideal study seeking to determine the relative effectiveness of alternative management strategies would initially define a homogeneous population of children with mild head trauma, and randomly assign such children to 1 of 2 or more potential approaches. Such approaches might include inpatient observation for a defined period of time without initial imaging, outpatient observation without imaging, or CT scanning followed by outpatient observation if scans are normal. No such study has been identified in the pediatric literature. The rarity of adverse outcomes would make such a study difficult to perform, and would require careful collaboration across multiple institutions.

One decision analysis has been published that assesses the cost-effectiveness of a particular strategy for the evaluation of head trauma. This analysis, although not limited to children, utilized much pediatric data in developing the probabilities required for the analysis. The authors recommend immediate CT scanning for patients with abnormal clinical signs; for patients who are otherwise normal, these authors recommend skull radiography, with CT if radiographs are abnormal. If such a strategy were followed for 10 000 persons presenting with mild head trauma, of 10 000 individuals with head injuries, the 9900 additional skull films and 250 CT scans would identify 6 or 7 additional cases of early intracranial hemorrhage.

Outcome of Mild Head Trauma

In an idealized decision analytic framework, the "utilities" to patients of the various clinical outcomes are incorporated in assessing the value of each potential treatment arm. We sought to identify through the literature the long-term outcome for the index case, assuming no significant intracranial abnormalities were identified.

Several studies did not specifically report on outcomes for pediatric patients, although authors typically commented that outcomes for children were better than those for adults. Four studies, however, did specifically examine outcomes for children. One large cohort study of children with "minimal" (or "trivial") head injury, ie, excluding children with skull fracture, loss of consciousness, or having been admitted to an inpatient unit, found physical health 1 month after injury to be identical to that of a normal population, but that role limitations, eg, school absenteeism, was substantially increased. Unfortunately, this study could not distinguish whether this effect was the result of the head injury, or associated either with the use of the emergency department or with whatever factors led to the injury. A smaller study of children with mild injury including "concussion" found a slight increase in teacher-reported hyperactivity (activity and inattentiveness) 10 years after the injury, with no other differences in school performance, cognitive ability, or behavioral symptoms. In this relatively small cohort, no differences in these outcomes between those patients who had been observed in inpatient or out-patient settings were identified. Two more recent studies also suggested some possible long-term impact of head injury. Comparing a cohort of 95 children followed up 1 year after hospitalization for head trauma of varying degree with population norms, investigators found that the children with head injuries had higher levels of physical and behavioral impairment; this investigation did not control for preexisting morbidity leading to the injury. Only patients at the most severe end of the spectrum (Abbreviated Injury Scale level 5) had demonstrably worse outcomes than those with milder injuries (Abbreviated Injury Scale level 2). A more compelling study from New Zealand compared children ages 2½ to 3½ years of age with mild head trauma (evaluated in an emergency department but not admitted to the hospital) with injury date-matched children with other forms of mild trauma 1, 6, and 12 months after the injury and when the children were 6½ years of age. The investigators found specific deficits in solving visual puzzles beginning 6 months after injury and persisting throughout the observation; these children were also more likely to have reading disabilities. We conclude from these investigations that children who present with head injuries or other types of injuries are different from the general population and more likely to have some functional impairment unrelated to the injury per se; at the same time, children with mild or minimal head injury may be more likely to experience subtle abnormalities in specific cognitive functions.

CONCLUSION

The literature on mild head trauma does not provide a sufficient scientific basis on which clinical management decisions can be made with certainty. The field remains burdened by inconsistent definitions of case severity, inadequate specification of the population base, and varied and incomplete definition of outcome. Nonetheless, the published data do indicate that 1) a small proportion of children with minimal and mild head injury will have significant intracranial injury; 2) the presence of either loss of consciousness or amnesia increases the probability that an injury is present in many, but not all studies; 3) CT scanning is the most sensitive, specific, and clinically safe mode of identifying such injury, whereas plain radiographs in this pediatric age group have neither sufficient sensitivity nor specificity to recommend their general use; 4) extremely rare children with normal examinations and CT scans will experience delayed bleeding or edema; and 5) long-term outcomes for children with minimal or mild head injury, in the absence of significant intracranial hemorrhage, are generally very good, with a suggestion of a small increase in risk for subtle specific deficits in particular cognitive skills.

The confusion in this field mandates that multicenter, collaborative investigations be performed that will begin to address the limited information base on which such a large volume of clinical care rests.

Practice Parameter: Neuroimaging of the Neonate

The following guideline for neuroimaging of the neonate, developed by the American Academy of Neurology, has been endorsed by the American Academy of Pediatrics.

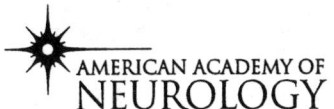
AMERICAN ACADEMY OF
NEUROLOGY

CME Practice parameter: Neuroimaging of the neonate

Report of the Quality Standards Subcommittee of the American Academy of Neurology and the Practice Committee of the Child Neurology Society

L.R. Ment, MD; H.S. Bada, MD; P. Barnes, MD; P.E. Grant, MD; D. Hirtz, MD; L.A. Papile, MD;
J. Pinto–Martin, PhD; M. Rivkin, MD; and T.L. Slovis, MD

Article abstract—*Objective:* The authors reviewed available evidence on neonatal neuroimaging strategies for evaluating both very low birth weight preterm infants and encephalopathic term neonates. *Imaging for the preterm neonate:* Routine screening cranial ultrasonography (US) should be performed on all infants of <30 weeks' gestation once between 7 and 14 days of age and should be optimally repeated between 36 and 40 weeks' postmenstrual age. This strategy detects lesions such as intraventricular hemorrhage, which influences clinical care, and those such as periventricular leukomalacia and low-pressure ventriculomegaly, which provide information about long-term neurodevelopmental outcome. There is insufficient evidence for routine MRI of all very low birth weight preterm infants with abnormal results of cranial US. *Imaging for the term infant:* Noncontrast CT should be performed to detect hemorrhagic lesions in the encephalopathic term infant with a history of birth trauma, low hematocrit, or coagulopathy. If CT findings are inconclusive, MRI should be performed between days 2 and 8 to assess the location and extent of injury. The pattern of injury identified with conventional MRI may provide diagnostic and prognostic information for term infants with evidence of encephalopathy. In particular, basal ganglia and thalamic lesions detected by conventional MRI are associated with poor neurodevelopmental outcome. Diffusion-weighted imaging may allow earlier detection of these cerebral injuries. *Recommendations:* US plays an established role in the management of preterm neonates of <30 weeks' gestation. US also provides valuable prognostic information when the infant reaches 40 weeks' postmenstrual age. For encephalopathic term infants, early CT should be used to exclude hemorrhage; MRI should be performed later in the first postnatal week to establish the pattern of injury and predict neurologic outcome.

NEUROLOGY 2002;58:1726–1738

Despite the development of sophisticated care techniques, the incidence of neurodevelopmental disability among the survivors of newborn intensive care remains high.[1-4] As newborn special care enters its fifth decade, survival rates for both severely compromised

term infants and very low birth weight (VLBW) preterm (PT) infants have increased.[5,6] However, the incidence of cerebral palsy (CP) has not changed during the past 10 years, the number of children with school-based problems is on the rise, and the population of infants at risk for disability is increasing.[7-13] Because the clinical evaluation of these infants may not provide either adequate diagnostic or prognostic information, neuroimaging is frequently used.[14-16]

Additional material related to this article can be found on the *Neurology* Web site. Go to www.neurology.org and scroll down the Table of Contents for the June 25 issue to find the title link for this article.

This statement has been endorsed by the American Academy of Pediatrics, the American Society of Pediatric Neuroradiology, and the Society for Pediatric Radiology.

Approved by the AAN Quality Standards Subcommittee December 8, 2001. Approved by the AAN Practice Committee January 28, 2002. Approved by the AAN Board of Directors February 23, 2002. Approved by the CNS Practice Committee January 30, 2002.

From the Departments of Pediatrics and Neurology (Dr. Ment), Yale University School of Medicine, New Haven, CT; Department of Pediatrics (Dr. Bada), Department of Radiology (Dr. Barnes), Stanford University School of Medicine, Stanford, CA; Departments of Radiology (Dr. Grant) and Neurology (Dr. Rivkin), Harvard University School of Medicine, Boston, MA; Clinical Trials Section, National Institute of Neurological Disorders and Stroke (Dr. Hirtz), Bethesda, MD; Department of Pediatrics (Dr. Papile), University of New Mexico Health Science Center, Albuquerque; Schools of Nursing and Medicine (Dr. Pinto–Martin), University of Pennsylvania, Philadelphia; and Department of Radiology (Dr. Slovis), Wayne State University School of Medicine, Detroit, MI.

Address correspondence and reprint requests to the American Academy of Neurology, 1080 Montreal Avenue, St. Paul, MN 55116.

Neuroimaging plays two important roles: 1) diagnosis of brain injury in the newborn at risk so that appropriate medical management can be provided and 2) detection of those lesions associated with long-term neurodevelopmental disability. Currently, cranial ultrasonography (US), CT, and MRI are the most available means for these tasks.

Goals. The Quality Standards Subcommittee of the American Academy of Neurology and the Practice Committee of the Child Neurology Society seek to develop scientifically sound, clinically relevant practice parameters for physicians for diagnostic procedures, treatment modalities, and clinical disorders. Practice parameters are strategies for patient management that might include diagnosis, symptom, treatment, or procedure evaluation. They make specific recommendations based on the analysis of evidence in the published literature.

This practice parameter provides recommendations in response to questions regarding brain imaging of PT and term infants. For PT infants: which PT infants should undergo routine screening US? When should these studies be performed? Do abnormalities shown by neonatal US require follow-up MRI? What is the ability of US to accurately predict long-term neurodevelopmental outcome for this patient population? For term infants: which imaging strategies are able to provide clinically important information for infants with neonatal encephalopathy? Can MRI provide prognostic information for these infants?

Description of the process. The committee consisted of neonatologists, pediatric neurologists, perinatal epidemiologists, and neonatal radiologists selected by five professional organizations (see the electronic version of this article for appendix 1 at www.neurology.org); we evaluated the quality of the evidence from the published literature. Evidence reviewed for this parameter was identified through literature searches using MEDLINE and EMBASE for the years 1990 to 2000 and CURRENT CONTENTS for 2000. This literature search was updated in June 2001. Relevant articles were chosen from the English-language literature using the following search terms: neonate, infant, brain, cerebral, MRI, MRS, diffusion-weighted imaging (DWI), diffusion tensor imaging, US, echoencephalography, Doppler ultrasonography, cranial axial tomography, near-infrared spectroscopy, SPECT, germinal matrix hemorrhage, intraventricular hemorrhage (IVH), periventricular leukomalacia (PVL), stroke, ischemia, ventriculomegaly, and echodensity. Because neonatal practices and imaging strategies have changed over the past decade,[12,17-21] we reviewed only those references from 1990 onward.

This search produced >1,320 citations, from which 90 met the predefined inclusion criteria: original clinical articles published since 1990, review articles, and reports of meta-analyses.

Each of the selected articles was reviewed, abstracted, and classified (appendix 2) by at least two reviewers. Abstracted data included patient number, mean birth weight (BW), mean gestational age (GA), age at the time of the neuroimaging study, primary neuroimaging measure, primary and secondary outcome measures, and timing of subject selection (prospective, retrospective, case-control, or case series study). We also noted both inclusion and exclusion criteria for patient selection and description of the neuroimaging strategy in addition to the results of the given study.

The strength of the evidence for each relevant article was ranked using the defined criteria shown in appendix 2. Recommendations were derived based on the strength of the evidence and stratified (level A, B, C, or U) as shown in appendix 3.

For the purposes of this practice parameter, a screening neuroimaging study was defined as one that is routinely applied to identify infants at sufficient risk of a specific disorder who would benefit from further investigation or direct action but who have no specific neurologic signs or symptoms requiring medical attention (e.g., infants born before 28 weeks of gestation).

Neuroimaging strategies. Although neuroimaging has proven to be extremely helpful for the assessment of injury to the PT brain and may provide useful information for evaluating the infant with neonatal encephalopathy, there are significant problems associated with imaging of the critically ill infant.[14,22,23] These include the choice of imaging technique, the timing of the imaging study, and regional variations in maturation of the developing brain. Further, transporting acutely ill neonates, many of whom require ventilatory assistance, multiple indwelling catheters, infusions, vasopressor support, and warming lights, represents a major challenge.

Currently, US, CT, and MRI represent the major imaging modalities most widely available for evaluating critically ill infants.

VLBW PT infants. Birth weight (BW) remains one of the most important predictors of infant mortality and morbidity. VLBW infants (BW <1,500 grams) now represent 1.45% of all live births in the United States.[5,6,24] In addition, the survival rates for this population are steadily increasing. In contrast, the handicap rates for surviving infants—particularly those with the lowest BW—are high. At 8 years of age, >50% of children with BW of <1,000 grams are educated in special education classrooms or resource rooms, 20% have repeated a grade in school, and 10% to 15% have spastic motor handicaps.[1,9,13]

Hemorrhage, hypoxia, and ischemia are the major causes of injury to the PT brain, and multiple studies over the past decade have used neuroimaging techniques to assess these injuries.[24-28]

US screening of the VLBW PT infant. Although cranial US of VLBW PT infants is routinely performed

Table 1 *Classification of cranial ultrasound findings for the preterm infant*

Classification		Findings
Intraventricular hemorrhage*	Grade 1	Germinal matrix hemorrhage
	Grade 2	Blood within the ventricular system but not distending it
	Grade 3	Intraventricular hemorrhage with ventricular dilatation
	Grade 4	Parenchymal involvement
Preterm white matter injury†	Cystic lesions	Periventricular
Ventriculomegaly‡	Mild	0.5–1.0 cm§
	Moderate	1.0–1.5 cm§
	Severe	>1.5 cm§

*Reference 30.
†References 29, 31–35.
‡References 36, 37.
§ Measurements at the midbody of the lateral ventricle on sagittal scan.

in newborn intensive care units, the target populations, number of examinations, and timing of these studies vary widely. Further, different institutions use different systems of nomenclature to describe IVH, white matter injury, and ventriculomegaly, the three major findings for the PT infant. For this parameter, the grading system for IVH of Papile et al.[29] will be used (table 1). In addition, because there is controversy surrounding the meaning of the periventricular echodensities routinely reported in US studies of PT infants,[28,30-32] injury to the PT white matter will include only periventricular cystic lesions.[114,115] There is a consensus in the field that the degree of ventriculomegaly (see table 1) predicts long-term neurodevelopmental outcome for PT infants studied at or near term.[33,34]

Correlation of US findings with neuropathologic data. Before reviewing data pertinent to the practice parameter questions, the committee reviewed the evidence correlating clinical US findings with neuropathologic data. In four class II studies[35-38] reporting results of a total of 87 autopsies performed on PT infants, US was 76% to 100% accurate in detecting grade 1 lesions of >5 mm and grade 3 and grade 4 hemorrhages (see the electronic version of this article for table 4 at www. neurology.org). Detection of grade 2 hemorrhages was much less accurate.

Correlation of US findings of cystic PVL with neuropathologic data was evaluated in three class II studies.[38-40] Each study found 100% correlation between US findings and neuropathologic data.

Which PT infants should undergo routine screening cranial US? Evidence. Seven class II studies evaluated the need for screening cranial US in low BW PT infants.[25,27,28,41-44] Review of these studies (ta-

ble 2; see the electronic version of this article for table 5 at www.neurology.org) suggests that although cranial US of 12% to 51% of infants with BW of <1,500 grams or GA of <33 weeks shows some abnormalities in the first 2 weeks of life, major US abnormalities such as grades 3 and 4 IVH or bilateral cystic PVL occur in ≤20% of infants. Furthermore, more severe abnormalities occur in those infants with the lowest BW.

Because infants with grades 3 and 4 IVH are at considerable risk for metabolic abnormalities, posthemorrhagic hydrocephalus, and its sequelae (e.g., apnea and obtundation), such a, US finding would in all likelihood alter the infant's care and thus was considered clinically significant.[16] In addition, cystic PVL and ventriculomegaly are risk factors for CP. These US findings might not only provide critical prognostic information but also influence long-term care strategies. Therefore, it is important to determine which infants are at high risk for grades 3 and 4 IVH, cystic PVL, and/or ventriculomegaly.

In only four studies, the data were presented by specific GA and/or BW groups.[25,28,41,43] In these studies, grades 3 and 4 IVH was noted in 11% of infants with BW of <1,000 grams and in 5% of infants with BW of 1,000 to 1,250 grams; when infants were compared by GA groups, 16% of those with GA of ≤25 weeks and 1% to 2% of infants with GA of >25 weeks had grades 3 and 4 IVH (see the electronic version of this article for table 5 at www.neurology.org). Likewise, cystic PVL was noted in 5% to 26% of infants weighing <1,000 grams, compared with 1% to 5% of infants with BW of >1,000 grams. Ventriculomegaly was described in 5% to 7% of infants weighing <1,000 grams. Conclusions. Twelve percent to 51% of infants with BW of <1,500 grams and/or GA of 33 weeks have cranial US abnormalities (class II evidence). However, major abnormalities such as grades 3 and 4 IVH, cystic PVL, and ventriculomegaly, which might alter treatment or provide prognostic information, are considerably more common (20%–25%) in infants with GA of <30 weeks.

Recommendations (level B). Close to 25% of infants with GA of <30 weeks have significant cranial US abnormalities that trigger important changes in acute and long-term care. Therefore, routine screening cranial US should be performed on all infants with GA of <30 weeks.

When should screening cranial US be performed? Evidence. Multiple class II studies performed before 1990 suggested that >90% of all IVH cases in VLBW PT infants were detected during postnatal days 4 to 5.[45-48]

Data from recent class II studies are shown in table 2 (see the electronic version of this article for table 6 at www.neurology.org). In one study,[28] 248 infants with BW of <1,500 grams underwent regular US at predefined times (1–5 days, 10–14 days, 28 days, and term). Approximately 65% of IVH cases were detected within the first week. The other cases

Table 2 *Incidence and timing of ultrasound abnormalities in preterm infants*

Reference no.	Class	Inclusion criteria	US abnormalities, incidence (%)	Major abnormalities, incidence (%)	No. (%) of major abnormalities	Incidence of major abnormalities by GA or BW	Timing of major abnormalities, incidence (%)
41	II	BW, <1,500 g; GA, <34 wk	IVH, 50/250 (20)	Grades 3 and 4 IVH, 13/250 (5)	13 (5)	GA of <25 wk, 9/57 (16); GA of >25 wk, 4/193 (2)	
42	II	BW, <1,500 g; 33 wk	IVH and/or PVL, 245/338 (43)	Grades 3 and 4 IVH and/or cystic PVL, 75/338 (22)	75 (22)		d 1–3, 27/75 (36); d 4–7, 36/75 (48); d 8–14, 12/75 (16)
43	II	BW, <1500 g	PVL, 14/115 (12)			BW of <1000 g, 12/46 (26)	wk 1, 6/14 (43); wk 3–15, 8/14 (57)
25	II	GA, <32 wk; BW, <1,500 g; or GA, <37 wk with ventilator	IVH, 106/800 (13)	Grades 2–4 IVH, 51/800 (6)	51 (6)	GA of <30 wk, 46/364 (13); GA of >30 wk, 5/436 (1)	
27	II	GA, <33 wk	PVL, 26/172 (15)				wk 1, 19/26 (73); wk 2–7, 7/26 (27)
44	II	GA, <36 wk	PVL, 11/53 (21)				wk 1, 10/11 (91); wk 2, 1/11 (9)
28	II	BW, <1,500 g	IVH, PVL and/or VM, 161/317 (51)	Grades 3 and 4 IVH, PVL and/or VM, 40/317 (13)	40 (12.6)	BW of <1,000 g; 13/114 (11.4); BW of >1,000 g; 4/203 (2)	BW of <1,000 g; wk 1 (52) wk 2 (12); wk 4 (16); term (20)

BW = birth weight; GA = gestational age; wk = week; IVH = intraventricular hemorrhage; PVL = periventricular leukomalacia; VM = ventriculomegaly; d = day.

occurred in the second and third postnatal weeks, and one infant developed severe IVH after postnatal day 28. When BW was <1,000 grams, severe IVH was detected in 10 (77%) of 13 infants on days 1 to 5; 13 (100%) of 13 cases of severe IVH were detected on day 28.

In a study designed to assess changes in US findings across time,[42] 144 infants with BW of <1,500 grams or GA of <33 weeks underwent US between days 1 and 7 and then between days 10 and 14. Fifteen infants (10%) had significant changes in US findings from the first to the second scan. Thirteen infants whose first US showed normal results or grades 1 and 2 IVH were found to have major abnormalities (i.e., grades 3 and 4 IVH and/or PVL) at the time of the second scan. For two infants, US findings changed from a major abnormality during the first US (i.e., PVL) to either normal results or a minor abnormality (i.e., grade 2 IVH) during the second US.

Cystic PVL has been detected in infants without previous US abnormalities as late as postnatal day 104.[27,43,44] In one report,[28] cystic PVL and ventriculomegaly were found in 8 (3%) of 256 neonates after previously normal US findings. For infants weighing <1,000 grams, 3 (50%) of 6 cases of PVL were noted at 36 to 40 weeks' postmenstrual age.

Conclusions. The timing at which US can detect injury in the developing brain may be changing. Grades 3 and 4 IVH, which may alter medical management and prognostic information, may be detected as late as the third postnatal week. Cystic PVL and ventriculomegaly, which may alter progno-

sis and treatment programs, may be first seen by US at term. Furthermore, these lesions may be detected in many infants after previously normal US findings.

Recommendation (level B). Screening cranial US should be performed on all infants with GA of <30 weeks at 7 to 14 days of age and should be optimally repeated at 36 to 40 weeks' postmenstrual age. This recommendation is designed to detect both clinically unsuspected IVH, which may require additional clinical and/or radiologic monitoring and changes in management plans, and evidence for PVL and/or ventriculomegaly, which are useful for prognosis and best seen when the infants are examined at term.

Do abnormalities of screening cranial US for the PT infant require follow-up MRI either to obtain information for patient management or to provide long-term prognostic data? Evidence. Three recent class II studies (see the electronic version of this article for table 7 at www.neurology.org) compared results of cranial US and MRI performed during the newborn period for PT infants.[26,49,50] Maalouf et al.[26] performed paired MRI and US studies on the same day for 32 infants with GA of <30 weeks. US accurately detected the presence of germinal matrix, IVH, and parenchymal hemorrhage confirmed by MRI (positive predictive values of 0.8, 0.85, and 0.96, respectively). However, in this study and others,[49,50] white matter injury detected by MRI was less well predicted by US (sensitivity of 0.56–0.89). Additional information provided by MRI included depiction of hemorrhagic lesions in 64% of infants and more numerous or extensive cysts in infants with

PVL diagnosed by US.[50] To date, there has not been correlation with neurodevelopmental follow-up.

Conclusions. Compared with US performed on the same day, MRI of PT neonates detects more white matter abnormalities in the first week of life, more hemorrhagic lesions, and more numerous or extensive cysts. There are insufficient data from follow-up studies to indicate whether these additional findings provide more information about the neurodevelopmental prognosis.

Recommendation (level C). Currently, available data from class II studies do not provide sufficient evidence that routine MRI should be performed on all VLBW PT infants for whom results of screening cranial US are abnormal.

What is the ability of neonatal cranial US to predict long-term neurodevelopmental outcome for VLBW PT infants? Evidence. VLBW PT infants are at high risk for neurodevelopmental handicap. Depending on the GA of the cohort and the year of birth, the previously reported incidence of mental retardation and/or CP among PT infants ranged from 7% to almost 50%.[1,4,51,52] Further, the timing of cranial US used to predict outcome in the reported literature varied from the first 2 weeks of life through term. For this reason, the lesions reported and the predictive values for these lesions were difficult to compare. Finally, in several studies, children deemed excessively impaired were omitted from the follow-up assessments, and in many, the outcome measures were reported in broad categories. Therefore, it was difficult to assess the nature of CP or mental retardation across cohorts.

Only reports containing the following data were included: GA and/or BW of the study population, postmenstrual age of the "predictor" US when recorded, neurodevelopmental follow-up rate, age at assessment, and outcome variables.

The six class II studies[34,53-57] (see the electronic version of this article for table 8 at www.neurology.org) compared US findings with the incidence of CP for almost 2,250 VLBW PT children at ages 2 to 9 years. Significant associations between grade 4 IVH, PVL, and/or ventriculomegaly and CP were noted in all six studies. In the largest of these studies,[58] both grade 4 IVH and PVL were associated with CP (odds ratio [OR], 15.4; 95% CI, 7.6–31.1); any grade IVH alone was also associated with CP (OR, 3.14; 95% CI, 1.5–6.5). Similar data were available from one class III study and three class IV studies (see the electronic version of this article for table 8 at www.neurology.org).[59-62]

When the same groups from class II and class III studies[53-55,57-59,63,64] assessed the correlation of neonatal US findings with the developmental quotient, grade 4 IVH and moderate to severe ventriculomegaly were strongly associated with the risk of mental retardation at 2 to 9 years of age (see the electronic version of this article for table 8 at www.neurology.org). In these prospective studies, OR ranged from 9.97 to 19.0. In addition, Whitaker et al.[65] demonstrated that for infants with BW of 500 to 2,000 grams who had grade 4 IVH and/or moderate to severe ventriculomegaly, the OR for the development of any neuropsychiatric disorder at the age 6 years was 4.4.

Conclusions. Grades 3 and 4 IVH, cystic PVL, and moderate to severe ventriculomegaly determined by US have all been shown to be significantly associated with CP at 2 to 9 years of age in VLBW PT infants (class II evidence). In addition, class II evidence, grade 4 IVH, and ventriculomegaly have been significantly associated with mental retardation and neuropsychiatric disorders at the same time points. The OR, which vary depending on the population under study, the lesion, and the outcome measure, all indicate at least a 10-fold elevation in the risk of adverse outcome for VLBW PT infants with US evidence of grades 3 and 4 IVH, cystic PVL, and moderate to severe ventriculomegaly.

Recommendation (level A). For VLBW PT infants, US should be used to predict long-term neurodevelopmental outcome. The findings of grades 3 and 4 IVH, periventricular cystic lesions, and moderate to severe ventriculomegaly are all associated with adverse outcome.

Term infants with neonatal encephalopathy. Clinical examination of the term infant with signs and symptoms of neonatal encephalopathy is often unable to determine the severity or extent of cerebral damage and frequently provides little information regarding the etiology of the insult. Although numerous reports suggest that hypoxic–ischemic encephalopathy (HIE) is a common cause of neonatal encephalopathy, the differential diagnosis of this condition is extensive, including a spectrum of abnormalities ranging from infectious to metabolic abnormalities and congenital malformations.[66,67] Even in those infants with documented HIE, the clinical presentation may vary widely.[68] Of those neonates with moderate to severe HIE, almost one-quarter have mental retardation, seizures, and CP, and promising intervention strategies are now becoming available.[69-71] Therefore, for diagnostic and prognostic reasons, early assessment and diagnosis of infants with neonatal encephalopathy is important.

For the definition of neonatal encephalopathy, the committee used the criteria set forth by the American Academy of Pediatrics and the American College of Obstetricians and Gynecologists in *Guidelines for Prenatal Care*.[72] For results of a study to be rated as class I evidence, infants described therein must meet all of the following conditions:

1. Profound metabolic or mixed acidemia (pH <7.00 [umbilical cord artery blood sample if obtained]).
2. Apgar score of 0 to 3 for >5 minutes.
3. Neonatal neurologic manifestations (e.g., seizures, coma, or hypotonia).
4. Multisystem organ dysfunction (e.g., cardiovascu-

lar, gastrointestinal, hematologic, pulmonary, or renal system).

Although these criteria were originally developed for those infants thought to have HIE, they also describe any infant who requires immediate neonatal evaluation—both to determine the underlying cause of encephalopathy and to provide therapeutic interventions, when available.[67,73,74] Studies in which the entry criteria of the infants evaluated were less rigorously defined received lower classification levels than did those in which infants met these conditions.

Which neonatal neuroimaging strategies can detect cerebral abnormalities that may affect the immediate and long-term management of the infant with neonatal encephalopathy? Evidence. One study discussed gray-scale US of the infant with neonatal encephalopathy.[75] A second study compared findings of gray-scale US and Doppler US with outcome,[76] and a third study compared results of gray-scale US and Doppler US with somatosensory evoked potentials, visual evoked potentials, and results of the cerebral function monitoring.[77] A fourth study compared findings of gray-scale US, Doppler US, and CT.[78] Three other studies compared results of gray-scale US and MRI for infants with neonatal encephalopathy.[79-81] Four studies reported CT findings for these infants.[82-85]

Gray-scale US, Doppler US, and studies comparing US with CT and/or MRI. In one class III study[75] (see the electronic version of this article for table 9 at www.neurology.org), US was performed on 104 encephalopathic term neonates and 70 control term neonates on the first postnatal day. A diffuse increase in echogenicity of the cerebral parenchyma and slit-like ventricles were significantly more common in infants with encephalopathy than in controls (39% versus 1% [$p < 0.001$] and 44% versus 9% [$p < 0.001$], respectively), but the investigators found no correlation between US findings on the first postnatal day and neurodevelopmental status at 1 year of age. Similar results were noted in a class II study evaluating term infants with neonatal encephalopathy on the first postnatal day.[76]

In the same class II study,[76] analysis of simultaneous Doppler US demonstrated resistive indices (resistive index = peak systolic velocity minus end diastolic velocity divided by peak systolic velocity) of <0.60 for all children with adverse neurodevelopmental outcome. In another class II study,[78] gray-scale US, Doppler US, and CT were performed on infants with neonatal encephalopathy (see the electronic version of this article for table 9 at www.neurology.org). Gray-scale US was not predictive of outcome, but a resistive index of ≤0.5 in the middle cerebral artery was associated with adverse neurodevelopmental outcome at 1 to 2 years (sensitivity, 82%; specificity, 89%). In addition, CT demonstrating generalized decreased density had 91% sensitivity and 100% specificity for adverse outcomes.

Three studies compared early US and MRI studies for infants with neonatal encephalopathy (see the electronic version of this article for table 9 at www.neurology.org).[79-81] An abnormal MRI signal in the basal ganglia in association with an abnormal US result for the basal ganglia was most frequently associated with an adverse neurodevelopmental outcome including CP, seizures, and developmental delay at 1 year of age, while normal findings of US and CT or US and MRI had low negative predictive values.

Conclusions. Seven studies (classes II and III) assessed the role of gray-scale US in the diagnosis of term infants with neonatal encephalopathy. Although gray-scale US can be easily performed at the bedside, there are little data to support the use of this modality in imaging of the encephalopathic term neonate. However, two class II studies of Doppler US suggested that resistive indices of <0.5–0.6 are consistent with the diagnosis of HIE.

CT studies. CT can be performed rapidly and without sedation of the neonate. Four studies used CT to evaluate term infants with neonatal encephalopathy. One study[84] reported basal ganglia changes; a second study[82] reported both basal ganglia and thalamic changes. Two studies[83,85] used CT to detect intracranial hemorrhages in infants with signs and symptoms of neonatal encephalopathy who also had low hematocrit or evidence of coagulopathy; in both studies, detection of intracranial hemorrhages altered clinical care.

Conclusions. One class II study and three class IV studies assessed the value of CT for encephalopathic term neonates. Two studies suggested that low attenuation in the basal ganglia and/or thalami indicates severe injury consistent with HIE. The other two studies demonstrated that CT plays a role in the detection of hemorrhagic lesions.

MRI studies. Two studies (see the electronic version of this article for table 9 at www.neurology.org) compared MRI findings with neuropathologic data for infants with neonatal encephalopathy believed attributable to HIE.[86,87] In the larger study,[87] imaging data were compared with results of neuropathologic analyses of the posterior limb of the internal capsule, thalamus, parietal cortex, hippocampus, and medulla. The posterior limb of the internal capsule was the most reliable region analyzed, and agreement of MRI findings was similar to that achieved by two pathologists reviewing the histologic sections ($\kappa = 0.66$). In this study, the MRI abnormality was predictive of the pathologic abnormality with a sensitivity of 0.70 and a positive predictive value of 1.0. The predictive value of a single MRI abnormality was 0.79 (95% CI, 0.61–0.96).

In eight class II studies (see the electronic version of this article for table 9 at www.neurology.org),[2,88-94] conventional T1- and T2-weighted MRI studies were performed for a total of 272 term neonates, most of whom were clinically suspected of having neonatal encephalopathy secondary to hypoxic–ischemic injury. Scans were obtained at ages ranging from 1 to 30 postnatal days, and the mean age range was 2 to

8 days. Three patterns of injury were detected by MRI: 1) injury to the thalami and/or posterior–lateral putamen with involvement of the subcortical white matter in the most severe injuries; 2) injury to the parasagittal gray matter and subcortical white matter, posteriorly typically more than anteriorly; and 3) focal or multifocal injury. Thalamic and basal ganglia damage was the most common abnormality reported. This pattern of injury was detected in almost 40% of infants and represented over one-half of all abnormalities (see the electronic version of this article for table 10 at www.neurology.org). In one class III study,[95] abnormal T1-weighted images showing hyperintensities in a characteristic distribution were demonstrated as early as 3 days after the injury; abnormal T2-weighted images showing hypointensities were demonstrated by 6 to 7 days.

Conclusions. Results of class II studies indicate that characteristic MR patterns of cerebral injury can be detected using conventional T1- and T2-weighted imaging sequences performed at mean ages of 2 to 8 days for encephalopathic term infants.

Diffusion weighted imaging. Studies of adult arterial infarcts have shown that DWI signal changes occur within minutes of symptom onset and hours before changes become apparent on T1- or T2-weighted images.[96] In one class II study[86] and four class III studies[97-100] that investigated the use of DWI in the evaluation of term neonates (see the electronic version of this article for table 11 at www.neurology.org), entrance criteria were not stated in enough detail to determine which infants met strict criteria for acute neonatal encephalopathy, and neonates with focal seizures were also included. MR studies were performed a mean of 2 to 4 days after birth, and DWI findings were compared with those of standard MRI sequences. Abnormal DWI results were reported for two-thirds of infants. For 7% to 58% of infants with abnormal DWI findings, T2- and/or T1-weighted images were also abnormal. Abnormal DWI results and normal T1- and/or T2- weighted images typically occurred when imaging was performed earlier than day 2 of life or when there was diffuse white matter involvement. Robertson et al.[99] described one patient for whom all imaging sequences including DWI and T1- and T2-weighted imaging sequences were normal when performed at 13 hours despite development of DWI and T1- and T2-weighted imaging abnormalities by 5 days. Robertson et al. also described one other patient for whom DWI results were normal at 8 days when T1- and T2-weighted images were abnormal; this decreased sensitivity of DWI in the subacute to chronic phase has also been noted for the adult population, suggesting that the maximum sensitivity of DWI is between 2 and 8 days.

Conclusions. Findings of one class II study and four class III studies suggest that DWI can provide evidence of cerebral injury before conventional MRI techniques for term infants with neonatal encephalopathy. However, DWI results may be negative if it is performed earlier than 24 hours of life or later than 8 days of life.

Proton MRS. A number of investigators have explored the utility of ¹H-MRS and 31P-MRS at field strengths of ≥1.5 T, but the recommendations for this parameter will be limited to ¹H-MRS at 1.5 T because this is the equipment most commonly available for neonatal imaging. All of the studies that evaluated ¹H-MRS at 1.5 T used single-voxel point resolved spectroscopy (PRESS) or stimulate echo acquisition mode (STEAM) MRS; although mutivoxel chemical shift imaging (CSI) allows high resolution evaluation of larger regions of tissue, there are no data at this time that assess the role of this modality in perinatal brain injury.

In a number of class II studies (see the electronic version of this article for table 12 at www.neurology.org), echo times of ≈136 msec and 272 msec were preferred over the shorter echo times of ≈36 msec because of the higher SD of metabolite concentrations measured at these shorter echo times.[20,93] An echo time of 136 msec has the additional advantage of an inverted lactate peak, making distinction from lipids (which can resonate in the same region) more accurate.

One class II study[101] used MRS at 1.5 T within the first 18 hours in 31 cases of suspected HIE and in 7 matched controls. Lactate/creatine ratios ranged from 0 to 0.6 (median, 0.05) for the seven controls. In contrast, the investigators demonstrated lactate/creatine ratios of >1.0 for 10 (32%) of the 31 infants with suspected HIE. In three additional class II studies,[93,102,103] proton MRS of the basal ganglia was performed within the first 2 weeks of life on 77 infants with neonatal encephalopathy. Elevated lactate/N-acetylaspartate ratios were the most consistent findings, although elevated lactate/creatine and lactate/choline ratios were also reported for infants with suspected neonatal encephalopathy.

Conclusions. Data from class II studies suggest that MRS can play an important role in the assessment of encephalopathic term infants. Lactate/creatine ratios of >1 in the first 18 hours are more common in those infants with later neurologic findings consistent with HIE. Elevated lactate/NAA, lactate/creatine, and lactate/choline ratios in the first 2 postnatal weeks are more common in infants with suspected neonatal encephalopathy than in age-matched controls.

Recommendations for diagnostic assessment.
1. For infants with a history of neonatal encephalopathy, significant birth trauma, and evidence for low hematocrit or coagulopathy:
a. Noncontrast CT should be performed to look for hemorrhage (level B).
b. If the CT findings cannot explain the clinical status of the neonate, MRI should be performed (level A).
2. For other neonates with acute encephalopathy:
a. MRI should be performed between days 2 and 8 of life (level A).

b. If single-voxel MRS is available, MRI should include MRS (level B).

c. At the time of MRI, DWI should also be performed if this modality is available (level C).

d. CT should be performed only if MRI is not available or if the neonate is too unstable for MRI (level A).

Can MRI provide prognostic data for term infants with neonatal encephalopathy? Evidence. Eight class II studies (table 3; see the electronic version of this article for table 9 at www.neurology.org) assessed the ability of conventional MRI performed between 2 and 8 days of age to predict neurodevelopmental handicap at postnatal ages of 12 to 24 months.[2,88-94] Although results of several studies suggested that abnormalities of the cerebral white matter are associated with adverse outcome in term infants with neonatal encephalopathy, 50% to 94% of infants with changes in the basal ganglia developed CP, mental retardation, and seizures at 1 to 2 years of age.[2,88,91,94] Barkovich et al.[89] correlated cognitive and motor outcome with timing of conventional MRI. Proton density MRI scans correlated best during the first 3 postnatal days, proton density and T1-weighted im-

ages correlated best during the first 7 postnatal days, and T2-weighted images correlated best after 7 to 8 postnatal days. Overall, proton density images during the first 7 postnatal days were the best predictor of outcome in this study.

Similarly, three studies using DWI (table 3; see the electronic version of this article for table 11 at www.neurology.org) performed at a mean age of 2 days in neonatal encephalopathy demonstrated a significantly elevated risk of adverse neurologic outcome, although the small sample sizes make predictions unreliable.[97-99]

Finally, review of the class II studies using proton MRS (table 3; see the electronic version of this article for table 12 at www.neurology.org) within the first 11 days of life demonstrated that lactate/creatine ratios of >1.0 and elevated lactate/NAA or lactate/choline ratios were highly predictive of adverse neurodevelopmental outcome at 1 to 2 years of age.[93,101-103] Infants with lactate/creatine ratios of >1.0 were found to have adverse neurodevelopmental outcome at 1 year of age (OR, 13.2; sensitivity, 66%; specificity, 95%; positive predictive value, 86%; negative predictive value, 88%).[101] Similarly, ele-

Table 3 *MRI studies of term neonatal encephalopathy*

Reference no.	Class	Number	Follow-up	Predictor study	Time study	Outcome measures	Age	Data
88	II	15	15/15	MRI	newborn	CP	1 yr	only BG predict CP (3/3)
102	II	31	31/31	MRS	newborn	CP, MR	1 yr	BG lac/CHO & lac/NAA associated with MR and/or CP p < 0.003 for all
90	II	25	25/25	MRI	> 7 days	DQ	1 yr	6/6 N MRI—Normal 12 abn BG—12/12 MR/CP
117	III	16	16/16	MRS	d 18	exam	1 yr	no significant differences
101	II	31 HIE & 7N	31/31	MRS	newborn	CP, MR	1 yr	if Lac/creat >1.0, OR 13.2; sens 66%, spec 95%
97	II	26	26	DWI	newborn	exam	6 mo	abn DWI: 10/12 abn examN DWI: 12/14 N exam
98	II	4	4 of 4	DWI	d 2	exam	3–21 mo	abn DWI: 4/4 abn exam
91	II	43	43/43	MRI	d 6	MR, CP		abn BG predict CP or MR p < 0.01
2	II	52	52/52	MRI	d 8–30	head growth	1 yr	N MRI: 11/12 N outcome abn WM: 5/5 abn outcomeabn BG: 5/7 abn outcome
93	II	21	18/18 survivors 3 deaths	MRI/MRS	d 8	outcome	2 yrs	N MRI: 8/9 N; abn MRI: 5/11 abn; abn BG/MRI: 4/7 abn; Lac/NAA assoc with outcome p < 0.05
99	II	43	43/43	MRS	<1 mo	outcome	1 yr	lac/creat predict outcome p = 0.001
94	II	75	73/75	MRI	d 1–17	DQ	1 yr	abn BG: sens 90%; spec 100%
104	II	18 HIE & 3 N	14/14 survivors 4 deaths	MRI	d 6	outcome	1–2 yrs	Lac/NAA predict outcome p = 0.05

vated lactate/NAA and lactate/choline or lactate/creatine ratios in the region of the basal ganglia were significantly associated with CP and mental retardation ($p < 0.001$ for all studies).[102,103] In another report, abnormalities of NAA/creatine, NAA/choline, and choline/creatine ratios in the occipital gray/parietal white matter regions were predictive of adverse outcome at a mean age of 15 months in infants with HIE.[104] Positive predictive values for abnormal neurodevelopmental outcome based on these metabolites were 0.64, 0.68, and 0.75 for values >2 SD from those of controls.

Conclusions. Class II MRI studies demonstrated that the incidence of neurodevelopmental handicap among those infants with abnormalities of the thalami and basal ganglia at mean postnatal ages of 2 to 8 days is significant at 1 to 2 years of age. Limited and predominantly class III DWI evidence demonstrates abnormalities in infants with neonatal encephalopathy at a time when results of conventional MRI are normal. Class II studies of proton MRS performed within the first 8 postnatal days also suggest good to excellent predictive values for this measure for neurodevelopmental outcome at 1 to 2 years of age.

Recommendation. MRI should be performed within the first 2 to 8 days of life to provide predictive data for neurodevelopmental outcome in encephalopathic term infants (level A). DWI (level C) and MRS (level B), when available, should also be performed within the first 2 to 8 days to provide additional prognostic data concerning neurodevelopmental outcome.

Future directions. As the number of infants cared for in neonatal intensive care units grows and survival statistics steadily increase, neuroimaging has become critical technology. Imaging of the developing brain is no longer a research goal; it has become clinically relevant. Neuroimaging can provide diagnostic information but also data used for clinical decision making as well as information on treatment efficacy and prognosis. This becomes particularly important in the anticipation of potential preventive, protective, and rehabilitative strategies for the management of critically ill newborn infants.

Several ongoing clinical trials are assessing the impact of neuroprotective strategies on long-term neurodevelopmental outcome.[105] For these studies, neuroimaging is critical—not only to provide diagnostic entry criteria but also to assess the effect of the intervention and to provide prognostic neurologic information.

Two sets of difficulties must be overcome to more fully incorporate neuroimaging into the newborn intensive care unit. MRI holds great promise; however, this imaging modality and others that may be soon developed must become more infant friendly, and imaging strategies should be developed to provide maximum information in minimum time. This would include the following: improved magnet technology that would allow easy placement of affordable MRI devices in newborn intensive care units, software and hardware advances that would minimize imaging time and allow DWI and/or MRS sequences to be easily performed on critically ill neonates, and MRI-compatible devices that improve our ability to monitor and maintain critically ill neonates. Further, it is important that results of these imaging studies, including processed DWI and MRI data, be available immediately for viewing by all involved specialties.

To provide more accurate information, these MR techniques must be optimized and standardized in terms of types of sequence, parameters for each imaging sequence, regions of brain evaluated, and timing of evaluations. Prospective imaging studies with centralized, blinded readers and well-defined cohorts of infants and matched controls should be performed to determine accurate diagnostic criteria. Similarly, prognostic data can be determined only from blinded standardized follow-up assessments of all infants imaged by the modality under study.

Although there is some recent control data on DWI for neonates,[106,107] the numbers of patients studied are small. There is also a strong need for MRS control data for neonates. For both of these modalities, serial studies are generally lacking, and the impact of timing of the study and regional variation on its result remains unknown. For example, although elevated lactate/NAA, lactate/creatine, and lactate/choline ratios are reported to be more common for infants with suspected HIE, more studies are required to determine the upper limits of these ratios for the normal population at various postnatal ages and to determine the sensitivity, specificity, and predictive values of these ratios. Studies are also needed to determine not only the optimal timing of DWI and MRS evaluation for term infants with neonatal encephalopathy but also the optimal region for investigation for MRS. Long-term follow-up data on the disability rate are of critical importance. Control data, timing studies, neuropathologic correlations, and ultimately outcome assessments are also needed before MRI becomes the standard of care for the VLBW PT neonate. MRS and DWI for this age group have the potential to provide much needed information concerning the timing of white matter injury in the developing brain and may lead to injury-specific interventions.[108]

Preliminary studies suggest that the more aggressive and timely use of advanced structural and functional prenatal imaging techniques to detect and characterize abnormalities may allow intervention to prevent postnatal neurologic morbidity and mortality.[109,110] Prenatal imaging may provide information for consideration of corrective prenatal surgical or medical interventions where appropriate and can assist with the planning of surgical or medical interventions in the intrapartum and postpartum periods. Therefore, studies that correlate prenatal US and MRI findings with results of postnatal neuroimaging and outcome are needed.

Near infrared spectroscopy, nuclear medicine (SPECT and PET), and fMRI are other major imaging technologies not discussed in this parameter because of lack of data; these technologies are under evaluation for use in the assessment of the developing brain.[111-115] The challenge is to develop and implement effective applications of these advanced neuroimaging techniques and to perform studies evaluating their diagnostic and predictive ability. As evidence becomes available,[116] it must be reviewed on a regular basis, and the practice parameter must be modified accordingly.

Disclaimer. This statement is provided as an educational service of the American Academy of Neurology and the Child Neurology Society. It is based on an assessment of current scientific and clinical information. It is not intended to include all possible proper methods of care for a particular neurologic problem or all legitimate criteria for choosing to use a specific procedure. Neither is it intended to exclude any reasonable alternative methodologies. The American Academy of Neurology and the Child Neurology Society recognize that specific patient care decisions are the prerogative of the family and the physician caring for the patient.

Appendix 1

Professional Organizations Represented: American Academy of Pediatrics, American Academy of Neurology, American Society of Pediatric Neuroradiology, Child Neurology Society, Society for Pediatric Radiology.

AAN Quality Standards Subcommittee Members: Gary Franklin, MD, MPH (Co-Chair); Catherine Zahn, MD (Co-Chair); Milton Alter, MD, PhD (ex-officio); Stephen Ashwal, MD; Rose M. Dotson, MD; Richard M. Dubinsky, MD; Jacqueline French, MD; Gary H. Friday, MD; Michael Glantz, MD; Gary Gronseth, MD; Deborah Hirtz, MD (facilitator); Robert G. Miller, MD; David J. Thurman, MD, MPH; and William Weiner, MD.

CNS Practice Committee Members: Carmela Tardo, MD (Chair); Bruce Cohen, MD (Vice-Chair); Elias Chalhub, MD; Roy Elterman, MD; Murray Engel, MD; Bhuwan P. Garg, MD; Brian Grabert, MD; Annette Grefe, MD; Michael Goldstein, MD; David Griesemer, MD; Betty Koo, MD; Edward Kovnar, MD; Leslie Anne Morrison, MD; Colette Parker, MD; Ben Renfroe, MD; Anthony Riela, MD; Michael Shevell, MD; Shlomo Shinnar, MD; Gerald Silverboard, MD; Russell Snyder, MD; Dean Timmns, MD; Greg Yim, MD; Mary Anne Whelan, MD.

Appendix 2

Definitions for classification of diagnostic evidence

Class I: Evidence provided by a prospective study in a broad spectrum of persons with the suspected condition, using a "gold standard" for case definition, where test is applied in a blinded evaluation, and enabling the assessment of appropriate tests of diagnostic accuracy.

Class II: Evidence provided by a prospective study of a narrow spectrum of persons with the suspected condition, or a well designed retrospective study of a broad spectrum of persons with an established condition (by "gold standard") compared to a broad spectrum of controls, where test is applied in a blinded evaluation, and enabling the assessment of appropriate tests of diagnostic accuracy.

Class III: Evidence provided by a retrospective study where either persons with the established condition or controls are of a narrow spectrum, and where test is applied in a blinded evaluation.

Class IV: Any design where test is not applied in blinded evaluation OR evidence provided by expert opinion alone or in descriptive case series (without controls).

Definitions for classification of prognostic evidence

Class I: Evidence provided by a prospective study of a broad spectrum of persons who may be at risk for developing the outcome (e.g., target disease, work status). The study measures the predictive ability using an independent gold standard for case definition. The predictor is measured in an evaluation that is masked to clinical presentation and the outcome is measured in an evaluation that is masked to the presence of the predictor.

Class II: Evidence provided by a prospective study of a narrow spectrum of persons who may be at risk for developing the outcome, or by a retrospective study of a broad spectrum of persons with the outcome compared to a broad spectrum of controls. The study measures the predictive ability using an acceptable independent gold standard for case definition. The risk factor is measured in an evaluation that is masked to the outcome.

Class III: Evidence provided by a retrospective study where either the persons with the condition or the controls are of a narrow spectrum. The study measures the predictive ability using an acceptable independent gold standard for case definition. The risk factor is measured in an evaluation that is masked to the outcome.

Class IV: Any design where the predictor is not applied in a masked evaluation OR evidence provided by expert opinion or case series without controls.

Appendix 3

Definitions for strength of recommendations

Level A: Established as useful/predictive or not useful/predictive for the given condition in the specified population (requires at least one convincing class I study or at least two consistent, convincing class II studies).

Level B: Probably useful/predictive or not useful/predictive for the given condition in the specified population (requires at least one convincing class II study or at least three consistent class III studies).

Level C: Possibly useful/predictive or not useful/predictive for the given condition in the specified population (requires at least two convincing and consistent class III studies).

Level U: Data inadequate or conflicting. Given current knowledge, test/predictor is unproven.

Acknowledgment

The authors thank Wendy Edlund, Alison Nakashima, Vicki Glascow, Marjorene Ainley, and Nancy DiMaio for bibliographic and editorial support and Karol Katz for computing assistance.

References

1. Hack M, Taylor HG, Klein N, Mercuri-Minich N. Functional limitations and special health care needs of 10- to 14-year-old children weighing less than 750 grams at birth. Pediatrics 2000;106:554–560.
2. Mercuri E, Ricci D, Cowan FM, et al. Head growth in infants with hypoxic-ischemic encephalopathy: correlation with neonatal magnetic resonance imaging. Pediatrics 2000;106:235–243.
3. Sreenan C, Bhargava R, Robertson CM. Cerebral infarction in the term newborn: clinical presentation and long-term outcome. J Pediatr 2000;137:351–355.
4. Wood NS, Marlow N, Costeloe K, Gibson AT, Wilkinson AR. Neurologic and developmental disability after extremely preterm birth. N Engl J Med 2000;343:378–384.
5. Guyer B, MacDorman MF, Martin JA, Peters KD, Strobino DM. Annual summary of vital statistics—1997. Pediatrics 1998;102:1333–1349.
6. Guyer B, Hoyert DL, Martin JA, Ventura SJ, MacDorman MF, Strobino DM. Annual summary of vital statistics—1998. Pediatrics 1999;104:1229–1246.
7. Allen MC. Developmental outcome of neonatal intensive care: what questions are we asking? Curr Opin Pediatr 2000; 12:116–122.

8. Hutton JL, Colver AF, Mackie PC. Effect of severity of disability on survival in a northeast England cerebral palsy cohort. Arch Dis Child 2000;83:468–474.

9. McCarton C, Brooks-Gunn J, Wallace I, Bauer C. Results at age 8 years of early intervention for low-birth-weight premature infants. JAMA 1997;277:126–132.

10. McCormick M, Workman-Daniels K, Brooks-Gunn J. The behavioral and emotional well-being of school-age children with different birth weights. Pediatrics 1996;97:18–25.

11. Salokorpi T, Rautio T, Sajaniemi N, Serenius-Sirve S, Tuomi H, von Wendt L. Neurological development up to the age of four years of extremely low birth weight infants born in southern Finland in 1991-94. Acta Paediatr 2001;90:218–221.

12. Stevenson DK, Wright LL, Lemons JA, et al. Very low birth weight outcomes of the National Institute of Child Health and Human Development Neonatal Research Network, January 1993 through December 1994. Am J Obstet Gynecol 1998;179:1632–1639.

13. Taylor HG, Klein N, Hack M. School-age consequences of birth weight less than 750 g: a review and update. Dev Neuropsychol 2000;17:289–321.

14. Barnes PD. Neuroimaging and the timing of fetal and neonatal brain injury. J Perinatol 2001;21:44–60.

15. Huppi PS, Barnes PD. Magnetic resonance techniques in the evaluation of the newborn brain. Clin Perinatol 1997;24:693–723.

16. Volpe JJ. Brain injury in the premature infant. Clin Perinatol 1997;24:567–587.

17. Hack M, Horbar JD, Malloy MH, Tyson JE, Wright E, Wright L. Very low birth weight outcomes of the National Institute of Child Health and Human Development Neonatal Network. Pediatrics 1991;87:587–597.

18. Hack M, Fanaroff AA. Outcomes of extremely immature infants—a perinatal dilemma. N Engl J Med 1993;329:1649–1650.

19. Hack M, Wright LL, Shankaran S, et al. Very-low-birth-weight outcomes of the National Institute of Child Health and Human Development Neonatal Network, November 1989 to October 1990. Am J Obstet Gynecol 1995;172:457–464.

20. Holshouser BA, Ashwal S, Shu S, Hinshaw DB Jr. Proton MR spectroscopy in children with acute brain injury: comparison of short and long echo time acquisitions. J Magn Reson Imaging 2000;11:9–19.

21. Novotny E, Ashwal S, Shevell M. Proton magnetic resonance spectroscopy: an emerging technology in pediatric neurology research. Pediatr Res 1998;44:1–10.

22. Barkovich AJ. The encephalopathic neonate: choosing the proper imaging technique. AJNR Am J Neuroradiol 1997;18:1816–1820.

23. Rivkin MJ. Developmental neuroimaging of children using magnetic resonance techniques. MRDD Res Rev 2000;6:68–80.

24. Lemons JA, Bauer CR, Oh W, et al. Very low birth weight outcomes of the National Institute of Child Health and Human Development Neonatal Research Network, January 1995 through December 1996. NICHD Neonatal Research Network. Pediatrics 2001;107:E1.

25. Harding D, Kuschel C, Evans N. Should preterm infants born after 29 weeks' gestation be screened for intraventricular haemorrhage? J Paediatr Child Health 1998;34:57–59.

26. Maalouf EF, Duggan PJ, Counsell SJ, et al. Comparison of findings on cranial ultrasound and magnetic resonance imaging in preterm neonates. Pediatrics 2001;107:719–727.

27. Hayakawa F, Okumura A, Kato T, Kuno K, Watanabe K. Determination of the timing of brain injury in preterm infants with periventricular leukomalacia with serial neonatal electroencephalography. Pediatrics 1999;104:1077–1081.

28. Perlman JM, Rollins N. Surveillance protocol for the detection of intracranial abnormalities in premature neonates. Arch Pediatr Adolesc Med 2000;154:822–826.

29. Papile LS, Burstein J, Burstein R. Incidence and evolution of the subependymal intraventricular hemorrhage: a study of infants with weights less than 1500 grams. J Pediatr 1978;92:529–534.

30. Dammann O, Leviton A. Duration of transient hyperechoic images of white matter in very low birth weight infants: a proposed classification. Dev Med Child Neurol 1997;39:2–5.

31. Maalouf EF, Duggan PJ, Rutherford MA, et al. Magnetic resonance imaging of the brain in a cohort of extremely preterm infants. J Pediatr 1999;135:351–357.

32. Paneth N, Rudelli R, Monte W, et al. White matter necrosis in very low birth weight infants: neuropathologic and ultrasonographic findings in infants surviving six days or longer. J Pediatr 1990;116:975–984.

33. Poland RL, Slovis TL, Shankaran S. Normal values for ventricular size as determined by real time sonographic techniques. Pediatr Radiol 1985;15:12–14.

34. Allan WC, Vohr B, Makuch RW, Ment LR. Antecedents of cerebral palsy in a multicenter trial of indomethacin for IVH. Arch Pediatr Adolesc Med 1997;151:580–585.

35. Babcock DS, Bove KE, Han BK. Intracranial hemorrhage in premature infants: sonographic-pathologic correlation. AJNR Am J Neuroradiol 1982;3:309–317.

36. Mack LA, Wright K, Hirsch JH, et al. Intracranial hemorrhage in premature infants: accuracy in sonographic evaluation. AJR Am J Roentgenol 1981;137:245–250.

37. Pape KE, Bennett-Britton S, Szymonowicz W, Martin DJ, Fitz CR, Becker LE. Diagnostic accuracy of neonatal brain imaging: a postmortem correlation of computed tomography and ultrasound scans. J Pediatr 1983;102:275–280.

38. Trounce JQ, Fagan D, Levene MI. Intraventricular haemorrhage and periventricular leukomalacia: ultrasound and autopsy correlation. Arch Dis Child 1986;61:1203–1207.

39. Behar R, Coen RW, Merrit TA, et al. Focal necrosis of the white matter (periventricular leukomalacia): sonographic, pathologic, and electroencephalographic features. AJNR Am J Neuroradiol 1986;7:1073–1080.

40. Levene MI, Wigglesworth JS, Dubowitz V. Hemorrhagic periventricular leukomalacia in the neonate: a real-time ultrasound study. Pediatrics 1983;71:794–797.

41. Batton DG, Holtrop P, DeWitte D, Pryce C, Roberts C. Current gestational age-related incidence of major intraventricular hemorrhage. J Pediatr 1994;125:623–625.

42. Boal DK, Watterberg KL, Miles S, Gifford KL. Optimal cost-effective timing of cranial ultrasound screening in low-birth-weight infants. Pediatr Radiol 1995;25:425–428.

43. Goetz MC, Gretebeck RJ, Oh KS, Shaffer D, Hermansen MC. Incidence, timing, and follow-up of periventricular leukomalacia. Am J Perinatol 1995;12:325–327.

44. Ito T, Hashimotor K, Kadowaki K, et al. Ultrasonographic findings in the periventricular region in premature newborns with antenatal periventricular leukomalacia. J Perinat Med 1997;25:180–183.

45. Dolfin T, Skidmore MB, Fong KW, Kosins EM, Shennan AT. Incidence, severity and timing of subependymal and intraventricular hemorrhage in preterm infants born in a perinatal unit as detected by serial real-time ultrasound. Pediatrics 1983;71:541–546.

46. McDonald MM, Koop BL, Johnson ML. Timing and antecedents of intracranial hemorrhage in the newborn. Pediatrics 1984;84:32–36.

47. Ment LR, Duncan CC, Ehrenkranz RA. Intraventricular hemorrhage of the preterm neonate: timing and cerebral blood flow changes. J Pediatr 1984;104:419–425.

48. Perlman JM, Volpe JJ. Intraventricular hemorrhage in extremely small premature infants. Am J Dis Child 1986;140:1122–1124.

49. Inder TE, Huppi PS, Warfield S, et al. Periventricular white matter injury in the premature neonate is followed by reduced cerebral cortical gray matter volume at term. Ann Neurol 1999;46:755–760.

50. Sie LT, vander Knapp MD, van Wezel-Meijler G, Taets van Aerongen AH, Lafeber HN, Valk J. Early MR features of hypoxic-ischemic brain injury in neonates with periventricular densities on sonograms. AJNR Am J Neuroradiol 2000;21:852–861.

51. Doyle LW. Outcome at 5 years of age of children 23-27 weeks GA: refining the prognosis. Pediatrics 2001;108:134–141.

52. Strathearn L, Gray PH, O'Callaghan MJ, Wood DO. Childhood neglect and cognitive development in extremely low birth weight infants: a prospective study. Pediatrics 2001;108:142–151.

53. Bass WT, Jones MA, White LE, Montgomery TR, Aiello FI, Karlowicz MG. Ultrasonographic differential diagnosis and

neurodevelopmental outcome of cerebral white matter lesions in premature infants. J Perinatol 1999;19:330–336.

54. deVries LS, Eken P, Groenendaal F, Rademaker KJ, Hoogervorst B, Bruines HW. Antenatal onset of haemorrhagic and/or ischaemic lesions in preterm infants: prevalence and associated obstetric variables. Arch Dis Child Fetal Neonatal Ed 1998;78:F51–F56.

55. Piecuch R, Leonard C, Cooper B, Sehring S. Outcome of extremely low birth weight infants (500-999 grams) over a 12-year period. Pediatrics 1997;100:633–639.

56. Pinto-Martin JA, Riolo S, Cnaan A, Holzman C, Susser MW, Paneth N. Cranial ultrasound prediction of disabling and nondisabling cerebral palsy at age two in a low birth weight population. Pediatrics 1995;95:249–254.

57. van de Bor M, Ens-Dokkum M, Schreuder AM, Veen S, Brand R, Verloove-Vanhorick SP. Outcome of periventricular-intraventricular hemorrhage at five years of age. Dev Med Child Neurol 1993;35:33–41.

58. Pinto-Martin JA, Whitaker AH, Feldman J, van Rossem R, Paneth N. Relation of cranial ultrasound abnormalities in low-birth-weight infants to motor or cognitive performance at ages 2, 6 and 9 years. Dev Med Child Neurol 1999;41:826–833.

59. Wilson-Costello D, Borawski E, Friedman H, Redline R, Fanaroff AA. Perinatal correlates of cerebral palsy and other neurologic impairment among very low birth weight children. Pediatrics 1998;102:315–322.

60. Bozynski ME, DiPietro MA, Meisels SJ, Plunkett JW, Burpee B, Claflin CJ. Cranial sonography and neurologic examination at term and motor performance through 19 months of age. Dev Behav Pediatr 1993;14:112–116.

61. Lai FF, Tsou KY. Transient periventricular echodensities and developmental outcome in preterm infants. Pediatr Neurol 1999;21:797–801.

62. Pierrat V, Eken P, DeVries LS. The predictive value of cranial ultrasound and of somatosensory evoked potentials after nerve stimulation for adverse neurological outcome in preterm infants. Dev Med Child Neurol 1997;39:398–403.

63. Ment LR, Vohr B, Allan W, et al. The etiology and outcome of cerebral ventriculomegaly at term in very low birth weight preterm infants. Pediatrics 1999;104:210–215.

64. Whitaker AG, Feldman JF, Rossem RV, et al. Neonatal cranial ultrasound abnormalities in low birth weight infants: relation to cognitive outcomes at six years of age. Pediatrics 1996;98:719–729.

65. Whitaker AH, van Rossem R, Feldman JF, et al. Psychiatric outcomes in low-birth-weight children at age 6 years: relation to neonatal cranial ultrasound abnormalities. Arch Gen Psychiatry 1997;54:847–856.

66. Edwards AD, Nelson KB. Neonatal encephalopathies. Time to reconsider the cause of encephalopathies [editorial]. BMJ 1998;317:1537–1538.

67. Nelson KB, Grether JK. Selection of neonates for neuroprotective therapies: one set of criteria applied to a population. Arch Pediatr Adolesc Med 1999;153:393–398.

68. Grether JK, Nelson KB. Maternal infection and cerebral palsy in infants of normal birth weight. JAMA 1998;279:207–211.

69. Johnston MV. Hypoxic-ischemic encephalopathy. Curr Treat Options Neurol 2000;2:109–116.

70. Whitelaw A. Systematic review of therapy after hypoxic-ischaemic brain injury in the perinatal period. Semin Neonatol 2000;5:33–40.

71. Rovertson NJ, Edwards AD. Recent advances in developing neuroprotective strategies for perinatal asphyxia. Curr Opin Pediatr 1998;10:575–580.

72. Hauth JC, Merenstein GB. Guidelines for perinatal care. 4th ed. Elk Grove Village, IL, American Academy of Pediatrics and American College of Obstetricians and Gynecologists, 1997:122–123.

73. Badawi N, Kurinczuk JJ, Keogh JM, et al. Antepartum risk factors for newborn encephalopathy: the Western Australian case-control study. BMJ 1998;317:1549–1555.

74. Perlman JM, Risser R. Can asphyxiated infants at risk for neonatal seizures be rapidly identified by current high-risk markers? Pediatrics 1996;97:456–462.

75. Boo N, Chandran V, Zulfiqar M, et al. Early cranial ultrasound changes as predictors of outcome during the first year of life in term infants with perinatal asphyxia. J Paediatr Child Health 2000;36:363–369.

76. Stark JE, Seibert JJ. Cerebral artery Doppler ultrasonography for prediction of outcome after perinatal asphyxia. J Ultrasound Med 1994;13:595–600.

77. Eken P, Toet MC, Groenendaal F, de Vries LS. Predictive value of early neuroimaging, pulsed Doppler and neurophysiology in full term infants with hypoxic-ischaemic encephalopathy. Arch Dis Child 1995;73:F75–F80.

78. Gray PH, Tudehope DI, Masel JP, et al. Perinatal hypoxic-ischemic brain injury: prediction of outcome. Dev Med Child Neurol 1993;35:965–973.

79. Rutherford MA, Pennock JM, Doubowitz LMS. Cranial ultrasound and magnetic resonance imaging in hypoxic-ischaemic encephalopathy: a comparison with outcome. Dev Med Child Neurol 1994;36:813–825.

80. Blankenberg FG, Loh N-N, Bracci P, et al. Sonography, CT, and MR imaging: a prospective comparison of neonates with suspected intracranial ischemia and hemorrhage. AJNR Am J Neuroradiol 2000;21:213–218.

81. Blankenberg FG, Norbash AM, Lane B, Stevenson DK, Bracci PM, Enzmann DR. Neonatal intracranial ischemia and hemorrhage: diagnosis with US, CT and MR imaging. Radiology 1996;199:253–259.

82. Okumura A, Hayakawa F, Kato T, Kuno K, Watanabe K. Bilateral basal ganglia-thalamic lesions subsequent to prolonged fetal bradycardia. Early Hum Dev 2000;58:111–118.

83. Perrin RG, Rutka JT, Drake JM, et al. Management and outcomes of posterior fossa subdural hematomas in neonates. Neurosurgery 1997;40:1190–2000.

84. Roland EH, Poskitt K, Rodriguez E, Lupton BA, Hill A. Perinatal hypoxic-ischemic thalamic injury: clinical features and neuroimaging. Ann Neurol 1998;44:161–166.

85. Odita JC, Hebi S. CT and MRI characteristics of intracranial hemorrhage complicating breech and vacuum delivery. Pediatr Radiol 1996;26:782–785.

86. Cowan FM, Pennock JM, Hanrahan JD, Manji KP, Edwards AD. Early detection of cerebral infarction and hypoxic ischemic encephalopathy in neonates using diffusion-weighted magnetic resonance imaging. Neuropediatrics 1994;25:172–175.

87. Jouvet P, Cowan FM, Cox P, et al. Reproducibility and accuracy of MR imaging of the brain after severe birth asphyxia. AJNR Am J Neuroradiol 1999;20:1343–1348.

88. Aida N, Nishimura G, Hachiya Y, Matsui K, Takeuchi M, Itani Y. MR imaging of perinatal brain damage: comparison of clinical outcome with initial and follow-up MR findings. AJNR Am J Neuroradiol 1998;19:1909–1921.

89. Barkovich AJ, Hajnal BL, Vigneron D, et al. Prediction of neuromotor outcome in perinatal asphyxia: evaluation of MR scoring systems. AJNR Am J Neuroradiol 1998;19:143–149.

90. Biagioni E, Mercuri E, Rutherford MA, et al. Combined use of electroencephalogram and magnetic resonance imaging in full-term neonates with acute encephalopathy. Pediatrics 2001;107:461–468.

91. Kuenzle C, Baenziger O, Martin E, et al. Prognostic value of early MR imaging in term infants with severe perinatal asphyxia. Neuropediatrics 1994;25:191–200.

92. Leth H, Toft PB, Herning M, Peitersen B, Lou HC. Neonatal seizures associated with cerebral lesions shown by magnetic resonance imaging. Arch Dis Child 1997;77:F105–F110.

93. Roelants-van Rijn AM, van der Grond J, DeVries LS, Groenendaal F. Value of ¹H-MRS using different echo times in neonates with cerebral hypoxia-ischemia. Pediatr Res 2001;49:356–362.

94. Rutherford MA, Pennock JM, Counsell SJ, et al. Abnormal magnetic resonance signal in the internal capsule predicts poor neurodevelopmental outcome in infants with hypoxic-ischemic encephalopathy. Pediatrics 1998;102:323–328.

95. Barkovich AJ, Westmark K, Partridge C. Perinatal asphyxia: MR findings in the first ten days. AJNR Am J Neuroradiol 1995;16:427–438.

96. Albers GW, Lansberg MG, Norbash AM, et al. Yield of diffusion-weighted MRI for detection of potentially relevant findings in stroke patients. Neurology 2000;54:1562–1567.

97. Johnson AJ, Lee BCP, Lin W. Echoplanar diffusion-weighted imaging in neonates and infants with suspected hypoxic-

ischemic injury: correlation with patient outcome. AJR Am J Roentgenol 1999;172:219–226.

98. Krishnamoorthy KS, Soman TB, Takeoka M, Schaefer PW. Diffusion-weighted imaging in neonatal cerebral infarction: clinical utility and follow-up. J Child Neurol 2000;15:592–602.

99. Robertson RL, Ben-Sira L, Barnes PD, et al. MR line-scan diffusion-weighted imaging of term neonates with perinatal brain ischemia. AJNR Am J Neuroradiol 1999;20:1658–1670.

100. Wolf RL, Zimmerman RA, Clancy RR, Haselgrove JH. Quantitative apparent diffusion coefficient measurements in term neonates for early detection of hypoxic-ischemic brain injury: initial experience. Radiology 2001;218:825–833.

101. Hanrahan JD, Cox IJ, Azzopardi D, et al. Relation between proton magnetic resonance spectroscopy within 18 hours of birth asphyxia and neurodevelopment at 1 year of age. Dev Med Child Neurol 1999;41:76–82.

102. Barkovich AJ, Baranski K, Vigneron D, et al. Proton MR spectroscopy for the evaluation of brain injury in asphyxiated, term neonates. AJNR Am J Neuroradiol 1999;20:1399–1405.

103. Robertson NJ, Cox IJ, Cowan FM, Counsell SJ, Azzopardi D, Edwards AD. Cerebral intracellular lactic alkalosis persisting months after neonatal encephalopathy measured by magnetic resonance spectroscopy. Pediatr Res 1999;46:287–296.

104. Shu SK, Ashwal S, Holshouser BA, Nystrom G, Hinshaw DB Jr. Prognostic value of ^{1}H-MRS in perinatal CNS insults. Pediatr Neurol 1997;17:309–318.

105. Nelson K. Can magnesium sulfate reduce the risk of cerebral palsy in very low birth weight infants? Pediatrics 1995;95:263–269.

106. Neil JJ, Shiran SI, McKinsstry RC, et al. Normal brain in human newborns: apparent diffusion coefficient and diffusion anisotropy measured by using diffusion tensor imaging. Radiology 1998;209:57–66.

107. Morriss MC, Zimmerman RA, Bilaniuk LT, Hunter JV, Haselgrove JC. Changes in brain water diffusion during childhood. Neuroradiology 1999;41:929–934.

108. Huppi PS, Maier SEP, Zientara GP, Barnes PD, Jolesz FA, Volpe JJ. Microstructural development of human newborn cerebral white matter assessed in vivo by diffusion tensor magnetic resonance imaging. Pediatr Res 1998;44:584–590.

109. Levine D, Barnes Madsen JR, Abbott J, et al. Fetal CNS anomalies revealed on ultrafast MR imaging. AJR Am J Roentgenol 1999;172:813–818.

110. Whitby E, Paley MN, Davies N, Sprigg A, Griffiths PD. Ultrafast magnetic resonance imaging of central nervous system abnormalities in utero in the second and third trimester of pregnancy: comparison with ultrasound. Br J Obstet Gynaecol 2001;108:519–526.

111. Anderson AW, Marois R, Colson ER, et al. Neonatal auditory activation detected by functional magnetic resonance imaging. Magn Reson Imaging 2001;19:1–5.

112. Born P, Leth H, Miranda MJ, et al. Visual activation in infants and young children studied by functional magnetic resonance imaging. Pediatr Res 1998;44:578–583.

113. Born AP, Miranda MJ, Rostrup E, et al. Functional magnetic resonance imaging of the normal and abnormal visual system in early life. Neuropediatrics 2000;31:24–32.

114. DeVries LS, Eken P, Dubowitz LMS. The spectrum of leucomalacia using cranial ultrasound. Behav Brain Res 1992;49:1–6.

115. Hesser U, Katz-Salamon M, Mortensson W, Flodmark O, Forssberg H. Diagnosis of intracranial lesions in very low birth weight infants by ultrasound: incidence and association with potential risk factors. Acta Paediatr 1997;419(suppl):116–126.

116. Am Acad Ped, Am Coll Obstet Gynecol. Neonatal encephalopathy and subsequent cerebral palsy: defining the pathogenesis and pathology. Elk Grove Village, IL, AAP: Washington, DC: ACOG. in press, 2002.

117. Chaterl JF, Quesson B, Brun M, et al. Localized proton magnetic resonance spectroscopy of the brain after perinatal hypoxia: a preliminary report. Pediatr Radiol 1999;29:199–205.

Guidelines for Referral of Children and Adolescents to Pediatric Rheumatologists

• •

The following guideline for referral of children and adolescents to pediatric rheumatologists, developed by the American College of Rheumatology, has been endorsed by the American Academy of Pediatrics.

AMERICAN COLLEGE OF RHEUMATOLOGY
POSITION STATEMENT

SUBJECT: Guidelines for Referral of Children and Adolescents to Pediatric Rheumatologists

PRESENTED BY: Pediatric Section of the American College of Rheumatology

BACKGROUND:

This document was developed to provide a general understanding of the reasons for involving a pediatric rheumatologist in patient care and to identify circumstances when referral to a pediatric rheumatologist is appropriate. The ultimate objective in providing medical care for children with rheumatic diseases is to achieve the best possible health outcome in the most cost-effective setting.

Rheumatic diseases are an important cause of disability in childhood. Proper diagnosis and early aggressive intervention can minimize both short and long term morbidity of these conditions. Without proper therapy, acute rheumatic fever, systemic lupus erythematosus, dermatomyositis, progressive systemic sclerosis, and many forms of vasculitis can be fatal. Other conditions such as juvenile rheumatoid arthritis and spondyloarthropathies which do not acutely threaten life, can be associated with lifetime disability. Rheumatic diseases in childhood differ from those in adults. There are important age related impacts of the diseases on the developing immune, neurologic and musculoskeletal systems. These chronic diseases have profound psychosocial effects on patients and their families.

The goals of treatment of childhood rheumatologic diseases are to control disease activity, preserve normal physical, social and emotional growth and development, minimize chronic disability and deformity, and achieve remission of disease. In pediatric rheumatic diseases, findings on physical examination often take precedence over laboratory findings in the establishment of a diagnosis and a treatment plan. Children and adolescents are often difficult to evaluate due to their development and behavioral stages; therefore the importance of a skilled examiner cannot be over emphasized.

Pediatric rheumatologists are physicians who specialize in providing comprehensive care to children with rheumatologic diseases and their families. They are pediatricians who have completed an additional 2-3 years of specialized training in pediatric rheumatology and are usually Board Certified in Pediatric Rheumatology. (In some cases these physicians may have been trained initially as internists rather than pediatricians). Pediatric rheumatologists are specifically trained to be highly skilled in: 1) differential diagnosis in children and adolescents; 2) efficient use of diagnostic interventions in children and adolescents; 3) selecting the most appropriate therapy (including other consultative services) for children and adolescents with rheumatic diseases; 4) monitoring long term therapy for effectiveness and side effects unique to children and adolescents; 5) achieving favorable outcomes in terms of control of rheumatologic diseases and prevention of disability; 6) coordination of care for children and adolescents with multisystem diseases; and 7) dealing with chronically ill children, adolescents and their families.

Most pediatric rheumatologists are located at University centers and work with a multi-disciplinary team that includes one or more pediatric rheumatologists and other health care professionals who specialize in the treatment of rheumatologic diseases, such as registered nursed, physical therapists, occupational therapists and social workers. A pediatric rheumatology center will also have available the services frequently needed by these patients such as nutrition, pediatric orthopedics, pediatric nephrology, pediatric ophthalmology, pediatric cardiology, child psychology/psychiatry, maxillo-facial surgery, pediatric dermatology, and physiatry.

The major strength of the multidisciplinary team is facilitating the achievement of the goals of treatment of childhood rheumatic diseases in the least costly setting In those geographic areas of the country where visits to a pediatric rheumatologist or center can only be accomplished one to two times per year, a local adult rheumatologist may be part of this treatment team as well. Due to the limited availability of pediatric rheumatology services in many areas of the country, adult rheumatologists who have training and experience in pediatric rheumatology should also be utilized as part of the multidisciplinary team to facilitate the achievement of the goals of treatment of childhood rheumatic diseases.

POSITION

Children and adolescents with the following diseases or in the following situations may benefit from referral to a pediatric rheumatologist:

1. Patients with unclear diagnoses
   - Prolonged fever
   - Loss of function
     - inability to attend school
     - regression in physical skills
   - Normal laboratory findings but local or generalized pain and/or swelling
   - Abnormal laboratory findings but symptoms and/or examination do not fit clinical criteria for a specific rheumatic disease
   - Complaints not consistent with laboratory findings or physical examination
   - Unexplained physical findings such as rash, fever, arthritis, anemia, weakness, weight loss, fatigue or anorexia
   - Unexplained musculoskeletal pain
   - Undefined autoimmune disease

2. Diagnostic evaluation and long-term management of:
   - Juvenile rheumatoid arthritis
   - Mixed connective tissue disease
   - Scleroderma—systemic and localized
   - Spondyloarthropathies
     - ankylosing spondylitis
     - Reiter's syndrome
     - psoriatic arthritis
     - arthritis associated with inflammatory bowel
   - Chronic vasculitis
     - Polyarteritis nodosa
     - Wegner's granulomatosis
     - Behcet's syndrome
     - Takayasu's arteritis
     - hypocomplementemic vasculitis
     - hypersensitivity vasculitis
   - Systemic lupus erythematosus

HEALTH SCIENCES BROOKE LIBRARY

- Anti-phospholipid syndrome
- Cerebral vasculitis
- Sarcoidosis
- Juvenile Dermatomyositis
- Lyme disease with arthritis
- Sjögren's Syndrome
- Chronic recurrent multifocal osteomyelitis
- Neonatal onset multisystem inflammatory disease
- Post-infectious arthritis
- Post-infectious vasculitis
- Relapsing polychondritis

3. Confirm diagnosis and help formulate and/or partici-
   pate in a treatment plan for the following conditions:
   - Henoch-Schonlein Purpura
   - Apophysitis
   - Reactive (post infectious) arthritis
   - Osteochondroses
   - Serum sickness
   - Growing pains
   - Kawasaki disease
   - Iritis
   - Acute rheumatic fever
   - Erythromelalgia
   - Fibromyalgia

- Raynaud's disease
- Reflex sympathetic dystrophy
- Cold induced injury
- Pain syndromes
- Osteoporosis
- Over use syndromes; hypermobility
- Osteoarthritis
- Complex autoimmune hemolytic anemia
- Periodic fever syndromes
- Complex autoimmune thrombocytopenia

4. Diagnostic or treatment plan evaluation for autoimmune
   disorders associated with other primary diseases such
   as: immunodeficiency, neoplasm, infectious disease,
   endocrine disorders, genetic and metabolic diseases,
   post-transplantation, cystic fibrosis and arthritis associated with birth defects.

5. Provide second opinion or confirmatory evaluation
   when requested in certain cases where primary care
   physicians request expert opinion for families requiring
   subspecialty input to cope with disease process, accept
   treatment plan, allay anxiety and provide education.

APPROVAL DATE: 11/11/97

Practice Parameter: Evaluating a First Nonfebrile Seizure in Children

● ●

The following guideline for evaluating a first nonfebrile seizure in children, developed by the Quality Standards Subcommittee of the American Academy of Neurology, the Child Neurology Society, and the American Epilepsy Society, has been endorsed by the American Academy of Pediatrics.

Practice parameter: Evaluating a first nonfebrile seizure in children

Report of the Quality Standards Subcommittee of the American Academy of Neurology, the Child Neurology Society, and the American Epilepsy Society

D. Hirtz, MD; S. Ashwal, MD; A. Berg, PhD; D. Bettis, MD; C. Camfield, MD; P. Camfield, MD; P. Crumrine, MD; R. Elterman, MD; S. Schneider, MD; and S. Shinnar, MD, PhD

Article abstract—*Objective:* The Quality Standards Subcommittee of the American Academy of Neurology develops practice parameters as strategies for patient management based on analysis of evidence. For this practice parameter, the authors reviewed available evidence on evaluation of the first nonfebrile seizure in children in order to make practice recommendations based on this available evidence. *Methods:* Multiple searches revealed relevant literature and each article was reviewed, abstracted, and classified. Recommendations were based on a three-tiered scheme of classification of the evidence. *Results:* Routine EEG as part of the diagnostic evaluation was recommended; other studies such as laboratory evaluations and neuroimaging studies were recommended as based on specific clinical circumstances. *Conclusions:* Further studies are needed using large, well-characterized samples and standardized data collection instruments. Collection of data regarding appropriate timing of evaluations would be important.

NEUROLOGY 2000;55:616–623

The Quality Standards Subcommittee (QSS) of the American Academy of Neurology (AAN) seeks to develop scientifically sound, clinically relevant practice parameters for physicians for diagnostic procedures, treatment modalities, and clinical disorders. Practice parameters are strategies for patient management that might include diagnosis, symptom, treatment, or procedure evaluation. They consist of one or more specific recommendations based on the analysis of evidence.

Every year, an estimated 25,000 to 40,000 US children experience their first nonfebrile seizure, a dramatic and frightening event.[1-4] This practice parameter reviews available evidence concerning the value of diagnostic testing after a first nonfebrile seizure in a child, and provides recommendations based on this evidence. It addresses the evaluation of children age 1 month to 21 years who have experienced a first nonfebrile seizure that cannot be explained by an immediate, obvious provoking cause such as head trauma or intracranial infection. Reports concerning serum laboratory studies, CSF examination, EEG, CT, and MRI are reviewed. This parameter concerns diagnostic evaluation; a subsequent parameter will focus on treatment of the first nonfebrile seizure.

The seizure types covered by this parameter include partial (simple or complex partial, or partial with secondary generalization), generalized tonic-clonic, or tonic seizures. We are specifically not including children diagnosed with epilepsy, defined as two or more seizures without acute provocation. For this reason, myoclonic and atonic seizures are excluded because they typically are not recognized until there have been multiple occurrences. We defined the first seizure using the International League Against Epilepsy (ILAE) criteria to include multiple seizures within 24 hours with recovery of conscious-

From the National Institute of Neurological Disorders and Stroke (Dr. Hirtz), National Institutes of Health, Bethesda, MD; Department of Pediatrics (Dr. Ashwal), Loma Linda University School of Medicine, Loma Linda, CA; Department of Biological Sciences (Dr. Berg), Northern Illinois University, Dekalb; Dr. David Bettis, Boise, ID; Department of Pediatric Neurology (Drs. C. Camfield and P. Camfield), IW Killam Hospital for Children, Halifax, Nova Scotia; Department of Neurology (Dr. Crumrine), Children's Hospital of Pittsburgh, PA; Dr. Roy Elterman, Dallas, TX; Dr. Sanford Schneider, Riverside, CA; and the Departments of Neurology and Pediatrics (Dr. Shinnar), Montefiore Medical Center, Albert Einstein College of Medicine, Bronx, NY.

Approved by the Quality Standards Subcommittee April 1, 2000. Approved by the Practice Committee May 3, 2000. Approved by the AAN Board of Directors June 9, 2000.

Received September 27, 1999. Accepted in final form June 13, 2000.

Address correspondence and reprint requests to QSS, American Academy of Neurology, 1080 Montreal Avenue, St. Paul, MN 55116; phone: 800-879-1960

ness between seizures.[5] Children with significant head trauma immediately preceding the seizure or those with previously diagnosed CNS infection or tumor or other known acute precipitating causes are excluded. We excluded neonatal seizures (28 days), first seizures lasting 30 minutes or more (status epilepticus), and febrile seizures, because these disorders are diagnostically and therapeutically different. The American Academy of Pediatrics has recently published recommendations for evaluation of children with a first simple febrile seizure.[6]

Description of process. An initial MEDLINE literature search was performed for relevant articles published from 1980 to August 1996, using the following key words: epilepsy, seizures, convulsions, magnetic resonance imaging, computed tomography, electroencephalography, blood chemical analysis, neurological examination, and diagnostic errors. Standard search procedures were used, and subheadings were applied as appropriate. In addition, the database provided by *Current Contents* was searched for the most recent 6-month period. These searches produced 279 titles of journal articles in English, and 79 in non-English languages. An updated MEDLINE search was performed in June 1997 and again in November 1998.

Titles and abstracts were reviewed for content regarding first nonfebrile seizures in children and adults. Articles from the searches were identified for review and additional articles from the references in these primary articles were included. Articles were excluded if they contained only data on adults with established epilepsy, but references were reviewed pertaining to adults with first seizures only, to both children and adults with first seizures, and to children with both new and established seizures. Two of the articles published in non-English languages met our criteria and were included. Of the articles reviewed from searches, bibliographies, and committee member suggestions, 66 met the above criteria and were included as references. The age ranges included in the studies were variable, and most pediatric studies included up to age 16 to 19 years. In most reports, results were not broken down according to subsets of age groups.

A new three-tiered scheme of classification of evidence was developed specifically to be used for evaluation of diagnostic studies (Appendix 1). This classification scheme was approved by the QSS of the AAN and differs from one that has been used for the assessment of treatment efficacy studies, which largely pertains to randomized trials.

Each of the selected articles was reviewed, abstracted, and classified by at least two reviewers. Abstracted data included patient numbers, ages and gender, timing of subject selection (prospective, retrospective, or referral), case-finding methods, exclusion criteria, seizure characteristics, neurologic abnormalities prior to or after the seizure, evalua-

tions and results, and recommendations of the authors. Methods of data analysis were also noted.

Goals of immediate evaluation. After stabilization of the child, a physician must determine if a seizure has occurred, and if so, if it is the child's first episode. It is critical to obtain as detailed a history as possible at the time of presentation. The determination that a seizure has occurred is typically based on a detailed history provided by a reliable observer (Appendix 2). A careful history and neurologic examination may allow a diagnosis without need for further evaluation. Children can present with seizure-like symptoms that may not in fact represent actual seizures, but rather breath-holding spells, syncope, gastro–esophageal reflux, pseudoseizures (psychogenic), and other nonepileptic events. No single clinical symptom can reliably discriminate between a seizure and a nonepileptic event.[7,8] Studies have investigated whether serum prolactin levels[9,10] or creatine kinase levels[11] may help distinguish seizures from nonepileptic events, but neither of these tests is sufficiently reliable to use routinely.

The next goal of assessment is to determine the cause of the seizure. In many children, the history and physical examination alone will provide adequate information regarding probable cause of the seizure[12] or the need for other tests including neuroimaging.[13] The etiology of the seizure may necessitate prompt treatment or provide important prognostic information. Provoked seizures are the result of an acute condition such as hypoglycemia, toxic ingestion, intracranial infection, trauma, or other precipitating factors. Unprovoked seizures occur in the absence of such factors; their etiology may be cryptogenic (no known cause), remote symptomatic (pre-existing brain abnormality or insult), or idiopathic (genetic).

Laboratory studies. *Evidence.* In one Class I study of 30 children ages 0 to 18 years, and 133 adults with seizures, of whom 24 (15%) had new onset seizures, the standard diagnostic laboratory workup, which included complete blood count (CBC), serum electrolytes, blood urea nitrogen (BUN), creatinine, glucose, calcium, and magnesium, revealed one case of hyperglycemia that was unsuspected clinically[14] (95% CI 0, 4.9%). This patient's age was not noted, nor were those with new onset seizures identified by age. Another prospective study of 136 new onset seizure patients found no clinically significant laboratory abnormalities in the 16 children in the study who were ages 12 to 19 years[15] (95% CI 0, 19%).

In two Class II studies including 507 children with both febrile and nonfebrile seizures, results of laboratory studies did not contribute to diagnosis or management.[12,16] In another Class II study including 65 children with new onset seizures not accompanied by fever, one had a positive cocaine screen, and seven had electrolyte abnormalities (additional data supplied by the author of reference 17). Of these, four children were hyponatremic and three were hypocalcemic. Of the four children with hyponatremia, three had a history of illness, lethargy, or diarrhea, and one had no specific symptoms. Of the three with hypocalcemia, one (age 4 months) had clinical signs of rickets, one (age 1 month) had multiple seizures, and one (age 5 years) had a prolonged focal seizure. An exception to the small number of abnormal laboratory findings in the absence of specific suggestive features is in the under 6 month age group. Hyponatremia (<125 mM/L) was found to be associated with seizures in 70% of 47 infants younger than 6 months in a Class II study.[18]

In a sample of 56 children with a first seizure, 40 of whom were febrile, there was one positive urine toxicology screen of the 11 performed. None of 53 hematology tests (95% CI 0, 6%) and two of 96 (2%) chemistry tests were found to be clinically significant (both hyponatremia) (95% CI 0, 11%).[19] In three studies that included a total of 400 adults,[19-21] only 27 (<7%) were found to have abnormalities of calcium, sodium, glucose, BUN, or arterial blood gas (ABG) determinations. Of these abnormalities, only three were unsuspected on a clinical basis.

Conclusions. The fact that a first nonfebrile seizure occurred in the absence of any suggestive history or symptoms in a child who is older than age 6 months and has returned to baseline has not been shown to be sufficient reason to perform routine laboratory testing in the child with a first nonfebrile seizure. However, the number of children reported is too small to be confident that in rare circumstances, routine laboratory screening such as blood glucose determination[12,15,16] might not provide important information, even without specific clinical indications. There were only two reports of positive toxicology screens, but no studies that systematically evaluated the yield from doing routine toxicology screening in children with first seizures. If no cause for the seizure has been identified, it is important to ask questions regarding possible toxic ingestions or exposures.[20]

Recommendations.

- Laboratory tests should be ordered based on individual clinical circumstances that include suggestive historic or clinical findings such as vomiting, diarrhea, dehydration, or failure to return to baseline alertness.[12,14,15,20] **(Option)**

- Toxicology screening should be considered across the entire pediatric age range if there is any question of drug exposure or substance abuse. **(Option)**

Lumbar puncture. *Evidence.* Lumbar puncture (LP) is frequently performed in children in the presence of fever and seizures to rule out CNS infection.[6,21,22] In the only report found giving the frequency of positive spinal fluid examinations in children with nonfebrile seizures, of 57 spinal fluid samples in children ages 2 to 24 months following nonfebrile seizures, 12.3% had >5 leukocytes/mm³ in the CSF.[23] These children did not have CNS infec-

tion. CSF glucose increased with seizure duration and the range of CSF glucose was 32 to 130 mg/dL; the range of CSF protein was 9 to 115 mg/dL.[23] A 1993 AAN practice parameter regarding the value of LP did not mention nonfebrile seizure as an indication for LP in either children or adults.[21]

Conclusions. There is no evidence regarding the yield of routine LP following a first nonfebrile seizure. The one study available (Class II) is limited in size and age range. Recommendations based on age and clinical symptoms are available from Class III publications. In the very young child (<6 months), in the child of any age with persistent (cause unknown) alteration of mental status or failure to return to baseline, or in any child with meningeal signs, LP should be performed.[6,21,22] If increased intracranial pressure is suspected, the LP should be preceded by an imaging study of the head.[20]

Recommendations.

- In the child with a first nonfebrile seizure, LP is of limited value and should be used primarily when there is concern about possible meningitis or encephalitis. **(Option)**

EEG. *Evidence.* Of 10 Class I studies reviewed[24-34] (references 26 and 27 were from the same study) and one meta analysis,[35] five studies addressed the prognostic value of EEG in a population of children with a first seizure.[25-27,30,32,33] In four of these studies, epileptiform discharges or focal slowing on the EEG were predictive of recurrence.[25,27,32,33] In children with a cryptogenic (cause unknown) first seizure, 54% of 103 children with an abnormal EEG had a recurrence compared with 25% of 165 children with a normal EEG ($p < 0.001$).[27] EEG abnormalities were reported to be the best predictors of recurrence in children who were neurologically normal; however, abnormal neurologic examination[25,26] and etiology[26,36] were also strong predictors of recurrence. Several of these studies indicated that the information provided by the EEG is useful for diagnosis of the event, identification of a specific syndrome, and prediction of long-term outcome.[26,27,32,33]

Of the four Class I studies of first seizures in adults only, or in both children and adults, an abnormal EEG was predictive for recurrence risk in three studies.[28,29,34] Inclusion of both an awake and a sleep tracing, as well as hyperventilation and photic stimulation,[27,31,32,37-39] are recommended by the American EEG Society,[38] as they increase the yield of abnormalities seen on EEG tracings.

A Class I study published in 1998 in children and adults concluded that an EEG obtained within 24 hours of a seizure was more likely to contain epileptiform abnormalities than one done later (51% versus 34%).[34] The value of an EEG performed in the emergency department shortly after a seizure was addressed in two Class II studies of adult first seizure patients.[40,41] In these studies, interpretation was difficult in the presence of diffuse postictal slowing,[42] and an EEG done at that time was not helpful in determining which patients should be admitted to the hospital.[40]

A recent analysis of selected findings from several of the Class I studies referred to above[25-27,30,31] concluded that an EEG should not be routinely performed after a first seizure because it does not yield sufficient information to alter treatment decisions.[43] To reach this conclusion, the authors did not consider evidence that the EEG result does in fact alter treatment decisions. They assumed a treatment threshold to be at an 80% risk of recurrence, and used a univariate analysis. However, where the EEG is used as one of several variables, it can identify children with very high and very low recurrence risks.[25,26,32,35] The EEG is not used solely to determine recurrence, but also helps differentiate a seizure from other events, is essential to the diagnosis of a syndrome, and provides information on long-term prognosis; it influences the decision to perform subsequent neuroimaging studies[44] and may influence counseling about management of the child.

Conclusions. The majority of evidence from Class I and Class II studies confirms that an EEG helps in determination of seizure type, epilepsy syndrome, and risk for recurrence, and therefore may affect further management decisions. Experts commonly recommend that an EEG be performed after all first nonfebrile seizures.[39,45-47] It is not clear what the optimal timing should be for obtaining an EEG. Although an EEG done within 24 hours of the seizure is most likely to show abnormalities,[34] physicians should be aware that some abnormalities such as postictal slowing that can be seen on EEG done within 24 to 48 hours of a seizure may be transient and must be interpreted with caution.

There is no evidence that the EEG must be done before discharge from the emergency department; the study may be arranged on an outpatient basis. Epileptiform EEG abnormalities may be useful in confirming that the event was a seizure; however, an EEG abnormality by itself is not sufficient to make a diagnosis that an epileptic seizure occurred, nor can its absence rule out a seizure.[46,47] The EEG is necessary to determine the epilepsy syndrome and the diagnosis of an epilepsy syndrome may be helpful in determining the need for imaging studies.[34] The EEG is also useful in predicting the prognosis for recurrences.[20,39,45-47]

It is not clear what the optimal timing should be for obtaining an EEG. Although an EEG done within 24 hours of the seizure is most likely to show abnormalities, physicians should be aware that some abnormalities such as postictal slowing that can be seen on EEG done within 24 to 48 hours of a seizure may be transient and must be interpreted with caution.

Recommendations.

- The EEG is recommended as part of the neurodiagnostic evaluation of the child with an apparent first unprovoked seizure. **(Standard)**

Neuroimaging studies. *Evidence—CT scans.* There were five Class I studies regarding imaging by CT scan after a first seizure; the data pertained to children[32] and adults[24,42,48] with first seizures, and to adults and children over age 6 with both new onset and established seizures.[14] In the single Class I study of first seizures in children, the abnormalities (mostly atrophy) found in 12 children were "without therapeutic consequences" (95% CI 0, 3%).[32] In one of the adult studies, 1.3% of the patients who had CT scans were diagnosed with tumors,[24] and in another, of 62 patients there were three tumors seen on CT, all in patients with abnormal neurologic examinations.[42] Of 119 adults who had CT scans after a first generalized seizure, 20 had abnormalities that warranted therapeutic intervention.[48] In the Class I study in which 19 CT scans were done in selective cases (first seizures if greater than age 6 years, head trauma, or focal seizure), there was one significant abnormality (age of the patient was not given), a subdural hematoma, not predicted by history and physical examination.[14]

Of the 14 Class II studies, nine involved children only (n = 2559),[17,19,49-56] four were of adults only (n = 666),[24,42,57,58] and one involved children and adults (n = 109).[59] Only a small percentage of children in these studies (0 to 7%) had lesions on CT that altered or influenced management. These were most commonly brain tumors, communicating or obstructive hydrocephalus, one subarachnoid and one porencephalic cyst, and three children with cysticercosis. The yield of abnormality on CT when the neurologic examination and EEG were normal was 5 to 10%.[50,54] In a Class II study in which seven children (14% of children with nonfebrile seizures) had CT scans that influenced management, five had focal or complex partial seizures. Abnormalities on neuroimaging were associated with a higher recurrence risk.[54] In one study of febrile and nonfebrile children, CT scans were always normal in the absence of defined risk factors such as known neurologic diagnosis, age <5 months, or focal deficit.[57] Focal lesions on CT scans tended to be more commonly found in adults (18 to 34%)[40,48,57,58] than in children (0 to 12%),[17,32,49,52,54-56] particularly when ordered for specific clinical indications. At least three studies provided evidence that MRI scanning was preferable to CT[51,54,60] in children following nonfebrile seizures.

Evidence—MRI. There was one Class I report regarding MRI in children presenting with a first seizure[54] and another Class I report of newly diagnosed epilepsy in children.[60] Of 411 children who presented with a first seizure, 218 had neuroimaging studies. Four had lesions seen on MRI or CT (two brain tumors, two neurocysticercosis) that potentially altered

Table Class I and II neuroimaging studies in children

Reference	No. children	Ages	Class	Method	No. imaged	No. abnormal (%)	95% CI (%)	No. significantly abnormal* (%)	95% CI (%)
Stroink et al., 1998[32]	156	1 mo to 16 y	I	CT	112	12 (11)	9–12	0	0–3
Berg et al., 1999[60]†	273	1 mo to 15 y	I	MRI/CT	236	27 (11)	10–13	0	0–1
King et al., 1998[34]†	59	5 to 16 y	I	MRI	43	3 (3.9)	0–2	0	0–7
O'Dell et al., 1997[54]	411	1 mo to 19 y	I	MRI/CT	218	44 (20)	18–22	4 (2)	2–2
Gibbs et al., 1993[49]	964	2 mo to 17 y	II	CT	121	26 (21)	18–24	2 (2)	1–2
Yang et al., 1979[50]	256	0 to 18 y	II	CT	256	84 (33)	30–36	7 (3)	2–3
McAbee et al., 1989[52]	81	1 mo to 18 y	II	CT	81	6 (7)	6–9	4 (5)	4–6
Warden et al., 1997[56]	158	Median 3.1 y	II	CT	158	10 (6)	5–7	0	0–2
Garvey et al., 1998[17]	65	2 wk to 16 y	II	CT	65	11 (17)	16–24	7 (11)	11–17
Total	2423				1290	223 (17.3)	15–19	24 (1.9)	1–3

* Influencing treatment or management decisions.
† The author provided data regarding analyses of the children who presented with a first nonfebrile seizure.

management.[54] When these four were excluded, 407 children remained in this Class I study. Of these, 58 children had an MRI scan, and 19 (33%) scans were abnormal, but none of the children required intervention on the basis of the neuroimaging findings. In the Class I study of 613 children with newly diagnosed epilepsy, 273 had partial, generalized tonic clonic, or generalized tonic seizures and came to medical attention at the time of their first unprovoked seizure[60] (additional data supplied by the author of reference 60). Of these, 86% had neuroimaging, and none had abnormalities influencing immediate treatment or management decisions. One Class I study of 300 adults and children with first seizures reported 43 MRI scans done in 59 children, one showing hippocampal sclerosis and two showing single gray matter heterotopic nodules (additional data supplied by the author of reference 34).[34] All patients with generalized epilepsy had normal MRI scans.[34] In two Class II reports of retrospective evaluations of MRI in children with seizures, one of which was limited to children with first seizures only, abnormalities on MRI scan such as localized atrophy, mesial temporal sclerosis, and brain malformation were common but did not mandate a change in management.[51,61] There were also six Class III reports.[39,46,62-65]

It was consistently reported in the literature cited above that the MRI was more sensitive than the CT scan.[39,51,54,60,62,63,65] MRI findings included atrophy, infarction, evidence of trauma, cerebral dysgenesis, and cortical dysplasia. Authors of review articles also emphasized a preference for MRI to exclude progressive lesions such as tumors and vascular malformations, or focal cortical dysplasia.[39,62,63,65,66] Neuroimaging was recommended if there is a postictal focal deficit not promptly resolving.[46,66] A recently published practice parameter on neuroimaging in the emergency patient presenting with seizures reviewed literature primarily from adults but included children. This parameter recommended "emergent" neuroimaging if there was suspicion of a serious structural lesion, and that "urgent" neuroimaging should be considered if there was no clear cause of the seizure. This parameter states that if an emergent imaging study is needed, it would be to detect hemorrhage, brain swelling, or mass effect, conditions that are typically adequately imaged on CT.[66] These recommendations were not restricted to any age bracket.

Conclusions. Although abnormalities on neuroimaging are seen in up to one third of children with a first seizure, most of these abnormalities do not influence treatment or management decisions such as the need for hospitalization or further studies (table). Of available reported imaging results, from Class I and Class II studies of children, an average of about 2% revealed clinically significant findings that contributed to further clinical management, the majority of which were performed because the seizure was focal or there were specific clinical findings beyond the fact that a seizure had occurred (see the table).

Thus, there is insufficient evidence to support a recommendation at the level of standard or guideline for the use of routine neuroimaging, i.e., imaging performed for which having had a seizure is the sole indication, after a first nonfebrile seizure in children. However, neuroimaging may be indicated under some circumstances either as an emergent or nonurgent procedure.

The purpose of performing an *emergent* neuroimaging study in the context of a child's first seizure is to detect a serious condition that may require immediate intervention. The possible effects of emergency medication used to treat the seizure must be taken into consideration.

The purpose of performing a *nonurgent* neuroimaging study, which can be deferred to the next several days or later, is to detect abnormalities that may affect prognosis and therefore have an impact on long-term treatment and management.[20,22] Factors to be considered include the age of the child, the need for sedation to perform the study, the EEG results, a history of head trauma, and other clinical circumstances such as a family history of epilepsy.

Recommendations.

- If a neuroimaging study is obtained, MRI is the preferred modality.[50,51,54,60,62,63,65] **(Guideline)**

Emergent neuroimaging should be performed in a child of any age who exhibits a postictal focal deficit (Todd's paresis) not quickly resolving, or who has not returned to baseline within several hours after the seizure.[46,66] **(Option)**

- Nonurgent imaging studies with MRI should be seriously considered in any child with a significant cognitive or motor impairment of unknown etiology, unexplained abnormalities on neurologic examination, a seizure of partial (focal) onset with or without secondary generalization, an EEG that does not represent a benign partial epilepsy of childhood or primary generalized epilepsy, or in children under 1 year of age.[20,34] **(Option)**

Summary. In the child with a first nonfebrile seizure, diagnostic evaluations influence therapeutic decisions, how families are counseled, and the need for hospital admission and/or specific follow-up plans. This practice parameter has reviewed the published literature concerning the usefulness of studies following a first nonfebrile seizure in children, and has classified the strength of the available evidence. There is sufficient Class I evidence, which involves a well executed prospective study, to provide a recommendation with the highest degree of clinical certainty—i.e., a **Standard**—that an EEG be obtained in all children in whom a nonfebrile seizure has been diagnosed, to predict the risk of recurrence and to classify the seizure type and epilepsy syndrome. The decision to perform other studies, including LP, laboratory tests, and neuroimaging, for the purpose of determining the cause of the seizure and detecting potentially treatable abnormalities, will depend on the age of the patient and the specific clinical circumstances. Children of different ages may require different management strategies.[20,22]

Future research. For most of the questions addressed by this parameter, evidence was insufficient for making a strong recommendation for a standard or guideline, particularly for laboratory studies. In order to generate definitive evidence regarding the value of routine (or selective) laboratory testing and the use of routine neuroimaging studies, sufficiently large samples allowing for adequate statistical power to provide precise estimates (i.e., with narrow confidence intervals) are needed. Neuroimaging studies are needed to understand the significance of neuronal migration defects in the context of a first seizure, and are important because of the improved technical

ability of current MRI. In addition, prospective collection of data using standardized treatment protocols and standardized data collection instruments is essential. Results of studies will only be helpful if the patient sample and factors that resulted in inclusion into or exclusion from the sample are well described and documented. Ideally, large consecutive series of well-characterized patients are needed for the results to be accurate and generalizable. Finally, future studies should present separate data from children and adults, and it would be optimal for results in children to be presented by age groupings.

Appropriate timing as well as the choice of evaluative studies have not been adequately studied. Children may present as actively having a seizure when brought to the emergency department, as postictal, or as alert with a history of a possible seizure episode having occurred hours, days, or weeks previously. Data regarding the appropriate timing of laboratory testing, neuroimaging, or EEG studies require adequate prospective studies of these specific questions, with clearly defined entry criteria and a common protocol for type and timing of evaluations.

Research studies with adequate sample sizes and appropriate protocols that provide answers to these questions may serve to reduce the expense and discomfort of unnecessary testing in children with first seizures, and, more importantly, by identifying appropriate candidates, may improve the care and management that these children receive.

Disclaimer. This statement is provided as an educational service of the American Academy of Neurology. It is based on an assessment of current scientific and clinical information. It is not intended to include all possible proper methods of care for a particular neurologic problem or all legitimate criteria for choosing to use a specific procedure. Neither is it intended to exclude any reasonable alternative methodologies. The AAN recognizes that specific patient care decisions are the prerogative of the patient and the physician caring for the patient, based on all of the circumstances involved.

Acknowledgment

The authors thank the members of the Quality Standards Subcommittee of the AAN, and Wendy Edlund, the AAN Clinical Policy Administrator, for their time, expertise, and efforts in developing this document.

Appendix 1

Classification of evidence

Class I. Must have all of a–d:

a. Prospective study of a well defined cohort which includes a description of the nature of the population, the inclusion/exclusion criteria, demographic characteristics such as age and sex, and seizure type.

b. The sample size must be adequate with enough statistical power to justify a conclusion or for identification of subgroups for whom testing does or does not yield significant information.

c. The interpretation of evaluations performed must be done blinded to outcome.

d. There must be a satisfactory description of the technology used for evaluations (e.g., EEG, MRI).

Class II. Must have a or b:

a. A retrospective study of a well-defined cohort which otherwise meets criteria for Class 1a, 1b, and 1d.

b. A prospective or retrospective study which lacks any of the following: adequate sample size, adequate methodology, a description of inclusion/exclusion criteria, and information such as age, sex, and characteristics of the seizure.

Class III. Must have a or b:

a. A small cohort or case report.

b. Relevant expert opinion, consensus, or survey.

A cost-benefit analysis or a meta-analysis may be Class I, II, or III, depending on the strength of the data upon which the analysis is based.

Appendix 2

Outline for seizure assessment

Features of a seizure:

Associated factors
Age
Family history
Developmental status
Behavior
Health at seizure onset
Precipitating events other than illness—trauma, toxins
Health at seizure onset—febrile, ill, exposed to illness, complaints of not feeling well, sleep deprived

Symptoms during seizure (ictal)
Aura: Subjective sensations
Behavior: Mood or behavioral changes before the seizure
Preictal symptoms: Described by patient or witnessed
Vocal: Cry or gasp, slurring of words, garbled speech
Motor: Head or eye turning, eye deviation, posturing, jerking (rhythmic), stiffening, automatisms (purposeless repetitive movements such as picking at clothing, lip smacking); generalized or focal movements
Respiration: Change in breathing pattern, cessation of breathing, cyanosis
Autonomic: Pupillary dilatation, drooling, change in respiratory or heart rate, incontinence, pallor, vomiting
Loss of consciousness or inability to understand or speak

Symptoms following seizure (postictal)
Amnesia for events
Confusion
Lethargy
Sleepiness
Headaches and muscle aches
Transient focal weakness (Todd's paresis)
Nausea or vomiting

Appendix 3

Strength of recommendations

Standards. Generally accepted principles for patient management that reflect a high degree of clinical certainty (i.e., based on Class I evidence or, when circumstances preclude randomized clinical trials, overwhelming evidence from Class II evidence that directly addresses the issue, decision analysis that directly addresses the issue, or strong consensus of Class III evidence).

Guidelines. Recommendations for patient management that may identify a particular strategy or range of management strategies and that reflect moderate clinical certainty (i.e., based on Class II evidence that directly addresses the issue, decision analysis that directly addresses the issue, or strong consensus of Class III evidence).

Practice options. Other strategies for patient management for which the clinical utility is uncertain (i.e., based on inconclusive or conflicting evidence or opinion).

Practice parameters. Results, in the form of one or more specific recommendations, from a scientifically based analysis of a specific clinical problem.

Appendix 4

Quality Standards Subcommittee Members: Gary Franklin, MD, MPH—Co-Chair; Catherine Zahn, MD—Co-Chair; Milton Alter, MD, PhD; Stephen Ashwal, MD; John Calverley, MD; Richard M. Dubinsky, MD; Jacqueline French, MD; Gary Gronseth, MD; Deborah Hirtz, MD; Robert G. Miller, MD; James Stevens, MD; and William Weiner, MD.

References

1. Kaufman L, Hesdorffer D, Mu Kherjee R, Hauser WA. Incidence of first unprovoked seizures among children in Washington Heights, New York City, 1990–1994. Epilepsia 1996; 37:85. Abstract.
2. Verity CM, Ross EN, Golding J. Epilepsy in the first ten years of life: findings of the child health and education study. BMJ 1992;305:857–861.
3. Camfield CS, Camfield PR, Gordon K, Wirrell E, Dooley JM. Incidence of epilepsy in childhood and adolescence: a population-based study in Nova Scotia from 1977 to 1985. Epilepsia 1996;37:19–23.
4. Hauser W, Annegers J, Kurland L. Incidence of epilepsy and unprovoked seizures in Rochester, Minnesota, 1935–1984. Epilepsia 1993;34:453–468.
5. Commission on Epidemiology and Prognosis, International League Against Epilepsy. Guidelines for epidemiologic studies on epilepsy. Epilepsia 1993;37:592–596.
6. Provisional Committee on Quality Improvement, Subcommittee on Febrile Seizures. Practice parameter: the neurodiagnostic evaluation of the child with a first simple febrile seizure. Pediatrics 1996;97:769–775.
7. Williams J, Grant M, Jackson M, et al. Behavioral descriptors that differentiate between seizure and nonseizure events in a pediatric population. Clin Pediatr 1996;35:243–249.
8. Van Donselaar CA, Geerts AT, Meulstee J, Habbema JDF, Staal A. Reliability of the diagnosis of a first seizure. Neurology 1989;39:267–271.
9. Fein JA, Lavelle JM, Clancy RR. Using age-appropriate prolactin levels to diagnose children with seizures in the emergency department. Acad Emerg Med 1997;4:202–205.
10. Kurlemann G, Heyen P, Menges E-M, Palm DG. Prolaktin im Serum nach zerebralen und psychogenen Krampfanfallen im Kindesund Jugendlichenalter—eine nutzliche Zusatzmethode zur Unterscheidung zwischen beiden Anfallsformen. Klin Paediatr 1992;204:150–154.
11. Neufeld MY, Treves TA, Chistik V, Korczyn AD. Sequential serum creatine kinase determination differentiates vaso-vagal syncope from generalized tonic-clonic seizures. Arch Neurol Scand 1997;95:137–139.
12. Smith RA, Martland T, Lowry MF. Children with seizures presenting to accident and emergency. J Accid Emerg Med 1996;13:54–58.
13. Bardy AH. Decisions after first seizure. Acta Neurol Scand 1991;83:294–296.
14. Eisner RF, Turnbull TL, Howes DS, Gold IW. Efficacy of a "standard" seizure workup in the emergency department. Ann Emerg Med 1986;15:69–75.
15. Turnbull TL, Vanden Hoek TL, Howes DS, Eisner RF. Utility of laboratory studies in the emergency department patient with a new-onset seizure. Ann Emerg Med 1990;19:373–377.
16. Nypaver MM, Reynolds SL, Tanz RR, Davis T. Emergency department laboratory evaluation of children with seizures: dogma or dilemma? Pediatr Emerg Care 1992;8:13–16.
17. Garvey MA, Gaillard WD, Rusin JA, et al. Emergency brain computed tomography in children with seizures: who is most likely to benefit? J Pediatr 1998;133:664–669.
18. Farrar HC, Chande VT, Fitzpatrick DF, Shema SJ. Hyponatremia as the cause of seizures in infants: a retrospective analysis of incidence, severity, and clinical predictors. Ann Emerg Med 1995;26:42–48.
19. Landfish N, Gieron-Korthals M, Weibley RE, Panzarino V. New onset childhood seizures: emergency department experience. J Fla Med Assoc 1992;79:697–700.
20. Nordli DR, Pedley TA. Evaluation of children with seizures. In: Shinnar S, Amir N, Branski D, eds. Childhood seizures. Pediatric and adolescent medicine. Basel: Karger, 1995:67–77.
21. American Academy of Neurology. Practice parameter: lumbar puncture. Neurology 1993;43:625–627.
22. Hirtz DG. First unprovoked seizure. In: Maria BL, ed. Current management in child neurology. London: B.C. Decker, 1999:125–129.
23. Rider LG, Thapa PB, Del Beccaro MA, et al. Cerebrospinal

fluid analysis in children with seizures. Pediatr Emerg Care 1995;11:226–229.

24. Hopkins A, Garman A, Clarke C. The first seizure in adult life: value of clinical features, electroencephalography, and computerised tomographic scanning in prediction of seizure recurrence. Lancet 1988;1:721–726.

25. Camfield PR, Camfield CS, Dooley JM, Tibbles JAR, Fung T, Garner B. Epilepsy after a first unprovoked seizure in childhood. Neurology 1985;35:1657–1660.

26. Shinnar S, Berg AT, Moshe SL, et al. The risk of seizure recurrence following a first unprovoked afebrile seizure in childhood: an extended follow-up. Pediatrics 1996;98:216–225.

27. Shinnar S, Kang H, Berg AT, Goldensohn ES, Hauser WA, Moshe SL. EEG abnormalities in children with a first unprovoked seizure. Epilepsia 1994;35:471–476.

28. van Donselaar CA, Schimsheimer RJ, Geerts AT, Declerck AC. Value of the electroencephalogram in adult patients with untreated idiopathic first seizures. Arch Neurol 1992;49:231–237.

29. Hauser WA, Anderson VE, Loewenson RB, McRoberts, SM. Seizure recurrence after a first unprovoked seizure. N Engl J Med 1982;307:522–528.

30. Boulloche J, Leloup P, Mallet E, Parain D, Tron P. Risk of recurrence after a single unprovoked generalized tonic-clonic seizure. Dev Med Child Neurol 1989;31:626–632.

31. Carpay JA, de Weerd AW, Schimsheimer RJ, et al. The diagnostic yield of a second EEG after partial sleep deprivation: a prospective study in children with newly diagnosed seizures. Epilepsia 1997;38:595–599.

32. Stroink H, Brouwer OF, Arts WF, Geerts AT, Peters ABC, Van Donselaar CA. The first unprovoked, untreated seizure in childhood: a hospital based study of the accuracy of diagnosis, rate of recurrence, and long term outcome after recurrence. Dutch study of epilepsy in childhood. J Neurol Neurosurg Psychiatry 1998;64:595–600.

33. Martinovic Z, Jovic N. Seizure recurrence after a first generalized tonic clonic seizure, in children, adolescents and young adults. Seizure 1997;6:461–465.

34. King MA, Newton MR, Jackson GD, et al. Epileptology of first seizure presentation: a clinical, electroencephalographic and magnetic resonance imaging study of 300 consecutive patients. Lancet 1998;352:1007–1011.

35. Berg AT, Shinnar S. The risk of seizure recurrence following a first unprovoked seizure: a quantitative review. Neurology 1991;41:965–972.

36. Shinnar S, Berg AT, Ptachewich Y, Alemany M. Sleep state and the risk of seizure recurrence following a first unprovoked seizure in childhood. Neurology 1993;43:701–706.

37. Verity CM. The place of the EEG and imaging in the management of seizures. Arch Dis Child 1995;73:557–562.

38. Guideline one: minimal technical requirements for performing clinical electroencephalography. J Clin Neurophysiol 1994;11:2–5.

39. Gilliam F, Wyllie E. Diagnostic testing of seizure disorders. Neurol Clin 1996;14:61–84.

40. Rosenthal RH, Heim ML, Waeckerie JF. First time major motor seizures in an emergency department. Ann Emerg Med 1980;9:242–245.

41. Tardy B, Lafond P, Convers P, et al. Adult first generalized seizure: etiology, biological tests, EEG, CT scan, in an ED. Am J Emerg Med 1995;13:1–5.

42. Russo LS, Goldstein KH. The diagnostic assessment of single seizures. Is cranial computed tomography necessary? Arch Neurol 1983;40:744–746.

43. Gilbert DL, Buncher RC. An EEG should not be obtained routinely after first unprovoked seizure in childhood. Neurology 2000;54:635–641.

44. Commission on Neuroimaging of the International League Against Epilepsy. Recommendations for neuroimaging of patients with epilepsy. Epilepsia 1997;38:1255–1256.

45. Panayiotopoulos CP. Significance of the EEG after the first afebrile seizure. Arch Dis Child 1998;78:575–577.

46. Vining EP, Freeman JM. Management of nonfebrile seizures. Pediatr Rev 1986;8:185–190.

47. Holmes GL. How to evaluate the patient after a first seizure. Postgrad Med 1988;83:199–209.

48. Schoenenberger RA, Heim SM. Indication for computed tomography of the brain in patients with first uncomplicated generalized seizure. BMJ 1994;309:986–989.

49. Gibbs J, Appleton RE, Carty H, Beirne M, Acomb BA. Focal electroencephalographic abnormalities and computerised tomography findings in children with seizures. J Neurol Neurosurg Psychiatry 1993;56:369–371.

50. Yang PJ, Berger PE, Cohen ME, Duffner PK. Computed tomography and childhood seizure disorders. Neurology 1979;29:1084–1088.

51. Resta M, Palma M, Dicuonzo F, et al. Imaging studies in partial epilepsy in children and adolescents. Epilepsia 1994;35:1187–1193.

52. McAbee GN, Barasch ES, Kurfist LA. Results of computed tomography in "neurologically normal" children after initial onset of seizures. Pediatr Neurol 1989;5:102–106.

53. Sachdev HPS, Shiv VK, Bhargava SK, Dubey AP, Choudhury P, Puri RK. Reversible computerized tomographic lesions following childhood seizures. J Trop Pediatr 1991;37:121–126.

54. O'Dell C, Shinnar S, Mitnick R, Berg AT, Moshe SL. Neuroimaging abnormalities in children with a first afebrile seizure. Epilepsia 1997;38(suppl 8):184. Abstract.

55. Aicardi J, Murnaghan K, Gandon Y, Beraton J. Efficacite de la tomodensiometrie dans les epilepsies de l'enfant. J Neuroradiol 1983;10:127–129.

56. Warden CR, Brownstein DR, DelBeccaro MA. Predictors of abnormal findings of computed tomography of the head in pediatric patients presenting with seizures. Ann Emerg Med 1997;29:518–523.

57. Gordon WH, Jabbari B, Dotty JR, Gunderson CH. Computed tomography and the first seizure of adults. Ann Neurol 1985;18:153. Abstract.

58. Ramirez-Lassepas M, Cipolle RJ, Morillo LR, Gumnit RJ. Value of computed tomographic scan in the evaluation of adult patients after their first seizure. Ann Neurol 1984;15:536–543.

59. Wood LP, Parisi M, Finch IJ. Value of contrast enhanced CT scanning in the non-trauma emergency room patient. Neuroradiology 1990;32:261–264.

60. Berg AT, Shinnar S, Levy SR, Testa FM. Status epilepticus in children with newly diagnosed epilepsy. Ann Neurol 1999;45:618–623.

61. Klug JM, deGrauw A, Taylor CNR, Eglehoff JC. Magnetic resonance evaluation in children with new onset of seizure. Ann Neurol 1996;40:71. Abstract.

62. Kuzniecky RI. Neuroimaging in pediatric epilepsy. Epilepsia 1996;37(suppl 1):S10–S21.

63. Iannetti P, Spalice A, Atzei G, Boemi S, Trasimeni G. Neuronal migrational disorders in children with epilepsy: MRI, interictal SPECT and EEG comparisons. Brain Dev 1996;18:269–279.

64. Greenberg MK, Barsan WG, Starkman S. Neuroimaging in the emergency patient presenting with seizure. Neurology 1996;47:26–32.

65. Radue EW, Scollo-Lavizzari G. Computed tomography and magnetic resonance imaging in epileptic seizures. Eur Neurol 1994;34(suppl 1):55–57.

66. Ferry PC. Pediatric neurodiagnostic tests: a modern perspective. Pediatr Rev 1992;13:248–256.

Long-term Treatment of the Child With Simple Febrile Seizures

· ·

- *Clinical Practice Guideline*
- *Technical Report Summary*

Readers of this clinical practice guideline are urged to review the technical report to enhance the evidence-based decision-making process. The full technical report is available on the enclosed CD-ROM.

AMERICAN ACADEMY OF PEDIATRICS

Committee on Quality Improvement, Subcommittee on Febrile Seizures

Practice Parameter: Long-term Treatment of the Child With Simple Febrile Seizures

ABSTRACT. The Committee on Quality Improvement, Subcommittee on Febrile Seizures, of the American Academy of Pediatrics, in collaboration with experts from the Section on Neurology, general pediatricians, consultants in the fields of child neurology and epilepsy, and research methodologists, developed this practice parameter. This guideline provides recommendations for the treatment of a child with simple febrile seizures. These recommendations are derived from a thorough search and analysis of the literature. The methods and results of the literature review can be found in the accompanying technical report. This guideline is designed to assist pediatricians by providing an analytic framework for the treatment of children with simple febrile seizures. It is not intended to replace clinical judgment or establish a protocol for all patients with this condition. It rarely will be the only appropriate approach to the problem.

The technical report entitled "Treatment of the Child With Simple Febrile Seizures" provides in-depth information on the studies used to form guideline recommendations. A complete bibliography is included as well as evidence tables that summarize data extracted from scientific studies. This report also provides pertinent evidence on the individual therapeutic agents studied including study results and dosing information. Readers of this clinical practice guideline are urged to review the technical report to enhance the evidence-based decision-making process. The report is available on the *Pediatrics electronic pages* website at the following URL: http://www.pediatrics.org/cgi/content/full/103/6/e86.

DEFINITION OF THE PROBLEM

This practice parameter provides recommendations for therapeutic intervention in neurologically healthy infants and children between 6 months and 5 years of age who have had one or more simple febrile seizures. A simple febrile seizure is defined as a brief (<15 minutes) generalized seizure that occurs only once during a 24-hour period in a febrile child who does not have an intracranial infec-

tion or severe metabolic disturbance. This practice parameter is not intended for patients who have had complex febrile seizures (prolonged, ie, >15 minutes, focal, or recurrent in 24 hours), nor does it pertain to children with previous neurologic insults, known central nervous system abnormalities, or a history of afebrile seizures.

TARGET AUDIENCE AND PRACTICE SETTING

This practice parameter is intended for use by pediatricians, family physicians, child neurologists, neurologists, emergency physicians, and other health care professionals who treat children with febrile seizures.

POSSIBLE THERAPEUTIC INTERVENTIONS

Possible therapeutic approaches to a child with simple febrile seizures include continuous anticonvulsant therapy with agents such as phenobarbital, valproic acid, carbamazepine, or phenytoin; intermittent therapy with antipyretic agents or diazepam; or no anticonvulsant therapy.

BACKGROUND

For a child who has experienced a simple febrile seizure, there are potentially 2 major adverse outcomes that may theoretically be altered by an effective therapeutic agent. These are the occurrence of subsequent febrile seizures or afebrile seizures, including epilepsy. The risk of having recurrent simple febrile seizures varies, depending on age. Children younger than 12 months at the time of their first simple febrile seizure have approximately a 50% probability of having recurrent febrile seizures. Children older than 12 months at the time of their first event have approximately a 30% probability of a second febrile seizure; of those that do have a second febrile seizure, 50% have a chance of having at least 1 additional recurrence.[1]

Children with simple febrile seizures have only a slightly greater risk for developing epilepsy by the age of 7 years than the 1% risk of the general population.[2,3] Children who have had multiple simple febrile seizures and are younger than 12 months at the time of the first febrile seizure are at the highest risk, but, even in this group, generalized afebrile seizures develop by age 25 in only 2.4%.[4] No study has demonstrated that treatment for simple febrile seizures can prevent the later development of epilepsy. Furthermore, there is no evidence that simple febrile seizures cause structural damage and no evi-

The recommendations in this statement do not indicate an exclusive course of treatment or serve as a standard of medical care. Variations, taking into account individual circumstances, may be appropriate.

This clinical practice guideline was reviewed by the appropriate councils, committees and sections of the American Academy of Pediatrics including the Committee on Practice and Ambulatory Medicine, the Committee on Pediatric Emergency Medicine, the Committee on Drugs and sections on Emergency Medicine, Clinical Pharmacology, and Neurology. It was also reviewed by the Chapter Review Group, a focus group of practicing pediatricians representing each AAP district: Thomas J. Herr, MD, Gene R. Adams, MD, Charles S. Ball, MD, Diane E. Fuquay, MD, Michael J. Heimerl, MD, Donald T. Miller, MD, Lawrence C. Pakula, MD, William R. Sexson, MD, and Howard B. Weinblatt, MD.

PEDIATRICS (ISSN 0031 4005). Copyright © 1999 by the American Academy of Pediatrics.

dence that children with simple febrile seizures are at risk for cognitive decline.[5]

Despite the frequency of febrile seizures (approximately 3%), there is no unanimity of opinion about therapeutic interventions.[3] The following recommendations are based on an analysis of the risks and benefits of continuous or intermittent therapy in children with simple febrile seizures. The recommendations reflect an awareness of the very low risk that a simple febrile seizure poses to the individual child and the large number of children who have this type of seizure at some time in early life.[1,3-5] To be commensurate, a proposed therapy would need to be exceedingly low in risks and adverse effects, inexpensive, and highly effective.

The expected outcomes of this practice parameter include the following:

1. Optimize practitioner understanding of the scientific basis for using or avoiding various proposed treatments for children with simple febrile seizures.
2. Improve the health of children with simple febrile seizures by avoiding therapies with high potential for side effects and no demonstrated ability to improve children's eventual outcomes.
3. Reduce costs by avoiding therapies that will not demonstrably improve children's long-term outcomes.
4. Help the practitioner educate caregivers about the low risks associated with simple febrile seizures.

METHODOLOGY

More than 300 medical journal articles reporting studies of the natural history of simple febrile seizures or the therapy of these seizures were reviewed and abstracted. Emphasis was placed on articles that differentiated simple febrile seizures from other types of febrile seizures, articles that carefully matched treatment and control groups, and articles that described adherence to the drug regimen. Tables were constructed from 62 articles that best fit these criteria. A more comprehensive review of the literature on which this report is based can be found in the technical report. The technical report also contains dosing information.

BENEFITS AND RISKS OF CONTINUOUS ANTICONVULSANT THERAPY

Phenobarbital

Phenobarbital is effective in preventing the recurrence of simple febrile seizures.[6-8] In a controlled, double-blind study, daily therapy with phenobarbital reduced the rate of subsequent febrile seizures from 25 per 100 subjects per year to 5 per 100 subjects per year.[6]

The adverse effects of phenobarbital include behavioral problems such as hyperactivity and hypersensitivity reactions.[6,9-11]

Valproic Acid

In randomized, controlled studies, only 4% of children taking valproate as opposed to 35% of control subjects had a subsequent febrile seizure. Therefore,

valproic acid seems to be at least as effective in preventing recurrent, simple febrile seizures as phenobarbital and significantly more effective than placebo.[7,12,13] Drawbacks to therapy with valproic acid include its rare association with fatal hepatotoxicity (especially in children younger than 3 years who also are at greatest risk for febrile seizures), thrombocytopenia, weight loss and gain, gastrointestinal disturbances, and pancreatitis.[14]

Carbamazepine

Carbamazepine has not been shown to be effective in preventing the recurrence of simple febrile seizures.[9]

Phenytoin

Phenytoin has not been shown to be effective in preventing the recurrence of simple febrile seizures.[15]

BENEFITS AND RISKS OF INTERMITTENT ORAL THERAPY

Antipyretic Agents

Antipyretic agents, in the absence of anticonvulsants, are not effective in preventing recurrent febrile seizures.[6,16]

Diazepam

A double-blind, controlled study in patients with a history of febrile seizures demonstrated that administration of oral diazepam (given at the time of a fever) could reduce the recurrence of febrile seizures. Children with a history of febrile seizures were given oral diazepam or a placebo at the time of fever. There was a 44% reduction in the risk of febrile seizures per person-year with diazepam.[17] A potential drawback to intermittent medication is that a seizure could occur before a fever is noticed. Adverse effects of oral diazepam include lethargy, drowsiness, and ataxia.[17] The sedation associated with this therapy could mask evolving signs of a central nervous system infection.

SUMMARY

The Subcommittee has determined that a simple febrile seizure is a benign and common event in children between the ages of 6 months and 5 years. Most children have an excellent prognosis. Although there are effective therapies that could prevent the occurrence of additional simple febrile seizures, the potential adverse effects of such therapy are not commensurate with the benefit. In situations in which parental anxiety associated with febrile seizures is severe, intermittent oral diazepam at the onset of febrile illness may be effective in preventing recurrence. There is no convincing evidence, however, that any therapy will alleviate the possibility of future epilepsy (a relatively unlikely event). Antipyretics, although they may improve the comfort of the child, will not prevent febrile seizures.

RECOMMENDATION

Based on the risks and benefits of the effective therapies, neither continuous nor intermittent anti-

convulsant therapy is recommended for children with 1 or more simple febrile seizures. The American Academy of Pediatrics recognizes that recurrent episodes of febrile seizures can create anxiety in some parents and their children, and, as such, appropriate education and emotional support should be provided.

ACKNOWLEDGMENTS

The Committee on Quality Improvement and Subcommittee on Febrile Seizures appreciate the expertise of Richard N. Shiffman, MD, Center for Medical Informatics, Yale School of Medicine, for his input and analysis in development of this practice guideline. Comments were also solicited and received from organizations such as the American Academy of Family Physicians, the American Academy of Neurology, the Child Neurology Society, and the American College of Emergency Physicians.

COMMITTEE ON QUALITY IMPROVEMENT, 1998–1999
David A. Bergman, MD, Chairperson
Richard D. Baltz, MD
James R. Cooley, MD
Gerald B. Hickson, MD
Paul V. Miles, MD
Joan E. Shook, MD
William M. Zurhellen, MD

LIAISONS
Betty A. Lowe, MD
    National Association for Childrens Hospitals and
    Related Institutions
Shirley Girouard, PhD, RN
    National Association for Children's Hospitals and
    Related Institutions
Michael J. Goldberg, MD
    AAP Sections
Charles J. Homer, MD
    AAP Section on Epidemiology
Jan E. Berger, MD
    AAP Committee on Medical Liability
Jack T. Swanson, MD
    AAP Committee on Practice and Ambulatory
    Medicine

SUBCOMMITTEE ON FEBRILE SEIZURES, 1998–1999
Patricia K. Duffner, MD, Chairperson
Robert J. Baumann, MD, Methodologist
Peter Berman, MD
John L. Green, MD
Sanford Schneider, MD

CONSULTANTS
Carole S. Camfield, MD, FRCP(C)
Peter R. Camfield, MD, FRCP(C)
David L. Coulter, MD
Patricia K. Crumrine, MD
W. Edwin Dodson, MD
John M. Freeman, MD
Arnold P. Gold, MD
Gregory L. Holmes, MD
Michael Kohrman, MD
Karin B. Nelson, MD
N. Paul Rosman, MD
Shlomo Shinnar, MD

REFERENCES

1. Nelson KB, Ellenberg JH. Prognosis in children with febrile seizures. *Pediatrics.* 1978;61:720–727
2. Nelson KB, Ellenberg JH. Predictors of epilepsy in children who have experienced febrile seizures. *N Engl J Med.* 1976;295:1029–1033
3. Verity CM, Golding J. Risk of epilepsy after febrile convulsions: a national cohort study. *Br Med J.* 1991;303:1373–1376
4. Annegers JF, Hauser WA, Shirts SB, Kurland LT. Factors prognostic of unprovoked seizures after febrile convulsions. *N Engl J Med.* 1987;316:493–498
5. Ellenberg JH, Nelson KB. Febrile seizures and later intellectual performance. *Arch Neurol.* 1978;35:17–21
6. Camfield PR, Camfield CS, Shapiro SH, Cummings C. The first febrile seizure: antipyretic instruction plus either phenobarbital or placebo to prevent recurrence. *J Pediatr.* 1980;97:16–21
7. Wallace SJ, Smith JA. Successful prophylaxis against febrile convulsions with valproic acid or phenobarbitone. *Br Med J.* 1980;280:353–380
8. Wolf SM. The effectiveness of phenobarbital in the prevention of recurrent febrile convulsions in children with and without a history of pre-, peri-, and postnatal abnormalities. *Acta Paediatr Scand.* 1977;66:585–587
9. Antony JH, Hawke S. Phenobarbital compared with carbamazepine in prevention of recurrent febrile convulsions. *Am J Dis Child.* 1983;137:892–895
10. Knudsen FU, Vestermark S. Prophylactic diazepam or phenobarbitone in febrile convulsions: a prospective, controlled study. *Arch Dis Child.* 1978;53:660–663
11. Vining EPG, Mellits ED, Dorsen MM, et al. Psychologic and behavioral effects of antiepileptic drugs in children: a double-blind comparison between phenobarbital and valproic acid. *Pediatrics.* 1987;80:165–174
12. Marmelle NM, Plasse JC, Revol M, Gilly R. Prevention of recurrent febrile convulsions: a randomized therapeutic assay: sodium valproate, phenobarbital and placebo. *Neuropediatrics.* 1984;:15:37–42
13. Ngwane E, Bower B. Continuous sodium valproate or phenobarbitone in the prevention of "simple" febrile convulsions. *Arch Dis Child.* 1980;55:171–174
14. Dreifuss FE. Valproic acid toxicity. In: Levy RH, Mattson RH, Meldrum BS, eds. *Antiepileptic Drugs.* New York, NY: Raven Press; 1995:641–648
15. Bacon CJ, Hierons AM, Mucklow JC, Webb J, Rawlins MD, Weightman D. Placebo-controlled study of phenobarbitone and phenytoin in the prophylaxis in febrile convulsions. *Lancet.* 1981;2:600–604
16. Uhari M, Rantala, H, Vainionpaa L, Kurttila R. Effect of acetaminophen and of low intermittent doses of diazepam on prevention of recurrence of febrile seizures. *J Pediatr.* 1995;126:991–995
17. Rosman NP, Colton T, Labazzo J, et al. A controlled trial of diazepam administered during febrile illnesses to prevent recurrence of febrile seizures. *N Engl J Med.* 1993;329:79–84

Technical Report Summary:
Treatment of the Child With
Simple Febrile Seizures

Author:
Robert J. Baumann, MD

American Academy of Pediatrics
PO Box 927, 141 Northwest Point Blvd
Elk Grove Village, IL 60009-0927

ABSTRACT

Overview

Simple febrile seizures that occur in children ages 6 months to 5 years are common events with few adverse outcomes. Those who advocate therapy for this disorder have been concerned that such seizures lead to additional febrile seizures, to epilepsy, and perhaps even to brain injury. Moreover, they note the potential for such seizures to cause parental anxiety. We examined the literature to determine whether there was demonstrable benefit to the treatment of simple febrile seizures and whether such benefits exceeded the potential side effects and risks of therapy. The therapeutic approaches considered included continuous anticonvulsant therapies, intermittent therapy, or no anticonvulsant therapy.

Methods

This analysis focused on the neurologically healthy child between 6 months and 5 years of age whose seizure is brief (<15 minutes), generalized, and occurs only once during a 24-hour period during a fever. Children whose seizures are attributable to a central nervous system infection and those who have had a previous afebrile seizure or central nervous system abnormality were excluded. A review of the current literature was conducted using articles obtained through searches in MEDLINE and additional databases. Articles were obtained following defined criteria and data abstracted using a standardized literature review form. Abstracted data were summarized into evidence tables.

Results

Epidemiologic studies demonstrate a high risk of recurrent febrile seizures but a low, though increased, risk of epilepsy. Other adverse outcomes either don't occur or occur so infrequently that their presence is not convincingly demonstrated by the available studies. Although daily anticonvulsant therapy with phenobarbital or valproic acid is effective in decreasing recurrent febrile seizures, the risks and potential side effects of these medications outweigh this benefit. No medication has been shown to prevent the future onset of recurrent afebrile seizures (epilepsy). The use of intermittent diazepam with fever after an initial febrile seizure is likely to decrease the risk of another febrile seizure, but the rate of side effects is high although most families find the perceived benefits to be low. Although antipyretic therapy has other benefits, it does not prevent additional simple febrile seizures.

Conclusions

The Febrile Seizures Subcommittee of the American Academy of Pediatrics' Committee on Quality Improvement used the results of this analysis to derive evidence-based recommendations for the treatment of simple febrile seizures. The outcomes anticipated as a result of the analysis and development of the practice guideline include: 1) to optimize practitioner understanding of the scientific basis for using or avoiding various proposed treatments for children with simple febrile seizures; 2) to improve the health of children with simple febrile seizures by avoiding therapies with high potential for side effects and no demonstrated ability to improve children's eventual outcomes;

3) to reduce costs by avoiding therapies that will not demonstrably improve children's long-term outcomes; and 4) to help the practitioner educate caregivers about the low risks associated with simple febrile seizures. *Key words: febrile seizures, epilepsy, valproic acid, carbamazepine, phenytoin, diazepam, phenobarbital, sodium valproate, pyridoxine.*

The debate over whether children with recurrent febrile seizures benefit from anticonvulsant therapy began early in this century. An important advance was the identification of the subgroup of children with simple febrile seizures; a subgroup that is large, remarkably homogeneous, and healthy at 7- and 10-year follow-ups. Furthermore, the recognition of such favorable outcomes has accentuated the need to balance the risk of any treatment with an expected benefit. Epidemiologic studies helped to identify this subgroup, demonstrated their predominantly favorable outcomes, and confirmed what has long been known: febrile seizures are common events. Of youngsters in a British birth cohort, 2.7% had febrile seizures, 88% of whom had simple febrile seizures.

DEFINITION OF THE PROBLEM

This parameter is limited to children with simple febrile seizures defined as neurologically healthy infants and children between 6 months and 5 years of age whose seizure is brief (<15 minutes), generalized, and occurs only once during a 24-hour period in a febrile child. This definition is easily applied in the usual clinical circumstances and has the additional advantages of encompassing most children with febrile seizures and defining a relatively homogeneous group of patients. This practice parameter excludes children whose seizures are attributable to a central nervous system infection (symptomatic febrile seizures) and those who have had a previous afebrile seizure or central nervous system abnormality (secondary febrile seizures).

BACKGROUND

Proponents of therapy for simple febrile seizures have worried that repeated simple febrile seizures will lead to more febrile seizures and possibly to afebrile seizures (epilepsy). They also have been apprehensive that these seizures will cause brain injury and thus diminish intelligence or impair motor coordination.

A child who has experienced a single simple febrile seizure is likely to experience another. As epidemiologic data indicate, this recurrence rate is strongly age-related. The younger the child at the time of the first event, the more likely there will be subsequent events. In the National Collaborative Perinatal Project (NCPP), half the subjects with onset of febrile seizures during the first year versus approximately 30% with onset after the first year had one or more additional febrile seizures. This project included 1706 prospectively studied children with febrile seizures from approximately 54 000 pregnancies.

The risk of experiencing a single afebrile seizure or two or more afebrile seizures (defined as epilepsy) is elevated when comparing children with simple febrile seizures with the general age-matched population. In the NCPP, the risk factors for epilepsy after a febrile seizure were a positive family history of afebrile seizures, preexisting neurologic abnormality, and a complicated initial febrile seizure. Interestingly, the age at first febrile seizure and the number of febrile seizures did not alter this risk. At age 7 years, only

1.9% of children with simple febrile seizures and negative family histories of epilepsy had experienced a single afebrile seizure, and epilepsy had developed in 0.9%. The comparable figures for study children who never experienced a febrile seizure were 0.9% for a single afebrile seizure and 0.5% for epilepsy. Similar rates were seen in the large British cohort study that included all surviving neonates born in the United Kingdom during 1 week in April 1970. These children were followed until age 10 years, and 305 had an initial simple febrile seizure. Of the 305 children, 8 (2.6%) subsequently had an afebrile seizure and epilepsy eventually developed in 5 (1.6%). The comparable number with epilepsy among the 14 278 children who never had febrile seizures was 53 (0.4%).

Although the risk of epilepsy among children with simple febrile seizures is elevated, the rate is still low, and the number of children in any given study is small. These numbers provide some understanding of the difficulty of designing a population-based study to determine if any treatment for the prevention of simple febrile seizures would subsequently prevent the development of epilepsy.

Investigators have attempted to look at this issue. The Kaiser Foundation Hospitals in Southern California studied 400 children who had febrile seizures (identified from lumbar puncture reports). They divided the children into three study groups: those who received phenobarbital daily, those who received phenobarbital only with fever, and those who received no therapy. Follow-up lasted a mean of 6.3 years. No difference was found in the rate of afebrile seizures. This study included children with complex as well as simple febrile seizures, many children did not receive the prescribed medication (approximately one third), and the study was small and could have missed a statistically valid effect.

In another study, 289 children with febrile seizures were randomized to rectal diazepam prophylaxis at the onset of any fever or rectal diazepam therapy during any febrile seizure. At age 14 years, there was no difference in intelligence, coordination, or occurrence of epilepsy between the two groups. The number of study patients was small, there are questions regarding compliance, and patients with complex and simple febrile seizures were included.

Evidence for adverse outcomes other than epilepsy has been sought. The NCPP had the benefit of longitudinal examination of a predefined group of children. No evidence of death in relation to asymptomatic febrile seizures was found, and examination of the children revealed no evidence for the development of motor deficits. There also has been concern about cognitive deficits in relation to febrile seizures. The NCPP found no effect on intelligence among 431 children with febrile seizures who were compared with their siblings. Comparisons of children with simple febrile seizures with the general population also have found no adverse effect. Smith and Wallace believed that they found an adverse effect of repeated febrile seizures on intelligence as measured by the Griffith Mental Development Scale. Because they studied children with simple and complex febrile seizures, it is possible that underlying neurologic disease predisposed to further seizures and to lower scores on retesting.

METHODS

Pertinent articles previously obtained by a medline search and a search of the Epilepsy Foundation of America database 4 were reviewed and supplemented by references suggested by members of the Committee and the Committee's consultants. More than 300 articles were reviewed.

The goal of the review was to identify articles that met the following criteria:

- The study children had simple febrile seizures that were convincingly differentiated from afebrile seizures and other types of febrile seizures.
- The subjects with simple febrile seizures were reasonably representative of children with simple febrile seizures.
- A suitable control group was included in the study. Preference was given to blinded protocols.

CONTINUOUS ANTICONVULSANT THERAPY

Phenobarbital

There are several studies in which phenobarbital administered daily successfully prevented recurrent febrile seizures. Camfield and associates randomized 79 children who had had a first simple febrile seizure to receive phenobarbital at 5 mg/kg per day in a single dose or a placebo. Compliance was monitored by use of the urine fluorescence of a riboflavin additive and by measurements of serum phenobarbital levels. There was a significant difference in the incidence of recurrent febrile seizures between the phenobarbital recipients (2/39 [5%]) and the placebo group (10/40 [25%]). Neither parents nor investigators knew which subjects received the active drug. Investigators found no significant difference in IQ (using Stanford-Binet or Bayley Scales) between the placebo and phenobarbital groups after 8 to 12 months of therapy. Nevertheless, phenobarbital was demonstrated to decrease memory and concentration in proportion to higher serum phenobarbital levels. Transient sleep disturbances and daytime fussiness were more common among phenobarbital recipients, but by 1 year, the two groups were indistinguishable. This was partially accounted for by 4 children receiving phenobarbital whose side effects resolved after the dosage was reduced.

In a controlled trial comparing phenobarbital (5 mg/kg per day) with phenytoin (8 mg/kg per day) and placebo, Bacon and associates also found phenobarbital to be effective. In younger children, the febrile seizure recurrence rate was 9% (2/22) for phenobarbital recipients versus 44% (12/27) placebo recipients. This trial included subjects with complicated febrile seizures who were stratified proportionally into the three groups. The study had major problems with compliance. All phenobarbital-treated children with a recurrence for whom drug levels were obtained at the time of recurrence had a plasma level <15 mg/L. Interestingly the reported behavioral changes were similar in the subjects treated with phenobarbital and a placebo.

Mamelle et al compared phenobarbital (3 to 4 mg/kg per day), valproate (30 to 40 mg/kg per day in 2 doses), and placebo in a randomized single-blind study of infants with a first simple febrile seizure. They found significantly fewer recurrences in the valproate (1/22 [4.5%]) and phenobarbital (4/21 [19%]) groups compared with the placebo group (9/26 [35%]). Compliance was measured by serum drug levels. Only 5 subjects were removed from therapy because of side effects; all were described as having agitation and all were receiving phenobarbital. Other studies, some with designs that were less rigorous, also found phenobarbital to be effective, including the previously mentioned Kaiser Foundation study.

Not all studies have found phenobarbital to be effective. Heckmatt et al found recurrent febrile seizures in 14 (19%) of 73 control subjects, 10 (11%) of 88 children for whom phenobarbital was prescribed, and 4 (8%) of 49 who actually took the prescribed phenobarbital (4 to 5 mg/kg per day in divided doses). These last 4 subjects had plasma phenobarbital levels >16 mg/L at the time of recurrence. Although the differences between the treatment groups are not statistically important, they seem to suggest that an effect favoring phenobarbital might have been evident had the numbers been larger or the duration of the study longer.

Children who had complicated febrile seizures analyzed by intention to treat experienced no difference in recurrence rate between phenobarbital-treated subjects and controls. The study described a poor rate of compliance and seemed to show that a medication is not effective if parents are unable to administer it. Early in the study when compliance was high, 56% of phenobarbital recipients (4 to 5 mg/kg once per day) and 35% of placebo recipients were reported to have side effects. The study found that the mean IQ was 8.4 points lower in the phenobarbital group than in the placebo group (95% CI: −3.3 − −3.5, $P = .0057$) at the end of the 2-year study, with an IQ differential that persisted 6 months after the taper of medication had begun. The analysis of these data was complicated by the low compliance rates, the fact that 24 (26%) of 94 placebo recipients and 53 (64%) of 83 phenobarbital recipients were prescribed phenobarbital after the study ended, and the inclusion of subjects with complicated febrile seizures.

Phenobarbital is associated with impairment of short-term memory and concentration and worsening of behavior. Most data on the effects of phenobarbital have been obtained from adults or from children with epilepsy. The drug's effect seems most prominent at the onset of therapy. The reported effect in children with simple febrile seizures varies among studies. In the study by Camfield et al, parents were only aware of side effects early in the study, but higher serum levels were associated with decreased memory concentration. Smith and Wallace found no effect of therapy but believed that repeated seizures in children with complicated febrile seizures were associated with lower mental development scores. Wolf and Forsythe reported hyperactivity in 46 (42%) of 109 children treated with phenobarbital (initial dose, 3 to 4 mg/kg per day, adjusted to give a serum level of 10 to 15 μg/mL) for febrile seizures compared with 21 (17.5%) of 120 not receiving phenobarbital. As in other studies, a substantial rate of improvement was noted in both groups with time. When 25 children from each group were extensively tested, no cognitive differences could be detected.

Valproic Acid

A number of studies have demonstrated the effectiveness of this agent in preventing recurrent febrile seizures. The study by Mamelle et al typifies the studies that found valproic acid to be more effective than phenobarbital.

Although no severe adverse effects are described among the children participating in the febrile seizure trials, the numbers in these trials are small. Valproic acid therapy is associated with fatal hepatotoxicity, pancreatitis, renal toxicity, hematopoietic disturbances, and other problems.

Carbamazepine

Carbamazepine was not effective for febrile seizures in preliminary trials and, thus, has not been studied widely. In a double-blind trial of carbamazepine (20 mg/kg per day in twice daily doses) vs phenobarbital (4 to 5 mg/kg per day) involving children with complicated febrile seizures, Antony and Hawke reported recurrent febrile seizures in 9 (47%) of 19 carbamazepine recipients and 2 (10%) of 21 phenobarbital recipients.

Phenytoin

As with carbamazepine, preliminary studies showed no evidence that phenytoin was effective for febrile seizures, so it has not been studied extensively. In a randomized, controlled study of children with simple and complex febrile seizures, the recurrence rate in the phenytoin group (8 mg/kg per day) of younger children was 33% (9/27) compared with 9% (2/22) for the phenobarbital group (5 mg/kg per day) and 44% (12/27) for the equivalent placebo group.

INTERMITTENT THERAPY

Antipyretic Agents

Because simple febrile seizures occur only in conjunction with a fever, it has seemed logical to try to prevent these seizures by using aggressive antipyretic therapy. In the randomized, double-blind study by Camfield and associates, all subjects received detailed instruction about temperature control, including antipyretic use with any rectal temperature higher than 37.2°C (99°F). Ten (25%) of 40 subjects using only temperature control had recurrences compared with 2 (5%) of 39 receiving continuous phenobarbital. A randomized, controlled trial using a complicated study design with placebo, low-dose diazepam, and acetaminophen also found no evidence that acetaminophen prevented recurrent febrile seizures. In this protocol, the diazepam-treated children who had previously experienced a febrile seizure received a rectal diazepam solution (if they weighed <7 kg, they received 2.5 mg; if 7 to 15 kg, 5 mg; and if >15 kg, 10 mg) followed in 6 hours by 0.2 mg/kg three times a day whenever they were febrile. The antipyretic treatment group received 10 mg/kg of acetaminophen four times per day.

In children hospitalized after a simple febrile seizure, Schnaiderman et al found that acetaminophen (15 to 20 mg/kg per dose) given every 4 hours did not prevent a second febrile seizure during that admission any better than giving acetaminophen sporadically. The two groups also had the same frequency, duration, and height of temperature elevations. There is no evidence that aggressive antipyretic therapy prevents recurrent febrile seizures.

Diazepam

The use of intermittent diazepam prophylaxis for febrile seizures is well-reported in the literature. Autret and colleagues, in a randomized, controlled multicenter study, found that oral diazepam (0.5 mg/kg initially, then 0.2 mg/kg every 12 hours) was no more effective than a placebo in preventing recurrent febrile seizures. Most of the children had simple febrile seizures, and the data were analyzed by intention to treat. Recurrence was experienced by 15 (16%) of 93 children in the diazepam group compared with 18 (20%) of 92 children in the placebo group. Although parents "were instructed verbally, in writing, and by demonstration," there were major problems with compliance. In children with recurrences, only 1 (7%) of /15 diazepam recipients and 7 (39%) of 18 placebo recipients received the medication or placebo as prescribed. The difference between these two groups is significant. The reasons that the subjects did not receive their assigned treatment included the following: 1) 7 in each group had a seizure as the first sign of illness, 2) 5 parents in the diazepam group and 4 in the placebo group did not give the medication, and 3) 2 children in the diazepam group would not take their medication. Because 14 (93%) of the 15 children for whom diazepam was prescribed who had a recurrence had not received their prescribed medication, these data demonstrate that a treatment is not effective if parents cannot or will not administer it before the febrile seizure occurs. The only noted side effect was hyperactivity, which was significantly more frequent in the diazepam group (138 vs 34 days).

By contrast, in a similarly well-designed, randomized, double-blind, placebo-controlled trial, Rosman et al found oral diazepam to be significantly more effective than placebo when analyzed by intention to treat. A 44% reduction in the risk of febrile seizures per person-year occurred with diazepam. Children in the diazepam group had 675 febrile episodes and 41 febrile seizures, of which 7 occurred while receiving the study medication. Comparable figures for the placebo group were 526 febrile episodes and 72 febrile seizures, of which 38 occurred while receiving the placebo. These investigators describe febrile seizures as "highly upsetting" to the parent population, which may have influenced adherence. Not surprisingly, they found that a higher rate of side effects accompanied their subjects' better compliance. Of the diazepam recipients, 59 (39%) had at least one "moderate" side effect and a similar number had a "mild" side effect.

The Neurodiagnostic Evaluation of the Child With a First Simple Febrile Seizure

• *Clinical Practice Guideline*
• *Technical Report Summary*

Readers of this clinical practice guideline are urged to review the technical report to enhance the evidence-based decision-making process. The full technical report is available on the enclosed CD-ROM.

Clinical Practice Guideline:
The Neurodiagnostic Evaluation of the Child
With a First Simple Febrile Seizure

Author:

Subcommittee on Febrile Seizures
Provisional Committee on Quality Improvement

American Academy of Pediatrics
PO Box 927, 141 Northwest Point Blvd
Elk Grove Village, IL 60009-0927

SUBCOMMITTEE ON DIAGNOSIS AND
TREATMENT OF FEBRILE SEIZURES
1992–1995

Thomas A. Riemenschneider, MD, Chairman

Robert J. Baumann, MD
Patricia K. Duffner, MD

John L. Green, MD
Sanford Schneider, MD

Consultants:

James R. Cooley, MD,
  Clinical Algorithm
David L. Coulter, MD
Patricia K. Crumrine, MD
Sandra D'Angelo, PhD,
  Methodology Consultant
W. Edwin Dodson, MD

John M. Freeman, MD
Michael Kohrman, MD
James O. McNamara, MD
Karin B. Nelson, MD
N. Paul Rosman, MD
Shlomo Shinnar, MD

PROVISIONAL COMMITTEE ON QUALITY IMPROVEMENT
1993–1996

David A. Bergman, MD, Chairman

Richard D. Baltz, MD
James R. Cooley, MD
John B. Coombs, MD
Lawrence F. Nazarian, MD

Thomas A. Riemenschneider, MD
Kenneth B. Roberts, MD
Daniel W. Shea, MD

Liaison Representatives:

Michael J. Goldberg, MD
  Sections Liaison
Charles J. Homer, MD, MPH
  Section on Epidemiology

Thomas F. Tonniges, MD
AAP Board of Directors

ABSTRACT

The American Academy of Pediatrics and its Provisional Committee on Quality Improvement, in collaboration with experts from the Section on Neurology, general pediatricians, consultants in the fields of neurology and epilepsy, and research methodologists, developed this practice parameter.

This parameter provides recommendations for the neurodiagnostic evaluation of a child with a first simple febrile seizure. These recommendations derive from both a thorough review of the literature and expert consensus. Interventions of direct interest include lumbar puncture, electroencephalography, blood studies, and neuroimaging. The methods and results of the literature review and data analyses can be found in the technical report that is available from the American Academy of Pediatrics. This parameter is designed to assist pediatricians by providing an analytic framework for the evaluation and treatment of this condition. It is not intended to replace clinical judgment or establish a protocol for all patients with this condition. It rarely will be the only appropriate approach to the problem.

DEFINITION OF THE PROBLEM

This practice parameter provides recommendations for the neurodiagnostic evaluation of neurologically healthy infants and children between 6 months and 5 years of age who have had their first simple febrile seizures and present within 12 hours of the event. This practice parameter is not intended for patients who have had complex febrile seizures (prolonged, focal, and/or recurrent), nor does it pertain to those children with previous neurologic insults, known central nervous system abnormalities, or histories of afebrile seizures.

TARGET AUDIENCE AND PRACTICE SETTING

This practice parameter is intended for use by pediatricians, family physicians, child neurologists, neurologists, emergency physicians, and other providers who treat children for febrile seizures.

INTERVENTIONS OF DIRECT INTEREST

1. Lumbar puncture;
2. Electroencephalography (EEG);
3. Blood studies—serum electrolytes, calcium, phosphorus, magnesium, and blood glucose, and a complete blood count (CBC); and
4. Neuroimaging—skull radiographs, computed tomography (CT), and magnetic resonance imaging.

BACKGROUND

A febrile seizure is broadly defined as a seizure accompanied by fever without central nervous system infection, occurring in infants and children between 6 months and 5 years of age. Febrile seizures occur in 2% to 5% of all children and, as such, make up the most common convulsive event in children younger than 5 years of age. In 1976, Nelson and Ellenberg,[1] using data from the National Collaborative Perinatal Project, further defined febrile seizures as being either simple or complex. Simple febrile seizures were defined as primary generalized seizures lasting less than 15 minutes and not recurring within 24 hours. Complex febrile seizures were defined as focal, prolonged

(>15 minutes), and/or occurring in a flurry. Those children who had simple febrile seizures had no evidence of increased mortality, hemiplegia, or mental retardation. During follow-up evaluation, the risk of epilepsy after a simple febrile seizure was shown to be only slightly higher than that of the general population, whereas the chief risk associated with simple febrile seizures was recurrence in one third of the children. The report concluded that simple febrile seizures are benign events with excellent prognoses, a conclusion reaffirmed in the 1980 National Institutes of Health Consensus Statement.[2]

Despite progress in understanding febrile seizures and the development of consensus statements about their diagnostic evaluation and management, a review of practice patterns of pediatricians indicates that a wide variation persists in physician interpretation, evaluation, and treatment of children with febrile seizures.[3]

This parameter is not intended for the evaluation of patients who have had complex febrile seizures, previous neurologic insults, or known brain abnormalities. The parameter also does not address treatment.

The expected outcomes of this practice parameter include the following.

1. Optimizing practitioner understanding of the scientific basis for the neurodiagnostic evaluation of children with simple febrile seizures;
2. Using a structured framework to aid the practitioner in decision making;
3. Optimizing evaluation of the child who has had a simple febrile seizure by ensuring that underlying diseases such as meningitis are detected, minimizing morbidity, and enabling the practitioner to reassure the anxious parents and child; and
4. Reducing costs of physician and emergency department visits, hospitalizations, and unnecessary testing.

METHODOLOGY

Two hundred three medical journal articles addressing the diagnosis and evaluation of febrile seizures were identified. Each article was subjected to formal, semistructured review by committee members. These completed reviews, as well as the original articles, were then reexamined by epidemiologic consultants to identify those population-based studies limited to children with simple febrile seizures that examined the usefulness of specific diagnostic studies. Given the scarcity of such studies, data from hospital-based studies and comparable groups were also reviewed. Tables were constructed using data from 28 articles. A second literature search failed to disclose pertinent articles containing data on brain imaging in children with febrile seizures.

A summary of the technical report describing the analyses used to prepare this parameter begins on page 263.

RECOMMENDATIONS

Lumbar Puncture

Recommendation. **The American Academy of Pediatrics (AAP) recommends, on the basis of the published evidence and consensus, that after the first seizures with fever in infants younger than 12 months, performance of a lumbar puncture be strongly considered, because the clinical signs and symptoms associated with meningitis may be minimal or absent in this age group. In a child between 12 and 18** months of age, a lumbar puncture should be considered, because clinical signs and symptoms of meningitis may be subtle. In a child older than 18 months, although a lumbar puncture is not routinely warranted, it is recommended in the presence of meningeal signs and symptoms (ie, neck stiffness and Kernig and Brudzinski signs), which are usually present with meningitis, or for any child whose history or examination result suggests the presence of intracranial infection. In infants and children who have had febrile seizures and have received prior antibiotic treatment, clinicians should be aware that treatment can mask the signs and symptoms of meningitis. As such, a lumbar puncture should be strongly considered.

The clinical evaluation of young febrile children requires skills that vary among examiners. Moreover, published data do not address the quantification of such skills adequately. Because this practice parameter is for practitioners with a wide range of training and experience, the committee chose a conservative approach with an emphasis on the value of lumbar puncture in diagnosing meningitis.

The committee recognizes the diversity of opinion regarding the need for routine lumbar puncture in children younger than 18 to 24 months with first febrile seizures. In approximately 13% to 16% of children with meningitis, seizures are the presenting sign of disease, and in approximately 30% to 35% of these children (primarily children younger than 18 months), meningeal signs and symptoms may be lacking.[4,5] On the basis of published evidence, cerebrospinal fluid is more likely to be abnormal in children initially seen with fevers and seizures who have had: (1) suspicious findings on physical and/or neurologic examinations (particularly meningeal signs); (2) complex febrile seizures; (3) physician visits within 48 hours before the seizures; (4) seizures on arrival to emergency departments; (5) prolonged postictal states (typically most children with simple febrile seizures recover quickly); and (6) initial seizures after 3 years of age.[6,7] An increased risk of failure to diagnose meningitis occurs in children: (1) younger than 18 months who may show no signs and symptoms of meningitis; (2) who are evaluated by a less-experienced health care provider; or (3) who may be unavailable for follow-up.[5-8] A recognized source of fever, eg, otitis media, does not exclude the presence of meningitis. All recommendations, including those for lumbar puncture, are also given in the Algorithm.

EEG

Recommendation. **The AAP recommends, based on the published evidence and consensus, that EEG not be performed in the evaluation of a neurologically healthy child with a first simple febrile seizure.**

No published study demonstrates that EEG performed either at the time of presentation after a simple febrile seizure or within the following month will predict the occurrence of future afebrile seizures. Although the incidence of abnormal EEGs increases over time after a simple febrile seizure, no evidence exists that abnormal EEGs after the first febrile seizure are predictive for either the risk of recurrence of febrile seizures or the development of epilepsy. Even studies that have included children with complex febrile seizures and/or those with preexisting neurologic disease (a group at higher risk of having epilepsy develop) have not shown EEG to be predictive of the development of epilepsy.[9-10]

Blood Studies

Recommendation. **On the basis of published evidence,[7,8,11] the AAP recommends that the following determinations not be performed routinely in the evaluation of a child with a first simple febrile seizure: serum electrolytes, calcium, phosphorus, magnesium, CBC, or blood glucose.**

There is no evidence to suggest that routine blood studies are of benefit in the evaluation of the child with a first febrile seizure. Although some children initially seen with febrile seizures are dehydrated and have abnormal serum electrolyte values, their conditions should be identifiable by obtaining appropriate histories and performing careful physical examinations. A blood glucose determination, although not routinely needed, should be obtained if the child has a prolonged period of postictal obtundation. CBCs may be useful in the evaluation of fever, particularly in young children, because the incidence of bacteremia in children younger than 2 years of age with or without febrile seizures is the same.[12]

When fever is present, the decision regarding the need for laboratory testing should be directed toward identifying the source of the fever rather than as part of the routine evaluation of the seizure itself.

Neuroimaging

Recommendation. **On the basis of the available evidence and consensus, the AAP recommends that neuroimaging not be performed in the routine evaluation of the child with a first simple febrile seizure.**

The literature does not support the use of skull films in the evaluation of the child with a first febrile seizure.[7,13] Although no data have been published that either support or negate the need for CT or magnetic resonance imaging in the evaluation of children with simple febrile seizures, extrapolation of data from the literature on the use of CT in children who have generalized epilepsy has shown that clinically important intracranial structural abnormalities in this patient population are uncommon.[14,15]

CONCLUSION

Physicians evaluating infants or young children after first simple febrile seizures should direct their evaluations toward the diagnosis of the causes of the children's fevers. A lumbar puncture should be strongly considered in a child younger than 12 months and should be considered in children between 12 and 18 months of age. In children older than 18 months, the decision to do a lumbar puncture rests on the clinical suspicion of meningitis. The seizure usually does not require further evaluation—specifically EEG, blood studies, or neuroimaging.

The practice parameter, "The Neurodiagnostic Evaluation of the Child With a First Simple Febrile Seizure," was reviewed by the appropriate committees and sections of the AAP, including the Chapter Review Group, a focus group of office-based pediatricians representing each AAP district: Gene R. Adams, MD; Robert M. Corwin, MD; Lawrence C. Pakula, MD; Barbara M. Harley, MD; Howard B. Weinblatt, MD; Thomas J. Herr, MD; Kenneth E. Mathews, MD; Diane Fuquay, MD; Robert D. Mines, MD; and Delosa A. Young, MD. Comments were also solicited from relevant outside organizations. The clinical algorithm was developed by Michael Kohrman, MD, Buffalo Children's Hospital, and James R. Cooley, MD, Harvard Community Health Plan.

The supporting data analyses are contained in the summary of the technical report, which begins on page 263.

REFERENCES

1. Nelson KB, Ellenberg JH. Predictors of epilepsy in children who have experienced febrile seizures. *N Engl J Med.* 1976;295:1029–1033

2. Consensus statement. Febrile seizures: long-term management of children with fever-associated seizures. *Pediatrics.* 1980;66:1009–1012

3. Hirtz DG, Lee YJ, Ellenberg JH, Nelson KB. Survey on the management of febrile seizures. *Am J Dis Child.* 1986;140:909–914

4. Ratcliffe JC, Wolf SM. Febrile convulsions caused by meningitis in young children. *Ann Neurol.* 1977;1:285–286

5. Rutter N, Smales OR. Role of routine investigations in children presenting with their first febrile convulsion. *Arch Dis Child.* 1977;52:188–191

6. Joffe A, McCormick M, DeAngelis C. Which children with febrile seizures need lumbar puncture? A decision analysis approach. *Am J Dis Child.* 1983;137:1153–1156

7. Jaffe M, Bar-Joseph G, Tirosh E. Fever and convulsions—indications for laboratory investigations. *Pediatrics.* 1981;57:729–731

8. Gerber MA, Berliner BC. The child with a "simple" febrile seizure: appropriate diagnostic evaluation. *Am J Dis Child.* 1981;135:431–433

9. Frantzen E, Lennox-Butchthal M, Nygaard A. Longitudinal EEG and clinical study of children with febrile convulsions. *Electroencephalogr Clin Neurophysiol.* 1968;24:197–212

10. Thorn I. The significance of electroencephalography in febrile convulsions. In: Akimoto H, Kazamatsuri H, Seino M, Ward A, eds. *Advances in Epileptology: XIIIth Epilepsy International Symposium.* New York, NY: Raven Press; 1982:93–95

11. Heijbel J, Blom S, Bergfors PG. Simple febrile convulsions: a prospective incidence study and an evaluation of investigations initially needed. *Neuropaediatrie.* 1980;11:45–56

12. Chamberlain JM, Gorman RL. Occult bacteremia in children with simple febrile seizures. *Am J Dis Child.* 1988;142:1073–1076

13. Nealis GT, McFadden SW, Asnes RA, Ouellette EM. Routine skull roentgenograms in the management of simple febrile seizures. *J Pediatr.* 1977;90:595–596

14. Yang PJ, Berger PE, Cohen ME, Duffner PK. Computed tomography and childhood seizure disorders. *Neurology.* 1979;29:1084–1088

15. Bachman DS, Hodges FJ, Freeman JM. Computerized axial tomography in chronic seizure disorders of childhood. *Pediatrics.* 1976;58:828–832

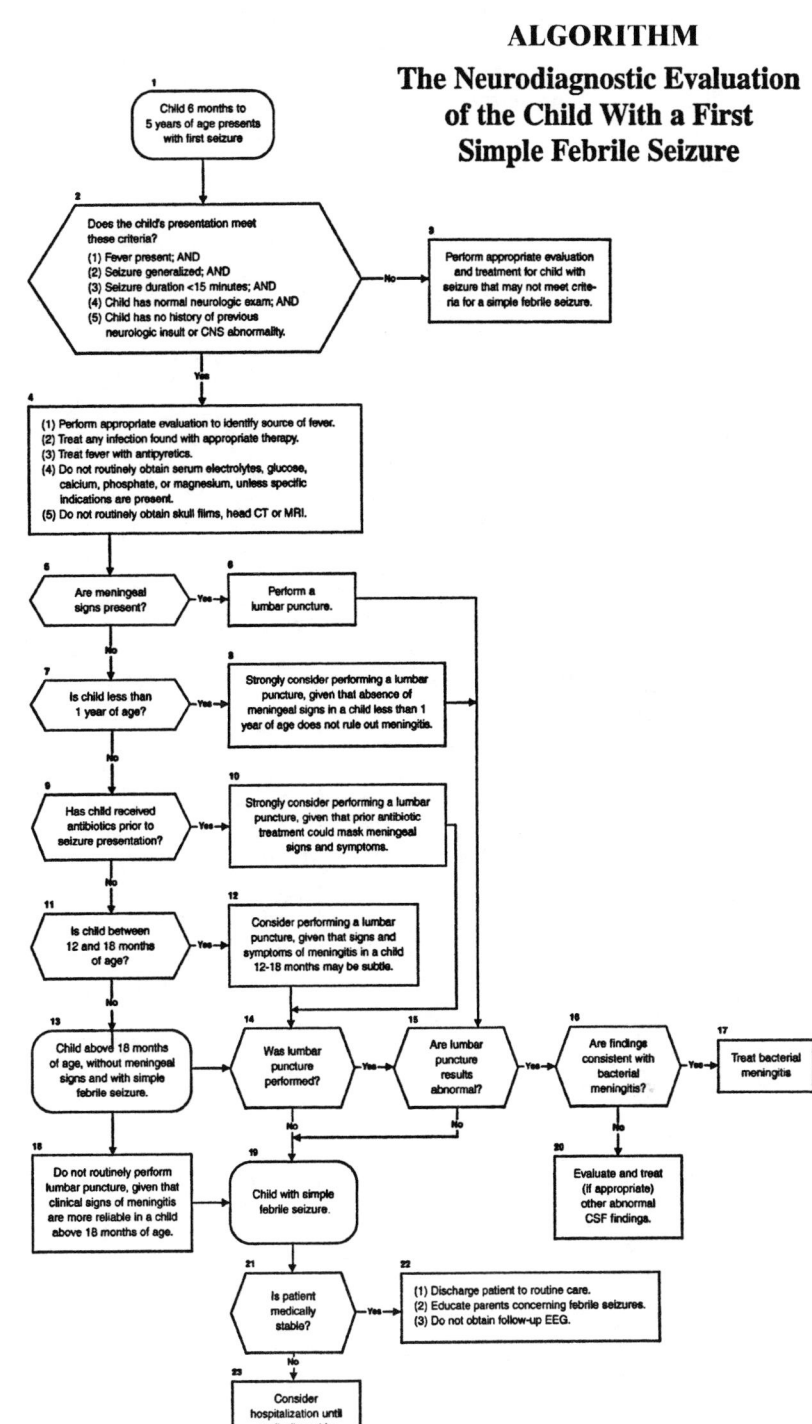

Technical Report Summary:
The Neurodiagnostic Evaluation of the Child
With a First Simple Febrile Seizure

Authors:

Robert J. Baumann, MD
Sandra L. D'Angelo, PhD

University of Kentucky
Lexington, Kentucky

consultants to the Subcommittee on Simple Febrile Seizures

American Academy of Pediatrics
PO Box 927, 141 Northwest Point Blvd
Elk Grove Village, IL 60009-0927

**SUBCOMMITTEE ON DIAGNOSIS AND
TREATMENT OF FEBRILE SEIZURES
1992 – 1995**

Thomas A. Riemenschneider, MD, Chairman

Robert J. Baumann, MD

Patricia K. Duffner, MD

John L. Green, MD

Sanford Schneider, MD

In Consultation With:

David L. Coulter, MD

Patricia K. Crumrine, MD

Sandra D'Angelo, PhD (methodology consultant)

W. Edwin Dodson, MD

John M. Freeman, MD

Michael Kohrman, MD

James O. McNamara, MD

Karin B. Nelson, MD

N. Paul Rosman, MD

Shlomo Shinnar, MD

**PROVISIONAL COMMITTEE ON QUALITY IMPROVEMENT
1993 – 1995**

David A. Bergman, MD, Chairman

Richard D. Baltz, MD

James R. Cooley, MD

John B. Coombs, MD

Michael J. Goldberg, MD
  Sections Liaison

Charles J. Homer, MD, MPH
  Section on Epidemiology Liaison

Lawrence F. Nazarian, MD

Thomas A. Riemenschneider, MD

Kenneth B. Roberts, MD

Daniel W. Shea, MD

Thomas F. Tonniges, MD
  AAP Board of Directors Liaison

INTRODUCTION

The scope of the practice parameter that is supported by this technical report was limited to the initial neurodiagnostic evaluation (within 12 hours of the event) of neurologically normal children with simple febrile seizures. Febrile seizures are a common problem in clinical practice, occurring in 2.7% of children in the British Birth Cohort study. Febrile seizures are also the most common epileptic events in children younger than 5 years. The subcommittee's efforts were focused on the large subgroup of children (88%)[1] who have simple febrile seizures because in the view of most clinicians and on the basis of the epidemiologic evidence, this is a relatively homogeneous clinical grouping in terms of age, clinical presentation, course, and outcome. It is appropriate, therefore, to help clinicians develop a common neurodiagnostic approach for their evaluation.

DEFINITION OF THE PROBLEM

Children younger than 5 years who experience their first seizure in association with a fever are commonly divided into three groups. Children with simple febrile seizures make up the largest group. The second group includes children whose seizures are secondary to a central nervous system (CNS) infection (symptomatic febrile seizures). In the third group, children whose seizures are neither simple nor secondary to CNS infection are classified as having complex febrile seizures.

The practice parameter supported by this technical report contains recommendations for the initial neurodiagnostic evaluation of a child who has experienced a simple febrile seizure. The parameter requires all of the following factors for inclusion: Children who were between 6 months and 5 years at the time of the seizure. Seizures were single, isolated, and generalized; associated with a fever in the absence of a CNS infection; and lasted less than 15 minutes. The study excluded any children experiencing focal or complex seizures or flurries of seizures, or children who had experienced a previous neurologic insult or who were not neurologically normal on examination.

This definition of a simple febrile seizure corresponds to that in usual clinical practice and is also supported by the analysis of data from the Collaborative Perinatal Project of the National Institute of Neurological and Communicative Disorders and Stroke. In that project, Nelson and Ellenberg analyzed the data of 1706 children aged 7 years who had had one or more febrile seizures. The risk of epilepsy (afebrile seizures) was significantly higher for children whose neurological development was not normal before the seizure, whose seizure occurred before 6 months of age, whose seizure lasted longer than 15 minutes, or who had more than one febrile seizure per day. Most recently Verity and Golding examined the records for 398 children who had had at least one febrile seizure. Follow-up continued until age 10 years. They found a higher rate of epilepsy after a complex febrile convulsion (lasting longer than 15 minutes, focal or multiple seizures) than after a simple febrile convulsion. The available data indicated that these children experienced adverse neurologic outcomes (such as early mortality or mental retardation) at rates similar to those of their peers. Nevertheless, their rate for single or repeated afebrile seizures (epilepsy is defined as having two or more afebrile seizures) exceeded that of the general age-matched population. The study concluded that chil-

dren with simple febrile seizures demonstrated a higher rate for afebrile seizures than that seen in the base population but had a lower rate than subjects who experienced complex febrile seizures.

The Commission on Epidemiology and Prognosis of the International League Against Epilepsy, which published a "Guidelines for Epidemiologic Studies on Epilepsy," suggested that the definition of febrile seizure include "childhood after age 1 month." No maximum age or definition of the duration of childhood was given. This Panel agreed that epidemiologic studies should examine the outcomes of febrile seizures among infants younger than 6 months as well as children older than 5 years. Nevertheless, existing studies as well as common clinical practice suggest that the practice parameter be limited to patients older than 6 months and younger than 5 years of age.

SELECTION OF INTERVENTIONS

The subcommittee further limited the parameter to the study of commonly used neurodiagnostic tests. These tests were evaluated on their potential to help the clinician decide whether children: had experienced a simple febrile seizure (as opposed to a complex or symptomatic febrile seizure) or were likely to have subsequent afebrile seizures or other adverse outcomes.

The following tests were included:
1. Lumbar puncture (to diagnose CNS infection).
2. Electroencephalography (EEG [to predict the likelihood of future afebrile seizures]).
3. Blood chemistries (to discover potential metabolic etiologies for the seizure).
4. Imaging studies of the head and brain, including skull x-ray films, computed tomography (CT), and magnetic resonance imaging (MRI) (to identify brain lesions).

METHODS

In an attempt to discover all pertinent articles, a Medline search was performed by staff of the American Academy of Pediatrics. An additional search from the Epilepsy Foundation of America using their database was also performed. Other articles that were obtained from bibliographies were suggested by subcommittee members; 203 articles were identified. Each article was reviewed by a subcommittee member using a semistructured review form. The completed forms and the articles were reviewed again by the epidemiologic consultants with the assistance of a graduate student.

The goal of this search was to identify population-based studies limited to patients with well-defined simple febrile seizures and in which neurodiagnostic tests were employed. The subcommittee attempted to use the method of Eddy and Woolf to develop these guidelines. Such a rigorous analysis requires well-designed population-based or case-comparison studies. The studies must adhere to a consistent definition of the study group, in this instance children with simple febrile seizures (as previously defined). The diagnostic test of interest must be applied in a standard way to all eligible subjects. The subjects must then be followed up for a sufficient period of time to discover important outcomes.

None of the previously cited population-based studies were designed to investigate the utility of neurodiagnostic testing. In all three studies, tests were selectively requested based on the physician's clinical judgment. Further retrospective analysis is unlikely to be fruitful.

Given the scarcity of population-based studies, data from hospital and clinic series were also analyzed. These studies had the following methodological problems.

Subject Selection. Most studies recruited subjects from clinics, emergency departments, or hospital admissions. The selection factors that influenced the constitution of these patient groups were difficult, if not impossible, to characterize. Moreover children from these patient groups usually have substantially higher rates of adverse outcomes than do children in population-based studies.

Disease Definition. Many studies either failed to define their criteria for febrile seizures, used a definition different from that used in the practice parameter, or did not rigorously follow any specific definition. Often there was no attempt to exclude (or at least identify) children with preexisting neurological disease.

Uniformity of Neurodiagnostic Testing. Many studies failed to apply the test(s) to all eligible subjects, raising serious questions about subject selection. An excess of positive tests and adverse outcomes could be expected based on physicians who exempt "healthier" children from testing.

Duration of Follow-up. Few studies had an extended follow-up period. The number of subjects experiencing afebrile seizures increases with age. Although the optimal duration of follow-up is uncertain, in the Rochester, Minnesota study most subjects were found to have experienced a seizure by age 9 years.

The consultants presented the abstracted data from 28 articles in tabular form, subsequently eliminating nine of them. These do not contain studies suitable for meta-analysis.

The subcommittee was concerned with the use of MRI and CT in evaluating children with febrile seizures. Because the initial literature search did not discover any suitable articles using these technologies, another literature search was conducted using MRI and CT MeSH terms, but again no pertinent articles were located.

Many articles not included in the study were reviews, commentaries, or editorials that lacked original data. Some of these articles reported disorders other than simple febrile seizures or intermingled children with simple seizures with children who were not neurologically normal or who had had complex febrile seizures. An additional 13 studies were eliminated because they did not define "febrile seizure" or used a definition different from that of the subcommittee.

SUBCOMMITTEE RECOMMENDATIONS AND LEVELS OF EVIDENCE

Recommendations were made based on the quality of scientific evidence. In the absence of high-quality scientific evidence, subcommittee consensus or a combination of evidence and consensus was used as the basis for recommendations.

Clinical options are actions for which the Panel failed to find compelling evidence for or against. A health care provider may or may not wish to implement clinical options, depending on the child.

No recommendation was made when scientific evidence was lacking and there was no compelling reason to make an expert judgment.

PANEL RECOMMENDATIONS

Lumbar Puncture

The goal of lumbar puncture is to identify children with CNS infection. A positive spinal fluid examination can have obvious treatment implications. In addition if the seizure is associated with an intracranial infection, the child is considered to have a symptomatic febrile seizure. Lumbar puncture with spinal fluid examination is not an effective neurodiagnostic technique for evaluating the febrile seizure per se.

An important concern is the number of children presenting with fever and seizures who have meningitis (for example, 4/119, or 3.4% [Heijbel et al], 28/562, or 5% [Jaffe et al], 13/241, or 5.4% [Joffe et al], 21/878, or 2.4% [Rossi et al], 6/328, or 1.8% [Rutter and Smales]). In the study by Jaffe et al, children with simple febrile seizures were less likely (2/323) to have meningitis than those with complex febrile seizures (26/239). None of the subjects with simple febrile seizures and 6 subjects with complex febrile seizures had bacterial meningitis. The previously described rates of meningitis (except those for the study by Heijbel et al) include children admitted to emergency departments or the hospital and thus are unlikely to typify the populations from which they come and are likely to vary with the factors that influence emergency department and hospital utilization.

Reviewing the emergency room records for 241 children who had a first seizure with fever and underwent lumbar puncture, Joffe et al found that the following five items were important in determining those with and without meningitis: 1) visiting a physician within 48 hours of the seizure, 2) seizure activity at the time of arrival in the emergency room, 3) a focal seizure, 4) suspicious findings on physical examination (rash or petechiae, cyanosis, hypotension, or grunting respirations), and 5) abnormal neurological examination results (stiff neck, increased tone, deviated eyes, ataxia, no response to voice, inability to fix and follow, no response to painful stimuli, positive doll's eye sign, floppy muscle tone, nystagmus, or bulging or tense fontanel).

Clearly the clinical evaluation of young febrile children requires skills that vary between examiners. Moreover, published data do not adequately address the quantification of such skills. Therefore the subcommittee relied on expert opinion and Panel consensus. Since this practice parameter is for practitioners with a wide range of training and experience, the committee chose a conservative approach with an emphasis on the value of lumbar puncture in diagnosing meningitis. This was not intended to ignore the occurrence of false-negative results (for example, Rutter and Smales found 2/310 false-negative spinal fluid examinations).

In the absence of other data, the Panel reviewed studies in which children with fever and seizures presented to medical institutions. The study of Heijbel et al was population-based, but lumbar puncture was performed selectively in 47 of 107 subjects.

EEG

The primary purpose of EEG in the evaluation of the children with simple febrile seizures is to predict the risk of future afebrile seizures. The subcommittee searched for but could not find a definitive study. In such a population-based study, EEGs would be obtained on children shortly after they experience their first simple seizure, with the EEG pattern being correlated with subsequent seizure occurrence. The study from Macedonia by Sofijanov et al seems to approximate this pattern. Initial EEG data were published; follow-up data, however, are not yet available. In this study 18% of 376 subjects with first febrile seizures had paroxysmal abnormalities on EEG, which were more likely when the seizure was either focal or lasted longer than 15 minutes (not a simple febrile seizure).

Given the high rate of simple febrile seizures and the low rate of subsequent afebrile seizures, obtaining routine EEGs would require a large number of tests to identify a small number of children destined to have these seizures. For example, in the British Birth Cohort study, only 2.6% of children who had experienced their first simple febrile seizure subsequently had a single afebrile seizure before their 10th birthday. Only 1.6% of the children had two or more afebrile seizures (ie, epilepsy). A number of well-known studies included patients with both simple and focal febrile seizures and did not exclude subjects with preexisting neurological disability. The results for subjects with simple febrile seizures from the published data could not be isolated. Heijbel et al limited their study to simple febrile seizures. Their two subjects who subsequently developed epilepsy had normal initial EEGs. Interpretation of their data is complicated by the small number of subjects (n=107) and the elimination of 5 potential subjects because they had epileptiform EEG activity interictally. These 5 subjects were not characterized further so it is unknown whether they fit the clinical criteria for having experienced simple febrile seizures. No follow-up data were given for these 5 children and follow-up was limited to 3 years for the other subjects. Koyama et al evaluated 133 subjects from a population of 490 children with a history of febrile seizures. It is unclear if the 133 subjects are typical of the 490. Moreover, the EEGs were obtained months after the initial seizure; 32% of the subjects had abnormal EEGs—in 9% of the subjects the abnormalities were paroxysmal compared with 7% of the control group (who had had EEGs for "other medical reasons"). Follow-up data were not available.

The study of Heijbel is population-based. Some of its limitations are discussed above. Without other population-based data, the Panel reviewed studies in which relatively large numbers of children with fever and seizures presented to medical institutions. In some studies only a subset of subjects had EEGs, introducing the additional issue of selection bias.

BLOOD CHEMISTRIES

In a population-based study that included 107 children with simple febrile seizures, Heijbel et al retrospectively reviewed the routine blood chemistries requested by the treating physicians. They found no clinically important abnormalities in serum calcium (n=92), phosphorus (n=85), or glucose (n=56) levels. One child with a low glucose level was reportedly asymptomatic on follow-up.

Other studies were hospital-based. For 100 consecutive admissions Gerber and Berliner reported normal values of serum glucose (n=82), calcium (n=58), electrolytes, and urea nitrogen.[7] The five children with elevated glucose levels were asymptomatic. Thirteen children had minimally reduced calcium levels (8.3 to 8.9 mg/dL) and were asymptomatic. Jaffe et al reviewed 323 records of children with simple febrile seizures. Three children had abnormalities (one each hyponatremia, hypocalcemia, and hypokalemia) and the authors thought that the abnormalities could have been anticipated on clinical grounds independent of the occurrence of the simple febrile seizure. One child was a compulsive water drinker, one had "florid" rickets, and one had dehydration due to gastroenteritis. Rutter and Smales[9] reviewed 328 children admitted to the hospital after their first febrile convulsion and found that determinations for serum sugar, calcium, urea, electrolytes, and blood counts were "commonly performed but were unhelpful." Among 269 subjects who had blood glucose measurements they found hyperglycemia to be common (14%) but clinically unimportant. The child who was hypoglycemic on admission (glucose level, 30 mg/dL) subsequently had a normal fasting blood glucose level; of the 232 children who had serum calcium determinations, three of the four children with levels below 8.0 mg/dL were normal on further evaluation and the fourth child was lost to follow-up.

Four authors determined that in their subjects with simple febrile seizures, the routine blood chemistries performed did not alter patient management in an important way. The child's clinical condition and underlying illness determined the need for routine blood chemistries. Otherwise, the management of a child after a simple febrile seizure was not improved.

NEUROIMAGING

To our knowledge, no study has been done in which children with simple febrile seizures have undergone imaging. We also searched (without success) for a related imaging study involving otherwise normal children after a first seizure. Three studies reviewing skull x-ray films in children with febrile seizures concluded that skull x-ray films were not of value.

Practice Parameter: Treatment of the Child With a First Unprovoked Seizure

The following guideline for treatment of the child with a first unprovoked seizure, developed by the American Academy of Neurology, has been endorsed by the American Academy of Pediatrics.

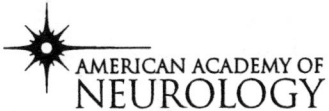

CME   Practice parameter: Treatment of the child with a first unprovoked seizure

Report of the Quality Standards Subcommittee of the American Academy of Neurology and the Practice Committee of the Child Neurology Society*

D. Hirtz, MD; A. Berg, PhD; D. Bettis, MD; C. Camfield, MD; P. Camfield, MD; P. Crumrine, MD; W.D. Gaillard, MD; S. Schneider, MD; and S. Shinnar, MD, PhD

Abstract—The Quality Standards Subcommittee of the American Academy of Neurology and the Practice Committee of the Child Neurology Society develop practice parameters as strategies for patient management based on analysis of evidence regarding risks and benefits. This parameter reviews published literature relevant to the decision to begin treatment after a child or adolescent experiences a first unprovoked seizure and presents evidence-based practice recommendations. Reasons why treatment may be considered are discussed. Evidence is reviewed concerning risk of recurrence as well as effect of treatment on prevention of recurrence and development of chronic epilepsy. Studies of side effects of anticonvulsants commonly used to treat seizures in children are also reviewed. Relevant articles are classified according to the Quality Standards Subcommittee classification scheme. Treatment after a first unprovoked seizure appears to decrease the risk of a second seizure, but there are few data from studies involving only children. There appears to be no benefit of treatment with regard to the prognosis for long-term seizure remission. Antiepileptic drugs (AED) carry risks of side effects that are particularly important in children. The decision as to whether or not to treat children and adolescents who have experienced a first unprovoked seizure must be based on a risk–benefit assessment that weighs the risk of having another seizure against the risk of chronic AED therapy. The decision should be individualized and take into account both medical issues and patient and family preference.

NEUROLOGY 2003;60:166–175

Population-based studies of the incidence of first unprovoked seizures suggest that there are between 25,000 and 40,000 children per year in the United States who experience a first unprovoked seizure.[1-4] Until relatively recently, it was common practice for physicians to begin long-term, daily antiepileptic drug (AED) therapy after a child or adolescent experienced a single seizure of any type. The rationale for this practice was based on the belief that all seizures were likely to recur and that seizures could be dangerous and cause brain damage. Furthermore, it was thought that if any recurrence were to take place,

this would lead to progressively more seizures. It was also assumed that AED were safe, had few side effects, and were effective in prevention of seizure recurrences. These assumptions have undergone substantial modification over the last 20 years, leading to a more optimistic view about the nature of seizures and a more conservative approach to the use of treatment. However, no clear evidence-based guidelines have emerged regarding the initiation of treatment after a first unprovoked seizure in the pediatric population.

Practice parameters are developed by the Quality

Approved by the Quality Standards Subcommittee on April 16, 2002. Approved by the Practice Committee on August 3, 2002. Approved by the AAN Board of Directors on October 19, 2002.

This statement has been endorsed by the American Epilepsy Society; the American Academy of Pediatrics; and the Child Neurology Society.

*See the Appendix for a list of Committee members.

From the National Institute of Neurological Disorders and Stroke (Dr. Hirtz), NIH, Bethesda, MD; Department of Biological Sciences (Dr. Berg), Northern Illinois University, Dekalb; Boise (Dr. Bettis), ID; Department of Pediatric Neurology (Drs. C. Camfield and P. Camfield), IWK Health Center, Halifax, Nova Scotia, Canada; Department of Neurology (Dr. Crumrine), Children's Hospital of Pittsburgh, PA; Department of Neurology (Dr. Gaillard), Children's National Medical Center, Washington, DC; Riverside (Dr. Schneider), CA; and Departments of Neurology and Pediatrics (Dr. Shinnar), Montefiore Medical Center, Albert Einstein College of Medicine, New York, NY.

Received April 14, 2002. Accepted in final form July 19, 2002.

Address correspondence and reprint requests to QSS, American Academy of Neurology, 1080 Montreal Ave., St. Paul, MN 55116; e-mail: wedlund@aan.com

Table 1 *Evidence classification scheme of the American Academy of Neurology: rating of therapeutic article*

Class I: Prospective, randomized, controlled clinical trial with masked outcome assessment, in a representative population. The following are required:

  a. Primary outcome(s) is/are clearly defined.

  b. Exclusion/inclusion criteria are clearly defined.

  c. Adequate accounting for dropouts and crossovers with numbers sufficiently low to have minimal potential for bias.

  d. Relevant baseline characteristics are presented and substantially equivalent among treatment groups or there is appropriate statistical adjustment for differences.

Class II: Prospective matched group cohort study in a representative population with masked outcome assessment that meets a–d above *or* a randomized, controlled trial in a representative population that lacks one criteria a–d.

Class III: All other controlled trials (including well-defined natural history controls or patients serving as own controls) in a representative population, where outcome assessment is independent of patient treatment.

Class IV: Evidence from uncontrolled studies, case series, case reports, or expert opinion.

Standards Subcommittee of the American Academy of Neurology and the Child Neurology Society and are evidence-based documents about diagnostic or prognostic evaluations and therapeutic interventions. These involve a systematic evaluation and classification of available evidence (table 1) that determine whether specific recommendations can be made and, if so, the strength of the recommendations (table 2).

This practice parameter reviews the current evidence about treatment with AED after a child experiences a first unprovoked seizure. We examine the risk of seizure recurrence and predictors that may affect that risk. We review and classify the published evidence on whether treatment prevents recurrences as well as chronic epilepsy. We also evaluate potential risks and side effects of AED commonly used to treat seizures in children.

This is the second of two parameters addressing a child's first unprovoked seizure; the first concerned the initial evaluation.[5] Febrile seizures have been addressed separately in recently published recommendations from the American Academy of Pediatrics[6] and are not included here. This parameter

pertains to children and adolescents with first seizures only and does not include children diagnosed with epilepsy, defined as the occurrence of two or more seizures without acute provocation. For this reason, absence, myoclonic, and atonic seizures were excluded because they typically are not recognized until there have been multiple occurrences. The seizure types covered by this parameter include all partial seizures as well as generalized onset tonic-clonic or tonic seizures.

We defined the first seizure using the International League Against Epilepsy criteria to include multiple seizures within 24 hours with recovery of consciousness between seizures.[7] Children with a known immediate precipitating head trauma or those with previously diagnosed CNS infection, tumor, or other known acute precipitating causes such as hypoglycemia were excluded. We also excluded neonatal seizures (≤ 28 days) and febrile seizures because these disorders are diagnostically and therapeutically different. Status epilepticus, defined as a seizure lasting >30 minutes without regaining of consciousness,[7] was included when data were available. Most articles describing pediatric studies covered up to age 18 years; studies including both adolescents and adults were also examined. The recommendations of this parameter pertain to children (excluding the neonate) and adolescents.

Before any treatment decisions are approached, it is critical to determine whether the event is truly a seizure and whether it is the child's first.[5] A detailed history from a reliable observer and careful medical history and neurologic examination may provide information allowing the physician to rule out nonepileptic events.

Description of process. A literature search was performed including Ovid Medline and Ovid Biosys and Current Contents for relevant articles published from 1980 to 2001 using the following key words: treatment, antiepileptics, medications, therapy, management, epilepsy, seizures, convulsions, child, newborn, and adolescent. Standard search procedures were used, and subheadings were applied as appropriate. These searches produced 948 titles of journal articles.

Titles and abstracts were reviewed for content re-

Table 2 *Evidence classification scheme of the American Academy of Neurology: recommendations*

Translation of evidence to recommendations	Rating of recommendation	
Level A rating requires at least one convincing Class I study or at least two consistent, convincing Class II studies.	A	established as effective, ineffective, or harmful for the given condition in the specified population.
Level B rating requires at least one convincing Class II study or overwhelming Class III evidence.	B	probably effective, ineffective, or harmful for the given condition in the specified population.
Level C rating requires at least two convincing Class III studies.	C	possibly effective, ineffective, or harmful for the given condition in the specified population.
— U		data inadequate or conflicting. Given current knowledge, treatment is unproven.

garding first unprovoked seizures in children and adults. Articles from the searches were identified as relevant, and additional articles from the references in these primary articles were included. Articles pertaining to children with both first seizures and established epilepsy were included but were excluded if they did not report data from either children or adults who had experienced only a single seizure. References were classified as to whether they contained data related to children and adults or just children. Articles were reviewed from searches, bibliographies, and suggestions by colleagues and committee members. In most reports pertaining to both children and adults, results were not categorized according to subsets of age groups.

A recently revised classification of evidence to determine the quality of data was used for the evaluation of reports of therapeutic studies (see table 1). Each article containing data regarding treatment was reviewed and classified by two or more reviewers. Abstracted data included numbers of subjects, study design, ages, seizure types, whether first seizures only or a mixture of single and multiple seizures, seizure recurrences, types of treatment, side effects, and measurement of compliance and length of follow-up. Methods of data analysis and power were noted when available. Recommendations were based on the level of evidence (see table 2).

What are the potential risks resulting from having a second seizure? Preventing seizure recurrences has been a concern ever since Gowers wrote: "The tendency of the disease is to self perpetuation; each attack facilitates the occurrence of another, by increasing the instability of the nerve elements."[8] This clinical belief has been supported by animal studies on kindling, an experimental technique for inducing epilepsy by a series of subclinical electrical stimulations of the temporal lobe that induce progressive intensification of evoked electrographic and behavioral seizures.[9-11] There is evidence from animal models that prolonged or recurrent seizures, under certain circumstances, cause neuronal injury and predispose to epilepsy.[12,13] There is recent evidence that seizures, some prolonged, that occur during critical periods of brain development in animals may alter neuronal activity and circuitry in a manner that may predispose to the later development of epilepsy.[14,15] The relevance of data from these animal models to seizures in humans is unclear.[10,11,16] Data from children indicate that even prolonged seizures rarely cause clinically discernible brain damage unless associated with an underlying acute neurologic insult.[17]

One reason why treatment may be considered is concern about the risk of physical injury or death from a subsequent seizure. Serious injury from a seizure in a child is a rare event, usually from a fall with loss of consciousness. To reduce that risk, restrictions are recommended that would apply to any young child, such as bicycling on a sidewalk rather than the street and always with a helmet and swimming only with a buddy. Showering rather than bathing is recommended for children and adolescents, unless they are supervised. Sudden unexpected death in children with epilepsy is, fortunately, very uncommon. When death occurs in children, it is nearly always related to an underlying neurologic handicap rather than the epilepsy.[18-20] One population-based study found that the risk of death in those with childhood-onset epilepsy is the same as that for the general population for children without significant neurologic handicap.[21] No studies were found that examined whether treating a child after a first unprovoked seizure would reduce the risk of either subsequent significant injury or sudden death.

Psychosocial considerations. The effect of taking daily medication on the child's self-perception may be a concern in some cases.[22,23] A child who is taking chronic medication is perceived to have a chronic illness by the child, family, and possibly others such as teachers. Additionally, chronic treatment to prevent seizure recurrence may affect the family's ability to obtain health insurance or day care. Issues in teenagers become more complicated as concerns about driving privileges and teratogenicity come into play.[24]

How likely is a second seizure? The probability of having a second seizure has been explored in several large, observational Class III studies with long-term follow-up. Results presented in table 3 are limited to studies that included children with or without adults. The cumulative risk of recurrence increases over time; however, in studies where the information is available, the majority of the recurrences occur early (within the first 1 to 2 years).[25-33] At any given time, the reported risk of recurrence is highly variable. For example, at 1 year, it ranges from a low of 14%[26] to a high of 65%.[33] In all these Class III studies, there is variability in the mix of patients, the nonrandomized use of treatment, and the distributions of important prognostic factors. Some methodologic differences in seizure identification, age ranges included, recruitment, and follow-up of study participants may also contribute to this variability.

How likely are multiple recurrences in children who present with a first unprovoked seizure? A minority of children will go on to experience not just one but many recurrences. One study that enrolled 207 children with follow-up for 2 years found that in addition to an overall recurrence rate of 54%, 26% of the enrolled children were still experiencing one or more seizures during the last 6 months of the study follow-up, that is, >18 months after the index event.[27] Another study with longer follow-up enrolled 407 children and followed them for an average of >10 years. Of these, 46% had one or more recurrences during that period of time. Over the extended follow-up period, 19% of the children

Table 3 *Risk of recurrence after a first seizure*

| Study | Age range | n | Treated, % | Risk of recurrence at different times since first seizure, % | | | | |
				6 mo	1 y	2 y	3 y	5 y
Children and adolescents only								
27	1–16 y	156	0	40	46	54	—	—
33	3–21 y	78	58	55	65	69	—	—
25,28	1 mo–19 y	407	14	22	29	37	—	42
29	2–16 y	119	61	22	29	—	32	—
30	1 mo–16 y	168	68	36	40	47	—	—
42	1 mo–7 y	284	—	—	—	—	—	69, up to 7 y
Children, adolescents, and adults								
31	All ages	424	?	30	36	45	48	—
32	All ages	564	?	27	37	43	46	—
26	All ages	208	80	—	14	25	29	34

enrolled experienced ≥ 4 seizures and only 10% experienced ≥ 10 seizure episodes.[28] Few of the children in either study met criteria for intractability.[34]

Are there factors that increase the recurrence risk? Certain factors may elevate the risk of experiencing a second seizure. The underlying etiology and whether the EEG is normal or abnormal are consistently related to the risk of recurrence.[35] The recurrence rate is higher in individuals who have a remote symptomatic etiology. In those with an idiopathic or cryptogenic etiology, it is significantly lower.[25-28,30,33] We use the term "remote symptomatic" to mean without immediate cause but with a prior identifiable major brain insult such as severe trauma or accompanying a condition such as cerebral palsy or mental retardation. Idiopathic seizures are not associated with a known CNS disorder and are of suspected genetic etiology (such as occur with benign rolandic epilepsy), and cryptogenic seizures occur in individuals otherwise normal with no clear etiology.[7] The estimates of risk at 2 years are highly variable. The extent to which treatment was used also varied and may have influenced, to some degree, the overall risk observed. For children with first seizures that are idiopathic/cryptogenic, the recurrence risk is generally between 30 and 50% by 2 years,[25,27-30] and for remote symptomatic seizures, the estimate of recurrence risk is generally above 50%.[25,27,28,30,33] An EEG performed after the initial seizure also helps to predict recurrence,[25-27,29-31,33] particularly if there is an epileptiform abnormality. Patients with remote symptomatic seizures and abnormal EEG were more likely to be treated than those with idiopathic/cryptogenic seizures and normal EEG. All of these studies addressing recurrence risk represent Class III evidence.

Are there special considerations if the first seizure is prolonged? Approximately 10 to 12% of children and adults with a first unprovoked seizure will present with a seizure lasting ≥ 30 minutes (status epilepticus) as their first seizure.[36] In the absence of an acute or progressive brain injury or disease, the morbidity and mortality of status epilepticus in children are relatively low.[17,37] Of 46 children with "idiopathic" seizures in a study of sequelae of status epilepticus in 193 children, 2 children had mental retardation, but they had been recruited retrospectively and details of the clinical circumstances were not clear. None of children studied prospectively had residual motor or cognitive disability.[17]

Evidence concerning the impact of status epilepticus on the risk of recurrence and, in particular, the risk of a prolonged recurrence is available from one Class III prospective observational study of 407 children with a first unprovoked seizure.[25,36] The overall recurrence risk following a prolonged first seizure was no different from the recurrence risk following a brief first seizure. However, if a child with an initial prolonged seizure did experience a seizure recurrence, it was more likely to be prolonged. Of 24 children with initial episodes of status epilepticus who had a recurrence, 5 (21%) had status epilepticus as a recurrence, whereas of 147 whose first seizures were brief and who had a recurrence, 2 (1%) had status epilepticus as their recurrence.[25] Thus, the risk of a recurrent seizure being prolonged is limited largely to those children whose first seizure was prolonged (Class III studies).

How effective is treatment after a first seizure in prevention of recurrences? *Evidence.* There are four randomized clinical trials including children and adolescents that have examined the efficacy of treatment after a first seizure.[38-41] Only one of these studies consisted solely of children randomized to treatment versus no treatment after a first nonfebrile seizure (Class II).[41] In this study with a total of 31 children, 2 of 14 children (14%) treated with carbamazepine (CBZ) experienced a recurrence compared with 9 of 17 (53%)

Table 4 Recurrence rate by treatment in studies of children

Study	Class	n	Recurrence rate, n (%)	Treated vs untreated	Length of follow-up, y
41	II	31	11/31	2/14 vs 9/17, 14.3% vs 52.9%	1
42	III	284	196/284 (69)	No difference	To 7
29	III	119	40/119 (32)	27% vs 38%, no difference	3
25	III	407	151/393 (38) at 2 y, 171/375 (46) at 5 y	No difference	6.3, mean
33	III	78, includes 12 symptomatic	54/78 at 2 y (69)	No difference	5.2

who were not treated. Follow-up was for 1 year, and compliance was monitored. Although the recurrence rate up to 1 year was significantly lower in the treated group, only 6 of 14 (43%) patients randomized to CBZ completed the year with no significant side effects or seizure recurrence and 7 of 17 (41%) assigned to no medication had no seizure recurrence.

In studies involving both children and adults, outcome was not provided based on age. One Class I study in which 228 subjects were randomized to valproic acid (VPA) or placebo included 33 adolescents between the ages of 16 and 19.[38] The follow-up period for this trial was between 9 months and 5 years. Five (4%) of the treated group experienced a recurrence compared with 63 (56%) of those treated with placebo. However, these results were not found in another Class II randomized study (n = 419), in which 114 subjects were between 2 and 16 years old. Twenty-four percent of patients treated after a first seizure and 42% untreated patients had a recurrence by 1 year, but no difference by initial treatment assignment was seen after 2 years; 32% of those treated and 40% of those untreated had a recurrence by 2 years.[39]

In other studies in children (Class III), although the cohorts are prospectively followed, treatment was not randomly assigned and therefore baseline factors affecting risk of recurrence were not comparable.[25,29,33,42] None of these studies found a significant difference in recurrence rate in the treated and untreated children (table 4).

Summary. Studies of children and adults in which treatment assignment was randomized usually indicate that treatment with AED after a first seizure reduces the risk of seizure recurrence. The magnitude of the impact is variable, and the evidence from pediatric studies alone is weak (see table 4). Differences among the studies, the populations targeted, and the method in which treatment was administered may explain some of the variability. In the only randomized study restricted to the pediatric age group, the sample size is small and the confidence intervals are accordingly wide, ranging from 0 to 93% efficacy.[41]

Does treatment with AED after a first seizure change the long-term prognosis for seizure remission? *Evidence.* Although treatment after a first unprovoked seizure may reduce the risk of a

second seizure, does treatment at this time make any difference in the patient's long-term prognosis for seizure control? This question is addressed in two randomized, prospective, but not placebo-controlled (Class II) first-seizure studies. One study had 419 subjects, of whom 114 were between 2 and 16 years of age.[39] This study compared the probability of experiencing a remission, that is, 1 or 2 seizure-free years, in patients treated after a first seizure versus in patients treated after a second seizure. Follow-up was for at least 3 years or a minimum of 2 years seizure-free. Patients treated after the first seizure and those treated after a second seizure had the same probability of achieving a 1- or 2-year seizure remission (68%, n = 215 versus 60%, n = 204) (risk of recurrence [RR] = 1.04, 95% CI = 1.30 to 0.82). Another smaller study[43] of 31 children randomized to CBZ (n = 14) or no treatment (n = 17) echoes the results of this large study. After a 15-year follow-up, the rate of 2-year terminal remission was the same in both the treated and the untreated groups (RR = 0.79, 95% CI = 0.3 to 2.1).

Summary. Two Class II studies provide no evidence of a difference when treatment is started after the first seizure versus after a second seizure in achieving a 1-or 2-year seizure remission.

What are the nature and frequency of side effects of AED commonly used after a first seizure in children? *Evidence.* AED may cause systemic side effects such as rash, hirsutism, and weight gain. Severe reactions such as hepatic toxicity, bone marrow toxicity, and Stevens–Johnson syndrome cannot be anticipated and require early recognition of symptoms. Side effects of AED occurring in children include effects on behavior and higher cortical function,[44] which are often dose related and may be under-recognized. Dose-related side effects may be highest initially and amenable to dosage reduction, but this may also limit the potential effectiveness of AED. If the patient is a teenage girl who may become pregnant, the risk of teratogenicity is an additional consideration.[24,45]

Trials that report data relating to efficacy do not always include data relating to side effects. Data regarding toxicity or side effects of AED are not specifically available for treatment after a first seizure. However, studies that include initial treatment of

Table 5 *Behavioral and cognitive side effects of antiepileptic drugs in children treated for epilepsy*

Study	Age, y	Follow-up	Medication (n)	Reported side effects
Class I				
50,51	5–14	1 y	CBZ (23)	Impaired recent recall, reported slow by teachers
			PHT (20)	Impaired information processing at 1 mo
			VPA (21)	No change
49	7–15	6 and 12 mo	CBZ (26)	No change
			PB (25)	Disturbed information processing (auditory event-related potentials prolonged)
			VPA (25)	No change
47	2–16	12 mo	CBZ (78)	29 of total of 116 had moderate/severe behavior problems
			PHT (38)	
48	6–14	6 mo	PB	Did less well on cognitive tests, more hyperactivity
			VPA	No change
53	—	None	CBZ (50)	No difference high vs. low level
54			VPA (46)	Low doses gave better accuracy and response time
55			PHT (50)	No difference high vs. low level
52	4–12	2 y	PB (51)	22% hyperactivity
			VPA (48)	13% hyperactivity
			PHT (52)	8% impaired school performance
Class 2				
56	3–16	3 y	PB (10)	6 withdrew owing to side effects
			PHT (50)	5 withdrew owing to side effects
			CBZ (54)	2 withdrew owing to side effects
			VPA (49)	2 withdrew owing to side effects
51	Average 9	12 mo	VPA (26)	Increase in IQ
			PB (23)	Significant impairment in learning
58	6–17	6 mo	CBZ (17)	No difference
			VPA (11)	No difference
			PHT (1)	No difference
59	7–12	12 mo	VPA (34)	No difference
			CBZ (29)	No difference
60	4–16	26–6 mo	CBZ (5)	No difference
		12–12 mo	VPA (3)	No difference
			Ethosuximide (4)	No difference

CBZ = carbamazepine; PHT = phenytoin; VPA = valproic acid; PB = phenobarbital.

children for epilepsy provide information that may be extrapolated to treatment after a first seizure.

Behavioral and cognitive side effects. Five Class I studies reported on behavioral and cognitive side effects in children with epilepsy treated with AED.[46-52] One study reported that 29 of 116 children treated with either CBZ or phenytoin (PHT) had moderate to severe behavioral or mood changes.[46,47] In a blinded, randomized, crossover study comparing phenobarbital (PB) with VPA, children taking PB had lower scores on four tests of cognitive function and had more behavior problems that were not dose related, particularly hyperactivity.[48] Although Wechsler Intelligence Scale for Children–Revised scores were not different, a study that included auditory event-related potentials found prolonged latencies indicating delayed information processing associated with PB.[49] In a Class I study of children with newly diagnosed epilepsy in which 23 children received CBZ, 20 received PHT, and 21 received VPA, those on CBZ and PHT were slower on tests of information processing, and children on CBZ showed increased irritability[50,51] (table 5).

A series of three Class I studies each designed to compare the cognitive effects of low versus high levels of one AED in children with epilepsy found no differences between low and high levels with either CBZ or PHT.[53,54] Children with a lower level of VPA performed better on specific cognitive tasks such as accuracy and response time than those with a higher level.[55] In one Class II study, 15 of 163 children assigned to AED withdrew because of intolerable side

Table 6 Systemic side effects of antiepileptic drugs in children treated for epilepsy

Study	n	Follow-up	Medication (n)	Side effects
Class I				
51	64	1 y	CBZ (23)	3 h/a, anorexia, nausea
			PHT (20)	1 depression, anorexia
			VPA (21)	0
47	116	1 y	CBZ (78)	9 n&v, 10 ataxia, 5 rash, 5 gingival hyperplasia
			PHT (38)	
52	151	29 mo, mean	PB (51)	17 patients including behavioral
			VPA (48)	15 patients, including behavioral
			PHT (52)	33 patients had at least 1, 30 gingival hyperplasia, 13 dose-related ataxia
Class II				
41	31	1 y	CBZ (14)	2 somnolence, 2 allergic rash
56	167	4 y	PB (10)	5 behavior, 1 drowsy
			PHT (54)	2 drowsy, 1 rash, 1 blood dyscrasia, 1 hirsutism
			CBZ (54)	1 drowsy, 1 blood dyscrasia
			VPA (49)	1 behavior problem, 1 tremor
61	260	1 y	VPA (130)	Half had adverse events, e.g., somnolence, ataxia, rash; 12% d/c owing to "adverse events" such as increased appetite, weight gain, alopecia
			CBZ (130)	7% d/c owing to side effects

CBZ = carbamazepine; PHT = phenytoin; VPA = valproic acid; PB = phenobarbital; h/a = headache; n&v = nausea and vomiting; d/c = discontinued.

effects,[56] and in another, children taking PB did not show an expected increase in IQ on retest.[57] In three other studies, which included 48 children taking VPA, 1 taking PHT, and 51 taking CBZ, evidence was not seen of behavioral or cognitive impairment[58-60] (see table 5).

A report from the American Academy of Pediatrics[44] regarding general recommendations for awareness of behavioral and cognitive effects of AED noted that high blood levels of some AED (PHT, PB, primidone) were significantly related to cognitive decline. Cognitive and behavioral effects of AED were described as subtle and affecting isolated functions. These effects were seen in conjunction with academic underachievement and neuropsychological impairment in children with epilepsy.

Systemic side effects. Systemic side effects other than behavioral or cognitive also occur in children placed on AED (table 6). In a Class I study of 116 children randomized to CBZ or PHT, 24 had one or more side effects including nausea and vomiting (9), ataxia (10), rash (5), gingival hyperplasia (3), and dizziness (3).[47] Another Class I study reported that of 23 children on CBZ, 3 experienced headache, anorexia, nausea or abdominal pain, and increased irritability. Systemic side effects were not reported for the 20 children on PHT or the 21 on VPA.[50,51] Dropout because of failure to comply with treatment, possibly due to side effects, occurred in several cases in all three groups.

In the one prospective, randomized, but not blinded study in children that pertains to first sei-

zures only, 2 of 14 children on CBZ discontinued medication because of rash and 2 of 14 because of excessive somnolence.[41] When four drugs were compared in a Class II study of 167 children with newly diagnosed epilepsy, PB was dropped after 6 of 10 children had unacceptable side effects. Side effects occurred at a rate of 9% for PHT, 4% for CBZ, and 4% for VPA.[56] Included were behavioral problems, drowsiness, sleep problems, blood dyscrasia, hirsutism, and tremor. A randomized and blinded prospective study of 151 children with epilepsy found that 32% of children on PB, 19% of children on VPA, and 40% of children on PHT had more than one toxic side effect. Fifty-eight percent of those on PHT experienced gingival hyperplasia, and 25% had dose-related ataxia or sedation. Follow-up was 2 years.[52] In a Class II study of 130 children assigned to VPA and 130 assigned to CBZ, by 1 year, 13% discontinued VPA and 7% discontinued CBZ owing to adverse effects such as somnolence, fatigue, weight gain, headache, nausea, vomiting, and rash.[61]

In a Class III study of first seizures, four AED were used and an overall rate of side effects of 24% was reported. These were noted as behavior disorders, hyperkinesias, and sleepiness.[29] The exacerbation of seizures by CBZ has been reported in 11 of 129 cases of new-onset epilepsy.[62]

Several of the newer AED carry warnings or precautions for Stevens–Johnson syndrome (lamotrigine, zonisamide, felbamate), hepatic toxicity (lamotrigine, felbamate), aplastic anemia (felbamate), renal stones (topiramate, zonisamide), and

other rare medical complications such as hyperther-
mia secondary to hypohidrosis and hyponatremia
(zonisamide and oxcarbazepine). The spectrum and
incidence of medical ill effects of the newer AED in
special populations such as children may not become
apparent until after several years of use.[63] There are
not yet adequate data on behavioral or cognitive side
effects of newer AED in children, and they are not
currently approved for monotherapy in children. A
new form of treatment for acute seizure activity that
may be used at home is diazepam administered in a
rectal solution, but this is approved for use in selected refractory patients to control acute, repetitive
seizure activity and is not used after a single unprovoked seizure.[64,65]

Summary. Whereas evidence from studies of
treatment after only a single unprovoked seizure is
lacking, Class I and II evidence concerning the AED
accepted for use as first-line anticonvulsants in children (PB, PHT, VPA, CBZ) indicates that clinically
relevant cognitive and behavioral effects may occur,
particularly with PB. Parents and teachers may often overlook such cognitive and behavioral effects. In
addition, one or more important systemic side effects
such as rash, hirsutism, weight gain, or nausea may
occur with a frequency ranging from 7 to 58%.

Conclusions. The majority of children who experience a first unprovoked seizure will have few or no
recurrences. Only approximately 10% will go on to
have many (10) seizures regardless of therapy.
Treatment with AED after a first seizure as opposed
to after a second seizure has not been shown to improve prognosis for long-term seizure remission
(Class II evidence).

Treatment has been shown in several studies combining both children and adults to reduce the risk of
seizure recurrence (Class II evidence). There is a
relative paucity of data from studies involving only
children after a first seizure. AED therapy in children who have epilepsy (at least two seizures) has
potential serious pharmacologic and psychosocial
side effects (Class I evidence). No separate data exist
specifically for treatment side effects in children who
have experienced only a single seizure.

There is no evidence about whether treatment
specifically after the first seizure alters the risk of
sudden unexpected death in epilepsy patients in
children.

Recommendations. The decision as to whether or
not to treat with AED following a first unprovoked
seizure in a child or adolescent must be based on a
risk–benefit assessment that weighs the risk of another seizure (both the statistical risk of recurrence
and the potential consequences of a recurrence)
against the risk (cognitive, behavioral, and physical
as well as psychosocial) of chronic AED therapy. This
decision must be individualized and take into account both medical issues and patient and family
preference. Therefore, the following recommenda-

tions are made for children and adolescents who
have experienced a first seizure:

1. Treatment with AED is not indicated for the prevention of the development of epilepsy (Level B).
2. Treatment with AED may be considered in circumstances where the benefits of reducing the risk of a
   second seizure outweigh the risks of pharmacologic
   and psychosocial side effects (Level B).

Future research recommendations. Although
evidence reviewed in this practice parameter does
not support the routine treatment of every child who
presents with a first unprovoked seizure, a minority
of children (approximately 10%) will develop
difficult-to-control and protracted epilepsy. Prediction of who these children will be is currently not
possible; the prognosis becomes evident only after
months or years have passed. Research is needed to
identify these children after a first seizure and to
determine which treatment and management options are best. Imaging studies may help determine
if and under what circumstances children may sustain neuronal injury due to seizure. Identifying genetic, immune, or imaging markers may improve
prediction of prognosis.

More research is needed on the efficacy and side
effects in children of the new AED. Behavioral and
cognitive side effects need to be better evaluated,
especially for new AED, and individual risks as well
as group differences assessed on tests of cognition. A
goal of pharmacogenetics will be to minimize the
likelihood of adverse events from medication. Identification of children at risk for idiosyncratic adverse
reactions to AED and understanding the pharmacogenetics of responders to specific AED may improve
our ability to identify those children who should be
treated and to use only those treatments to which
they are likely to respond.

Determinants of psychosocial factors involved in
seizures and AED therapy must be better understood for the different ages of children and their families, so that overall best possible quality of life is the
goal of management. Research on seizure disorders
in the next decade will be focused on "no seizures, no
side effects" and, most importantly, toward strategies for prevention and cure of the underlying
process.[66]

Acknowledgment

The authors thank Wendy Edlund and Alison Nakashima at the
American Academy of Neurology for their superb assistance in
coordinating this project and Francine Hill for preparing the
manuscript.

Disclaimer: This statement is provided as an educational service of the American Academy of Neurology
(AAN) and the Child Neurology Society (CNS). It is
based on an assessment of current scientific and clinical information. It is not intended to include all
possible proper methods of care for a particular neurologic problem or all legitimate criteria for choosing

to use a specific procedure. Neither is it intended to exclude any reasonable alternative methodologies. The AAN and CNS recognize that specific patient care decisions are the prerogative of the patient and the physician caring for the patient, based on all of the circumstances involved.

Appendix

American Academy of Neurology Quality Standards Subcommittee members: Gary Franklin, MD, MPH (co-chair); Catherine Zahn, MD (co-chair); Milton Alter, MD, PhD (ex officio); Stephen Ashwal, MD; Richard M. Dubinsky, MD; Jacqueline French, MD; Gary H. Friday, MD; Michael Glantz, MD; Gary Gronseth, MD; Deborah Hirtz, MD; Robert G. Miller, MD; David J. Thurman, MD, MPH; and William J. Weiner, MD. *Child Neurology Society Practice Committee members:* Carmela Tardo, MD (chair); Bruce Cohen, MD (vice-chair); Elias Chalhub, MD; Roy Elterman, MD; Murray Engel, MD; Bhuwan P. Garg, MD; Brian Grabert, MD; Annette Grefe, MD; Michael Goldstein, MD; David Griesemer, MD; Betty Koo, MD; Edward Kovnar, MD; Leslie Anne Morrison, MD; Colette Parker, MD; Ben Renfroe, MD; Anthony Riela, MD; Michael Shevell, MD; Shlomo Shinnar, MD; Gerald Silverboard, MD; Russell Snyder, MD; Dean Timmns, MD; Greg Yim, MD; Mary Anne Whelan, MD.

References

1. Verity CM, Ross EN, Golding J. Epilepsy in the first ten years of life: findings of the child health and education study. Br Med J 1992;305: 857–861.
2. Camfield CS, Camfield PR, Gordon K, Wirrell E, Dooley JM. Incidence of epilepsy in childhood and adolescence: a population-based study in Nova Scotia from 1977 to 1985. Epilepsia 1996;37:19–23.
3. Hauser W, Annegers J, Kurland L. Incidence of epilepsy and unprovoked seizures in Rochester, Minnisota, 1935–1984. Epilepsia 1993;34: 453–468.
4. Jallon P, Goumaz M, Haenggeli C, Morabia A. Incidence of first epileptic seizures in the canton of Geneva, Switzerland. Epilepsia 1997;38: 547–552.
5. Hirtz D, Ashwal S, Berg A, et al. Practice parameter: evaluating a first nonfebrile seizure in children. Neurology 2000;55:616–623.
6. Academy of Pediatrics, Committee on Quality Improvement, Subcommittee on Febrile Seizures. Practice parameter: long-term treatment of the child with simple febrile seizures. Pediatrics 1999;103:1307–1309.
7. Commission on Epidemiology and Prognosis, International League Against Epilepsy. Guidelines for epidemiologic studies on epilepsy. Epilepsia 1993;37:592–596.
8. Gowers WR. Epilepsy and other chronic convulsive diseases: their causes, symptoms and treatment. London: J & A Churchill, 1881:242.
9. Goddard GV, Mc Intyre DC, Leech CK. A permanent change in brain function resulting from daily electrical stimulation. Exp Neurol 1969; 25:295–330.
10. Berg AT, Shinnar S. Do seizures beget seizures? An assessment of the clinical evidence in humans. J Clin Neurophysiol 1997;14:102–110.
11. Wasterlain CG. Recurrent seizures in developing brain are harmful. Epilepsia 1997;38:728–734.
12. Meldrum B. Physiological changes during prolonged seizures and epileptic brain damage. Neuropaediatrie 1978;9:203–212.
13. Cavazos JE, Das I, Sutula TP. Neuronal loss induced in limbic pathways by kindling: evidence for induction of hippocampal sclerosis by repeated brief seizures. J Neurosci 1994;14:3106–3121.
14. Chen K, Baram TZ, Soltesz I. Febrile seizures in the developing brain result in persistent modification of neuronal excitability in limbic circuits. Nat Med 1999;5:888–894.
15. Schmid R, Tandon P, Stafstrom CE, Holmes GL. Effects of neonatal seizures on subsequent seizure-induced brain injury. Neurology 1999; 53:1754–1761.
16. Camfield PR. Recurrent seizures in the developing brain are not harmful. Epilepsia 1997;38:735–737.
17. Maytal J, Shinnar S, Moshé SL, Alvarez LA. Low morbidity and mortality of status epilepticus in children. Pediatrics 1989;83:323–331.
18. Harvey AS, Nolan T, Carlin JB. Community-based study of mortality in children with epilepsy. Epilepsia 1993;34:597–603.
19. Callenbach PM, Westendorp RG, Geerts AT, et al. Mortality risk in children with epilepsy: the Dutch study of epilepsy in childhood. Pediatrics 2001;107:1259–1263.
20. Donner EJ, Smith CR, Snead OC. Sudden unexplained death in children with epilepsy. Neurology 2001;57:430–434.
21. Camfield CS, Camfield PR, Veugelers P. Death in children with epilepsy: a population-based study. Lancet 2002;315:1891–1895.
22. Austin JK, Dunn DW. Assessing children's concerns about epilepsy. Clin Nurs Practice Epilepsy 1996;3:11–12.
23. Austin JK. Concerns and fears of children with seizures. Clin Nurs Practice Epilepsy 1993;1:4–10.
24. O'Dell C, Shinnar S. Initiation and discontinuation of antiepileptic drugs. Neurol Clin 2001;19:289–311.
25. Shinnar S, Berg AT, Moshe SL, et al. The risk of seizure recurrence after a first unprovoked febrile seizure in childhood: an extended follow-up. Pediatrics 1996;98:216–225.
26. Hauser WA, Rich SS, Annegers JF, Anderson VE. Seizure recurrence after a first unprovoked seizure: an extended follow-up. Neurology 1990;40:1163–1170.
27. Stroink H, Brouwer OF, Arts WF, Geerts AT, Peters AC, van Donselaar CA. The first unprovoked, untreated seizure in childhood: a hospital based study of the accuracy of the diagnosis, rate of recurrence, and long term outcome after recurrence. Dutch Study of Epilepsy in Childhood. J Neurol Neurosurg Psychiatry 1998;64:595–600.
28. Shinnar S, Berg AT, O'Dell C, Newstein D, Moshe SL, Hauser WA. Predictors of multiple seizures in a cohort of children prospectively followed from the time of their first unprovoked seizure. Ann Neurol 2000;48:140–147.
29. Boulloche J, Leloup P, Mallet E, Parain D, Tron P. Risk of recurrence after a single, unprovoked, generalized tonic-clonic seizure. Dev Med Child Neurol 1989;31:626–632.
30. Camfield PR, Camfield CS, Dooley JM, Tibbles JAR, Fung T, Garner B. Epilepsy after a first unprovoked seizure in childhood. Neurology 1985; 35:1657–1660.
31. Annegers JF, Shirts SB, Hauser WA, Kurland LT. Risk of recurrence after an initial unprovoked seizure. Epilepsia 1986;27:43–50.
32. Hart YM, Sander JWAS, Johnson AL, Shorvon SD. National general practice study of epilepsy: recurrence after a first seizure. Lancet 1990; 336:1271–1274.
33. Martinovic Z, Jovic N. Seizure recurrence after a first generalized tonic-clonic seizure in children, adolescents and young adults. Seizure 1997; 6:461–465.
34. Berg AT, Shinnar S, Levy SR, Testa FM, Smith-Rapaport S, Beckerman B. Early development of intractable epilepsy in children: a prospective study. Neurology 2001;56:1445–1452.
35. Berg AT, Shinnar S. The risk of seizure recurrence following a first unprovoked seizure: a quantitative review. Neurology 1991;41:965–972.
36. Shinnar S, Berg AT, Moshe SL, Shinnar R. How long do new-onset seizures in children last? Ann Neurol 2001;49:659–664.
37. Dodson WE, De Lorenzo RJ, Pedley TA, Shinnar S, Treiman DM, Wannamaker DB. The treatment of convulsive status epilepticus: recommendations of the Epilepsy Foundation of America's Working Group on Status Epilepticus. JAMA 1993;270:854–859.
38. Chandra B. First seizure in adults: to treat or not to treat. Clin Neurol Neurosurg 1992;94:S61–S63.
39. Musicco M, Beghi E, Solari A, Viani F. Treatment of first tonic-clonic seizure does not improve the prognosis of epilepsy. Neurology 1997;49: 991–998.
40. Das CP, Sawhney IMS, Lal V, Prabhakar S. Risk of recurrence of seizures following single unprovoked idiopathic seizure. Neurol India 2000;48:357–360.
41. Camfield P, Camfield C, Dooley J, Smith E, Garner B. A randomized study of carbamazepine versus no medication after a first unprovoked seizure in childhood. Neurology 1989;39:851–852.
42. Hirtz DG, Ellenberg JH, Nelson KB. The risk of recurrence of nonfebrile seizures in children. Neurology 1984;34:637–641.
43. Camfield PR, Camfield CS, Dooley JM, Smith S, Smith E. Long-term outcome is unchanged by anti-epileptic drug treatment after a first seizure: a 15-year follow-up from a randomized trial in childhood. Epilepsia 2002;43:662–663.
44. American Academy of Pediatrics. Behavioral and cognitive effects of anticonvulsant therapy (RE9537). Pediatrics 1995;96:538–540.
45. Yerby MS. Teratogenic effects of antiepileptic drugs: what do we advise patients? Epilepsia 1997;38:957–958.
46. Canadian Study Group for Childhood Epilepsy. The cognitive and behavioral effects of clobazam and standard monotherapy are comparable. Epilepsy Res 1999;33:133–143.
47. Canadian Study Group for Childhood Epilepsy. Clobazam has equivalent efficacy to carbamazepine and phenytoin as monotherapy for childhood epilepsy. Epilepsia 1998;39:952–959.
48. Vining EP, Mellits ED, Dorsen MM, et al. Psychologic and behavioral effects of antiepileptic drugs in children: a double-blind comparison between phenobarbital and valproic acid. Pediatrics 1987;80:165–174.
49. Chen YJ, Kang WM, So WCM. Comparison of antiepileptic drugs on cognitive function in newly diagnosed epileptic children: a psychometric and neurophysiological study. Epilepsia 1996;37:81–86.
50. Berg I, Butler A, Ellis M, Foster J. Psychiatric aspects of epilepsy in childhood treated with carbamazepine, phenytoin or sodium valproate: a random trial. Dev Med Child Neurol 1993;35:149–157.
51. Forsythe I, Butler R, Berg I, McGuire R. Cognitive impairment in new cases of epilepsy randomly assigned to carbamazepine, phenytoin and sodium valproate. Dev Med Child Neurol 1991;33:524–534.
52. Thilothammal N, Banu K, Tatnam RS. Comparison of phenobarbitone, phenytoin with sodium valproate: Randomized, double-blind study. Indian Pediatr 1996;33:549–555.
53. Aman MG, Werry JS, Paxton JW, Turbott SH. Effects of phenytoin on cognitive–motor performance in children as a function of drug concen-

tration, seizure type, and time of medication. Epilepsia 1994;35:172–180.

54. Aman MG, Werry JS, Paxton JW, Turbott SH, Steward AW. Effects of carbamazepine on psychomotor performance in children as a function of drug concentration, seizure type, and time of medication. Epilepsia 1990;31:51–60.

55. Aman MG, Werry JS, Paxton JW, Turbott SH. Effect of sodium valproate on psychomotor performance in children as a function of dose, fluctuations in concentration, and diagnosis. Epilepsia 1987;28:115–124.

56. De Silva M, MacArdle B, McGowan M, et al. Randomised comparative monotherapy trial of phenobarbitone, phenytoin, carbamazepine, or sodium valproate for newly diagnosed childhood epilepsy. Lancet 1996;347:709–713.

57. Calandre EP, Dominguez-Granados R, Gomez-Rubio M, Molina-Font JA. Cognitive effects of long-term treatment with phenobarbital and valproic acid in school children. Acta Neurol Scand 1990;81:504–506.

58. Williams J, Bates S, Griebel ML, et al. Does short-term antiepileptic drug treatment in children result in cognitive or behavioral changes? Epilepsia 1998;39:1064–1069.

59. Stores G, Williams PL, Styles E, Zaiwalla Z. Psychological effects of sodium valproate and carbamazepine in epilepsy. Arch Dis Child 1992;67:1330–1337.

60. Mandelbaum DE, Burack GD. The effect of seizure type and medication on cognitive and behavioral functioning in children with idiopathic epilepsy. Dev Med Child Neurol 1997;39:731–735.

61. Verity CM, Hosking G, Easter DJ. A multicentre comparative trial of sodium valproate and carbamazepine in pediatric epilepsy. Dev Med Child Neurol 1995;37:97–108.

62. Prasad AN, Setfanelli M, Nagarajan L. Seizure exacerbation and developmental regression with carbamazepine. Can J Neurol Sci 1998;25:287–294.

63. Dreifuss FE, Langer DH, Moline KA, Maxwell JE. Valproic acid hepatic fatalities. II. US experience since 1984. Neurology 1989;39:201–207.

64. Dreifuss FE, Rosman NP, Cloyd JC, et al. A comparison of rectal diazepam gel and placebo for acute repetitive seizures. N Engl J Med 1998;338:1869–1875.

65. Morton LD, Rizkallah E, Pellock J. New drug therapy for acute seizure management. Semin Pediatr Neurol 1997;4:51–63.

66. Jacobs MP, Fischbach GD, Davis MR, et al. Future directions for epilepsy research. Neurology 2001;57:1536–1542.

Management of Sinusitis

• *Clinical Practice Guideline*
• *Technical Report*

AMERICAN ACADEMY OF PEDIATRICS

Subcommittee on Management of Sinusitis and Committee on Quality Improvement

Clinical Practice Guideline: Management of Sinusitis

ABSTRACT. This clinical practice guideline formulates recommendations for health care providers regarding the diagnosis, evaluation, and treatment of children, ages 1 to 21 years, with uncomplicated acute, subacute, and recurrent acute bacterial sinusitis. It was developed through a comprehensive search and analysis of the medical literature. Expert consensus opinion was used to enhance or formulate recommendations where data were insufficient.

A subcommittee, composed of pediatricians with expertise in infectious disease, allergy, epidemiology, family practice, and pediatric practice, supplemented with an otolaryngologist and radiologist, were selected to formulate the practice parameter. Several other groups (including members of the American College of Emergency Physicians, American Academy of Otolaryngology-Head and Neck Surgery, American Academy of Asthma, Allergy and Immunology, as well as numerous national committees and sections of the American Academy of Pediatrics) have reviewed and revised the guideline. Three specific issues were considered: 1) evidence for the efficacy of various antibiotics in children; 2) evidence for the efficacy of various ancillary, nonantibiotic regimens; and 3) the diagnostic accuracy and concordance of clinical symptoms, radiography (and other imaging methods), and sinus aspiration.

It is recommended that the diagnosis of acute bacterial sinusitis be based on clinical criteria in children ≤6 years of age who present with upper respiratory symptoms that are either persistent or severe. Although controversial, imaging studies may be necessary to confirm a diagnosis of acute bacterial sinusitis in children >6 years of age. Computed tomography scans of the paranasal sinuses should be reserved for children who present with complications of acute bacterial sinusitis or who have very persistent or recurrent infections and are not responsive to medical management.

There were only 5 controlled randomized trials and 8 case series on antimicrobial therapy for acute bacterial sinusitis in children. However, these data, plus data derived from the study of adults with acute bacterial sinusitis, support the recommendation that acute bacterial sinusitis be treated with antimicrobial therapy to achieve a more rapid clinical cure. Children with complications or suspected complications of acute bacterial sinusitis should be treated promptly and aggressively with antibiotics and, when appropriate, drainage. Based on controversial and limited data, no recommendations are made about the use of prophylactic antimicrobials, ancillary therapies, or complementary/alternative medicine for prevention and treatment of acute bacterial sinusitis.

The recommendations in this statement do not indicate an exclusive course of treatment or serve as a standard of medical care. Variations, taking into account individual circumstances, may be appropriate.
PEDIATRICS (ISSN 0031 4005). Copyright © 2001 by the American Academy of Pediatrics.

This clinical practice guideline is not intended as a sole source of guidance in the diagnosis and management of acute bacterial sinusitis in children. It is designed to assist pediatricians by providing an analytic framework for evaluation and treatment. It is not intended to replace clinical judgment or establish a protocol for all patients with this condition.

ABBREVIATION. CT, computed tomography.

BACKGROUND

The ethmoid and the maxillary sinuses form in the third to fourth gestational month and, accordingly, are present at birth. The sphenoid sinuses are generally pneumatized by 5 years of age; the frontal sinuses appear at age 7 to 8 years but are not completely developed until late adolescence. The paranasal sinuses are a common site of infection in children and adolescents.[1] These infections are important as a cause of frequent morbidity and rarely may result in life-threatening complications. It may be difficult to distinguish children with uncomplicated viral upper respiratory infections or adenoiditis from those with an episode of acute bacterial sinusitis.[2] Most viral infections of the upper respiratory tract involve the nose and the paranasal sinuses (viral rhinosinusitis).[3] However, bacterial infections of the paranasal sinuses do not usually involve the nose. When the patient with bacterial infection of the paranasal sinuses has purulent (thick, colored, and opaque) nasal drainage, the site of infection is the paranasal sinuses; the nose is simply acting as a conduit for secretions produced in the sinuses.

The common predisposing events that set the stage for acute bacterial sinusitis are acute viral upper respiratory infections that result in a viral rhinosinusitis (a diffuse mucositis that predisposes to approximately 80% of bacterial sinus infections) and allergic inflammation (that predisposes to 20% of bacterial sinus infections).[4] Children have 6 to 8 viral upper respiratory infections each year; it is estimated that between 5% to 13% of these infections may be complicated by a secondary bacterial infection of the paranasal sinuses.[5–7] Acute bacterial otitis media and acute bacterial sinusitis are the most common complications of viral upper respiratory infections and are probably the most common indications for the prescription of antimicrobial agents.[8] The middle ear cavity connects to the nasopharynx via the eustachian tube. In a sense then, the middle ear cavity is also a paranasal sinus.[9] The pathogenesis and microbiology of acute otitis media and acute bacterial sinusitis are similar.[9] This similarity allows us to extrapolate information known about the treatment of acute otitis media and apply it to the treatment of acute bacterial sinusitis. This is especially helpful when considering antimicrobials and antibacterial resistance. Data on antimicrobial efficacy and antibacterial resistance also may be derived from the study of adult patients with acute sinusitis, in whom there have been more recent systematic inquiry.[10,11]

This practice guideline focuses on the diagnosis, evaluation, and treatment of children, ages 1 to 21 years, with uncomplicated acute, subacute, and recurrent acute bacterial sinusitis. Neonates and children younger than 1 year of age are not considered. Although bacterial sinusitis does occur rarely in children less than 1 year of age, their exclusion reflects, in part, the difficulty in conducting clinical investigation in this age group. This is a consequence of the small size of the paranasal sinuses and the difficulty in safely performing sinus aspiration.[12] This practice parameter does not apply to children with previously recognized anatomic abnormalities of their paranasal sinuses (facial dysmorphisms or trauma), immunodeficiencies, cystic fibrosis, or immotile cilia syndrome.

A discussion of chronic sinusitis (defined by the presence of symptoms for 90 days) and acute exacerbations of chronic sinusitis are not included in this guideline. The role of bacterial infection as a primary cause of chronic sinusitis is controversial.[11,13] Chronic inflammation of the paranasal sinuses may be a consequence of noninfectious conditions such as allergy, environmental pollutants, cystic fibrosis, or gastroesophageal reflux.

This guideline is intended for use by clinicians who treat children and adolescents in a variety of clinical settings including the office and emergency department. The purpose of the guideline is to encourage accurate diagnosis of bacterial sinusitis, appropriate use of imaging procedures, and judicious use of antibiotics.

DEFINITIONS

<u>Acute bacterial sinusitis:</u> Bacterial infection of the paranasal sinuses lasting less than 30 days in which symptoms resolve completely.

<u>Subacute bacterial sinusitis:</u> Bacterial infection of the paranasal sinuses lasting between 30 and 90 days in which symptoms resolve completely.

<u>Recurrent acute bacterial sinusitis:</u> Episodes of bacterial infection of the paranasal sinuses, each lasting less than 30 days and separated by intervals of at least 10 days during which the patient is asymptomatic.

<u>Chronic sinusitis:</u> Episodes of inflammation of the paranasal sinuses lasting more than 90 days. Patients have persistent residual respiratory symptoms such as cough, rhinorrhea, or nasal obstruction.

<u>Acute bacterial sinusitis superimposed on chronic sinusitis:</u> Patients with residual respiratory symptoms develop new respiratory symptoms. When treated with antimicrobials, these new symptoms resolve, but the underlying residual symptoms do not.[14]

METHODS

To develop the clinical practice guideline on the management of acute bacterial sinusitis, the American Academy of Pediatrics subcommittee partnered with the Agency for Healthcare Research and Quality and colleague organizations from family practice and otolaryngology. The Agency for Healthcare Research and Quality worked with the New England Medical Center Evidence-based Practice Center, as one of several centers that focus on conducting systematic reviews of the literature. A full report was produced by the New England Medical Center on the diagnosis and management of acute sinusitis.[15] However, because there were only 5 randomized studies in children, a supplemental analysis was conducted that included nonrandomized pediatric trials. The subcommittee used both reports to form the practice guideline recommendations but relied heavily on the pediatric supplement.[16]

For the pediatric supplement, the major research questions to be analyzed through the literature on acute bacterial sinusitis in childhood were 1) evidence for the efficacy of various antibiotics in children; 2) evidence for the efficacy of various ancillary, nonantibiotic regimens; and 3) the diagnostic accuracy and concordance of clinical symptoms, radiography (and other imaging methods), and sinus aspiration.

The literature was searched in Medline, complemented by Excerpta Medica, from 1966 through March 1999, using the word "sinusitis." Search criteria were limited to human studies and English language and appropriate pediatric terms. More than 1800 citations were reviewed. One hundred thirty-eight articles were fully examined, resulting in 21 qualifying studies. These studies included 5 controlled randomized trials and 8 case series on antimicrobial therapy, 3 controlled randomized trials on ancillary treatments, and 8 studies with information on diagnostic tests. The heterogeneity and paucity of the data did not allow for formal meta-analysis. When possible, rates were pooled across different studies and heterogeneity assessed.

The draft clinical practice guideline underwent extensive peer review by committees and sections within the American Academy of Pediatrics and by numerous outside organizations. Liaisons to the committee also distributed the draft within their organizations. Comments were compiled and reviewed by the subcommittee and relevant changes incorporated into the guideline.

The recommendations contained in this practice guideline are based on the best available data. Where data are lacking, a combination of evidence and expert opinion was used. Strong recommendations were based on high-quality scientific evidence or, when such was unavailable, strong expert consensus. Fair and weak recommendations are based on lesser-quality or limited data and expert consensus. Clinical options are identified as interventions for which the subcommittee could not find compelling positive or negative evidence. These clinical options are interventions that a reasonable health care professional may or may not wish to consider.

RECOMMENDATIONS

Methods of Diagnosis

Under normal circumstances the paranasal sinuses are assumed to be sterile.[17–19] However, the paranasal sinuses are in continuity with surface areas, such as the nasal mucosa and nasopharynx, which are heavily colonized with bacteria. Although it is reasonable to assume that the paranasal sinuses are frequently and transiently contaminated by bacteria from neighboring surfaces, these bacteria, which are present in low density, are probably removed by the normal function of the mucociliary apparatus. Accordingly, the gold standard for the diagnosis of acute bacterial sinusitis is the recovery of bacteria in high density ($\geq 10^4$ colony-forming units/mL) from the cavity of a paranasal sinus.[20] Although sinus aspiration is the gold standard for the diagnosis of acute bacterial sinusitis,[11] it is an invasive, time-consuming, and potentially painful procedure that should only be performed by a specialist (otolaryngologist). It is not a feasible method of diagnosis for the primary care practitioner and is not recommended for the routine diagnosis of bacterial sinus infections in children. However, the results of sinus aspiration have been correlated with clinical and radiographic findings in children with acute respiratory symptoms.[21,22]

Recommendation 1

The diagnosis of acute bacterial sinusitis is based on clinical criteria in children who present with upper respiratory symptoms that are either persistent or severe (strong recommendation based on limited scientific evidence and strong consensus of the panel).

Acute bacterial sinusitis is an infection of the paranasal sinuses lasting less than 30 days that presents with either persistent or severe symptoms.[4,23] Patients are asymptomatic after recovery from episodes of acute bacterial sinusitis.

Persistent symptoms are those that last longer than 10 to 14, but less than 30, days. Such symptoms include nasal or postnasal discharge (of any quality), daytime cough (which may be worse at night), or both.

Severe symptoms include a temperature of at least 102°F (39°C) and purulent nasal discharge present concurrently for at least 3 to 4 consecutive days in a child who seems ill. The child who seems toxic should be hospitalized and is not considered in this algorithm.

Uncomplicated viral upper respiratory infections generally last 5 to 7 days but may last longer.[24,25] Although the respiratory symptoms may not have completely resolved by the 10th day, almost always they have peaked in severity and begun to improve. Therefore, the persistence of respiratory symptoms without any evidence that they are beginning to resolve suggests the presence of a secondary bacterial infection. Significant fever or complaints of facial pain or headache are variable. It is important for the practitioner to attempt to differentiate between sequential episodes of uncomplicated viral upper respiratory tract infections (which may seem to coalesce in the mind of the patient or parent) from the onset of acute sinusitis with persistent symptoms. The objective of treatment of acute bacterial sinusitis is to foster rapid recovery, prevent suppurative complications, and minimize exacerbations of asthma (reactive airways diseases).[26]

Children with acute bacterial sinusitis who present with severe symptoms need to be distinguished from those with uncomplicated viral infections who are moderately ill. If fever is present at all in uncomplicated viral infections of the upper respiratory tract, it tends to be present early in the illness, usually accompanied by other constitutional symptoms such as headache and myalgias.[24] Generally, the constitutional symptoms resolve in the first 48 hours and then the respiratory symptoms become prominent. In most uncomplicated viral infections, purulent nasal discharge does not appear for several days. Accordingly, it is the concurrent presentation with high fever and purulent nasal discharge for at least 3 to 4

consecutive days that helps to define the severe presentation of acute bacterial sinusitis.[23] Children with severe onset of acute bacterial sinusitis may have an intense headache that is above or behind the eye; in general, they seem to be moderately ill.

Unfortunately, the physical examination does not generally contribute substantially to the diagnosis of acute bacterial sinusitis. This is explained by the similarity of physical findings in the patient with an uncomplicated viral rhinosinusitis and the patient with acute bacterial sinusitis.[2] In both instances, examination of the nasal mucosa may show mild erythema and swelling of the nasal turbinates with mucopurulent discharge. Facial pain is an unusual complaint in children. Facial tenderness is a rare finding in small children and may be unreliable as an indicator of acute bacterial sinusitis in older children and adolescents. Reproducible unilateral pain, present on percussion or direct pressure over the body of the frontal and maxillary sinuses, may indicate a diagnosis of acute bacterial sinusitis.[27] Likewise, observed or reported periorbital swelling is suggestive of ethmoid sinusitis. Examination of the tympanic membranes, pharynx, and cervical lymph nodes does not usually contribute to the diagnosis of acute bacterial sinusitis.

The value of the performance of transillumination of the sinuses to assess whether fluid is present in the maxillary and frontal paranasal sinuses is controversial. The technique is performed in a completely darkened room (after the examiner's eyes are adapted to the dark) by placing a transilluminator (high-intensity light beam) either in the mouth or against the cheek (for the maxillary sinuses) or under the medial aspect of the supraorbital ridge area (for the frontal sinuses) to assess the transmission of light through the sinus cavity.[27] Transillumination is difficult to perform correctly and has been shown to be unreliable in children younger than 10 years.[22,28] In the older child it may be helpful at the extremes of interpretation; if transillumination is normal, sinusitis is unlikely; if the transmission of light is absent, the maxillary or frontal sinus is likely to be filled with fluid.[18]

Subacute sinusitis is defined by the persistence of mild to moderate and often intermittent respiratory symptoms (nasal discharge, daytime cough, or both) for between 30 and 90 days. The nasal discharge may be of any quality, and cough is often worse at night. Low-grade fever may be periodic but is usually not prominent. The microbiology of subacute sinusitis is the same as that observed in patients with acute bacterial sinusitis.[29]

Patients with recurrent acute bacterial sinusitis are defined as having had 3 episodes of acute bacterial sinusitis in 6 months or 4 episodes in 12 months. The response to antibiotics is usually brisk and the patient is completely free of symptoms between episodes.

The most common cause of recurrent sinusitis is recurrent viral upper respiratory infection, often a consequence of attendance at day care or the presence of an older school-age sibling in the household. Other predisposing conditions include allergic and nonallergic rhinitis, cystic fibrosis, an immunodeficiency disorder (insufficient or dysfunctional immunoglobulins), ciliary dyskinesia, or an anatomic problem.[23]

Recommendation 2a

Imaging studies are not necessary to confirm a diagnosis of clinical sinusitis in children ≤6 years of age (strong recommendation based on limited scientific evidence and strong consensus of the panel).

In 1981, children between the ages of 2 and 16 years presenting with either persistent or severe symptoms were evaluated with sinus radiographs.[21,22] When children with persistent or severe symptoms were found to have abnormal sinus radiographs (complete opacification, mucosal thickening of at least 4 mm, or an air-fluid level), an aspiration of the maxillary sinus was performed. Bacteria in high density (≥10[4] colony-forming units/mL) were recovered in 70% to 75% of the children. This proportion of positive cultures (75%) is similar to the likelihood that a tympanocentesis will yield middle ear fluid with a positive culture for bacteria in children with otoscopic evidence of acute otitis media.[30]

In children with persistent symptoms, the history of protracted respiratory symptoms (>10 but <30 days without evidence of improvement) predicted significantly abnormal radiographs (complete opacification, mucosal thickening of at least 4 mm, or an air-fluid level) in 80% of children.[31] For children 6 years of age or younger, the history predicted abnormal sinus radiographs in 88% of children. For children older than 6 years, the history of persistent symptoms predicted abnormal sinus radiographs in 70%. The peak age for acute bacterial sinusitis is in children 6 years of age or younger. Accordingly, in this age group, because a positive history predicts the finding of abnormal sinus radiographs so frequently (and because history plus abnormal radiographs results in a positive sinus aspirate in 75% of cases), radiographs can be safely omitted and a diagnosis of acute bacterial sinusitis can be made on clinical criteria alone. Approximately 60% of children with symptoms of sinusitis (persistent or severe) will have bacteria recovered from an aspirate of the maxillary sinus.

In contrast to the general agreement that radiographs are not necessary in children 6 years of age or younger with persistent symptoms, the need for radiographs as a confirmatory test of acute sinusitis in children older than 6 years with persistent symptoms and for all children (regardless of age) with severe symptoms is controversial.[32,33] Some practitioners may elect to perform sinus radiographs with the expectation or suspicion that the study may be normal. A normal radiograph is powerful evidence that bacterial sinusitis is not the cause of the clinical syndrome.[34] However, the American College of Radiology has taken the position that the diagnosis of acute uncomplicated sinusitis should be made on clinical grounds alone.[35] They support this position by noting that plain radiographs of the paranasal sinuses are technically difficult to perform, particularly in

very young children. Correct positioning may be difficult to achieve and therefore the radiographic images may overestimate and underestimate the presence of abnormalities within the paranasal sinuses.[36,37] The college would reserve the use of images for situations in which the patient does not recover or worsens during the course of appropriate antimicrobial therapy. Similarly, a recent set of guidelines generated by the Sinus and Allergy Health Partnership (representing numerous constituencies) does not recommend either radiographs or computed tomography (CT) or magnetic resonance imaging scans to diagnose uncomplicated cases of acute bacterial sinusitis in any age group.[1]

It is essential to recognize that abnormal images of the sinuses (either radiographs, CT, or magnetic resonance imaging) cannot stand alone as diagnostic evidence of acute bacterial sinusitis under any circumstances. Images can serve only as confirmatory measures of sinus disease in patients whose clinical histories are supportive of the diagnosis. Numerous investigations have demonstrated the high frequency of abnormal images in the paranasal sinuses of children undergoing imaging for indications other than suspected sinusitis.[38-40] In a study by Glasier et al,[39] almost 100% of young children who were undergoing CT examination for reasons other than sinus disease and who had an upper respiratory tract infection in the previous 2 weeks demonstrated soft tissue changes in their sinuses. A study by Gwaltney et al in 1994[3] found that abnormalities of the paranasal sinuses on CT scan are extremely common in young adults with acute (<72 hours) uncomplicated viral upper respiratory infections. This study and others serve to underscore that when abnormalities of the mucosa are present on images they indicate the presence of inflammation but do not disclose whether the inflammatory process is caused by viral infection, bacterial infection, allergy, or chemical irritation (eg, chlorine exposure in the swimmer).

Recommendation 2b

CT scans of the paranasal sinuses should be reserved for patients in whom surgery is being considered as a management strategy (strong recommendation based on good evidence and strong panel consensus).

Despite the limitations of CT scans,[3,38-40] they offer a detailed image of sinus anatomy and, when taken in conjunction with clinical findings, remain a useful adjunct to guide surgical treatment. Computed tomography scans are indicated in children who present with complications of acute bacterial sinus infection or those who have very persistent or recurrent infections that are not responsive to medical management.[33] In these instances, the image, preferably a complete CT scan of the paranasal sinuses, is essential to provide precise anatomic information to the clinician. These are instances in which the physician may be contemplating surgical intervention, including aspiration of the paranasal sinuses.

Recommendation 3

Antibiotics are recommended for the management of acute bacterial sinusitis to achieve a more rapid clinical cure (strong recommendation based on good evidence and strong panel consensus).

To promote the judicious use of antibiotics, it is essential that children diagnosed as having acute bacterial sinusitis meet the defining clinical presentations of "persistent" or "severe" disease as described previously.[41] This will minimize the number of children with uncomplicated viral upper respiratory tract infections who are treated with antimicrobials.

In a study comparing antimicrobial therapy with placebo in the treatment of children with the clinical and radiographic diagnosis of acute bacterial sinusitis, children receiving antimicrobial therapy recovered more quickly and more often than those receiving placebo.[31] On the third day of treatment, 83% of children receiving an antimicrobial were cured or improved compared with 51% of the children in the placebo group. (Forty-five percent of children receiving antimicrobial therapy were cured [complete resolution of respiratory symptoms] compared with 11% receiving placebo.) On the 10th day of treatment, 79% of children receiving an antimicrobial were cured or improved compared with 60% of children receiving placebo. Approximately 50% to 60% of children will improve gradually without the use of antimicrobials; however, the recovery of an additional 20% to 30% is delayed substantially compared with children who receive appropriate antibiotics.

A recent study by Garbutt et al[42] has challenged the notion that children identified as having acute sinusitis on clinical grounds alone (without the performance of images) will benefit from antimicrobial therapy. When children randomized to low-dose antibiotic therapy were compared with those receiving placebo there were no differences observed in outcome, either in the timing or frequency of recovery. The discrepancy in results between this investigation and the Wald[31] study may be attributable to the inclusion in this study of a larger cohort of older children (who may not have had sinusitis) and the exclusion of more seriously ill children with a temperature > 39°C or facial pain. Current recommendations for antibiotic management of uncomplicated sinusitis vary depending on a previous history of antibiotic exposure (in the previous 1–3 months), attendance at day care, and age. Some of the children in the Garbutt study might have qualified for high-dose amoxicillin-clavulanate to overcome antimicrobial resistant pathogens.

Comparative bacteriologic cure rates in studies of adults with acute sinusitis indicate the efficacy of antimicrobial treatment.[11,43] The findings of these studies indicate that antimicrobials in adequate doses with appropriate antibacterial spectra are highly effective in eradicating or substantially reducing bacteria in the sinus cavity, whereas those with inadequate spectrum or given in inadequate doses are not (Table 1).

TABLE 1. Comparative Bacteriologic Cure Rates (as Determined by Sinus Puncture) Among Adult Patients With Acute Community-Acquired Bacterial Sinusitis*

Comment Regarding Treatment	Number (%) of Bacteriologic Cures
Antibiotic concentration was ≥ MIC of causative bacteria	19/21 (90)
Antibiotic concentration was < MIC of causative bacteria	15/33 (45)
Appropriate antimicrobial and dose given	278/300 (93)
Suboptimal dose given	53/76 (70)

MIC indicates minimum inhibitory concentration.
* Adapted from Gwaltney.[11]

The microbiology of acute, subacute, and recurrent acute bacterial sinusitis has been outlined in several studies.[20–22] The principal bacterial pathogens are *Streptococcus pneumoniae*, nontypeable *Haemophilus influenzae*, and *Moraxella catarrhalis*. *S pneumoniae* is recovered from approximately 30% of children with acute bacterial sinusitis, whereas *H influenzae* and *M catarrhalis* are each recovered from about 20%.[23] In the remaining 30% of children, aspirates of the maxillary sinus are sterile. It is noteworthy that neither *Staphylococcus aureus* nor respiratory anaerobes are likely to be recovered from children with acute bacterial sinusitis.[22]

Currently, approximately 50% of *H influenzae* and 100% of *M catarrhalis* are likely to be ß-lactamase positive nationwide.[44,45] Upper respiratory tract isolates of *S pneumoniae* are not susceptible to penicillin in 15% to 38% (average 25%) of children; approximately 50% are highly resistant to penicillin and the remaining half are intermediate in resistance.[1,46,47] The mechanism of penicillin resistance in *S pneumoniae* is an alteration of penicillin binding proteins. This phenomenon, which varies considerably according to geographic location, results in resistance to penicillin and cephalosporin. Table 2 shows the calculation for the likelihood that a child with acute bacterial sinusitis will harbor a resistant pathogen and not respond to treatment with amoxicillin. The following should be considered: the prevalence of each bacterial species as a cause of acute bacterial sinusitis, the prevalence of resistance among each bacterial species, and the rate of spontaneous improvement. Extrapolating from data derived from patients with acute otitis media, 15% of children with acute bacterial sinusitis caused by *S pneumoniae* will recover spontaneously, half of the children with acute bacterial sinusitis caused by *H influenzae* and half to three-quarters of the children infected with *M catarrhalis* also will recover spontaneously.[48] Furthermore, only *S pneumoniae* that are highly resistant to penicillin will not respond to conventional doses of amoxicillin. Accordingly, in the absence of any risk factors, approximately 80% of children with acute bacterial sinusitis will respond to treatment with amoxicillin. Risk factors for the presence of bacterial species that are likely to be resistant to amoxicillin include 1) attendance at day care, 2) recent receipt (< 90 days) of antimicrobial treatment, and 3) age less than 2 years.[49,50]

TABLE 2. Calculation of the Likelihood that a Child With Acute Bacterial Sinusitis Will Fail Treatment With Standard Doses of Amoxicillin*†

Bacterial Species	Prevalence	Spontaneous Cure Rate (%)	Prevalence of Resistance (%)	Failure to Amoxicillin (%)
Streptococcus pneumoniae	30	15	25	3
Haemophilus influenzae	20	50	50	5
Moraxella catarrhalis	20	50–75	100	5–10

* This table is based on data obtained from treatment of acute otitis media.
† Consider that 50% of resistant strains are highly resistant to penicillin and only highly resistant isolates will fail to respond to standard doses of amoxicillin (45 mg/kg/day); Minimum inhibitory concentration (MIC) of susceptible *S pneumoniae* ≤0.1 μg/mL; MIC of moderately resistant *S pneumoniae* = 0.1–1.0 μg/mL; MIC of highly resistant *S pneumoniae* ≥2.0 μg/mL.

The desire to continue to use amoxicillin as first-line therapy in patients suspected of having acute bacterial sinusitis relates to its general effectiveness, safety, and tolerability; low cost; and narrow spectrum. For children younger than 2 years of age with uncomplicated acute bacterial sinusitis that is mild to moderate in degree of severity, who do not attend day care, and have not recently been treated with an antimicrobial, amoxicillin is recommended at either a usual dose of 45 mg/kg/d in 2 divided doses or a high dose of 90 mg/kg/d in 2 divided doses (Fig 1). If the patient is allergic to amoxicillin, either cefdinir (14 mg/kg/d in 1 or 2 doses), cefuroxime (30 mg/kg/d in 2 divided doses), or cefpodoxime (10 mg/kg/d once daily) can be used (only if the allergic reaction was not a type 1 hypersensitivity reaction). In cases of serious allergic reactions, clarithromycin (15 mg/kg/d in 2 divided doses) or azithromycin (10 mg/kg/d on day 1, 5 mg/kg/d × 4 days as a single daily dose) can be used in an effort to select an antimicrobial of an entirely different class. The Food and Drug Administration has not approved azithromycin for use in patients with sinusitis. Alternative therapy in the penicillin-allergic patient who is known to be infected with a penicillin-resistant *S pneumoniae* is clindamycin at 30 to 40 mg/kg/d in 3 divided doses.

Most patients with acute bacterial sinusitis who are treated with an appropriate antimicrobial agent respond promptly (within 48–72 hours) with a diminution of respiratory symptoms (reduction of nasal discharge and cough) and an improvement in general well-being.[11,23,31] If a patient fails to improve, either the antimicrobial is ineffective or the diagnosis of sinusitis is not correct.

If patients do not improve while receiving the usual dose of amoxicillin (45 mg/kg/d), have recently been treated with an antimicrobial, have an illness that is moderate or more severe, or attend day care, therapy should be initiated with high-dose amoxicillin-clavulanate (80–90 mg/kg/d of amoxicillin component, with 6.4 mg/kg/d of clavulanate in 2 divided doses). This dose of amoxicillin will yield sinus fluid levels that exceed the minimum inhibitory concentration of all *S pneumoniae* that are intermediate in resistance to penicillin and most, but not all, highly resistant *S pneumoniae*. There is sufficient potassium clavulanate to inhibit all β-lactamase producing *H influenzae* and *M catarrhalis*. Alternative therapies include cefdinir, cefuroxime, or cefpo-

doxime. A single dose of ceftriaxone (at 50 mg/kg/d), given either intravenously or intramuscularly, can be used in children with vomiting that precludes administration of oral antibiotics. Twenty-four hours later, when the child is clinically improved, an oral antibiotic is substituted to complete the therapy. Although trimethoprim-sulfamethoxazole and erythromycin-sulfisoxazole have traditionally been useful in the past as first- and second-line therapy for patients with acute bacterial sinusitis, recent pneumococcal surveillance studies indicate that resistance to these 2 combination agents is substantial.[51,52] Therefore, when patients fail to improve while receiving amoxicillin, neither trimethoprim-sulfamethoxazole nor erythromycin-sulfisoxazole are appropriate choices for antimicrobial therapy. For patients who do not improve with a second course of antibiotics or who are acutely ill, there are 2 options. It is appropriate to consult an otolaryngologist for consideration of maxillary sinus aspiration to obtain a sample of sinus secretions for culture and sensitivity so that therapy can be adjusted precisely. Alternatively, the physician may prescribe intravenous cefotaxime or ceftriaxone (either in hospital or at home) and refer to an otolaryngologist only if the patient does not improve on intravenous antibiotics. Some authorities recommend performing cultures of the middle meatus instead of aspiration of the maxillary sinus to determine the cause of acute bacterial sinusitis.[53] However, there are no data in children that have correlated cultures of the middle meatus with cultures of the maxillary sinus aspirate.[54]

The optimal duration of therapy for patients with acute bacterial sinusitis has not received systematic study. Often empiric recommendations are made for 10, 14, 21, or 28 days of therapy. An alternative suggestion has been made that antibiotic therapy be continued until the patient becomes free of symptoms and then for an additional 7 days.[23] This strategy, which individualizes treatment for each patient, results in a minimum course of 10 days and avoids prolonged courses of antibiotics in patients who are asymptomatic and thereby unlikely to be compliant.

Adjuvant Therapies

No recommendations are made based on controversial and limited data.

Adjuvant therapies used to supplement the effect of antimicrobials have received relatively little systematic investigation.[55] Available agents include sa-

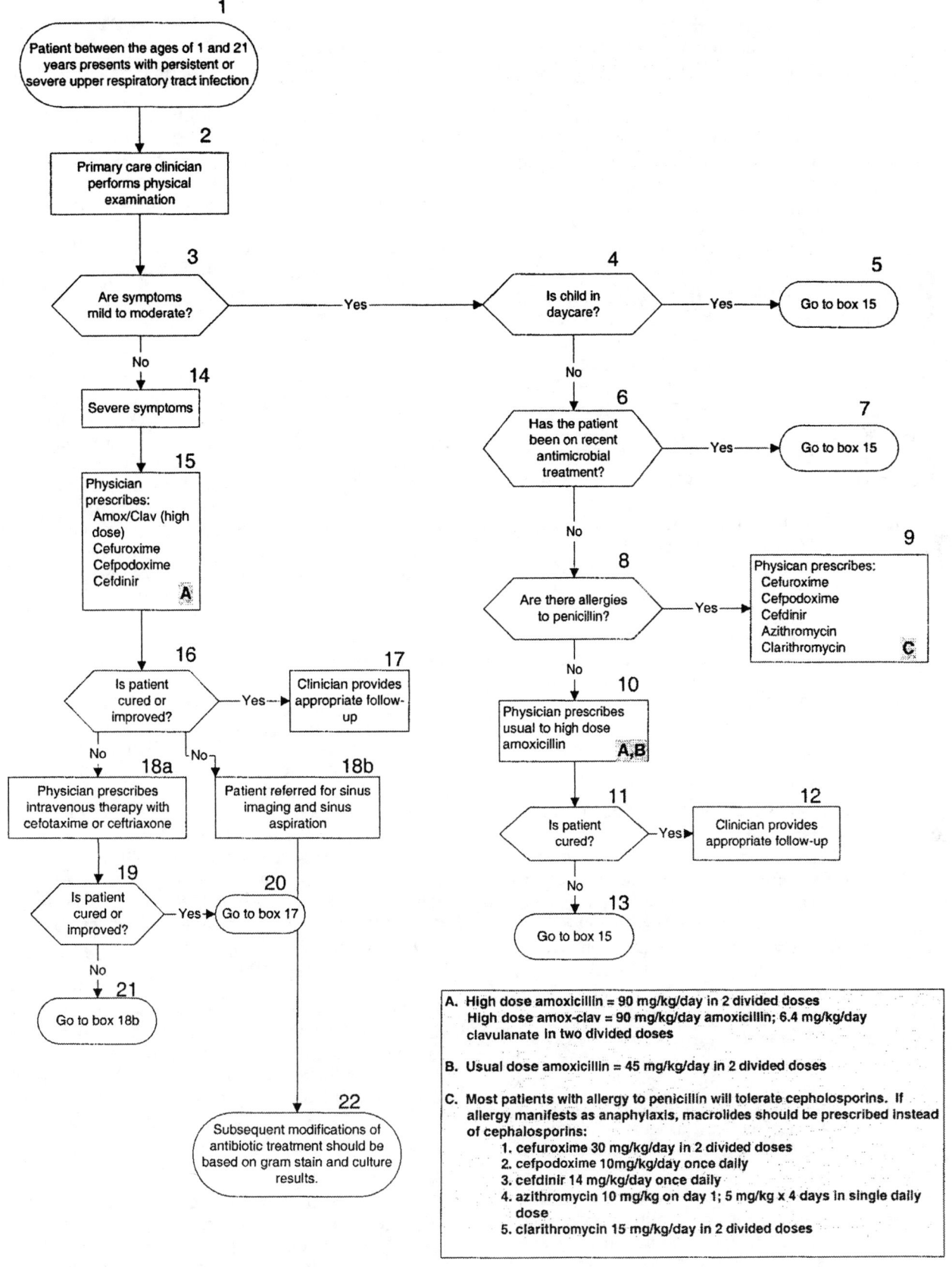

Fig 1. Management of children with uncomplicated acute bacterial sinusitis.

line nasal irrigation (hypertonic or normal saline), antihistamines, decongestants (topical or systemic), mucolytic agents, and topical intranasal steroids.

Currently there are no data to recommend the use of H1 antihistamines in nonallergic children with acute bacterial sinusitis. There is a single prospective study in which children with presumed acute bacterial sinusitis were randomized to receive either decongestant-antihistamine or placebo in addition to amoxicillin. The active treatment group received topical oxymetazoline and oral decongestant-antihistamine syrup (brompheniramine and phenylpropanolamine). No difference in clinical or radiographic resolution was noted between groups.[56]

There has been a single study of intranasal steroids as an adjunct to antibiotics in young children with presumed acute bacterial sinusitis. Intranasal budesonide spray had a modest effect on symptoms only during the second week of therapy.[57] A multicenter, double-blind, randomized, parallel trial evaluating flunisolide spray as an adjunct to oral antibiotic therapy was reported in patients at least 14 years of age.[58] The benefit of flunisolide was marginal and of minimal clinical importance. There is little reason to expect a substantial benefit from intranasal steroids in patients with acute bacterial sinusitis when antibiotics work effectively in the first 3 to 4 days of treatment.

No clinical trials of mucolytics have been reported in nonatopic children or adults with acute bacterial sinusitis.[59] Neither saline nose drops nor nasal spray have been studied in patients with acute bacterial sinusitis. However, by preventing crust formation and liquefying secretions, they may be helpful. In addition, saline also may act as a mild vasoconstrictor of nasal blood flow.[59] A method for performing a nasal saline flush was reported anecdotally by Schwartz.[60]

Antibiotic Prophylaxis

No recommendations are made based on limited and controversial data.

Antibiotic prophylaxis as a strategy to prevent infection in patients who experience recurrent episodes of acute bacterial sinusitis has not been systematically evaluated and is controversial.[59] Although previously successful in children who experience recurrent episodes of acute otitis media,[61,62] there is little enthusiasm for this approach in light of current concerns regarding the increasing prevalence of antibiotic-resistant organisms. Nonetheless, it may be used in a few highly selected patients whose infections have been defined meticulously (always fulfilling criteria for persistent or severe presentation) and are very frequent (at least 3 infections in 6 months or 4 infections in 12 months). Amoxicillin (20 mg/kg/d given at night) and sulfisoxazole (75 mg/kg/d in 2 divided doses) have been used successfully to prevent episodes of acute otitis media. Usually prophylaxis is maintained until the end of the respiratory season. It is appropriate to initiate an evaluation for factors that commonly predispose to episodes of recurrent acute bacterial sinusitis such as atopy, immunodeficiency, cystic fibrosis, and dysmotile cilia syndrome. Children with craniofacial abnormalities also are at risk to develop acute bacterial sinusitis.

Complementary/Alternative Medicine for Prevention and Treatment of Rhinosinusitis

No recommendations are made based on limited and controversial data.

A substantial number of children, adolescents, and their parents use nonprescription cold medicines or simple home-based remedies such as soups, fruit juices, or teas as alternatives or complements to conventional therapy for the treatment of upper respiratory infections including rhinosinusitis.[63,64] Others use herbal remedies and nutritional supplements or seek care from acupuncturists, chiropractors, homeopaths, naturopaths, aromatherapists, massage and therapeutic touch practitioners, and a variety of other healing modalities.[64-67]

Few of these therapies for upper respiratory tract infection or rhinosinusitis have been validated in randomized controlled trials. Claims that homeopathic medicines,[68-70] vitamin C preparations,[71] or zinc lozenges[72] prevent upper respiratory infections or hasten their resolution are controversial. A recently published study provides evidence that zinc nasal gel is effective in shortening the duration of symptoms of the common cold when taken within 24 hours of their onset.[73] Studies performed among adults indicating efficacy of *Echinacea* preparations in stimulating the immune system, thereby reducing the incidence, duration, or severity of respiratory infections, are debated[74,75]; however, a recent meta-analysis suggested a predominance of generally positive effects.[76]

Physicians treating children and young adults should be aware that many of their patients are using complementary therapies, often without informing them. Most of these remedies are harmless and, whether through pharmacologic or placebo effect, a perception of efficacy in providing relief from symptoms has stood the test of time. Nevertheless, many herbal medicines sold in the United States are of uncertain efficacy, content, and toxicity and carry a potential for serious adverse effects.[77] Of particular concern is the ability of the botanicals, either by direct interaction or by altering excretion mechanisms, to magnify or oppose the effect of conventional medicines that patients may be using concurrently.[78] Physicians should inquire about the use of complementary medicine for upper respiratory tract infections among their patients, particularly those on long-term medication for chronic conditions. Information on dietary supplements is available on a regularly updated Internet site.[79]

Recommendation 4

Children with complications or suspected complications of acute bacterial sinusitis should be treated promptly and aggressively. This should include referral to an otolaryngologist usually with the consultation of an infectious disease specialist, ophthalmologist, and neurosurgeon (strong recommendation based on strong consensus of the panel).

The complications of acute bacterial sinusitis usually involve either the orbit, the central nervous system, or both. Although rare, complications can result in permanent blindness or death if not treated promptly and appropriately.

Periorbital and intraorbital inflammation and infection are the most common complications of acute sinusitis and most often are caused by acute ethmoiditis. These disorders are commonly classified in relation to the orbital septum. The orbital septum is a sheet of connective tissue continuous with the periosteum of the orbital bones that separates tissues of the eyelid from those of the orbit. Preseptal inflammation involves only the eyelid, whereas postseptal inflammation involves structures of the orbit. Complications can be classified as 1) periorbital (or preseptal) cellulitis or sympathetic edema (periorbital cellulitis is not a true orbital complication. The periorbital swelling is attributable to passive venous congestion; infection is confined to the paranasal sinuses), 2) subperiosteal abscess, 3) orbital abscess, 4) orbital cellulitis, or 5) cavernous sinus thrombosis.

Mild cases of periorbital cellulitis (eyelid <50% closed) may be treated with appropriate oral antibiotic therapy as an outpatient with daily patient encounters. However, if the patient has not improved in 24 to 48 hours or if the infection is progressing rapidly, it is appropriate to admit the patient to the hospital for antimicrobial therapy consisting of intravenous ceftriaxone (100 mg/kg/d in 2 divided doses) or ampicillin-sulbactam (200 mg/kg/d in 4 divided doses). Vancomycin (60 mg/kg/d in 4 divided doses) may be added in children in whom infection is either known or likely to be caused by *S pneumoniae* that are highly resistant to penicillin.

If proptosis, impaired visual acuity, or impaired extraocular mobility are present on examination, a CT scan (preferably coronal thin cut with contrast) of the orbits/sinuses is essential to exclude a suppurative complication. In such cases, the patient should be evaluated by an otolaryngologist and an ophthalmologist. Suppurative complications generally require prompt surgical drainage. An exception to this is the patient with a small subperiosteal abscess and minimal ocular abnormalities for whom intravenous antibiotic treatment for 24 to 48 hours is recommended while performing frequent visual and mental status checks. Patients who have changes in visual acuity or mental status or who fail to improve within 24 to 48 hours require prompt surgical intervention and drainage of the abscess. Antibiotics can be altered, if inappropriate, when results of culture and sensitivity studies become available.

In patients with altered mental status, neurosurgical consultation is indicated. Signs of increased intracranial pressure (headache and vomiting) or nuchal rigidity require immediate CT scanning (with contrast) of the brain, orbits, and sinuses to exclude intracranial complications such as cavernous sinus thrombosis, osteomyelitis of the frontal bone (Pott's puffy tumor), meningitis, subdural empyema, epidural abscess, and brain abscess. Central nervous system complications, such as meningitis and empyemas, should be treated either with intravenous cefotaxime or ceftriaxone and vancomycin pending the results of culture and susceptibility testing.

AREAS FOR FUTURE RESEARCH

The extensive Medline searches to review the literature for the diagnosis and treatment of acute bacterial sinusitis in children uncovered the fact that there are scant data on which to base recommendations. Accordingly, areas for future research include the following:

1. Conduct more and larger studies correlating the clinical findings of acute bacterial sinusitis with findings of sinus aspiration, imaging, and treatment outcome.
2. Develop noninvasive strategies to accurately diagnose acute bacterial sinusitis in children.
   a. Correlate cultures obtained from the middle meatus of the maxillary sinus of infected individuals with cultures obtained from the maxillary sinus by puncture of the antrum.
   b. Develop imaging technology that differentiates bacterial infection from viral infection or allergic inflammation.
   c. Develop rapid diagnostic methods to image the sinuses without radiation.
3. Determine the optimal duration of antimicrobial therapy for children with acute bacterial sinusitis.
4. Determine the causes and treatment of subacute and recurrent acute bacterial sinusitis.
5. Determine the efficacy of prophylaxis with antimicrobials to prevent recurrent acute bacterial sinusitis.
6. Determine the impact of bacterial resistance among *S pneumoniae*, *H influenzae*, and *M catarrhalis* on outcome of treatment with antibiotics by the performance of randomized, double-blind, placebo-controlled studies in well-defined populations of patients.
7. Determine the role of adjuvant therapies (mucolytics, decongestants, antihistamines, etc) in patients with acute bacterial sinusitis by the performance of prospective, randomized, clinical trials.
8. Determine the role of complementary and alternative medicine strategies in patients with acute bacterial sinusitis by performing systematic, prospective, randomized clinical trials.
9. Assess the effect of the pneumococcal conjugate vaccine on the epidemiology of acute bacterial sinusitis.
10. Develop new bacterial and viral vaccines to reduce the incidence of acute bacterial sinusitis.

CONCLUSION

This clinical practice guideline provides evidence-based recommendations for the management of bacterial rhinosinusitis in children ages 1 to 21 years. The guideline emphasizes 1) appropriate diagnosis in children who present with persistent or severe upper respiratory symptoms; 2) the utility of imaging studies to confirm a diagnosis; 3) treatment therapies such as antibiotic use including prophylaxis, adjuvant treatment, and alternative interventions; and 4) management of complications. The guideline provides decision-making strategies for managing sinusitis to assist primary care providers in diagnosing and treating children with this common health problem.

ACKNOWLEDGMENTS

The subcommittee wishes to acknowledge the Agency for Healthcare Research and Quality and the New England Medical Center Evidence-based Practice Center for their work in developing the evidence report. We especially thank John P. A. Ioannidis, MD, and Joseph Lau, MD, for their work on the technical report.

SUBCOMMITTEE ON MANAGEMENT OF SINUSITIS
Ellen R. Wald, MD, Chairperson
W. Clayton Bordley, MD, MPH
David H. Darrow, MD, DDS
Katherine Teets Grimm, MD
Jack M. Gwaltney, Jr, MD
S. Michael Marcy, MD
Melvin O. Senac, Jr, MD
Paul V. Williams, MD

LIAISONS
Larry Culpepper, MD, MPH
    American Academy of Family Physicians
David L. Walner, MD
    American Academy of Otolaryngology-Head and
    Neck Surgery

STAFF
Carla Herrerias, MPH

COMMITTEE ON QUALITY IMPROVEMENT, 2000–2001
Charles J. Homer, MD, MPH, Chairperson
Richard D. Baltz, MD
Michael J. Goldberg, MD
Gerald B. Hickson, MD
Paul V. Miles, MD
Thomas B. Newman, MD, MPH
Joan E. Shook, MD
William M. Zurhellen, MD

LIAISONS
Charles H. Deitschel, Jr, MD
    Committee on Medical Liability
Denise Dougherty, PhD
    Agency for Healthcare Research and Quality
    Institutions
F. Lane France, MD
    Committee on Practice and Ambulatory Medicine
Kelly J. Kelleher, MD, MPH
    Section on Epidemiology
Betty A. Lowe, MD
    National Association of Children's Hospitals and
    Related Institutions
Ellen Schwalenstocker, MBA
    National Association of Children's Hospitals and
    Related Institutions
Richard N. Shiffman, MD
    Section on Computers and Other Technology

REFERENCES

1. Sinus and Allergy Health Partnership. Antimicrobial treatment guidelines for acute bacterial rhinosinusitis. *Otolaryngol Head Neck Surg.* 2000; 123:5–31

2. Lusk RP, Stankiewicz JA. Pediatric rhinosinusitis. *Otolaryngol Head Neck Surg.* 1997;117:S53–S57

3. Gwaltney JM Jr, Phillips CD, Miller RD, Riker DK. Computed tomographic study of the common cold. *N Engl J Med.* 1994;330:25–30

4. Fireman P. Diagnosis of sinusitis in children: emphasis on the history and physical examination. *J Allergy Clin Immunol.* 1992;90:433–436

5. Aitken M, Taylor JA. Prevalence of clinical sinusitis in young children followed up by primary care pediatricians. *Arch Pediatr Adolesc Med.* 1998;152:244–248

6. Ueda D, Yoto Y. The ten-day mark as a practical diagnostic approach for acute paranasal sinusitis in children. *Pediatr Infect Dis J.* 1996;15:576–579

7. Wald ER, Guerra N, Byers C. Upper respiratory tract infections in young children: duration of and frequency of complications. *Pediatrics.* 1991;87:129–133

8. McCaig LF, Hughes JM. Trends in antimicrobial drug prescribing among office-based physicians in the United States [published erratum in *JAMA.* 1998;11:279]. *JAMA.* 1995;273:214–219

9. Parsons DS, Wald ER. Otitis media and sinusitis: similar diseases. *Otolaryngol Clin North Am.* 1996;29:11–25

10. Gwaltney JM Jr, Scheld WM, Sande MA, Sydnor A. The microbial etiology and antimicrobial therapy of adults with acute community-acquired sinusitis: a fifteen-year experience at the University of Virginia and review of other selected studies. *J Allergy Clin Immunol.* 1992;90:457–462

11. Gwaltney JM Jr. Acute community-acquired sinusitis. *Clin Infect Dis.* 1996;23:1209–1223

12. Wald ER. Purulent nasal discharge. *Pediatr Infect Dis J.* 1991;10:329–333

13. Wald ER. Chronic sinusitis in children. *J Pediatr.* 1995;127:339–347

14. International Rhinosinusitis Advisory Board. Infectious rhinosinusitis in adults: classification, etiology and management. *Ear Nose Throat J.* 1997;76(suppl):1–22

15. Lau J, Ioannidis JP, Wald ER. *Diagnosis and Treatment of Uncomplicated Acute Sinusitis in Children. Evidence Report/Technology Assessment: Number 9.* Rockville, MD: Agency for Healthcare Research and Quality, US Department of Health and Human Services; 2000. AHRQ Contract No. 290-97-0019. Available at: http://www.ahrq.gov/clinic/sinuschsum.htm. Accessed February 23, 2001

16. Lau J, Zucker D, Engels EA, et al. *Diagnosis and Treatment of Acute Bacterial Rhinosinusitis. Summary, Evidence Report/Technology Assessment: Number 9.* Rockville, MD: Agency for Healthcare Research and Quality, US Department of Health and Human Services; 1999. AHRQ Contract No. 290–97-0019. Available at: http://hstat.nlm.nih.gov/ftrs/tocview. Accessed February 23, 2001

17. Arruda LK, Mimica IM, Sole D, et al. Abnormal maxillary sinus radiographs in children: do they represent infection? *Pediatrics.* 1990;85:553–558

18. Evans FO, Sydnor JB, Moore WE, et al. Sinusitis of the maxillary antrum. *N Engl J Med.* 1975;293:735–739

19. Shapiro ED, Wald ER, Doyle WJ, Rohn D. Bacteriology of the maxillary sinus of rhesus monkeys. *Ann Otol Rhinol Laryngol.* 1982;91:150–151

20. Wald ER. Microbiology of acute and chronic sinusitis in children. *J Allergy Clin Immunol.* 1992;90:452–456

21. Wald ER, Milmoe GJ, Bowen A, Ledesma-Medina J, Salamon N, Bluestone CD. Acute maxillary sinusitis in children. *N Engl J Med.* 1981;304:749–754

22. Wald ER, Reilly JS, Casselbrant M, et al. Treatment of acute maxillary sinusitis in childhood: a comparative study of amoxicillin and cefaclor. *J Pediatr.* 1984;104:297–302

23. Wald ER. Sinusitis. *Pediatr Ann.* 1998;27:811–818

24. Gwaltney JM Jr, Hendley JO, Simon G, Jordan WS. Rhinovirus infection in an industrial population. II. Characteristics of illness and antibody response. *JAMA.* 1967;202:494–500

25. Gwaltney JM Jr, Buier RM, Rogers JL. The influence of signal variation, bias, noise, and effect size on statistical significance in treatment studies of the common cold. *Antiviral Res.* 1996;29:287–295

26. Slavin RG. Asthma and sinusitis. *J Allergy Clin Immunol.* 1992;90:534–537

27. Williams JW, Simel DL. Does this patient have sinusitis? Diagnosing acute sinusitis by history and physical examination. *JAMA.* 1993;270:1242–1246

28. Otten FW, Grote JJ. The diagnostic value of transillumination for maxillary sinusitis in children. *Int J Pediatr Otorhinolaryngol.* 1989;18:9–11

29. Wald ER, Byers C, Guerra N, Casselbrant M, Beste D. Subacute sinusitis in children. *J Pediatr.* 1989;115:28–32

30. Kline MW. Otitis media. In: McMillan JA, DeAngelis CD, Feigin RD, Warshaw JB, eds. *Oski's Pediatrics: Principles and Practice.* Philadelphia, PA: Lippincott Williams & Wilkins; 1999:1301–1304

31. Wald ER, Chiponis D, Ledesma-Medina J. Comparative effectiveness of amoxicillin and amoxicillin-clavulanate potassium in acute paranasal sinus infections in children: a double-blind, placebo-controlled trial. *Pediatrics.* 1986;77:795–800

32. Diament MJ. The diagnosis of sinusitis in infants and children: x-ray,

computed tomography and magnetic resonance imaging. *J Allergy Clin Immunol.* 1992;90:442–444

33. McAlister WH, Kronemer K. Imaging of sinusitis in children. *Pediatr Infect Dis J.* 1999;18:1019–1020

34. Kovatch AL, Wald ER, Ledesma-Medina J, Chiponis DM, Bedingfield B. Maxillary sinus radiographs in children with nonrespiratory complaints. *Pediatrics.* 1984;73:306–308

35. McAlister WH, Parker BR, Kushner DC, et al. Sinusitis in the pediatric population. In: *ACR Appropriateness Criteria.* Reston, VA: American College of Radiology; 2000. Available at: http://www.acr.org/departments/appropriateness_criteria/toc.html. Accessed February 23, 2001

36. Lazar RH, Younis RT, Parvey LS. Comparison of plain radiographs, coronal CT, and interoperative findings in children with chronic sinusitis. *Otolaryngol Head Neck Surg.* 1992;107:29–34

37. McAlister WH, Lusk R, Muntz HR. Comparison of plain radiographs and coronal CT scans in infants and children with recurrent sinusitis. *AJR Am J Roentgenol.* 1989;153:1259–1264

38. Kronemer KA, McAlister WH. Sinusitis and its imaging in the pediatric population. *Pediatr Radiol.* 1997;27:837–846

39. Glasier CM, Mallory GB, Steele RW. Significance of opacification of the maxillary and ethmoid sinuses in infants. *J Pediatr.* 1989;114:45–50

40. Diament MJ, Senac MO, Gilsanz V, Baker S, Gillespie T, Larsson S. Prevalence of incidental paranasal sinuses opacification in pediatric patients: a CT study. *J Comput Assist Tomogr.* 1987;11:426–431

41. Dowell SF, Marcy SM, Phillips WR, Gerber MA, Schwartz B. Principles of judicious use of antimicrobial agents for pediatric upper respiratory tract infections. *Pediatrics.* 1998;101(suppl):163–165

42. Garbutt JM, Goldstein M, Gellman E, Shannon W, Littenberg B. A randomized, placebo-controlled trial of antimicrobial treatment for children with clinically diagnosed acute sinusitis. *Pediatrics.* 2001;107:619–625

43. Gwaltney JM Jr. Acute community acquired bacterial sinusitis: to treat or not to treat. *Can Respir J.* 1999;6(suppl):46A–50A

44. Doern GV, Brueggemann AB, Pierce G, Holley HP, Rauch A. Antibiotic resistance among clinical isolates of *Haemophilus influenzae* in the United States in 1994 and 1995 and detection of beta-lactamase-positive strains resistant to amoxicillin-clavulanate; results of a national multicenter surveillance study. *Antimicrob Agents Chemother.* 1997;41:292–297

45. Doern GV, Jones RN, Pfaller MA, Kugler K. *Haemophilus influenzae* and *Moraxella catarrhalis* from patients with community-acquired respiratory tract infections: antimicrobial susceptibility patterns from the SENTRY antimicrobial Surveillance Program (United States and Canada, 1997). *Antimicrob Agents Chemother.* 1999;43:385–389

46. Centers for Disease Control and Prevention. Geographic variation in penicillin resistance in *Streptococcus pneumoniae*-selected sites, United States, 1997. *MMWR Morb Mortal Wkly Rep.* 1999;48:656–661

47. Dowell SF, Butler JC, Giebink GS, et al. Acute otitis media: management and surveillance in an era of pneumococcal resistance—a report from the Drug-resistant *Streptococcus pneumoniae* Therapeutic Working Group. *Pediatr Infect Dis J.* 1999;18:1–9

48. Howie VM, Ploussard JH. The "in vivo sensitivity test"—bacteriology of middle ear exudate during antimicrobial therapy in otitis media. *Pediatrics.* 1969;44:940–944

49. Block SL, Harrison CJ, Hedrick JA, et al. Penicillin-resistant *Streptococcus pneumoniae* in acute otitis media: risk factors, susceptibility patterns and antimicrobial management. *Pediatr Infect Dis J.* 1995;14:751–759

50. Levine OS, Farley M, Harrison LH, Lefkowitz L, McGeer A, Schwartz B. Risk factors for invasive pneumococcal disease in children: a population-based case-control study in North America. *Pediatrics.* 1999;103(3). Available at: http://www.pediatrics.org/cgi/content/full/103/3/e28. Accessed February 28, 2001

51. Jacobs MR, Bajaksouzian S, Zilles A, Lin G, Pankuch GA, Appelbaum PC. Susceptibilities of *Streptococcus pneumoniae* and *Haemophilus influenzae* to 10 oral antimicrobial agents based on pharmacodynamic parameters: 1997 US Surveillance study. *Antimicrob Agents Chemother.* 1999;43:1901–1908

52. Doern GV, Pfaller MA, Kugler K, Freeman J, Jones RN. Prevalence of antimicrobial resistance among respiratory tract isolates of *Streptococcus pneumoniae* in North American: 1997 results from the SENTRY antimicrobial surveillance program. *Clin Infect Dis.* 1998;27:764–770

53. Gold SM, Tami TA. Role of middle meatus aspiration culture in the diagnoses of chronic sinusitis. *Laryngoscope.* 1997;107:1586–1589

54. Gordts F, Abu Nasser I, Clement PA, Pierard D, Kaufman L. Bacteriology of the middle meatus in children. *Int J Pediatr Otorhinolaryngol.* 1999;48:163–167

55. Zeiger RS. Prospects for ancillary treatment of sinusitis in the 1990s. *J Allergy Clin Immunol.* 1992;90:478–495

56. McCormick DP, John SD, Swischuk LE, Uchida T. A double-blind, placebo-controlled trial of decongestant-antihistamine for the treatment of sinusitis in children. *Clin Pediatr (Phila).* 1996;35:457–460

57. Barlan IB, Erkan E, Bakir M, Berrak S, Basaran MM. Intranasal budesonide spray as an adjunct to oral antibiotic therapy for acute sinusitis in children. *Ann Allergy Asthma Immunol.* 1997;78:598–601

58. Meltzer EO, Orgel HA, Backhaus JW, et al. Intranasal flunisolide spray as an adjunct to oral antibiotic therapy for sinusitis. *J Allergy Clin Immunol.* 1993;92:812–823

59. Spector SL, Bernstein IL, Li JT, et al. Parameters for the diagnosis and management of sinusitis. *J Allergy Clin Immunol.* 1998;102:S107–S144

60. Schwartz RH. The nasal saline flush procedure. *Pediatr Infect Dis J.* 1997;16:725

61. Perrin JM, Charney E, MacWhinney JB, McInerny TK, Miller RL, Nazarian LF. Sulfisoxazole as chemoprophylaxis for recurrent otitis media: a double-blind crossover study in pediatric practice. *N Engl J Med.* 1974;291:664–667

62. Casselbrant ML, Kaleida PH, Rockette HE, et al. Efficacy of antimicrobial prophylaxis and of tympanostomy tube insertion for prevention of recurrent acute otitis media: results of a randomized clinical trial. *Pediatr Infect Dis J.* 1992;11:278–286

63. Krouse JH, Krouse HJ. Patient use of traditional and complementary therapies in treating rhinosinusitis before consulting an otolaryngologist. *Laryngoscope.* 1999;109:1223–1227

64. Pachter LM, Sumner T, Fontan A, Sneed M, Bernstein BA. Home-based therapies of the common cold among European American and ethnic minority families: the interface between alternative/complementary and folk medicine. *Arch Pediatr Adolesc Med.* 1998;152:1083–1088

65. Kemper KJ. *The Holistic Pediatrician: A Parent's Comprehensive Guide to Safe and Effective Therapies for the 25 Most Common Childhood Ailments.* New York, NY: Harper Perennial; 1996

66. Lee ACC, Kemper KJ. Homeopathy and naturopathy: practice characteristics and pediatric care. *Arch Pediatr Adolesc Med.* 2000;154:75–80

67. Spigelblatt L, Laine-Ammara G, Pless IB, Guyver A. The use of alternative medicine by children. *Pediatrics.* 1994;94:811–814

68. de Lange de Klerk ES, Blommers J, Kuik DJ, Bezemer PD, Feenstra L. Effect of homeopathic medicines on daily burden of symptoms in children with recurrent upper respiratory tract infections. *BMJ.* 1994;309:1329–1332

69. Langman MJ. Homeopathy trials: reason for good ones but are they warranted? *Lancet.* 1997;350:825

70. Vandenbroucke JP. Homeopathy trials: going nowhere. *Lancet.* 1997;350:824

71. Hemila H. Does vitamin C alleviate the symptoms of the common cold?—a review of current evidence. *Scand J Infect Dis.* 1994;26:1–6

72. Macknin ML, Piedmonte M, Calendine C, Janosky J, Wald E. Zinc gluconate lozenges for treating the common cold in children: a randomized controlled trial. *JAMA.* 1998;279:1962–1967

73. Hirt M, Novel S, Barron E. Zinc nasal gel for the treatment of common cold symptoms; a double-blind, placebo-controlled trial. *Ear Nose Throat J.* 2000;79:778–782

74. Grimm W, Muller HH. A randomized controlled trial of the effect of fluid extract of *Echinacea purpurea* on the incidence and severity of colds and respiratory infections. *Am J Med.* 1999;106:138–143

75. Turner RB, Riker DK, Gangemi JD. Ineffectiveness of echineacea for prevention of experimental rhinovirus colds. *Antimicrob Agents Chemother.* 2000;44:1708–1709

76. Barret B, Vohmann M, Calabrese C. Echinacea for upper respiratory infection. *J Fam Pract.* 1999;48:628–635

77. Angell M, Kassirer JP. Alternative medicine—the risks of untested and unregulated remedies. *N Engl J Med.* 1998;339:839–841

78. Fugh-Berman A. Herb-drug interactions. *Lancet.* 2000;355:134–138

79. Office of Dietary Supplements. International Bibliographic Information on Dietary Supplements (IBIDS) Database. Available at: http://ods.od.nih.gov/databases/ibids.html. Accessed February 23, 2001

Technical Report:
Evidence for the Diagnosis and Treatment of
Acute Uncomplicated Sinusitis in Children:
A Systematic Overview

Authors:
John P. A. Ioannidis, MD
Joseph Lau, MD

American Academy of Pediatrics
PO Box 927, 141 Northwest Point Blvd
Elk Grove Village, IL 60009-0927

AMERICAN ACADEMY OF PEDIATRICS

Technical Report: Evidence for the Diagnosis and Treatment of Acute Uncomplicated Sinusitis in Children: A Systematic Overview

John P. A. Ioannidis, MD*‡§, and Joseph Lau, MD*§

ABSTRACT. *Objective.* To evaluate and analyze the existing evidence for the diagnosis and treatment of acute uncomplicated sinusitis in children.

Design. A systematic overview and meta-analysis considered all pertinent studies with at least 10 children younger than 18 years with acute symptoms of <30 days and without serious complications.

Outcomes. Clinical improvement rates for intervention studies of antibiotics or ancillary measures; concordance of diagnostic tests (expressed as likelihood ratios).

Results. Of 1857 citations originally reviewed, we identified 21 qualifying studies, compared with 450 reports on complications of acute sinusitis and 233 nonsystematic reviews of the subject. The qualifying studies included 5 randomized, controlled trials and 8 case series on antibiotic therapy, 3 randomized, controlled trials on ancillary treatments, and 8 studies with information on diagnostic tests (including 3 therapeutic trials). Definitions and inclusion criteria were heterogeneous across studies. The pooled clinical improvement rate with antibiotics was 88% (177/202) in randomized, controlled trials and 92% (318/345) in nonrandomized studies; the improvement rates on no antibiotics were 60% and 80%, respectively. Improvement rates were significantly higher in nonrandomized studies (Mantel-Haenszel odds ratio: 1.79; 95% CI: 1.05–3.04, stratified for use of antibiotics). Data on ancillary measures were sparse and heterogeneous. In studies comparing clinical findings with plain film radiography, the pooled rate of abnormal radiographic findings against a clinical diagnosis of sinusitis was 73% (596/814; range: 55% to 96% between studies). There was poor concordance between clinical criteria, plain radiographs, ultrasonography, computed tomography, and fluid on aspiration in all available paired assessments (all positive likelihood ratios were ≤4 and all negative likelihood ratios were ≥0.2).

Conclusions. Good, high-quality evidence for acute uncomplicated sinusitis in children is limited. Diagnostic modalities show poor concordance, and treatment options are based on inadequate data. More evidence is needed for defining the optimal treatment and diagnostic methods for this common condition. *Pediatrics* 2001;108(3). URL: http://www.pediatrics.org/cgi/content/full/108/3/e57; *clinical practice guideline, bacterial sinusitis, literature review.*

ABBREVIATIONS. OR, odds ratio; CT, computed tomography.

INTRODUCTION

Acute sinusitis is one of the most common community-acquired infections.[1–6] One investigator estimated that there are as many as 1 billion episodes (viral, bacterial, or other) occurring each year in the US population.[2] The condition is even more common in children than in adults. Given the frequency of this condition, the costs associated with its diagnosis and medical treatment (either antibiotics or ancillary measures) are large.[3] However, evidence on the diagnosis and management of this common condition is limited and fragmented.

In 1997, the Agency for Healthcare Research and Quality contracted with the New England Medical Center Evidence-based Practice Center to produce an evidence report, titled "Diagnosis and Management of Acute Sinusitis." A supplemental analysis to include nonrandomized trials for the pediatrics population was added to this contract when only 2 relevant randomized studies were found that studied exclusively pediatric populations. Although randomized studies are more likely to provide unbiased information, nonrandomized evidence may provide additional information and is needed when randomized data are sparse.

In this study, we systematically identified and analyzed all the accumulated evidence that pertains to the diagnosis and therapeutic management of acute uncomplicated sinusitis in children. The main questions addressed in this study are: 1) What is the evidence for the efficacy of various antibiotics in children with a diagnosis of acute sinusitis? 2) What is the evidence for the efficacy of various ancillary, nonantibiotic regimens in children with acute sinusitis? 3) What is the diagnostic accuracy and concordance of clinical symptoms, radiography, and other imaging methods and sinus aspiration for the diagnosis of acute sinusitis in children?

METHODS

Definitions

The definition of uncomplicated sinusitis excludes cases in which clinically evident neurologic, soft tissue, or other complications were present. Acute sinusitis is defined typically by a duration of symptoms of <30 days. We did not attempt to sepa-

From the *New England Medical Center Evidence-based Practice Center, Boston, Massachusetts; ‡Clinical Trials and Evidence-Based Medicine Unit, Department of Hygiene and Epidemiology, University of Ioannina School of Medicine, Ioannina, Greece; and §Division of Clinical Care Research, New England Medical Center, Tufts University School of Medicine, Boston, Massachusetts.

The recommendations in this statement do not indicate an exclusive course of treatment or serve as a standard of medical care. Variations, taking into account individual circumstances, may be appropriate.
PEDIATRICS (ISSN 0031 4005). Copyright © 2001 by the American Academy of Pediatrics.

rate bacterial from nonbacterial cases in the considered reports. Cures and failures were recorded as defined by each individual study: "cure" generally meant resolution of all signs and symptoms, and "failure" generally signified no change or worsening of signs and symptoms. "Improvement" was typically used for intermediate changes, although some studies used the term without a distinction from "cure."

The reference standard for the diagnosis of acute uncomplicated bacterial sinusitis is sinus aspiration and culture; this is infrequently used because it is invasive, cumbersome to perform, and time-consuming. Other diagnostic parameters (clinical presentation, plain-film, and ultrasound) were compared to assess concordance rather than as proof of diagnostic accuracy.

Inclusion Criteria

Published reports on acute sinusitis qualified for inclusion regardless of study design if they studied at least 10 children younger than 18 years, or if subgroups of age younger than 18 years could be readily identified in the presented data. Studies of subacute and chronic sinusitis were excluded. Subgroup data on acute sinusitis (with at least 10 children) from reports in which chronic and acute sinusitis or other infections were considered, qualified for inclusion. Studies limited to complications (neurologic, local soft tissue, or other) of acute sinusitis were excluded.

Search Strategy

We searched Medline using a broad search strategy covering from January 1966 through March 1999. The word sinusitis was used in the search as a text word and as a medical subject heading. We then limited the search results to human studies and English language that included pediatric patients using the terms "infant, newborn," "infant," "child, preschool," "child," and "adolescence." The titles and abstracts of the citations produced by the search were screened for articles that may have data on treatment of acute sinusitis in the pediatric population.

As part of a previous project,[7,8] we also had retrieved all published randomized, controlled trials on the management of acute uncomplicated sinusitis in all age groups. This collection of randomized, controlled trials had been generated based on Medline searches complemented by Excerpta Medica searches, perusal of the Abstracts for the Interscience Conference on Antimicrobial Agents and Chemotherapy, review of bibliographies of retrieved studies, and communication with technical experts and colleagues in the field. Randomized, controlled trials were included in this collection with no foreign language restrictions. All identified randomized, controlled trials were screened for the presence of data in children.

Statistical Analysis

Given the paucity and heterogeneity of the data for specific questions, we did not attempt the application of formal meta-analytic techniques in most circumstances.[9] When possible, rates

were combined across different studies and heterogeneity was assessed with a χ^2 statistic. Odds ratios (ORs) for efficacy (clinical improvement) also were estimated by the Mantel-Haenszel formula stratified per antibiotic use.

For diagnostic modalities, we expressed concordance by using the positive likelihood ratio, which is calculated as

$$\text{positive likelihood ratio} = \text{sensitivity}/(1 - \text{specificity})$$

and the negative likelihood ratio, which is calculated as

$$\text{negative likelihood ratio} = (1 - \text{sensitivity})/\text{specificity}.$$

The positive likelihood ratio gives an estimate of how much more common a specific diagnostic finding in the positive group is versus the negative group, when positive and negative are defined by a different diagnostic standard. For example, a sensitivity of 50% with specificity of 90% corresponds to a positive likelihood ratio of 5. The higher the positive likelihood ratio, the better the concordance of the 2 diagnostic modalities. A positive likelihood ratio of 1 indicates that there is no concordance at all. There are no absolute cutoffs, but positive likelihood ratios between 1 and 5 are generally suggestive of poor concordance, while positive likelihood ratios >20 suggest strong concordance. The positive likelihood ratio can take values up to infinity. The inverse considerations hold true for the negative likelihood ratio, where good concordance is shown by diminishing values. A negative likelihood ratio of 1 also shows lack of concordance. Again, there are no absolute cutoffs, but negative likelihood ratios between 0.2 and 1 are generally suggestive of poor concordance, while negative likelihood ratios <0.05 suggest strong concordance.

All reported P values are 2-tailed.

RESULTS

Retrieved Reports

The Medline strategy produced 1857 articles (Fig 1). Of those, 1719 were rejected on the basis of their title and abstracts. Notably, these included 450 articles on complications of acute sinusitis and 233 nonsystematic review articles without apparent primary original data. One hundred thirty-eight articles were retrieved in full and examined because the possibility that they might qualify could not be excluded from the title and/or abstract alone. A total of 21 studies qualified for inclusion.[10–30]

Of 68 randomized, controlled trials on antibiotic treatment of acute sinusitis that we identified in the more extended search, only 5 dealt with exclusively a pediatric population.[10–14] These 5 trials are among the 21 identified qualifying reports. For 30 additional

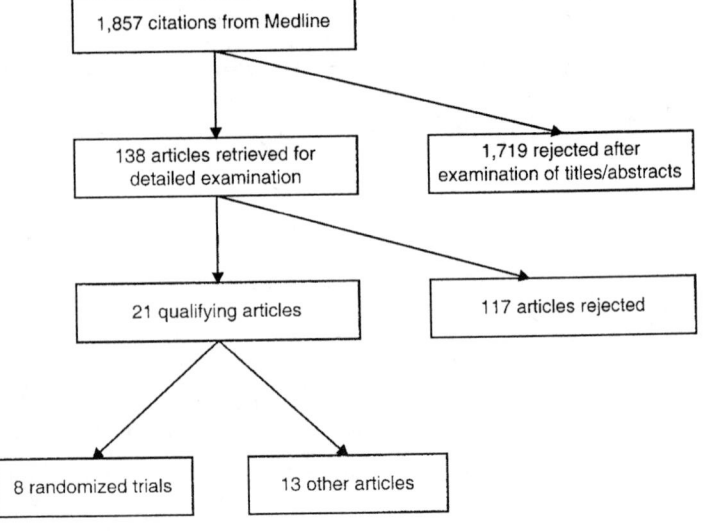

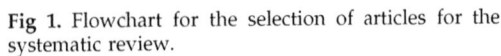

Fig 1. Flowchart for the selection of articles for the systematic review.

randomized, controlled trials, the age range of the enrolled patients extended to younger than 18 years, but no separate data on children younger than 18 years were available, and the majority of the patients were presumably adults. For 23 of these 30 trials, the lower age limit was between 12 and 17 years, and for another 5 trials it was 10 or 11 years.

Of the 12 randomized, controlled trials on ancillary measures identified as part of the extended search, there were only 3 trials (with a total of 243 patients) that studied the efficacy of ancillary measures in the treatment of acute sinusitis in exclusively pediatric populations.[15–17] The age range of the remaining 9 trials extended to as young as 9 to 20 years (younger than 12 years in 7 of them), but no separate data on the pediatric population were provided and the majority of the enrolled patients were presumably adults (upper age limit: 62 years to undefined).

Efficacy of Antibiotic Interventions

The efficacy of various antibiotic interventions was addressed in 5 randomized, controlled trials[10–14] and 8 nonrandomized studies[18–25] (Table 1). These 13 qualifying studies were published between 1970 and 1997 and with 2 exceptions had been conducted at single centers by pediatricians or otolaryngologists. Nine of the 13 reports, including 6 of the 8 nonrandomized studies, originated outside the United States. Pharmaceutical sponsorship was clearly mentioned in 4 reports. The largest case series had 106 patients, and the largest randomized, controlled trial had 93 patients. Overall, 255 children had been studied in the 5 randomized, controlled trials, and 418 children had been studied in the 8 nonrandomized studies. Eight of the 13 reports did not specify the duration of symptoms. Puncture for aspiration/irrigation was performed in 6 studies in selected children. Positive radiographic findings (typically combinations of air-fluid level, opacification, and/or mucosal thickening criteria) were required for the diagnosis of acute sinusitis in 9 of the 13 studies. Clinical symptoms and signs were typically the other mainstay of diagnosis, but there was large variability on how sinusitis was diagnosed as well as on the

TABLE 1. Studies of Antibiotic Treatment and Ancillary Measures in the Management of Acute Sinusitis in Children*

Author (Year)	N	Age (Years)	Abnormal Radiograph	Clinical Symptoms and Signs	Antibiotic	Duration (Days)	Ancillary Measures
ANTIBIOTICS							
Randomized							
Ficnar (1997)[10]	27	½–12	Required	Yes, but not specified	Azithromycin	3	ND
	18				Azithromycin	5	ND
Careddu (1993)[11]	25	2–14	ND	Not mentioned how diagnosed	Brodimoprim	8	ND
	27				Amoxicillin/clavulanate	8?	ND
Wald (1986)[12]	28	2–16	Required	Nasal discharge or cough >10 d required	Amoxicillin/clavulanate	10	Antihistamines
	30				Amoxicillin		
	35				Placebo		
Wald (1984)[13]	27	1–16	Required	Specified severe or persistent symptoms	Amoxicillin	10	Antihistamines
	23				Cefaclor		
Jeppesen (1972)[14]	7†	6–10	Required	Secretions, edema, dilated vessels on sinoscopy	Pivampicillin	7–30	Decongestant + lavage
	8†				Placebo		
Case series							
Hager (1980)[18]	30	1–12	Required	Red and swollen mucosa with discharge	Co-trimazine	10	ND
Helin (1982)[19]	61	1–15	Required	Various reported	Penicillin v	10	Nose drops and PPA
	16				Pivampicillin	10	Nose drops and PPA
	15				Erythromycin	10	Nose drops and PPA
Nylen (1972)[20]	25	5–15	Not required	Yes, but not specified	Penicillin	10	Decongestants for 7 d
Gurses (1996)[21]	39	5–14	Required	Various reported	Cefuroxime	7	ND
Herz (1977)[22]	106	6–17	Required	Various reported	Doxycycline	10–28	ND
Puhakka (1986)[23]	14	0–15	Not required	Purulent drainage; transillumination (required?)	Cefadroxil	7–17	ND
McLean (1970)[24]	25	4–15	Required	Various reported	Various	14–21	ND
Aitken (1998)[25]	68	1–5	Not required	Nasal congestion/drainage ± cough >9 d required	Various	various	ND
	19				None		
ANCILLARY							
Barlan (1997)[15]	43	2–14	Not required‡	Required specified major and minor criteria§	Amoxicillin/clavulanate	21	Budenoside
	46	1–15					Placebo
Revonta (1982)[16]	50	4–10	Not required‖	No symptoms of sinusitis except for rhinnorhea	Amoxicillin	10	PPA + lavage
	36						PPA only
McCormick (1996)[17]	34	1–18	Required	Symptom score used; components not mentioned	Amoxicillin	14	Triple combination
	34						Placebo

* PPA indicates phenylpropanolamine; ND, no data available.
† Number of sinuses.
‡ Abnormal in 68/89 of patients performed.
§ At least 2 of 3 major criteria (purulent nasal discharge, pharyngeal drainage, cough) or 1 major and 2 of 9 prespecified minor criteria were required for the diagnosis.
‖ Radiograph abnormalities were seen in 168/452 children who came for adenoidectomy or adenotonsillectomy without having any clinical symptoms of sinusitis.

prevalence of various specific symptoms and signs as reported in the various studies.

An array of antibiotics were tested, while a placebo arm was present in 2 randomized, controlled trials and a "no antibiotic" treatment group was considered in 1 of the case series. The duration of treatment varied between 3 and 28 days. The 2 shorter courses (3 and 5 days) were with azithromycin, which retains high drug levels for several days after its discontinuation.[10] All other studies used at least 7 days of therapy. Decongestants were either reported to be routinely prescribed or their use was not mentioned at all.

The response to treatment typically was assessed after 7 to 14 days, but it also was assessed at 21 days and 1 month in 2 early studies.[19,24] Cure, improvement, and failure rates are shown in Table 2. Overall, using the available data we estimated that the clinical improvement rate with antibiotics was 88% in randomized, controlled trials (177/202) and 92% (318/345) in nonrandomized studies. The rate of improvement on no antibiotics was 66% (33/50). It was 60% (21/35) in a randomized trial and 80% (12/15) in an observational study. The only randomized trial that compared antibiotics with placebo and provided

cure rates found significantly better efficacy for antibiotics.[12] There were no significant differences in the efficacy of various antibiotic regimens in direct randomized comparisons. Overall, there was a trend for higher improvement rates in the nonrandomized studies compared with the randomized studies (OR: 1.79; 95% CI: 1.05–3.04; $P = .03$ stratified for antibiotic use). Improvement rates were higher in nonrandomized studies versus randomized studies in the stratum of patients receiving antibiotics (OR: 1.66) and in the stratum of patients not receiving antibiotics (OR: 2.67). Improvement rates did not differ significantly between the various individual studies.

Data on outcome as documented by the performance of follow-up images were available from 5 studies; overall 81% (269/333) of images (plain film radiography or ultrasound) improved. Reporting of safety data were limited; the frequency of discontinuations of treatment attributable to side effects was mentioned per arm in only 5 studies.[11,12,18,22,23] In all, there were 7 discontinuations attributable to side effects among 233 (3%) patients treated with antibiotics. In 1 placebo-controlled trial, the discontinuation rate attributable to side effects was 6 of 58

TABLE 2.   Clinical and Imaging Outcome Measures for Studies of Antibiotic and Ancillary Interventions*

Author Year	Antibiotic	Ancillary Measures	Cure	Improvement	Failure	Imaging Improved
ANTIBIOTICS						
Randomized						
Ficnar (1997)[10]	Azithromycin (3 d)	ND	23/24	23/24	1/24 (relapse)	ND
	Azithromycin (5 d)	ND	18/18	18/18	0/18	ND
Careddu (1993)[11]	Brodimoprim	ND	24/25	24/25	1/25	ND
	Amox/clavulanate	ND	23/27	23/27	4/27	ND
Wald (1986)[12]	Amox/clavulanate	Antihistamines	ND	21/28	7/28	ND
	Amoxicillin		ND	25/30	5/30	ND
	Placebo		ND	21/35	14/35	ND
Wald (1984)[13]	Amoxicillin	Antihistamines	ND	23/27	4/27	16/22
	Cefaclor		ND	20/23	3/23	18/22
Jeppesen (1972)[14]	Pivampicillin	Ephedrine chloride and lavage	ND†	ND†	ND†	ND
	Placebo		ND‡	ND‡	ND‡	ND
Case series						
Hager (1980)[18]	Co-trimazine	ND	23/28	26/28	2/28	ND
Helin (1982)[19]	Penicillin V	Nose drops and PPA	53/61	53/61	8/61	51/61
	Pivampicillin	Nose drops and PPA	14/16	14/16	2/16	14/16
	Erythromycin	Nose drops and PPA	12/15	12/15	3/15	12/15
Nylen (1972)[20]	Penicillin	Decongestants for 7 d	12/25	ND	ND	ND
Gurses (1996)[21]	Cefuroxime	ND	ND	36/39	3/39	ND
Herz (1977)[22]	Doxycycline	ND	77/106	100/106	6/106	80/106
Puhakka (1986)[23]	Cefadroxil	ND	13/14	13/14	1/14	ND
McLean (1970)[24]	Various	ND	20/21	20/21	1/21	14/14
Aitken (1998)[25]	Various	ND	37/43	44/45	1/45	ND
	None		10/14	12/15	3/15	ND
ANCILLARY						
Barlan (1997)[15]	Amox/clavulanate	Budenoside	ND§	ND§	ND§	ND
	Placebo		ND§	ND§	ND§	ND
Revonta (1982)[16]	Amoxicillin	PPA + lavage	No SX	No SX	No SX	62/72‖
		PPA only	No SX	No SX	No SX	36/49‖
McCormick (1996)[17]	Amoxicillin	Triple combination	ND¶	ND¶	ND¶	ND
	Placebo		ND¶	ND¶	ND¶	ND

* PPA indicates phenylpropanolamine; ND, no data available; SX, symptoms.
† Outcome data provided as mean (standard deviation) time to recovery: 7.86 (3.69) days in the antibiotic group.
‡ Outcome data provided as mean (standard deviation) time to recovery: 6.38 (1.45) days in the control group.
§ Outcome data given as cough and nasal discharge scores per week in the 2 groups (budenoside was superior to placebo only at the second week).
¶ Outcome data given as clinical and radiography scores (there was no difference at 3 and 14 days from onset of treatment).
‖ Outcomes based on ultrasound (all other studies in the table used plain radiographs to assess improvement of imaging).

patients with antibiotics versus 2 of 35 patients with placebo (risk ratio: 1.8; 95% CI: 0.4–8.5).

Bacteriologic response with sinus aspirates obtained before and after treatment was assessed only in 2 studies. In the study by Ficnar et al,[10] eradication was achieved with azithromycin in 3 of 3 patients who had isolated pathogens. Puhakka et al[23] used sinus aspirates and exudates from sinus ostia for culture; information on the 2 sampling modes is not presented separately. In addition, the results on eradication are mixed with those of other infections and thus are not interpretable.

Efficacy of Ancillary Measures

Of the 3 trials qualifying for inclusion regarding the efficacy of ancillary measures (Table 1), 1 trial enrolled children who had sinusitis on the basis of ultrasonography, in the absence of any symptoms, and addressed the value of lavage as adjunctive therapy to amoxicillin and a decongestant.[16] The other 2 trials addressed, in a double-blind fashion, the efficacy of steroid or combination agents (nasal spray budenoside[15] and a combination of nasal oxymetazoline in addition to oral liquid brompheniramine and phenylpropanolamine,[17] respectively) against placebo.

None of the 3 studies used the categorization "cure-improvement-failure" for clinical outcomes (Table 2). The study on lavage used strictly ultrasonographic criteria. The other 2 studies used composite clinical and/or radiologic scores, and there was no statistically significant difference found at any of the addressed time points, except for a superiority of budenoside over placebo at the end of 2 weeks in terms of the clinical score. It should be noted that in this study,[15] only 89 of the 151 enrolled patients were followed up adequately to be included in the analysis.

Concordance of Diagnostic Methods

We were able to identify only 5 studies that addressed the comparative diagnostic accuracy of at least 2 procedures used as diagnostic tools in children with acute sinusitis (Table 3). In addition, 2 of the randomized, controlled trials on therapeutic measures provided data on percentage of abnormal radiographs among children with a clinical diagnosis of sinusitis[12,15]; a third trial[16] addressed the presence of aspiration fluid in the setting of abnormal ultrasonography without any symptoms being present. Thus, a total of 8 studies qualified for considerations pertaining to diagnostic concordance.

These diagnostic studies were very heterogeneous. Five of the 8 originated outside the United States. In several of them, radiology and/or otolaryngology specialists authored the reports, rather than general pediatricians. The study population was usually not adequately defined in terms of duration of symptoms, except in 2 randomized, controlled trials.[12,15]

Of the 7 studies in which some or all patients had clinical symptoms or signs, plain film radiography was performed in 6, while plain films were considered to be worthless in a study of infants. In these 6 studies, the rate of abnormal plain film radiography findings (typically opacification, mucosal thickening, and/or air-fluid level) against a clinical diagnosis of sinusitis ranged from 55% to 96%. These rates were statistically significantly different across the various studies ($P < .001$). The pooled rate was 73% (596/814). The largest component of this variability is probably attributable to variability in the clinical definition of sinusitis. This could be discerned easily in the only study that used different thresholds for the clinical definition.[30] When the subgroup of children who had only 1 of the 3 criteria of purulent secretion, history of upper respiratory secretion, and sinus pain or tenderness were considered, radiographic abnormalities were present only in 22/79 cases (28%). When 2 or 3 of these criteria were present, radiographic abnormalities were noted in 75/96 cases (78%). The likelihood ratios are shown in Table 4.

Similar rates of abnormal radiographs also were seen in the 2 randomized, controlled trials that used

TABLE 3. Studies of Concordance of Diagnostic Tests for Acute Uncomplicated Sinusitis in Children*

Author	N	Age (Years)	Aspiration	Abnormal Plain Radiograph	Other Imaging	Clinical Diagnosis
Kogutt[26]	100	1/2–14	Not done	96/100†	Not done	Various signs and SX reported
Watt-Boolsen[27]	86 (155 sinuses)	3–12	Done	114/155	Not done	Not specified
Van Buchem[28]	79 ("sinusitis")	2–12	Done	80/124	Ultrasound	Clinical impression of "sinusitis"
	68 ("rhinitis")		Not done	Not done	Not done	Clinical impression of "rhinitis"
Glasier[29]‡	15 with URI SX	<1	Not done	Not done	CT scan	Upper respiratory infection SX
	85 without URI SX			Not done	CT scan	No upper respiratory infection SX
Revonta[16]§	86	4–10	Done	Not done	Ultrasound	No children had sinusitis-specific SX
Jannert[30]	175	0–15	Not done	97/175	Not done	Purulent secretion, URI in previous 2 weeks, sinus pain or tenderness
Wald[12]	171	2–16	Not done	136/171	Not done	Nasal discharge or cough not improving >10 d
Barlan[15]	89	1–15	Not done	69/89	Not done	Major criteria: purulent nasal discharge, pharyngeal drainage, cough; 9 minor criteria‖

* URI indicates upper respiratory infection; SX: symptoms.

† Includes 5 children with pansinusitis in the setting of immunodeficiency.

‡ CT scan was performed on infants for unrelated reason, none were diagnosed a priori with "sinusitis" per se, but a subgroup was clinically diagnosed with upper respiratory infection.

§ Ultrasound was performed in the absence of clinical symptoms for sinusitis in 452 children referred for adenoidectomy or adenotonsillectomy.

‖ Two major or 1 major and 2 minor criteria required.

strict clinical criteria for the diagnosis of acute sinusitis. Wald et al[12] defined sinusitis by the presence of any nasal discharge and/or cough that were not improving for 10 to 30 days. Barlan et al[15] defined sinusitis by the presence of at least 2 of 3 major criteria (purulent nasal discharge, pharyngeal discharge, cough) or 1 of them plus 2 of 9 minor ones with duration of at least 7 days. In these 2 randomized, controlled trials, abnormal radiographs were seen in 136/171 (80%) and 69/89 (78%) of children with a clinical diagnosis, respectively.

The other 3 studies that offer data on radiography and clinical diagnosis do not specify a priori explicit criteria for the clinical diagnosis of acute sinusitis. One study simply lists the percentage of various symptoms,[26] while another[27] does not give any clinical information on signs and symptoms. The third study[28] states that the distinction between "sinusitis" and "rhinitis" was left to the impression of the clinician. Interestingly, the "rhinitis" group did not differ from the "sinusitis" group in the prevalence of fever, purulent secretion, sinus tenderness, or headache.

In a study of infants (newborn to 12 months of age), plain film radiographs were considered worthless and thus only computed tomography (CT) scans were evaluated.[29] Excluding cases of sinus hypoplasia, evidence of CT involvement of the maxillary sinus(es) had an 87% (13/15) sensitivity, but only 41% (28/69) specificity against the clinical impression of upper respiratory infection symptoms. The positive predictive value is only 13/54 (24%), and the negative predictive value is 28/30 (93%). The respective figures for the ethmoid sinus(es) were sensitivity of 67% (10/15) and specificity of 61% (46/75), positive predictive value of 10/39 (26%) and negative predictive value of 46/51 (90%). Thus the concordance of CT scan and clinical impression in infants is very poor.

One study[16] found good correlation between ultrasonographic findings and retrieval of fluid on aspiration: 68 of 72 sinuses with ultrasonographic abnormalities yielded fluid on aspiration, but aspiration was not attempted in any control group with-

out ultrasonographic abnormalities. Cultures of the aspirate from 59 sinuses yielded microbial pathogens in less than half the cases (26/59). The only study[28] to compare ultrasonography with plain film radiography and sinus fluid abnormalities among children with a clinical picture of sinusitis[28] found very low concordance between these diagnostic techniques (Table 4). Finally, abnormalities of plain film radiography had a poor concordance even with the simple presence of fluid in one study[27] (Table 4).

DISCUSSION

This study evaluated the available randomized and nonrandomized evidence on the diagnosis and management of acute sinusitis in children. Compared with the frequency of this common condition, the amount of high-quality evidence regarding diagnosis and treatment is remarkably limited. Most randomized data on adolescents may have been inextricably merged with data on adults in previous studies, and it is unclear whether adolescents should differ from adults in the diagnosis and management of acute sinusitis. However, for children younger than 12 years, evidence is sparse. Furthermore, it is hazardous to extrapolate evidence from adults to children given that children have a different and continuously changing anatomy and a higher incidence of viral upper respiratory tract infections.

There are few data on how to accurately diagnose acute sinusitis in childhood. Clinical criteria may not be very reliable. Plain film radiography shows only modest concordance with clinical diagnosis, and the concordance depends largely on how a clinical diagnosis is defined. Other imaging modalities have no clear role in the diagnosis of uncomplicated acute bacterial sinusitis. A decision analysis suggests that imaging studies may not be cost-effective for any level of previous suspicion of acute bacterial sinusitis.[7]

Although 1 small trial has shown superiority of antibiotics over placebo,[12] its applicability to settings where sinusitis is defined by different criteria is uncertain. The available evidence also suggests that the

TABLE 4.   Concordance of Diagnostic Findings on Imaging and Aspiration Tests: Positive and Negative Likelihood Ratios*

Study	Evaluated Diagnostic Test and Finding	Reference Test and Finding	Positive Likelihood Ratio	Negative Likelihood Ratio
Jannert	Plain radiograph: any abnormality†	Clinical criteria: 2–3 vs 1 of pus, upper respiratory secretion, sinus pain/tenderness	2.8	0.3
Glasier	CT scan of maxillary sinuses in infants: opacification‡	Clinical diagnosis: upper respiratory infection	1.5	0.3
Glasier	CT scan of ethmoid sinuses in infants: opacification‡	Clinical diagnosis: upper respiratory infection	1.7	0.5
Van Buchem	Ultrasound: any abnormality	Plain radiograph: any abnormality†	1.7	0.9
Van Buchem	Ultrasound: any abnormality	Sinus aspirate: nonclear fluid	0.5	1.2
Van Buchem	Plain radiograph: any abnormality†	Sinus aspirate: nonclear fluid	1.1	0.9
Van Buchem	Sinus aspirate: nonclear fluid	Sinus aspirate: pathogenic microorganisms	0.9	1.0
Van Buchem	Sinus aspirate: >3 leukocytes per visual field	Sinus aspirate: pathogenic microorganisms	4.0	0.9
Watt-Boolsen	Plain radiograph: any abnormality†	Sinus aspirate: any fluid	2.7	0.2

* (See "Methods" for details on the calculation of positive and negative likelihood ratios).
† Typically including mucous thickening, opacification, or air-fluid level.
‡ Excluding hypoplasia.

various antibiotics, among the several used for children with sinusitis, do not differ in their efficacy; nevertheless, given the sparse evidence and the high rate of spontaneous resolution, modest differences could have been missed. Furthermore, no studies have been reported in the era of increased resistance among isolates of *Streptococcus pneumoniae* and bacteriologic response data are almost nonexistent. There is no convincing evidence to support the use of ancillary treatment with decongestant-antihistamines and limited evidence on the use of steroids.

Therapy for children with acute uncomplicated sinusitis is controversial. The rates of spontaneous resolution are high. Antibiotics have been shown to be superior to placebo in a population defined by symptoms of nasal discharge or cough that were not improving for at least 10 days and positive radiographs.[12] Perhaps obtaining a radiograph would not be necessary if these clinical criteria exist for >10 days because almost 80% of these children would have a positive radiograph. Empirical treatment with antibiotics may be warranted in such cases. However, there is no evidence to support the use of antibiotics in other groups of children, such as those without nasal discharge or cough, those with shorter duration of symptoms, or those with improving symptoms. Spontaneous recovery rates in these groups are likely to be too high for antibiotics to offer any meaningful benefit. Finally, if antibiotic treatment is prescribed in acute, uncomplicated cases of sinusitis, evidence supports the use of amoxicillin, unless there is a history of allergy to β-lactams. Currently, there is insufficient evidence to support the use of newer, broad-spectrum antibiotics,[31] although increasing rates of antibiotic resistance should prompt the performance of properly designed studies.

Finally, the current evidence does not offer any clear indication for the use of ancillary measures. Although routinely used, there is no strong evidence from randomized, controlled trials to justify the use of antihistamines and decongestants in children. Evidence for the use of steroids comes from a single small trial.[15] More data are needed to evaluate the usefulness of these agents.

The strongest message emanating from this report is the lack of standardized clinical criteria for defining acute bacterial sinusitis in children as well as the paucity of high-quality evidence for establishing the diagnosis and optimal management of this condition. Despite the presence of an extensive bibliography on sinusitis in children, actual evidence and primary data on the diagnosis and management of acute uncomplicated sinusitis are limited. We encountered 450 reports on complications of sinusitis, mostly case reports or case series. Although it is important to know about the rare complications of this disease, it is questionable whether all these case reports and small case series give us useful information when there is comparatively only a handful of studies that deal with the common uncomplicated forms of the infection. In addition, there were 233 nonsystematic review articles compared with approximately 20 primary studies with analyzable

original data. The paucity of primary data may be attributable to the difficulties in applying the necessary rigorous diagnostic methodologies to generate high-quality information in children. Additional well-designed prospective studies are much needed to establish optimal diagnostic procedures and management of children suspected to have acute bacterial sinusitis.

ACKNOWLEDGMENT

This work was supported by a contract from the Agency for Healthcare Research and Quality (formerly known as the Agency for Health Care Policy and Research), US Public Health Service (New England Medical Center Evidence-based Practice Center Contract No. 0019, Task Order No. 05).

REFERENCES

1. National Center for Health Statistics. *National Ambulatory Medical Care Survey* [serial on CD-ROM]. Hyattsville, MD: Centers for Disease Control and Prevention, National Center for Health Statistics; 1990–1995: series 13
2. Gwaltney JM. Acute community-acquired sinusitis. *Clin Infect Dis.* 1996; 23:1209–1223
3. McCaig LF, Hughes JM. Trends in antimicrobial drug prescribing among office-based physicians in the United States. *JAMA.* 1995;273: 214–219
4. Lund VJ, Kennedy DW. Quantification for staging sinusitis. The staging and therapy group. *Ann Otol Rhinol Laryngol Suppl.* 1995;167:17–21
5. Gwaltney JM, Phillips CD, Miller RD, Riker DK. Computed tomographic study of the common cold. *N Engl J Med.* 1994;330:25–30
6. Lanza DC, Kennedy DW. Adult rhinosinusitis defined. *Otolaryngol Head Neck Surg.* 1997;117(suppl 3, pt 2):S1–S7
7. Lau J, Zucker D, Engels E, et al. *Diagnosis and Treatment of Acute Rhinosinusitis: Evidence Report/Technology Assessment Number 9.* Rockville, MD: Agency for Healthcare Policy and Research, US Department of Health and Human Services; March 1999, AHCPR Contract No. 0019. Available at: http://hstat.nlm.nih.gov/ftrs/tocview. Accessed February 23, 2001
8. Ioannidis JPA, Lau J. State of the evidence: current status and prospects of meta-analysis in infectious diseases. *Clin Infect Dis.* 1999;29: 1178–1185
9. Fleiss JL. The statistical basis of meta-analysis. *Stat Methods Med Res.* 1993;2:121–145
10. Ficnar B, Huzjak N, Oreskovic K, Matrapazovski M, Klinar I. Azithromycin: 3-day versus 5-day course in the treatment of respiratory tract infections in children. *J Chemother.* 1997;9:38–43
11. Careddu P, Bellosta C, Tonelli P, Boccazzi A. Efficacy and tolerability of brodimoprim in pediatric infections. *J Chemother.* 1993;5:543–545
12. Wald ER, Chiponis D, Ledesma-Medina J. Comparative effectiveness of amoxicillin and amoxicillin-clavulanate potassium in acute paranasal sinus infections in children: a double-blind, placebo-controlled trial. *Pediatrics.* 1986;77:795–800
13. Wald ER, Reilly JS, Casselbrant M, et al. Treatment of acute maxillary sinusitis in childhood: a comparative study of amoxicillin and cefaclor. *J Pediatr.* 1984;104:297–302
14. Jeppesen F, Illum P. Pivampicillin (Pondocillin) in the treatment of maxillary sinusitis. *Acta Otolaryngol.* 1972;74:375–382
15. Barlan IB, Erkan E, Bakir M, Berrak S, Basaran MM. Intranasal budenoside spray as an adjunct to oral antibiotic therapy for acute sinusitis in children. *Ann Allergy Asthma Immunol.* 1997;78:598–601
16. Revonta M, Suonpaa J. Diagnosis and follow-up of ultrasonographical sinus changes in children. *Int J Pediatr Otorhinolaryngol.* 1982;4:301–308
17. McCormick DP, John SD, Swischuk LE, Uchida T. A double-blind, placebo-controlled trial of decongestant-antihistamine for the treatment of sinusitis in children. *Clin Pediatr (Phila).* 1996;35:457–460
18. Hager C, Bamberg P, Dorn G, Adam D. The use of co-trimazine once daily in acute otitis media and maxillary sinusitis in children. *J Int Med Res.* 1980;8:413–416
19. Helin I, Andreasson L, Jannert M, Pettersson H. Acute sinusitis in children—results of different therapeutic regimens. *Helv Paediatr Acta.* 1982;37:83–88
20. Nylen O, Jeppsson PH, Branefors-Helander P. Acute sinusitis. A clinical bacteriological and serological study with special reference to *Haemophilus influenzae. Scand J Infect Dis.* 1972;4:43–48
21. Gurses N, Kalayci AG, Islek I, Uysal S. Cefuroxime axetil in the treat-

ment of acute sinusitis in childhood. *J Antimicrob Chemother.* 1996;38:547–550

22. Herz G, Gfeller J. Sinusitis in paediatrics. *Chemotherapy.* 1977;23:50–57

23. Puhakka H, Virolainen E. Cefadroxil in the treatment of susceptible infections in infants and children. *Drugs.* 1986;32(suppl 3):21–28

24. McLean DC. Sinusitis in children. Lessons from twenty-five patients. *Clin Pediatr (Phila).* 1970;9:342–345

25. Aitken M, Taylor JA. Prevalence of clinical sinusitis in young children followed up by primary care pediatricians. *Arch Pediatr Adolesc Med.* 1998;152:244–248

26. Kogutt MS, Swischuk LE. Diagnosis of sinusitis in infants and children. *Pediatrics.* 1973;52:121–124

27. Watt-Boolsen S, Karle A. The clinical use of radiological examination of the maxillary sinuses. *Clin Otolaryngol.* 1977;2:41–243

28. Van Buchem FL, Peeters MF, Knottnerus JA. Maxillary sinusitis in children. *Clin Otolaryngol.* 1992;17:49–53

29. Glasier CM, Mallory GB, Steele RW. Significance of opacification of the maxillary and ethmoid sinuses in infants. *J Pediatr.* 1989;114:45–50

30. Jannert M, Andreasson L, Helin I, Pettersson H. Acute sinusitis in children—symptoms, clinical findings and bacteriology related to initial radiologic appearance. *Int J Pediatr Otorhinolaryngol.* 1982;4:139–148

31. de Ferranti SD, Ioannidis JP, Lau J, Anninger WV, Barza M. Are amoxycillin and folate inhibitors as effective as other antibiotics for acute sinusitis? A meta-analysis. *BMJ.* 1998;317:632–637

Diagnosis and Management of
Childhood Obstructive Sleep Apnea Syndrome

● ●

- *Clinical Practice Guideline*
- *Technical Report Summary*

Readers of this clinical practice guideline are urged to review the technical report to enhance the evidence-based decision-making process. The full technical report is available on the enclosed CD-ROM.

AMERICAN ACADEMY OF PEDIATRICS

Section on Pediatric Pulmonology, Subcommittee on Obstructive Sleep Apnea Syndrome

Clinical Practice Guideline: Diagnosis and Management of Childhood Obstructive Sleep Apnea Syndrome

ABSTRACT. This clinical practice guideline, intended for use by primary care clinicians, provides recommendations for the diagnosis and management of obstructive sleep apnea syndrome (OSAS).

The Section on Pediatric Pulmonology of the American Academy of Pediatrics selected a subcommittee composed of pediatricians and other experts in the fields of pulmonology and otolaryngology as well as experts from epidemiology and pediatric practice to develop an evidence base of literature on this topic. The resulting evidence report was used to formulate recommendations for the diagnosis and management of childhood OSAS.

The guideline contains the following recommendations for the diagnosis of OSAS: 1) all children should be screened for snoring; 2) complex high-risk patients should be referred to a specialist; 3) patients with cardiorespiratory failure cannot await elective evaluation; 4) diagnostic evaluation is useful in discriminating between primary snoring and OSAS, the gold standard being polysomnography; 5) adenotonsillectomy is the first line of treatment for most children, and continuous positive airway pressure is an option for those who are not candidates for surgery or do not respond to surgery; 6) high-risk patients should be monitored as inpatients postoperatively; 7) patients should be reevaluated postoperatively to determine whether additional treatment is required.

This clinical practice guideline is not intended as a sole source of guidance in the evaluation of children with OSAS. Rather, it is designed to assist primary care clinicians by providing a framework for diagnostic decision-making. It is not intended to replace clinical judgment or to establish a protocol for all children with this condition and may not provide the only appropriate approach to this problem. *Pediatrics* 2002;109:704–712; *obstructive sleep apnea, infant, child, adenoidectomy, tonsillectomy, meta-analysis, polysomnography, sleep disorders, snoring.*

ABBREVIATIONS. OSAS, obstructive sleep apnea syndrome; PS, primary snoring; REM, rapid eye movement; CPAP, continuous positive airway pressure; PPV, positive predictive value; NPV, negative predictive value.

INTRODUCTION

Obstructive sleep apnea syndrome (OSAS) is a common condition in childhood and can result in severe complications if left untreated. Nevertheless, there is no consensus on the best methods of evaluation and management of this syndrome in children. Therefore, the American Academy of

---

The recommendations in this statement do not indicate an exclusive course of treatment or serve as a standard of medical care. Variations, taking into account individual circumstances, may be appropriate.
PEDIATRICS (ISSN 0031 4005). Copyright © 2002 by the American Academy of Pediatrics.

Pediatrics has supported the development of a practice guideline for the diagnosis and management of childhood OSAS.

The purpose of this clinical practice guideline is to 1) increase the recognition of OSAS by pediatricians to decrease diagnostic delay and avoid serious sequelae of OSAS; 2) evaluate diagnostic techniques; 3) describe treatment options; 4) provide guidelines for follow-up; and 5) discuss areas requiring additional research.

This practice guideline focuses on uncomplicated childhood OSAS, that is, the otherwise healthy child with OSAS associated with adenotonsillar hypertrophy and/or obesity who is being treated in the primary care setting. This guideline specifically excludes infants younger than 1 year, patients with central apnea or hypoventilation syndromes, and patients with OSAS associated with other medical disorders, including but not limited to Down syndrome, craniofacial anomalies, neuromuscular disease (including cerebral palsy), chronic lung disease, sickle cell disease, metabolic disease, or laryngomalacia. These important patient populations are too complex to discuss within the scope of this paper and require specialist consultation. In addition, patients with life-threatening OSAS who present in cardiorespiratory failure will not be covered here, because these patients require urgent treatment.

METHODS OF GUIDELINE DEVELOPMENT

Details of the methods of guideline development are included in the accompanying technical report published online.[1] Committee members signed forms confirming that they did not have a conflict of interest. The guidelines were based on data available from the medical literature. A computerized search of the National Library of Medicine's PubMed database (http://www.ncbi.nlm.nih.gov/entrez/query.fcgi?db=PubMed) from 1966–1999 (later updated to include 2000) was performed using the following keywords: sleep apnea syndrome, apnea, sleep disorders, snoring, polysomnography, airway obstruction, adenoidectomy, tonsillectomy (adverse effects, mortality), and sleep-disordered breathing. The search was limited to articles involving children. Studies involving infants, animal studies, and articles written in languages other than English were excluded. Reviews, case reports, letters to the editor, and abstracts were not included. A total of 2110 articles were found. Committee members then screened the articles, first by title and then by abstract, to obtain articles relevant to the guideline.

After screening, a total of 278 articles were reviewed in full by committee members. An additional 6 articles, primarily from foreign publications, could not be obtained from local libraries. None of these were considered particularly germane to the guideline. In addition to the literature search, committee members supplemented the articles with additional publications thought to be relevant and with those published after 1999. Details of the literature grading system are available in the accompanying technical report published online. Review of the literature revealed that there were very few randomized controlled studies. When the evidence was poor or lacking, there was extensive discussion among committee members to achieve consensus. The guideline notes whether a decision was based on objective evidence or on consensus decision.

DEFINITION

OSAS in children is a "disorder of breathing during sleep characterized by prolonged partial upper airway obstruction and/or intermittent complete obstruction (obstructive apnea) that disrupts normal ventilation during sleep and normal sleep patterns."[2] Symptoms include habitual (nightly) snoring (often with intermittent pauses, snorts, or gasps), disturbed sleep, and daytime neurobehavioral problems. Daytime sleepiness may occur but is uncommon in young children. Complications include neurocognitive impairment, behavioral problems, failure to thrive, and cor pulmonale, particularly in severe cases. Risk factors include adenotonsillar hypertrophy, obesity, craniofacial anomalies, and neuromuscular disorders. Only the first 2 risk factors are discussed in this guideline.

OSAS needs to be distinguished from primary snoring (PS), which is defined as snoring without obstructive apnea, frequent arousals from sleep, or gas exchange abnormalities.[3] Although PS is usually considered benign, this has not been well evaluated, because most studies of snoring children did not discriminate between PS and OSAS.

PREVALENCE

OSAS occurs in children of all ages, from neonates to adolescents. It is thought to be most common in preschool-aged children, which is the age when the tonsils and adenoids are the largest in relation to the underlying airway size.[4] Three studies have evaluated the prevalence of childhood OSAS. These studies did not use conventional polysomnography, used adult rather than pediatric polysomnographic criteria, or studied only a selected high-risk sample of the population; thus, a definitive epidemiologic study has not yet been performed. Despite these limitations, the 3 studies showed similar prevalence rates of approximately 2%.[5–7] In contrast, PS is more common; habitual snoring occurs in 3% to 12% of preschool-aged children.[5,6,8–10] Thus, the clinician needs a method to distinguish OSAS from PS. OSAS occurs equally among boys and girls.[7] One study indicated that the prevalence is higher among African American individuals than among white individuals.[7]

SEQUELAE OF OSAS

Untreated OSAS can result in serious morbidity. Early reports documented such complications as failure to thrive, cor pulmonale, and mental retardation.[11] These severe sequelae appear to be less common now, probably because of earlier diagnosis and treatment. Although failure to thrive is the exception these days, children with OSAS still tend to have a growth spurt after adenotonsillectomy.[12–14] In the past, cor pulmonale with heart failure was not an uncommon mode of presentation for OSAS in children, but it is now rare. Although overt right heart failure now occurs less often, asymptomatic degrees of pulmonary hypertension may be common.[15] Systemic hypertension can occur.[16–18] Many reports have suggested that children with OSAS are at risk of neurocognitive deficits, such as poor learning, behavioral problems, and attention-deficit/hyperactivity disorder.[19–22] However, many of these studies were case series based on histories obtained from parents of snoring children without objective evaluation, control groups, or sleep studies to distinguish PS from OSAS. One recent study showed that children with sleep-disordered breathing were more likely to do poorly at school, and many improved after adenotonsillectomy.[23] If untreated, OSAS may result in death. Early OSAS literature described children who presented with cardiorespiratory failure or coma, some of whom died.[24–26]

METHODS OF DIAGNOSIS

Diagnostic methods that have been scientifically evaluated include history and physical examination, audiotaping or videotaping, pulse oximetry, abbreviated polysomnography, and full polysomnography. The goals of diagnosis are to 1) identify patients who are at risk for adverse outcomes; 2) avoid unnecessary intervention in patients who are not at risk for adverse outcomes; and 3) evaluate which patients are at increased risk of complications resulting from adenotonsillectomy so that appropriate precautions can be taken.

History and Physical Examination

A sleep history screening for snoring should be part of routine health care visits. In children, OSAS is very unlikely in the absence of habitual snoring. If a history of nightly snoring is elicited, a more detailed history regarding labored breathing during sleep, observed apnea, restless sleep, diaphoresis, enuresis, cyanosis, excessive daytime sleepiness, and behavior or learning problems (including attention-deficit/hyperactivity disorder) should be obtained. Findings on physical examination during wakefulness are often normal. There may be nonspecific findings related to adenotonsillar hypertrophy, such as mouth breathing, nasal obstruction during wakefulness, adenoidal facies, and hyponasal speech. Evidence of complications of OSAS may be present. These include systemic hypertension, an increased pulmonic component of the second heart sound indicating pulmonary hypertension, and poor growth (although conversely, some children with OSAS are obese).

Although history and physical examination are useful to screen patients and determine which patients need additional investigation for OSAS, there is controversy about their roles in determining which patients require treatment. A number of studies have shown that there is no relation between the size of the tonsils and adenoids and presence of OSAS.[27–30] This is because OSAS is thought to be attributable to a combination of adenotonsillar hypertrophy and the neuromuscular tone of the upper airway during sleep rather than to structural abnormalities alone. Thus, the presence of large tonsils and adenoids does not necessarily indicate that the patient has OSAS.

An accurate diagnosis is required not only to ensure that appropriate treatment is provided and to avoid unnecessary treatment, but also to determine which children are at risk of complications resulting from treatment. Several studies have objectively evaluated the utility of a standardized history alone; history and physical examination; or history, physical examination, and audiotaping or videotaping to diagnose OSAS. In 1984, a study evaluated the efficacy of a questionnaire-derived OSAS score.[31] The questionnaire was administered first to patients with polysomnographically proven OSAS and controls without OSAS and then prospectively to snoring patients being evaluated for suspected OSAS. The score was able to distinguish between patients with known OSAS and controls. However, three quarters of subjects had an indeterminate score. A more recent study by the same authors with a much larger sample found that the score had a sensitivity of 35% and specificity of 39%.[32] A number of other studies have shown that this score has limited utility when applied to snoring children being evaluated for OSAS[33,34] or when applied to obese patients.[35,36] Thus, this questionnaire has minimal usefulness in the evaluation of OSAS.

Other studies have evaluated the utility of history and physical examination in distinguishing children with PS from those with OSAS.[33,34,37–41] None of these studies were able to reliably discriminate between OSAS and PS.

There are a number of reasons why the history can be misleading. The loudness of snoring does not necessarily correlate with the degree of obstructive apnea. Thus, children may have very noticeable snoring without apnea. Children with OSAS experience obstruction primarily during rapid eye movement (REM) sleep, which occurs predominantly in the early morning hours when their parents are not observing them,[42] thus leading to an underestimation of apnea. Some children have a pattern of persistent partial upper airway obstruction associated with gas exchange abnormalities, rather than discrete, cyclic apneas ("obstructive hypoventilation"[2]). These children will not manifest pauses and gasps in their snoring, and therefore, the condition may be misdiagnosed as PS.

Nocturnal Polysomnography

Nocturnal polysomnography (sleep study) is the only diagnostic technique shown to quantitate the ventilatory and sleep abnormalities associated with sleep-disordered breathing and is currently the gold standard. Polysomnography can be performed satisfactorily in children of any age, providing that appropriate equipment and trained staff are used. Furthermore, pediatric studies should be scored and interpreted using age-appropriate criteria as outlined in the American Thoracic Society consensus statement on pediatric polysomnography.[2] Polysomnography, by definition, can distinguish PS from OSAS. It can objectively determine the severity of OSAS and related gas exchange and sleep disturbances. As such, it can help determine the risk of postoperative complications (Table 1). However, although it is generally believed that children with severely abnormal results of sleep studies are at increased risk for complications of OSAS, formal studies have not been performed to evaluate the correlation between polysomnographic parameters and adverse outcomes in children with OSAS.[43] Thus, although we know which polysomnographic parameters are statistically abnormal,[44] studies have not definitively evaluated which polysomnographic criteria predict morbidity. In addition, there is currently a shortage of facilities that perform pediatric polysomnography. The availability of pediatric polysomnography is expected to improve, especially with the computerized equipment currently available.

Audiotaping or Videotaping

Two studies have examined the use of audiotaping,[33,41] and 1 study has examined the use of videotaping,[45] alone or combined with clinical findings, in establishing a diagnosis. In these studies, sensitivity ranged from 71% to 94%, and specificity ranged from 29% to 80%. Positive predictive values (PPVs) were 50%[41] and 75%[33] for audiotaping and 83% for videotaping.[45] Sounds of struggle on audiotapes were found to be more predictive of OSAS than were pauses.[33] The negative predictive value (NPV) ranged from 73% to 88%. Although these techniques may have promise, the discrepancies in results from different centers indicate that additional study is necessary.

Abbreviated Polysomnography

Several studies have evaluated abbreviated polysomnographic techniques. Overnight oximetry can be useful if it shows a pattern of cyclic desaturation. Brouillette et al[32] performed oximetry in a group of

TABLE 1. Risk Factors for Postoperative Respiratory Complications in Children With OSAS Undergoing Adenotonsillectomy

Age younger than 3 years
Severe OSAS on polysomnography
Cardiac complications of OSAS (eg, right ventricular hypertrophy)
Failure to thrive
Obesity
Prematurity
Recent respiratory infection
Craniofacial anomalies*
Neuromuscular disorders*

* Not discussed in these guidelines.

children with suspected OSAS and compared it with simultaneous full polysomnography. Patients with complex medical conditions were excluded. Compared with polysomnography, they found a PPV of 97% and an NPV of 47%, indicating that oximetry was useful when results were positive. However, patients with negative results of oximetry required full polysomnography for definitive diagnosis. False-positive results were found in patients with mild coexistent medical problems, such as obesity and asthma, suggesting that this technique is useful only in otherwise healthy children.

Nap polysomnography is appealing, because it can be performed in the daytime and is, therefore, more convenient for patients and laboratory staff. Studies have shown a PPV of 77% to 100% and an NPV of 17% to 49%.[46,47] In children with OSAS, overnight polysomnograms demonstrate more severe abnormalities than do nap studies. Thus, nap polysomnography may be useful if results are positive, although it may underestimate the severity of OSAS. An overnight study should be performed if the results of the nap study are negative. The difference in predictive value between nap and overnight studies is probably attributable to the decreased amount of REM sleep during nap studies as well as the decreased total sleep time.

Unattended home polysomnography in children has been evaluated by only 1 center.[48] Home polysomnography yielded similar results to laboratory studies. However, it should be noted that the equipment used in this study was relatively sophisticated and included respiratory inductive plethysmography (a method for determining ventilation without using oronasal sensors), oximeter pulse wave form, and videotaping. The utility of unattended home studies in children using commercially available 4- to 6-channel recording equipment has not been studied.

Summary of Diagnostic Techniques

In summary, history and physical examination are poor at predicting OSAS. Most studies have shown that abbreviated or screening techniques, such as videotaping, nocturnal pulse oximetry, and daytime nap polysomnography tend to be helpful if results are positive but have a poor predictive value if results are negative. Thus, children with negative study results should undergo a more comprehensive evaluation. The cost efficacy of these screening techniques is unclear and would depend, in part, on how many patients eventually required full polysomnography. In addition, the use of these techniques in evaluating the severity of OSAS (which is important in determining management, such as whether outpatient surgery should be performed) has not been evaluated.

TREATMENT OPTIONS
Tonsillectomy and Adenoidectomy

Adenotonsillectomy is the most common treatment for children with OSAS. Adenoidectomy alone may not be sufficient.[38,49] In otherwise healthy chil-

dren with adenotonsillar hypertrophy, polysomnographic resolution occurs in 75% to 100%[37,49-51] after adenotonsillectomy; this is associated with symptom resolution.[37] Although obese children may have less satisfactory results, many will be adequately treated with adenotonsillectomy,[52] and it is generally the first-line therapy for these patients.

Potential complications of adenotonsillectomy include anesthetic complications; immediate postoperative problems, such as pain and poor oral intake; and hemorrhage. In addition, patients with OSAS may develop respiratory complications, such as worsening of OSAS or pulmonary edema, in the immediate postoperative period. Death attributable to respiratory complications in the immediate postoperative period has been reported in patients with severe OSAS. Identified risk factors are shown in Table 1.[53-58] High-risk patients should be hospitalized overnight after surgery and monitored continuously with pulse oximetry.

Continuous Positive Airway Pressure (CPAP)

For patients with specific surgical contraindications, minimal adenotonsillar tissue, or persistent OSAS after adenotonsillectomy or for those who prefer nonsurgical alternatives, CPAP therapy is an option.[59-61] However, unlike adenotonsillectomy, which is a 1-time procedure that is usually curative, CPAP will need to be used indefinitely. CPAP is delivered using an electronic device that delivers constant air pressure via a nasal mask, leading to mechanical stenting of the airway and improved functional residual capacity in the lungs. The pressure requirement varies among individuals; thus, CPAP must be titrated in the sleep laboratory before prescribing the device and periodically readjusted thereafter.[59] CPAP is a long-term therapy and requires frequent clinician assessment of adherence and efficacy. It is generally tolerated in older children.[59,60] Young children or older children with learning or behavioral problems may require behavioral or desensitization techniques to accept this form of therapy.[62] Attention to compliance with this therapy is crucial.

Other Treatment Modalities

Most adjunctive measures in the treatment of childhood OSAS have not been prospectively evaluated. Avoidance of environmental tobacco smoke and other indoor pollutants, avoidance of indoor allergens, and treatment of accompanying rhinitis may be helpful. In obese patients, weight loss strategies should be used. However, implementation of adjunctive therapies should not delay specific treatment of OSAS.

Oxygen therapy is sometimes prescribed in special cases to alleviate nocturnal hypoxemia in children with OSAS. However, there are few, if any, indications for its use in the otherwise healthy child with OSAS. Oxygen therapy does not prevent sleep-related upper airway obstruction and resultant problems, such as sleep fragmentation and increased work of breathing. Furthermore, it may worsen hy-

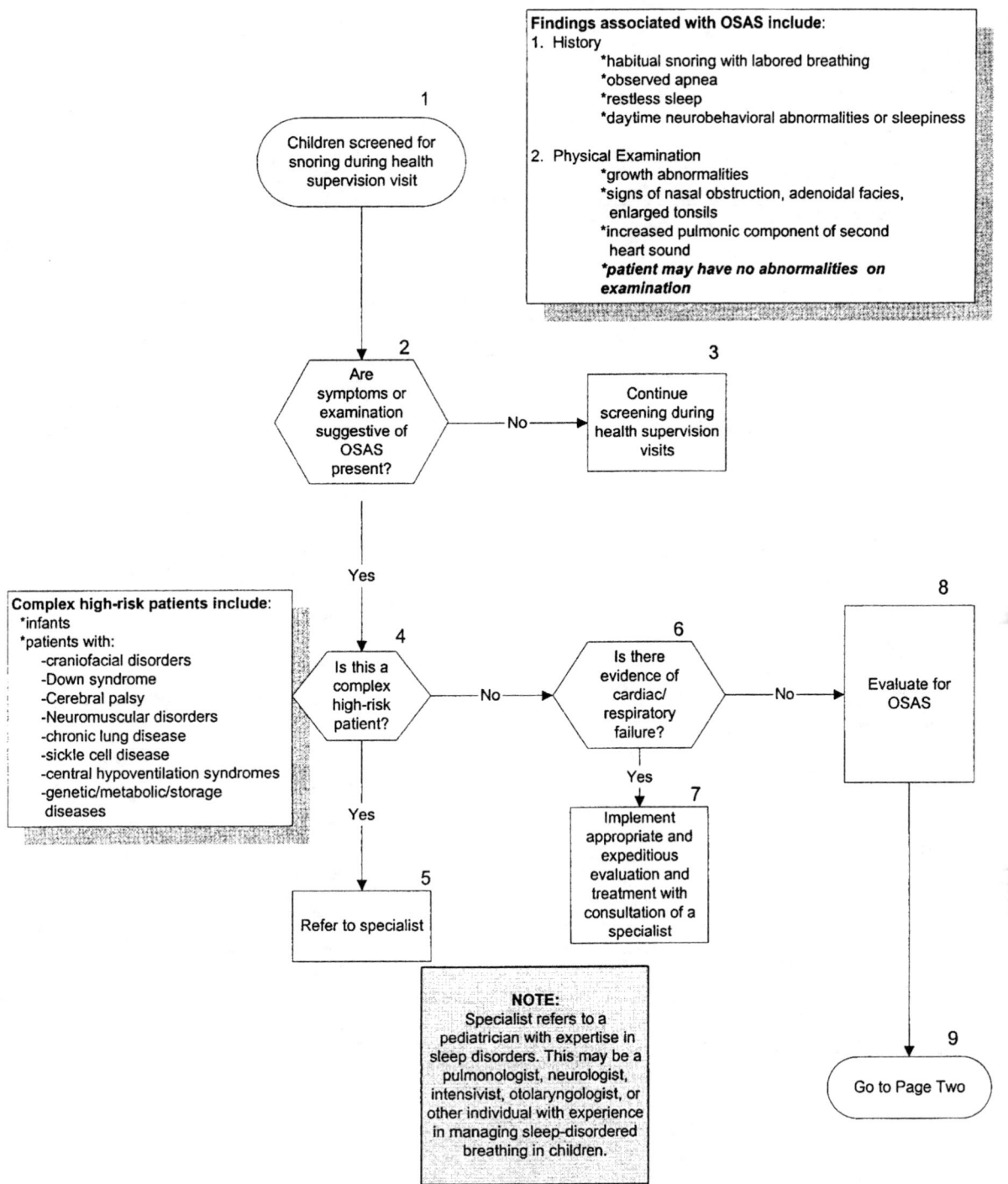

Fig 1. Diagnosis and management of uncomplicated childhood OSAS.

poventilation.[63] If oxygen therapy is to be used in children with OSAS, it should be evaluated during continuous Pco_2 monitoring to assess its effect on hypoventilation.

Other surgical options are available for patients not responding to usual treatment. These patients require care from pediatric surgical specialists. Surgical treatment options include uvulopharyngopalatoplasty, craniofacial surgery, and in severe cases, tracheostomy.

Follow-up of Patients Undergoing Surgical Treatment for OSAS

All patients should have clinical follow-up for reassessment of symptoms and signs associated with OSAS after initial treatment. Patients with mild to moderate OSAS who have complete resolution of symptoms and signs do not require objective testing to document resolution. Patients who have continued symptoms or signs, who have severe OSAS,[37] or

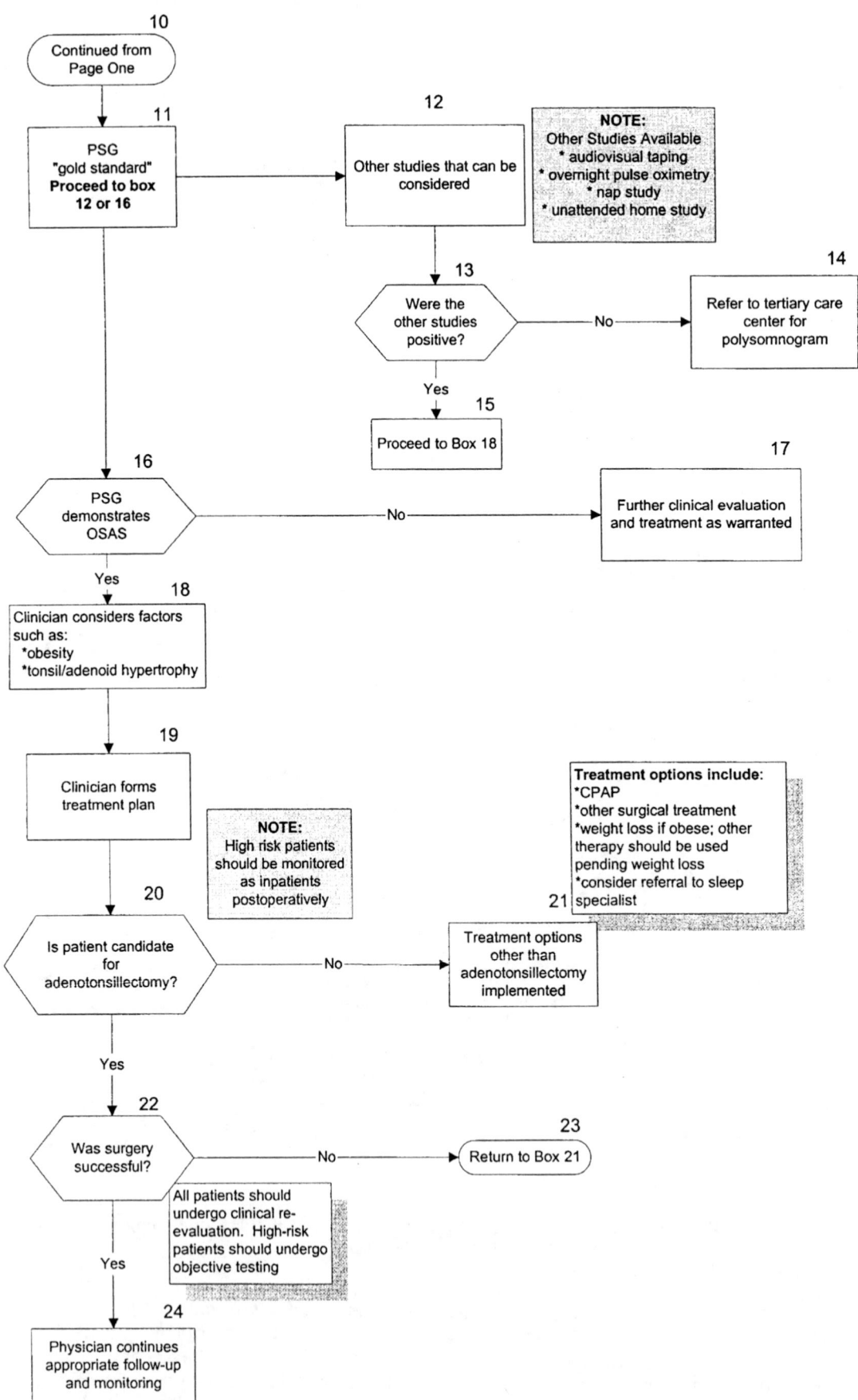

Fig 1. (continued)

who are obese require objective reevaluation to determine whether additional therapy, such as CPAP, is required. Objective data regarding timing of postoperative evaluation are not available. Most clinicians recommend waiting 6 to 8 weeks before reevaluation to ensure that upper airway, cardiac, and central nervous system remodeling is complete.

SUMMARY OF RECOMMENDATIONS FOR THE DIAGNOSIS AND MANAGEMENT OF UNCOMPLICATED CHILDHOOD OSAS

The following recommendations accompany an algorithm (Fig 1). As previously noted, these recommendations relate to otherwise healthy children older than 1 year with OSAS secondary to adenotonsillar hypertrophy and/or obesity and who are not in cardiorespiratory failure.

1. All children should be screened for snoring. As part of routine health care maintenance for all children, pediatricians should ask whether the patient snores. An affirmative answer should be followed by a more detailed evaluation. (Evidence for this recommendation is good, and the strength of the recommendation is strong.)
2. Complex, high-risk patients (Fig 1) should be referred to a specialist. (Evidence is good that these children are at increased surgical risk and require more complex management; the strength of the recommendation is strong.)
3. Patients with cardiorespiratory failure cannot await elective evaluation. It is expected that these patients will be in an intensive care setting and will be treated by a specialist; thus, these patients are not covered in this practice guideline.
4. Thorough diagnostic evaluation should be performed. History and physical examination have been shown to be poor at discriminating between PS and OSAS (evidence is strong). Polysomnography is the only method that quantifies ventilatory and sleep abnormalities and is recommended as the diagnostic test of choice. Other diagnostic techniques, such as videotaping, nocturnal pulse oximetry, and daytime nap studies, may be useful in discriminating between PS and OSAS if results of polysomnography are positive. However, they do not assess the severity of OSAS, which is useful for determining treatment and follow-up. In any case, because of their high rate of false-negative results, polysomnography should be performed in the event of negative results of the other diagnostic techniques. Additional study of audiotaping is necessary. (Evidence for and strength of the recommendation are strong.)
5. Adenotonsillectomy is the first line of treatment for most children. CPAP is an option for those who are not candidates for surgery or do not respond to surgery. (Evidence for and strength of the recommendation are strong.)
6. High-risk patients should be monitored as inpatients postoperatively. (Evidence that these patients are at high risk of postoperative complications is strong. Strength of the recommendation is strong.)

7. Patients should be reevaluated postoperatively to determine whether additional treatment is required. All patients should undergo clinical reevaluation. High-risk patients should undergo objective testing. (Evidence is good, strength of the recommendation is strong.)

RESEARCH RECOMMENDATIONS

Specific research questions have been delineated by an American Thoracic Society workshop.[43] Areas requiring additional investigation include:

1. Accurate prevalence data.
2. Identification of risk factors of complications resulting from OSAS, including the relationship of OSAS severity to specific outcomes.
3. Development and evaluation of low-cost, high-sensitivity, and high-specificity screening methods for OSAS.
4. Delineation of the natural history of treated and untreated PS and OSAS.
5. Assessment of long-term efficacy of adenotonsillectomy, CPAP, and other OSAS treatments.

SUBCOMMITTEE ON OBSTRUCTIVE SLEEP APNEA SYNDROME
Carole L. Marcus, MBBCh, Chairperson
Dale Chapman, MD
Sally Davidson Ward, MD
Susanna A. McColley, MD

LIAISONS
Lee J. Brooks, MD
    American College of Chest Physicians
Jacqueline Jones, MD
    Section on Otolaryngology and Bronchoesophagology
Michael S. Schechter, MD, MPH
    Epidemiologist

STAFF
Carla T. Herrerias, MPH

SECTION ON PEDIATRIC PULMONOLOGY, 2001–2002
Paul C. Stillwell, MD, Chairperson
Dale L. Chapman, MD
Sally L. Davidson Ward, MD
Michelle Howenstine, MD
Michael J. Light, MD
Susanna A. McColley, MD
David A. Schaeffer, MD
Jeffrey S. Wagener, MD

STAFF
Laura N. Laskosz, MPH

REFERENCES

1. Schechter MS, and the American Academy of Pediatrics, Section on Pediatric Pulmonology, Subcommittee on Obstructive Sleep Apnea Syndrome. Technical report: diagnosis and management of childhood obstructive sleep apnea syndrome. *Pediatrics.* 2002;109(4). Available at: http://www.pediatrics.org/cgi/content/full/109/4/e69
2. American Thoracic Society. Standards and indications for cardiopulmonary sleep studies in children. *Am J Respir Crit Care Med.* 1996;153:866–878
3. American Sleep Disorders Association. *International Classification of Sleep Disorders, Revised: Diagnostic and Coding Manual.* Rochester, MN: American Sleep Disorders Association; 1997:195–197

4. Jeans WD, Fernando DC, Maw AR, Leighton BC. A longitudinal study of the growth of the nasopharynx and its contents in normal children. *Br J Radiol.* 1981;54:117–121

5. Ali NJ, Pitson DJ, Stradling JR. Snoring, sleep disturbance, and behaviour in 4–5 year olds. *Arch Dis Child.* 1993;68:360–366

6. Gislason T, Benediktsdottir B. Snoring, apneic episodes, and nocturnal hypoxemia among children 6 months to 6 years old. *Chest.* 1995;107:963–966

7. Redline S, Tishler PV, Schluchter M, Aylor J, Clark K, Graham G. Risk factors for sleep-disordered breathing in children. Associations with obesity, race, and respiratory problems. *Am J Respir Crit Care Med.* 1999;159:1527–1532

8. Teculescu DB, Caillier I, Perrin P, Rebstock E, Rauch A. Snoring in French preschool children. *Pediatr Pulmonol.* 1992;13:239–244

9. Hultcrantz E, Lofstrand-Tidestrom B, Ahlquist-Rastad J. The epidemiology of sleep related breathing disorder in children. *Int J Pediatr Otorhinolaryngol.* 1995;32(suppl):S63–S66

10. Owen GO, Canter RJ, Robinson A. Overnight pulse oximetry in snoring and non-snoring children. *Clin Otolaryngol.* 1995;20:402–406

11. Brouillette RT, Fernbach SK, Hunt CE. Obstructive sleep apnea in infants and children. *J Pediatr.* 1982;100:31–40

12. Marcus CL, Carroll JL, Koerner CB, Hamer A, Lutz J, Loughlin GM. Determinants of growth in children with the obstructive sleep apnea syndrome. *J Pediatr.* 1994;125:556–562

13. Lind M, Lundell B. Tonsillar hyperplasia in children: a cause of obstructive sleep apneas, CO_2 retention, and retarded growth. *Arch Otolaryngol Head Neck Surg.* 1982;108:650–654

14. Bar A, Tarasiuk A, Segev Y, Phillip M, Tal A. The effect of adenotonsillectomy on serum insulin-like growth factor-I and growth in children with obstructive sleep apnea syndrome. *J Pediatr.* 1999;135:76–80

15. Tal A, Leiberman A, Margulis G, Sofer S. Ventricular dysfunction in children with obstructive sleep apnea: radionuclide assessment. *Pediatr Pulmonol.* 1988;4:139–143

16. Guilleminault C, Eldridge FL, Simmons FB, Dement WC. Sleep apnea in eight children. *Pediatrics.* 1976;58:23–30

17. Serratto M, Harris VJ, Carr I. Upper airways obstruction. *Arch Dis Child.* 1981;56:153–155

18. Marcus CL, Greene MG, Carroll JL. Blood pressure in children with obstructive sleep apnea. *Am J Respir Crit Care Med.* 1998;157:1098–1103

19. Ali NJ, Pitson D, Stradling JR. Natural history of snoring and related behaviour problems between the ages of 4 and 7 years. *Arch Dis Child.* 1994;71:74–76

20. Weissbluth M, Davis AT, Poncher J, Reiff J. Signs of airway obstruction during sleep and behavioral, developmental, and academic problems. *J Dev Behav Pediatr.* 1983;4:119–121

21. Chervin RD, Dillon JE, Bassetti C, Ganoczy DA, Pituch KJ. Symptoms of sleep disorders, inattention, and hyperactivity in children. *Sleep.* 1997;20:1185–1192

22. Goldstein NA, Post C, Rosenfeld RM, Campbell TF. Impact of tonsillectomy and adenoidectomy on child behavior. *Arch Otolaryngol Head Neck Surg.* 2000;126:494–498

23. Gozal D. Sleep-disordered breathing and school performance in children. *Pediatrics.* 1998;102:616–620

24. Ross RD, Daniels SR, Loggie JM, Meyer RA, Ballard ET. Sleep apnea-associated hypertension and reversible left ventricular hypertrophy. *J Pediatr.* 1987;111:253–255

25. Kravath RE, Pollak CP, Borowiecki B, Weitzman ED. Obstructive sleep apnea and death associated with surgical correction of velopharyngeal incompetence. *J Pediatr.* 1980;96:645–648

26. Massumi RA, Sarin RK, Pooya M, et al. Tonsillar hypertrophy, airway obstruction, alveolar hypoventilation, and cor pulmonale in twin brothers. *Dis Chest.* 1969;55:110–114

27. Fernbach SK, Brouillette RT, Riggs TW, Hunt CE. Radiologic evaluation of adenoids and tonsils in children with obstructive apnea: plain films and fluoroscopy. *Pediatr Radiol.* 1983;13:258–265

28. Mahboubi S, Marsh RR, Potsic WP, Pasquariello PS. The lateral neck radiograph in adenotonsillar hyperplasia. *Int J Pediatr Otorhinolaryngol.* 1985;10:67–73

29. Laurikainen E, Erkinjuntti M, Alihanka J, Rikalainen H, Suonpaa J. Radiological parameters of the bony nasopharynx and the adenotonsillar size compared with sleep apnea episodes in children. *Int J Pediatr Otorhinolaryngol.* 1987;12:303–310

30. Brooks LJ, Stephens BM, Bacevice AM. Adenoid size is related to severity but not the number of episodes of obstructive apnea in children. *J Pediatr.* 1998;132:682–686

31. Brouillette RT, Hanson D, David R, et al. A diagnostic approach to suspected obstructive sleep apnea in children. *J Pediatr.* 1984;105:10–14

32. Brouillette RT, Morielli A, Leimanis A, Waters KA, Luciano R, Ducharme FM. Nocturnal pulse oximetry as an abbreviated testing modality for pediatric obstructive sleep apnea. *Pediatrics.* 2000;105:405–412

33. Lamm C, Mandeli J, Kattan M. Evaluation of home audiotapes as an abbreviated test for obstructive sleep apnea syndrome (OSAS) in children. *Pediatr Pulmonol.* 1999;27:267–272

34. Carroll JL, McColley SA, Marcus CL, Curtis S, Loughlin GM. Inability of clinical history to distinguish primary snoring from obstructive sleep apnea syndrome in children. *Chest.* 1995;108:610–618

35. Marcus CL, Curtis S, Koerner CB, Joffe A, Serwint JR, Loughlin GM. Evaluation of pulmonary function and polysomnography in obese children and adolescents. *Pediatr Pulmonol.* 1996;21:176–183

36. Mallory GB, Fiser DH, Jackson R. Sleep-associated breathing disorders in morbidly obese children and adolescents. *J Pediatr.* 1989;115:892–897

37. Suen JS, Arnold JE, Brooks LJ. Adenotonsillectomy for treatment of obstructive sleep apnea in children. *Arch Otolaryngol Head Neck Surg.* 1995;121:525–530

38. Nieminen P, Tolonen U, Lopponen H, Lopponen T, Luotonen J, Jokinen K. Snoring children: factors predicting sleep apnea. *Acta Otolaryngol Suppl.* 1997;529:190–194

39. Leach J, Olson J, Hermann J, Manning S. Polysomnographic and clinical findings in children with obstructive sleep apnea. *Arch Otolaryngol Head Neck Surg.* 1992;118:741–744

40. Wang RC, Elkins TP, Keech D, Wauquier A, Hubbard D. Accuracy of clinical evaluation in pediatric obstructive sleep apnea. *Otolaryngol Head Neck Surg.* 1998;118:69–73

41. Goldstein NA, Sculerati N, Walsleben JA, Bhatia N, Friedman DM, Rapoport DM. Clinical diagnosis of pediatric obstructive sleep apnea validated by polysomnography. *Otolaryngol Head Neck Surg.* 1994;111:611–617

42. Goh DY, Galster P, Marcus CL. Sleep architecture and respiratory disturbances in children with obstructive sleep apnea. *Am J Respir Crit Care Med.* 2000;162:682–686

43. American Thoracic Society. Cardiorespiratory sleep studies in children: establishment of normative data and polysomnographic predictors of morbidity. *Am J Respir Crit Care Med.* 1999;160:1381–1387

44. Marcus CL, Omlin KJ, Basinki DJ, et al. Normal polysomnographic values for children and adolescents. *Am Rev Respir Dis.* 1992;146:1235–1239

45. Sivan Y, Kornecki A, Schonfeld T. Screening obstructive sleep apnoea syndrome by home videotape recording in children. *Eur Respir J.* 1996;9:2127–2131

46. Saeed MM, Keens TG, Stabile MW, Bolokowicz J, Davidson WS. Should children with suspected obstructive sleep apnea syndrome and normal nap sleep studies have overnight sleep studies? *Chest.* 2000;118:360–365

47. Marcus CL, Keens TG, Ward SL. Comparison of nap and overnight polysomnography in children. *Pediatr Pulmonol.* 1992;13:16–21

48. Jacob SV, Morielli A, Mograss MA, Ducharme FM, Schloss MD, Brouillette RT. Home testing for pediatric obstructive sleep apnea syndrome secondary to adenotonsillar hypertrophy. *Pediatr Pulmonol.* 1995;20:241–252

49. Zucconi M, Strambi LF, Pestalozza G, Tessitore E, Smirne S. Habitual snoring and obstructive sleep apnea syndrome in children: effects of early tonsil surgery. *Int J Pediatr Otorhinolaryngol.* 1993;26:235–243

50. Nieminen P, Tolonen U, Lopponen H. Snoring and obstructive sleep apnea in children: a 6-month follow-up study. *Arch Otolaryngol Head Neck Surg.* 2000;126:481–486

51. Agren K, Nordlander B, Linder-Aronsson S, Zettergren-Wijk L, Svanborg E. Children with nocturnal upper airway obstruction: postoperative orthodontic and respiratory improvement. *Acta Otolaryngol.* 1998;118:581–587

52. Kudoh F, Sanai A. Effect of tonsillectomy and adenoidectomy on obese children with sleep-associated breathing disorders. *Acta Otolaryngol.* 1996;523(suppl):216–218

53. McColley SA, April MM, Carroll JL, Loughlin GM. Respiratory compromise after adenotonsillectomy in children with obstructive sleep apnea. *Arch Otolaryngol Head Neck Surg.* 1992;118:940–943

54. Rosen GM, Muckle RP, Mahowald MW, Goding GS, Ullevig C. Postoperative respiratory compromise in children with obstructive sleep apnea syndrome: can it be anticipated? *Pediatrics.* 1994;93:784–788

55. Ruboyianes JM, Cruz RM. Pediatric adenotonsillectomy for obstructive sleep apnea. *Ear Nose Throat J.* 1996;75:430–433

56. Rothschild MA, Catalano P, Biller HF. Ambulatory pediatric tonsillectomy and the identification of high-risk subgroups. *Otolaryngol Head Neck Surg.* 1994;110:203–210

57. Wiatrak BJ, Myer CM, Andrews TM. Complications of adenotonsillectomy in children under 3 years of age. *Am J Otolaryngol.* 1991;12:170–172

58. Biavati MJ, Manning SC, Phillips DC. Predictive factors for respiratory complications after tonsillectomy and adenoidectomy in children with OSA. *Arch Otolaryngol Head Neck Surg.* 1997;123:517–521

59. Marcus CL, Ward SL, Mallory GB, et al. Use of nasal continuous positive airway pressure as treatment of childhood obstructive sleep apnea. *J Pediatr.* 1995;127:88–94

60. Waters KA, Everett FM, Bruderer JW, Sullivan CE. Obstructive sleep apnea: the use of nasal CPAP in 80 children. *Am J Respir Crit Care Med.* 1995;152:780–785

61. Guilleminault C, Pelayo R, Clerk A, Leger D, Bocian RC. Home nasal continuous positive airway pressure in infants with sleep-disordered breathing. *J Pediatr.* 1995;127:905–912

62. Rains JC. Treatment of obstructive sleep apnea in pediatric patients. *Clin Pediatr (Phila).* 1995;34:535–541

63. Marcus CL, Carroll JL, Bamford O, Pyzik P, Loughlin GM. Supplemental oxygen during sleep in children with sleep-disordered breathing. *Am J Respir Crit Care Med.* 1995;152:1297–1301

Technical Report Summary:
Diagnosis and Management of Childhood
Obstructive Sleep Apnea Syndrome

Authors:
Michael S. Schechter, MD, MPH,
and the Section on Pediatric Pulmonology,
Subcommittee on Obstructive Sleep Apnea Syndrome

American Academy of Pediatrics
PO Box 927, 141 Northwest Point Blvd
Elk Grove Village, IL 60009-0927

ABSTRACT.

Objective

This technical report describes the procedures involved in developing the recommendations of the Subcommittee on Obstructive Sleep Apnea Syndrome in children. The group of primary interest for this report was otherwise healthy children older than 1 year who might have adenotonsillar hypertrophy or obesity as underlying risk factors of obstructive sleep apnea syndrome (OSAS). The goals of the committee were to enhance the primary care clinician's ability to recognize OSAS, identify the most appropriate procedure for diagnosis of OSAS, identify risks associated with pediatric OSAS, and evaluate management options for OSAS.

Methods

A literature search was initially conducted for the years 1966–1999 and then updated to include 2000. The search was limited to English language literature concerning children older than 2 and younger than 18 years. Titles and abstracts were reviewed for relevance, and committee members reviewed in detail any possibly appropriate articles to determine eligibility for inclusion. Additional articles were obtained by a review of literature and committee members' files. Committee members compiled evidence tables and met to review and discuss the literature that was collected.

Results

A total of 2115 titles were reviewed, of which 113 provided relevant original data for analysis. These articles were mainly case series and cross-sectional studies; overall, very few methodologically strong cohort studies or randomized, controlled trials concerning OSAS have been published. In addition, a minority of studies satisfactorily differentiated primary snoring from true OSAS. Reports of the prevalence of habitual snoring in children ranged from 3.2% to 12.1%, and estimates of OSAS ranged from 0.7% to 10.3%; these studies were too heterogeneous for data pooling. Children with sleepdisordered breathing are at increased risk for hyperactivity and learning problems. The combined odds ratio for neurobehavioral abnormalities in snoring children compared with controls is 2.93 (95% confidence interval: 2.23– 3.83). A number of case series have documented decreased somatic growth in children with OSAS; right ventricular dysfunction and systemic hypertension also have been reported in children with OSAS. However, the risk growth and cardiovascular problems cannot be quantified from the published literature. Overnight polysomnography (PSG) is recognized as the gold standard for diagnosis of OSAS, and there are currently no satisfactory alternatives. The diagnostic accuracy of symptom questionnaires and other purely clinical approaches is low. Pulse oximetry appears to be specific but insensitive. Other methods, including audiotaping or videotaping and nap or home overnight PSG, remain investigational. Adenotonsillectomy is curative in 75% to 100% of children with OSAS, including those who are obese. Up to 27% of children undergoing adenotonsillectomy for OSAS have postoperative respiratory complications, but estimates are varied. Risk factors for persistent OSAS after adenotonsillectomy include continued snoring and a high apnea-hypopnea index on the preoperative PSG.

Conclusions

OSAS is common in children and is associated with significant sequelae. Overnight PSG is currently the only reliable diagnostic modality that can differentiate OSAS from primary snoring. However, the PSG criteria for OSAS have not been definitively validated, and it is not clear that primary snoring without PSG-defined OSAS is benign. Adenotonsillectomy is the first-line treatment for OSAS but requires careful postoperative monitoring because of the high risk of respiratory complications. Adenotonsillectomy is usually curative, but children with persistent snoring (and perhaps with severely abnormal preoperative PSG results) should have PSG repeated postoperatively.

INTRODUCTION

This technical report describes in detail the procedures involved in developing recommendations as given in the accompanying practice guideline on obstructive sleep apnea syndrome (OSAS). A description of the process, methods of data compilation and analysis, and summaries of the conclusions of the committee will be given.

FORMULATION AND ARTICULATION OF THE QUESTION ADDRESSED BY THE COMMITTEE

Target Audience

The practice guideline is primarily aimed at office-based pediatricians and other primary care clinicians who treat children (family physicians, nurse practitioners, physician assistants). The secondary audience for the guideline includes pediatric pulmonologists, neurologists, otolaryngologists, and developmental/behavioral pediatricians.

Definitions

The primary focus of the committee was on OSAS in childhood. The committee agreed to use the definition provided in a statement from the American Thoracic Society with some additional elaboration of associated symptoms:

> OSAS in children is a disorder of breathing during sleep characterized by prolonged partial upper airway obstruction and/or intermittent complete obstruction (obstructive apnea) that disrupts normal ventilation during sleep and normal sleep patterns. It is associated with symptoms including habitual (nightly) snoring, sleep difficulties, and/or daytime neurobehavioral problems. Complications may include growth abnormalities, neurologic disorders, and cor pulmonale, especially in severe cases. Various risk factors have been identified and are defined.

The committee sought to focus on otherwise healthy children who might have adenotonsillar hypertrophy or obesity as underlying risk factors and to specifically exclude infants younger than 1 year, children with central hypoventilation syndromes, and children at risk because of underlying abnormalities, such as craniofacial disorders; Down syndrome; cerebral palsy; neuromuscular disorders; chronic lung disease; sickle cell disease; genetic, metabolic, and storage diseases; and laryngomalacia.

Goals of the Committee

The committee sought to address several specific goals and questions:

1. *To enhance the primary care clinician's ability to recognize OSAS.* The committee believed that a certain amount of consciousness raising would be appropriate to alert the clinician to suspect the presence of OSAS. Thus, a catalog of associated signs and symptoms is provided in the accompanying practice guideline but will not be addressed in this technical report.

2. *To identify the most appropriate procedure for diagnosis of OSAS.* Approaches evaluated by the committee included history and physical examination, questionnaires, audiotaping or videotaping, nocturnal pulse oximetry, nap polysomnography (PSG), and ambulatory PSG, all of which would be compared with the gold standard, comprehensive overnight PSG, as defined by the American Thoracic Society. In view of the fact that overnight PSG is not readily available to children in all geographic areas, consideration was given to alternative diagnostic approaches even if their accuracy is suboptimal.

3. *To identify risks associated with pediatric OSAS.* In adults, OSAS is associated with excessive daytime sleepiness (leading to cognitive defects and increased mortality attributable to susceptibility to motor vehicle crashes), pulmonary hypertension, and systemic hypertension. The committee wished to evaluate the strength of pediatric data in this area.

4. *To evaluate management options for OSAS.* The committee sought to find data relating to adenotonsillectomy and alternative treatment modalities in the management of OSAS. The committee set out to evaluate the risk of complications after adenotonsillectomy in children with OSAS, especially given the fact that patients not suspected to have OSAS might undergo adenotonsillectomy for other indications. The postoperative complication of particular concern was respiratory compromise. Other complications of surgery, such as bleeding and pain, were not specifically addressed in relation to OSAS. In addition, data on postoperative recurrence and persistence of OSAS was sought.

METHODS

Literature Search

A literature search of the National Library of Medicine's PubMed database (http://www.ncbi.nlm.nih.gov/entrez/query. fcgi?db_PubMed) for the years 1966–1999 was conducted in August 1999 by staff at the American Academy of Pediatrics. The search was limited to English language literature concerning children older than 2 and younger than 18 years. The following search terms were used: sleep apnea syndrome; apnea; sleep disorders; snoring; polysomnography; airway obstruction; adenoidectomy; tonsillectomy (adverse effects, mortality); and sleep-disordered breathing.mp. This search was updated in November 2000 before preparation of this technical report.

Article Review

Titles and abstracts (when available) of articles found by the literature search were reviewed by committee members, and all those considered to be possibly relevant were marked for detailed review. Recent review articles were included to compare their bibliographies with the result of the automated literature search. Articles deemed possibly relevant were then printed and distributed to committee members for more detailed review. A literature review form was developed for this project to standardize this part of the process. Because there was a large number of articles requiring evaluation, some committee members recruited residents and fellows to assist in the performance of these reviews under their supervision. Although it became clear at this point that the number of articles that could be considered high quality by conventional epidemiologic standards was small, a low threshold was used to allow inclusion of any possibly relevant articles into the next level of review. At this point, articles were compiled and divided by the committee chair, additional articles were obtained by a review of literature, committee members' files were added, and committee members were assigned specific topics (as discussed previously in "Goals of the Committee") for detailed review and compilation of evidence tables. The findings of committee members were then presented at a follow-up meeting of the entire committee. A final review and compilation into evidence tables was performed by the lead author of this technical report (M.S.S.).

Calculation of prevalence, diagnostic test characteristics, and odds ratios were performed independently of the authors' reports, using data provided in the original articles. In 2 cases, authors were contacted for clarification of data. Where applicable, odds ratios from different studies were combined, using Mantel-Haenszel weights in stratified tables. Tests for heterogeneity are reported. All statistical calculations were performed using Stata 5.0 software (Stata Corporation, College Station, TX).

RESULTS

The literature search identified 2067 articles for initial review. Titles and abstracts (when available) of these articles were divided among the 7 committee members for perusal as an initial screening, and of those, 278 (16.2%) were retained for more detailed scrutiny. An additional 48 relevant publications were found outside this initial review. Articles were read in full if they appeared to have any relevance to childhood OSAS; included in this group were 70 general reviews and case reports or descriptive case series, which were used to allow committee members to gain a general sense of the literature and access their bibliographies. Among various committee members, the percentage of articles chosen for more detailed review ranged from 12.7% to 23.4%. This variability was statistically significant ($P = .007$ by Pearson χ^2). Excluding the methodologist, whose approach was the most permissive (23.4% acceptance rate), the range was 12.7% to 19.4%, and variability was not statistically significant ($P = .143$ by Pearson χ^2) among remaining committee members.

A total of 113 articles were found that contained original data relevant to the specific aims of this committee. Most of the publications that were reviewed in detail provided little quantitative data for analysis. In particular, most papers that were older than 5 years presented case series or poor-quality cohort studies or omitted important details. These lower-quality studies provide the background for current expert opinion but are otherwise of limited value and will not be listed in detail for this report. Studies that were of quantitative value are tabulated and were given quality ratings in the tables. Briefly, rating levels of studies on treatment efficacy were assigned as follows:

Level I—Randomized trials with low rates of false-positive (α) and/or false-negative (β) results (high power).

Level II—Randomized trials with high rates of false-positive(α) and/or false-negative (β) results (low power).

Level III—Nonrandomized concurrent cohort comparisons between contemporaneous patients who did and did not receive an intervention, or casecontrol or cross-sectional studies with appropriate control group.

Level IV—Nonrandomized historical cohort comparisons between current patients who received an intervention and former patients (from the same institution or from the literature) who did not, or casecontrol or cross-sectional studies for which control groups were suboptimally chosen.

Level V—Case series without controls.

Rating levels for diagnostic tests were assigned as follows:

Level 1—Independent blind comparison of patients from an appropriate spectrum of patients, all of whom have undergone both the diagnostic test and the reference standard.

Level 2—Independent blind or objective comparison performed in a set of nonconsecutive patients or confined to a narrow spectrum of study individuals (or both), all of whom have undergone both the diagnostic test and the reference standard.

Level 3—Independent blind or objective comparison of an appropriate spectrum of patients, but the reference standard was not applied to all.

Level 4—Reference standard was unobjective, unblinded, or not independent; positive and negative tests were verified using separate reference standards; or study was performed in an inappropriate spectrum of patients.

Prevalence of Snoring and OSAS

We found 7 studies that attempted to establish prevalence of snoring in childhood. These studies came from a variety of European countries, and all ascertained data via parent questionnaire. The prevalence of snoring in these studies ranged from 3.2% to 12.1%, which was significantly heterogeneous (P < .0001). The study by Gislason and Benediktsdottir seemed to be somewhat of an outlier, especially because the frequency of OSAS they reported was nearly the same as that of snoring, but with omission of that study, the heterogeneity remains significant (P < .001).

Three studies reported on prevalence of OSAS, and estimates ranged from 0.7% to 10.3%. All used very different criteria, including 1 that gave estimates based on 2 different criteria. The variability of these estimates was so great that no attempt was made to combine the data.

Sequelae of OSAS

Most published articles on complications of OSAS are reports of retrospective case series or prospectively collected, uncontrolled data comparing measures before and after surgical treatment. These articles are summarized in this report and in evidence tables.

Cognitive and Behavioral Abnormalities

The committee found 12 publications that evaluated the association of behavioral problems, especially hyperactivity or attention-deficit/hyperactivity disorder (ADHD), with sleep-disordered breathing. In an early case series of 50 children with OSAS documented by PSG, 84% had excessive daytime sleepiness, 76% had some behavior disturbance, 42% were hyperactive, and 16% had decreased school performance. A number of crosssectional studies have been done that compare the risk of behavioral problems in children who snore with that of a control population. None of these studies distinguish children with OSAS from those with primary snoring (PS). For the study of Weissbluth et al, parents of children attending a general pediatric practice were surveyed, and 71 children were reported to have behavioral or academic problems. Snoring, mouth breathing, and labored breathing when asleep were reported to be more than twice as common in these children as in the comparison group. The study of Chervin et al reported that 33% of children with ADHD were habitual snorers, compared with 11% of children attending a general psychiatric clinic and 9% attending a general pediatric clinic. A previously mentioned prevalence study by Ali et al found that children who were reported to snore during most nights were also reported to have more daytime sleepiness and hyperactivity than were children in a comparison group. Children were evaluated using Conners scales, and those with more severe sleep disturbance were also more likely to be at the 95th percentile on Conners subscales relating to hyperactive, inattentive, and aggressive behaviors. In a follow-up report, 29 of 60 children reported to snore 2 years previously no longer snored (weighted κ 0.52), although habitual snoring was again found to be associated with daytime sleepiness and hyperactivity. In another publication, the same authors identified 12 children with sleep-disordered breathing (by overnight pulse oximetry and videotaping), 11 snoring children without sleep-disordered breathing, and a control group not undergoing adenotonsillectomy and administered Conners scales, the Continuous Performance Test (a test of attention), and the Matching Familiar Figures Test (a test of vigilance). Significant improvement was found in Conners parent scale scores for aggressive, inattentive, and hyperactive behaviors; attention; and vigilance in the sleep-disordered breathing group after adenotonsillectomy, and similar changes were found in the primary snorers postoperatively, but not in control groups. In a recent population-based cross-sectional study of 988 Portuguese children, Ferreira et al found that habitual snorers were twice as likely as nonsnorers to have an abnormal score on the Children's Behavioral Questionnaire. Finally, Blunden et al compared 16 children referred for adenotonsillectomy or snoring with a control group and found impaired selective and sustained attention scores only in the children who snored. They also reported that the snoring children had significantly lower average IQ scores. PSG was done in these children, but for purposes of analysis, the PS and OSAS groups were combined because preliminary analyses revealed no significant group differences on any neurocognitive or behavioral parameter (all $P > .05$). The authors pointed out that even patients with OSAS had very mild abnormalities (mean respiratory disturbance index [RDI] <1). Although it is possible that lack of power and selection bias may have contributed to their findings, the implication is that snoring without overt OSAS might be associated with neurocognitive abnormalities.

Although the 6 cross-sectional studies described previously all reported on slightly different behavioral and cognitive phenomena, their findings were pooled, and the results of this are shown. The Mantel-Haenszel test for heterogeneity was not significant ($P=.4577$). The combined odds ratio for neurobehavioral abnormalities in snoring children is 2.93 (95% confidence interval [CI], 2.23–3.83).

Several other papers are of interest but cannot be quantitatively combined. Goldstein et al had parents of 36 children who were referred for adenotonsillectomy because of clinically significant obstructive symptoms complete the Child Behavior Checklist and found that 10 (28%) had abnormal results. Postoperatively, 15 had a repeat evaluation, and only 2 (13%) still had abnormal results. This finding was not clinically significant, presumably because of lack of statistical power, but there was a clinically significant improvement in mean test scores postoperatively ($P < .001$).

Four studies used overnight PSG testing to establish a diagnosis of OSAS. Rosen reported on a series of 326 children referred for evaluation of snoring, of whom 59% met PSG criteria for OSAS. Daily tiredness was reported in 19%; excessive daytime sleepiness was reported in 10%; and behavior, school, or mood problems were reported in 9%, with no difference between the OSAS and non-OSAS groups. Gozal conducted an interesting study in which 297 first graders who were in the lowest 10th percentile academically were evaluated for sleepdisordered breathing by parent questionnaire combined with overnight (home) oximetry. Adenotonsillectomy was recommended in the 54 children (18.1%) with abnormal test results; 24 accepted surgery, and 30 did not. Mean grades increased from 2.43 ± 0.17 to 2.87 ± 0.19 in the children who had surgery, with no change in the untreated OSAS group or the non-OSAS group ($P < .001$).

The findings of an Australian study contrasted with the aforementioned papers. Thirty-nine children with PSG evidence of OSAS were followed 6 months after the initial PSG, and 24 had received adenotonsillectomy. These were compared with children who were waiting for intervention ($n = 5$; median apnea-hypopnea index [AHI] = 5.5) or didn't require intervention ($n = 10$; median AHI = 3.1). Information on AHI was not given for the surgical group. At follow-up, children in the surgical and nonsurgical groups had improved sleep behavior. Intervention did not result in any statistically significant improvement in development or temperament, although the study was probably underpowered.

In summary, studies generally show a nearly threefold increase in behavior and neurocognitive abnormalities in children with sleep-disordered breathing. Most of these

studies did not definitively differentiate children with PS from those with OSAS, so the true prevalence of behavior and learning problems in children with OSAS versus PS is not clear. It is possible, however, that PS, even in the absence of clear-cut OSAS, might place children at risk.

Growth

Four studies evaluating growth and OSAS were found. Marcus et al evaluated 14 prepubertal children with a mean age of 4 years ± 1 standard deviation who had OSAS documented by overnight PSG and measured caloric intake and sleeping energy expenditure as well as anthropomorphic measurements before and after adenotonsillectomy. Average sleeping energy expenditure decreased, and mean weight z score increased postoperatively without any change in caloric intake. Bar et al evaluated changes in growth and also measured insulin-like growth factor (IGF)-I and IGF-binding protein-3 levels before and 18 months after adenotonsillectomy. Both studies showed statistically significant increases in weight but not height; IGF-I levels increased and IGF-binding protein levels did not. An interesting report on the effect of adenotonsillectomy on growth included a group of obese and morbidly obese children and documented postoperative increases in weight and height, even in those children who were initially obese. The other 2 studies, which had poorer documentation of OSAS, reported similar results. None of these studies reported a comparison with a nonsurgical control group, comparison with children operated on for indications other than OSAS, or comparison with children who had PS.

Cardiovascular

Eight case reports or small series were found that documented cor pulmonale or hypertension, which reversed with adenotonsillectomy or other surgical correction in patients with clinically diagnosed OSAS. Two case series reported children with adenotonsillar hypertrophy with or without clinical airway obstruction who were found to have right ventricular dysfunction that reversed after adenotonsillectomy. One study described pulsus paradoxus and leftward shift of the interventricular septum secondary to snoring in 3 of 6 children with OSAS. This correlated with negative esophageal pressures but not with oxygen desaturation, and it reversed with nasal continuous positive airway pressure (CPAP). Tal et al used radionuclide ventriculography to evaluate ventricular function in 27 children referred for oropharyngeal obstruction who had abnormal Brouillette questionnaire scores for OSAS; PSG was not performed. They found decreased right ventricular ejection fraction in 37% of these children and abnormal wall motion in 67%. All of the 11 patients who had a repeat evaluation after adenotonsillectomy showed improvement. Systemic blood pressure was evaluated in a study of children referred for PSG. Higher diastolic pressures (adjusted for body mass index and age) were found in children with OSAS, compared with those with PS. The prevalence of blood pressure measurements >95th percentile was high in both groups (32% vs 19%, respectively), with a nonsignificant difference that may have been attributable to low power. The response after adenotonsillectomy was not reported. This was the only study that compared cardiovascular complications in children with OSAS versus those with PS.

Miscellaneous

One study reported on 115 enuretic children undergoing adenotonsillectomy for any indication. There was a 66% reduction in enuretic nights 1 month after surgery and a 77% decrease 6 months after surgery. In the group with secondary enuresis, 100% were dry 6 months after surgery.

Diagnosis of OSAS

Polysomnography

One of the problems in evaluating various methods of diagnosing OSAS in children is that the gold standard, overnight PSG, has not been well standardized in its performance or interpretation. Although recent consensus statements pertaining to standards and normative data should lessen this problem, the question of definition remains problematic. Pediatric sleep specialists use the adult model in describing a continuum of sleep-disordered breathing from PS to upper airway resistance syndrome to obstructive hypoventilation and OSAS. It is assumed that PS is a benign condition and OSAS is associated with undesirable complications. Normative standards for their polysomnographic determination have been chosen on the basis of statistical distribution of data, but it has not been established that those standards have any validity as predictors of the occurrence of complications. In other words:

"On the basis of normative data, an obstructive apnea index of 1 is often chosen as the cutoff for normality. However, while an apnea index of 1 is statistically significant (ie, at the 97.5th percentile for an asymptomatic, normative population), it is not known what level is clinically significant."

Of the few studies that compare children with polysomnographically defined OSAS with those with PS in regard to prevalence of complications, only 1 found a clear difference between the 2 groups. This is an important point, because with a poorly validated gold standard, statements regarding diagnostic accuracy of alternative methods of diagnosis become dubious. Finally, the test-retest reliability of overnight PSG, which in adults is no greater than 91% and possibly somewhat lower, has never been evaluated in children.

Having stated these points, additional analysis of the validity of alternative diagnostic approaches will be done assuming PSG as the gold standard. One additional benefit of overnight PSG is that in addition to establishing the diagnosis of OSAS, PSG also may be used to determine its severity. It has been suggested that the severity of OSAS is an important predictor of complications, particularly in the immediate postoperative period. None of the alternative diagnostic techniques discussed below have been evaluated for this purpose.

Questionnaires

In 1984, Brouillette et al reported high accuracy for a diagnostic questionnaire for OSAS in children with adenotonsillar hypertrophy. This questionnaire was initially tested on 23 children with OSAS and 46 controls. On the basis of this questionnaire, a 3-variable discriminant function was calculated as follows:

$$OSAS\ score = 1.42D + 1.41A + 0.71S - 3.83$$

where D is difficulty during sleep, A is apnea observed during sleep, and S is snoring. Values assigned to D and S were: 0 = never; 1 = occasionally; 2 = frequently; and 3 = always. Values assigned to A were: 0 = no; and 1 = yes. This system was then applied to a prospective group of 23 patients referred for evaluation of possible OSAS. The authors demonstrated that a score of >3.5 perfectly predicted the presence of OSAS by PSG; a score of <-1 perfectly predicted absence of OSAS; and a score in between was indeterminate. Unfortunately, there were 5 children who were believed to have a borderline PSG, confusing the issue somewhat. It appears that the choices of 3.5 and -1 as breakpoints in the score were made posthoc and were, thus, somewhat arbitrary. Since the initial publication of the questionnaire, 3 additional studies have been published detailing the results of its use. All of these studies prospectively evaluated similar groups of pediatric patients with a similar prevalence of OSAS; PSG with similar evaluation criteria was performed on all subjects, and all completed the same questionnaire applied in similar ways. This scoring system is sufficiently simple and straightforward, so its application can be expected to be fairly standard and replicable. Thus, data from these studies was combined, and conclusions were drawn accordingly.

The OSAS questionnaire by Brouillette et al performed much less well in subsequent applications. The 4 studies (including a later study by the same authors) included a total of 765 patients with an overall prevalence of OSAS confirmed by PSG of 60%. Applied to these patients, the score was indeterminate in 47%; in subjects who were categorized (ie, not indeterminate), its positive predictive value (PPV) was 65% and negative predictive value (NPV) was 46%. Using the pooled data for calculation, the likelihood ratio of positive questionnaire results is 1.24, and the likelihood ratio of negative questionnaire results is 0.78. Overall, the use of the questionnaire by Brouillette et al as a substitute for PSG would clearly be fraught with error, leading to numerous false-positive and falsenegative results in the diagnosis of OSAS.

Other publications reporting attempts at creating questionnaires or developing other purely clinical criteria to substitute for PSG are uninterpretable because of their failure to compare their criteria with PSG50–53 or unsuccessful in developing any reliable predictive criteria.

Audiotaping and Videotaping

Two studies have evaluated the use of home audiotaping, and 1 evaluated home videotaping, as a screening test for OSAS. The methods used to evaluate these techniques were different, so the data do not lend themselves to pooling. Sivan et al scored a 30-minute videotape in 58 children using 7 variables, including loudness and type of inspiratory noise, movements during sleep, number of waking episodes, number of apneas, chest retractions, and mouth breathing. The PSG results were abnormal in 62%. They reported a sensitivity of 94%, specificity of 68%, PPV of 83%, and NPV of 88%. Posthoc analysis (similar to what was done in the 1984 study by Brouillette et al) was performed in 2 ways, leading to the development of an indeterminate score and better test characteristics in the categorizable group. As might be expected, a scoring system that places a greater number of subjects into the indeterminate group leads to better NPV and PPV.

Goldstein et al developed a 7-item predictive score that considered the presence of snoring, respiratory pauses, gasping, sleeping with neck extended, daytime sleepiness, adenoid facies, and the presence of pauses in breathing of at least 5 seconds on an audiotape recorded by the parents. The criteria used to score each category were not precisely described, and there seemed to be significant variability in the evaluation of the audiotapes, which were reviewed for "at least 2 minutes...for each child, and an average of 10 minutes were generally reviewed. Various parts of the tape were sampled." Patients were categorized as definitely, possibly, or not likely having OSAS on the basis of these items, but no description was provided of how these items were scored and combined, and no measure of interobserver vari- ability was attempted, so reproducibility is unknown. A total of 30 children were studied prospectively, of whom 13 (43%) had OSAS confirmed by PSG. The authors reported a sensitivity of 92.3%, specificity of 29.4%, PPV of 50.0%, and NPV of 83.3%, which they calculated by combining the "definite" and "possible" groups into a positive screening category. If their possible group was eliminated from consideration (analogous to the way Brouillette et al treated indeterminate scores), a mild decrease in sensitivity (91%) and mild increases in specificity (38%) and PPV (56%) are seen.

Goldstein et al concluded that children whose results of evaluation for sleep apnea (as performed using their technique, including audiotaping) are negative do not need PSG, because the sensitivity of their clinical assessment is high. They recommended PSG for children who appear to have OSAS, because the specificity of clinical assessment is low. It is important to note that the percentage of positive results of PSG in their study (43%) was somewhat lower than the prevalence of approximately 60% reported in most studies of children referred for evaluation of possible OSAS. This is probably (at least in part) because they used more restrictive PSG criteria for diagnosing OSAS (AHI >15). If a population with a higher prevalence of OSAS were studied, it is likely that the PPV of the clinical evaluation by Goldstein et al would be higher and the NPV would be lower. In addition, the higher AHI as a diagnostic criterion might have biased the study toward the more severe end of the OSAS spectrum. The possibility of spectrum bias and the undocumented reproducibility of the tape evaluation raise the question of whether test characteristics will be as good if applied to a large, general population.

A second study of the use of home audiotaping as an abbreviated test for OSAS used 7 observers to analyze audiotapes of 29 children referred for evaluation; 48% were subsequently found to have positive PSG. Observers listened to 15 minutes of audiotape and specifically scored the presence of struggle sounds and respiratory pauses. A mean κ statistic of 0.70 (range, 0.50–0.93) was calculated, indicating moderately good interobserver agreement. The presence of a struggle sound on the audiotape gave the best posthoc test characteristics, with a sensitivity of 0.71, specificity of 80%, NPV of 73%, and PPV of 75%.

To summarize, the use of home audiotaping and videotaping has been inadequately investigated. Additional studies are necessary. It should be pointed out that there was no consensus of the committee regarding acceptable rates of false-negative and false-positive results for tests used as an alternative to PSG.

Pulse Oximetry

Seven studies were found that reported on pulse oximetry in children suspected of having OSAS. However, only 1 compared pulse oximetry to PSG. In this study involving 349 children, pulse oximetry was performed during PSG and was evaluated independently of the PSG interpretation, with well-defined criteria and excellent interobserver agreement. There were 89 PSGs (25.5%) performed in a sleep lab; the others were done at home, so the gold standard was not identical for all subjects. In this group, with a 60.2% prevalence of OSAS, the PPV was 97% (90 of 93). However, the NPV of the test (calculated by the authors by combining subjects with either inconclusive or negative tests) was only 53%. When the analysis was limited to subjects without any medical diagnoses other than adenotonsillar hypertrophy, the PPV was 100%, with an insubstantial change in NPV.

Given the test characteristic described, it appears that overnight pulse oximetry could provide an accurate screen for OSAS, insofar as a positive result may be a good predictor of an abnormal PSG result. However, the findings of the single study described in this report need to be replicated.

Nap Polysomnography

Two papers from the same institution have evaluated the utility of brief (1 hour) daytime nap studies in comparison with full overnight PSGs. The conclusions of both are generalizable to only a limited degree, however. Marcus et al studied 40 children referred for evaluation of possible OSAS, but this group was not representative of the type of patient addressed by this practice guideline, because only 35% had adenotonsillar hypertrophy as the underlying cause of their sleep disturbances. Other diagnoses included Down syndrome (40% of subjects), various upper airway abnormalities, and other neurologic and respiratory problems. Furthermore, 95% (38 of 40) of the patients studied had abnormal overnight PSG results, providing little opportunity to evaluate the test performance of nap studies in children with normal PSG results. The study by Saeed et al limited itself to children addressed by this practice guideline (age, 1–18 years; adenotonsillar hypertrophy; absence of other significant disease). They reported on the results of overnight PSG in children with normal and mildly abnormal nap study results. Patients with severely abnormal nap study results were excluded; they were assumed to have significant OSAS and, therefore, referred directly for tonsillectomy without overnight PSG (S.D. Ward, personal communication). In this group, for which prevalence of PSG-documented OSAS was 66%, the nap studies had a PPV of 77% and NPV of 49%. In fact, if children with more severely abnormal nap study results were included in the analysis and the investigators are correct in their assumption that these children all have abnormal overnight PSG results, then the sensitivity and PPV of nap studies is actually higher than that reported in this paper. Thus, it is possible that abnormal nap study results might provide a predictive value adequate to allow the recommendation for surgery without corroborative overnight PSG, but confirmation of this conclusion (asserted by the authors) is lacking. On the other hand, a nap study with negative results would still require a follow-up overnight PSG for confirmation.

Home Polysomnography

One group has published data comparing the results of PSG performed in children at home with those performed at the sleep laboratory. In a report of 21 children between the ages of 2 and 12 years who were studied in both environments, the sensitivity and specificity of home PSG varied depending on the severity of OSA. When an AHI >1 was used as the criterion for diagnosing OSAS, the sensitivity of home PSG was 100% and the specificity was 62%; for AHI >3, sensitivity was 88% and specificity was 77%; for AHI >5, sensitivity and specificity were both 100%. This group uses a sophisticated type of ambulatory PSG that is not commercially available and is not analogous to commercial systems. Also, their system did not allow for detection of obstructive hypoventilation. Furthermore, the subjects used in their report were not chosen sequentially or at random, and the authors describe a complex process for specifically selecting children for inclusion in the study. Nonetheless, the comparability of the results of home and sleep laboratory overnight PSG appears good; additional study using commercially available equipment in a more representative population would be helpful.

Treatment of OSAS

Tonsillectomy and/or Adenoidectomy

There are many published papers, primarily case reports and case series, that support the efficacy of tonsillectomy with or without adenoidectomy as treatment for OSAS. Most of these studies use relief of snoring and other clinical symptoms as their endpoint. Others cite improvement in growth, behavior, cardiovascular complications, or enuresis after surgery. Several papers suggest that adenotonsillectomy is effective treatment of OSAS even in children who are morbidly obese. Many of these studies are anecdotal and methodologically uninterpretable.

Frank et al were the first to use PSG to analyze the effect of surgery on OSAS in children. Of an initial group of 32 children referred for suspected OSAS, they reported on 7 who had PSG before and after adenotonsillectomy. These children had an average of 194 obstructive apneas per night preoperatively and 7 postoperatively ($P < .025$). They provide no breakdown of individual cure rate. Zucconi et al, using nocturnal or nap PSG, reported a 100% cure rate of OSAS in 29 children receiving adenotonsillectomy or adenoidectomy and monotonsillectomy and a 0% cure rate in 5 children receiving only adenoidectomy. Two more recent studies were methodologically superior regarding diagnosis of OSAS. Suen et al reported on 69 children referred for evaluation of possible OSAS; 35 (51%) had a RDI >5 and were referred for adenotonsillectomy, and 30 had the procedure. Follow-up PSG was performed in 26; all showed improvement, although 4 (15%) still had an RDI >5. All children with persistently high RDIs continued to snore, although 3 children with RDIs that had normalized continued to snore. Thus, adenotonsillectomy resulted in a cure rate of 85%, and the absence of postoperative snoring was associated with no treatment failures (NPV of postoperative snoring = 100%), whereas 57% of children who still snored continued to have abnormal PSG results (PPV = 57%). The authors of that paper emphasized that a high preoperative RDI was a strong predictor of abnormal postoperative RDI and suggested 19.1 as a cutoff.

However, their data shows that the PPV of preoperative RDI ≥19.1 for a postoperative RDI >5 was 43% and the NPV was 95%, neither of which are as high as the predictive values afforded by the presence of persistent snoring postoperatively. The findings of Nieminen were similar, although their criteria for positive PSG results were slightly different (AHI >1). They reported a 95% cure rate for a group of 21 children after adenotonsillectomy or tonsillectomy; 1 of 5 children who continued to snore had postoperative PSG results that remained abnormal (PPV = 20%), and none of the children who stopped snoring had abnormal PSG results (NPV = 100%). The authors pointed out that 73% of this group had previously had their adenoids removed, implying confirmation of the lack of efficacy of adenoidectomy alone for relief of OSAS. This paper also mentioned in passing that 2 children with abnormal results of PSG did not have surgery; in 1, the follow-up PSG results were unchanged, and in the other, the results had normalized. Although no generalizations can be made on the basis of these data, it represents the only published report of follow-up PSG in children with OSAS who were not treated.

Several other papers reported PSG results in association with adenotonsillectomy, but these reports were somewhat less clearly written. Wiet et al reported a series of 48 patients in whom sleep studies were performed because of unclear history or physical findings, or complicated OSA. An AHI >5 was considered abnormal. Thirteen patients had no complicating medical factors, and of the 35 remaining, 20 were morbidly obese. All 13 uncomplicated patients had adenotonsillectomy. They had a significant decrease in mean AHI (from 23 to 6 [$P < .01$]); it was not stated whether any had residual abnormal postoperative PSG results. Of the obese patients, 12 of 20 had adenotonsillectomy alone, and the rest had uvulopharyngopalatoplasty in addition. It was not specified how the decision to perform uvulopharyngopalatoplasty was made, and the report of results for this group was not broken down by surgical procedure. Mean AHI in the obese group decreased from 33 to 4 ($P < .001$). Agren et al reported on a group of 20 children with "unequivocal anamnestic nocturnal obstructive breathing." The preoperative AHI was >5 in 10 children, and the apnea index (AI) was >1 in 17. Five of these patients had an adenoidectomy in the past. The terminology used in that paper was confusing, and it was not entirely clear whether AI meant apnea index or apnea-hypopnea index. Postoperatively, no AHI (or AI) was reported; it was stated that 5 patients still had some partial obstruction postoperatively, but all had a normal oxygen desaturation index (which had been abnormal in 13 preoperatively). Shintani et al described 134 children referred for snoring and clinical sleep apnea; 74 had a preoperative AHI >10, but for the rest of the group, the AHI was unspecified. Of this group, 114 had adenotonsillectomy, 13 had adenoidectomy, 4 had adenoidectomy with monotonsillectomy, and 3 had tonsillectomy alone, all presumably at the discretion of the surgeon. Using the authors' criterion for improvement of a postoperative decrease in AHI by 50%, 84.5% of children who had adenoidectomy and 75.4% of those who had adenotonsillectomy were improved postoperatively (difference between adenotonsillectomy and adenoidectomy, $P = .732$). In contrast to the findings of Suen et al, the preoperative AHI in this report did not predict the likelihood of treatment failure.

To summarize these studies, all of which were case series that were reported with variable rigor, it appears that adenotonsillectomy is curative in 75% to 100% of children, even if obese. The role of adenoidectomy alone is unclear. Postoperatively, children should be retested for OSAS if they continue to snore and possibly if the preoperative AHI was high.

*Postoperative Complications and the
Need for Inpatient Monitoring*

A number of publications have catalogued postoperative complications of adenotonsillectomy in large series of patients, but these will not be discussed further here. An additional large group of papers have described the risk of complications associated with outpatient adenotonsillectomy in the general population; these case series have generally excluded children with upper airway obstruction from consideration and also will not be discussed further. However, several papers provide data pertaining to complications of surgery in children undergoing adenotonsillectomy for upper airway obstruction, all specifically addressing the risk of postoperative respiratory obstruction. These authors define respiratory compromise in various ways but generally consider the need for supplemental oxygen as a minimum criterion. The papers report a wide range for the rate of postoperative respiratory complications (0%–27%), primarily because their populations include different proportions of children with neuromuscular, chromosomal, and craniofacial disorders. This variation makes the study groups too heterogeneous for pooling of the data, and their inclusion of complex patients makes them less valid in estimating the risk of postoperative respiratory compromise in the population being addressed by this practice guideline. Young age (younger than 3 years) and associated medical problems were found in most papers to define the highest risk groups. High preoperative RDI also seems to be a risk factor for postoperative complications. Time to onset of respiratory compromise appears to be brief, although McColley et al reported that 1 patient took 14 hours to manifest respiratory symptoms.

All in all, children with OSAS clearly seem to be at high risk of postoperative respiratory compromise, and increased vigilance in postoperative monitoring is warranted.

Nasal CPAP

Several papers report on the successful use of CPAP in childhood. In children, CPAP is usually used when adenotonsillectomy is unsuccessful or contraindicated rather than as a primary treatment. Thus, most cases in the above reports describe children with complicated OSAS who are not the target group for this practice guideline. For example, of 80 children reported by Waters et al, 70 had previous adenotonsillar surgery; the 10 who did not were younger than 6 months or had other significant medical conditions. Of 94 patients reported by Marcus et al, only 2 of 18 patients whose OSAS was idiopathic (ie, not associated with another predisposing cause) had not had previous adenotonsillectomy; 1 of these patients had cystic fibrosis. All of the patients described by Guilleminault et al (1995) were younger than 1 year. All of the patients described by Rains et al and by Guilleminault et al (1986) had under-

lying predisposing abnormalities. All of the subjects described by Tirosh et al had previous adenotonsillectomy. These studies do confirm, however, that CPAP is efficacious in children.

CONCLUSIONS

Prevalence of Childhood OSAS

Snoring is a common occurrence in childhood, with reported prevalence between 3.2% and 12.1%. The prevalence of childhood OSAS is difficult to estimate, largely because published studies use different PSG criteria for its ascertainment. Reports range from 0.7% to 10.3%.

Sequelae of Childhood OSAS

Childhood OSAS is associated with several important sequelae and complications for which prevalence is unclear because of a lack of population-based cohort studies.

Neurobehavioral Complications

Cross-sectional studies suggest a nearly threefold increase in behavior problems and neurocognitive abnormalities in children with sleep-disordered breathing. Most of these studies did not definitively differentiate children with PS from those with OSAS, so the true prevalence of behavior and learning problems in children with OSAS versus PS is not clear.

Growth Inhibition

No systematic studies exist, but case series suggest that growth (especially weight gain) accelerates after surgery for OSAS, even in children with preexisting obesity, so it appears that OSAS has an inhibitory effect on growth. One study suggests that this effect is attributable to increased metabolic expenditures associated with OSAS.

Cardiovascular Complications

Cor pulmonale, right ventricular dysfunction, and pulmonary hypertension all have been reported in case reports and series, but their prevalence is unknown. These appear to be reversible after adenotonsillectomy. Systemic hypertension is a known complication of adult OSAS, and elevated diastolic blood pressure has been found in children with OSAS.

Diagnosis of OSAS

Overnight Polysomnography

The gold standard for diagnosis of OSAS is overnight PSG performed in a sleep lab. Methodologic standards and population-based normal ranges have recently been published, so although older published studies reflect a problem of variability in methods and interpretation, this has diminished in recent years. However, current normative standards for PSG determination of OSAS have been chosen on the basis of statistical distribution of data, and it has not been established that those standards have any validity as predictors of the occurrence of complications. Nonetheless, at the very least, it appears that the severity of PSG abnormality is an important predictor of complications in the immediate postoperative period after adenotonsillectomy.

Alternatives to PSG

Clinical evaluation, including the use of questionnaires such as the one published by Brouillette et al, has unacceptably low sensitivity and specificity for predicting OSAS. The use of home audiotaping and videotaping to supplement the clinical evaluation has been inadequately investigated. Additional studies are necessary before any statements about their validity can be made. Pulse oximetry and nap PSG appear to have high specificity and low sensitivity, meaning that positive test results are probably true, but negative test results would need to be confirmed using overnight PSG. The comparability of the results of home and sleep laboratory overnight PSG appears good, but additional study using commercially available equipment in a representative population is necessary for confirmation.

Treatment of OSAS

On the basis of case series that were reported with variable rigor, it appears that adenotonsillectomy is curative in 75% to 100% of children, even if the children are obese. The role of adenoidectomy alone is unclear. Postoperatively, children should be retested for OSAS if they continue to snore and possibly if the preoperative AHI was high. Children with OSAS clearly seem to be at high risk of postoperative respiratory compromise, and increased vigilance in postoperative monitoring is warranted, particularly in those with a high preoperative RDI. CPAP is effective in children, but it is usually used when adenotonsillectomy is delayed, contraindicated, or unsuccessful rather than as a primary treatment.

Concussion in Sports

· ·

The following guideline for evaluation and treatment of concussion in sports, developed by the American Orthopaedic Society for Sports Medicine, has been endorsed by the American Academy of Pediatrics.

0363-5465/99/2727-0676$02.00/0
THE AMERICAN JOURNAL OF SPORTS MEDICINE, Vol. 27, No. 5
© 1999 American Orthopaedic Society for Sports Medicine

Current Concepts

Concussion in Sports*

Edward M. Wojtys,† MD, David Hovda, PhD, Greg Landry, MD, Arthur Boland, MD,
Mark Lovell, PhD, Michael McCrea, PhD, and Jeffrey Minkoff, MD

From the AOSSM Concussion Workshop Group, Rosemont, Illinois

This is a special report of the findings of the Concussion Workshop, sponsored by the AOSSM in Chicago in December 1997. Here follows a listing of the members of the workshop: Julian Bailes, MD, American Association of Neurological Surgeons; Arthur Boland, MD, AOSSM; Charles Burke III, MD, National Hockey League; Robert Cantu, MD, American College of Sports Medicine; Letha "Etty" Griffin, MD, National Collegiate Athletic Association; David Hovda, PhD, Neuroscientist, UCLA School of Medicine; Mary Lloyd Ireland, MD, American Academy of Orthopaedic Surgeons; James Kelly, MD, American Academy of Neurology; Greg Landry, MD, American Academy of Pediatrics; Mark Lovell, PhD, Neuropsychology Specialist, Henry Ford Health Systems; James Mathews, MD, American College of Emergency Physicians; Michael McCrea, PhD, Neuropsychology Specialist, Waukesha Memorial Hospital; Douglas McKeag, MD, American Medical Society for Sports Medicine; Dennis Miller, ATC, National Athletic Trainers Association; Jeffrey Minkoff, MD, AOSSM; Stephen Papadopoulus, MD, Congress of Neurological Surgeons; Elliott Pellman, MD, National Football League; Richard Quincy, MS, PT, ATC, Sports Physical Therapy, El Pomar Sports Center; Herbert Ross, DO, American Osteopathic Academy of Sports Medicine; Bryan Smith, MD, National Collegiate Athletic Association; and Edward Wojtys, MD, Workshop Chairman, AOSSM.

The views in this report do not necessarily represent the views of the entire group comprising the Concussion Workshop Group.

One of the most challenging problems faced by medical personnel responsible for the health care of athletes is the recognition and management of concussions.[40,53] Concussions can be defined as any alteration in cerebral function caused by a direct or indirect (rotation) force transmitted to the head resulting in one or more of the following acute signs or symptoms: a brief loss of consciousness, light-headedness, vertigo, cognitive and memory dysfunction, tinnitus, blurred vision, difficulty concentrating, amnesia, headache, nausea, vomiting, photophobia, or a balance disturbance. Delayed signs and symptoms may also include sleep irregularities, fatigue, personality changes, an inability to perform usual daily activities, depression, or lethargy. Although many concussions are mild, the range of injury is wide. Nevertheless, concussions are a form of traumatic brain injury.

In recent years, these injuries have captured many news headlines as several professional football and hockey players have retired because of the effects of concussions. Interestingly, depending on the nature of the sport and the type (for example, rotation) and degree of contact expected, these injuries are many times viewed as just "part of the game." While many of these injuries are minor, some can be quite serious, with long-term consequences. Therefore, early detection through a thorough knowledge of the signs and symptoms and specific documentation of the injury is critical to the management of concussion and the monitoring of the natural history of the injury.[36,40] Unfortunately, attempts to characterize and classify the spectrum of concussions by stratifying the signs and symptoms as indicators of relative severity have been difficult.[7,10] Yet the need to accurately diagnose the severity of these injuries is obvious, especially at the time of injury when the triage decision could be critical to the patient's future. Returning an injured athlete to competition when the brain needs time to recover is an obvious concern. One of the reasons for concern is the second-impact syndrome,[24,29,52,59] a rare but ominous consequence of an untimely blow to a vulnerable central nervous system. While recent reviews cast a shadow of doubt on the occurrence and frequency,[51] the catastrophic nature of these events requires its consideration in the evaluation and treatment of concussions. Also, the cumulative effects of repeated injuries, even mild injuries, over time remains a serious concern to those involved in sports medicine.[15] The fact that some athletes do not recover as

* Address correspondence and reprint requests to Edward M. Wojtys, MD, University of Michigan, MedSport, Domino Farms, POB 363, Ann Arbor MI 48106.

No author or related institution has received financial benefit from research in this study. See "Acknowledgment" for funding information.

expected from concussions and are hampered by persistent symptoms for weeks or months is troublesome. In 1999, a complete understanding of the pathobiology of cerebral concussion is still lacking,[66] as is an explanation as to why the brain of some athletes may become so vulnerable to secondary injury after a seemingly mild insult.

Because of these lingering concerns, an American Orthopaedic Society for Sports Medicine-sponsored Concussion Workshop was held in December 1997 to assemble representatives from the medical community who routinely diagnose and treat these injuries in athletes. Invited participants included health-care professionals who perform research on brain injuries, a variety of clinicians responsible for the care of the athlete, and representatives of organized contact sports (NFL, NHL, NCAA). These representatives met with the hope of defining areas of agreement and disagreement in the detection and management of concussion in sports.

Realizing that differences do exist among clinicians regarding the safety of return-to-play at various time points after concussion, defining areas of disagreement was also a goal of the concussion workshop so that these differences could be subjected to discussion and investigation. Lastly, participants focused on the key elements of the initial evaluation of concussion so that data collection, future studies, and follow-up reports could benefit from the use of common terminology and evaluation tools.

NEUROBIOLOGY OF CEREBRAL CONCUSSION: WHY IS THE BRAIN SO VULNERABLE AFTER A CONCUSSION?

Cerebral concussion has been and continues to be defined primarily in neurologic terms related to an altered state of consciousness and to neuropsychologic variables associated with transient (or lasting) deficits in cognition and various other symptoms. Unfortunately, at this time there are no objective neuroanatomic or physiologic measurements that can be used to determine if a patient has sustained a concussion or to assess the severity of the insult. Neurologic and neurophysiologic studies have gone to great lengths to garner measurement instruments through an understanding of traumatic brain injury unconsciousness and the corresponding cognitive disruption that is associated with concussion.[15,17,38,41,54] These studies have provided information regarding the clinical indications of the degree of severity while highlighting the incident rate of minor head injury in sporting activities. However, at present, we lack a complete understanding of the pathobiology of cerebral concussion and an explanation of why, after a seemingly mild insult, the brain may become so vulnerable to secondary injury in some patients.

Essential to this discussion is the fact that during the minutes to few days after concussion injury, brain cells that are not irreversibly destroyed remain alive but exist in a vulnerable state. This concept of injury-induced vulnerability has been put forth to describe the fact that patients suffering from head injury are extremely vulnerable to the consequences of even minor changes in cerebral blood flow and/or increases in intracranial pressure and apnea.[13,24,53] In animal models of head injury, experiments have indicated that up to 3 days after either a concussion or a cerebral contusion, a reduction in cerebral blood flow, which would normally be well tolerated, now produces extensive neuronal cell loss.[29,30,42,43,63] Although not understood in terms of its underlying cellular mechanism, this concept of injury-induced vulnerability is a major concern in the management of all patients with head injuries and is not confined to second-impact syndrome.[13]

Experimental studies have identified metabolic dysfunction as the key postconcussion physiologic event that produces and maintains this state of vulnerability. This period of enhanced vulnerability is characterized by both an increase in the demand for glucose (fuel) and an inexplicable reduction in cerebral blood flow (fuel delivery).[58] The result is an inability of the neurovascular system to respond to increasing demands for energy to reestablish its normal chemical and ionic environments. This is dangerous because these altered environments can kill brain cells.

This initial injury-induced increase in the demand for glucose is primarily the response of cells activating sodium-potassium pumps.[1,33,72] This increased demand for energy occurs immediately on injury as brain cells are exposed to a massive ionic flux, including the resultant increased levels of extracellular potassium ($[K^+]_e$).[32] The $[K^+]_e$ elevation is linked to the stimulation of excitatory amino acid receptors since it can be drastically attenuated by blocking glutamatergic receptors before injury.[31] Furthermore, this injury-induced increase in $[K^+]_e$ activates ATP-dependent sodium-potassium pumps, resulting in a tremendous metabolic stress to already damaged neural tissue.[33,72]

The acute increase in glycolytic energy demand after traumatic brain injuries has been demonstrated experimentally, both in animals[2,25,27,33,71,72] and in severely injured patients.[5] In addition, this injury-induced increase in glucose metabolism has been shown to occur in the presence of low cerebral blood flow.[55,69,70,73] These findings provide compelling evidence that the ratio between the use of fuel (glucose) and fuel delivery (cerebral blood flow) is out of balance. Moreover, in studies using animals, this mismatch between glucose demand and fuel availability can be seen after mild concussion brain injury.[26,32] From these studies it appears that in virtually all types and severity of head injuries, the dramatic increase in glucose metabolism during the first minutes to days after injury is a fundamental part of a cellular pathophysiologic cascade seen after cerebral concussion. Correlating these cellular changes to clinical manifestations is a continuous challenge for researchers and clinicians alike.

The increase in cerebral glucose metabolism after human head injury has been demonstrated recently in severe head injuries.[5] Using positron-emission tomography for assessing the local cerebral metabolic rate for glucose (intracerebral metabolic rate glucose [ICMRglu], measured in milligrams per 100 grams per minute), the ICMRglu is markedly increased during the first few days after head injury, with evidence of increases lasting up to 1 week. This is all part of a disturbance in metabolic autoregulation that includes the experimentally proven increase in glucose metabolism and the relative reduction in cerebral blood flow seen in some concussion patients. In an attempt to establish a theory of prognostication, it is of value to note that outcomes in animal studies vary with the rate of cerebral blood flow recovery. Unfortunately, the acute increase in glucose metabolism in some patients is associated with a relative reduction in cerebral blood flow.[60] However, as in animal studies, the patients with the greatest degree and rate of cerebral blood flow recovery achieve the best outcome. Given the experimental data described, it is not surprising that the duration of reduced cerebral blood flow is an important prognostic factor in the outcome of patients with head injury. Consequently, the sustained reduction in cerebral blood flow due to the loss of metabolic autoregulation can potentiate the adverse effects of subsequent injuries, leading to more pronounced neural degeneration and a worse outcome.

Interestingly, there appears to be a strong relationship between the concentration of Ca^{2+} and regional control of cerebral blood flow and, in fact, a close association has been shown between the regions of the brain exhibiting Ca^{2+} flux and the area of reduced cerebral blood flow after traumatic brain injury. To better understand the altered physiology present, autoradiographic images of $^{45}Ca^{2+}$ have been compared with those obtained via $[^{14}C]$iodoantipyrine for the assessment of cerebral blood flow.[57] In rats, cerebral blood flow was measured at various times after fluid percussion ("closed-head") and cortical impact ("open-head") brain injuries.[14,42] These results indicated that for all cortical, hippocampal, and basal forebrain structures assessed, there were immediate decreases in cerebral blood flow that gradually resolved over 3 days. The magnitude in the reduction of cerebral blood flow was correlated with the amount of Ca^{2+} influx near the site of injury. This finding, coupled with the well-documented effect that Ca^{2+} channel blockers (nimodipine and dextromethorphan) have on the ability to increase cerebral blood flow under various brain injury conditions,[28,44,45,62] lend strong support to the contention that the reduction in cerebral blood flow after traumatic brain injury is due to the effect that Ca^{2+} has on cerebral blood flow.

The reduction in cerebral blood flow after traumatic brain injury is likely due to an increased vasoconstriction caused by endothelial accumulation of Ca^{2+}. Recently, several laboratories have reported that the elevation of extracellular Ca^{2+} potentiates the neurovascular constriction of central and peripheral arterioles.[19,22,64,65] These studies demonstrate that the twofold elevation of extracellular Ca^{2+} (from 2 to 4 mM) dramatically enhances the vasoconstriction induced by increased capillary pressure,[22] neuropeptide Y,[16] angiotensin II,[65] and endothelins.[65] Although the mechanism by which Ca^{2+} mediates vasoconstriction remains unknown, it appears to involve protein kinase C as an intermediate step.[65] Additional evidence derived from binding studies suggests that the levels of extracellular Ca^{2+} facilitate the extent of vaso-

constriction. These studies revealed high levels of L-type calcium channels in arteriole branch points.[19]

Whatever the mechanism, it is now quite clear that although cerebral concussion may not, in and of itself, produce extensive neuroanatomic damage, the surviving cells are placed in a state of vulnerability. This vulnerability is perhaps best characterized in terms of a metabolic dysfunction. The cascade of events leading to this dysfunction is multidimensional, resulting initially in acute periods of hyperglycolysis, followed by a more chronic period of metabolic depression. However, in general terms, this dysfunction may be thought of as a breakdown in the harmony between energy demand, production, and delivery.

The fact that this energy crisis exists after severe head injury is now documented.[5] However, the critical question for sports medicine is, does this metabolic alteration occur with lesser degrees of injury in humans and, if so, how long does the crisis last? Only a few experiments have addressed this question.[12,23] Work with a cerebral concussion model in the rodent indicates that a state of metabolic dysfunction can last for as long as 10 days. Whether this period correlates with the period of cellular vulnerability in man or with the results of neuropsychologic testing is not yet known, nor is it clear that the time frame would be similar in man.

When comparing head injury-induced pathophysiology in animals to what is seen clinically, the time course of events appears to be longer in human patients. This is particularly true for changes in cerebral metabolism and alterations in extracellular neurochemistry. For example, cerebral hyperglycolysis has been observed for as long as 2 weeks after human head injury, with the subsequent metabolic depression being present for over 1 year. In contrast, experimental studies using animals rarely report hyperglycolysis after 6 hours, and the recovery from metabolic depression typically occurs within a few weeks. As already reviewed, these physiologic changes after cerebral concussion play an important role in terms of cellular vulnerability. Consequently, when trying to estimate the length of time after clinical concussion during which the brain is vulnerable, extrapolation from animal studies will most likely result in estimates that are too short.

INITIAL EVALUATION—ANTICIPATION, AWARENESS, PREPARATION

The goal of this workshop section on initial evaluation was to define and prioritize the steps that should be taken by medical personnel responding to an athlete who has sustained a potential concussion. The evaluation process has been subdivided into those measures that should be addressed on the playing field, when an athlete is down, and those that can be performed on the sideline after the player has either been removed from the playing surface or has come off the field independently.

On-the-Field Evaluation

The most important objective of on-the-field evaluation is to make an accurate and complete diagnosis of the level of consciousness and to rule out the presence of significant associated injuries, especially to the cervical spine. Those responsible for the care of athletic teams must have a plan formulated in advance that should include a routine protocol for assessing athletes with head injuries. This should include the presence of adequately trained personnel, appropriate equipment, and an emergency back-up plan to evacuate a critically injured player safely and promptly, should it become necessary. Medical personnel must review these procedures before the season and be assured that all responsible persons understand the routine.

Medical personnel must understand the mechanisms of head injury, realizing that concussions may occur either by direct contact of the head against a hard surface or from sudden rotational or shear forces transmitted to the brain. Rapid acceleration or deceleration of the head and neck from a whiplash type of force can be as harmful as direct contact with a hard surface. Whereas a brief attempt to determine the mechanism of injury is advisable, prolonged questioning about the mechanism should not delay the initial assessment on the field. When approaching a player who is injured, observing the posture of the athlete and noting any spontaneous motion or verbalization from the player is the first step. Total lack of motion in the extremities should always alert those at the scene to the potential for a cervical spine injury. Incoherent speech would suggest a significant concussion. The player's helmet should not be removed initially unless a cervical spine injury can be ruled out. The face guard may require removal in emergent situations.

The ABCs of Evaluation. The respondents' initial obligation is to determine whether the injured player is breathing spontaneously, has an unobstructed airway, and has a pulse. Second, medical personnel should quickly determine whether further evaluation on the sidelines is appropriate or whether emergent transport to a hospital is needed. For the cardiovascular assessment, the carotid and radial pulses are usually the most accessible. If the patient has an adequate airway, respiration, and pulse, the initial assessment of the level of consciousness should be performed in the position in which the athlete lies. If the player is unconscious, one must assume that the athlete has an associated cervical spine injury until proven otherwise.

In the absence of a pulse and adequate respiration, the neck should be stabilized by an experienced person. With the assistance of two or three trained personnel, the athlete may then be log-rolled into a supine position so that cardiopulmonary resuscitation can be initiated effectively.

Athletes with closed-head injuries frequently have a blank expression, may appear confused, exhibit delayed verbal responses, and seem emotionally labile. The standard method of assessing the level of consciousness is by establishing a Glasgow Coma Scale[57] rating (Table 1). By observing the patient's eyes and motor and verbal responses, one can quantify the level of consciousness. A Glasgow Coma Scale of 11 or higher is usually associated with an excellent prognosis for recovery. On the other hand, a Glasgow Coma Scale of 7 or less is considered very serious.

TABLE 1
Glasgow Coma Scale[a]

Response	Point/s	Action
Eye opening		
Spontaneously	4	Reticular activity system is intact; patient may not be aware
To verbal command	3	Opens eyes when told to do so
To pain	2	Opens eyes in response to pain
None	1	Does not open eyes to any stimuli
Verbal		
Oriented, converses	5	Relatively intact CNS; aware of self and environment
Disoriented, converses	4	Well articulated, organized, but disoriented
Inappropriate words	3	Random, exclamatory words
Incomprehensible	2	Moaning, no recognizable words
No response	1	No response or intubated
Motor		
Obeys verbal commands	6	Readily moves limbs when told to
Localizes to painful stimuli	5	Moves limb in an effort to avoid pain
Flexion withdrawal	4	Pulls away from pain in flexion
Abnormal flexion	3	Decorticate rigidity
Extension	2	Decerebrate rigidity
No response	1	Hypotonic, flaccid: suggests loss of medullary function or concomitant cord injury

[a] Normal, 15.

The athlete's orientation to time, place, and person should be determined by asking the date, month, day of the week, the score, the period of the game, or the play in which he or she was injured. It is also important to establish the presence of retrograde amnesia, which is associated with a more significant injury. This can be done by asking about events earlier in the day, such as what was consumed for breakfast, how the athlete traveled to the game, or the location of the locker room. The presence of symptoms such as dizziness, blurring of vision, and head or neck pain should be noted before moving the patient.

When an associated cervical spine injury has been ruled out and the level of confusion and orientation has improved to the point where the athlete can understand and follow commands, the patient may be assisted into a sitting position. This position will often decrease intracranial pressure and help to relieve the patient's confusion and apprehension. Keep the patient in the sitting position until you are satisfied that the symptoms are improving and that the athlete has adequate strength, coordination, and orientation to follow instructions. At this point, the athlete may be assisted into the standing position with people on either side for support. If the athlete is unsteady in the upright position, it is safer to remove him or her from the field seated in a motorized cart or on a stretcher. However, if the athlete does have adequate strength and coordination, he or she can be assisted from the field, being sure there are people on either side for assistance, if necessary.

On-the-Bench Evaluation

When a player with a head injury is brought to the sidelines, he or she should be thoroughly evaluated in a routine manner to further define the level of injury. This should include a review of symptoms, a careful neurologic examination, and neuropsychologic testing. Players with concussion are frequently confused, irritable, and, at times, even combative. They frequently ask to be left alone. It is preferable to take the player to a quiet spot on the sidelines near the end of the bench or into the locker room. The player should be questioned about the symptoms of dizziness, light-headedness, vertigo, blurring or double vision, photophobia, ringing in the ears, headache, nausea, and vomiting. Many of these symptoms may be present initially after an acute head injury, while headache, nausea, and vomiting may not become evident for several minutes after the precipitating trauma. Vomiting is not very common after athletic injuries, but when it is present, it suggests a significant injury with elevated intracranial pressure and should be cause for concern.

The initial clinical examination should also include careful inspection and palpation of the head and neck followed by a careful neurologic evaluation. A baseline evaluation is important to accurately appreciate any changing clinical signs and symptoms in a deteriorating situation. In all contact injuries to the head or facial region, particularly those in which a helmet is not worn, the scalp, skull, and facial bones should be palpated, in search of lacerations and tenderness. If there is a laceration, it should be cleansed and then inspected carefully with a sterile glove for crepitus, which is indicative of an underlying skull fracture. The periorbital, mandibular, and maxillary areas should be carefully palpated after blunt trauma. Having an athlete open and close the mouth and clench the teeth will often lead to detection of a malocclusion or pain secondary to a mandibular fracture. The nose should also be observed for deformity and palpated for crepitus and tenderness in facial injuries. The presence of clear fluid around the nose (rhinorrhea) is indicative of a skull fracture in the cribriform plate region.

The neurologic examination should include a careful eye examination. About 3% of the population has one pupil larger than the other (anisocoria). This should have been detected on a preparticipation physical examination and the information should be available in the athlete's record. A direct blow to the face can result in a unilateral dilation of the pupil due to sympathetic nerve response. Serious head injuries, such as a skull fracture or subdural hematoma, may damage the third cranial nerve (oculomotor), but this is generally evident later in the clinical course. It is, therefore, essential to have a baseline evaluation of the size and symmetry of the pupils to appreciate subsequent changes that may result from increasing intracranial pressure. Visual acuity (ability to read small print), visual fields, extraocular motion, the level of the eyes (asymmetric with infraorbital blow-out fracture), and the presence of nystagmus should be part of the initial assessment. Nystagmus may be seen after a sudden rotational or shearing injury to the brain stem. It may be transient and is most frequently detected by the initial observer. A baseline evaluation of the 7th cranial nerve (facial) is also essential because paralysis of the 7th nerve may be the result of a basilar skull fracture, resulting in increasing intracranial pressure. The tympanic membrane should be visualized while looking for a spinal fluid leak (otorrhea) from a fracture in the petrous region of the temporal bone. Bleeding behind the tympanic membrane may be seen with skull fractures. Ecchymosis posterior to the ear over the mastoid region (Battle's sign) is a subsequent finding indicative of skull fractures in the posterior region of the head.

The cervical spinous processes and the brachial plexus in the supraclavicular region should be palpated. Pain with movement or tenderness warrants further assessment. Even though neck pain is common after head injuries, radiographic examination of the cervical spine is indicated in the presence of pain and tenderness.

Upper extremity strength should be thoroughly assessed, including the rotator cuff muscles, biceps, triceps, deltoid, wrist extensors and flexors, and the intrinsic muscles. Sensation in the arms and legs should be tested, and a baseline Hoffman test performed. Functional lower extremity strength and coordination can be evaluated by observing the athlete while standing, toe and heel walking, and squatting. Coordination can be evaluated by the finger-nose test, tandem walking, and the Romberg test.

On the sidelines, neuropsychologic testing can be performed to document defects in orientation, concentration, and memory. Orientation and retrograde amnesia are usually evaluated on the field. If the player has come off the field under his or her own power and was not examined on the field, these functions should be assessed immediately. Memory can be tested by asking the player to recall three words or three objects at 0 and 5 minutes. Detailed concentration can be evaluated by asking the player to repeat three, four, and five digits backward, to recite the months of the year in reverse order, or to do serial 7s. Knowledge of the player's capabilities through preseason testing is usually necessary in evaluating cognitive performance.

A player should be initially observed for a minimum of 15 minutes on the sidelines and reevaluated as needed. If any symptoms develop, the athlete should not return to competition that day. If the player has not lost consciousness, is oriented, and is asymptomatic, provocative testing should be performed next to determine whether symptoms will occur with physical stress. A 40-yard dash, five sit-ups, five push-ups, or five deep knee bends are usually adequate to increase intracranial pressure. Having the patient recline supine with the feet elevated for several seconds may also increase intracranial pressure sufficiently to cause symptoms. If there are any symptoms after these maneuvers, the player should not be allowed to return to play.

If a player is asymptomatic and returns to the game, it is essential that the athlete be reevaluated repeatedly during the contest to detect any change in clinical course. These subsequent evaluations are preferably performed by the same person who performed the initial examination. It is also helpful to communicate to the player the importance of being extremely honest about symptoms, realizing that many players will deny symptoms to be able to return to competition. The seriousness of the second-impact syndrome and postconcussion syndrome should be explained to the player before he or she is allowed to return to competition. A conservative approach would be to not allow the athlete who has had a head injury back into the game because of the potential risk.

NEUROPSYCHOLOGIC ASSESSMENT OF THE ATHLETE

Although the majority of athletes who experience a concussion are likely to recover completely, an unknown number of these athletes may experience chronic cognitive sequelae. In some cases, these difficulties can be permanent and disabling. At the current time, there are no curative medical treatments for concussion and the best approach to management of concussion emphasizes early recognition of postconcussion symptoms and prevention of additional concussion injury. While most clinicians are aware of the fact that suffering a second blow to the head while symptomatic from a previous concussion can have severe consequences, as in the case of second-impact syndrome,[34] many may not realize that concussions can lead to impairment of cognitive processes, mood, and behavior.[46]

If preinjury evaluations have been performed, neuropsychologic testing may be the most sensitive method of detecting postconcussive dysfunction. These test instruments are sensitive to even subtle changes in attention, concentration, memory, information processing, and motor speed or coordination.[46] Unlike other neurodiagnostic procedures that provide information on brain structure, such as computed tomography or magnetic resonance imaging, neuropsychologic testing provides information on the athlete's functional status. Unfortunately, traditional comprehensive approaches to neuropsychologic assessment that involve hours of testing are not applicable to the evaluation of large groups of athletes and are cost-prohibitive for most teams.

However, the usefulness of neuropsychologic assessment in clinical decision-making should not be short-changed. The use of shortened neuropsychologic assessment procedures in organized athletics may lead to the resolution of a number of important clinical issues. In particular, the long-term impact of multiple concussions in athletes needs further clarification and may be successfully investigated through the longitudinal systematic neuropsychologic evaluation of athletes. The study of athletes who participate in contact sports provides an excellent opportunity to create baselines of cognitive function and to longitudinally investigate the single or cumulative effects of mild concussions. These studies may eventually lead to the development of more sensitive evaluation strategies and more effective treatment programs.

Baseline Neuropsychologic Assessment of the Athlete

The approach used by the Pittsburgh Steelers since 1993 is based on the University of Virginia study[47] and involves the systematic testing of the athlete at set times before and after a suspected concussion. This approach involves the formal evaluation of each player before the beginning of the season to provide the basis for comparison, in the event of a concussion during the season. Testing is then repeated within 24 hours after a suspected concussion, and again approximately 5 days after the injury.

If neuropsychologic testing is going to be used to evaluate the athlete with concussion, preseason baseline evaluation of the athletes is recommended whenever possible for several reasons. First, individual players vary tremendously with regard to their level of performance on tests of memory, attention, concentration, mental processing speed, and motor speed. Therefore, without the benefit of knowing how players perform before suffering a concussion, it is very difficult to determine whether any testing deficits are due to the effects of that concussion or are secondary to other factors that have nothing to do with the concussion. Some players may perform poorly on the more demanding tests because of preinjury learning disabilities, attention deficit disorder, or other factors such as test-taking anxiety. Since similar patterns of cognitive difficulties may be observed after a concussion, if the player has not been evaluated before the concussion, there is no sure way of determining whether the deficits predated the injury. Additionally, if the player has a history of previous concussions, it may not be clear whether the postconcussion assessment is identifying cognitive difficulties that are secondary to a recent concussion or to a previous event.[3]

Important Characteristics of the Neuropsychologic Evaluation

It is very important to emphasize that the neuropsychologic tests that are selected for the evaluation of athletes must be carefully constructed and researched before their actual clinical use. Each test should be thoroughly researched with regard to the reliability (the extent to which the test produces uniform results) and validity (the extent to which the test accurately measures what it is supposed to measure). Whenever possible, tests should be used that have multiple equivalent forms to limit the impact of practice effects due to repeated exposure to the tests.

Timeline for the Evaluation of the Athlete with Concussion

The initial evaluation of the athlete with concussion begins on the playing field and should continue until symptoms have completely resolved. When formal neuropsychologic evaluations of the athlete are performed, they should take place within 24 hours of the suspected concussion, whenever possible. Many athletes who have suffered very mild concussions may appear to be symptom-free by this time, but a neuropsychologic evaluation to determine more subtle aspects of cognitive functioning can be very revealing, even if the player denies persistent difficulties. If the athlete displays any deficits on neuropsychologic testing, a follow-up evaluation should be undertaken within 48 hours. The interval of 5 days represents a useful and practical follow-up interval. Currently, research is underway that should better clarify the expected recovery curve for athletes with different severity levels.

Neuropsychologic Assessment Instruments

A large number of neuropsychologic test instruments have been successfully employed for the assessment of sports-related brain injuries. The selection of these test instruments has generally followed the previous application of these tests with brain-injured nonathletes. Limitations regarding the time that is typically available for the evaluation of athletes has also been an important factor in the selection and use of neuropsychologic assessment with athletes.

The tests listed here have been found to be useful in the assessment of sports-related head injury. This is a limited list of tests that are currently in use at both the professional and college levels that have been shown to have predictive use. Computerized versions of neuropsychologic tests are now under development and should result in increased access to testing by sports medicine physicians in the near future.

The current test procedures are the Trail making test, Parts A and B[56]; Stroop test[18]; Digit span from the Wechsler Memory Scale, Revised[68]; Symbol Digit modalities test[61]; Controlled oral word association test[4]; Hopkins verbal learning test[6]; Letter and number sequencing from Wechsler Memory Scale—III[67]; Grooved pegboard test[39]; and Ruff's Figural Fluency test.[47]

STANDARDIZED ASSESSMENT OF CONCUSSION: SIDELINE EVALUATION OF THE ATHLETE

The Standardized Assessment of Concussion (SAC) (Appendix 1) was developed to establish a valid, standardized, systematic sideline evaluation for the immediate assessment of concussion in athletes.[36] An objective quantifiable initial assessment of the injury is essential to evaluating a player's readiness to return to competition.[54] Close observation and reliable clinical assessment of the injured athlete are thought to be critical to the prevention of a more serious or catastrophic brain injury,[35,53,59] second-impact syndrome,[8] or cumulative neuropsychologic impairment.[20,31] Clinicians point out that it is often difficult to assess athletes without objective test measures because of the subtlety of concussion symptoms and a tendency on the part of the injured player to deny symptoms to be able to return to play.[40] The importance of objectively assessing orientation, concentration, and memory as part of the

on-field mental status examination of athletes suspected of having suffered concussion has been emphasized.[11,36]

The Standardized Assessment of Concussion

The SAC[50] was developed in line with the neuropsychologic research documenting the impairment that occurs with concussions.[9] The SAC includes measures of orientation, immediate memory, concentration, and delayed recall. The SAC was intended to be a standardized means of objectively documenting the presence and severity of neurocognitive impairment associated with concussion to provide immediate information to athletic trainers and other medical personnel responsible for clinical decision-making in the care of athletes. The SAC is not, however, intended as a substitute for formal clinical or neuropsychologic evaluation of the injured athlete, although correlations will be drawn between the result of the SAC and the latter.

The SAC takes approximately 5 minutes to administer and is designed for use by a nonneuropsychologist with no prior expertise in psychometric testing. Three alternate forms (A, B, and C) of the SAC were designed to allow for follow-up testing of injured players with minimal practice effects to track postconcussion recovery. The SAC is printed on pocket-sized cards for convenient use by athletic trainers and other medical personnel on the sideline.

Orientation is assessed by asking the subject to provide the day of the week, month, year, and time of day to within 1 hour. A five-word list is used to measure immediate memory; the list is read to the subject for immediate recall and the procedure is repeated for three trials. Concentration is tested by having the subject repeat, in reverse order, strings of digits that increase in length from three to six numbers. Reciting the months of the year in reverse order is also used to assess concentration. Delayed recall of the original five-word list is also assessed. A composite total score is computed to derive an index of the subject's overall level of impairment after concussion.

Research efforts have focused on use of the SAC with high school and college football players because of the relatively high incidence rate of concussion at these levels (Ref. 37; J. Powell, personal communication, 1998). The results of separate studies in 1995[48] and 1996[49] support the clinical use of the SAC in the evaluation of concussion in football players. In those studies, athletic trainers administered the SAC to 568 normal, noninjured high school and college players before the start of the football season and immediately after concussion of any player during the 1995 and 1996 football seasons. Research findings revealed that 33 players suspected of having sustained a concussion scored statistically significantly below the group of normal, noninjured players on the SAC. Further analysis revealed that players with concussion, as a group, also scored significantly below their own normal baseline in terms of the SAC total score. On average, players with concussion dropped 3.5 points (maximum of 30) from preinjury baseline, which falls 1.48 SDs below their own mean and 1.58 SDs below the normal mean for the control group, indicating that the SAC total score appears to be sensitive in detecting cognitive defects in the injured players that were tested. These injuries were initially classified by athletic trainers as mild concussions without observable evidence of significant neurologic dysfunction. The SAC demonstrated a preliminary, but useful, trend in tracking recovery from concussion. Follow-up testing on 28 of the 33 injured players indicated that all players had returned to baseline on all SAC measures within 48 hours.

In addition to SAC total score, each of the individual domains (orientation, immediate memory, concentration, and delayed recall) assessed as part of the SAC also yielded useful clinical information in recognizing the concussion, which may further our understanding of the immediate effects of mild forms of brain injury. Players with concussion scored significantly below normal controls on the orientation, immediate memory, concentration, and delayed recall sections of the SAC, despite the fact that none of the injured players were obviously disoriented or neurologically impaired. This finding suggests that the SAC may be able to detect subtle cognitive changes associated with concussion in the absence of other symptoms. Because all of the subjects with concussion in these studies[48,49] suffered what appeared to be mild injuries, further research is required to identify which SAC domain scores are most sensitive to change during injury and to characterize how orientation, concentration, and memory are affected in more severe forms of concussion.

An evaluation of the psychometric properties of the SAC showed no significant differences between scores of high school and college players, suggesting that age and education within the population studied have minimal effects on performance. There were no meaningful differences between forms A, B, and C of the SAC, thereby allowing for the reassessment of mental status and tracking recovery with minimal practice effects. There were no significant differences between examinations conducted during games or practice, suggesting that the emotion of athletic competition does not significantly confound test performance.

The important implication here is that baseline testing can be conducted during the off-season or preseason to establish a valid and reliable marker against which change associated with concussion can be detected. The finding that the average score for normal subjects fell 1.60 SDs below the ceiling and that only 7% of controls managed a perfect score of 30 on the SAC suggests that the instrument is reasonably free of significant ceiling effects. Collection of normal test-retest data on the SAC is underway to clarify the presence of any practice effects. The issue of interrater reliability is also being addressed by additional research, but is difficult to empirically assess. A number of factors are often encountered by brief screening instruments, including a limited range in scores by controls and the need for clinical data. These factors present problems because of the dynamic and unpredictable nature of concussion.

An important practical finding from research on the SAC is that athletic trainers thought that the instrument was convenient for use on the sideline during sporting events. A survey of several athletic trainers indicated that the SAC was easy to administer and score.

Research thus far on the SAC has involved comparing an injured player's score with his or her own preinjury baseline performance to detect change that is likely indicative of concussion. Further research is underway regarding the sensitivity, specificity, validity, and reliability of the SAC in detecting concussion when baseline data are not available for comparison. Sufficient data are not available at this point to determine if the SAC can be used clinically if baseline data are not available. Additional research is also being conducted on the clinical application of the SAC in assessing concussion in sports other than football, including soccer, hockey, lacrosse, and wrestling.

Empirical research data support the further testing of the SAC by medical personnel as an objective and quantifiable measure of the immediate neurocognitive effects of concussion. The SAC appears to be sensitive in evaluating athletes with concussion immediately after the injury and may be helpful in making decisions as to a player's readiness to return to play. The SAC is not, however, meant as a substitute for formal neurologic or neuropsychologic examination of the injured athlete. Rather, the SAC is intended to detect cognitive defects immediately so that further evaluation and proper management techniques can be implemented, if needed. Use of an objective, standardized mental status examination such as the SAC, in combination with a thorough clinical examination, may represent the most sensitive and informative approach to the sideline assessment of concussion. However, for the SAC to become an integral and unconditional component of the evaluation of an athlete with concussion, further statistical validation is necessary.

RECOMMENDATIONS FOR CONCUSSION WORK-UP AND RETURN TO PLAY

In general, if an athlete has any symptoms on the field that are related to a concussion, the athlete should not be allowed to continue to play. Additionally, athletes with concussions should always be evaluated by a physician before return to athletic play. Parameters for return to activity in the asymptomatic athlete should be the same for all sports, regardless of the degree of contact or use of protective equipment such as helmets. A small number of symptomatic athletes may require subsequent evaluation by a neurosurgeon or a neurologist because of persistent symptoms. Caution should always be exercised by the medical staff responsible for making return-to-play decisions because the athlete's motivation as well as peer or coaching pressure may be significant factors.

Most importantly, any athlete who is symptomatic after a concussion requires serial neurologic evaluations. These examinations should be performed, as needed, for as long as symptoms persist to determine if the athlete's condition is deteriorating. If a neurologic evaluation at any time reveals any deterioration in mental status or a loss of consciousness after a concussion, immediate transport to an appropriate emergency facility is indicated where a neurosurgeon or neurologist and diagnostic neuroimaging are available. No other abnormalities on the neurologic examination would be needed to warrant such emergent treatment.

When a concussion occurs, the athlete should be observed and evaluated for a minimum of 15 minutes. The medical personnel at the competition may allow the athlete to return to play if there was no loss of consciousness and all signs and symptoms are normal. If the athlete's symptoms do not abate during the initial 15 to 20 minutes of observation, the athlete should be disqualified from that day's competition. Only when the athlete is totally asymptomatic, passes memory and concentration tests, and has no symptoms after provocative testing, may the athlete be returned to play. Once the athlete has returned to competition, medical personnel should continue to observe and reexamine the athlete carefully for any signs that the athlete is not 100% recovered. The increased stress of competition may produce signs and symptoms that are not produced by the provocative maneuvers off the field. If the athlete is not 100% recovered, the athlete should be disqualified. This is especially important in sports where breaks in the action are infrequent and frequent reevaluations off the field are not possible.

Several clinical rules are important to keep in mind when evaluating athletes with concussion. Any observed period of unconsciousness is significant and should always preclude return to play. Even brief episodes of loss of consciousness are usually associated with other symptoms that will preclude play. While a brief loss of consciousness is only one factor to consider in the clinical evaluation, it should be evaluated in context with other signs and symptoms. As with any other injury, careful serial follow-up examinations are always recommended.

Return-To-Play Classifications

Return to Play (Same Day).
1. Signs and symptoms cleared within 15 minutes or less both at rest and exertion
2. Normal neurologic evaluation
3. No documented loss of consciousness
Delayed Return to Play (Not the Same Day).
1. Signs and symptoms did not clear in 15 minutes at rest or with exertion
2. Documented loss of consciousness
Any new headache in the first 48 to 72 hours after a concussion or an unusual headache should be considered a significant symptom and should preclude play; either is also an indication that further medical evaluation is needed. Caution should always be exercised in the younger athlete with headache, particularly a unilateral headache.

The other symptoms that should preclude play at any time are dizziness, slowness in responding to questions, evidence of difficulty concentrating, physical sluggishness, and memory loss, especially if there is a loss of memory of events before the injury (retrograde amnesia). Athletes who experience retrograde amnesia do not usually recover during the athletic contest. If the player has had any symptoms or difficulty with concentration tests,

that player should not return to play. While a loss of consciousness usually receives a lot of attention by those attending an injured athlete, a brief loss of consciousness, such as a matter of a couple of seconds during the time it takes medical personnel to reach the athlete on the playing surface, may not be as significant as other symptoms that do not clear in the first 15 minutes.

While some concussion scenarios present challenges to the clinician, there is no question about a symptomatic athlete's status: the athlete should not return to play. However, the clinical decisions become more difficult when symptoms clear after 20 to 30 minutes, after the game, or the next day. All of these situations should be classified as prolonged symptoms and are cause for concern. Unfortunately, at the present time, it is not known if neurocognitive function returns to normal when symptoms subside in humans. Therefore, it cannot be assumed that an athlete is normal when he or she "feels fine." The return to play for a young (for example, high school) athlete who experienced symptoms for longer than 15 minutes continues to be a difficult decision and represents a gray zone in the medical literature. Current medical knowledge does not adequately address this situation. While some athletes may benefit from 5 to 7 days of rest after experiencing initial symptoms in excess of 15 minutes,[59] others may be able to safely return to play much sooner.

Until neuropsychologic testing can be done on enough asymptomatic athletes in the first 48 hours after symptoms resolve, correlation between the absence of symptoms and neurocognitive function in humans cannot be drawn, and even if it could, it may still not mean the player is safe to return to play. Presently, the NHL is performing neuropsychologic testing on all players after concussion. The relationship between neurofunction and symptoms in this group of athletes may soon be known. However, these same correlative studies, between symptoms and cognitive function, will have to be repeated in all age ranges and athletic groups to determine the safety of a return to play. It is very important not to generalize the results of these correlative studies. What is medically acceptable in adults may not be safe in teenagers or adolescents. Further studies in the various age groups and sports will be needed to answer these clinical problems safely. Unfortunately, as far as we know, there are no ongoing studies in child or adolescent athletes such as those being conducted by the NHL and the NFL.

Recommendations

1. Every athlete with concussion should be evaluated by a physician.
2. Loss of consciousness precludes return to play that day.
3. Persistence of (longer than 15 minutes) or delayed onset of any symptoms such as headache, dizziness, malaise, slowness to respond mentally or physically at rest, or with provocation (supine with legs elevated) or with exercise precludes return to play that day.

4. Any deterioration in physical or mental status after the initial trauma, such as increasing headache, dizziness, or nausea, warrants immediate transport to an emergency facility where neurologic or neurosurgical consultation and neuroimaging are available.

5. When prolonged symptoms (greater than 15 minutes) are experienced after a concussion, great care must be exercised in returning an asymptomatic athlete to practice or competition. Without at least 5 to 7 days of rest, neurofunction may not yet be normal. Further research is needed to demonstrate the association, or lack of association, between symptoms, neurocognitive function, and injury susceptibility. Until this age-specific information is available, such decisions must be approached with great concern. Repeated examinations of the athlete are needed during a gradual increase in physical exertion to determine if these stresses trigger symptoms. If symptoms recur, the athlete is not ready to return to play. Current neuroscience knowledge in humans does not give a safe, firm timetable for return to play after concussion in most circumstances. Therefore, each athlete with prolonged symptoms (more than 15 minutes) must be evaluated individually. Repeated and thorough evaluations, preferably by the same clinician, are most helpful in determining readiness to play.

6. Newer tools, such as balance testing,[21] cannot be recommended for clinical decision-making after concussion at this time. However, their use for further data collection is encouraged. The balance test may prove to be a useful tool for identifying impairment associated with concussion.

7. We recommend further study of the SAC[48-50] as part of the initial evaluation of an athlete with concussion to gain experience with its use. Furthermore, wide-scale examination of this instrument is needed at all levels of competition and in different athletic groups. While recognizing its clinical potential, we believe it is premature to recommend its generalized use as the sole determinant of clinical decisions after concussion. We do recommend continued wide-scale clinical testing of this instrument.

8. We recognize the need for continued clinical and basic science research of sports-induced concussions. The clinical use of neuropsychologic assessments in the study of athletes has been limited by a current lack of research studies that have specifically investigated the use of these assessments in sports. We recommend the establishment of cooperative studies across athletic organizations at the junior, high school, college, and professional levels that would promote the longitudinal study of large groups of athletes.

9. We specifically promote the establishment of databases on all athletes with concussions. If similar neuropsychologic instruments are used at all levels, longitudinal analysis of test results for specific athletes will be possible as the athlete progresses from one level to the next. This type of information would be particularly useful to athletes, their families, and physicians to assess the risk of future injury and further difficulties.

ACKNOWLEDGMENT

This research was funded by a grant from the Foundation for Sports Medicine Education and Research, Rosemont, Illinois.

REFERENCES

1. Ackermann RF, Lear JL: Glycosis-induced discordance between glucose metabolic rates measured with radiolabeled fluorodeoxyglucose and glucose. *J Cereb Blood Flow Metab 9:* 774–785, 1989
2. Andersen BJ, Marmarou A: Post-traumatic selective stimulation of glycolysis. *Brain Res 585:* 184–189, 1992
3. Barth JT, Alves WM, Ryan TV, et al: Mild head injury in sports: Neuropsychological sequelae and recovery of function, in Levin HS, Eisenberg HM, Benton AL (eds): *Mild Head Injury.* New York, Oxford University Press, 1989, pp 257–275
4. Benton A, Hamsher K: *Multilingual Aphasia Examination.* Iowa City, University of Iowa Press, 1978
5. Bergsneider M, Hovda DA, Shalman E, et al: Cerebral hyperglycolysis following severe traumatic brain injury in humans: A positron emission tomography study. *J Neurosurg 86:* 241–251, 1997
6. Brandt J: The Hopkins verbal learning test: Development of a new memory test with six equivalent forms. *Clin Neuropsychology 5:* 125–142, 1991
7. Cantu RC: Guidelines for return to contact sports after cerebral concussion. *Physician Sportsmed 14:* 75–83, 1986
8. Cantu RC, Voy R: Second impact syndrome: A risk in any contact sport. *Physician Sportsmed 23(6):* 172–177, 1995
9. Capruso DX, Levin HS: Cognitive impairment following closed head injury. *Neurol Clin 10:* 879–893, 1992
10. Clifton GL, Hayes RL, Levin HS, et al: Outcome measures for clinical trials involving traumatically brain-injured patients: Report of a conference. *Neurosurgery 31:* 975–978, 1992
11. Colorado Medical Society. Report of the Sports Medicine Committee: *Guidelines for the Management of Concussion in Sports (Revised).* Denver, Colorado Medical Society, 1991
12. Cosgrove JW, Atack JR, Rapoport SI: Regional analysis of rat brain proteins during senescence. *Exp Gerontol 22:* 187–198, 1987
13. Doberstein CE, Hovda DA, Becker DP: Clinical considerations in the reduction of secondary brain injury. *Ann Emerg Med 22:* 993–997, 1993
14. Doberstein CE, Vlarde F, Badie H, et al: Changes in local cerebral blood flow following concussive brain injury [abstract]. *Soc Neurosci 18:* 175, 1992
15. Evans RW: The postconcussion syndrome: 130 years of controversy. *Semin Neurol 14:* 32–39, 1994
16. Fallgren B, Arlock P, Edvinsson L: Neuropeptide Y potentiates noradrenaline-evoked vasoconstriction by an intracellular calcium-dependent mechanism. *J Auton Nerv Syst 44:* 151–159, 1993
17. Fick DS: Management of concussion in collision sports: Guidelines for the sidelines. *Postgrad Med 97:* 53–56, 59–60, 1995
18. Golden CJ: *The Stroop Color and Word Test. A Manual for Clinical and Experimental Use.* Chicago, Stoelting, 1978
19. Goligorsky MS, Colflesh D, Gordienko D, et al: Branching points of renal resistance arteries are enriched in L-type calcium channels and initiate vasoconstriction. *Am J Physiol 268:* F251–F257, 1995
20. Gronwall D, Wrightson P: Cumulative effects of concussion. *Lancet 2:* 995–997, 1975
21. Guskiewicz KM, Riemann BL, Perrin DH, et al: Alternative approaches to the assessment of mild head injury in athletes. *Med Sci Sports Exerc 29 (7 Suppl):* S213–S221, 1997
22. Harder DR: Pressure-induced myogenic activation of cat cerebral arteries is dependent on intact endothelium. *Circ Res 60:* 102–107, 1987
23. Hovda DA: Metabolic dysfunction, in Narayan RK, Wilberger JE, Povlishock JT (eds): *Neurotrauma.* New York, McGraw Hill, 1995, pp 1459–1478
24. Hovda DA, Badie H, Karimi S, et al: Concussive brain injury produces a state of vulnerability for intracranial pressure perturbation in the absence of morphological damage, in Avezaat CJJ, Van Eijndhoven JHM, Maas AIR, et al (eds): *Intracranial Pressure VIII.* New York, Springer-Verlag, 1993, pp 469–472
25. Hovda DA, Katayama Y, Yoshino A, et al: Pre or postsynaptic blocking of glutamatergic functioning prevents the increase in glucose utilization following concussive brain injury, in Globus M, Dietrich WD (eds): *The Role of Neurotransmitters in Brain Injury.* New York, Plenum Press, 1992, pp 327–332
26. Hovda DA, Le HM, Lifshitz J, et al: Long-term changes in metabolic rates for glucose following mild, moderate and severe concussive head injuries in adult rats [abstract]. *J Neurosurg 376A,* 1995

27. Hovda DA, Yoshino A, Kawamata T, et al: The increase in local cerebral glucose utilization following fluid percussion brain injury is prevented with kynurenic acid and is associated with an increase in calcium. *Acta Neurochir Suppl 51*: 331–333, 1990

28. Jacewicz M, Brint S, Tanabe J, et al: Nimodipine pretreatment improves cerebral blood flow and reduces brain edema in conscious rats subjected to focal cerebral ischemia. *J Cereb Blood Flow Metab 10*: 903–913, 1990

29. Jenkins LW, Marmarou A, Lewelt W, et al: Increased vulnerability of the traumatized brain to early ischemia, in Baethmann A, Go GK, Unterberg A (eds): *Mechanisms of Secondary Brain Damage*. Wien, Springer, 1996, pp 273–282

30. Jenkins LW, Moszynski K, Lyeth BG, et al: Increased vulnerability of the mildly traumatized rat brain to cerebral ischemia: The use of controlled secondary ischemia as a research tool to identify common or different mechanisms contributing to mechanical and ischemic brain injury. *Brain Res 477*: 211–224, 1989

31. Jordan BD, Zimmerman RD: Computed tomography and magnetic resonance imaging comparison in boxers. *JAMA 263*: 1670–1674, 1990

32. Katayama Y, Becker DP, Tamura T, et al: Massive increases in extracellular potassium and the indiscriminate release of glutamate following concussive brain injury. *J Neurosurg 73*: 889–900, 1990

33. Kawamata T, Katayama Y, Hovda DA, et al: Administration of excitatory amino acid antagonists via microdialysis attenuates the increase in glucose utilization seen following concussive brain injury. *J Cereb Blood Flow Metab 12*: 12–24, 1992

34. Kelly J: Concussion, in Torg JS, Shephard RJ (eds): *Current Therapy in Sports Medicine*. Third edition. St. Louis, Mosby, 1995

35. Kelly JP, Nichols JS, Filley CM, et al: Concussion in sports: Guidelines for the prevention of catastrophic outcome. *JAMA 266*: 2867–2869, 1991

36. Kelly JP, Rosenberg J: Practice parameter: The management of concussion in sport: Report of the Quality Standards Subcommittee. *Neurology 48*: 581–585, 1997

37. Kelly JP, Rosenberg J: Diagnosis and management of concussion in sports. *Neurology 48*: 575–580, 1997

38. King NS, Crawford S, Wenden FJ, et al: The Riverhead Post Concussion Symptoms Questionnaire: A measure of symptoms commonly experienced after head injury and its reliability. *J Neurol 242*: 587–592, 1995

39. Klove H, Matthews C: Neuropsychological studies of patients with epilepsy, in *Clinical Neuropsychology: Current Status and Applications*, published by Hemisphere (available from Lafayette Instrument Co, Lafayette, Indiana), 1974

40. Landry G: Mild brain injury in athletes, in National Athletic Trainers Association Research and Education Foundation: *Proceedings from Mild Brain Injury Summit*. Washington, DC, April 16–18, 1994

41. Leblanc KE: Concussions in sports: Guidelines for return to competition. *Am Fam Physician 50*: 801–808, 1994

42. Lee SM, Lifshitz, J, Hovda DA, et al: Focal cortical-impact injury produces immediate and persistent deficits in metabolic autoregulation [abstract]. *J Cereb Blood Flow Metab 15*: 722, 1995

43. Lifshitz J, Pinanong P, Le HM, et al: Regional uncoupling of cerebral blood flow and metabolism in degenerating cortical areas following a lateral cortical contusion [abstract]. *J Neurotrauma 12*: 129, 1995

44. Lo EH, Steinberg GK: Effects of dextromethorphan on regional cerebral blood flow in focal cerebral ischemia. *J Cereb Blood Flow Metab 11*: 803–809, 1991

45. Lo EH, Sun GH, Steinberg GK: Effects of NMDA and calcium channel antagonists on regional cerebral blood flow. *Neurosci Lett 131*: 17–20, 1991

46. Lovell MR, Collins MW: Neuropsychological assessment of the college football player. *J Head Trauma Rehabil 13(2)*: 9–26, 1998

47. Macciocchi SN, Barth JT, Alves WM, et al: Neuropsychological functioning and recovery after mild head injury in collegiate athletes. *Neurosurgery 39*: 510–514, 1996

48. McCrea M, Kelly JP, Kluge J, et al: Standardized assessment of concussion in football players. *Neurology 48*: 586–588, 1997

49. McCrea M, Kelly JP, Randolph C, et al: Standardized assessment of concussion (SAC): On-site mental status evaluation of the athlete. *J Head Trauma Rehabil 13(2)*: 27–35, 1998

50. McCrea M, Kelly JT, Randolph C: *The Standardized Assessment of Concussion (SAC): Manual for administration, scoring, and interpretation.* Clinical Instrument and Manual published and distributed by Brain Injury Association (BIA), Washington, DC, 1997

51. McCrory PR, Berkovic SF: Second impact syndrome. *Neurology 50*: 677–683, 1998

52. McQuillen JB, McQuillen EN, Morrow P: Trauma, sports, and malignant cerebral edema. *Am J Forensic Med Pathol 9*: 12–15, 1988

53. Muizelaar JP: Cerebral blood flow, cerebral blood volume, and cerebral metabolism after severe head injury, in Becker DP, Gudeman SK (eds): *Textbook of Head Injury*. Philadelphia, WB Saunders, 1989, pp 221–240

54. Parkinson D: Evaluating cerebral concussion. *Surg Neurol 45*: 459–462, 1996

55. Pfenninger EG, Reith A, Breitig D, et al: Early changes of intracranial pressure, perfusion pressure, and blood flow after acute head injury. Part 1. An experimental study of the underlying pathophysiology. *J Neurosurg 70*: 774–779, 1989

56. Reitan R: Validity of the trail making test as an indicator of organic brain damage. *Percept Motor Skills 8*: 271–276, 1958

57. Rosen P, Barkin RM: *Emergency Medicine: Concepts of Clinical Practice.* Fourth edition. St. Louis, Mosby Year Book, 1998

58. Sakurada O, Kennedy C, Jehle J, et al: Measurement of local cerebral blood flow with iodo[14c] antipyrine. *Am J Physiol 234*: H59–H66, 1978

59. Saunders RL, Harbaugh RE: The second impact in catastrophic contact sports head trauma. *JAMA 252*: 538–539, 1984

60. Shalman E, Bergsneider M, Kelly DG, et al: Existence of regional coupling between cerebral blood flow and glucose metabolism following brain injury [abstract]. *J Neurotrauma 12*: 141, 1995

61. Smith A: *Symbol Digit Modalities Test Manual*. Los Angeles, Western Psychological Services, 1982

62. Steinberg GK, Lo EH, Kunis DM, et al: Dextromethorphan alters cerebral blood flow and protects against cerebral injury following focal ischemia. *Neurosci Lett 133*: 225–228, 1991

63. Sutton RL, Hovda DA, Adelson PD, et al: Metabolic changes following cortical contusion: Relationships to edema and morphological changes. *Acta Neurochir Suppl (Wien) 60*: 446–448, 1994

64. Tabrizchi R: Role of intracellular and extracellular calcium in alpha 1-adrenoceptor-mediated vasoconstriction in the rat perfused hindquarters. *Arch Int Pharmacodyn Ther 328*: 26–38, 1994

65. Takenaka T, Forster H, Epstein M: Protein kinase C and calcium channel activation as determinants of renal vasoconstriction by angiotensin II and endothelin. *Circ Res 73*: 743–750, 1993

66. Walker AE: The physiological basis of concussion: 50 years later [Commemorative Article]. *J Neurosurg 81*: 493–494, 1994

67. Wechsler D: *Wechsler Memory Scale—III*. Third edition. San Antonio, TX, Psychological Corporation, 1997

68. Wechsler D: *Wechsler Memory Scale-Revised Manual*. San Antonio, TX, Psychological Corporation, 1987

69. Yamakami I, McIntosh TK: Effects of traumatic brain injury on regional cerebral blood flow in rats as measured with radiolabeled microspheres. *J Cereb Blood Flow Metab 9*: 117–124, 1989

70. Yamakami I, Yamaura A, Makino H, et al: Effects of traumatic brain injury on regional cerebral blood flow and electroencephalogram [abstract]. *J Neurotrauma 7*: 101, 1990

71. Yoshino A, Hovda DA, Katayama Y, et al: Hippocampal CA3 lesion prevents postconcussive metabolic dysfunction in CA1. *J Cereb Blood Flow Metab 12*: 996–1006, 1992

72. Yoshino A, Hovda DA, Kawamata T, et al: Dynamic changes in local cerebral glucose utilization following cerebral concussion in rats: Evidence of a hyper- and subsequent hypometabolic state. *Brain Res 561*: 106–119, 1991

73. Yuan XQ, Prough DS, Smith TL, et al: The effects of traumatic brain injury on regional cerebral blood flow in rats. *J Neurotrauma 5*: 289–301, 1988

This work was endorsed by the following organizations: American Orthopaedic Society for Sports Medicine, American Academy of Orthopaedic Surgeons, American Academy of Pediatrics, American Osteopathic Academy for Sports Medicine, National Academy of Neuropsychology, and International Neuropsychological Society.

Appendix 1   The SAC form for evaluating concussion.

1. Orientation

Month: _____	0	1
Date: _____	0	1
Day of week: _____	0	1
Year: _____	0	1
Time (within 1 hr): _____	0	1

Orientation Total Score _____ / 5

2. Immediate Memory (all 3 trials are completed regardless of score on trial 1 & 2; total score equals sum across all 3 trials)

List	Trial 1	Trial 2	Trial 3
Word 1	0 1	0 1	0 1
Word 2	0 1	0 1	0 1
Word 3	0 1	0 1	0 1
Word 4	0 1	0 1	0 1
Word 5	0 1	0 1	0 1
Total			

Immediate Memory Total Score __ / 15

(Note: Subject is not informed of Delayed Recall testing of memory)

NEUROLOGICAL SCREENING:

Recollection if injury (pre- or post-traumatic amnesia)

Strength:

Sensation:

Coordination:

Loss of Consciousness:

3. Concentration

Digits Backward (If correct, go to next string length. If incorrect, read trial 2. Stop after incorrect on both trials.)

4-9-3	6-2-9 _____	0	1
3-8-1-4	3-2-7-9 _____	0	1
6-2-9-7-1	1-5-2-8-6 ____	0	1
7-1-8-4-6-2	5-3-9-1-4-8 ___	0	1

Months in reverse order (entire sequence correct for 1 point)
Dec-Nov-Oct-Sep-Aug-Jul
Jun-May-Apr-Mar-Feb-Jan ___   0   1

Concentration Total Score __ / 5

EXERTIONAL MANEUVERS:

(when appropriate):	
5 jumping jacks	5 push-ups
5 sit-ups	5 knee bends

4. Delayed Recall

Word 1	0	1
Word 2	0	1
Word 3	0	1
Word 4	0	1
Word 5	0	1

Delayed Recall Total Score __ / 5

Summary of Total Scores:

Orientation _____	/	5
Immediate Memory _____	/	15
Concentration _____	/	5
Delayed Recall _____	/	5
Overall Total Score _____	/	30

National Athletic Trainers' Association Position Statement: Lightning Safety for Athletics and Recreation

The following guideline for lightning safety for athletics and recreation, developed by the National Athletic Trainers' Association, has been endorsed by the American Academy of Pediatrics.

Journal of Athletic Training 2000;35(4):471–477
© by the National Athletic Trainers' Association, Inc
www.journalofathletictraining.org

National Athletic Trainers' Association Position Statement: Lightning Safety for Athletics and Recreation

Katie M. Walsh, EdD, ATC-L*; Brian Bennett, MEd, ATC†;
Mary Ann Cooper, MD‡; Ronald L. Holle, MS§; Richard Kithil, MBA¶;
Raul E. López, PhD§

*East Carolina University, Greenville, NC; †The College of William and Mary, Williamsburg, VA; ‡The University of Illinois at Chicago, Chicago, IL; §National Severe Storms Laboratory, Norman, OK; ¶The National Lightning Safety Institute, Louisville, CO

Objective: To educate athletic trainers and others about the dangers of lightning, provide lightning-safety guidelines, define safe structures and locations, and advocate prehospital care for lightning-strike victims.

Background: Lightning may be the most frequently encountered severe-storm hazard endangering physically active people each year. Millions of lightning flashes strike the ground annually in the United States, causing nearly 100 deaths and 400 injuries. Three quarters of all lightning casualties occur between May and September, and nearly four fifths occur between 10:00 AM and 7:00 PM, which coincides with the hours for most athletic or recreational activities. Additionally, lightning casualties from sports and recreational activities have risen alarmingly in recent decades.

Recommendations: The National Athletic Trainers' Association recommends a proactive approach to lightning safety, including the implementation of a lightning-safety policy that identifies safe locations for shelter from the lightning hazard. Further components of this policy are monitoring local weather forecasts, designating a weather watcher, and establishing a chain of command. Additionally, a flash-to-bang count of 30 seconds or more should be used as a minimal determinant of when to suspend activities. Waiting 30 minutes or longer after the last flash of lightning or sound of thunder is recommended before athletic or recreational activities are resumed. Lightning-safety strategies include avoiding shelter under trees, avoiding open fields and spaces, and suspending the use of land-line telephones during thunderstorms. Also outlined in this document are the prehospital care guidelines for triaging and treating lightning-strike victims. It is important to evaluate victims quickly for apnea, asystole, hypothermia, shock, fractures, and burns. Cardiopulmonary resuscitation is effective in resuscitating pulseless victims of lightning strike. Maintenance of cardiopulmonary resuscitation and first-aid certification should be required of all persons involved in sports and recreational activities.

Key Words: lightning, policies and procedures, lightning casualties, severe-storm hazards, environmental hazards, emergency action plan, thunderstorms, lightning-safety policy, athletics, recreation

Over the past century, lightning has consistently been 1 of the top 3 causes of weather-related deaths in this country.[1,2] It kills approximately 100 people and injures hundreds more each year.[2–5] Lightning is an enormous and widespread danger to the physically active population, due in part to the prevalence of thunderstorms in the afternoon to early evening during the late spring to early fall and a societal trend toward outdoor physical activities.[2,3,6] Certain areas of the United States have higher propensities for thunderstorm activity, and thus, higher casualty rates: the Atlantic seaboard, southwest, southern Rocky Mountains, and southern plains states.[2,7]

Worldwide, approximately 2000 thunderstorms and 50 to 100 lightning flashes occur every second.[8] In 1997, the National Lightning Detection Network recorded nearly 27 000 000 cloud-to-ground lightning strikes in the United States (Christoph Zimmerman, Global Atmospherics, Inc, Tucson, AZ, unpublished data). Many of these strikes caused fires, power outages, property damage, loss of life, and disabling injuries. Property damage from lightning is estimated to cost $5 000 000 000 to $6 000 000 000 annually in this country.[9] While print and television news reports of lightning-strike incidents to recreational athletes are frequent during the thunderstorm season, many people are unsure about what to do and where to go to improve their safety during thunderstorms. It is incumbent on all individuals, particularly those who are leaders in athletics and recreation, to appreciate the lightning hazard, learn the published lightning-safety guidelines, and act prudently, wisely, and in a spirit that will encourage safe behavior in others.

The guidelines presented in this article govern all outdoor activities, as well as indoor swimming-pool activities. The purpose of this position statement is to recommend lightning-safety policy guidelines and strategies and to educate athletic trainers and others involved with athletic or recreation activities about the hazards of lightning.

Address correspondence to National Athletic Trainers' Association, Communications Department, 2952 Stemmons Freeway, Dallas, TX 75247.

RECOMMENDATIONS

1. Formalize and implement a comprehensive, proactive lightning-safety policy or emergency action plan specific to lightning safety.[1,7,10–14] The components of this policy should include the following:

    A. An established chain of command that identifies who is to make the call to remove individuals from the field or an activity.

    B. A designated weather watcher (ie, a person who actively looks for the signs of threatening weather and notifies the chain of command if severe weather becomes dangerous).

    C. A means of monitoring local weather forecasts and warnings.

    D. A listing of specific safe locations (for each field or site) from the lightning hazard.

    E. The use of specific criteria for suspension and resumption of activities (refer to recommendations 4, 5, and 6).

    F. The use of the recommended lightning-safety strategies (refer to recommendations 7, 8, and 9).

2. The primary choice for a safe location from the lightning hazard is any substantial, frequently inhabited building. The electric and telephone wiring and plumbing pathways aid in grounding a building, which is why buildings are safer than remaining outdoors during thunderstorms. It is important not to be connected to these pathways while inside the structure during ongoing thunderstorms.

3. The secondary choice for a safer location from the lightning hazard is a fully enclosed vehicle with a metal roof and the windows closed.[1,7,10,11,13,14] Convertible cars and golf carts do not provide protection from lightning danger. It is important not to touch any part of the metal framework of the vehicle while inside it during ongoing thunderstorms.

4. Seeking a safe structure or location at the first sign of lightning or thunder activity is highly recommended. By the time the flash-to-bang count approaches 30 seconds (or is less than 30 seconds), all individuals should already be inside or should immediately seek a safe structure or location.[1,13–15] To use the flash-to-bang method, the observer begins counting when a lightning flash is sighted. Counting is stopped when the associated bang (thunder) is heard. Divide this count by 5 to determine the distance to the lightning flash (in miles). For example, a flash-to-bang count of 30 seconds equates to a distance of 6 miles (9.66 km).

5. Postpone or suspend activity if a thunderstorm appears imminent before or during an activity or contest (regardless of whether lightning is seen or thunder heard) until the hazard has passed. Signs of imminent thunderstorm activity are darkening clouds, high winds, and thunder or lightning activity.

6. Once activities have been suspended, wait at least 30 minutes after the last sound of thunder or lightning flash before resuming an activity or returning outdoors.[1,13–15] A message should be read over the public address system and lightning-safety tips should be placed in game programs alerting spectators and competitors about what to do and where to go to find a safer location during thunderstorm activity.[13,15]

7. Extremely large athletic events are of particular concern with regard to lightning safety. Consider using a multidisciplinary approach to lessen lightning danger, such as integrating weather forecasts, real-time thunderstorm data, a weather watcher, and the flash-to-bang count to aid in decision making.

8. Avoid being in contact with, or in proximity to, the highest point of an open field or on the open water. Do not take shelter under or near trees, flag poles, or light poles.[1,8,10,13–15]

9. Avoid taking showers and using plumbing facilities (including indoor and outdoor pools) and land-line telephones during thunderstorm activity.[1,8,10,13–15] Cordless or cellular telephones are safer to use when emergency help is needed.

10. Individuals who feel their hair stand on end or skin tingle or hear crackling noises should assume the lightning-safe position (ie, crouched on the ground, weight on the balls of the feet, feet together, head lowered, and ears covered). Do not lie flat on the ground.[1,8,10,13–15]

11. Observe the following basic first-aid procedures, in order, to manage victims of lightning strike[16]:

    A. Survey the scene for safety. Ongoing thunderstorms may still pose a threat to emergency personnel responding to the situation.

    B. Activate the local emergency management system.

    C. Move the victim carefully to a safer location, if needed.

    D. Evaluate and treat for apnea and asystole.

    E. Evaluate and treat for hypothermia and shock.

    F. Evaluate and treat for fractures.

    G. Evaluate and treat for burns.

12. All persons should maintain current cardiopulmonary resuscitation (CPR) and first-aid certification.

13. All individuals should have the right to leave an athletic site or activity, without fear of repercussion or penalty, in order to seek a safe structure or location if they feel they are in danger from impending lightning activity.[13,15]

BACKGROUND

Lightning-Flash Development

Within a developing thunderstorm cloud, updrafts promote the collision of rising and descending ice and water particles, and the positive and negative charges are separated into distinct layers. Positive charges are taken via updrafts to the top of the cloud, while negative charges accumulate in the bottom of the cloud, creating the equivalent of a giant atmospheric battery.[8]

A cloud-to-ground lightning flash is the product of the buildup and discharge of static electric energy between the charged regions of the cloud and the earth. The negatively charged lower region of the cloud induces a positive charge on the ground below. The tremendous electric forces between these 2 opposite charges initiate the lightning flash, which begins as a barely visible step leader moving in a series of steps downward from the cloud. Various objects on the ground (trees, chimneys, people, etc) can produce positively charged, upward streamers. The connection of the step leader with an upward streamer determines the connection point on the ground. After contact, a bright return stroke propagates upward from the ground, while electrons move downward toward the earth.[8] This entire phenomenon happens in less than a fraction of a second,[8] but a large amount of charge is transferred to the earth from the cloud.

Most lightning flashes have several return strokes, separated by only 0.004 to 0.005 seconds.[8] The human eye can barely resolve the intervals between the strokes that cause the lightning flash to appear to flicker. A lightning flash is essentially a brief spark, similar to that received from touching a doorknob after walking across a carpeted room. The lightning channel is approximately 2.54 cm (1 inch) in diameter and averages 4.83 to 8.05 km (3 to 5 miles) in vertical height but can be 9.66 km (6 miles) or higher.[8] Cloud-to-ground lightning flashes typically have peak currents ranging from 10 000 to 200 000 Å, and the electric potential between the cloud and ground can be 10 000 000 to 100 000 000 V.[8]

Thunder is created when lightning quickly heats the air around it, sometimes to temperatures greater than approximately 27 800°C (50 000°F), which is about 5 times hotter than the surface of the sun.[8] The rapidly heated air around a lightning channel explodes, which in turn creates the sound we hear as a clap of thunder.[8] The audible range of thunder is about 16.09 km (10 miles) but can be more or less depending on local conditions.[1] Heat lightning is intracloud or intercloud lightning that is too distant for the accompanying thunder to be heard.[8] Although it is possible to have lightning without thunder, thunder never occurs in the absence of lightning.

Lightning Casualty Demographics

On average, lightning kills approximately 100 people each year in this country, while many hundreds more are injured.[2-5] The death toll from lightning for 1940 to 1973 was greater than that from tornadoes and hurricanes combined.[17] Ninety-two percent of lightning casualties occur between May and September, while July has the greatest number of casualties.[2,3,7,18] Furthermore, 45% of the deaths and 80% of the casualties occurred in these months between 10:00 AM and 7:00 PM,[2,3,7,8] which coincides with the most likely time period for athletic or recreational events. For these reasons, it is accurate to say that lightning is the most dangerous and frequently encountered severe-storm hazard that most people experience each year.[10,11]

The statistics on lightning casualty demographics compiled from the National Oceanographic and Atmospheric Administration publication *Storm Data* for the state of Colorado over the last few decades demonstrate an increase in the number of lightning casualties in persons involved in sports and outdoor recreation.[7,10,18,19] Fifty-two percent of lightning casualties were people involved in outdoor recreation.[7,18] In addition, these authors noted that the highest number of casualties from lightning was recorded in recreational and sports activities for each year of the study.[18] During the 1960s, more than 30% of lightning casualties occurred during outdoor recreation activities; during the 1970s, that figure rose to 47%.[17] Furthermore, the rate of increase of lightning casualties during sports was higher than the general United States population rate of increase during the same time period.[7,18]

Lightning casualty statistics from Colorado demonstrate that the most common sites for fatalities were open fields (27%), near trees (16%), and close to water (13%).[7,8,18] Statistics from the country as a whole mimic the numbers from Colorado. Open fields, ballparks, and playgrounds accounted for nearly 27% of casualties, and under trees (14%), water-related (8%), and golf-related (5%) deaths associated with lightning followed.[19] All these fatalities had 1 common denominator: being near the highest object or being the tallest object in the immediate area. This single factor accounted for 56% of all fatalities from Colorado. Thus, it is imperative to

avoid high ridges and high points on the terrain, and conversely, it is important to seek low-lying points on the terrain.[1,3,8,13-15]

The height above ground has been demonstrated to play a prominent role in determining the strike probability. Therefore, it is important to understand why minimizing vertical height is critical in decreasing the chances of becoming a victim of lightning. Warning signs of a high electromagnetic field and imminent lightning strike include hair standing on end and sounds similar to bacon sizzling or cloth tearing.[8] If these conditions occur, a cloud-to-ground lightning flash could strike in the immediate area. Therefore, one should immediately crouch in the lightning-safe position: feet together, weight on the balls of the feet, head lowered, and ears covered.[1] This position is intended to minimize the probability of a direct strike by both lowering the person's height and minimizing the area in contact with the surface of the ground. Taller objects are more likely to be struck (but not always) because their upward streamer occurs first, so that it is closer in proximity to the step leader coming downward from the cloud.

The ultimate message is that individuals in dangerous lightning situations should never wait to seek a safe location and pursue safety measures. It is important to be proactive by having all individuals inside a safe structure or location long before the lightning is close enough to be threatening.

Mechanisms of Lightning Injury

Injury from lightning can occur via 5 mechanisms.[16] A direct strike most commonly occurs to the head, and lightning current enters the orifices. This mechanism explains why eye and ear injuries in lightning-strike victims are abundantly reported in the literature.[16] The shock wave created by the lightning channel can also produce injuries, such as rupture of the tympanic membrane, a common clinical presentation in the lightning-strike victim.[16,23,24] Recommending that individuals cover their ears while in the lightning-safe position may help to mitigate this type of injury.

The second mechanism, contact injury, occurs when the lightning victim is touching an object that is in the pathway of a lightning current.[16] Side flash, the third mechanism, occurs when lightning strikes an object near the victim and then jumps from that object to the victim. This is the main danger to a person who is sheltered under an isolated, tall tree.[6] An upward streamer is triggered by the tree but when this connects with the step leader, the resulting stroke jumps to the victim, who represents an additional pathway to ground.

The fourth mechanism, a step voltage or ground current, occurs when the lightning current flowing in the ground radiates outward in waves from the strike point. If 1 of the individual's feet is closer to the strike than the other, a step voltage is created.[6,16] Humans are primarily salt minerals in an aqueous solution, and a lightning current preferentially travels up from the earth through this solution (that is, the person) rather than through the ground. The greater the differential step voltage (ie, the greater the distance between the 2 feet), the greater the likelihood of injury. Placing one's feet close together while in the crouched position and not lying flat on the ground are crucial in reducing the likelihood of injury from a step voltage or ground current.

Blunt injury is the fifth mechanism for lightning-strike injuries. Lightning current can cause violent muscular contractions that throw its victims many meters from the strike point.

Explosive and implosive forces created by the rapid heating and cooling by the lightning current are also enough to produce traumatic injuries.[16]

Common Effects of Lightning Injury

While lightning kills nearly 100 people annually in this country, the protracted suffering of the survivors should not be underestimated. Although the only acute cause of death from lightning injury is cardiac arrest,[20] the anoxic brain damage that can occur if the person is not rapidly resuscitated can be devastating. In addition, even for the survivor who did not sustain a cardiac arrest, permanent sequelae can include common brain-injury symptoms such as deficits in short-term memory and processing of new information, as well as severe and ongoing headaches, hyperirritability, sleep disturbances, and distractibility.[21,22] Others may develop chronic pain syndromes or absence-type seizures. Frequently, survivors are unable to return to their previous level of function. They may not be able to continue in their jobs or in their educational pursuits and may be permanently disabled.

Components of a Lightning-Safety Policy

The purpose of formalizing a policy on lightning safety is to provide written guidelines for safety during lightning storms. Ninety-two percent of National Collegiate Athletic Association Division I athletics departments responding to a survey did not have a formal, written lightning-safety policy.[12] The best means of reducing the lightning hazard to people is to be proactive. Athletic and recreational personnel should formalize and implement an emergency action plan specific to lightning safety before the thunderstorm season.[1,11,13–15] Dissemination of the plan is paramount, so that all persons will know what to do and where to go to improve their own safety during thunderstorms. The 6 components of a lightning-safety policy or emergency action plan for lightning are discussed in the following paragraphs.

The first component in an emergency action plan or policy for lightning safety is the establishment of a specific chain of command that identifies the person who has the authority to remove participants from athletic venues or activities. The second is to appoint a weather watcher who actively looks for signs of developing local thunderstorms, such as high winds, darkening clouds, and any lightning or thunder.

The third element of a lightning-safety policy is the stipulation for monitoring local weather forecasts. One method is to use weather radios that broadcast information on daily forecasts and approaching storm systems. Weather radios are an excellent informational tool for general storm movement and strength. While this information is extremely important in decision making, the National Weather Service does not broadcast information on specific storm cells or lightning. Therefore, in addition to monitoring weather radios, it is essential that the weather watcher be on constant lookout for conditions in the immediate vicinity of the athletic event and compare these conditions with the weather radio information.

When a local area is placed under a severe-storm watch or warning by the National Weather Service, weather radios can be programmed to give audible alert tones. A watch indicates conditions are favorable for severe weather; a warning means severe weather has been detected in the locale, and all persons should take the necessary precautions to preserve their own

safety. If severe storms are in the vicinity, all individuals should more intently monitor thunderstorm activity, such as severity and direction of movement of the storm. It may also mean that steps should be taken to remove athletes from the field or perhaps to postpone or suspend athletic or recreational activities during the event or before the storm begins.

Safe Locations

The fourth aspect of a lightning-safety policy, defining and listing safe structures or locations to evacuate to in the event of lightning, is of utmost importance. While there are reports of people being injured by lightning inside buildings,[8] evacuating to a substantial building can considerably lower the risks of lightning injury compared with those of remaining outside during the thunderstorm. The lightning-safety policy should identify the safe structure or location specific to each venue. This information will enable individuals to know where to go in advance of any thunderstorm situation and appreciate how long it takes to get to the specific safe location from each field or event site.

The primary choice for a safe structure is any fully enclosed, substantial building.[1,3,8,13–15] Ideally, the building should have plumbing, electric wiring, and telephone service. The lightning current is more likely to follow these pathways to ground, which aids in electrically grounding the structure.[8] If a substantial building is not available, a fully enclosed vehicle with a metal roof and the windows completely closed is a reasonable alternative.[1,3,13–15] It is not the rubber tires that make the vehicle safe but the metal enclosure that guides the lightning current around the passengers, rather than through them. Do not touch any part of the metal framework while inside the vehicle.[8] Convertible vehicles and golf carts do not provide a high level of protection and cannot be considered safe from lightning.

Unsafe Locations

Unfortunately, those properties that serve to define a safe structure and improve the safety of its inhabitants also present a potential risk. Lightning current can enter a building via the electric or telephone wiring. It can also enter via a ground current through the incoming plumbing pipelines. This condition makes locker-room shower areas, swimming pools (indoor and outdoor), telephones, and electric appliances unsafe during thunderstorms because of the possible contact with current-carrying conduction. While such reports are rare, people have been killed or injured by lightning in their homes while talking on the telephone, taking a shower, or standing near household appliances such as dishwashers, stoves, or refrigerators.[1,3,8,13–15]

From 1959 through 1965, lightning killed 4 people and injured 36 others while they were talking on the telephone. These numbers comprised 0.42% (n = 960) of deaths and 2.1% (n = 1736) of injuries for the period.[5] Studying reports from *Storm Data*, researchers found that between 1959 and 1994, 2.4% of lightning casualties were telephone related.[2] Because they are not connected directly to a land-line phone, cellular and cordless telephones are reasonably safe alternatives for summoning help during a thunderstorm. It should be noted that injury from acoustic damage can occur via explosive static from the earpiece caused by a nearby lightning strike.

Even though a swimming pool may be indoors and apparently safe, it can be a dangerous location during thunderstorms.[25] The current can be propagated through plumbing and electric connections via the underwater lights and drains of most swimming pools. Lightning current can also enter the building, either into the electric wiring inside the building or through underground plumbing pipelines that enter the building.[8] If lightning strikes the building or ground nearby, the current will most likely follow these pathways to the swimmers through the water. Thus, indoor-pool activities are potentially dangerous and should be avoided during thunderstorms.[25]

Small structures, such as rain or picnic shelters or athletic storage sheds, are generally not properly protected and should be avoided during thunderstorms. These locations may actually increase the risk of lightning strike via a side flash and cause injury to the occupants.

Criteria for Postponement and Resumption of Activities

The fifth component of any lightning-safety policy is to clearly describe criteria for both the suspension and resumption of athletic or recreational activities. Various technologies currently on the market propose to assist in determining when lightning is in the immediate area. Within the developing area of this lightning technology, data-based research is insufficient to either support or dispute companies' claims regarding establishing when one is in danger of a lightning strike. Therefore the National Athletic Trainers' Association promotes the flash-to-bang standard to warn people of imminent lightning danger. The flash-to-bang method is the easiest and most convenient means for determining the distance to a lightning flash and can also be used to determine when to suspend or postpone activities. The flash-to-bang method is based on the fact that light travels faster than sound, which travels at a speed of approximately 1.61 km (1 mile) every 5 seconds.[1,8,13,14] To use the flash-to-bang method, begin counting on the lightning flash, and stop counting when the associated clap of thunder is heard. When storms have a high flash rate, it is important to correlate a specific flash with the thunder it produced. Divide the time to thunder (in seconds) by 5 to determine the distance (in miles) to the lightning flash.[1,8,13,14] For example, an observer obtains a count of 30 seconds from the time he or she spots the flash to when the thunder is heard. Thirty divided by 5 equals 6; therefore, that lightning flash was 6 miles (9.66 km) from the observer.

The 30-second rule is not an arbitrary guideline. López and Holle[26] studied storms in Oklahoma, Colorado, and Florida and found that in larger thunderstorms, the distance between successive flashes can be up to 6 miles (9.66 km) (ie, a flash-to-bang count of 30 seconds) in approximately 80% of the flash pairs. The authors also found the distance between successive flashes may be as great as 9 miles (14.48 km) or more, depending on local geography and atmospheric conditions. If a flash-to-bang count of 30 seconds is observed, the next flash could conceivably be at the observer's location.

Another important factor to consider when using the flash-to-bang method is that, although a relatively rare occurrence, lightning has been reported to strike 16.09 km (10 miles) or more from where it is raining.[1] Therefore, a flash-to-bang count of at least 30 seconds is strongly recommended as a determinant of when to suspend or postpone athletic or recreational activities.[13–15] As the flash-to-bang count approaches 30 seconds, all persons should be seeking, or already inside, a safe structure or location. This is the minimal guideline when using the flash-to-bang method to halt athletic or recreational activities. Seeking a safe location at the first sign of thunder or lightning activity is also highly recommended.

Another facet of the lightning-safety policy is embodied in the "30–30 rule" (Table 1), which relies on the flash-to-bang method. If a game, practice, or other activity is suspended or postponed due to lightning activity, it is important to establish strict criteria in the lightning-safety policy for resumption of activities. Waiting at least 30 minutes after the last lightning flash or sound of thunder is recommended.[13–15] When storm reports and flash data at the time of death or injury were compared, researchers found that the end of the storm, when the flash-rate frequency began to decline, was as deadly as the middle of the storm, when the lightning flash rate was at its peak. The authors postulated that once the flash rate begins to decline, people do not perceive the thunderstorm as dangerous and are struck by lightning when they return outdoors prematurely.[1] An important adage for athletic trainers, coaches, and officials to remember is, "if you see it (lightning) flee it, if you hear it (thunder), clear it."

The 30-minute rule can also be explained in another way. A typical thunderstorm moves at a rate of approximately 40.23 km (25 miles) per hour. Experts believe that 30 minutes allow the thunderstorm to be about 16.09 to 19.31 km (10 to 12 miles) from the area, minimizing the probability of a nearby, and therefore dangerous, lightning strike.[15] Blue sky in the local area or a lack of rainfall are not adequate reasons to breach the 30-minute return-to-play rule. Lightning can strike far from where it is raining, even when the clouds begin to clear and show evidence of blue sky.[1] This situation is often referred to as a "bolt out of the blue." Each time lightning is observed or thunder is heard, the 30-minute clock should be reset.

Obligation to Warn

The recommendation for reading lightning-safety messages over public address systems and placing placards conspicuously around each venue resulted from a fatal lightning strike in Washington, DC, in May 1991.[27] During a high school lacrosse game, a dangerous thunderstorm swept into the local area, and the game was suspended. Lightning killed 1 young person and injured 10 others who sought refuge under a tree. Many people stated that they did not know what to do or where to go to protect themselves from the dangers of lightning.

According to the basic principles of tort law, an individual has a duty to warn others of dangers that may not be obvious to a guest or subordinate of that person.[28] Black et al[29] defined the legal principle of "foreseeability" as "the ability to see or

Table 1. The 30-30 Rule[15]

Criteria for suspension of activities	By the time the flash-to-bang count approaches 30 seconds, all individuals should already be inside a safe shelter.
Criteria for resumption of activities	Wait at least 30 minutes after the last sound (thunder) or observation of lightning before leaving the safe shelter to resume activities.

know in advance, eg, reasonable anticipation, that harm or injury is a likely result from certain acts or omissions." With regard to dangerous lightning situations, it could be argued that an institution (or athletic department) has the duty to warn spectators, invited guests, and participants if conditions are such that lightning activity may be an imminent danger in the immediate area. Whereas lightning is understood by all to be a dangerous phenomenon, the importance of seeking safe shelter and the specific time that one should vacate to safety are generally not known. Based on research presented in this article regarding the number of lightning casualties resulting from the erroneous tendency of people to seek shelter under trees, it would be wise for an organization to promote lightning safety to its clientele and participants, including a list of specific safe locations or structures.

Warnings should be commensurate with the age and understanding of those involved. Announcements should be repeated over the public address system and colorful notices and safety instructions both placed in the event programs and posted in visible, high-traffic areas. Safety instructions should include the location of the nearest safe shelter, similar to airline pocket diagrams of nearest emergency exits. Being proactive with regard to the lightning threat demands not putting individuals at risk if a hazardous situation could have been prevented. If thunderstorm activity looks menacing before or during an event, consider canceling or postponing the event until the complete weather situation can be ascertained and determined to no longer be a threat. The first lightning flash from the thunderstorm cloud and storms that produce only a few flashes still pose a potential threat and should be treated as such. Every cloud-to-ground lightning flash is dangerous and potentially deadly and should not be taken lightly or viewed complacently. Therefore, it is the recommendation of the National Athletic Trainers' Association to postpone or suspend athletic and recreational activities before their onset, if thunderstorm activity appears imminent.

Prehospital Care of Victims

If a lightning-strike victim presents in asystole or respiratory arrest, it is critical to initiate CPR as soon as safely possible.[23] Because lightning-strike victims do not remain connected to a power source, they do not carry an electric charge and are safe to assess.[30] However, during an ongoing thunderstorm, lightning activity in the local area still poses a deadly hazard for the medical team responding to the incident. The athletic trainer or other medical personnel should consider his or her own personal safety before venturing into a dangerous situation to render care.

If medical personnel assume the risk of entering a dangerous lightning situation to render care, the first priority should be to move the victim to a safe location. In this way, a hazardous situation can be neutralized for the athletic trainer, as well as the victim. It is unlikely that moving a victim to an area of greater safety for resuscitation will cause any serious injury to the victim.[16] The primary and secondary survey of the victim's condition can then be conducted once safety is reached.

It is not uncommon to find a lightning-strike victim unconscious, with fixed and dilated pupils and cold extremities and in cardiopulmonary arrest. Case studies of individuals with prolonged apnea and asystole after a lightning strike have demonstrated successful resuscitations using CPR.[23,24,31] Once stopped, the heart will most likely spontaneously restart, but

Table 2. Recommended Prehospital Care for Treating Lightning-Strike Victims[16]

Perform the following steps in order:
1. Survey the scene for safety.
2. Activate the local emergency management system.
3. Carefully move the victim to a safe area, if needed.
4. Evaluate and treat for apnea and asystole.
5. Evaluate and treat for hypothermia and shock.
6. Evaluate and treat for fractures.
7. Evaluate and treat for burns.

breathing centers in the brain may be damaged. Respiratory arrest lasts longer than cardiac arrest, leading to secondary asystole from hypoxia.[16] Therefore, the basic principle of triage, "treat the living first," should be reversed in cases involving casualties from a lightning strike. It is imperative to treat those persons who are "apparently dead" first by promptly initiating CPR. See Table 2 for quick-reference guidelines in evaluating and treating victims of lightning strike.

CONCLUSIONS

Due to its pervasiveness during the times that most athletic events occur, lightning is a significant hazard to the physically active population. Lightning-casualty statistics show an alarming rise in the number of lightning casualties in recreational and sports settings in recent decades.[2,3,9] Each person must take responsibility for his or her own personal safety during thunderstorms.[10] However, because people are often under the direction of others, whether they are children or adults participating in organized athletics, athletic trainers, coaches, teachers, and game officials must receive education about the hazards of lightning and become familiar with proved lightning-safety strategies. A policy is only as good as its compliance and unwavering, broad-based enforcement.

It is important to be much more wary of the lightning threat than the rain. Lightning can strike in the absence of rain, as well as from apparently clear blue skies overhead, even though a thunderstorm may be nearby. The presence of lightning or thunder should be the determining factor in postponing or suspending games and activities, not the amount of rainfall on the playing field. Lightning should be the only critical factor in decision making for athletic trainers, umpires, officials, referees, and coaches.

Athletic trainers, umpires, officials, referees, coaches, teachers, and parents can make a difference in reducing the number of lightning casualties if they (1) formalize and implement a lightning-safety policy or emergency action plan specific to lightning safety; (2) understand the qualifications of safe structures or locations, in addition to knowing where they are in relation to each athletic field or activity site; (3) understand the 30–30 rule as a minimal determinant of when to suspend activities and follow it; being conservative and suspending activities at the first sign of lightning or thunder activity is also prudent and wise; (4) practice and follow the published lightning-safety guidelines and strategies; (5) and maintain CPR and standard first-aid certification.

ACKNOWLEDGMENTS

This position statement was reviewed for the National Athletic Trainers' Association by the Pronouncements Committee, Richard Ray, PhD, ATC, and Philip Krider, PhD.

REFERENCES

1. Holle RL, López RE, Howard KW, Vavrek J, Allsopp J. Safety in the presence of lightning. *Semin Neurol.* 1995;15:375–380.
2. López RE, Holle RL, Heitkamp TA, Boyson M, Cherington M, Langford K. The underreporting of lightning injuries and deaths in Colorado. *Bull Am Meteorol Soc.* 1993;74:2171–2178.
3. Duclos PJ, Sanderson LM. An epidemiological description of lightning-related deaths in the United States. *Int J Epidemiol.* 1990;19:673–679.
4. Craig SR. When lightning strikes: pathophysiology and treatment of lightning injuries. *Postgrad Med.* 1986;79:109–112,121–123.
5. Zegel FH. Lightning deaths in the United States: a seven-year survey from 1959 to 1965. *Weatherwise.* 1967;20:169.
6. Andrews CJ, Cooper MA, Darveniza M. *Lightning Injuries: Electrical, Medical, and Legal Aspects.* Boca Raton, FL: CRC Press; 1992.
7. López RE, Holle RL. Demographics of lightning casualties. *Semin Neurol.* 1995;15:286–295.
8. Uman MA. *All About Lightning.* New York, NY: Dover Publications; 1986.
9. Kithil R. Annual USA lightning costs and losses. National Lightning Safety Institute. Available at: www.lightningsafety.com/nlsi_lls/nlsi_annual_usa_losses.htm. Accessed January 19, 1999.
10. Holle RL, López RE. Lightning: impacts and safety. *World Meteorol Bull.* 1998;47:148–155.
11. Holle RL, López RE, Vavrek J, Howard KW. Educating individuals about lightning. In: *Preprints of the American Meteorological Society 7th Symposium on Education*; January 11–16, 1998; Phoenix, AZ.
12. Walsh KM, Hanley MJ, Graner SJ, Beam D, Bazluki J. A survey of lightning policy in selected Division I colleges. *J Athl Train.* 1997;32:206–210.
13. Bennett BL. A model lightning safety policy for athletics. *J Athl Train.* 1997;32:251–253.
14. Bennett BL, Holle RL, López RE. Lightning safety guideline 1D. *1997–98 National Collegiate Athletic Association Sports Medicine Handbook.* Overland Park, KS: National Collegiate Athletic Association; 1997–1998:12–14.
15. Vavrek JR, Holle RL, López RE. Updated lightning safety recommendations. In: *Preprints of the American Meteorological Society 8th Symposium on Education*; January 10–15, 1999; Dallas, TX.
16. Cooper MA. Emergent care of lightning and electrical injuries. *Semin Neurol.* 1995;15:268–278.
17. Weigel EP. Lightning: the underrated killer. *NOAA [National Oceanographic and Atmospheric Administration].* 1976;6:4–11.
18. López RE, Holle RL, Heitkamp TA. Lightning casualties and property damage in Colorado from 1950 to 1991 based on storm data. *Weather Forecast.* 1995;10:114–126.
19. Curran EB, Holle RL, López RE. *Lightning Fatalities, Injuries, and Damage Reports in the United States: 1959–1994.* Washington, DC: National Oceanic and Atmospheric Administration; 1997. Technical Memorandum NWS SR-193.
20. Cooper MA. Lightning: prognostic signs for death. *Ann Emerg Med.* 1980;9:134–138.
21. Primeau M, Engelstatter GH, Bares KK. Behavioral consequences of lightning and electrical injury. *Semin Neurol.* 1995;15:279–285.
22. Andrews CJ, Darveniza M. Telephone-mediated lightning injury: an Australian survey. *J Trauma.* 1989;29:665–671.
23. Fontanarosa PB. Electrical shock and lightning strike. *Ann Emerg Med.* 1993;22(Pt 2):378–387.
24. Steinbaum S, Harviel JD, Jaffin JH, Jordan MH. Lightning strike to the head: case report. *J Trauma.* 1994;36:113–115.
25. Wiley S. Shocking news about lightning and pools. *USA Swimming Safety Q.* 1998;4:1–2.
26. López RE, Holle RL. The distance between subsequent lightning flashes. In: *Preprints of the International Lightning Detection Conference*; November 17–18, 1998; Tucson, AZ.
27. Sanchez R, Wheeler L. Lightning strike at St. Albans game kills Bethesda student, injures 10. *Washington Post.* May 18, 1991;A1.
28. Keeton WP, Dobbs DB, Keeton RE, Owen DG. *Prosser and Keeton on Torts.* 5th ed. St. Paul, MN: West Publishing; 1984.
29. Black HC, Nolan JR, Nolan-Haley JM. *Black's Law Dictionary.* 6th ed. St. Paul, MN: West Publishing; 1990.
30. Cooper MA. Myths, miracles, and mirages. *Semin Neurol.* 1995;15:358–361.
31. Jepsen DL. How to manage a patient with lightning injury. *Am J Nurs.* 1992;92:38–42.

Prehospital Care of the Spine-Injured Athlete

- *Clinical Practice Guideline*

Prehospital Care of the Spine-Injured Athlete

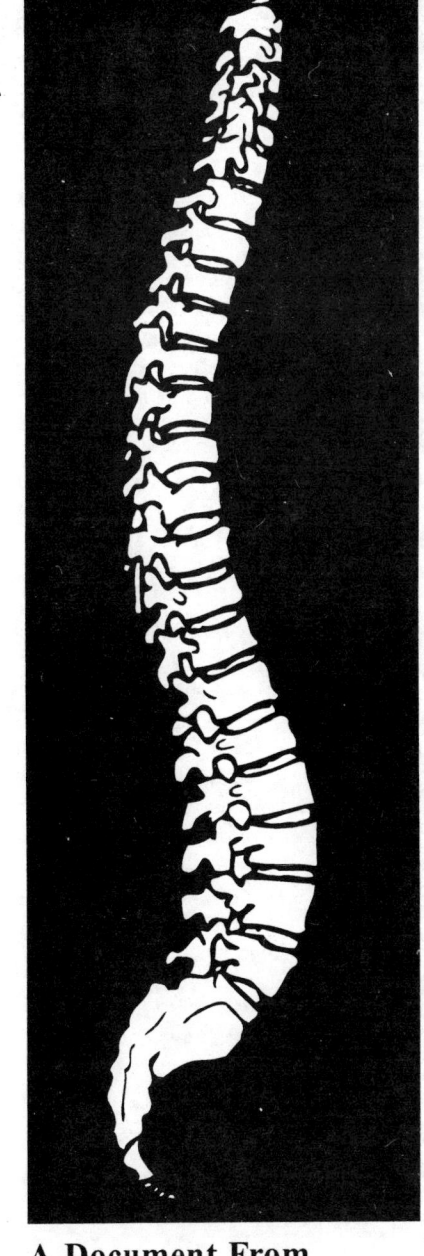

A Document From

the Inter-Association

Task Force For

Appropriate Care of

the Spine-Injured Athlete

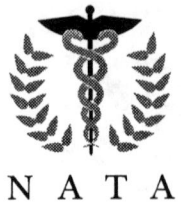

Proper on-the-field management of an athlete with a suspected spinal injury has long been a topic of discussion among certified athletic trainers and other allied healthcare professionals. Because each group has its expertise in a particular area, the question of correct technique or appropriate procedure has been the subject of much debate.

Recognizing a uniform set of guidelines for handling possible spine injuries was needed, the National Athletic Trainers' Association formed the Inter-Association Task Force for Appropriate Care of the Spine-Injured Athlete in 1998. More than 30 emergency medicine and sports medicine organizations were invited to participate in two summits to develop recommendations for all healthcare providers who might be involved in the care of this kind of injury.

The result: a complete set of guidelines and recommendations were created and unanimously approved by the members of the task force. This document expands on those guidelines and offers an extensive look at the many aspects of caring for an athlete with a suspected spinal injury.

As certified athletic trainers, we must manage potentially life threatening and catastrophic injuries. This paper provides a resource for our community to use as a reference if ever faced with a situation involving a spine-injured athlete. Although we hope you will never have to utilize the procedures delineated in this document, you must be prepared to meet any eventuality.

We would like to express our thanks to the individuals who served on the Inter-Association Task Force for Appropriate Care of the Spine-Injured Athlete for their dedication and commitment to this important project.

Sincerely,

Julie Max, ATC, MEd   Kent Falb, ATC, PT   Doug Kleiner, PhD, ATC
President   Immediate Past President   Chair, Inter-Association Task
NATA   NATA   Force for Appropriate Care of
                                                             the Spine-Injured Athlete

Credits

This manuscript was written by:

Douglas M. Kleiner, PhD, ATC, EMT, FACSM (Chair)
National Athletic Trainers' Association

Jon L. Almquist, ATC
NATA Secondary School Athletic Trainers' Committee

Julian Bailes, MD
American Association of Neurological Surgeons

T. Pepper Burruss, ATC, PT
Professional Football Athletic Trainers' Society

Henry Feuer, MD
National Football League Physicians Society

Letha Y. Griffin, MD
NCAA Committee on Competitive Safeguards and Medical
Aspects of Sports

Stanley Herring, MD, FACSM
American College of Sports Medicine/North American Spine
Society

Connie McAdam, MICT
National Association of EMTs

Dennis Miller, ATC, PT
National Athletic Trainers' Association

David Thorson, MD
American Academy of Family Physicians

Robert G. Watkins, MD
American Academy of Orthopaedic Surgeons – Committee on
the Spine

Stuart Weinstein, MD, FACSM
American College of Sports Medicine/Physiatric Association
of Spine, Sports & Occupational Rehabilitation

*The task force would like to thank the following individuals
for their input on this paper. Their suggestions and advice
have greatly improved its content and presentation.*

**Edward C. Benzel, MD representing American Academy of
Neurological Surgeons**

**Robert C. Cantu, MD, FACSM representing National
Athletic Trainers' Association**

**Joel M. Press, MD, FACSM representing American
College of Sports Medicine**

**Joseph S. Torg, MD, FACSM representing National
Athletic Trainers' Association**

**Edward Wojtys, MD representing American Orthopaedic
Society for Sports Medicine**

**Members of the National Athletic Trainers' Association
Pronouncements Committee**

**Members of the National Athletic Trainers' Association
Board of Directors**

*The provision of input on this document in no way implies
endorsement by these individuals or organizations.*

CREDITS

The Inter-Association Task Force for Appropriate Care of the Spine-Injured Athlete was comprised of representatives from the following organizations:

American Academy of Family Physicians
David Thorson, MD

American Academy of Neurology
Jay Rosenberg, MD

**American Academy of Orthopaedic Surgeons –
Committee on the Spine**
Robert Watkins, MD

**American Academy of Pediatrics – Committee on Sports
Medicine and Fitness**
Bernard Griesemer, MD, FAAP
Robert Hannemann, MD

**American Academy of Physical Medicine and
Rehabilitation**
Stuart Weinstein, MD, FACSM

American Association of Neurological Surgeons
Julian Bailes, MD

American Chiropractic Board of Sports Physicians
Jay Greenstein, DC

American College of Emergency Physicians
Joe Waeckerle, MD

American College of Sports Medicine
Stanley Herring, MD, FACSM
Stuart Weinstein, MD, FACSM

American College of Surgeons – Committee on Trauma
Jack Wilberger, MD

American Medical Society for Sports Medicine
Daniel Kraft, MD

American Orthopaedic Society for Sports Medicine
Kevin Black, MD, MS
Kevin Shea, MD

American Osteopathic Academy of Sports Medicine
John Biery, DO, FAOASM, FACSM

**American Physical Therapy Association – Sports Physical
Therapy Section**
Dan Smith, DPT, ATC, SCS, OCS

National Association of EMS Physicians
Robert Domeier, MD

National Association of EMTs
Connie McAdam, MICT

National Association of Intercollegiate Athletics
Patrick Trainor, ATC

National Athletic Trainers' Association
Douglas Kleiner, PhD, ATC, EMT, FACSM, Chair
Kent Falb, ATC, PT
Denny Miller, ATC, PT

NATA College & University Athletic Trainers' Committee
Michael Hanley, ATC
James Laughnane, ATC

NATA Secondary School Athletic Trainers' Committee
Jon Almquist, ATC

**NCAA Committee on Competitive Safeguards and
Medical Aspects of Sports**
Letha Griffin, MD

National Federation of State High School Associations
Jerry Diehl, Assistant Director

National Football League Physicians Society
Henry Feuer, MD

National Operating Committee on Safety and Equipment
Michael Oliver, Executive Director

National Registry of EMTs
Alexander Butman, DSc, NREMT-P

National Safety Council
Robb Rehberg, ATC, CSCS, NREMT

North American Spine Society
Stanley Herring, MD, FACSM

Orthopaedic Trauma Association
Andrew Pollak, MD

**Physiatric Association of Spine, Sports & Occupational
Rehabilitation**
Stuart Weinstein, MD, FACSM

Professional Football Athletic Trainers' Society
T. Pepper Burruss, ATC, PT

United States Olympic Committee
Margaret Hunt, MS, ATC

Abstract

Kleiner DM, Almquist JL, Bailes J, Burruss P, Feuer H, Griffin LY, Herring, S, McAdam C, Miller D, Thorson D, Watkins RG, Weinstein S. *Prehospital Care of the Spine-Injured Athlete: A Document from the Inter-Association Task Force for Appropriate Care of the Spine-Injured Athlete.* **Dallas, Texas, National Athletic Trainers' Association, March 2001.**

Objective: The primary purpose of this paper is to provide guidelines for the prehospital management of a physically active person with a suspected spinal injury. A secondary purpose is to provide additional information that, although beyond the scope of prehospital care, may prove to be useful in understanding the need for a comprehensive approach when treating the spine and is valuable to the different types of clinicians for whom this document is intended.

Background: For many years, disagreements have occurred among various healthcare professionals as to the proper management of a spine-injured athlete, because each group of professionals had their own protocols. In 1998, the National Athletic Trainers' Association formed an inter-association task force to develop guidelines for the appropriate management of the catastrophically spine-injured athlete. Although not all catastrophic injuries are spine injuries and not all spine injuries are catastrophic, it is believed that the improper management of a suspected spinal injury can result in a secondary injury. Thus, it was important to develop standard guidelines to be used by all providers of prehospital care that ensured the safe management of the spine-injured athlete.

Recommendations: The Inter-Association Task Force for Appropriate Care of the Spine-Injured Athlete developed guidelines that were endorsed by the representatives of various healthcare specialties, including certified athletic trainers, physicians, and providers of emergency medical services. This paper provides more details and more thorough information on the guidelines that were developed and endorsed by the task force.

> In 1998, the National Athletic Trainers' Association formed an inter-association task force to develop guidelines for the appropriate management of the spine-injured athlete.

TABLE OF CONTENTS

This statement is only a general practice guide for the healthcare professional. Individual treatment decisions should not be based solely on the information contained in this statement. Individual treatment must be tailored to specific facts and circumstances.

The mention of name brands in this statement in no way implies endorsement of the product.

Introduction

Neither the work of the task force nor the information given here is specific to football, but football players sustain a relatively higher incidence of spine injuries than other athletes and the sport of football often poses unique complications, such as the presence of protective equipment.

In 1998, the National Athletic Trainers' Association (NATA) formed the Inter-Association Task Force for Appropriate Care of the Spine-Injured Athlete to develop guidelines for the appropriate management of the catastrophically injured athlete.[1,2] The guidelines developed by and the recommendations made by the Inter-Association Task Force are presented in Tables 1 and 2, respectively. Every effort was made to base these recommendations on current research. Where data were inadequate or unavailable, recommendations were based on the consensus and expertise of task force members. Techniques that have been scientifically validated have been referenced where appropriate.

Neither the work of the task force nor the information given here is specific to football, but football players sustain a relatively higher incidence of spine injuries than other athletes and the sport of football often poses unique complications, such as the presence of protective equipment.[3-7] Protective equipment has always been a source of controversy, in part because athletic protective equipment is so different from other protective equipment. Motorcycle helmets do not usually have a removable face mask, are not always snugly fit to the head, are worn without shoulder pads, and have other limitations, so after trauma they are routinely removed before transportation as to achieve spinal immobilization.[8,9] However, a properly fitted football helmet holds the head and spine in position, provided the athlete is wearing shoulder pads.[10,11] Thus, the information presented here is specific to the spine-injured athlete and can be applied not only to football but also to a variety of other sports.[12-26]

This document contains guidelines to follow regarding on-the-field management and immediate care, including:

• who should provide prehospital care of the injured athlete

• equipment removal

• immobilization and transportation

• injuries and possible mechanisms

• return-to-play criteria

• prevention

• development of an emergency plan

Some of this information is beyond the scope of prehospital care, but is useful information and is valuable in understanding the complete process of caring for a spine-injured athlete.

On-the-Field Management and Immediate Care

The ideal care of a specific athletic incident begins with observation of the event that leads to the possibility of a spinal injury.[27] The certified athletic trainers and medical staff should make every attempt to closely observe all of the plays because knowledge of the mechanism of injury and degree of contact are often helpful in understanding the likelihood of significant injury (see *Injuries and Possible Mechanisms*).

Initial Assessment. The initial assessment of an injured player begins by forming a general impression of the athlete's condition,[28] which includes the consideration of basic life support.[29-32] If any concerns regarding basic life support are present at this time, the emergency medical services (EMS) system should be activated immediately.[33] The athlete should not be moved unless it is absolutely essential to maintain the airway, breathing, or circulation.[34]

Airway. The evaluation and maintenance of a functional airway are rapidly performed with full consideration for the potential of a spinal injury.[29,31,32,34] Any athlete who is suspected of having a spinal injury should not be moved until the appropriate personnel are present, and he or she should be managed as though a spinal injury exists. If unconscious, the player is presumed to have an unstable fracture until it is proved otherwise.[35] If it is necessary to move the athlete, he or she should be placed in a supine position while the spine is safeguarded. However, as in any instance of trauma response, whatever method necessary to achieve an adequate airway must be used. If a jaw thrust maneuver is unsuccessful, an oral airway or endotracheal intubation may be required. The team physician and/or EMS personnel should be available if such intervention is required.

Breathing. Next, the presence of sufficient ventilatory exchange is confirmed through either observation of the chest respiratory excursions or listening and feeling for air movement at the upper airway. Ineffective breathing patterns, the use of accessory breathing muscles, or even apnea can be caused by a cervical spinal cord injury. High cervical cord damage may inhibit the output of the phrenic nerve, which controls the diaphragm and arises from the third, fourth, and fifth cervical nerves.

Circulation. Circulation is evaluated. A circulation abnormality with inadequate peripheral perfusion is rare and unlikely to be present in the absence of a primary cardiac event.

Level of Consciousness. The athlete's level of consciousness is assessed.[29,31,32] The athlete should be oriented to person, place, time, and incident. A fully conscious player is questioned regarding the presence of pain, particularly in the spinal region or a limb, altered sensation or strength of any body part, weakness, and visual and hearing function. In the unconscious player or one who exhibits any abnormal neurological function, the Glasgow Coma Scale may be helpful as a rapid, objective, and reproducible measure of cerebral function and should be used until a more formal neurological examination is carried out.

Neurological Screening. A screening examination is performed to assess motor and sensory function in the four extremities. In a cooperative player, an accurate initial neurological examination of the extremities can be achieved and is vital for a full evaluation of the injury. A cranial nerve assessment should be performed as completely as possible while the helmet is left in place.

Transportation. If the athlete is suspected of having a vertebral column or spinal cord injury, he or she should be transported to an emergency department, where a more formal neurological examination can be conducted and serial assessments can be completed.[27,36-38] When it becomes necessary to move the athlete, the head and trunk must be moved as one unit, which can be accomplished by manually splinting the head to the trunk as the body is moved (see *Immobilization and Transportation*).[39,40] Due to the difficulty in attaining a definitive exclusion regarding the possibility of spinal injury in an on-field setting, the Inter-Association Task Force recommends that any player suspected of such be evaluated in a controlled environment, and that any athlete with significant neck or spine pain, diminished level of consciousness, or significant neurological deficits be transported, in an appropriate manner, to a medical receiving facility with definitive diagnostic and medical resources.

ON-THE-FIELD MANAGEMENT AND IMMEDIATE CARE

To transport the athlete, he or she should be secured to a suitable backboard (specific steps for this vary from situation to situation and are discussed later in *Immobilization and Transportation*). Should the airway, breathing, or circulation be compromised, spinal immobilization must be maintained when removing the face mask (see *Equipment Management*).

Emergency Plan Activation. On-the-field management procedures might include the presence of the team physician and the initiation of additional medical assistance, such as activation of the EMS system (see *The Emergency Plan*). When other medical or allied healthcare personnel arrive on the scene, a briefing of the situation must be completed efficiently and effectively. History, signs, and symptoms obtained by the first responder must be shared with all those involved. However, it is imperative that only proper medical or allied health personnel be involved. Good Samaritans who come down from the stands and who are unfamiliar with the protocols should not be allowed to participate. A potential on-the-field disagreement on protocol can be detrimental to the health and welfare of the injured athlete and should be avoided. Administrative personnel and coaches can be helpful in restricting the access of individuals other than the previously established appropriate personnel on the field while care is being given by the first responders and follow-up personnel.

> **When other medical or allied healthcare personnel arrive on the scene, a briefing of the situation must be completed efficiently and effectively.**

A defined delegation of duties is essential to maintain on-the-field management and crowd control during a medical emergency. The primary athletic healthcare provider must work quickly and efficiently with full focus on the athlete in distress. Coaches and administrative personnel should immediately step into action, instructing teammates and bystanders to move away from the injured athlete.[41,42] If a spinal injury is suspected, athletes and onlookers should be directed to an area away from the injured athlete. It is recommended that athletic teams be educated on the dangers of moving an injured player (well in advance of the onset of contact practices or contests). It is a common response to offer assistance to an injured teammate or an opponent. However, all participants on the field must be cognizant of the dangers of moving a player with a suspected spinal injury and must refrain from moving any player who shows signs of a severe injury.

The National Football League has developed guidelines for its game officials to use during a serious on-field player injury, such as a spinal injury (Table 3).[41] These guidelines are the first of their kind and show the importance of on-the-field management.[43] In August 1999, the Inter-Association Task Force for Appropriate Care of the Spine-Injured Athlete commended the National Football League for these guidelines.[43] The Inter-Association Task Force recommends that teammates and coaches be reminded to not move an injured player. A coach or game official should keep concerned teammates and family away from the injured athlete.[41]

Skilled and practiced medical care should be readily available at the athletic event. When this is not possible, such as in many rural areas, a plan to obtain this type of care at the scene when needed must be in place. Deviation from a standard and practiced protocol should be avoided (see *The Emergency Plan*).

Equipment Removal. The face mask should be removed at the earliest opportunity, before transportation and regardless of current respiratory status (see *Equipment Management*). Specific guidelines for helmet removal should be followed (see *Equipment Management*).

Equipment Management

The emergency management of an injured athlete can be made more difficult because of the protective equipment worn by the athlete.[44-47] This is especially true in collision sports such as football and hockey, but it can also occur in other sports.[17,20-25,44,48,49] In much of this section on equipment management, football protective equipment is used as the example, but these guidelines can be applied to other sports as well. In addition, specialized equipment, such as appropriate-size spine boards, cervical collars, accessories, and tools for face mask removal must also be available.[50]

FACE MASK

When to Remove the Face Mask. The face mask should be removed as quickly as possible any time a player is suspected of having a spinal injury, even if the player is still conscious. The Inter-Association Task Force recommends the face mask be removed immediately when the decision is made to transport, regardless of current respiratory status. Formerly the face mask was removed only when cardiopulmonary resuscitation had to be initiated. However, the Inter-Association Task Force recommends that EMS providers not wait until the player stops breathing to begin the task of face mask removal because at that point, time becomes more critical.[51]

How to Remove the Face Mask. Regardless of the tools selected, those involved in the prehospital care of injured football players should have the tools for face mask removal readily available and must be familiar with updated equipment. The face mask of the football helmet is usually secured to the helmet with four or more plastic loop-straps that can be cut or removed, thus allowing the face mask to be retracted or taken off completely (removed). This procedure enables rescue personnel to gain access to the airway and vital areas of the face for examination and to administer prehospital care to the football player without having to remove the helmet. When the two lateral loop-straps are cut or removed, the face mask is said to be "retracted," or "swung away," using the two anterior loop-straps as a hinge. Face mask retraction has been the protocol used by certified athletic trainers in the past; however, it has been reported that more head and neck movement occurs while the face mask is being retracted than while the straps are being cut.[52,53]

Reduction in movement of the football player's head and neck is of primary importance since it is believed that any additional movement that occurs during face mask retraction can cause secondary damage to the football player with an injury to the cervical spine. Therefore, the Inter-Association Task Force recommends that all loop-straps of the face mask be cut and that the face mask be removed from the helmet, rather than being retracted.[52]

Tools for Removal. Several tools for removing the loop-straps that secure the face mask to the helmet have been cited in the athletic training literature, including saws, the FM Extractor, the Trainer's Angel, Dremel tools, knives, PVC pipe cutters, pruning shears, and scissors.[54-65] A screwdriver seems appropriate, because the loop-straps are fastened to the helmet by a T-bolt, a washer, and a screw. In fact, compared with other tools, the screwdriver has been shown to be very efficient.[53,66] However, during the length of a football season, moisture can rust the screws and T-bolts, making them difficult to remove with a screwdriver. Other cases have been reported in which the T-bolt that holds the screw turns as the screw is loosened.[56,67] The screw can also be damaged beyond repair by the screwdriver being used, thus rendering it impossible to remove the face mask. This has even been reported during a research study in a controlled laboratory, with new hardware.[53] Hence, the effectiveness of a screwdriver has been deemed limited and unreliable. Because it has been proved to be unreliable, the Inter-Association Task Force does not recommend the screwdriver as the *primary* tool for loop-strap removal.

Another recommendation has been to use a sharp knife, scalpel, or box cutter to cut the loop-straps. However, new-generation loop-straps are being made of harder plastics and are more difficult to cut.[68,69] Injuries to subjects (the rescuers) during research studies have been reported when the knife slipped while the rescuers tried to cut through the loop-straps.[53] Because of the risk of injury to the victim and the rescuer, the Inter-Association Task Force does not recommend the use of knives or similar products to cut loop-straps.

EQUIPMENT MANAGEMENT

DuraShears, or "EMT scissors," are popular tools in the field for cutting seat belts, shoulder pad straps, clothing, and so on but are not recommended for cutting loop-straps.[60] It has been previously shown that the time it takes to remove the face mask with the DuraShears is unacceptable, with most times being greater than 8 minutes and one subject taking as long as 35 minutes in one study.[60]

At the present time, the most popular and widely used tool for face mask removal is the Trainer's Angel, which was the first tool specifically designed to cut the loop-straps that secure the face mask to the helmet.[54,59] However, compared with other tools, the Trainer's Angel was found to cause more head movement. In addition, many individuals are unaware of the recommended technique for the use of this tool.[59] The Trainer's Angel was the gold standard tool for many years but appears to be less effective with new-generation loop-straps.[62,68,70]

Face mask removal should be accomplished as quickly as possible and with as little movement of the head and neck as possible. The best tool that is used for face mask removal should be efficient with regard to both time and movement.[53,58] The anvil pruner, which is commonly used for gardening, has been shown, repeatedly, to be the most efficient tool for removal of the loop-straps.[51-53,57,68,69,71-75] Regardless of the tool selected, the Inter-Association Task Force recommends that those involved in the prehospital care of injured football players have the tools they select for face mask removal readily available, and be practiced in their use.[54,76]

Difficulties Encountered. Face mask removal can be a difficult task under the best of circumstances.[70] However, many other factors can complicate the efficient removal of the face mask,[65,69,72,74,76] including hardware that has been exposed to the elements, the effects of environmental temperature on the loop-strap, the effects of hand size and gender, and the sharpness of the rescue tools.

For example, many equipment managers modify the loop-strap arrangement and frequently use four loop-straps to secure the face mask to the lateral sides of the helmet (two on each side).[70] This arrangement makes it very difficult, if not impossible, to remove the loop-straps with the tools that are currently available.

Cra-Lite Face Mask. The Cra-Lite face mask is a solid plastic face mask (as opposed to the usual plastic-coated metal) supplied by Riddell, and it must be secured to the helmet with four lateral loop-straps. As indicated by the manufacturer, this unique face mask should be removed with a PVC pipe cutter (also sold by Riddell) rather than by cutting or removing the loop-straps.

Another complication occurs when the face mask is not secured by loop-straps but rather is bolted directly to the helmet. This is the way face masks were originally secured to the helmet, before loop-straps came into existence. Today, many youth leagues, such as Pop Warner, use helmets that are not approved by the National Operating Committee on Standards for Athletic Equipment (NOCSAE) and have a face mask bolted directly to the helmet. The Inter-Association Task Force recommends that football helmet face guards be attached by loop straps, and not bolted on, to facilitate appropriate emergency management by medical personnel. Additional recommendations regarding equipment are provided in Table 2.

> **The Inter-Association Task Force recommends that football helmet face guards be attached by loop straps, and not bolted on, to facilitate appropriate emergency management by medical personnel.**

Summary. *Certified athletic trainers and other initial responders should have the appropriate removal equipment available at all times and should be familiar with the use of this equipment before an emergency occurs.*[54] *They should also practice face mask removal with the tools they intend to use and on the helmets used in the competition.*[55,56,67,70,71,73,75]

HELMET

Most football helmets consist of a polycarbonate shell (approximately 4 mm thick) lined with either padding, air cells, or a combination of both to provide a secure fit to the athlete's head.[10] A chin strap further secures the helmet to the head. The helmet and chin strap should be left in place unless they do not hold the head securely enough for immobilization. The helmet should only be removed if the airway cannot be maintained or if the face mask cannot be removed. If the helmet is removed, spinal immobilization and alignment must be maintained. The potential for injury during helmet removal can be further complicated by the presence of shoulder pads that elevate the trunk; proper alignment is maintained by removing the shoulder pads simultaneously with the helmet.

When to Remove the Helmet. Because motorcycle helmets do not usually have a removable face mask, are not snugly fit to the head, and are worn without shoulder pads, they are routinely removed before transportation to achieve neutral spinal alignment and adequate stabilization of the injured motorcyclist on a spine board while access to the airway and chest is obtained for resuscitation efforts.[8,9] However, a properly fitted football helmet holds the head in a position of neutral spinal alignment, provided the athlete is wearing shoulder pads.[10,11] Therefore, the Inter-Association Task Force recommends that neither the football helmet nor the shoulder pads be removed before transportation (see *Guidelines for Removal*).[1,77-80]

In the management of a football player with a suspected spinal injury, both NATA and the American College of Sports Medicine have promoted statements that advise against the removal of football helmets in an uncontrolled environment.[78] Reduction in the amount of head and neck movement that occurs during helmet removal is very important because any additional motion can cause further damage to the football player with a cervical spine injury.[51]

The Inter-Association Task Force recommends that only the face mask be removed from the helmet. The helmet itself should not be removed unless the rescuer is unable to access the airway by all other means (or if the helmet does not adequately secure the head).[80]

Furthermore, by removing only the face mask and not the entire helmet, the spine will remain in a neutral position. If the helmet is removed, the athlete's head hyperextends, particularly when the athlete is wearing shoulder pads.[81] Unless the shoulder pads are removed at the same time, it would be very difficult to maintain in-line neutral stabilization. Spinal immobilization and alignment must be maintained during removal of the helmet. The design and fit of the helmet and shoulder pads require careful removal of each to maintain spinal alignment. The helmet and shoulder pads significantly elevate the athlete's trunk and head when in the supine position; the removal of only one piece of equipment can cause a significant change in spinal alignment.

Guidelines for Removal. In general, any athletic helmet should be removed on the field only under any of the following circumstances:

- If after a reasonable period of time, the face mask cannot be removed to gain access to the airway[1,79]
- If the design of the helmet and chin strap is such that even after removal of the face mask, the airway cannot be controlled or ventilation provided[1,10,77,83,84]
- If the helmet and chin straps do not hold the head securely such that immobilization of the helmet does not also immobilize the head[1,10,83,85]
- If the helmet prevents immobilization for transport in an appropriate position[1,10]

How to Remove the Helmet. The Inter-Association Task Force acknowledges that specific guidelines for helmet removal need to be developed and, in the interim, offer the following general guidelines. The Inter-Association Task Force recommends that the helmet be removed in a controlled environment after radiographs have been obtained and only by qualified medical personnel with training in equipment removal.[42,86] Helmet removal should never be attempted without thorough communication among all involved parties. One person should stabilize the head, neck, and helmet while another person cuts the chin strap. Accessible internal helmet padding, such as cheek pads, should be removed, and air padding should be deflated before removal of the helmet, while a second assistant manually stabilizes the chin and back of the neck, in a cephalad direction, making sure to maintain the athlete's position.[87] The pads are removed through

EQUIPMENT MANAGEMENT

the insertion of a tongue depressor or a similar stiff, flat-bladed object between the snaps and helmet shell to pry the cheek pads away from their snap attachment.[1,88,89] If an air cell--padding system is present, deflate the air inflation system by releasing the air at the external port with an inflation needle or large-gauge hypodermic needle. The helmet should slide off the occiput with slight forward rotation of the helmet.[11,77,88] In the event the helmet does not move, slight traction can be applied to the helmet which can then be gently maneuvered anteriorly and posteriorly, although the head/neck unit must not be allowed to move.[46] The helmet should not be spread apart by the ear holes[42,87] as this maneuver only serves to tighten the helmet on the forehead and occiput region.

> If an air cell--padding system is present, deflate the air inflation system by releasing the air at the external port with an inflation needle or large-gauge hypodermic needle.

SHOULDER PADS

The padded plastic shell of a football player's shoulder pads is of sufficient thickness that the pads elevate the torso of the supine player to the same height as the helmeted head.[11,83,90,91] It is important to note that shoulder pads used in lacrosse, ice hockey and field hockey are not as thick as those used in football. As such, the removal of equipment from a spine-injured athlete in any of these sports could vary. Shoulder pads are held in place with straps that clip to the front sternal plate. Neck rolls may be attached to the shoulder pads or be independent of them. In most cases, the front of the shoulder pads can be opened to allow the rescuer access to the athlete's chest for evaluation, auscultation of breath and cardiac sounds, and chest compression during cardiopulmonary resuscitation and for defibrillation (or automated external defibrillator pad placement) when necessary.

When to Remove the Shoulder Pads. Spinal immobilization must be maintained while the helmet is removed; therefore, during helmet removal, the shoulder pads must be removed simultaneously.[82] The helmet/shoulder pad unit should be thought of as an all-or-none scenario with regard to spinal immobilization. Studies have shown excess movement in the cervical spine when helmet or shoulder pads are removed alone.[82,92-94]

In the athlete with a potential cervical spine injury, controversy has arisen over whether the helmet, shoulder pads, or both should be removed before transport from the field to an emergency facility. Concerns regarding the removal of equipment include

1. The ability to maintain neutral spinal alignment
2. The ability to secure rigid fixation of the athlete to the board
3. A guarantee of access to the airway and to the chest for resuscitation efforts[94]

Possible situations in which removal of shoulder pads would be necessary before transport to an emergency facility may include, but are not limited to, the following situations:

1. The helmet is removed
2. Multiple injuries require full access to shoulder area
3. Ill-fitting shoulder pads caused the inability to maintain spinal immobilization

The helmet and shoulder pads elevate an athlete's trunk in the supine position. Should either be removed or if only one is present, appropriate spinal alignment must be maintained. With removal of only the face mask, and not the entire helmet, the spine is able to remain in the existing position. If the helmet is removed, the athlete's head will hyperextend, particularly if the player is wearing shoulder pads.[82,92-98] Research with fluoroscopy and kinetic magnetic resonance imaging shows that unless the shoulder pads are removed simultaneously, it is not possible to maintain in-line neutral stabilization.[82,90-94,96-98] Therefore, removal of the helmet and shoulder pads, if required only as a last resort, must be coordinated to avoid cervical hyperextension. Head/shoulder stabilization must be maintained during any manipulation of equipment. The Inter-Association Task Force recommends that neither the football helmet nor the shoulder pads be removed before transportation.[1,77-80] Furthermore, the simultaneous removal of the helmet and shoulder pads is best done in a controlled atmosphere, such as the emergency department, with many trained hands.[51,82,94]

How to Remove the Shoulder Pads. The Inter-Association Task Force recommends that shoulder pads be removed only in conjunction with the athlete's helmet and only when removal is warranted (see *When to Remove the Shoulder Pads*). Whenever the decision is made to remove the shoulder pads, it is favorable to follow the following steps:

1. Cut jersey and all other shirts from neck to waist and from the midline to the end of each arm sleeve.
2. Cut all straps used to secure the shoulder pads to the torso. Attempts to unbuckle or unsnap any fasteners should be avoided due to the potential for unnecessary movement.
3. Cut all straps used to secure the shoulder pads (and extenders) to the arms.
4. Cut laces or straps over the sternum. A consistent manufactured characteristic of shoulder pads is the mechanism to attach the two halves of the shoulder pad unit on the anterior aspect. This lace or strap system allows for quick and efficient access to the anterior portion of the chest.
5. Cut and/or remove any and all accessories such as neck rolls or collars, so they can be removed simultaneously with the shoulder pads. The shoulder pads can now be released with full access to chest, face, neck, and arms. The posterior portion of the shoulder pads helps to maintain spinal alignment when the helmet and shoulder pads are in place.
6. A primary responder maintains cervical stabilization in a cephalad direction by placing his or her forearms on the athlete's chest while holding the maxilla and occiput. This is a skilled position that requires personnel who are practiced in this technique.

7. With responders at each side of the patient, their hands are placed directly against the skin in the thoracic region of the back.
8. Additional support is placed at strategic locations down the body as deemed appropriate in consideration of the size of the patient.
9. While the patient is lifted, the individual who was in charge of head/shoulder stabilization should remove the helmet and then immediately remove the shoulder pads by spreading apart the front panels and pulling them around the head.
10. All shirts, jerseys, neck rolls, extenders, and so on should be removed at this time.
11. The patient is lowered.

Shoulder pads have consistent design characteristics that allow removal procedures to be relatively uniform. It is highly recommended these procedures be practiced with all necessary rescue and medical personnel using the equipment commonly worn by the athletes.[1,79,99] It is also suggested that all equipment be properly maintained. It is the integrity of the shoulder pads and helmet working together that provide spinal immobilization and safe removal of equipment when it is necessary to do so.[93] Poorly maintained or modified equipment may hamper the safe removal process, which may lead to an increase in the severity of the initial injury.

> The Inter-Association Task Force recommends that shoulder pads be removed only in conjunction with the athlete's helmet and only when removal is warranted.

Immobilization and Transportation

For initial stabilization of an injured athlete, see *On-the-Field Management* and *Immediate Care*.

Manual stabilization of the head, neck, and shoulders should be performed as the patient is being assessed. In most cases, the football helmet and shoulder pads should not be removed during evaluation, immobilization, and transportation, but when the helmet must be removed, the shoulder pads should be removed as well (see *Equipment Management*).

When a determination is made that transportation to an emergency receiving facility is imminent, the athlete will have to be secured to an appropriate immobilization device (see *Immobilization Equipment*). Controversy has arisen over whether the athlete whose spine is found in a less than anatomically correct position should be repositioned. In the past, when an athlete could actively reposition his or her head into a neutral position without encountering resistance or pain, they were encouraged to do so. Recently, a more cautious approach has been observed since it is assumed that an unstable spinal injury can be converted to an injury with more severe damage if the athlete is mishandled.[100]

The Inter-Association Task Force recommends only that stabilization of the head and spine be maintained. In most cases, this means that the head and spine are repositioned into a neutral position so in-line stabilization can be accomplished with appropriate immobilization devices.[101-103] However, in some instances, it may be best for the athlete's head and neck to be immobilized in the position in which they are found. The appropriateness of repositioning the head into a spine-neutral position should be assessed on an individual basis. Techniques for spinal immobilization and the determination of whether in-line stabilization is required for transportation should be left to local protocols or the clinical judgment, expertise, and training of the individuals on-site.

The Inter-Association Task Force recognize that it may not be possible to apply a rigid cervical collar when the helmet and shoulder pads are left in place or when spinal immobilization is being accomplished in a position other than neutral. Other methods of padding, such as towels or blanket rolls, must then be used to secure the head to the spine board.[28] It has also been suggested that a cervical vacuum splint is an effective immobilizer in the athlete wearing protective equipment.[104] If the athlete's spine is being immobilized in a neutral (in-line) position, every attempt should be made to apply a rigid cervical collar.[14,105-110] When the athlete is anchored to the spine board, the body should be secured using standard techniques.[8,111-117] The application of a spine board should always include straps to secure the pelvis, shoulders, legs, and, last, the head.[118] After removal of the face mask, with the chin strap left in place, the helmeted head is secured to the board with adhesive tape or straps. At least two straps should be used to secure the torso, pelvis, and legs. The straps must be applied snugly so the athlete does not move if rolled onto his or her side due to vomiting. Any gaps must be filled in with towels or rigid foam.[9,42,80,119] Once the athlete is completely stabilized, the person at the head relinquishes his or her control, and the athlete is transported to an emergency medical facility.[100] The Inter-Association Task Force recommends some form of acceleration/deceleration, or "trauma strapping", to prevent axial loading in the ambulance during braking. It is also a common practice and a local protocol in some districts to load the stretcher in the ambulance with the athlete's head at the rear to avoid axial loading during ambulance braking.

Patients with spinal injuries often have a component of head injury that can lead to vomiting. Athletes who are vomiting or bleeding from the oral cavity must be kept prone or placed on their side to prevent aspiration of blood or vomitus into the airway.[9] However, this can be performed after the athlete is immobilized (see above). Furthermore, proper equipment, such as a suction apparatus, should be readily available (see *The Emergency Plan*). These procedures should be identified and practiced often to ensure a smooth transfer to a spine board when an emergency occurs.

TRANSFER OF THE ATHLETE

To transfer a *supine athlete*, the Inter-Association Task Force recommends using a six-plus--person lift along with a scoop stretcher to lift the athlete onto a rigid long spine board rather than a log roll technique.[80] A six-plus--person lift is recommended due to the size of many athletes and the interference by protective equipment. To transfer a *prone athlete*, the Inter-Association Task Force recommends log rolling the athlete directly onto a rigid long spine board. Movement of the athlete from the prone to the supine position should be done with a minimum of four persons, with one designated to maintain stabilization of the head and neck. All movement should be carefully coordinated to avoid shifting the head, neck, and torso.[8]

Log Roll of a Prone Athlete. Due to the urgency of establishing an airway in the athlete, assessment must be made very quickly and efficiently. If a prone athlete is not breathing, a log roll should be performed immediately. Unless the immobilization device is readily available, the athlete must be log rolled into a supine position on the playing surface and then moved (lifted) a second time onto the long back board. Obviously, with each movement the chances of a secondary injury increase. If the athlete is conscious and stable, the log roll should be delayed until the backboard is available.

To immobilize the prone athlete, the rescuer at the head (rescuer 1) should maintain the athlete's head/neck complex in the position in which it was found until it is completely splinted on the full body splint. When possible, the athlete should be treated with a rigid cervical collar to ensure the immobilization of all segmental levels.[78,109,120] Next, position the immobilization device by the injured athlete on the side of rescuer 1's lower hand. When the athlete is wearing protective equipment, the athlete's arms should be maintained at his or her side (with palm inward). Rescuers 2 and 3 will then roll the athlete onto his or her arm, which should be kept to the side during the log roll maneuver. An injury that involves the arm calls for the athlete to be log rolled to the opposite side, which may be difficult in the presence of shoulder pads. Shoulder pads are not easy

to remove, especially if worn with a neck collar; thus, they should be only removed in the most extenuating of circumstances.

Rescuer 1 is in charge and will give every command to move the athlete. Rescuer 1 must continue to maintain the position of the head/neck complex until the athlete is completely immobilized. Rescuers 2 and 3 position themselves adjacent to the athlete. On the opposite side of the athlete, rescuer 4 positions himself or herself and the splinting device. Rescuer 2 is positioned at the chest area, and rescuer 3 is positioned at thigh level. Rescuer 3 is expected to control both legs during the log roll maneuver. To roll the athlete, rescuer 1 gives the command "prepare to roll, roll." The other rescuers should then roll the athlete onto his or her side, toward the rescuers. By rolling the athlete onto his or her arm, the head, shoulders, and pelvis are kept in anatomical alignment. Rescuer 4 places the splinting device against the athlete's back at a 30-degree angle. While positions are maintained, rescuer 1 gives the command "prepare to lower, lower," and the athlete is lowered onto the splint.[99]

Six-Plus--Person Lift. Heavy persons, including many athletes, can be handled more efficiently with a six-plus--person lift; this is also preferred for suspected spine injuries. The Inter-Association Task Force recommends that the six-plus--person lift be used along with a scoop stretcher whenever possible. In the athletic arena, there are usually a sufficient number of certified athletic trainers, physicians, and EMS personnel on hand to effectively administer the six-plus--person lift.

For the six-plus--person lift, rescuer 1 immobilizes the neck. The rescuer's hands are placed on the athlete's shoulders (under the shoulder pads) with the thumbs pointed away from the athlete's face. The athlete's head will then be resting between the rescuer's forearms.

The other six rescuers position themselves along the athlete's sides: one on each side of the chest, pelvis, and legs. The hands are slid under the athlete and equipment, if any, to provide a firm, coordinated lift. To lift, rescuer 1 gives the command "prepare to lift, lift." The assistants lift the athlete 4 to 6 inches off the ground. It is imperative to maintain a coordinated lift

IMMOBILIZATION AND TRANSPORTATION

and to prevent any movement of the spine. One of the rescuers at the thigh level must control the legs with his or her arms toward the feet so the splint can be slid into place from the foot end. After the splint is in place, while positions are maintained, rescuer 1 gives the command "prepare to lower, lower," and the athlete is lowered onto the splint.

In the case of larger athletes, as many as 10 individuals should participate in the lift, with one on each side of the chest and pelvis, two at the legs, one at the head, and one with the splint. The Inter-Association Task Force does not recommend the use of fewer than four-plus--persons to lift athletes suspected of having a spinal injury, even smaller athletes and children, in part due to the weight of the athlete while wearing protective equipment.

IMMOBILIZATION EQUIPMENT

Any injured athlete who may have a cervical spine injury should be immobilized on a suitable full-body splint. The equipment used for splinting athletes with head or neck injuries will depend on the appliances that are available, as well as the training and knowledge of EMS personnel.

Certified athletic trainers should know how to use the equipment that is available and should be familiar with the equipment EMS providers will bring to the scene. EMS providers should take the lead in the immobilization of an athlete for transportation because they are far more practiced in immobilization techniques and will be responsible for the athlete during transportation. However, team physicians and certified athletic trainers are more familiar with athletic protective equipment and should therefore direct and assist the EMS providers in the immobilization process of the athlete with protective equipment. Certified athletic trainers and team physicians should familiarize themselves and rehearse the handling of such equipment on a regular basis because of their infrequent use of such equipment.

Equipment for spinal immobilization includes the Miller full-body splint, the standard rigid spine board, the vacuum mattress, and the scoop stretcher.

Miller Full-Body Splint. To use the Miller full-body splint, move the splint next to the athlete. Open the harness, and fold all straps onto themselves to prevent entanglement of the Velcro. Lift or log roll the athlete onto the Miller full-body splint. Align the athlete's shoulders with the shoulder pins on the Miller full-body splint. Place the chest straps loosely over the athlete's chest. Place the shoulder strap onto the chest strap. Thread the chest strap through the pins on the Miller full-body splint. Adjust the chest strap, and then adjust the shoulder straps. Do not overtighten either of the straps. Adjust the torso and the leg and ankle straps to secure the athlete to the Miller full-body splint.

If the athlete is wearing a protective helmet, tape the helmet directly to the Miller full-body splint headpiece. Apply the chin strap snugly but loose enough to allow the mouth to open.

Rigid Spine Board. Once the athlete has been placed on the board (by six-plus--person lift or log roll), apply blankets, rolled towels, or commercial head immobilizers, and strap the athlete into position. At least two straps should be used to secure the torso, pelvis, and legs. The Inter-Association Task Force recommends some form of acceleration/deceleration, or "trauma strapping". With the helmet and shoulder pads in place, towels or other padding is usually sufficient to fill the voids. Finally, the helmet should be secured to the backboard with adhesive tape. When completed, the athlete with protective equipment is said to be immobilized.

Vacuum Mattress. The vacuum mattress is one of the newest methods of immobilization. Unlike the rigid spine board, the vacuum splints consist of Styrofoam beads encapsulated in a vacuum nylon covering. When air is released, the splint provides support to the axial spine or total body. The splint includes wooden slats posteriorly for head-to-toe stability.

To prepare the splint for use, remove from the case at the beginning of each practice or game. Create a semirigid splint through partial removal of air. In the event of an injury, the semirigid splint can be moved into place as needed.

When an injury occurs that necessitates total body immobilization, those who are providing care must decide how to move the athlete onto the splint. Always protect the athlete with a suspected spinal injury. Athletes in awkward positions may be moved onto the rigid spine board or vacuum splint with a scoop stretcher. When the vacuum mattress is used, release the buckles on the mattress before moving the athlete onto the splint. The person at the head maintains firm support, or pressure, to the head. Pressure includes gentle, in-line traction. When preparing the athlete for the vacuum mattress, use standard commands of "prepare to lift, lift" or "prepare to roll, roll." Once the athlete is positioned onto the mattress, continue stabilization of the head and neck. Open the valves at the head and foot ends to allow air to enter the mattress. Bunch the beads around the head and into the body to mold the splint. At this point, screw the valve at the head to the locked position. Continue the application of pressure so the beads form around the head and helmet. The person at the head works with the second rescuer to accomplish this molding around the head/helmet. Reattach the straps by connecting color-coded buckles. Take care not to twist the straps, which could create uncomfortable pressure points for the athlete. Move the excess strap down the body from head to toe. As tightened, attach the pump to the foot end and release air from the splint. As the splint becomes rigid, recheck the straps in a head-to-toe direction to remove any excess slack from the belt. Apply adhesive tape across the head area to secure the helmet to the splint. Screw all valves to the locked position.

Scoop Stretcher. The scoop stretcher, or split litter, is adjusted to the correct length and then separated, inserted, and fastened according to its design. The patient is lifted 4 to 6 inches off the ground while a rigid long board is slid underneath. The split litter should not be picked up from the head and foot ends or used to carry the patient before it has been placed on a long board because it can sag without center support. The scoop stretcher can be left in place or removed before the athlete is secured to the long board, but keep in mind that these devices are usually made of aluminum and x-rays do not penetrate easily. The Inter-Association Task Force recommends using a scoop stretcher along with the six-plus--person lift to facilitate the transfer of the supine athlete onto a long spine board for definitive immobilization.

ADVANCED TRANSPORTATION AND CARE

Team physicians, certified athletic trainers, and EMS personnel who are caring for an athlete with a potential spinal injury should be familiar with local trauma networks and protocols. If the patient is hemodynamically stable, transport should be directed to a designated hospital with special capabilities for spinal injury. Critical patients may need to be stabilized at the closest appropriate hospital before transfer to a more definitive care facility. In remote areas where the distance to a trauma center is very long, the physician may elect to accompany the athlete to the hospital and participate in the treatment.

Any athlete who is suspected of having a spinal injury is to be transported by trained professionals in an ambulance. Transportation in a private vehicle is never to be attempted. In certain settings, air transportation may be preferred to ground transportation. A trauma center should be the first-choice destination for spine-injured athletes. Trauma center designation levels and capabilities will vary by state, so it is important to be familiar with the facilities available in your area.

Methylprednisolone. Methylprednisolone is used in cases of spinal cord injury, but it must be administered as soon as possible and over 24 hours. The dosage of this medication is 30 mg/kg body weight administered over 1 hour. The subsequent dosage is 5.6mg/kg body weight, administered over the next 23 hours. The first dose of intravenous methylprednisolone should be administered within 4 hours of the injury to be most effective. Therefore, team physicians in rural areas or those who travel substantial distances may elect to carry methylprednisolone or to ensure that the emergency receiving facilities and/or EMS providers have the medication on hand. Many local EMS providers are able to begin this treatment while transporting the patient.

Injuries and Possible Mechanisms

Injuries can be classified as direct or indirect.[27,121] Direct injuries occur as a result of sports participation and include closed head injuries and cervical spine trauma as a result of contact/collision. Indirect injuries can include heart attack, heat illness, or other preexisting medical conditions. Direct injuries are more common in contact/collision sports such as football, hockey, and rugby.[12,13,48,122,123]

All of the anatomic components of the cervical spine are subject to traumatic injury, including soft tissues, bone and joint structures, and neurological elements.[124,125] Within each category, these tissues are variably susceptible to both compressive and tensile overload, which will result in specific injury patterns and clinical presentations.[36,126] Not all spinal injuries are catastrophic, although many of the same signs and symptoms can appear in catastrophic and noncatastrophic injuries. Therefore, an understanding of all of the possible injuries to the spine is warranted.

SOFT TISSUE INJURIES

Soft tissue injuries to the cervical spine, including muscle, ligament, and tendon injuries, probably occur most frequently.[29] *Muscle contusions* can result from direct impact in the neck region or can occur indirectly via forces transmitted through protective equipment (i.e., the shoulder pads and helmet). *Tensile* overload to the musculotendinous unit occurs most commonly and is often associated with tackling in football. This is particularly true with a blind-side tackle when the player is not prepared for the collision, which can result in a forceful eccentric muscle contraction that places the musculotendinous unit at risk. This risk is often increased when muscle fatigue is present.

Acute muscular spasm often develops secondary to an underlying spinal injury, so a spinal injury should be considered whenever an initial assessment reveals spasm, tenderness or loss of active range of motion.[127,128]

Ligamentous injuries typically result from tensile overload with varying degrees of disruption. The innervation of the ligamentous structures in the cervical spine includes receptors that respond to slow tonic input, which is important in postural control, rather than ballistic movement.[129] Thus, ligaments are susceptible to sudden loads. Ligament injury may lead to instability patterns specific for the segmental location of the particular ligament and may be associated with neurological impairment. Instability must be considered in any player with neurological symptoms, especially if the symptoms are persistent.

SKELETAL INJURIES

The spatial and geometric orientation of the cervical *zygapophyseal joints* (also known as facet joints, or z-joints) allows a high degree of mobility of the cervical spine, which places all anatomic structures at risk for injury. The z-joints are loaded when the head and neck are moved into the posterior and posterolateral quadrants. Acute compressive overload or chronic repetitive loading of these structures may result in synovitis of the z-joint and, depending on the force, may have an impact on injury and microfracture of the articular cartilage and subchondral bone of the facet processes. Tensile overload injuries lead to a spectrum of capsular damage, from strain to complete disruption. Greater degrees of capsular incompetence contribute to segmental hypermobilities and instabilities. Whether resulting in hypomobility or hypermobility, z-joint injury at one segmental level may lead to a cascading effect of segmental motion abnormalities elsewhere in the cervical spine.

Fractures of the cervical spine can occur when a player's head unexpectedly strikes another object and the force of impact exceeds the compressive or tensile limit of the bony structure.[130-132] Both the anterior column (i.e., vertebral body) and the posterior column (i.e., pedicle, lamina, or facet) structures are at risk.[133,134] Fractures can be associated with instability, which must always be considered if neurological sequelae develop, but can also exist without neurological symptoms or signs. It is important to note that some fractures, particularly in the posterior column, can be difficult, if not impossible, to identify on plain radiography and require some type of advanced imaging technique.[135,136]

Acute cervical fracture-dislocations occur most commonly as the result of an axial load to the top of the helmet with the neck slightly flexed, the so-called segmented column.[131,137-140] The straightened spine buckles in the center in an accordion-type mechanism, which produces a fracture dislocation or a transitory subluxation.[141,142] It is for this reason that spearing is illegal in football. However, inadvertent contact with another player, or even the ground, also can produce this injury.[85,138,143,144] Catastrophic injuries almost universally result from the axial load mechanism, of which an understanding is important for injury prevention. Other injuries that can occur from axial loading include the following[137,145,146]:

- Flexion rotation fracture dislocation of the midcervical spine
- Jefferson fracture of the ring of C1
- An anterior subluxation injury that involves a rupture of the posterior longitudinal ligament and ligamentum flavum
- Bilateral and unilateral facet dislocation
- Cervical disc herniation
- Vertebral body fracture
- Intervertebral facet fracture
- A rupture of the atlantoaxial ligament

A variety of other mechanisms can also result in fracture-dislocation or in dislocation without fracture (i.e., unilateral or bilateral facet dislocation), including forceful rotation with flexion or extension.[147,148] These types of injuries usually result in an intervertebral disc injury, as well as a disc rupture or herniation.[124] Less severe disc injury also can occur, due to excessive torque to the cervical spine and excessive shear force across the annulus fibrosus, leading to annular tears and possibly disc herniations.

Predisposing Conditions. Numerous injuries can be acquired from head contact. Predisposing conditions can make certain players more vulnerable even though they are unaware of this predisposition. The most common abnormality is congenital stenosis, in which the spinal canal is too small for the spinal cord. Klippel-Feil syndrome is a congenital abnormality that involves the fusion of different segments of the neck to produce compensatory hypermobility in other areas. Most players and physicians are not aware of congenital abnormalities until some symptoms develop. These findings can be a major factor in

determining potential risk and in decisions concerning continued play after an injury.[149-154]

Spinal stenosis, whether congenital or acquired, means the player is more likely
- To have an episode of transient quadriplegia[153,154]
- To have "stingers"[146,154]
- To require surgery after a cervical disc herniation[152,153]
- To run the risk of potential paralysis without a fracture-dislocations[152,156,157]
- To develop paralysis and a greater degree of paralysis after a fracture-dislocation[154,156,157]

NEUROLOGICAL INJURIES

From a mechanical basis, the neurological contents of the spinal canal can be compromised by bone or disc fragment, malalignment, or instability.[131,155,157,158] Vascular insult also may contribute to various neurological syndromes. The three main neurological elements at risk are the spinal cord, nerve root/spinal nerve complex, and brachial plexus. Catastrophic injury that results in transient or permanent quadriplegia is rare, with an incidence of approximately 0.6 to 1.5 per 100,000 participants in high school and college, respectively, during the 19-year period of 1977 to 1995.[6,7]

As previously described, *central spinal canal compromise* is associated with fracture-dislocation and other instability patterns. The spinal cord is deformable and can accommodate some change in the length of the spinal canal without injury. However, the presence of spinal stenosis, developmental or acquired, decreases the chances for full neurological recovery if an athlete develops quadriplegia due to cervical spine trauma.[160-162] Spinal cord injury may be neurapraxic (a reversible concussive event) with motor and sensory function returning within approximately 24 hours.[163]

The most typical pattern of incomplete spinal cord injury is the central cord syndrome.[164] Due to the lamination of the corticospinal tracts located toward the center of the spinal cord, the upper extremities are most susceptible to impairment with swelling or contusion to the cord. A variety of incomplete spinal cord injuries can develop due to a combination of mechanical and vascular effects on the spinal cord.

INJURIES AND POSSIBLE MECHANISMS

Burners and Stingers. The more common neurological injury is the *"stinger,"* or *"burner."*[165] The stinger is a peripheral nerve injury, not a spinal cord injury. It is characterized by burning dysesthesias that usually begin in the shoulder and radiate unilaterally into the arm and hand. Weakness, numbness, or both are occasionally associated in a C5-6 nerve root distribution. Recovery from an initial stinger usually occurs in minutes, but the symptoms and signs (most commonly numbness or weakness) can persist for several days to a few weeks, particularly if it is a recurrent condition.

Stingers typically result from one of two mechanisms of injury, which can vary depending on the skill and physical maturity of the athlete. A *compressive mechanism* develops when the head and neck are forcibly moved into a posterolateral direction toward the symptomatic upper limb.[166] The other mechanism, a *tensile mechanism*, occurs when the involved arm and neck are forced in opposite directions. With either pathomechanism (tension or compression), the cervical spine nerve is probably at greater risk than the brachial plexus.[124,145] Thus, stingers are more appropriately considered a cervical radiculopathy than a brachial plexopathy, although a brachial plexopathy can occur from a direct blow to the upper thorax or from tension. Cervical radiculopathy also can occur due to a cervical disc herniation, cervical foraminal stenosis, and instability.

Burners and stingers typically produce loss of function and pain only for a limited period of time.[167-170] Often the player will flex and laterally bend his or her head and neck away from the involved arm. As the pain decreases, the player will gradually demonstrate improved range of motion. There can be a great deal of posterior cervical tenderness with the stinger because the posterior primary ramus of the nerve innervates the skin in that area and comes directly off the dorsal ganglion.

The symptoms of a stinger should be distinguished from those of a spinal cord injury to initiate an appropriate treatment relative to the severity of the injury.[127] The key clinical distinction between spinal cord injury and a stinger is that the spinal cord injury results in multiple limb involvement (i.e., two to four),

whereas the stinger always results in unilateral upper extremity impairment. The determination of whether an injury is related to the spinal cord or is a stinger should be made with great caution due to the importance of initial management of the injury.[171] Unlike the consequences of a spinal cord injury, players with burners and stingers often are headed off the field when their symptoms are discovered.[167,168]

Transient quadriplegia is a temporary paralysis that is characterized by a loss of motor or sensory function, or both. It is current neurosurgical thinking that a common mechanism of transient quadriplegia is a contusion of the spinal cord that produces a temporary restriction of blood flow to a portion of the cervical spinal cord. The extent of neurological deficit and how long it lasts are critical and determine prognosis. The mechanism of injury may be varied and complex.[163,172] The most significant factor is the initial head-first contact. If subsequent neck flexion follows, the spinal cord becomes taut and is stretched over the floor of the spinal canal, producing a transitory plastic deformation of the cord. This produces a collapse of blood vessels and an interruption of blood supply to the cord. Neck extension after head contact produces the opposite effect, or slackening of the cord. Further extension narrows the central spinal canal, and the posterior disc, osteophytes, and ligamentum flavum protrude into the spinal canal and compress the spinal cord. In addition, the intervertebral foramen diameter narrows and becomes smaller in extension as the two articular facets slide into a small relative subluxation. Conversely, flexion produces a larger central canal diameter through removal of the relative infolding of ligamentum flavum and posterior disc bulging from the canal. Extension and flexion can produce a pincer effect between the posterior edge of one vertebral body and the lamina of another. This is a relative subluxation between two vertebral segments that squeezes the spinal cord producing a contusion and localized deformation of the cord. Transient quadriplegia is, by definition, a temporary condition, a neurapraxia, but the player initially presents with paralysis and must be managed accordingly.[173]

Return-to-Play Criteria

There is not a simple algorithm that determines return to play after a cervical spine injury.[174] Medical factors are paramount, although a variety of nonmedical factors (e.g., age of the athlete, level of competition, psychosocial issues) can influence return-to-play decisions.[175-180] Although the decision to return to play can be complex, some medical sequelae of certain cervical spine injuries do represent absolute contraindications to return to contact or collision sports. These include neck injuries resulting in permanent central nervous system (i.e., spinal cord) dysfunction, permanent and significant peripheral nerve (i.e., nerve root) dysfunction, and injuries resulting in a spinal fusion at the C4 level or above. Some other conditions, which include anatomic abnormalities such as spinal stenosis, represent relative contraindications to return to play, even in the clinical setting of "full" recovery.[156,181] The Inter-Association Task Force recommends that any athlete who sustains a cervical spinal injury be evaluated individually and completely by a licensed, well-trained sports medicine physician who is then responsible for making the final return-to-play decision.[182-191]

Prevention

Many believe that prevention is the most important aspect of this topic. Over the years, many strategies have been used to reduce spine injuries, including rules changes,[55,142,192-198] changes in equipment and equipment standards,[193,198-200] and conditioning and strengthening programs.[192,201,202] However, the heart and soul of the preventive program should be teaching the proper technique. The majority of catastrophic spine injuries are a result of the axial loading mechanism.

Tackling Techniques. Proper tackling techniques are the key. Although some players have hit their head into their teammate after missing the tackle they were attempting, many simply lower their head in an attempt to deliver a blow to their opponents. Smaller players occasionally develop a head tackling technique to be successful against larger players. This is also evident by the fact that fracture dislocations with paralysis occur in a higher incidence in defensive backs.

Proper instruction in blocking and tackling techniques has, and can continue to, significantly decrease the incidence of axial loading injuries to the cervical spine through purposeful head contact.[203] Although hard tackling and hard blocking are a part of football and other sports, a certain number of these injuries may be unavoidable. A proper preventative approach educates players about the potential risk for catastrophic injury when tackling an opponent with a lowered head and teaches athletes alternate ways to be effective on the playing field.[76,199]

The Inter-Association Task Force recommends that players, parents, and coaches all participate in educational programs. These educational programs in youth leagues and other developmental programs should emphasize a "see what you hit" approach to blocking and tackling. Educational programs at all levels should remind players, parents, and coaches about the dangers of moving an injured player. Everyone should be cognizant of the dangers of moving a player with a suspected spinal injury and must be instructed and reminded not to move any player who shows signs of a severe injury. Educational programs should also include a picture of the potential for catastrophe.[199,200] The Inter-Association Task Force recommends that educational programs be held at regular intervals.

Having an emergency plan in place is also an important part of the prevention program.

The Emergency Plan

Although professional organizations, including NATA, have specific documents detailing the components of an emergency plan, the Inter-Association Task Force believes that a comprehensive document regarding the care of the spine-injured athlete should contain at least basic information regarding an emergency plan.

OVERVIEW

A quick review established procedures with all parties involved should take place before every contest due to the possibility of a personnel change in any component of the athletic healthcare delivery system. This review may include the determination of who should be on the field (team physician, certified athletic trainer, etc.), who will be responsible for completing the initial evaluation, when EMS personnel are to be summoned, and what special equipment should be brought onto the field. A review that is specific to the activity being covered should occur as often as possible and

> A review that is specific to the activity being covered should occur as often as possible and especially before every competition.

especially before every competition. For example, exact procedures for back boarding an equipment-laden football player will differ from that for the soccer player with no heavy equipment. Follow-up plans, such as determining who accompanies the athlete to the hospital, who notifies a family member, and who completes all appropriate documentation, should be discussed and agreed on by all responsible parties before the start of the sports season.

Essential to the smooth operation of any emergency situation is proper planning; all athletic healthcare providers must work together as a team, and a well-conceived plan must be followed. This plan is frequently called an emergency plan.[204] Although it is not the purpose of this paper to discuss the emergency plan, it is important to emphasize that following an organized plan is critical to the emergency

management of an athlete with a suspected head or cervical spine injury. Furthermore, the emergency plan should address equipment issues specific to the management and packaging of suspected head or cervical spine injuries.

The emergency plan should be thought of as a blueprint for handling emergencies. It should contain the roles and responsibilities of each member of the sports medicine team, and it should include steps to properly activate the EMS system.[205] A good emergency plan is easily understood and establishes accountability.[204]

Emergency plans should be comprehensive and practical, yet flexible enough to adapt to any emergency situation. The emergency plan must be established, approved, revised, and rehearsed on a regular basis.[204] Emergency plans must be written documents that are distributed to key personnel and approved by administrators.[205-207]

Each emergency plan can vary but should include information on education, emergency equipment, personnel, and communication and a rehearsal schedule.[205]

EDUCATION

It is likely that each member of the prehospital emergency care team will have a different type or level of education, have different levels of knowledge, and possess different skills.[208] These differences should be considered a positive circumstance. Individually, each member brings strengths to the team. Collectively, these differences become complementary to one another.

EMERGENCY EQUIPMENT AND SUPPLIES

Each member of the emergency team should be knowledgeable and practiced in the function and operation of emergency equipment.[50] It would be helpful for each member of the sports medicine team to be multi-skilled and cross-trained in the use of all emergency equipment. For example, it is common for certified athletic trainers to know how to remove a football helmet face mask, whereas physicians and emergency medical technicians may not have this skill.[208] Likewise, emergency medical technicians are more familiar with the operation of automated external defibrillators and are more practiced in packaging an individual for transportation (athlete or not) than are certified athletic trainers.[208]

In addition, many certified athletic trainers do not have ready access to the types of emergency care equipment to which EMS providers have access, particularly in the high school setting.[208]

Access to and familiarity with the equipment is only part of being prepared. Having sufficiently practiced with the equipment is the other part. It has been suggested that practice with the tools required for face mask removal of the catastrophically injured football player is essential.[51-53,55,59,60,71,73]

Equipment must be properly maintained and readily accessible.[50,205,206] Each member of the sports medicine team should be aware of the location of all emergency equipment and know how to use it. More importantly, each member should be practiced and skilled in its use. However, each state may have specific guidelines regarding the use of emergency equipment and who is legally authorized to use the equipment.[205] The Inter-Association Task Force advise individuals to become aware of the regulations in their particular state.

EMERGENCY PERSONNEL

When an athlete sustains an on-the-field cervical spine injury, potentially devastating and even life-threatening consequences can occur. These serious injuries are complex and happen in a difficult environment, significantly challenging the medical team. Well-rehearsed preparation and cooperation among all of the personnel involved in the prehospital care of the cervical spine injured athlete are essential to ensure the best chance for recovery.

Certified athletic trainers, physicians, emergency medical technicians, paramedics, and all other participants must be comprehensively trained and completely clear regarding their duties and responsibilities. This is best achieved through the repeated practice of all aspects of on-the-field triage, initial treatment, and transport of the injured athlete

until every component is automatic. Remember there must also be a plan in place for both practice and event situations.

> It is the opinion of the task force that no one discipline should have entitlement to supervision or performance of any particular aspect of the rescue.

Responsibilities for care may vary among different medical teams based on individual qualifications, skills, and availability. It is the opinion of the task force that no one discipline should have entitlement to supervision or performance of any particular aspect of the rescue. By working together, the knowledge and experience of individual team members can best be used to provide care for the athlete in this critical situation.

Certified athletic trainers play a critical role in the emergency management of athletic injuries.[207] The certified athletic trainer should take responsibility for better communication among all emergency personnel, which includes educating other professionals about the training and the roles and responsibilities of certified athletic trainers.[208] It is also advisable to get to know other members of the emergency care team on a personal basis and to establish a good working relationship at the athletic contest.[209] Each healthcare provider has individual expertise and deserves the respect of the other.[209]

Each member of the emergency team has his or her role in the emergency plan.[210] For example, it is not the responsibility of the certified athletic trainer or the team physician to transport injured athletes, and emergency medical technicians are generally more practiced at securing an individual to a spine board. In each case, the roles and responsibilities of the team members may change, based on the situation and the participants. The most qualified individual should always be in charge but should also respect the qualifications and expertise of his or her coworkers.[208]

THE EMERGENCY PLAN

COMMUNICATION

A physical means of communication must be available, including the use of telephones and radios.[99] This is necessary to activate the EMS system or to communicate with team physicians, parents, and so on. However, communication is a much broader topic and includes interaction between individuals.

Many individuals are unaware of the qualifications of certified athletic trainers in providing emergency care.[196-199] Furthermore, because of the changes in the educational process for certified athletic trainers, there can be great variability in knowledge and qualifications among certified athletic trainers.[208,211] Communication is the key to identifying who is present at the game and their roles and responsibilities.[208,209,212,213] It is important to establish this communication before the game starts and before an emergency situation arises.[210,212,213]

The lack of communication and role delineation has made for difficult and embarrassing situations for athletic healthcare providers, particularly with regard to differences in protocol on helmet removal in potential cervical spine injuries.[205,208,210,214,215] The best way to avoid this type of conflict in an emergency situation is to discuss the protocols and roles of each member of the medical team before the event and to familiarize the team members with the emergency plan.[206] Emergency plans should be detailed and should be reviewed and practiced. Forming a written emergency plan together with local EMS providers may also help to modify existing EMS protocols.

REHEARSAL SCHEDULE

To avoid potential conflicts, a meeting should be scheduled before a problem arises.[212,214] All providers of prehospital care, such as emergency medical technicians and EMS medical directors, should meet with team physicians, certified athletic trainers, coaches, and concerned parents to agree on an emergency plan.[204,208] Planning should take place before the start of the sports season and should be approved through all appropriate administrative channels.[204]

Certified athletic trainers should meet with coaches and game officials to review basic safety issues regarding spine injuries. Within the first few days of practice, certified athletic trainers should also meet with athletes to review the dangers of moving an injured player (see Table 3 for the guidelines of the National Football League).

Certified athletic trainers should conduct a meeting with the team's emergency care providers, including student athletic trainers, and with EMS personnel and medical directors to discuss all aspects of the emergency plan, including the protocol for spine-injured athletes.[210] All aspects of emergency spine care should be agreed on in concept and then practiced to perfection before the need for implementation on the field.[76] Formal rehearsal, such as mock emergency drills, should be conducted with all members of the emergency care team.

> **All aspects of emergency spine care should be agreed on in concept and then practiced to perfection before the need for implementation on the field.**

The Inter-Association Task Force recommends that the education, practice, and rehearsal of the protocol for managing a spine-injured athlete be scheduled at regular intervals and followed.

Summary and Conclusions

Injuries to the spine are relatively rare in athletics. However, when they do occur, they must be treated promptly and correctly. Certified athletic trainers and other providers of prehospital care must know which procedures to use in these situations. They must have the necessary equipment readily available and be proficient in its use. The regular practice of immobilization of athletes with potential cervical spine injuries is a must for individuals who expect to perform these important tasks in an actual emergency.

Care of the injured athlete should follow a carefully designed protocol. The athlete's airway, breathing, and circulation; neurological status; and level of consciousness should be assessed, and the EMS system should be activated.

Because unconscious individuals are unable to speak, they are unable to tell the rescuer whether they have a spinal injury. Therefore, all unconscious athletes in a situation that may have included a collision or a fall and conscious athletes with any sign or symptoms that suggest cervical spine trauma must be treated as if they have a cervical spine injury.

Any athlete suspected of having a head or spinal injury should not be moved unless absolutely essential to maintain airway, breathing, and circulation. If the athlete must be moved to maintain airway, breathing, and circulation, the athlete should be placed in a supine position while spinal immobilization is maintained.

In the conscious athlete, a possible cervical spine injury must be identified early. Athletes who display spasm, tenderness or loss of active range of motion should be suspected of having significant cervical spine trauma and should be treated accordingly. Cervical spine injuries are usually orthopedic in nature and may or may not have immediately observable neurological sequelae.

Athletes with no neurological signs or symptoms and no findings that suggest trauma to the cervical spine can be safely moved to a more suitable site for further evaluation. However, if there is any question as to medical status, it is best to err on the side of safety and to treat the injury as if it were a significant cervical spine injury.

When it becomes necessary to transport the athlete, the head and trunk should be moved as a unit. It takes many people to correctly move an injured athlete, with one rescuer responsible for stabilizing the athlete's head and cervical spine; as a general rule, this should be the most qualified and experienced person on the scene. It is imperative that this rescuer maintains cervical stabilization throughout the procedure. The rescuer who is stabilizing the head must continue to keep it stabilized until the athlete is completely immobilized with an appropriate device.

Injuries to the head and neck are difficult to evaluate and treat in the athletic environment. To adequately prepare for these and other critical injuries to athletes, an emergency plan should be developed. Providers of emergency care must make sure to have the proper equipment readily available and that it is in good working order.

The sports medicine team must be prepared for any emergency; preparation includes education and training, maintenance of appropriate emergency equipment and supplies, utilization of appropriate personnel (including certified athletic trainers), and the formation and implementation of an emergency plan.

Emergency plans should be comprehensive and practical, yet flexible enough to adapt to any emergency situation. The emergency plan must be established, approved, revised, and rehearsed on a regular basis. Each emergency plan may vary but should include information on education, emergency equipment, personnel, and communication and a rehearsal schedule. The emergency plan should also address equipment issues, which are particularly important in managing and packaging persons with suspected head or cervical spine injuries. Each member of the emergency team should be knowledgeable and practiced in the function and operation of emergency equipment. It would be helpful for each member of the sports medicine team to be multi-skilled and cross-trained in the use of all emergency equipment. For example, it has been suggested that practice with tools required for face mask removal of the catastrophically injured football player is essential.

Emergency medical personnel must take extreme caution when evaluating and treating an athlete with a suspected head or spinal injury. The proper management of head and neck injuries can prevent further damage from occurring.

References

1. Hunt V. Question of caution: task force examines spine care, helmet removal. *NATA News*. August 1998:10-12.
2. Inter-Association Task Force for Appropriate Care of the Spine-Injured Athlete. General guidelines. Presented at the Inter-Association Task Force for Appropriate Care of the Spine-Injured Athlete Summit; May 30--31, 1998; Indianapolis, Ind.
3. Mueller FO. Fatalities from head and cervical spine injuries occurring in tackle football: 50 years' experience. *Clin Sports Med*. 1998;17:169-182.
4. Mueller FO. Fatalities from intercranial and cervical spine injuries occurring in tackle football: 1945--1988. In: Torg JS, ed. *Athletic Injuries to the Head, Neck, and Face*. St Louis, Mo: Mosby--Year Book Inc; 1991:112-123.
5. Mueller FO, Blyth CS. Fatalities from head and cervical spine injuries occurring in tackle football: 40 years' experience. *Clin Sports Med*. 1987;6:185-196.
6. Torg JS, Vegso JJ, Sennett B. The National Football Head and Neck Injury Registry: 14-year report on cervical quadriplegia, 1971--1984. *Clin Sports Med*. 1987;6:61-72.
7. Torg JS, Vegso JJ, Sennett B, Das M. The National Football Head and Neck Injury Registry: 14-year report on cervical quadriplegia, 1971--1984. *JAMA*. 1985;254:3439-3443.
8. Mistovich JJ, Hafen BQ, Karren KJ. *Prehospital Emergency Care*, 6th ed. Upper Saddle River, NJ: Prentice-Hall; 2000:651-688.
9. O'Keefe MF, Limmer D, Grant HD, Murray RH, Bergeron JD. *Emergency Care*, 8th ed. Upper Saddle River, NJ: Brady/Prentice-Hall; 1998:595-630.
10. Feld F, Blanc R. Immobilizing the spine-injured football player. *J Emerg Med Serv*. 1987;12:38-40.
11. Patel MN, Rund DA. Emergency removal of football helmets. *Phys Sportsmed*. 1994;22:57-59.
12. Biasca N, Simmen HP, Bartolozzi AR, Trentz O. Review of typical ice hockey injuries: survey of the North American NHL and Hockey Canada versus European leagues. *Unfallchirurg*. 1995;98:283-288.
13. Deady B, Brison RJ, Chevrier L. Head, face and neck injuries in hockey: a descriptive analysis. *J Emerg Med*. 1996;14:645-649.
14. Graziano AF, Scheidel EA, Cline JR, Baer LJ. A radiographic comparison of prehospital cervical immobilization methods. *Ann Emerg Med*. 1987;16:1127/63, 1131/67.
15. Murray TM, Livingston LA. Hockey helmets, face masks, and injurious behavior. *Pediatrics*. 1995;95:419-421.
16. Noguchi T. A survey of spinal cord injuries resulting from sport. *Paraplegia*. 1994;32:170-173.
17. Reynen PD, Clancy WG Jr. Cervical spine injury, hockey helmets, and face masks. *Am J Sports Med*. 1994;22:167-170.
18. Scher AT. Rugby injuries to the cervical spine and spinal cord: a 10-year review. *Clin Sports Med*. 1998;17:195-206.
19. Scher AT. Spinal cord concussion in rugby players. *Am J Sports Med*. 1991;19:485-488.
20. Tator CH. Neck injuries in ice hockey: a recent, unsolved problem with many contributing factors. *Clin Sports Med*. 1987;6:101-114.
21. Tator CH, Carson JD, Edmonds VE. New spinal injuries in hockey. *Clin J Sports Med*. 1997;7:17-21.
22. Tator CH, Carson JD, Edmonds VE. Spinal injuries in ice hockey. *Clin Sports Med*. 1998;17:183-194.
23. Tator CH, Edmonds VE. National survey of spinal injuries in ice hockey players. *Can Med Assoc J*. 1984;130:875-880.
24. Tator CH, Edmonds VE. Sports and recreation are a rising cause of spinal cord injury. *Phys Sportsmed*. 1986;14:157-167.
25. Tator CH, Edmonds VE, Lapczak L, Tator IB. Spinal injuries in ice hockey players, 1966--1987. *Can J Surg*. 1991;34:63-69.
26. Wetzler MJ, Akpata T, Foster TE, Levy AS. A retrospective study of cervical spine injuries in American rugby, 1970 to 1994. *Am J Sports* Med. 1996;24:454-458.
27. Torg JS. Athletic Injuries to the Head, Neck and Face, 2nd ed. St Louis, Mo: Mosby--Year Book Inc; 1991.

28. Feuer H. History, physical examination, and acute management of spinal injury. In: Nicholas JA, Hershman EB, eds. *The Lower Extremity and Spine in Sports Medicine*, 2nd ed. St Louis, Mo: Mosby; 1995:1083-1094.
29. Cantu R. Head and neck injuries. In: Mueller FO, Ryan AJ, eds. *Prevention of Athletic Injuries: The Role of the Sports Medicine Team*. Philadelphia, Pa: FA Davis; 1991:201-213.
30. Lowery DW. Soft tissue trauma of the head and neck. *Phys Sportsmed*. 1991;19:21-24.
31. Romeo JH. The critical minutes after spinal cord injury. *RN*. April 1988:61-67.
32. Wiesenfarth J, Briner W Jr. Neck injuries: urgent decisions and actions. *Phys Sportsmed*. 1996;24:35-41.
33. Butman AM, Schelble DT, Vomacka RW. The relevance of the occult cervical spine controversy and mechanism of injury to prehospital protocols: a review of the issues and literature. *Prehosp Disaster Med*. 1996;11:228-233.
34. Warren WL Jr, Bailes JE. On the field evaluation of athletic neck injury. *Clin Sports Med*. 1998;17:99-110.
35. Hodge B. Common spinal injuries in athletes. *Nurs Clin North Am*. 1991;26:211-221.
36. Torg JS, Wiesel SW, Rothman RH. Diagnosis and management of cervical spine injuries. In: Torg JS, ed. *Athletic Injuries to the Head, Neck, and Face*. Philadelphia, Pa: Lea & Febiger; 1982:181-209.
37. Vegso JJ, Lehman RC. Field evaluation and management of head and neck injuries. *Clin Sports Med*. 1987;6:1-15.
38. Vegso JJ, Torg JS. Field evaluation and management of cervical spine injuries. In: Torg JS, ed. *Athletic Injuries to the Head, Neck, and Face*. St Louis, Mo: Mosby--Year Book Inc; 1991:426-437.
39. Watkins RG. Neck injuries in football. In: Watkins R, ed. *The Spine in Sports*. St Louis, Mo: Mosby--Year Book Inc; 1996:314-336.
40. Watkins RG. Cervical spine injuries. In: Watkins R, ed. The Spine in Sports. St Louis, Mo: Mosby--Year Inc; 1996:126-136.
41. National Football League. *Guidelines for Game Officials to Use During a Serious On-Field Player Injury*. New York, NY; National Football League; 1999.
42. Almquist JL. Spine injury management: a comprehensive plan for managing the cervical spine-injured football player. *Sports Med Update*. 1998;13:8-11.
43. Kleiner DM. Task force commends NFL. *NATA News*. August 1999:10-12.
44. Bahr R, Bendiksen F, Engebretsen L. 'Tis the season: diagnosing and managing ice hockey injuries. *J Musculoskeletal Med*. 1995;2:48-50, 52-56.
45. Arnheim DD, *Prentice WE. Principles of Athletic Training*, 9th ed. St Louis, Mo: Mosby--Year Book Inc; 1993:185-213.
46. Bailes JE, Maroon JC. Management of cervical spine injuries in athletes. *Clin Sports Med*. 1989;8:43-58.
47. Mundt DJ, Kelsey JL, Golden AL, Panjabi MM, Pastides H, Berg AT, et al. An epidemiologic study of sports and weight lifting as possible risk factors for herniated lumbar and cervical discs. The Northeast Collaborative Group on Low Back Pain. *Am J Sports Med*. 1993;21:854-860.
48. Golden IJ. Commentary on head and neck injuries in soccer. *ENA's Nursing Scan in Emerg Care*. 1993;3:12.
49. Torg JS. Epidemiology, pathomechanics, prevention of athletic injuries to the cervical spine. *Med Sci Sports Exerc*. 1985;17:295-303.
50. Rubin A. Emergency equipment: what to keep on the sidelines. *Phys Sportsmed*. 1993;21:47-54.
51. Kleiner DM. Football helmet face mask removal. *Athl Ther Today*. 1996;1:11-13.
52. Kleiner DM. Face mask removal vs face mask retraction. *J Athl Train*. 1996;31(suppl 2):32.
53. Knox K, Kleiner DM. The efficiency of tools used to retract a football helmet face mask. *J Athl Train*. 1997;32:211-215.
54. Almquist JL, Rehberg RS, Kleiner DM. An assessment of the response time prior to face mask removal. *J Athl Train*. 2000;35(suppl 2):S61.
55. Angotti DD, Hoenshel RW, Kleiner DM. The most efficient technique for using the FM Extractor™. *J Athl Train*. 2000;35(suppl 2):S60.
56. Clover J. Letter to the editor. *J Athl Train*. 1992;27:198.

57. Hoenshel RW, Angotti DD, Kleiner DM. An objective evaluation of the FM Extractor™. *J Athl Train.* 2000;35(suppl 2):S61.

58. Kleiner DM. Author's response to Mr Porter's letter regarding football helmet face mask removal. *Athl Ther Today.* 1996;1:52-53.

59. Kleiner DM, Knox KE. An evaluation of the techniques used by athletic trainers when removing a facemask with the Trainers Angel™. *J Athl Train.* 1995;30(suppl 2):7.

60. Knox KE, Kleiner DM. The effectiveness of EMT shears for face mask removal. *J Athl Train.* 1996;31(suppl 2):17.

61. Putman LA. Alternative methods for football helmet face mask removal. *J Athl Train.* 1992;27:170-172.

62. Ray RR, Luchies C, Bazuin D, Farrell R. Airway preparation techniques for the cervical spine-injured football player. *J Athl Train.* 1995;30:217-221.

63. Rehberg RS. Facemask removal tools come in all shapes, styles. *NATA News.* August 1999:8-9.

64. Rehberg RS. Rating facemask removal tools. *NATA News.* January 1995:26-27.

65. Schiess PK. Letter to the editor. J Athl Train. 1992;27:198.

66. AF, Goldfuss AJ, Hauth JM, Wagner LE. Effect on selected tools on face mask removal time and head motion. *J Athl Train.* 2000;35(suppl 2):S62.

67. Baker DA. Letter to the editor. *J Athl Train.* 1992;27:198.

68. Block JJ, Kleiner DM, Knox KE. Football helmet face mask removal with various tools and straps. *J Athl Train.* 1996;31(suppl 2):11.

69. Kleiner DM, Greenwood LD. The influence of hand size and grip strength on the ability to remove a football helmet face mask. *J Athl Train.* 1997;32(suppl 2):50.

70. Knight KL.Removing football helmet face masks. *J Athl Train.* 1992;27:197. Editorial.

71. Kleiner DM, Almquist JL, Hoenshel RW, Angotti DD. The effects of practice on face mask removal skills. *J Athl Train.* 2000;35(suppl 2):S60.

72. Kleiner DM, Sonnenberg R. The influence of temperature on the ability to cut the football helmet face mask loop-strap attachment. *J Athl Train.* 1999;34(suppl 2):84.

73. Knox KE, Kleiner DM, McCaw ST, Ryan MA. The effects of qualifications on the efficiency of football helmet facemask removal with various tools. *J Athl Train.* 1995;30(suppl 2):7.

74. Redden WW, Kleiner DM, Holcomb WR. The effects of gender, hand size and grip strength on the ability to remove a football helmet face mask. *J Athl Train.* 1998;33(suppl 2):43.

75. Sanville M, Hoenshel RW, Angotti DD, Kleiner DM. The sharpness of face mask removal tools and performance. *J Athl Train.* 2000;35(suppl 2):S60.

76. Almquist JL. Potential spine injury in football...what to do? *Athl Ther Today* 1998;3:42-43. Benson M, ed. *National Collegiate Athletic Association 1996--1997 Sports Medicine Handbook,* 8th ed. Overland Park, Ks: NCAA; 1997:65-66.

77. Cantu RC. Transportation/immobilization. In: Cantu RC, Micheli LJ, eds. ACSM's *Guidelines for the Team Physician.* Philadelphia, Pa: Lea & Febiger; 1991:151-152.

78. Denegar CR, Saliba E. On the field management of the potentially cervical spine injured football player. *Athl Train.* 1989;24:108-111.

79. Kleiner DM, Cantu RC. *Football Helmet Removal.* Current Comment. Indianapolis, Ind: The American College of Sports Medicine; 1996.

80. Wilkerson GB. Cervical immobilization of a football player on a scoop stretcher. *Athl Train.* 1983;18:207-209.

81. Waninger KN. On-field management of potential cervical spine injury in helmeted football players: leave the helmet on! Clin *J Sports Med.* 1998;8:124-129.

82. Donaldson WF III, Lauerman WC, Heil B, Blanc R, Swenson T. Helmet and shoulder pad removal from a player with suspected cervical spine injury: a cadaveric model. *Spine.* 1998;23:1729-1732, discussion 1732-1733.

83. Segan RD, Cassidy C, Bentkowski J. A discussion of the issue of football helmet removal in suspected cervical spine injuries. *J Athl Train.* 1993;28:294-305.

84. Knox KE, Kleiner DM. A description of how chin straps are attached to high school football helmets. *J Athl Train.* 2000;35(suppl 2):S61.

85. Blanchard BM, Castaldi CR. Injuries in youth hockey: on-ice emergency care. *Phys Sportsmed.* 1991;19:54-71.

86. Stenger A. Preparation key in treating Dennis Byrd. *Phys Sportsmed.* 1993;21:19-20.

87. Almquist JL, Schuler TC. *Cervical Spine Injured Athlete Transfer Protocol* [videotape]. Reston, Va: Northern Virginia Spine Institute; 1993.

88. Vegso JJ, Lehman RC. Field evaluation and management of head and neck injuries. *Clin Sports Med.* 1987;6:1-15.

89. Feld F. Management of the critically injured football player. *J Athl Train.* 1993;28:206-212.

90. Palumbo MA, Hulstyn MJ, Fadale PD, O'Brien T, Shall L. The effect of protective football equipment on alignment of the injured cervical spine: radiographic analysis in a cadaveric model. *Am J Sports Med.* 1996;24:446-453.

91. Blanc RO. Swenson TM, Fu FH. Cervical spine alignment in the immobilized football player: radiographic analysis before and after helmet removal. *J Athl Train.* 1996;31(suppl 2):6.

92. Gastel JA, Palumbo MA, Hulstyn MJ, Fadale PD, Lucas P. Emergency removal of football equipment: a cadaveric cervical spine injury model. *Ann Emerg Med.* 1998;32:411-417.

93. Prinsen RK, Syrotuik DG, Reid DC. Position of the cervical vertebrae during helmet removal and cervical collar application in football and hockey. *Clin J Sports Med.* 1995;5:155-161.

94. Bailes JE. Management of cervical spine sports injuries. *Athl Train.* 1990;25:156-159.

95. Metz CM, Kuhn JE, Greenfield ML. Cervical spine alignment in immobilized hockey players: radiographic analysis with and without helmets and shoulder pads. *Clin J Sports Med.* 1998;8:92-95.

96. Stephenson A, Horodyski MB, Meister K, Kaminski TW. Cervical spine alignment in the immobilized ice hockey player: radiographic analysis before and after helmet removal. *J Athl Train.* 1999;34(suppl):27.

97. Swenson TM, Lauerman WC, Blanc RO, Donaldson WF III, Fu FH. Cervical spine alignment in the immobilized football player: radiographic analysis before and after helmet removal. *Am J Sports Med.* 1997;25:226-230.

98. Walters R. Spinal immobilization. *Athl Ther Today.* 1996;1:16-20.

99. Walters R, Kleiner DM. Management of the critically injured athlete: packaging of head and cervical-spine injuries. In Courson R, Robinson JB, Davis G, eds. *Athletic Training Emergency Care.* Boston, Mass: Jones and Bartlett. In press.

100. Schriger DL. Immobilizing the cervical spine in trauma: should we seek an optimal position or an adequate one? *Ann Emerg Med.* 1996;28:351-353.

101. Schriger DL, Larmon B, Legassick T, Blinman T. Spinal immobilization on a flat backboard: does it result in neutral position of the cervical spine? *Ann Emerg Med.* 1991;20:878-881.

102. DeLorenzo RA, Olson JE, Boska M, et al. Optimal positioning for cervical immobilization. *Ann Emerg Med.* 1996;28:301-308.

103. Colachis SC, Strohm BR, Ganter EL. Cervical spine motion in normal women: radiographic study of effect of cervical collars. *Arch Phys Med Rehabil.* 1973;54:161-169.

104. Ransone J, Kersey R, Walsh K. The efficacy of the rapid form cervical vacuum immobilizer in cervical spine immobilization of the equipped football player. *J Athl Train.* 2000;35:65-69.

105. McCabe JB, Nolan DJ. Comparison of the effectiveness of different cervical immobilization collars. *Ann Emerg Med.* 1986;15:50-53.

106. McSwain NE. Proper C-spine immobilization. *Emerg Med.* 1995;2:120- 107. Nypaver M, Treolar D. Neutral cervical spine positioning in children. *Ann Emerg Med.* 1994;23:208-211.

108. Podolsky S, Baraff LJ, Simon RR, Hoffman JR, Larmon B, Ablon W. Efficacy of cervical spine immobilization methods. *J Trauma.* 1983;23:461-464.

109. Rosen PB, McSwain NE, Arata M, Stahl S, Mercer D. Comparison of two new immobilization collars. *Ann Emerg Med.* 1992;21 :1189-1195.

REFERENCES

110. Chandler DR, Nemejc C, Adkins RH, Waters RL. Emergency cervical-spine immobilization. *Ann Emerg Med.* 1992;21:1185/19-1188/22.

111. Cline JR, Scheidel E, Rigsby EF. A comparison of methods of cervical immobilization used in patient extrication and transport. *J Trauma.* 1985;25:649-653.

112. Herzenberg JE, Hensinger RN, Dedrick DK, Phillips WA. Emergency transport and positioning of young children who have an injury of the cervical spine. *J Bone Joint Surg.* 1989;71A:15-22.

113. Howell JM, Burrow R, Dumontier C, Hillyard A. A practical radiographic comparison of short board technique and Kendrick extrication device. *Ann Emerg Med.* 1989;18:943/79-946/82.

114. Karbi OA, Caspari DA, Tator CH. Extrication, immobilization and radiologic investigation of patients with cervical spine injuries. *CMAJ.* 1988;139:617-620.

115. Mazolewski MS, Manix TH. The effectiveness of strapping techniques in spinal immobilization. *Ann Emerg Med.* 1994;23:1290-1295.

116. Sumchai AP, Sternbach GL, Laufer M. Cervical spine traction and immobilization. *Top Emerg Med.* 1988;10:9-22.

117. DeLorenzo RA. A review of spinal immobilization techniques. *J Emerg Med.* 1996;14:603-613.

118. Bourn S. Put me in the game, coach: evaluation and management of sports injuries. *J Emerg Med Serv.* December 1993:26-38.

119. Curran C, Dietrich AM, Bowman MJ, Ginn-Pease ME, King DR, Kosnik E. Pediatric cervical-spine immobilization: achieving neutral position? *J Trauma Injury Infect Crit.* 1995;39:729-732.

120. Cantu RC. Head and spine injuries in the young athlete. *Clin Sports Med.* 1988;7:459-472.

121. Waeckerle JF. Planning for emergencies. *Phys Sportsmed.* 1991;19:35-38.

122. Cantu RC, Mueller FO. Catastrophic spine injuries in football (1977-1989). *J Spinal Discord.* 1990;3:227-231.

123. Odor J, Watkins RG, Dillin WH. Degenerative disorders of the cervical spine. In: Watkins R, ed. *The Spine in Sports.* St Louis, Mo: Mosby--Year Book Inc; 1996:164-176.

124. Otis JC, Burstein AH, Torg JS. Mechanisms and pathomechanics of athletic injuries to the cervical spine. In: Torg JS, ed. *Athletic Injuries to the Head, Neck, and Face.* St Louis, Mo: Mosby--Year Book Inc; 1991:438-456.

125. Myers BS, Winklestein BA. Epidemiology, classification, mechanism, and tolerance of human cervical spine injuries. *Crit Rev Biomed* Eng. 1995;24:235-239.

126. Akau CK, Press JM, Gooch JL. Sports medicine: spine and head injuries: part 4. *Arch Phys Med Rehabil.* 1993;74(suppl 5):443-446.

127. BenEliyahu DJ. Conservative management of post-traumatic cervical intersegmental hypermobility and anterior subluxation. *J Manipulative Physiol Ther.* 1995;18:315-321.

128. McClain RF. Mechanoreceptor endings of the cervical, thoracic and lumbar spine. *Iowa Orthop J.* 1995;15:147-155.

129. Jacobs B. Cervical fractures and dislocations. *Clin Orthop.* 1975;109:18-32.

130. Torg JS, Sennett B, Vegso JJ. Spinal injury at the third and fourth cervical vertebrae resulting from the axial loading mechanism: an analysis and classification. *Clin Sports Med.* 1987;6:159-185.

131. Trupiano TP, Sampson ML, Weise MW. Fracture of the first cervical vertebra in a high school football player: a case report. *J Athl Train.* 1997;32:159-162.

132. Kokkino AJ, Lazio BE, Perin NI. Vertical fracture of the odontoid process: case report. *Neurosurgery.* 1996;38:200-203.

133. Rappoport LH, Cammisa FP Jr, O'Leary PF. Fractures and dislocations of the cervical spine. In: Jordan BD, Tsairis P, Warren RF, eds. *Sports Neurology,* 2nd ed. Philadelphia, Pa: Lippincott-Raven; 1998:157-179.

134. Beirne JC, Butler PE, Brady FA. Cervical spine injuries in patients with facial fractures: a 1-year prospective study. *Int J Oral Maxillofac Surg.* 1995;24(pt 1):26-29.

135. Borock EC, Gabram SGA, Lenworth FM, Murphy MA. A prospective analysis as an adjunct for cervical spine clearance. *J Trauma.* 1991;31:1001-1006.

136. Torg JS, Sennett B, Vegso JJ, Pavlov H. Axial loading injuries to the middle cervical spine segment. *Am J Sports Med.* 1991;19:6-20.

137. Torg JS, Vegso JJ, O'Neill MJ, Sennett B. The epidemiologic, pathologic, biomechanical, and cinematographic analysis of football induced cervical spine trauma. *Am J Sports Med.* 1990;18:50-57.

138. Torg JS. The epidemiologic, biomechanical and cinematographic analysis of football induced cervical spine trauma. *Athl Train.* 1990;25:147-155.

139. Tator CH, Edmonds VE. Acute spinal cord injury: analysis of epidemiologic factors. *Can J Surg.* 1979;22:575-578.

140. Torg JS. *Prevent Paralysis: Don't Hit With Your Head* [videotape]. Philadelphia, Pa: Penn Sports Medicine; 1992.

141. Benda C. Catastrophic head and neck injuries in amateur hockey. *Phys Sportsmed.* 1989;17:115-122.

142. Anderson C. Neck injuries: backboard, bench or return to play? *Phys Sportsmed.* 1993;21:23-28,31-32,34.

143. Chalmers DJ, Hume PA, Wilson BD. Trampolines in New Zealand: a decade of injuries. *Br J Sports Med.* 1994;28:234-238.

144. Torg JS. Epidemiology, pathomechanics, prevention of football-induced cervical spinal cord trauma. *Exerc Sports Sci Rev.* 1992;20:321-38.

145. Torg JS, Pavlov H, O'Neill MJ, Nichols CE, Sennett B. The axial load teardrop fracture: a biomechanical, clinical, and roentgenographic analysis. *Am J Sports Med.* 1991;19:355-364.

146. Carter DR, Frankel VH. Biomechanics of hyperextension injuries to the cervical spine in football. *Am J Sports Med.* 1980;8:302-309.

147. Cantu RC. Stingers, transient quadriplegia, and cervical spinal stenosis: return to play criteria. *Med Sci Sports Exerc.* 1997;29(suppl):233-235.

148. Virgin H. Cineradiographic study of football helmets and the cervical spine. *Am J Sports Med.* 1980;8:310-317.

149. Cantu RC. The cervical spinal stenosis controversy. *Clin Sports Med.* 1998;17:121-126.

150. Cantu RC, Bailes JE, Wilberger JE Jr. Guidelines for return to contact or collision sport after a cervical spine injury. *Clin Sports Med.* 1998;17:137-146.

151. Cantu RC. Cervical spinal stenosis: challenging an established detection method. *Phys Sportsmed.* 1993;21:57-63

152. Cantu RC. Functional spinal stenosis: a contraindication to participation in contact sports. *Med Sci Sports Exerc.* 1993;25:316-317.

153. Cantu RV, Cantu RC. Guidelines for return to contact sports after transient quadriplegia. *J Neurosurg.* 1994;80:592-594.

154. Cantu RC. Transient quadriplegia: to play or not to play. *Sports Med Digest.* 1994;16:1-4 Torg JS. Cervical spine stenosis with cord neurapraxia and transient quadriplegia. *Athl Train.* 1990;25:138-146.

155. Riggins RS, Kraus JF. The risk of neurologic damage with fractures of the vertebrae. *J Trauma.* 1977;17:126-132.

156. Eismont FJ, Clifford S, Goldberg M, Green B. Cervical sagittal spinal canal size in spine injury. *Spine.* 1984;9:663-666.

157. Firooznia H, Ahn JH, Rafii M, Ragnarsson KT Sudden quadriplegia after a minor trauma: the role of preexisting spinal stenosis. *Surg Neurol.* 1985;23:165-168.

158. White AA, Johnson RM, Panjabi MM, Southwick WO. Biomechanical analysis of clinical stability in the cervical spine. *Clin Orthop.* 1975;109:85-95.

159. Winkelstein BA, Myers BS. The biomechanics of cervical spine injury and implications for injury prevention. *Med Sci Sports Exerc.* 1997;29(suppl 7):246-255.

160. Matsuura P, Waters RL, Adkins RH, Rothman S, Gurbani N, Sie I. Comparison of computerized tomography parameters of the cervical spine in normal control subjects and spinal-cord injured patients. *J Bone Joint Surg.* 1989;71A:183-188.

161. Odor J, Watkins R, Dillin W, et al. Incidence of cervical spinal stenosis in professional and rookie football players. *Am J Sports Med.* 1990;18:507-509.

REFERENCES

162. Torg JS, Sennett B, Pavlov H, Levelthal MR, Glasgow SG. Spear tackler's spine: an entity precluding participation in tackle football and collision activities that expose the cervical spine to axial energy inputs. *Am J Sports Med.* 1993;21:640-649.
163. Torg JS, Corcoran TA, Thibault LE, et al. Cervical cord neuropraxia: classification, pathomechanic, morbidity, and management guidelines. *J Neurosurg.* 1997;87:843-50.
164. Schneider RC, Cherry G, Pantek H. The syndrome of acute central cervical spinal cord injury with special reference to mechanisms involved in hyperextension injuries of the cervical spine. *J Neurosurg.* 1954;11:546-577.
165. Weinstein SM. Assessment and rehabilitation of the athlete with a "stinger": a model for the management of noncatastrophic athletic cervical spine injury. *Clin Sports Med.* 1998;17:127-135.
166. Levitz CL, Reilly PJ, Torg JS. The pathomechanics of chronic, recurrent cervical nerve root neurapraxia: the chronic burner syndrome. *Am J Sports Med.* 1997;25:73-76.
167. American Academy of Orthopedic Surgeons. *Athletic Training and Sports Medicine*, 2nd ed. Chicago, Ill: American Academy of Orthopedic Surgeons; 1991:513-535.
168. Cibulka MT. Evaluation and treatment of cervical spine injuries. *Clin Sports Med.* 1989;8:691-701.
169. Dossett A, Watkins RG. Stinger injuries in football. In: Watkins R, ed. *The Spine in Sports.* St Louis, Mo: Mosby--Year Book Inc; 1996:337-342.
170. El-Khoury GY. Cervical spinal stenosis and stingers in collegiate football players. *Am J Sports Med.* 1994;22:158-166.
171. Garth WP Jr. Evaluating and treating brachial plexus injuries. *J Musculoskeletal Med.* 1994;11:55-56, 59-61, 65-67.
172. Torg JS, Naranja RJ Jr, Palov H, Galinat BJ, Warren R, Stine RA. The relationship of developmental narrowing of the cervical spinal canal to reversible and irreversible injury of the cervical spinal cord in football players. *J Bone Joint Surg Am.* 1996;78:1308-1314.
173. Torg JS, Fay CM. Cervical spinal stenosis with cord neuropraxia and transient quadriplegia. In: Torg JS, ed. *Athletic Injuries to the Head, Neck, and Face.* St Louis, Mo: Mosby--Year Book Inc; 1991:533-552.
174. Hopkins TJ, White AA. Rehabilitation of athletes following spine injury. *Clin Sports Med.* 1993;12:603-619.
175. Bailes JE, Hadley MN, Quigley MR, Sonntag VKH, Cerullo LJ. Management of athletic injuries of the cervical spine and spinal cord. *Neurosurgery.* 1991;29:491-497.
176. Maroon JC, Bailes JE. Athletes with cervical spine injury. *Spine.* 1996;21:2294-2299.
177. Bailes JE, Herman JM, Quigley MR, et al. Diving injuries of the cervical spine. *Surg Neurol* 1990;34:155-158.
178. Torg JS, Ramsey-Emrhein JA. Management guidelines for participation in collision activities with congenital, developmental, or post-injury lesions involving the cervical spine. *Clin Sports Med.* 1997;16:501-530.
179. Munnings F. Should athletes return to play after transient quadriplegia? *Phys Sportsmed.* 1991;19:127-132.
180. Torg JS, Ramsey-Emrhein JA. Suggested management guidelines for participation in collision activities with congenital, developmental, or post-injury lesions involving the cervical spine. *Med Sci Sports Exerc.* 1997;29(suppl 7):256-272.
181. Andrish JT, Bergfeld JA, Romo L. A method for the management of cervical injuries in football: a preliminary report. *Am J Sports Med.* 1977;5:89-92.
182. Meyer SA, Schulte KR, Callaghan JJ, et al. Cervical spinal stenosis and stingers in collegiate football players. *Am J Sports Med.* 1994;22:158-166.
183. Acheson MB, Livingston RR, Richardson ML, Stimac GK. High-resolution CT scanning in the evaluation of cervical spine fractures: comparison with plain film examinations. *J Radiol.* 1987;148:1179-1185.
184. Dorwart RH, LaMasters DL. Applications of computed tomographic scanning of the cervical spine. *Orthop Clin North Am.* 1985;16:381-393.
185. Greenan TJ. Diagnostic imaging of sports-related spinal disorders. *Clin Sports Med.* 1993;2:487-505.

186. Schlechauf K, Ross SE, Civil ID, Schwab CW. Computed tomography in the initial evaluation of the cervical spine. *Ann Emerg Med.* 1989;18:815-817.
187. Tress BM, Hare WSC. CT of the spine: are plain spine radiographs necessary? *Clin Radiol.* 1990;41:317-320.
188. Cantu RC. Head and spine injuries in youth sports. *Clin Sports Med.* 1995;14:517-532.
189. Fourre M. On-site management of cervical spine injuries. *Phys Sportsmed.* 1991;19:53-56.
190. Malanga GA. The diagnosis and treatment of cervical radiculopathy. *Med Sci Sports Exerc.* 1997;29(suppl 7):236-245.
191. Patterson D. Legal aspects of athletic injuries to the head and cervical spine. *Clin Sports Med.* 1987;6:197-210.
192. Heck JF. The incidence of spearing by high school football ball carriers and their tacklers. *J Athl Train.* 1992;27:120-124.
193. Cole AJ, Farrell JP, Stratton SA. Cervical spine athletic injuries: a pain in the neck. *Phys Med Rehabil Clin North Am.* 1994;5:37-68.
194. Fine KM, Vegso JJ, Sennett B, Torg JS. Prevention of cervical spine injuries in football. *Phys Sportsmed.* 1991;19 :54-62.
195. Heck JF. A survey of New Jersey high school football officials regarding spearing rules. *J Athl Train.* 1994;30:63-68.
196. Heck JF. The incidence of spearing during a high school's 1975 and 1990 football seasons. *J Athl Train.* 1996;31:31-38.
197. Heck JF. The state of spearing in football: incidence of cervical spine injuries doesn't indicate the risks. *Sports Med Update.* 1998;13:4-7.
198. Bishop PJ. Factors relating to quadriplegia in football and the implications for intervention strategies. *Am J Sports Med.* 1996;24:235-239.
199. Davis PM, McKelvey MK. Medicolegal aspects of athletic cervical spine injury. *Clin Sports Med.* 1998;17:147-154.
200. Heck JF, Weis MP, Gartland JM, Weis CR. Minimizing liability risks of head and neck injuries in football. *J Athl Train.* 1994;29:128-139.
201. Bland JH. Helping athletes avoid neck injuries: conditioning provides protection. *J Musculoskeletal Med.* 1996;13:30-32, 35-36, 38.
202. Funk FJ, Wells RE. Injuries of the cervical spine in football. *Clin Orthop.* 1975;109:50-58.
203. Albright JP, McAuley E, Martin RK, Crowley ET, Foster DT. Head and neck injuries in college football: an eight-year analysis. *Am J Sports Med.* 1985;13:147-152.
204. Andersen JC, Courson R, Kleiner DM, McLoda T. *Emergency Planning in Athletics.* Position Stand. Dallas, Tex: The National Athletic Trainers Association; 2000.
205. Dolan MG. Emergency care: planning for the worst. *Athl Ther Today.* 1998;3:12-13.
206. Nowlan WP, Davis GA, McDonald B. Preparing for sudden emergencies. *Athl Ther Today.* 1996;1:45-47.
207. Shea JF. Duties of care owed to university athletes in light of Kleinecht. *J Coll Univ Law.* 1995;21:591-614.
208. Kleiner DM. Prehospital treatment of catastrophic football injuries. *Emerg Med Serv.* 1998;27:27-32.
209. Mastrangelo FA. Letter to the editor. *J Athl Train.* 1993;28:101.
210. Establishing communication with EMTs. *NATA News.* June 1994:4-9.
211. National Athletic Trainers' Association Board of Certification, Inc. *Role Delineation Study*, 3rd ed. Philadelphia, Pa: FA Davis; 1995:18-62.
212. McAdam CA, Kleiner DM. Spinal injuries, helmet removal: what a dilemma! *NAEMT News.* 1998;10:6-7.
213. Roberts WO. Helmet removal in head and neck trauma. *Phys Sportsmed.* 1998;26:77-78.
214. Rehberg RS. Football helmets: to remove or not to remove... should there be a question? *NATA News.* June 1993:4-6.
215. Vieson M, Wimer JW. Attitudes about football helmet removal procedures from students in a paramedic education classroom. *J Athl Train.* 1998;33(suppl):61.

Table 1

GUIDELINES FOR APPROPRIATE CARE OF THE SPINE-INJURED ATHLETE

General Guidelines
- Any athlete suspected of having a spinal injury should not be moved and should be managed as though a spinal injury exists.
- The athlete's airway, breathing, circulation, neurological status and level of consciousness should be assessed.
- The athlete should not be moved unless absolutely essential to maintain airway, breathing and circulation.
- If the athlete must be moved to maintain airway, breathing and circulation, the athlete should be placed in a supine position while maintaining spinal immobilization.
- When moving a suspected spine-injured athlete, the head and trunk should be moved as a unit. One accepted technique is to manually splint the head to the trunk.
- The Emergency Medical Services system should be activated.

Face Mask Removal
- The face mask should be removed prior to transportation, regardless of current respiratory status.
- Those involved in the prehospital care of injured football players should have the tools for face mask removal readily available.

Football Helmet Removal
The athletic helmet and chin strap should only be removed:

- if the helmet and chin strap do not hold the head securely, such that immobilization of the helmet does not also immobilize the head;
- if the design of the helmet and chin strap is such that, even after removal of the face mask, the airway cannot be controlled nor ventilation provided;

- if the face mask cannot be removed after a reasonable period of time;
- if the helmet prevents immobilization for transportation in an appropriate position.

Helmet Removal
Spinal immobilization must be maintained while removing the helmet.

- Helmet removal should be frequently practiced under proper supervision.
- Specific guidelines for helmet removal need to be developed.
- In most circumstances, it may be helpful to remove cheek padding and/or deflate air padding prior to helmet removal.

Equipment
Appropriate spinal alignment must be maintained.

- There needs to be a realization that the helmet and shoulder pads elevate an athlete's trunk when in the supine position.
- Should either the helmet or shoulder pads be removed – or if only one of these is present – appropriate spinal alignment must be maintained.
- The front of the shoulder pads can be opened to allow access for CPR and defibrillation.

Additional Guidelines
- This task force encourages the development of a local emergency care plan regarding the prehosptial care of an athlete with a suspected spinal injury. This plan should include communication with the institution's administration and those directly involved with the assessment and transportation of the injured athlete.
- All providers of prehospital care should practice and be competent in all of the skills identified in these guidelines before they are needed in an emergency situation.

These guidelines were developed as a consensus statement by the Inter-Association Task Force of Appropriate Care of the Spine-Injured Athlete:
Douglas M. Kleiner, PhD, ATC. FACSM, (Chair), *National Athletic Trainers' Association;* Jon L. Almquist, ATC, *National Athletic Trainers' Association Secondary School Athletic Trainers' Committee;* Julian Bailes, MD. *American Association of Neurological Surgeons;* John C. Biery, DO, FAOASM, FACSM, *American Osteopathic Academy of Sports Medicine;* Kevin Black, MD, MS. *American Orthopaedic Society for Sports Medicine;* T. Pepper Burruss, ATC, PT, *Professional Football Athletic Trainers' Society;* Alexander M. Butman, DSc. NREMT-P, *National Registry of EMTs;* Jerry Diehl, *National Federation of State High School Associations;* Robert Domeier, MD, *National Association of EMS Physicians;* Kent Falb, ATC, PT, *National Athletic Trainers' Association;* Henry Feuer, MD, *National Football League Physicians Society;* Jay Greenstein, DC, *American Chiropractic Board of Sports Physicians;* Letha Y. Griffin, MD, *National Collegiate Athletic Association Committee on Competitive Safeguards and Medical Aspects of Sports;* Robert E. Hannemann, MD, *American Academy of Pediatrics Committee on Sports Medicine and Fitness;* Stanley Herring, MD, FACSM, *American College of Sports Medicine, North American Spine Society;* Margaret Hunt, ATC, *United States Olympic Committee;* Daniel Kraft, MD, *American Medical Society for Sports Medicine;* James Laughnane, ATC, *National Athletic Trainers' Association College and University Athletic Trainers' Committee;* Connie McAdam. MICT, *National Association of Emergency Medical Technicians;* Dennis A. Miller, ATC, PT, *National Athletic Trainers' Association;* Michael Oliver, *National Operating Committee on Safety and Equipment;* Andrew N. Pollak, MD, *Orthopaedic Trauma Association;* Jay Rosenberg, MD, *American Academy of Neurology;* Dan Smith, DPT, ATC, *American Physical Therapy Association Sports Physical Therapy Section;* David Thorson, MD, *American Academy of Family Physicians;* Patrick R. Trainor, ATC, *National Association of Intercollegiate Athletics;* Joe Waeckerle, MD, *American College of Emergency Physicians;* Robert G. Watkins, MD. *American Academy of Orthopaedic Surgeons Committee on the Spine;* Stuart Weinstein, MD, FACSM, *Physiatric Association of Spine, Sports & Occupational Rehabilitation; American Academy of Physical Medicine and Rehabilitation. American College of Sports Medicine;* Jack Wilberger, MD, *American College of Surgeons - Committee on Trauma*

Table 2

RECOMMENDATIONS FOR APPROPRIATE CARE OF THE SPINE-INJURED ATHLETE

- The Inter-Association Task Force for Appropriate Care of the Spine-Injured Athlete commends the current and ongoing commitment of helmet and face guard manufacturers for integrating safety in the development of their products.
- The Inter-Association Task Force for Appropriate Care of the Spine-Injured Athlete encourages manufacturers to continue to support research promoting helmet and face guard safety.
- The Inter-Association Task Force for Appropriate Care of the Spine-Injured Athlete recommends that manufacturers provide information to purchasers on the best methods for the emergency removal of the face guard.
- The Inter-Association Task Force for Appropriate Care of the Spine-Injured Athlete recommends that NOCSAE develop equipment standards that would allow for the emergency removal of helmets and face guards.
- The Inter-Association Task Force for Appropriate Care of the Spine-Injured Athlete recommends that helmets and face guards that meet current NOCSAE standards be worn by all football, lacrosse, baseball, and softball players.
- The Inter-Association Task Force for Appropriate Care of the Spine-Injured Athlete recommends that football helmet face guards be attached by loop straps and not bolted on, in order to facilitate appropriate emergency management by medical personnel (from the May 1998 meeting in Indianapolis, Indiana).
- The Inter-Association Task Force for Appropriate Care of the Spine-Injured Athlete recommends that loop straps be made of material that is easily cut, and that the producers of loop straps provide appropriate tools to cut/remove the loop straps that they manufacture (from the May 1998 meeting in Indianapolis, Indiana).

These guidelines were developed as a consensus statement by the Inter-Association Task Force of Appropriate Care of the Spine-Injured Athlete:
Douglas M. Kleiner, PhD, ATC, FACSM. (Chair), *National Athletic Trainers' Association;* Jon L. Almquist, ATC, *National Athletic Trainers' Association Secondary School Athletic Trainers' Committee;* Julian Bailes, MD. *American Association of Neurological Surgeons;* John C. Biery. DO, FAOASM, FACSM. *American Osteopathic Academy of Sports Medicine;* T. Pepper Burruss. ATC, PT, *Professional Football Athletic Trainers' Society;* Alexander M. Butman, DSc, NREMT-P, *National Registry of EMTs;* Michael Cendoma, MS, ATC, *Sports Medicine Concepts;* Ron Courson, ATC, PT, *Athletic Training Emergency Care;* Jerry Diehl, *National Federation of State High School Associations;* Robert Domeier, MD. *National Association of EMS Physicians;* Kent Falb, ATC, PT, *National Athletic Trainers' Association;* Henry Feuer. MD, *National Football League Physicians Society;* Jay Greenstein, DC, *American Chiropractic Board of Sports Physicians;* Bernard A. Griesemer, MD, FAAP, *American Academy of Pediatrics Committee on Sports Medicine and Fitness;* Letha Y. Griffin, MD, *National Collegiate Athletic Association Committee on Competitive Safeguards and Medical Aspects of Sports;* Michael Hanley, ATC, *National Athletic Trainers' Association College and University Athletic Trainers' Committee;* Stanley Herring, MD, FACSM, *American College of Sports Medicine, North American Spine Society;* Margaret Hunt, ATC, *United States Olympic Committee;* Daniel Kraft, MD, *American Medical Society for Sports Medicine;* Connie McAdam, MICT, *National Association of Emergency Medical Technicians;* Dennis A. Miller, ATC, PT, *National Athletic Trainers' Association;* Michael Oliver, *National Operating Committee on Safety and Equipment;* Andrew N. Pollak, MD, *Orthopaedic Trauma Association;* Robb Rehberg, ATC, CSCS, NREMT, *Athletic Training Emergency Care;* Jay Rosenberg, MD, *American Academy of Neurology;* Kevin Shea, MD, *American Orthopaedic Society for Sports Medicine;* Dan Smith, DPT, ATC, *American Physical Therapy Association Sports Physical Therapy Section;* David Thorson, MD, *American Academy of Family Physicians;* Patrick R. Trainor, ATC, *National Association of Intercollegiate Athletics;* Joe Waeckerle, MD, *American College of Emergency Physicians;* Robert G. Watkins, MD, *American Academy of Orthopaedic Surgeons Committee on the Spine;* Stuart Weinstein, MD, FACSM, *Physiatric Association of Spine, Sports & Occupational Rehabilitation; American Academy of Physical Medicine and Rehabilitation, American College of Sports Medicine;* Jack Wilberger, MD, *American College of Surgeons - Committee on Trauma*

Table 3

NATIONAL FOOTBALL LEAGUE GUIDELINES[41]

The guides set forth by the NFL for game officials to use during serious on-field injuries include:

- Players and coaches must go to and remain in the bench area. Direct all players and coaches accordingly. Always ensure adequate lines of vision between the medical staff and all available emergency personnel.
- Attempt to keep players a significant distance away from the seriously injured player(s).
- Do not allow a player to roll an injured athlete over.
- Do not allow players to assist a teammate who is lying on the field; i.e. removing the helmet or chin strap or attempting to assist breathing by elevating the waist.
- Do not allow players to pull an injured teammate or opponent from a pile-up.
- Once the medical staff begins to work on an injured player, all members of the officiating crew should control the total playing field environment and team personnel and allow the medical staff to perform services without interruption or interference.
- Players and coaches should be appropriately controlled to avoid dictating medical services to the certified athletic trainers or team physicians or taking up their time to perform such service.

Note: Officials should have a reasonable knowledge of the location of emergency personnel and equipment at all stadiums.

Treating Tobacco Use and Dependence

• •

The following guideline for treating tobacco use and dependence, developed by the Surgeon General, has been endorsed by the American Academy of Pediatrics. Full text of this guideline is available on the enclosed CD-ROM or on the Surgeon General Web site at http://www.surgeongeneral.gov/tobacco/default.htm. In addition, consumer information and other educational materials can be accessed either through the Surgeon General Web site or through the Agency for Healthcare Research and Quality Web site at http://www.ahrq.gov.

Treating Tobacco Use and Dependence
Summary

This Summary is from the updated guideline, Treating Tobacco Use and Dependence, which reflects new, effective clinical treatments for clinical treatment of tobacco dependence.

Findings include: Multiple efficacious treatments exist, these treatments can double or triple the likelihood of long-term cessation, many cessation treatments are appropriate for primary care settings, and the use and impact of cessation treatments can be increased by supportive health system policies.

OVERVIEW

In America today, tobacco stands out as the agent most responsible for avoidable illness and death. Millions of Americans consume this toxin on a daily basis. Its use brings premature death to almost half a million Americans each year, and it contributes to profound disability and pain in many others. Approximately one-third of all tobacco users in this country will die prematurely because of their dependence on tobacco. Unlike so many epidemics in the past, there is a clear, contemporaneous understanding of the cause of this premature death and disability—the use of tobacco.

It is a testament to the power of tobacco addiction that millions of tobacco users have been unable to overcome their dependence and save themselves from its consequences: perpetual worry, unceasing expense, and compromised health. Indeed, it is difficult to identify any other condition that presents such a mix of lethality, prevalence, and neglect, despite effective and readily available interventions.

Despite high, sustained tobacco use prevalence, the response of both clinicians and the U.S. health care delivery system is disappointing. Studies show that most smokers present at primary care settings, and they are not offered effective assistance in quitting. The smoker's lack of success in quitting, and the clinician's reluctance to intervene, can be traced to many factors. Until recently, few effective treatments existed, effective treatments had not been identified clearly, and health care systems had not supported their consistent and universal delivery. To single-out the clinician for blame would be inappropriate, when he or she has typically received neither the training nor support necessary to treat tobacco use successfully.

Current treatments for tobacco dependence offer clinicians their greatest single opportunity to staunch the loss of life, health, and happiness caused by this chronic condition. It is imperative, therefore, that clinicians actively assess and treat tobacco use. In addition, it is imperative that health care administrators, insurers, and purchasers adopt and support policies and practices that are aimed at reducing tobacco use prevalence. The chief purpose of this document is to provide clinicians, tobacco dependence specialists, health care administrators, insurers, and purchasers, and even tobacco users, with evidence-based recommendations regarding clinical and systems interventions that will increase the likelihood of successful quitting.

GUIDELINE ORIGINS

Treating Tobacco Use and Dependence, a Public Health Service-sponsored Clinical Practice Guideline, is the product of the Tobacco Use and Dependence Guideline Panel ("the panel"), consortium representatives, consultants, and staff. These 30 individuals were charged with the responsibility of identifying effective, experimentally validated, tobacco dependence treatments and practices. This guideline updates the 1996 *Smoking Cessation, Clinical Practice Guideline No. 18* that was sponsored by the Agency for Health Care Policy and Research, U.S. Department of Health and Human Services. The original guideline reflected the extant scientific research literature published between 1975 and 1994.

This guideline was written in response to new, effective clinical treatments for tobacco dependence that have been identified since 1994, and these treatments promise to enhance the rates of successful tobacco cessation. The accelerating pace of tobacco research that prompted the update is reflected by the fact that 3,000 articles on tobacco published between 1975 and 1994 were collected and screened as part of the original guideline. Another 3,000 were published between 1995 and 1999 and contributed to the updated guideline. These 6,000 articles were reviewed to identify a much smaller group of articles that served as the basis for guideline data analyses and panel opinion.

The updated guideline was sponsored by a consortium of seven Federal Government and nonprofit organizations:

- Agency for Healthcare Research and Quality (AHRQ).
- Centers for Disease Control and Prevention (CDC).
- National Cancer Institute (NCI).
- National Heart, Lung, and Blood Institute (NHLBI).
- National Institute on Drug Abuse (NIDA).
- Robert Wood Johnson Foundation (RWJF).
- University of Wisconsin Medical School's Center for Tobacco Research and Intervention (CTRI).

All of these organizations have the mission to reduce the human costs of tobacco use. Given the importance of this issue to the health of all Americans, the updated guideline is published by the U.S. Public Health Service.

GUIDELINE STYLE AND STRUCTURE

This guideline was written to be relevant to all tobacco users—those using cigarettes as well as other forms of tobacco. Therefore, the terms "tobacco user" and "tobacco dependence" will be used in preference to "smoker" and "cigarette dependence." However, in some cases the evidence for a particular recommendation consists entirely of studies using smokers as subjects. In these instances, the recommendation and evidence refers to "smoking" to communicate the parochial nature of the evidence. In most cases though, guideline recommendations are relevant to all types of tobacco users.

The updated guideline is divided into eight chapters:

Chapter 1, Overview and Methods: Provides the clinical practice and scientific context of the guideline update project and describes the methodology used to generate the guideline findings.

Chapter 2, Assessment of Tobacco Use: Describes how each patient presenting at a health care setting should have his or her tobacco use status determined, and how tobacco users should be assessed for willingness to make a quit attempt.

Chapter 3, Brief Clinical Interventions: Summarizes effective brief interventions that can easily be delivered in a primary care setting. In this chapter, separate interventions are described for the patient who is *willing* to try to quit at this time, for the patient who is *not yet willing* to try to quit, and for the patient who has recently quit.

Chapter 4, Intensive Clinical Interventions: Outlines a prototype of an intensive tobacco cessation treatment that comprises strategies shown to be effective in this guideline. Because intensive treatments produce the highest success rates, they are an important element in tobacco intervention strategies.

Chapter 5, Systems Interventions Relevance to Health Care Administrators, Insurers, and Purchasers: Offers a blueprint to guideline changes in health care coverage and health care administration such that tobacco assessment and intervention become "default options" in health care delivery.

Chapter 6, Evidence: Presents the results of guideline statistical analyses and the recommendations that emanate from them. Guideline analyses address topics such as:
- The efficacy of different pharmacotherapies and counseling strategies.
- The relation between treatment intensities and treatment success.
- Whether screening for tobacco use in the clinic setting enhances tobacco user identification.

The guideline panel made specific recommendations regarding future research on these topics.

Chapter 7, Special Populations: Evaluates evidence on tobacco intervention strategies and efficacy with special populations (e.g., women, pregnant smokers, racial and ethnic minorities, hospitalized smokers, smokers with psychiatric comorbidity and chemical dependency, children and adolescents, and older smokers). The guideline panel made specific recommendations for future research on topics relevant to these populations.

Chapter 8, Special Topics: Presents information and recommendations relevant to weight gain after smoking cessation, noncigarette tobacco products, clinician training, economics of tobacco treatment, and harm reduction. The guideline panel formulated specific recommendations regarding future research on these topics.

FINDINGS AND RECOMMENDATIONS

The key recommendations of the updated guideline, *Treating Tobacco Use and Dependence*, based on the literature review and expert panel opinion, follow:

Tobacco dependence is a chronic condition that often requires repeated intervention.

However, effective treatments exist that can produce long-term or even permanent abstinence.

Because effective tobacco dependence treatments are available, every patient who uses tobacco should be offered at least one of these treatments.
- Patients *willing* to try to quit tobacco use should be provided treatments identified as effective in this guideline.

- Patients *unwilling* to try to quit tobacco use should be provided a brief intervention designed to increase their motivation to quit.

It is essential that clinicians and health care delivery systems (including administrators, insurers, and purchasers) institutionalize the consistent identification, documentation, and treatment of every tobacco user seen in a health care setting.

Brief tobacco dependence treatment is effective, and every patient who uses tobacco should be offered at least brief treatment.

There is a strong dose-response relation between the intensity of tobacco dependence counseling and its effectiveness.

Treatments involving person-to-person contact (via individual, group, or proactive telephone counseling) are consistently effective, and their effectiveness increases with treatment intensity (e.g., minutes of contact).

Three types of counseling and behavioral therapies were found to be especially effective and should be used with all patients attempting tobacco cessation:
- Provision of practical counseling (problem-solving/skills training).
- Provision of social support as part of treatment (intra-treatment social support).
- Help in securing social support outside of treatment (extra-treatment social support).

Numerous effective pharmacotherapies for smoking cessation now exist. Except in the presence of contraindications, these should be used with all patients attempting to quit smoking.

Five *first-line* pharmacotherapies were identified that reliably increase long-term smoking abstinence rates:
- Bupropion SR.
- Nicotine gum.
- Nicotine inhaler.
- Nicotine nasal spray.
- Nicotine patch.

Two *second-line* pharmacotherapies were identified as efficacious and may be considered by clinicians if first-line pharmacotherapies are not effective:
- Clonidine.
- Nortriptyline.

Over-the-counter nicotine patches are effective relative to placebo, and their use should be encouraged.

Tobacco dependence treatments are both clinically effective and cost-effective relative to other medical and disease prevention interventions.

As such, insurers and purchasers should ensure that:
- All insurance plans include as a reimbursed benefit the counseling and pharmacotherapeutic treatments identified as effective in this guideline.
- Clinicians are reimbursed for providing tobacco dependence treatment just as they are reimbursed for treating other chronic conditions.

GUIDELINE UPDATE: ADVANCES

A comparison of the findings of the year 2000 guideline with the previous 1996 guideline reveals the considerable progress made in tobacco research over the brief period separating these two works. Among many important differences between the two documents, the following deserve special note:

- The updated guideline has produced even stronger evidence of the association between counseling intensity and successful treatment outcomes, and also has revealed evidence of additional efficacious counseling strategies. These include telephone counseling and counseling that helps smokers enlist support outside the treatment context.
- The updated guideline offers the clinician many more efficacious pharmacologic treatment strategies than were identified in the previous guideline. There are now seven different efficacious smoking cessation medications, allowing the clinician and patient many more treatment options. Further information also is available on the efficacy of combinations of nicotine replacement therapies and pharmacotherapies that are obtained over-the-counter.
- The updated guideline contains strong evidence that smoking cessation treatments shown to be efficacious in this guideline (both pharmacotherapy and counseling) are *cost-effective* relative to other routinely reimbursed medical interventions (e.g., treatment of hyperlipidemia and mammography screening).

The guideline panel concluded, therefore, that smoking cessation treatments should not be withheld from patients when other less cost-effective medical interventions are routinely delivered.

COORDINATION OF CARE: INSTITUTIONALIZING THE TREATMENT OF TOBACCO DEPENDENCE

There is increasing evidence that the success of any tobacco dependence treatment strategy cannot be divorced from the health care system in which it is embedded. Data strongly indicate that the consistent and effective delivery of tobacco interventions requires *coordinated interventions*. Just as a clinician must intervene with his or her patient, so must the health care administrator, insurer, and purchaser foster and support tobacco dependence treatment as an integral element of health care delivery. Health care purchasers should demand that tobacco intervention be a contractually covered obligation of insurers and providers. Health care administrators and insurers should ensure that clinicians have the training and support, and receive the reimbursement necessary to achieve consistent, effective intervention with tobacco users.

FUTURE PROMISE

About 20 years ago, data indicated that clinicians too frequently failed to intervene with their patients who smoke. Recent data confirm that this picture has not changed markedly over the past two decades. One recent study reported that only 15 percent of smokers who saw a physician in the past year were offered assistance with quitting, and only 3 percent were given a followup appointment to address this topic. These data are disheartening.

The updated guideline reports a family of findings that creates tremendous tension for change. This guideline reveals that multiple efficacious treatments exist, these treatments can double or triple the likelihood of long-term cessation, many cessation treatments are appropriate for the primary care setting, cessation treatments are more cost-effective than many other reimbursed clinical interventions, and the utilization and impact of cessation treatments can be increased by supportive health system policies (e.g., coverage through insurance plans). In sum, the updated guideline identifies and describes scientifically validated treatments and offers clear guidance on how such treatments can be consistently and effectively integrated into health care delivery.

The guideline panel is optimistic that this updated guideline is a harbinger of a new and very promising era in the treatment of tobacco use and dependence. The guideline codifies an evolving culture of health care—one in which every tobacco user has access to effective treatments for tobacco dependence. This new standard of care provides clinicians and health care delivery systems with their greatest opportunity to improve the current and future health of their patients by assisting those addicted to tobacco. Tobacco users and their families deserve no less.

The Diagnosis, Treatment, and Evaluation of the Initial Urinary Tract Infection in Febrile Infants and Young Children

●●

- *Clinical Practice Guideline*
- *Technical Report Summary*

Readers of this clinical practice guideline are urged to review the technical report to enhance the evidence-based decision-making process. The full technical report is available on the enclosed CD-ROM.

AMERICAN ACADEMY OF PEDIATRICS

Committee on Quality Improvement

Subcommittee on Urinary Tract Infection

Practice Parameter: The Diagnosis, Treatment, and Evaluation of the Initial Urinary Tract Infection in Febrile Infants and Young Children

ABSTRACT. *Objective.* To formulate recommendations for health care professionals about the diagnosis, treatment, and evaluation of an initial urinary tract infection (UTI) in febrile infants and young children (ages 2 months to 2 years).

Design. Comprehensive search and analysis of the medical literature, supplemented with consensus opinion of Subcommittee members.

Participants. The American Academy of Pediatrics (AAP) Committee on Quality Improvement selected a Subcommittee composed of pediatricians with expertise in the fields of epidemiology and informatics, infectious diseases, nephrology, pediatric practice, radiology, and urology to draft the parameter. The Subcommittee, the AAP Committee on Quality Improvement, a review panel of office-based practitioners, and other groups within and outside the AAP reviewed and revised the parameter.

Methods. The Subcommittee identified the population at highest risk of incurring renal damage from UTI—infants and young children with UTI and fever. A comprehensive bibliography on UTI in infants and young children was compiled. Literature was abstracted in a formal manner, and evidence tables were constructed. Decision analysis and cost-effectiveness analyses were performed to assess various strategies for diagnosis, treatment, and evaluation.

Technical Report. The overall problem of managing UTI in children between 2 months and 2 years of age was conceptualized as an evidence model. The model depicts the relationship between the steps in diagnosis and management of UTI. The steps are divided into the following four phases: 1) recognizing the child at risk for UTI, 2)

The recommendations in this statement do not indicate an exclusive course of treatment or serve as a standard of medical care. Variations, taking into account individual circumstances, may be appropriate.

"Practice Parameter: The Diagnosis, Treatment, and Evaluation of the Initial Urinary Tract Infection in Febrile Infants and Young Children" was reviewed by the appropriate committees and sections of the American Academy of Pediatrics (AAP), including the Committee on Infectious Diseases, the Committee on Medical Liability, and the Committee on Practice and Ambulatory Medicine; the Sections on Infectious Diseases, Nephrology, Radiology, and Urology; and the Chapter Review Group, a focus group of office-based pediatricians representing each AAP District: Gene R. Adams, MD; Charles S. Ball, MD; Robert M. Corwin, MD; Diane Fuquay, MD; Barbara M. Harley, MD; Michael J. Heimerl, MD; Thomas J. Herr, MD; Kenneth E. Matthews, MD; Robert D. Mines, MD; Lawrence C. Pakula, MD; Howard B. Weinblatt, MD; and Delosa A. Young, MD. The COQI and Subcommittee on UTI greatly appreciate the expertise of Richard N. Shiffman, MD, Center for Medical Informatics, Yale School of Medicine, for his input and analysis in the development of this practice guideline.

Comments also were solicited and received from the American Academy of Family Physicians, the American College of Emergency Physicians, and the American Urological Association.

PEDIATRICS (ISSN 0031 4005). Copyright © 1999 by the American Academy of Pediatrics.

making the diagnosis of UTI, 3) short-term treatment of UTI, and 4) evaluation of the child with UTI for possible urinary tract abnormality.

Phase 1 represents the recognition of the child at risk for UTI. Age and other clinical features define a prevalence or a prior probability of UTI, determining whether the diagnosis should be pursued.

Phase 2 depicts the diagnosis of UTI. Alternative diagnostic strategies may be characterized by their cost, sensitivity, and specificity. The result of testing is the division of patients into groups according to a relatively higher or lower probability of having a UTI. The probability of UTI in each of these groups depends not only on the sensitivity and specificity of the test, but also on the prior probability of the UTI among the children being tested. In this way, the usefulness of a diagnostic test depends on the prior probability of UTI established in Phase 1.

Phase 3 represents the short-term treatment of UTI. Alternatives for treatment of UTI may be compared, based on their likelihood of clearing the initial UTI.

Phase 4 depicts the imaging evaluation of infants with the diagnosis of UTI to identify those with urinary tract abnormalities such as vesicoureteral reflux (VUR). Children with VUR are believed to be at risk for ongoing renal damage with subsequent infections, resulting in hypertension and renal failure. Prophylactic antibiotic therapy or surgical procedures such as ureteral reimplantation may prevent progressive renal damage. Therefore, identifying urinary abnormalities may offer the benefit of preventing hypertension and renal failure.

Because the consequences of detection and early management of UTI are affected by subsequent evaluation and long-term management and, likewise, long-term management of patients with UTI depends on how they are detected at the outset, the Subcommittee elected to analyze the entire process from detection of UTI to the evaluation for, and consequences of, urinary tract abnormalities. The full analysis of these data can be found in the technical report. History of the literature review along with evidence-tables and a comprehensive bibliography also are available in the report. This report is published in *Pediatrics electronic pages* and can be accessed at the following URL: http://www.pediatrics.org/cgi/content/full/103/4/e54.

Results. Eleven recommendations are proposed for the diagnosis, management, and follow-up evaluation of infants and young children with unexplained fever who are later found to have a diagnosed UTI. Infants and young children are of particular concern because UTI in this age group (approximately 5%) may cause few recognizable signs or symptoms other than fever and has a higher potential for renal damage than in older children. Strategies for diagnosis and treatment depend on the clinician's assessment of the illness in the infant or young child. Diagnosis is based on the culture of a properly collected specimen of urine; urinalysis can only suggest the diagnosis. A sonogram should be performed on all infants and young children with fever and their first documented UTI; voiding cystourethrography or radionuclide cystography should be strongly considered.

ABBREVIATIONS. UTI, urinary tract infections; SPA, suprapubic aspiration; VUR, vesicoureteral reflux; WBC, white blood cell; TMP–SMX, trimethoprim–sulfamethoxazole; VCUG, voiding cystourethrography; RNC, radionuclide cystography.

The urinary tract is a relatively common site of infection in infants and young children. Urinary tract infections (UTIs) are important because they cause acute morbidity and may result in long-term medical problems, including hypertension and reduced renal function. Management of children with UTI involves repeated patient visits, use of antimicrobials, exposure to radiation, and cost. Accurate diagnosis is extremely important for two reasons: to permit identification, treatment, and evaluation of the children who are at risk for kidney damage and to avoid unnecessary treatment and evaluation of children who are not at risk, for whom interventions are costly and potentially harmful but provide no benefit. Infants and young children with UTI are of particular concern because the risk of renal damage is greatest in this age group and because the diagnosis is frequently challenging: the clinical presentation tends to be nonspecific and valid urine specimens cannot be obtained without invasive methods (suprapubic aspiration [SPA], transurethral catheterization).

Considerable variation in the methods of diagnosis, treatment, and evaluation of children with UTI was documented more than 2 decades ago.[1] Since then, various changes have been proposed to aid in diagnosis, treatment, and evaluation, but no data are available to suggest that such innovations have resulted in reduced variation in practice. This practice parameter focuses on the diagnosis, treatment, and evaluation of febrile infants and young children (2 months to 2 years of age). Excluded are those with obvious neurologic or anatomic abnormalities known to be associated with recurrent UTI and renal damage. Neonates and infants younger than 2 months have been excluded from consideration in this practice parameter. Children older than 2 years experiencing their first UTI also are excluded because they are more likely than younger children to have symptoms referable to the urinary tract, are less likely to have factors predisposing them to renal damage, and are at lower risk of developing renal damage.

This parameter is intended for use by clinicians who treat infants and young children in a variety of clinical settings (eg, office, emergency department, hospital).

METHODS

A comprehensive literature review was conducted to provide data for evidence tables that could be used to generate a decision tree. More than 2000 titles were identified from MEDLINE and bibliographies of current review articles from 1966 to 1996, and the authors' files. Of these, 402 articles contained relevant original data that were abstracted in a formal, standardized manner. An evidence-based model was developed using quantitative outcomes derived from the literature and cost data from the University of North Carolina. Decision analysis was used to perform risk analyses and cost-effectiveness analyses of alternative strategies for the diagnosis, management, and evaluation of UTI, using hypertension and end-stage renal disease as the undesirable outcomes. The calculated probability of undesirable outcome is the product of the probabilities of several steps (diagnosis, treatment, evaluation) and therefore is an estimate, influenced by approximations at each step. Cost-effectiveness of various strategies was assessed using the methods of Rice and associates[2] in which the break-even cost to prevent a chronic condition, such as hypertension or end-stage renal disease, is considered to be $700 000, an amount based on the estimated lifetime productivity of a healthy, young adult. Once this cost is assigned to the untoward clinical outcome (ie, hypertension or end-stage renal disease), it is possible to use the threshold method of decision-making.[3] The threshold approach to decision-making involves changing the value of a variable in the decision analysis to determine the value at which one strategy of diagnosis, treatment, and evaluation exceeds the break-even cost and an alternative strategy is preferred. Based on the results of these analyses and consensus, when necessary, an Algorithm was developed representing the strategies with the greatest benefit–risk characteristics. The strength of evidence on which recommendations were based was rated by the Subcommittee methodologist as strong, good, fair, or opinion/consensus. A detailed description of the methods by which the parameter was derived is available in a technical report from the American Academy of Pediatrics.

DIAGNOSIS

Recommendation 1

The presence of UTI should be considered in infants and young children 2 months to 2 years of age with unexplained fever (strength of evidence: strong).

The prevalence of UTI in infants and young children 2 months to 2 years of age who have no fever source evident from history or physical examination is high, ~5%.[4–8] The genders are not affected equally, however. The prevalence of UTI in febrile girls age 2 months to 2 years is more than twice that in boys (relative risk, 2.27). The prevalence of UTI in girls younger than 1 year of age is 6.5%; in boys, it is 3.3%. The prevalence of UTI in girls between 1 and 2 years of age is 8.1%; in boys it is 1.9%. The rate in circumcised boys is low, 0.2% to 0.4%.[9–13] The literature suggests that the rate in uncircumcised boys is 5 to 20 times higher than in circumcised boys.

Infants and young children are at higher risk than are older children for incurring acute renal injury with UTI. The incidence of vesicoureteral reflux (VUR) is higher in this age group than in older children (Fig 1), and the severity of VUR is greater, with the most severe form (with intrarenal reflux or pyelotubular backflow) virtually limited to infants.

Infants and young children with UTI warrant special attention because of the opportunity to prevent kidney damage. First, the UTI may bring to attention a child with an obstructive anomaly or severe VUR. Second, because infants and young children with UTI may have a febrile illness and no localizing findings, there may be a delay in diagnosis and treatment of the UTI. Clinical and experimental data support the concept that delay in instituting appro-

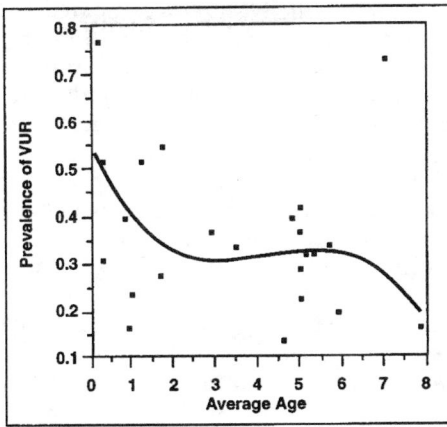

Fig 1. Prevalence of VUR by age. Plotted are the prevalences reported in 54 studies of urinary tract infections in children (references in Technical Report). The studies are weighted by sample size. The line is a third order polynomial fit to the data.

priate treatment of acute pyelonephritis increases the risk of kidney damage.[14,15] Third, the risk of renal damage increases as the number of recurrences increases[16] (Fig 2).

The presence of fever has long been considered a finding of special importance in infants and young children with UTI, because it has been accepted as a clinical marker of renal parenchymal involvement (pyelonephritis). The concept that otherwise unexplained fever in a child with UTI indicates that renal parenchymal involvement is based on comparison of children with high fever (39°C) and the clinical diagnosis of acute pyelonephritis with those with no fever (38°C) and a clinical diagnosis of cystitis.[17] Indirect tests for localization of the site of UTI, such as the presence of a reversible defect in renal concentrating ability and high levels of antibody titer to the infecting strains of *Escherichia coli*, and nonspecific tests of inflammation, such as elevated white blood cell (WBC) count, C-reactive protein, or sedimentation rate, are encountered more frequently in children with clinical pyelonephritis than in those with clinical cystitis. However, the indirect tests for localization of the site of infection and the nonspecific indicators of inflammation do not provide confirmatory evidence that the febrile infant or young child

with UTI has pyelonephritis. Cortical imaging studies using technetium 99 m Tc-dimercaptosuccinic acid (DMSA) or 99 m Tc-glucoheptonate may prove useful in determining whether the presence of high fever does identify children with pyelonephritis and distinguish them from those with cystitis; currently available studies with data that can be used to assess fever as a marker of pyelonephritis (defined by a positive scan) provide a wide range of sensitivity (53% to 84%) and specificity (44% to 92%).[18-20]

The likelihood that UTI is the cause of the fever may be increased if there is a history of crying on urination or of foul-smelling urine. An altered voiding pattern may be recognized as a symptom of UTI as early as the second year after birth in some children. Dysuria, urgency, frequency, or hesitancy may be present but are difficult to discern in this age group. Nonspecific signs and symptoms, such as irritability, vomiting, diarrhea, and failure to thrive, also may reflect the presence of UTI, but data are not available to assess the sensitivity, specificity, and predictive value of these clinical manifestations.

Decision analysis and cost-effectiveness analyses were performed, considering the different prevalences for age, gender, and circumcision status, and the prevalence of VUR by age. For girls and uncircumcised boys, it is cost-effective to pursue the diagnosis of UTI by invasive means and to perform imaging studies of the urinary tract. For circumcised boys younger than 1 year, the cost–benefit analysis is equivocal, but the Subcommittee supports the same diagnostic and evaluation measures as for girls and uncircumcised boys. Circumcised boys older than 1 year have a lower prevalence of UTI, and the prevalence of reflux is lower than that in those younger than 1 year. As a result, the cost-effectiveness analysis does not support invasive diagnostic procedures for all circumcised boys older than 1 year with unexplained fever. Analysis of a bag-collected specimen is a reasonable screening test in these boys, as long as they do not appear so ill as to warrant the initiation of antimicrobial therapy. Those who will be given antimicrobials on clinical grounds should have a specimen obtained for culture that is unlikely to be contaminated.

Recommendation 2

In infants and young children 2 months to 2 years of age with unexplained fever, the degree of toxicity, dehydration, and ability to retain oral intake must be carefully assessed (strength of evidence: strong).

In addition to seeking an explanation for fever, such as a source of infection, clinicians make a subjective assessment of the degree of illness or toxicity. Attempts have been made to objectify this assessment, using the prediction of bacteremia or serious bacterial infection as the outcome measure.[21] This clinical assessment, operationalized as whether antimicrobial therapy will be initiated, affects the diagnostic and therapeutic process regarding UTI as follows. If the clinician determines that the degree of illness warrants antimicrobial therapy, a valid urine

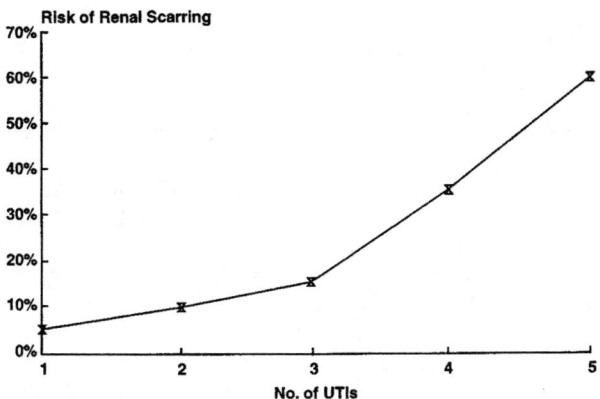

Fig 2. Relationship between renal scarring and number of urinary tract infections.[16]

specimen should be obtained before antimicrobials are administered, because the antimicrobials commonly prescribed in such situations will be effective against the usual urinary pathogens; invasive means are required to obtain such a specimen. If the clinician determines that the degree of illness does not require antimicrobial therapy, a urine culture is not essential immediately. In this situation, some clinicians may choose to obtain a specimen by noninvasive means (eg, in a collection bag attached to the perineum). The false-positive rate with such specimens dictates that before diagnosing UTI, all positive results be confirmed with culture of a urine specimen unlikely to be contaminated (see below).

Recommendation 3

If an infant or young child 2 months to 2 years of age with unexplained fever is assessed as being sufficiently ill to warrant immediate antimicrobial therapy, a urine specimen should be obtained by SPA or transurethral bladder catheterization; the diagnosis of UTI cannot be established by a culture of urine collected in a bag (strength of evidence: good).

Urine obtained by SPA or transurethral catheterization is unlikely to be contaminated and therefore is the preferred specimen for documenting UTI. In a clinical setting in which the physician has determined that immediate antimicrobial therapy is appropriate, the use of a bag-collected urine specimen is insufficient to document the presence of UTI.

Establishing a diagnosis of UTI requires a strategy that minimizes false-negative and false-positive results. Urine obtained by SPA is the least likely to be contaminated; urine obtained by transurethral bladder catheterization is next best. Either SPA or transurethral bladder catheterization should be used to establish the diagnosis of UTI. Cultures of urine specimens collected in a bag applied to the perineum have an unacceptably high false-positive rate; the combination of a 5% prevalence of UTI and a high rate of false-positive results (specificity, ~70%) results in a positive culture of urine collected in a bag to be a *false*-positive result 85% of the time. If antimicrobial therapy is initiated before obtaining a specimen of urine for culture that is unlikely to be contaminated, the opportunity may be lost to confirm the presence or establish the absence of UTI. Therefore, in the situation in which antimicrobial therapy will be initiated, SPA or catheterization is required to establish the diagnosis of UTI.

SPA has been considered the "gold standard" for obtaining urine for detecting bacteria in bladder urine accurately. The technique has limited risks. However, variable success rates for obtaining urine have been reported (23% to 90%),[16,22-24] technical expertise and experience are required, and many parents and physicians perceive the procedure as unacceptably invasive compared with catheterization. There may be no acceptable alternative in the boy with moderate or severe phimosis, however.

Urine obtained by transurethral catheterization of the urinary bladder for urine culture has a sensitivity of 95% and a specificity of 99% compared with that obtained by SPA.[23,25] Catheterization requires some skill and experience to obtain uncontaminated specimens, particularly in small infants, girls, and uncircumcised boys. Early studies in adults provided widely varying estimates of risk of introducing infection by a single, in-out catheterization. Turck and colleagues[26] demonstrated that the rate of bacteriuria secondary to transurethral catheterization in healthy young adults was considerably lower than that in hospitalized, older adults. Of the 200 healthy young adults studied, 100 men and 100 women, bacteriuria ultimately developed in only 1 woman—2 weeks after catheterization; bacteriuria was documented not to be present during the first 1 to 2 weeks after her catheterization. The risk of introducing infection in infants by transurethral catheterization has not been determined precisely, but it is the consensus of the Subcommittee that the risk is sufficiently low to recommend the procedure when UTI is suspected.

The techniques required for transurethral bladder catheterization and SPA are well described.[27] When SPA or transurethral catheterization is being attempted, the clinician should have a sterile container ready to collect a urine specimen voided because of the stimulus of the patient by manipulation in preparation for or during the procedure.

Recommendation 4

If an infant or young child 2 months to 2 years of age with unexplained fever is assessed as not being so ill as to require immediate antimicrobial therapy, there are two options (strength of evidence: good).

Option 1

Obtain and culture a urine specimen collected by SPA or transurethral bladder catheterization.

Option 2

Obtain a urine specimen by the most convenient means and perform a urinalysis. If the urinalysis suggests a UTI, obtain and culture a urine specimen collected by SPA or transurethral bladder catheterization; if urinalysis does not suggest a UTI, it is reasonable to follow the clinical course without initiating antimicrobial therapy, recognizing that a negative urinalysis does not rule out a UTI.

The option with the highest sensitivity is to obtain and culture a urine specimen collected by SPA or transurethral bladder catheterization; however, this approach may be resisted by some families and clinicians. In infants and young children assessed as *not* being so ill as to require immediate antimicrobial therapy, a urinalysis may help distinguish those with higher and lower likelihood of UTI. The urinalysis can be performed on any specimen, including one collected from a bag applied to the perineum, and has the advantage of convenience. The major disadvantage of collecting a specimen in a bag is that it is unsuitable for quantitative culture. In addition, there may be a delay of 1 hour or longer for the infant or young child to void; then, if the urinalysis suggests

UTI, a second specimen is required. The sensitivity of the bag method for detecting UTI is essentially 100%, but the false-positive rate of this method is also high, as demonstrated in several studies.[23,25,28] If the prevalence of UTI is 5%, 85% of positive cultures will be false-positive results; if the prevalence of UTI is 2% (febrile boys), the rate of false-positive results is 93%; if the prevalence of UTI is 0.2% (circumcised boys), the rate of false-positive results is 99%. The use of bag-collected urine specimens persists because collection of urine by this method is noninvasive and requires limited personnel time and expertise. Moreover, a negative (sterile) culture of a bag-collected urine specimen effectively eliminates the diagnosis of UTI, provided that the child is not receiving antimicrobials and that the urine is not contaminated with an antibacterial skin cleansing agent. Based on their experience, many clinicians believe that this collection technique has a low contamination rate under the following circumstances: the patient's perineum is properly cleansed and rinsed before application of the collection bag; the urine bag is removed promptly after urine is voided into the bag; and the specimen is refrigerated or processed immediately. Nevertheless, even if contamination from the perineal skin is minimized, there may be significant contamination from the vagina in girls or the prepuce in uncircumcised boys. Published results demonstrate that although a negative culture of a bag-collected specimen effectively rules out UTI, a positive culture does not document UTI. Confirmation requires culture of a specimen collected by transurethral bladder catheterization or SPA. Transurethral catheterization does not eliminate completely the possibility of contamination in girls and uncircumcised boys.

Of the components of urinalysis, the three most useful in the evaluation of possible UTI are leukocyte esterase test, nitrite test, and microscopy. A positive result on a leukocyte esterase test seems to be as sensitive as the identification of WBCs microscopically, but the sensitivity of either test is so low that the risk of missing UTI by either test alone is unacceptably high (Table 1). The nitrite test has a very high specificity and positive predictive value when urine specimens are processed promptly after collection. Using either a positive leukocyte esterase or nitrite test improves sensitivity at the expense of specificity; that is, there are many false-positive results. The wide range of reported test characteristics for microscopy indicates the difficulty in ensuring quality performance; the best results are achieved

with skilled technicians processing fresh urine specimens.

The urinalysis cannot substitute for a urine culture to document the presence of UTI, but the urinalysis can be valuable in selecting individuals for prompt initiation of treatment while waiting for the results of the urine culture. Any of the following are suggestive (although not diagnostic) of UTI: positive result of a leukocyte esterase or nitrite test, more than 5 white blood cells per high-power field of a properly spun specimen, or bacteria present on an unspun Gram-stained specimen.

In circumcised boys, whose low a priori rate of UTI (0.2% to 0.4%) does not routinely justify an invasive, potentially traumatic procedure, a normal urinalysis reduces the likelihood of UTI as the cause of the fever still further, to the order of 0.1%.

Recommendation 5
Diagnosis of UTI requires a culture of the urine (strength of evidence: strong).

All urine specimens should be processed as expediently as possible. If the specimen is not processed promptly, it should be refrigerated to prevent the growth of organisms that can occur in urine at room temperature. For the same reason, specimens requiring transportation to another site for processing should be transported on ice.

The standard test for the diagnosis of UTI is a quantitative urine culture; no element of the urinalysis or combination of elements is as sensitive and specific. A properly collected urine specimen should be inoculated on culture media that will allow identification of urinary tract pathogens.

UTI is confirmed or excluded based on the number of colony-forming units that grow on the culture media. Defining significant colony counts with regard to the method of collection considers that the distal urethra is commonly colonized by the same bacteria that may cause UTI; thus, a low colony count may be present in a specimen obtained by voiding or by transurethral catheterization when bacteria are not present in bladder urine. As noted in Table 2, what constitutes a significant colony count depends on the collection method and the clinical status of the patient; definitions of positive and negative cultures are operational and not absolute. Significance also depends on the identification of the isolated organism as a pathogen. Organisms such as *Lactobacillus* species, coagulase-negative staphylococci, and *Corynebacterium* species are not considered clinically relevant urine isolates in the otherwise healthy 2-month to 2-year-old. Alternative culture methods such as the dipslide may have a place in the office setting; sensitivity is reported in the range of 87% to 100%, and specificity, 92% to 98%.

TREATMENT
Recommendation 6
If the infant or young child 2 months to 2 years of age with suspected UTI is assessed as toxic, dehydrated, or unable to retain oral intake, initial anti-

TABLE 1. Sensitivity and Specificity of Components of the Urinalysis, Alone and in Combination (References in Text)

Test	Sensitivity % (Range)	Specificity % (Range)
Leukocyte esterase	83 (67–94)	78 (64–92)
Nitrite	53 (15–82)	98 (90–100)
Leukocyte esterase *or* nitrite positive	93 (90–100)	72 (58–91)
Microscopy: WBCs	73 (32–100)	81 (45–98)
Microscopy: bacteria	81 (16–99)	83 (11–100)
Leukocyte esterase *or* nitrite *or* microscopy positive	99.8 (99–100)	70 (60–92)

TABLE 2.   Criteria for the Diagnosis of UTI[53]

Method of Collection	Colony Count (Pure Culture)	Probability of Infection (%)
SPA	Gram-negative bacilli: any number	>99%
	Gram-positive cocci: more than a few thousand	
Transurethral catheterization	$>10^5$	95%; Infection likely suspicious;
	10^4–10^5	repeat infection unlikely
	10^3–10^4	
	$<10^3$	
Clean void		
Boy	$>10^4$	Infection likely
Girl	3 Specimens $\geq 10^5$	95%
	2 Specimens $\geq 10^5$	90%
	1 Specimen $\geq 10^5$	80%
	5×10^4 – 10^5	Suspicious, repeat
	10^4 – 5×10^4	Symptomatic: suspicious, repeat
		Asymptomatic: infection unlikely
	$<10^4$	infection unlikely

microbial therapy should be administered parenterally and hospitalization should be considered (strength of evidence: opinion/consensus).

The goals of treatment of acute UTI are to eliminate the acute infection, to prevent urosepsis, and to reduce the likelihood of renal damage. Patients who are toxic-appearing, dehydrated, or unable to retain oral intake (including medications) should receive an antimicrobial parenterally (Table 3) until they are improved clinically and are able to retain oral fluids and medications. The parenteral route is recommended because it ensures optimal antimicrobial levels in these high-risk patients. Parenteral administration of an antimicrobial also should be considered when compliance with obtaining and/or administering an antimicrobial orally cannot be ensured. In patients with compromised renal function, the use of potentially nephrotoxic antimicrobials (eg, aminoglycosides) requires caution, and serum creatinine and peak and trough antimicrobial concentrations need to be monitored. The clinical conditions of most patients improve within 24 to 48 hours; the route of antimicrobial administration then can be changed to oral (Table 4) to complete a 7- to 14-day course of therapy.

Hospitalization is necessary if patients have clinical urosepsis or are considered likely to have bacteremia based on clinical or laboratory evaluation. These patients need careful monitoring and repeated clinical examinations.

For children who do not appear toxic but who are vomiting, or when noncompliance is a concern, options include beginning therapy in the hospital or administering an antimicrobial parenterally on an outpatient basis. The route of administration is changed to oral when the child is no longer vomiting, and compliance appears to be ensured.

Recommendation 7

In the infant or young child 2 months to 2 years of age who may not appear ill but who has a culture confirming the presence of UTI, antimicrobial therapy should be initiated, parenterally or orally (strength of evidence: good).

The usual choices for treatment of UTI orally include amoxicillin, a sulfonamide-containing antimicrobial (sulfisoxazole or trimethoprim–sulfamethoxazole [TMP–SMX]), or a cephalosporin (Table 4). Emerging resistance of *E coli* to ampicillin appears to have rendered ampicillin and amoxicillin less effective than alternative agents. Studies comparing amoxicillin with TMP–SMX have demonstrated consistently higher cure rates with TMP–SMX (4% to 42%), regardless of the duration of therapy (1 dose, 3 to 4 days, or 10 days).[29–45]

Agents that are excreted in the urine but do not achieve therapeutic concentrations in the bloodstream, such as nalidixic acid or nitrofurantoin, should not be used to treat UTI in febrile infants and young children in whom renal involvement is likely.

Recommendation 8

Infants and young children 2 months to 2 years of age with UTI who have not had the expected clinical response with 2 days of antimicrobial therapy

TABLE 3.   Some Antimicrobials for Parenteral Treatment of UTI

Antimicrobial	Daily Dosage
Ceftriaxone	75 mg/kg every 24 h
Cefotaxime	150 mg/kg/d divided every 6 h
Ceftazidime	150 mg/kg/d divided every 6 h
Cefazolin	50 mg/kg/d divided every 8 h
Gentamicin	7.5 mg/kg/d divided every 8 h
Tobramycin	5 mg/kg/d divided every 8 h
Ticarcillin	300 mg/kg/d divided every 6 h
Ampicillin	100 mg/kg/d divided every 6 h

TABLE 4.   Some Antimicrobials for Oral Treatment of UTI

Antimicrobial	Dosage
Amoxicillin	20–40 mg/kg/d in 3 doses
Sulfonamide	
TMP in combination	6–12 mg TMP, 30–60 mg
with SMX	SMX per kg per d in 2 doses
Sulfisoxazole	120–150 mg/kg/d in 4 doses
Cephalosporin	
Cefixime	8 mg/kg/d in 2 doses
Cefpodixime	10 mg/kg/d in 2 doses
Cefprozil	30 mg/kg/d in 2 doses
Cephalexin	50–100 mg/kg/d in 4 doses
Loracarbef	15–30 mg/kg/d in 2 doses

should be reevaluated and another urine specimen should be cultured (strength of evidence: good).

Routine reculturing of the urine after 2 days of antimicrobial therapy is generally not necessary if the infant or young child has had the expected clinical response and the uropathogen is determined to be sensitive to the antimicrobial being administered. Antimicrobial sensitivity testing is determined most commonly by the application of disks containing the usual serum concentration of the antimicrobial to the culture plate. Because many antimicrobial agents are excreted in the urine in extremely high concentrations, an intermediately sensitive organism may be fully eradicated. Studies of minimal inhibitory concentration may be required to clarify the appropriateness of a given antimicrobial. If the sensitivity of the organism to the chosen antimicrobial is determined to be intermediate or resistant, or if sensitivity testing is not performed, a "proof-of-bacteriologic cure" culture should be performed after 48 hours of treatment. Data are not available to determine that clinical response alone ensures bacteriologic cure.

Recommendation 9

Infants and young children 2 months to 2 years of age, including those whose treatment initially was administered parenterally, should complete a 7- to 14-day antimicrobial course orally (strength of evidence: strong).

In 8 of 10 comparisons of long treatment duration (7 to 10 days) and short duration (1 dose or up to 3 days), results were better with long duration, with an attributable improvement in outcome of 5% to 21%.[33,38,41,44-48] Most uncomplicated UTIs are eliminated with a 7- to 10-day antimicrobial course, but many experts prefer 14 days for ill-appearing children with clinical evidence of pyelonephritis. Data comparing 10 days and 14 days are not available.

Recommendation 10

After a 7- to 14-day course of antimicrobial therapy and sterilization of the urine, infants and young children 2 months to 2 years of age with UTI should receive antimicrobials in therapeutic or prophylactic dosages until the imaging studies are completed (strength of evidence: good).

Although this practice parameter deals with the acute UTI, it is important to recognize the significance of recurrent infections. The association between recurrent bouts of febrile UTI and renal scarring follows an exponential curve[16] (Fig 2). Because the risk of recurrence is highest during the first months after UTI, children treated for UTI should continue antimicrobial treatment or prophylaxis (Table 5) until the imaging studies are completed and assessed. Additional treatment is based on the imaging findings assuming sterilization of the urine.

EVALUATION: IMAGING

Recommendation 11

Infants and young children 2 months to 2 years of age with UTI who do not demonstrate the expected clinical response within 2 days of antimicrobial therapy should undergo ultrasonography promptly, and either voiding cystourethrography (VCUG) or radionuclide cystography (RNC) should be performed at the earliest convenient time. Infants and young children who have the expected response to antimicrobials should have a sonogram and either VCUG or RNC performed at the earliest convenient time (strength of evidence: fair).

UTI in young children serve as a marker for abnormalities of the urinary tract. Imaging of the urinary tract is recommended in every febrile infant or young child with a first UTI to identify those with abnormalities that predispose to renal damage. Imaging should consist of urinary tract ultrasonography to detect dilatation secondary to obstruction and a study to detect VUR.

Ultrasonography

Urinary tract ultrasonography consists of examination of the kidneys to identify hydronephrosis and examination of the bladder to identify dilatation of the distal ureters, hypertrophy of the bladder wall, and the presence of ureteroceles. Previously, excretory urography (commonly called intravenous pyelography) was used to reveal these abnormalities, but now ultrasonography shows them more safely, less invasively, and often less expensively. Ultrasonography does have limitations, however. A normal ultrasound does not exclude VUR. Ultrasonography may show signs of acute renal inflammation and established renal scars, but it is not as sensitive as other renal imaging techniques.

Usually the timing of the ultrasound is not crucial, but when the rate of clinical improvement is slower than anticipated during treatment, ultrasonography should be performed promptly to look for a cause such as obstruction or abscess.

VUR

The most common abnormality detected in imaging studies is VUR (Fig 1). The rate of VUR among children younger than 1 year of age with UTI exceeds 50%. VUR is not an all-or-none phenomenon; grades of severity are recognized, designated I to V in the

TABLE 5. Some Antimicrobials for Prophylaxis of UTI

Antimicrobial	Dosage
TMP in combination with SMX	2 mg of TMP, 10 mg of SMX per kg as single bedtime dose *or* 5 mg of TMP, 25 mg of SMX per kg twice per week
Nitrofurantoin	1–2 mg/kg as single daily dose
Sulfisoxazole	10–20 mg/kg divided every 12 h
Nalidixic acid	30 mg/kg divided every 12 h
Methenamine mandelate	75 mg/kg divided every 12 h

International Study Classification (International Reflux Study Committee, 1981), based on the extent of the reflux and associated dilatation of the ureter and pelvis. The grading of VUR is important because the natural history differs by grade, as does the risk of renal damage. Patients with high-grade VUR are 4 to 6 times more likely to have scarring than those with low-grade VUR and 8 to 10 times more likely than those without VUR.[16,49]

VCUG; RNC

Either traditional contrast VCUG or RNC is recommended for detecting reflux. Although children may have pyelonephritis without reflux, the child with reflux is at increased risk of pyelonephritis and of scarring from UTI. With VCUG and RNC, a voiding phase is important because some reflux occurs only during voiding. If the predicted bladder capacity is not reached, the study may underestimate the presence or degree of reflux.

VCUG with fluoroscopy characterizes reflux better than does RNC. In addition, RNC does not show urethral or bladder abnormalities; for this reason, boys, whose urethra must be examined for posterior urethral valves, or girls, who have symptoms of voiding dysfunction when not infected, should have a standard fluoroscopic contrast VCUG as part of their initial studies. RNC has a lower radiation dose and therefore may be preferred in follow-up examinations of children with reflux. However, the introduction of low-dose radiographic equipment has narrowed the gap in radiation between the VCUG and RNC.[50]

There is no benefit in delaying performance of these studies as long as the child is free of infection and bladder irritability is absent. While waiting for reflux study results, the child should be receiving an antimicrobial, either as part of the initial treatment or as posttreatment prophylaxis (Table 5).

Radionuclide Renal Scans

Renal cortical scintigraphy (with 99 m Tc-DMSA or 99 m Tc-glucoheptonate) and enhanced computed tomography are very sensitive means of identifying acute changes from pyelonephritis or renal scarring. However, the role of these imaging modalities in the clinical management of the child with UTI still is unclear.

CONCLUSIONS

Eleven recommendations are proposed for the diagnosis, management, and evaluation of infants and young children with UTI and unexplained fever. Infants and children younger than 2 years of age with unexplained fever are identified for particular concern because UTI has a high prevalence in this group (~5%), may cause few recognizable signs or symptoms other than fever, and has a greater potential for renal damage than in older children. Strategies of diagnosis and treatment depend on how ill the clinician assesses the infant or young child to be, ie, whether antimicrobial therapy is warranted immediately or can be delayed safely until the results of urine culture are available. Diagnosis is based on the culture of an appropriately collected specimen of urine; urinalysis can only suggest the diagnosis. Imaging studies should be performed on all infants and young children with a documented initial UTI.

AREAS FOR FUTURE RESEARCH

The relationship between UTI in infants and young children and reduced renal function in adults has been established but is not well characterized in quantitative terms. The ideal prospective cohort study from birth to age 40 to 50 years has not been conducted and is unlikely to be conducted. Thus, estimates of undesirable outcomes in adulthood, such as hypertension and end-stage renal disease, are based on the mathematical product of probabilities at several steps, each of which is subject to bias and error. Other attempts at decision analysis[51] and thoughtful literature review[52] have recognized the same limitations. Until recently, imaging tools available to assess the effect of UTI have been insensitive. With the imaging techniques available now, it may be possible to follow a cohort of infants and young children who present with fever and UTI to assess the development of scars and functional impairment. Research is underway in this area.

The development of noninvasive methods of obtaining a urine specimen or of techniques that obviate the need for invasive sampling would be valuable for general use. One component of the urinalysis that merits particular attention is the assessment of WBCs in the urine. Bacteriuria can occur without pyuria, but it is not clear whether pyuria is a specific marker for renal inflammation, obviating the need for culture if WBCs are not present in the urine. Research is underway in this area under conditions that optimize the detection of WBCs in the urine by microscopy. If studies continue to demonstrate usefulness of microscopy, the general applicability of the test will need to be studied, particularly in offices without on-site laboratories or trained laboratory staff. Special attention will need to be given to specimens from girls and from uncircumcised boys, particularly infants, because transurethral catheterization may be difficult and produce a contaminated specimen. An alternative to SPA, which is not commonly performed anymore, would be welcome in clinical practice and in research to clarify such issues as the true prevalence of UTI in young uncircumcised boys.

There is consensus about the antimicrobial treatment of infants and young children with acute UTI, but questions remain relating to the specific duration and route of therapy. Currently, the efficacy of orally administered treatment is being compared with parenterally administered treatment under controlled conditions. If orally administered therapy is as efficacious as that administered parenterally, concern about variable adherence to a prescribed regimen will remain and influence the decision of whether to hospitalize and whether to administer the antimicrobial(s) parenterally or orally.

As noted in the section "Evaluation: Imaging," ultrasonography is recommended to detect dilatation associated with obstruction and is preferred over other modalities because it is noninvasive and does not expose the child to radiation. Data defining the yield of positive findings were generated before the widespread use of fetal ultrasonography, and it is not clear that they are applicable today. The absence of extensive data from modern studies and variations in the frequency and quality of fetal ultrasonography do not permit a determination of whether ultrasonography can reasonably be omitted. Further complicating the assessment is the changing utilization of fetal ultrasonography under the financial pressures of managed care. Studies in this area will need to be defined carefully so that the generalizability and applicability to individual patients can be assessed.

A study to determine the presence and severity of VUR also is recommended. It is recognized, however, that pyelonephritis (defined by cortical scintigraphy) can occur in the absence of VUR (defined by VCUG or RNC) and that progressive renal scarring (defined by cortical scintigraphy)

can occur in the absence of demonstrated VUR. Whether children with pyelonephritis (defined clinically or by cortical scintigraphy) who have normal results on VCUG or RNC benefit from antimicrobial prophylaxis is unknown but is being studied.

The role of cortical scintigraphy in the imaging examination of infants and young children with initial UTI is unclear and requires additional study. The demonstration by cortical scintigraphy of "cold" areas of decreased perfusion has led to the development of alternative imaging techniques, such as enhanced computed tomography and power Doppler ultrasonography. These modalities also can demonstrate hypoperfusion and have advantages, particularly power Doppler ultrasonography, which is noninvasive and does not expose the child to radiation. Studies are now in progress.

COMMITTEE ON QUALITY IMPROVEMENT, 1999
David A. Bergman, MD, Chairperson
Richard D. Baltz, MD
James R. Cooley, MD

LIAISON REPRESENTATIVES
Michael J. Goldberg, MD, Sections Liason
Gerald B. Hickson, MD

Algorithm

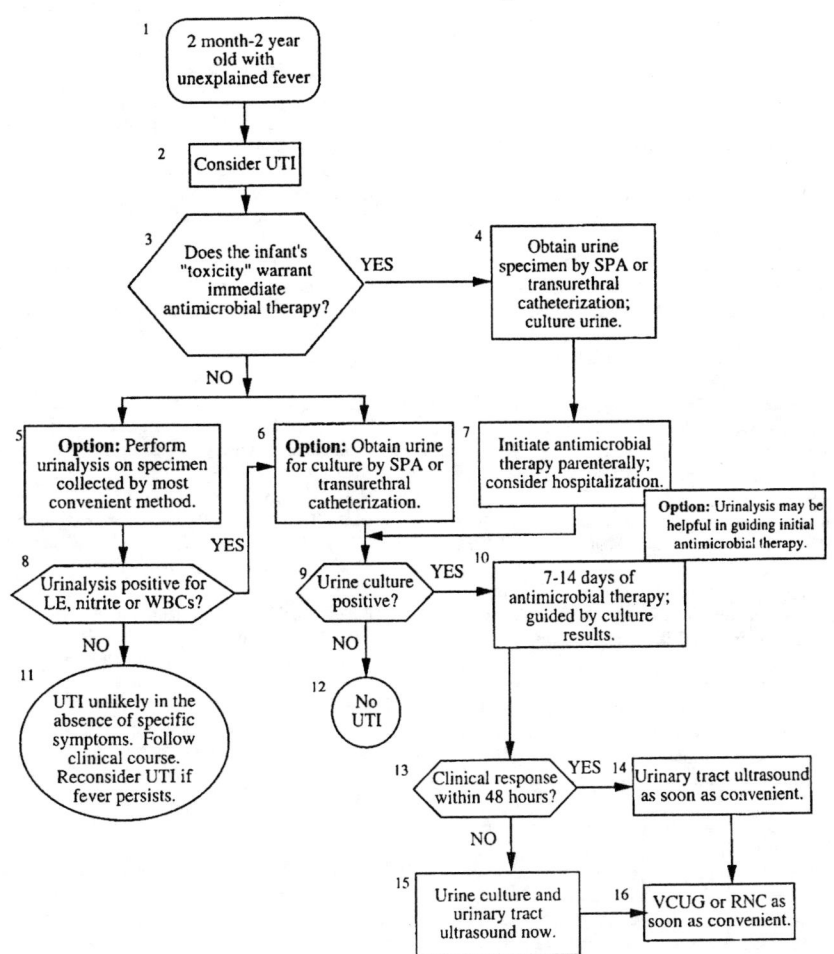

Charles J. Homer, MD, MPH, Section on
    Epidemiology Liaison
Paul V. Miles, MD
Joan E. Shook, MD
William M. Zurthellen, MD

LIAISON REPRESENTATIVE
Betty A. Lowe, MD, NACHRI Liaison

SUBCOMMITTEE ON URINARY TRACT
Kenneth B. Roberts, MD, Chairperson
Stephen M. Downs, MD, MS
Stanley Hellerstein, MD
Michael J. Holmes, MD, PhD
Robert L. Lebowitz, MD
Jacob A. Lohr, MD
Linda D. Shortliffe, MD
Russell W. Steele, MD

REFERENCES

1. Dolan TF Jr, Meyers A. A survey of office management of urinary tract infections in childhood. *Pediatrics.* 1973;52:21–24
2. Rice DP, Hodgeson TA, Kopstein AN. The economic costs of illness: a replication and update. *Health Care Financ Rev.* 1985;7:61–80
3. Pauker SG, Kassirer JP. The threshold approach to clinical decision making. *N Engl J Med.* 1980;302:1109–1117
4. Hoberman A, Chao HP, Keller DM, et al. Prevalence of urinary tract infection in febrile infants. *J Pediatr.* 1993;123:17–23
5. Roberts KB, Charney E, Sweren RJ, et al. Urinary tract infection in infants with unexplained fever: a collaborative study. *J Pediatr.* 1983;103:864–867
6. Bauchner H, Philipp B, Dahefsky G, Klein JO. Prevalence of bacteriuria in febrile children. *Pediatr Infect Dis J.* 1987;6:239–242
7. Bonadio WA. Urine culturing technique in febrile infants. *Pediatr Emerg Care.* 1987;3:75–78
8. North AF. Bacteriuria in children with acute febrile illnesses. *J Pediatr.* 1963;63:408–411
9. Ginsburg CM, McCracken GH Jr. Urinary tract infections in young infants. *Pediatrics.* 1982;69:409–412
10. Wiswell TE, Smith FR, Bass JW. Decreased incidence of urinary tract infections in circumcised male infants. *Pediatrics.* 1985;75:901–903
11. Wiswell TE, Roscelli JD. Corroborative evidence for the decreased incidence of urinary tract infections in circumcised male infants. *Pediatrics.* 1986;78:96–99
12. Wiswell TE, Hachey WE. Urinary tract infections and the uncircumcised state: an update. *Clin Pediatr.* 1993;32:130–134
13. Craig JC, Knight JF, Sureshjumar P, Mantz E, Roy LP. Effect of circumcision on incidence of urinary tract infection in preschool boys. *J Pediatr.* 1996;128:23–27
14. Winter AL, Hardy BE, Alton DJ, Arbus GS, Churchill BM. Acquired renal scars in children. *J Urol.* 1983;129:1190–1194
15. Smellie JM, Poulton A, Prescod NP. Retrospective study of children with renal scarring associated with reflux and urinary infection. *Br Med J.* 1994;308:1193–1196
16. Jodal U. The natural history of bacteriuria in childhood. *Infect Dis Clin North Am.* 1987;1:713–729
17. Winberg J, Andersen HJ, Bergstrom T, et al. Epidemiology of symptomatic urinary tract infection in childhood. *Acta Paediatr Scand.* 1974;252:1–20. Supplement
18. Tappin DM, Murphy AV, Mocan H, et al. A prospective study of children with first acute symptomatic *E coli* urinary tract infection: early 99 m technetium dimercaptosuccinic acid scan appearances. *Acta Paediatr Scand.* 1989;78:923–929
19. Verboven M, Ingels M, Delree M, Piepsz A. 99 mTc-DMSA scintigraphy in acute urinary tract infection in children. *Pediatr Radiol.* 1990;20:540–542
20. Rosenberg AR, Rossleigh MA, Brydon MP, Bass SJ, Leighton DM, Farnsworth RH. Evaluation of acute urinary tract infection in children by dimercaptosuccinic acid scintigraphy: a prospective study. *J Urol.* 1992;148:1746–1749. Part II
21. McCarthy PL, Sharpe MR, Spiesel SZ, et al. Observation scales to identify serious illness in febrile children. *Pediatrics.* 1982;70:802–809
22. Pryles CV, Atkin MD, Morse TS, Welch KJ. Comparative bacteriologic study of urine obtained from children by percutaneous suprapubic aspiration of the bladder and by catheter. *Pediatrics.* 1959;24:983–991
23. Leong YY, Tan KW. Bladder aspiration for diagnosis of urinary tract infection in infants and young children. *J Singapore Paediatr Soc.* 1976;18:43–47
24. Djojohadipringgo S, Abdul Hamid RH, Thahir S, Karim A, Darsono I. Bladder puncture in newborns—a bacteriological study. *Paediatr Indonesia.* 1976;16:527–534
25. Sorensen K, Lose G, Nathan E. Urinary tract infection and diurnal incontinence in girls. *Eur J Pediatr.* 1988;148:146–147
26. Turck M, Goffe B, Petersdorf RG. The urethral catheter and urinary tract infection. *J Urol.* 1962;88:834–837
27. Lohf J. *Pediatric Outpatient Procedures.* Philadelphia, PA: JB Lippincott Co; 1991:142–152
28. Shannon F, Sepp E, Rose G. The diagnosis of bacteriuria by bladder puncture in infancy and childhood. *Aust Paediatr J.* 1969;5:97–100
29. Cohen M. The first urinary tract infection in male children. *Am J Dis Child.* 1976;130:810–813
30. Ellerstein NS, Sullivan TD, Baliah T, Neter E. Trimethoprim/sulfamethoxazole and ampicillin in the treatment of acute urinary tract infections in children: a double-blind study. *Pediatrics.* 1977;60:245–247
31. Khan AJ, Ubriani RS, Bombach E, Agbayani MM, Ratner H, Evans HE. Initial urinary tract infection caused by *Proteus mirabilis* in infancy and childhood. *J Pediatr.* 1978;93:791–793
32. Howard JB, Howard JE. Trimethoprim–sulfamethoxazole vs sulfamethoxazole for acute urinary tract infections in children. *Am J Dis Child.* 1978;132:1085–1087
33. Wientzen RL, McCracken GH Jr, Petruska ML, Swinson SG, Kaijer B, Hanson LA. Localization and therapy of urinary tract infections of childhood. *Pediatrics.* 1979;63:467–474
34. Sullivan TD, Ellerstein NS, Neter E. The effects of ampicillin and trimethoprim/sulfamethoxazole on the periurethral flora of children with urinary tract infection. *Infection.* 1980;8:S339–S341. Supplement 3
35. Fennell RS, Luengnaruemitchai M, Iravani A, Garin EH, Walker RD, Richard GA. Urinary tract infections in children: effect of short course antibiotic therapy on recurrence rate in children with previous infections. *Clin Pediatr.* 1980;19:121–124
36. Shapiro ED, Wald ER. Single-dose amoxicillin treatment of urinary tract infections. *J Pediatr.* 1981;99:989–992
37. Helin I. Short-term treatment of lower urinary tract infections in children with trimethoprim/sulphadiazine. *Infection.* 1981;9:249–251
38. Pitt WR, Dyer SA, McNee JL, Burke JR. Single dose trimethoprim-sulphamethoxazole treatment of symptomatic urinary infection. *Arch Dis Child.* 1981;57:229–231
39. Avner ED, Ingelfinger JR, Herrin JT, et al. Single-dose amoxicillin therapy of uncomplicated pediatric urinary tract infections. *J Pediatr.* 1983;102:623–627
40. Aarbakke J, Opshaug O, Digranes A, Hoylandskjaer A, Fluge G, Fellner H. Clinical effect and pharmacokinetics of trimethoprim–sulphadiazine in children with urinary tract infections. *Eur J Clin Pharmacol.* 1983;24:267–271
41. Stahl G, Topf P, Fleisher GR, Normal ME, Rosenblum HW, Gruskin AB. Single-dose treatment of uncomplicated urinary tract infections in children. *Ann Emerg Med.* 1984;13:705–708
42. Hashemi G. Recurrent urinary tract infection. *Indian J Pediatr.* 1985;52:401–403
43. Rajkumar S, Saxena Y, Rajogopal V, Sierra MF. Trimethoprim in pediatric urinary tract infection. *Child Nephrol Urol.* 1988;9:77–81
44. Madrigal G, Odio CM, Mohs E, Guevara J, McCracken GH Jr. Single dose antibiotic therapy is not as effective as conventional regimens for management of acute urinary tract infections in children. *Pediatr Infect Dis J.* 1988;7:316–319
45. Nolan T, Lubitz L, Oberklaid F. Single dose trimethoprim for urinary tract infection. *Arch Dis Child.* 1989;64:581–586
46. Bailey RR, Abbott GD. Treatment of urinary tract infection with a single dose of trimethoprim–sulfamethoxazole. *Can Med Assoc J.* 1978;118:551–552
47. Bailey RR, Abbott GD. Treatment of urinary tract infection with a single dose of amoxycillin. *Nephron.* 1977;18:316–320
48. Copenhagen Study Group of Urinary Tract Infections in Children. Short-term treatment of acute urinary tract infection in girls. *Scand J Infect Dis.* 1991;23:213–220
49. McKerrow W, Davidson-Lamb N, Jones PF. Urinary tract infection in children. *Br Med J.* 1984;289:299–303
50. Kleinman PK, Diamond DA, Karellas A, Spevak MR, Nimkin K, Belanger P. Tailored low-dose fluoroscopic voiding cystourethrography for the reevaluation of vesicoureteral reflux in girls. *AJR Am J Roentgenol.* 1994;162:1151–1154
51. Kramer MS, Tange SM, Drummond KN, Mills EL. Urine testing in young febrile children: a risk–benefit analysis. *J Pediatr.* 1994;125:6–13
52. Dick PT, Feldman W. Routine diagnostic imaging for childhood urinary tract infections: a systematic overview. *J Pediatr.* 1996;128:15–22
53. Hellerstein S. Recurrent urinary tract infections in children. *Pediatr Infect Dis.* 1982;1:271–281

Technical Report Summary:
Urinary Tract Infections in Febrile Infants and Young Children

Author:
Stephen M. Downs, MD, MS

ABSTRACT

Overview

The Urinary Tract Infection Subcommittee of the American Academy of Pediatrics' Committee on Quality Improvement has analyzed alternative strategies for the diagnosis and management of urinary tract infection (UTI) in children. The target population is limited to children between 2 months and 2 years of age who are examined because of fever without an obvious cause. Diagnosis and management of UTI in this group are especially challenging for these three reasons: 1) the manifestation of UTI tends to be nonspecific, and cases may be missed easily; 2) clean voided midstream urine specimens rarely can be obtained, leaving only urine collection methods that are invasive (transurethral catheterization or bladder tap) or result in nonspecific test results (bag urine); and 3) a substantial number of infants with UTI also may have structural or functional abnormalities of the urinary tract that put them at risk for ongoing renal damage, hypertension, and end-stage renal disease (ESRD).

Methods

To examine alternative management strategies for UTI in infants, a conceptual model of the steps in diagnosis and management of UTI was developed. The model was expanded into a decision tree. Probabilities for branch points in the decision tree were obtained by review of the literature on childhood UTI. Data were extracted on standardized forms. Cost data were obtained by literature review and from hospital billing data. The data were collated into evidence tables. Analysis of the decision tree was used to produce risk tables and incremental cost-effectiveness ratios for alternative strategies.

Results

Based on the results of this analysis and, when necessary, consensus opinion, the Committee developed recommendations for the management of UTI in this population. This document provides the evidence the Subcommittee used in the development of its recommendations.

Conclusions

The Subcommittee agreed that the objective of the practice guideline would be to minimize the risk of chronic renal damage within reasonable economic constraints. Steps involved in achieving these objectives are: 1) identifying UTI; 2) short-term treatment of UTI; and 3) evaluation for urinary tract abnormalities.

METHODS

Analysis of the data on UTI consisted of several steps. The Subcommittee met to define the target population, setting, and providers for whom the practice parameter is intended. Subcommittee members identified the outcomes of interest for the analysis. A conceptual evidence model of the diagnosis and management of UTI was developed. The evidence model was used to generate a decision tree. A comprehensive review of the literature determined the probability estimates used in the tree. The tree was used to conduct risk analyses and cost-effectiveness analyses of alternative strategies for the diagnosis and management of UTI. Based on the results of these analyses and consensus when necessary, an algorithm representing the strategies with acceptable risk-benefit trade-offs was developed.

EVIDENCE MODEL

The overall problem of managing UTI in children between 2 months and 2 years of age was conceptualized as an evidence model. The model depicts the relationships between the steps in the diagnosis and management of UTI. The steps are divided into the following four phases: 1) recognizing the child at risk for UTI, 2) making the diagnosis of UTI, 3) short-term treatment of UTI, and 4) evaluation of the child with UTI for possible urinary tract abnormality.

Phase 1 represents the recognition of the child at risk for UTI. Age and other clinical features define a prevalence or *a priori* probability of UTI, determining whether the diagnosis should be pursued. If children at sufficiently high risk for UTI are not identified for diagnostic evaluation, the potential benefit of treatment will be lost. However, children with a sufficiently low likelihood of UTI should be saved the cost of diagnosis (and perhaps misdiagnosis) of UTI when the potential for benefit is minimal.

Phase 2 depicts the diagnosis of UTI. Alternative diagnostic strategies may be characterized by their cost, sensitivity, and specificity. The result of testing is the division of patients into groups according to a relatively higher or lower probability of having a UTI. The probability of UTI in each of these groups depends not only on the sensitivity and specificity of the test, but also on the prior probability of the UTI among the children being tested. In this way, the usefulness of a diagnostic test depends on the prior probability of UTI established in phase 1. Overdiagnosis of UTI may result in unnecessary treatment and unnecessary imaging evaluation for urinary tract abnormalities. Underdiagnosis will result in missing the opportunity to treat the acute infection and the consequences of possible underlying urinary tract abnormalities.

Phase 3 represents the short-term treatment of UTI. Alternatives for treatment of UTI may be compared, based on their likelihood of clearing the initial UTI (IUTI).

Phase 4 depicts the imaging evaluation of infants with the diagnosis of UTI to identify those with urinary tract abnormalities such as vesicoureteral reflux (VUR). Children with VUR are believed to be at risk for ongoing renal damage with subsequent infections, resulting in hypertension and renal failure. Prophylactic antibiotic therapy or surgical procedures such as ureteral reimplantation may prevent progressive renal damage. Therefore, identifying urinary abnormalities may offer the benefit of preventing hypertension and renal failure. Each alternative strategy for imaging evaluation can be characterized according to its cost, invasiveness, and test characteristics (sensitivity and specificity). The potential yield of an imaging evaluation will be affected by the accuracy of the initial diagnosis of UTI. If the probability of UTI is low because a nonspecific test was used to make the diagnosis, the cost of an imaging study will yield little benefit. Therefore, the value of imaging strategies depends on the accuracy of the diagnosis of UTI in phase 2.

Because the consequences of detection and early management of UTI are affected by subsequent evaluation and long-term management and, likewise, long-term management of patients with UTI depends on how they are detected at the outset, the Subcommittee elected to analyze the entire process from detection of UTI to the evaluation for, and consequences of, urinary tract abnormalities.

Decision Tree

The conceptual model was used to develop a decision tree. The tree quantifies the relationship between alternative strategies for the diagnosis and treatment of UTI, the evaluation of children for abnormalities of the urinary tract, and the anticipated consequences of these alternative diagnostic and treatment strategies.

In the diagnosis and treatment of UTI, four alternatives are represented. As anchor points, the alternatives of treating all or treating none of the patients at risk are represented. Two alternative tests are represented in the other branches. The test characteristics and costs of these tests were adjusted to correspond with the tests the Subcommittee chose to evaluate. In this way, the Subcommittee compared alternative testing strategies.

In the decision tree, if a testing strategy is used, the result is positive or negative. A positive result was assumed to lead to a decision to treat and a negative result to a decision to observe without treatment. If treatment is chosen, presumptively or based on the results of a diagnostic test, a treatment complication may result. Rarely, as in the case of anaphylaxis, the complication may result in death.

For all other patients, there is a risk of urosepsis. This risk is the probability of UTI multiplied by the prevalence of urosepsis among infants with UTI. Assuming urosepsis behaves like bacteremia from other sources in infants, the infection may clear spontaneously in those who have urosepsis. The probability of clearing the infection is increased among those who receive antimicrobials. If urosepsis does not clear, hospitalization will result, and the child has a risk of dying.

Once the short-term outcome of the UTI has been resolved, the second decision is whether and how to image the urinary tract for structural and functional abnormalities. The three following options are modeled: 1) a full evaluation, including ultrasonography or an intravenous pyelogram and voiding cystourethrography (VCUG) or radionuclide cystourethrography (RCG); 2) ultrasonography alone; and 3) no evaluation.

The results of the evaluation are determined separately for each patient type. For patients who have no UTI (false-positive diagnosis of UTI), it is assumed that abnormalities are not present and the infant is not at increased risk of renal damage. Patients who have a true UTI may or may not have VUR. Among those with VUR, the reflux may be low grade (1 or 2) or high grade (3, 4, or 5).

The probability of having a positive result when imaging an abnormal urinary tract depends on the sensitivity of the imaging modality for the abnormality. For example, ultrasonography is much more sensitive to high-grade VUR than to low-grade VUR. The analysis assumes that all imaging modalities have 100% specificity (ie, no false-positive diagnoses).

The result of the imaging evaluation would be used to select a treatment (surgical correction or antibiotic prophylaxis as appropriate) to prevent recurrent infections. An evaluation with normal results or no evaluation would lead to no therapy. Identifying the optimal therapy for a given urinary tract abnormality is beyond the scope of the present analysis.

Patients may or may not have recurrent UTI, defined as more than three infections in a 5-year period. Recurrent infections lead to progressive renal scarring. The risk of scarring is highest among those with high-grade VUR and lowest among those with no VUR. Therapeutic interventions reduce the risk of renal scarring by reducing VUR in the case of surgery or preventing infection in the case of antimicrobial prophylaxis.

Patients with progressive renal scarring are at increased risk of hypertension and ESRD. Those who do not experience these outcomes may have decreased renal function but will not have clinically important outcomes.

At the terminal nodes of each branch, the outcomes are tabulated as costs and clinical outcomes. Costs considered include the cost of diagnostic testing, treatment, complications of treatment, hospitalization for urosepsis, imaging studies, surgery or prophylaxis, management of hypertension, and ESRD. Clinical outcomes include chronic hypertension, renal failure, and death.

The decision tree was encoded and evaluated using the Decision Maker software Version 6.0 (Sonnenberg and Pauker, New England Medical Center, Boston, MA).

Literature Review

Articles for review were obtained from four sources in two rounds of searching. In the first round, the MEDLINE database was searched using four separate search strategies corresponding with the four phases of the diagnosis and treatment of UTI: recognition, diagnosis, short-term treatment, and imaging evaluation. The titles and abstracts resulting from these searches were distributed among the Subcommittee members who identified those that were definitely or potentially useful. These articles were reproduced in full.

In a second round of searching, articles were identified from three additional sources: the bibliographies of two recent reviews; a survey of the members of the Subcommittee, soliciting the articles they identified as most important and relevant to the analysis; and articles sought specifically to estimate costs for the management of chronic hypertension and ESRD. At each of the two rounds of searching, the articles were reviewed by the epidemiology consultant, and articles with no original data were removed.

The remaining articles were reviewed and data extracted using a data extraction form designed to identify estimates necessary to evaluate the decision model. In addition, the quality of each article was rated on a scale from 0 to 1 by using quality criteria adapted from Sackett and colleagues. Reviewers also provided a subjective rating of "good," "fair," or "poor" to each article. Data extracted were recorded in evidence tables, using an Excel (Microsoft Corporation, Redmond, WA) spreadsheet. A subset of 24 articles was reviewed twice by different reviewers to check interrater reliability. At the time of analysis of the decision models, the articles were reviewed again by the epidemiology consultant.

RESULTS

Literature Review

In the initial MEDLINE search, 1949 articles were identified. The title and abstract of each of these was reviewed by two members of the Subcommittee and identified as "useful," "potentially useful," or "not useful." After this review and elimination of duplicates, 430 articles were reproduced in full for data extraction. Of these, 105 were rejected because they contained no original data relevant to the analysis. In the second round, an additional 133 articles were identified. Twenty-six of these were rejected for lack of original data. A total of 432 articles were reviewed at least once.

The quality of the articles in this area is highly variable, but most articles met 50% or fewer of the quality criteria. Interrater reliability for quality scores was tested using a subset of the articles. Correlation of scores among reviewers was only fair ($r = 0.43$). Correlation among the readers' subjective ratings was less good ($r = 0.29$).

Age and Gender

The data indicate that the probability of finding UTI in febrile male infants is less than half that in females, and just greater than one third for males between 1 and 2 years of age. Findings from two studies report the prevalence of UTI by gender in an unbiased sample of febrile infants younger than 1 year. The studies show inconsistent results among males younger than 1 year. Among females, the prevalence was similar, 7.4% and 8.8%, respectively. Other studies also suggest a lower risk among males in older age groups.

Other studies used to estimate the effect of age and gender on the prevalence of UTI examined only children with confirmed UTI. Relative risk of UTI for a given gender was estimated from these studies using the odds ratio (OR), $P(\text{male} \mid \text{UTI}) / P(\text{female} \mid \text{UTI})$. Because this prevalence in males and females in the general population is ~50%, the OR is essentially the same as the ratio of the prevalence of UTI among males to the prevalence among females. The prevalence itself can be derived by assuming an overall prevalence of 5% for both genders and a 50% prevalence of males in the population, using the formula, $P(\text{UTI} \mid \text{male}) = P(\text{male} \mid \text{UTI}) \cdot P(\text{UTI}) / P(\text{male})$. The comparable formula was used for females.

Studies also were stratified by age. These data and the data for prevalence by gender were used to make crude estimates of the effect of age and gender on the prevalence of UTI in four subgroups: males younger than 1 year (3%), males older than 1 year (2%), females younger than 1 year (7%), and females older than 1 year (8%).

Circumcision

Several studies show a dramatic risk reduction among circumcised males. Most (but not all) of these data are retrospective, and the studies are plagued with missing data, but the findings are quite consistent. In all these studies, the probability of circumcision given UTI [$P(\text{circ} \mid \text{UTI})$] was reported. Relative risk was estimated by the OR, $P(\text{circ} \mid \text{UTI}) / P(\text{no circ} \mid \text{UTI})$. Estimates of prevalence of UTI given circumcision [$P(\text{UTI} \mid \text{circ})$] were calculated by assuming the previous probability of UTI regardless of circumcision status [$P(\text{UTI})$] is 5%, and the probability of circumcision (among males) is 70%. Prevalences are calculated using these estimates and Bayes' formula, $P(\text{UTI} \mid \text{circ}) = P(\text{circ} \mid \text{UTI}) \cdot P(\text{UTI}) / P(\text{circ})$. The results suggest that the prevalence of UTI among febrile male infants who are circumcised would be ~0.2%.

Most data come from studies of infants younger than 1 year, but the effect seems to persist even beyond infancy. Making the (reasonable) assumption that circumcision status is independent of age, circumcised males older than 1 year are at lowest risk.

Interestingly, circumcision could account for the gender differences in prevalence. If one assumes that febrile females and uncircumcised males have a UTI prevalence of 7%, that circumcised males have a prevalence of 0.2%, and that 70% of males are circumcised, then the prevalence of UTI among males would be $(0.3 \cdot 0.07) + (0.7 \cdot 0.002) = 0.022$ or 2%, a figure consistent with the data.

Tests for UTI

When an infant is considered to be at significant risk for UTI, the next step is to make the diagnosis. Choosing diagnostic criteria for UTI involves two competing considerations. A false-negative diagnosis will leave patients with UTI at risk for serious complications. A false-positive diagnosis may lead to unnecessary, invasive, and expensive testing. In evaluating alternative diagnostic tests for UTI, the Subcommittee defined as a "gold standard" any bacterial growth on a culture of urine obtained by suprapubic bladder aspiration (tap), ie, any bacterial growth on a culture of a urine specimen obtained by tap defines a UTI.

For the analysis, a culture of a urine specimen obtained by a tap was considered to have 100% sensitivity and specificity. However, this was not always used for comparisons in studies of other diagnostic strategies. Alternative diagnostic strategies fall into the three following areas: 1) urine analysis (UA) for immediate diagnostic information, 2) culture of a urine specimen obtained by urine bag or transurethral catheterization, and 3) culture of a urine specimen using the dipslide culture technique.

UA

The various components of the UA include the reagent slide tests, ie, LE, nitrite, blood, and protein, and microscopic examination for leukocytes or bacteria. The diagnostic characteristics of these tests have been evaluated individually and in combination. Tests can be combined serially, meaning all test results must be positive for the combination to be positive or, in parallel, meaning a positive result on any one of the tests defines a positive result for the combination. The serial strategy maximizes specificity at the expense of sensitivity, whereas parallel testing maximizes sensitivity at the expense of specificity.

Perhaps the most commonly used component of the UA used to evaluate a child who may have a UTI is the reagent strip (dipstick). Tests for UTI that are available on most reagent strips include the LE, nitrite, blood, and protein. The LE is the most sensitive single test. Its reported sensitivity ranges from 67% in a screening setting in which symptoms and, therefore, inflammation, would not be expected, to 94% in settings in which UTI is suspected. The specificity of LE generally is not as good. However, because the specificity describes the performance of the test on specimens from patients without a UTI, it is highly dependent on patient characteristics. The reported specificity varies from 63% to 92%.

The test for nitrite has a much higher specificity (90% to 100%) and lower sensitivity (16% to 82%). For this reason, nitrite may be useful for "ruling in" UTI when it is positive, but it has little value in ruling out UTI. Dipstick tests for blood and protein have poor sensitivity and specificity with respect to UTI. Therefore, the use of results for blood or protein from dipstick testing has a high likelihood of being misleading.

Carefully performed microscopic examination of the urine has high sensitivity and specificity in many studies. However, the wide range of reported test characteristics of microscopy for leukocytes or bacteria presumably reflects the difficulty of performing these tests well and the hazards of performing them poorly. In studies that have shown the best test characteristics, tests were performed by on-site laboratory technicians who often used counting chambers.

When examining the urine for bacteria, unstained and Gram-stained specimens seem to be effective. However, centrifugation of the specimen reduces the specificity of the test. The number of bacteria also is important. Using heavy bacterial counts as a diagnostic criterion results in low sensitivity and high specificity. The reverse applies when observation of any bacteria is considered a positive test.

Microscopy for leukocytes is variably sensitive (32% to 100%) and specific (45% to 97%). Studies with accurate results generally used mirrored counting chambers, on-site technicians, or both. Specimens also must be examined shortly after collection. A 3-hour delay results in a 35% drop in sensitivity. Finally, if the number of leukocytes considered abnormal is high, the test will be insensitive, if the number is low, it will be highly sensitive. The reverse is true for specificity.

A number of special tests have been evaluated for the diagnosis of UTI. The first is a modified nitrite test. This involves incubating a urine specimen for several hours with added nitrite before testing for nitrate. The reported sensitivity and specificity are 93% and 88%, respectively. However, comparable results have not been reported.

Immunochemical studies for early detection of bacterial growth have not had impressive results.

Obtaining a Urine Specimen

The Subcommittee defined the gold standard definition of a UTI to be growth on a culture of a urine specimen obtained by tap. Often, however, performance of a bladder tap is resisted because it is invasive. Moreover, bladder taps may not yield urine specimens. Success rates for obtaining urine specimens vary between 23% and 90%. Although 100% success has been achieved when using ultrasonographic guidance, practitioners often use transurethral catheterization or urine bags to obtain urine specimens for culture.

Cultures of urine specimens obtained by catheterization have a specificity of 83% to 89% compared with cultures of urine specimens obtained by tap. However, if only cultures yielding >1000 CFU/mL are considered positive, catheterization cultures have a 95% sensitivity with a specificity of 99%.

Cultures of bag urine specimens are 100% sensitive, but they have a specificity between 14% and 84%. Therefore, because UTI is present in a small minority (5%) of patients tested, use of culture results from urine specimens obtained from the bag to rule in UTI is likely to result in large numbers of false-positive results. Specifically, with a prevalence of 5% and specificity of 70%, the positive predictive value of a positive culture of bag urine specimens would be 15%. That is, 85% of positive cultures of urine specimens obtained from a bag would be false-positive results.

Culturing Techniques

The standard culturing technique involves streaking on blood agar and MacConkey media. More recently, dipslide methods have been developed. The few studies of dipslide cultures that were reviewed reported sensitivities between 87% and 100% and specificities between 92% and 98%.

Consequences of a Missed Diagnosis of UTI

If the diagnosis of UTI is not made because it was not suspected or a test of insufficient sensitivity was used, three consequences may result. The first (see "Prevalence of Urinary Tract Abnormalities") is the lost opportunity to find a urinary tract abnormality that could result in renal damage. The second is the formation of new renal scars. Although repeated UTI lead to scarring (see "Progressive Renal Damage") and progressive scarring is associated with hypertension and ESRD, the role of scarring from a single UTI in long-term clinical consequences is unknown. Nevertheless, timely treatment of febrile UTI in children appears to be important in preventing scars.

The third consequence of missing the diagnosis of UTI results from the urosepsis that occurs in a small proportion of febrile infants with UTI. Among patients with febrile UTI, in the age group to which this analysis applies, the risk of concurrent bacteremia is between 2.2% and 9%. The natural history of bacteremia in infants with febrile UTI is not described. Common pediatric experience is that septic shock and death are rarely seen in this situation, suggesting that spontaneous resolution of bacteremia occurs in this situation as it does in others. However, evidence exists that among infants with bacteremia attributable to *Escherichia coli* in the presence of a UTI, fatality rates may be as high as 10% to 12%.

Short-term Treatment of UTI

In studying the short-term treatment of UTI, the two following issues were addressed: 1) What do the data suggest about the duration of outpatient antibiotic therapy? and 2) What is the best choice for presumptive oral antibiotic therapy for the infant with suspected UTI before culture results are available? From the data presented subsequently in this report, it may be reasonable to conclude the following. 1) Single-dose to 3-day therapy is not as effective as therapy of 7 days or longer (perhaps because of more rapid metabolism of antimicrobials in children), but that the minimal acceptable duration of therapy has not been demonstrated. 2) Cotrimoxazole appears to be superior to amoxicillin for presumptive antibiotic therapy of UTI, but local antibiotic susceptibility patterns should ultimately dictate the antibiotic choice.

Duration of Therapy

Several studies have compared treatment of pediatric UTI with varying durations of therapy. The data have been analyzed in two ways. First, studies that directly compared different durations of therapy were examined. Then, data were pooled by antibiotic and duration of therapy, and the pooled values were compared.

None of the studies of duration of therapy compared 7 days with 10 days. In seven studies with 10 comparisons between long duration (7 to 10 days) and short duration (one dose to 3 days), 8 of 10 comparisons showed better results with an attributable improvement in outcome of 5% to 21%.

When the data were pooled by agent and duration, no discernible differences were found in initial cure or relapse among one-dose, 3-day, and 10-day courses of amoxicillin. However, single-dose cotrimoxazole was 10% less effective than 1-, 3-, 7-, or 10-day therapy. Differences among the latter regimens were not discernible.

Agent

The data pooled by agent and duration of therapy were used to compare amoxicillin and cotrimoxazole. For therapies of one dose, 3 to 4 days, or 10 days, cotrimoxazole consistently shows better cure rates (4% to 42%).

Data comparing parenteral and oral therapy were not found. However, intramuscular ceftriaxone (one dose) or gentamicin (10 days) was 100% effective in resolving UTI in children in whom oral therapy had failed. No data are available that clarify the role of oral vs parenteral therapy for bacteremia in association with UTI. Drawing on analyses of unsuspected bacteremia in children without UTI, parenteral antibiotic therapy is 95% effective in clearing bacteremia.

Prevalence of Urinary Tract Abnormalities

UTI in young children is a marker for abnormalities of the urinary tract. By far, the most common abnormality is VUR, which may be present with different degrees of severity that are graded I to V according to whether the reflux reaches the kidney and the degree of dilation of the collecting system. The grade of VUR is important because it determines the likelihood of detecting VUR on radiologic evaluation and the probability of renal damage, hypertension, or renal failure.

VUR

The Subcommittee identified 77 studies that reported the prevalence of VUR among children with UTI. The range of reported values is wide which may be primarily attributed to small sample size. As the sample size grows, the prevalence reported converges at 30% to 40%. The prevalence appears to decrease with age.

Specific studies of the relationship between age and prevalence of VUR show similar results. For example, one study reported a 68% prevalence among boys younger than 1 year and 25% among boys 1 to 3 years. Another study of boys found some type of abnormality in 76% of boys younger than 10 years (~54% of these were VUR) and 15% in boys older than 10 years. A population-based study showed a peak prevalence of VUR among girls 1 to 3 years of age and a rapid drop-off (perhaps by half) by age 5. A much smaller study found VUR in 100% of 9 boys younger than 1 year of age with a UTI and in 74% of 34 boys 1 to 5 years of age.

This relationship was fitted to a third-degree polynomial and a spline. Although the data are insufficient to define a particular functional relationship, they suggest a decline in the prevalence of VUR with age that seems to be most rapid during the first year of life. It levels off somewhat between 1 and 5 years of age, then drops off again after age 5. When studies of children younger than 3 years were pooled, the prevalence was 50%.

For this analysis, grades of VUR were grouped into low grade (grades I and II) and high grade (grades III to V). This grouping reduces the precision of the analysis slightly because higher grade reflux is easier to detect with ultrasonography and poses a greater risk of subsequent renal damage than do the lower grades. However, these effects were represented in this model, making this a more detailed analysis than has been reported previously. Some studies grouped patients in a similar manner, but grade III VUR was variably grouped as high grade or low grade. For classification of results, the classification used in the articles was (by necessity) used in this analysis. Pooling the data gives a 51.1% prevalence of low-grade (grades I to II) VUR among patients with VUR.

Tests for VUR

The Subcommittee identified the gold standard test for detecting VUR as the VCUG or RCG. These studies have, by definition, 100% sensitivity and specificity. The Subcommittee also believed that renal ultrasonography or intravenous pyelography should be performed to identify obstructions or other structural renal abnormalities.

VCUG and RCG are expensive and invasive. Data were collected on the sensitivity and specificity of renal ultrasonography alone in the detection of VUR. Overall, renal ultrasonography has poor sensitivity (30% to 62%) and good specificity (85% to 100%) for VUR. The sensitivity is better, however, for high-grade VUR than for low-grade VUR (82% to 100% vs 14% to 30%). The Subcommittee members believed that renal ultrasonography in young infants was less reliable than this. However, data supporting this point were not found.

Progressive Renal Damage

The evidence that links the presence of VUR to important clinical outcomes can only be assembled in a piecemeal way. The data link VUR to renal scarring in the presence of recurrent infection, and renal scarring is associated with subsequent hypertension and ESRD. The data support this model indirectly. However, there are no longitudinal data that link directly the presence of VUR in infants with febrile UTI and normal kidneys to the subsequent development of hypertension or ESRD. Therefore, it is difficult to quantify the strength of the relationship or the risk to such patients. The following discussion reviews evidence supporting each step in the hypothesized progression to renal damage.

Reflux and Scarring

The data demonstrate an association between VUR and subsequent renal scarring. More than 48 references reviewed reported renal scarring at rates between 1% and 40% in association with febrile UTI and VUR. Higher grades of VUR are associated with higher risk of scar progression. Patients with high-grade VUR are four to six times more likely to have scarring than those with low-grade VUR and eight to 10 times as likely as those without VUR. In one study of 84 consecutive children 2 to 70 months of age with their first recognized febrile UTI, the presence of VUR was 80% sensitive and 74% specific in predicting subsequent scarring in a follow-up period of 2 years or more. Of those with VUR, 30% had progressive renal scarring. Of those without VUR, only 4% did.

Recurrent Infections and Scarring

The association of VUR with renal scarring seems to be mediated through recurrent symptomatic infections. The association between recurrent bouts of febrile UTI and the risk of renal scarring in one study followed an exponential curve. Patients with no VUR or low-grade VUR and patients with no recurrences of UTI are at low risk for renal scarring. Thus, prophylactic antibiotic treatment of patients with VUR to prevent recurrences or surgical treatment to prevent VUR would be expected to prevent renal scarring.

ESRD and Hypertension

Retrospective examination of the causes of ESRD in registries of patients with renal failure shows that in 36% (of 9250 patients), the cause of ESRD is obstructive uropathy, renal hypoplasia or dysplasia, pyelonephritis, or a combination of these. Unfortunately, it is not possible to determine which patients originally had normal kidneys in whom disease progressed to ESRD because of VUR and recurrent infection. In the North American Renal Transplant Cooperative Study, the fraction of transplant recipients with reflux nephropathy is 102/2033, or 5%. Patients with pyelonephritis or interstitial nephritis make up another 2% of transplant recipients.

Most cohort studies to quantify the risk of ESRD and hypertension among patients with renal scarring and VUR are based on highly selected patients in whom extensive scarring already has occurred. Long-term studies show that

ESRD develops in 3% to 10% of these patients. In addition, 10% may require nephrectomy, and 0.4% renal transplantation. One study followed women from their first UTI in childhood and found that abnormal renal function could be documented in 21% of those with severe scarring. However, this study also had a selected population and did not provide data on VUR.

The rate of hypertension in these and similar studies varies between 0% and 50%. It is apparently lowest in those with low-grade VUR and those with the least scarring. However, the quality of the studies relating VUR nephropathy with ESRD and hypertension was rated poor, and quantification of the relationship is weak. One study identified retrospectively a cohort of children 1 month to 16 years of age with VUR and measured blood pressure levels 5 months to 21 years (average, 9.6 years) after VUR was identified. There was an increase in the blood pressure level associated with increasing grades of VUR. However, none of the patients had hypertension.

Effectiveness of Prophylactic Antimicrobials and Surgical Correction

Ultimately the value of identifying VUR depends on the potential to prevent its long-term consequences. This depends on reducing recurrent infections with antibiotic prophylaxis or eliminating VUR surgically. The efficacy of these procedures is not well documented because controlled studies have not been performed. Studies in which patients receiving antibiotic prophylaxis are compared with those not taking antimicrobials suggest a 50% effectiveness whether comparing rates of reinfection or progression of scarring.

Cost Data

Cost data were derived from literature where available, the accounting department of the University of North Carolina (UNC) Hospital, and the physicians' fee schedule from the UNC Physicians and Associates. Estimates used in the decision model are given below.

UA and Culture

Based on the cost data from the UNC Hospital, the cost of a urine culture is $21.53 (charge, $26.00). The cost of a UA is $6.77 (charge, $15.00).

Treatment

The cost of short-term treatment of UTI varies substantially depending on the treatment chosen. Standard oral therapy, such as amoxicillin or trimethoprim-sulfamethoxazole, costs about $10 for a course. Newer, broad-spectrum oral therapy costs about $40 for a 10-day course. If parenteral therapy, such as intramuscular ceftriaxone, is given, the cost of the drug and the injection may be $125.

Complications of Therapy

For the analysis, only complications requiring a return visit to the physician were considered. This visit would cost a $50 clinic fee, plus a $50 professional fee, for a total of $100. Death attributable to anaphylaxis is rare. The additional cost of this complication was not added.

Cost of Urosepsis

It is assumed that sepsis that does not clear spontaneously or with antibiotic therapy will require hospital admission for intravenous antibiotic therapy at a cost of $10 000.

Imaging Evaluation

The two following imaging strategies were considered: 1) a full work-up, including renal ultrasonography and VCUG, and 2) renal ultrasonography alone. The cost of renal ultrasonography includes the hospital cost of $104 and the physician fee of $200, for a total of $304. The cost of the VCUG is the hospital cost of $123 plus the physician fee of $200, totaling $323. Thus, the full work-up costs $627.

Cost of Treatment of VUR

The estimated cost of antibiotic prophylaxis was based on low-dose nitrofurantoin. The weekly cost was $6 for an average of 3 years. The total is $1040. It was assumed that the cost of ureteral reimplantation surgery was similar.

Complications of VUR

Patients with VUR are at increased risk for recurrent UTI, at least until the VUR resolves. The period the child is at risk was assumed to be 3 years. The cost of these recurrences was based on the average cost of a clinic visit related to a diagnosis of UTI or pyelonephritis in infants at UNC, $134, plus the physician fee of $70. This was multiplied by three, the average number of infections expected over 3 years, for a total of $612.

The cost of ESRD was derived from data in previous analyses. Based on a 10-year period, including 10 years of dialysis or a year in which transplantation occurs followed by 8 years with a functioning graft, followed by 1 year of a failed graft, the cost of ESRD is ~$300 000. The cost of managing severe hypertension and its complications was estimated at $100 000 based on $2000 per year for 50 years.

Analysis of the Decision Model

Using data extracted from the literature as described in "Evidence Tables," probabilities and costs were inserted into the decision tree. Using baseline estimates, three types of analysis were conducted. First, a risk analysis was performed to determine the average cost and frequency of outcomes expected with each of four strategies. Next, a cost-effectiveness analysis was used to determine the incremental cost per major clinical outcome averted by the strategies. Finally, sensitivity and threshold analyses were performed to examine alternative strategies for evaluation and management of UTI.

Risk Analysis

Two risk analyses were performed. The first examined the costs and clinical outcomes expected with different strategies for making the diagnosis of UTI. The second compared alternative strategies for imaging the urinary tract of patients with UTI.

Diagnosis of UTI

The risk analysis of diagnostic strategies examines two anchor states. The first, "treat all," is presumptive antibiotic therapy for occult infection without testing. The second,

"observe," is clinical observation without testing or treatment. Neither of these anchor strategies involves subsequent imaging of the urinary tract. Three testing strategies are evaluated. The first is the gold standard, culture of urine specimens obtained by suprapubic tap or transurethral catheter. The second is using a culture of the urine specimen obtained from the urine bag. Culture of bag urine specimens has 100% sensitivity and 70% specificity in the baseline analysis. The third strategy uses the cheaper but less reliable reagent strip as a test for UTI. A positive LE test result, a positive nitrite test result, or both, is considered a positive test result. The sensitivity and specificity of this strategy are 92% and 70%, respectively, based on median values. All three testing strategies include antibiotic therapy and imaging of the urinary tract of patients with positive test results.

The results of the risk analysis are presented as the number of outcomes expected per 100 000 infants treated by using each strategy. To observe patients without testing or treatment is the least expensive strategy. However, it results in inferior clinical outcomes, including death and hospitalization from urosepsis, hypertension, and ESRD. Presumptive treatment of all infants without testing costs slightly more than observing, but prevents hospitalization and death from urosepsis. Under the treat all strategy, it is impossible to select patients for imaging, and it is unreasonably expensive to image the urinary tracts of all patients (see "Cost-effectiveness Analysis"). Therefore, no patient in the treat all strategy undergoes imaging evaluation. As a result, there is no improvement in the rates of hypertension or ESRD.

Using culture of urine specimens obtained by catheterization or tap offers the lowest risk of death, because all children at risk for urosepsis are identified and there are no unnecessary treatments or treatment-related deaths. Moreover, because all children with UTI are identified for imaging evaluation, this strategy minimizes the risk of hypertension and ESRD.

Using a culture of bag urine specimens as a criterion for the diagnosis of UTI also identifies correctly all children with UTI. However, its poor specificity also results in many false-positive results. As a consequence, there are slightly more deaths (3 per million) attributable to unnecessary antibiotic treatment and many more imaging work-ups. This means an additional $47.2 million per 100 000 febrile infants with no improvement in clinical outcomes.

Using LE and nitrite as diagnostic criteria for UTI leaves a small number of UTIs undiagnosed and results in 2½ times as many imaging work-ups compared with a culture of urine specimens obtained by catheterization or tap. The result is poorer clinical outcomes at greater expense despite the lower cost of UA.

A fourth diagnostic strategy also was evaluated that used a full UA (reagent strip and microscopy) as an initial diagnostic test and treated any positive UA component as a positive result. A positive result would lead to presumptive treatment. However, positive results would be confirmed by a culture of urine specimens obtained by tap or catheterization before imaging was performed. This strategy has a sensitivity of virtually 100% and a specificity of 60% for making a treatment decision. Because positive results are confirmed with a culture of urine specimens obtained by catheterization or tap, the specificity is 100% for imaging. The cost of testing is higher for positive results because UA and culture are performed. Also, the false-positive results lead to more unnecessary treatment and the resulting costs and complications. However, there is a cost saving for patients with negative results of the UA because the UA costs less than the culture. Compared with a culture of specimens from all patients, there is a small net decrease in cost using UA followed by a culture of positive results. Moreover, this strategy has the advantage of allowing immediate treatment of patients at risk of UTI. The benefit of early treatment is difficult to quantify, but evidence suggests it reduces the risk of renal scarring. Although this strategy appears to be nearly as effective as (or perhaps more than) the culture of urine specimens obtained by catheterization or tap, its effectiveness depends on the accuracy of the urine microscopy. As noted above, the accuracy of urine microscopy is highly variable and apparently depends on the presence of an on-site technician. In many settings, this may be impossible or so expensive as to offset the benefits.

Imaging Strategies

Three imaging alternatives were evaluated by risk analysis. The first strategy was renal ultrasonography and VCUG. The second was renal ultrasonography alone, and the third was no imaging evaluation at all. The total cost associated with each strategy includes the cost of the imaging studies, the cost of treating abnormalities identified, and the cost of any complications incurred. Together, renal ultrasonography and VCUG will identify all cases of renal abnormalities. Renal ultrasonography alone detects ~42% of all abnormalities. However, most abnormalities (87%) missed by renal ultrasonography alone are low-grade VUR, which carries a lower risk of renal scarring. As a result, the differences in clinical outcomes (cases of hypertension and ESRD) are smaller between renal ultrasonography alone and the full evaluation.

Cost-effectiveness Analysis

Cost-effectiveness analysis was used to quantify the trade-offs between cost and clinical effect when moving from one clinical strategy to another. When one strategy offers a better clinical effect at a lower cost, it is said to be a dominant strategy. However, in most cases, the strategy with better clinical effect also has a higher cost. Cost-effectiveness analysis depicts the additional cost per unit of improvement in clinical effect. For this analysis, the units of effect were defined as cases of death, ESRD, or hypertension prevented.

Strategies were compared using the incremental (or marginal) cost-effectiveness ratio, ie, the difference in cost among strategies divided by the difference in effect. The mathematical term is as follows:

$$\frac{Cost_b - Cost_a}{Effect_b - Effect_a}.$$

Diagnosis of UTI

The least expensive strategy for the diagnosis of UTI is to do nothing. This also is the least effective strategy. By com-

parison, treating all febrile 2-month to 2-year-olds for UTI without diagnostic testing or urinary tract imaging improves clinical effect at a cost of $61 000 per death prevented. However, it does not prevent ESRD or hypertension.

As an alternative, one could obtain a dipstick UA on all patients, culturing specimens from those for whom the results of UA were positive. Because UA costs less than culture, this strategy has the potential to save money. However, because UA does not have perfect sensitivity, a few cases will be missed. In addition, patients for whom the results of UA are positive will incur the costs of UA and culture. To evaluate this strategy, a new branch was added to the decision tree. The new branch is a dipstick UA. If results are positive, it is linked to the "test" branch; if results are negative, it is linked to the "observe" branch. Positive results involve the cost of the UA plus culture; negative results, only the cost of the UA. This strategy prevents an additional two cases of death or serious complication per 10 000 at a cost of $261 000 per case.

Culturing catheterization or tap urine specimens on all patients and then treating and imaging the urinary tracts of all patients with positive results is the most effective and most expensive strategy. It prevents an additional 2.5 cases of death or serious complication per 100 000 over culture-confirmed positive dipstick results at an additional cost of $434 000 per case prevented. Compared with the no testing strategy, culturing specimens from all patients prevents three cases of death or serious complication per 10 000 at a cost of $200 000 per case prevented.

The optimal strategy depends on the decision-maker's willingness to pay for each additional case prevented. For example, if that willingness to pay is between $261 000 and $434 000, then the positive results of the dipstick confirmed by culture is the best strategy. Culturing specimens from all patients will prevent a few additional cases, but the cost to prevent each of these additional cases exceeds the decision-maker's willingness to pay. If the decision-maker is willing to pay >$434 000 to prevent a case of death or serious complication, then culturing specimens from all patients is the right strategy.

Imaging Strategies

The cost-effectiveness of the alternative imaging strategies also was calculated. The least expensive alternative is to perform no evaluation. Renal ultrasonography alone will prevent almost three cases of ESRD or hypertension per 1000 studies done at a cost of $260 000 per case prevented. A VCUG prevents an additional one case of ESRD or hypertension per 1000 studies over renal ultrasonography at a cost of $353 000 per case.

Again, the optimal strategy depends on the decision-maker's willingness to pay for each additional case prevented. For example, if that willingness to pay is between $260 000 and $353 000, then renal ultrasonography alone is the best strategy. A VCUG will prevent a few additional cases, but the cost to prevent each of these additional cases exceeds the decision-maker's willingness to pay. If the decision maker is willing to pay >$353 000 to prevent a case, then renal ultrasonography and VCUG is the right strategy.

Sensitivity and Threshold Analysis

Choosing one alternative over another from the risk analyses involves striking a balance between the cost of an intervention and the improvement in clinical outcomes. When comparing alternatives, if one alternative provides better clinical outcomes at lower costs, it is the dominant alternative and is the obvious choice. However, in most circumstances, choosing an alternative requires a trade-off between costs and clinical benefit. For example, obtaining a urine specimen for culture by catheterization or tap on all febrile infants, treating those with positive cultures, and imaging their urinary tracts with VCUG and renal ultrasonography improve clinical outcome but at a substantially higher cost than doing none of these evaluations.

To select the optimal alternative and, moreover, to identify different clinical circumstances in which different alternatives may be better, it is first necessary to make explicit the trade-off between costs and clinical outcomes. This means identifying a "willingness to pay" for each untoward clinical outcome avoided. For the following analyses, a value of $700 000 was placed on each case of ESRD or hypertension prevented. This figure is based loosely on the life-time productivity of a healthy, young adult. Once this cost is assigned to each untoward clinical outcome, it is possible to use the threshold method of decision-making.

The threshold approach to decision-making involves changing the value of a variable in the decision analysis to determine the value at which one alternative becomes too expensive and another would be preferred. In the case of UTI, if the prior probability of UTI is sufficiently high, it costs <$700 000 to prevent a case of ESRD or hypertension by screening all febrile children. However, if the probability that a particular patient has a UTI is sufficiently low, the yield of a urine culture will be extremely low and a positive result of a UA will almost certainly be a false-positive. Under these circumstances, a strategy involving the evaluation of this child's urinary tract would cost >$700 000 per case of ESRD or hypertension prevented. Threshold analysis identifies the threshold probability of UTI above which evaluation would be cost-effective and below which it would not. A number of threshold analyses follow.

Prevalence of UTI and Prevalence of VUR

Because fever without an obvious cause is common in pediatric practice, culturing the urine of all febrile 2-month to 2-year-old children represents a substantial investment. The Subcommittee was interested in determining whether there were some clinical subpopulations in which the prevalence of UTI was low enough that culture was unnecessary. A threshold analysis was used to examine this question.

Cost of Culturing Urine Obtained by Urine Bag

Many practitioners prefer to culture urine specimens obtained by urine bag rather than by transurethral catheter or suprapubic tap because the urine bag is less invasive. However, culture of a urine specimen obtained by bag has low specificity. When the prevalence of UTI is low, as it is in febrile infants, the result is a large number of false-positive urine cultures. False-positive cultures lead to unnecessary antibiotic treatment and urinary tract evaluation. The result

is additional costs with no clinical benefit. To examine these additional costs, the difference in costs between a strategy involving urine specimens obtained by catheterization or tap and a strategy involving specimens from bag urine was calculated at different levels of specificity for the urine bag. Results of the analysis imply that culturing urine specimens from bag urine in this setting can only be justified if one is willing to pay between $293 and $1340 per patient to use a urine bag rather than to obtain urine specimens by catheterization or tap.

Sensitivity and Specificity for UA

As an alternative to obtaining urine specimens for culture from all febrile children between 2 months and 2 years of age, one could use a UA to make the diagnosis of UTI. As noted previously, a carefully performed UA has high sensitivity and specificity. Two-way sensitivity analysis was used to determine the minimal sensitivity and specificity that would be necessary to justify the use of UA rather than culture. The results imply that a test must have a sensitivity >92% and a specificity >99% to be preferred over urine culture. This level of sensitivity and specificity is unlikely to be obtained in most clinical settings. Alternatively, several studies demonstrated that combinations of LE, nitrite, microscopy of fresh urine, in which any abnormality constituted a positive test result, yielded a sensitivity of >92%. If one of these tests were used to rule out UTI, and culture of urine specimens obtained by catheterization or tap were used to confirm UTI in positive results, the requisite sensitivity and specificity would be obtained.

Probability of UTI and Urinary Tract Imaging

The decision to image the urinary tracts of infants with documented UTI presumes that the diagnosis of UTI is certain. If an imperfect test (eg, using a bag urine specimen) is used to make the diagnosis of UTI, a substantial number of these patients in fact may not have had a UTI and, therefore, the yield of the imaging will be lower. Threshold analysis was used to determine the minimal probability of UTI that justified a full imaging evaluation. The analysis indicates that if the probability of UTI is <49%, imaging becomes too expensive. Bayes's theorem shows that among patients with a prevalence of UTI that is 5%, those who have a positive urine culture obtained by bag have a probability (positive predictive value) of UTI that is 15%, well below 49%. This implies that if the best evidence of the UTI available in a given patient is a positive culture of urine obtained by bag, additional imaging of the urinary tract is not justified.

Sensitivity of Renal Ultrasonography for VUR

Because VCUG is invasive and expensive, a threshold analysis was used to explore the possible use of renal ultrasonography alone in evaluating the urinary tracts of children with UTI. Renal ultrasonography has low sensitivity for low-grade VUR, but relatively higher sensitivity for high-grade VUR. Based on the professional opinion of the UTI Subcommittee, a sensitivity of 14% for low-grade VUR and 82% for high-grade VUR is a better reflection of the situation in children 2 months to 2 years of age. This implies that renal ultrasonography alone is an inadequate imaging evaluation for infants with UTI.

Risk of Renal Scarring With UTI

One area of relative uncertainty, in which quality data are lacking, is the risk of scarring in undetected or untreated VUR. This risk is higher for children with high-grade VUR than for those with low-grade VUR. Threshold analysis was used to explore how this risk of scarring affects the decision to culture urine specimens from all children 2 months to 2 years of age with fever and no obvious cause for the fever. Figure 14 plots the risk of scar progression given low-grade VUR on the x-axis and the risk of scar progression given high-grade VUR on the y-axis. For values that plot above and to the right of the threshold line, culture of urine specimens from all febrile infants is the preferred strategy. For values that plot below and to the left of the threshold line, no urine culture is the preferred strategy. The baseline estimates used in the analysis, 14% for low-grade VUR and 53% for high-grade VUR, are plotted on the graph. The risk of scarring because of untreated VUR seems to be high enough to justify culturing specimens from all febrile infants.

Risk of Hypertension and ESRD

The weakest probability estimates in the present analysis relate to the risk of ESRD and hypertension among patients who have progressive renal scarring attributable to VUR. Two-way sensitivity analysis was used to determine the effect of varying these estimates on the results of the analysis. Our best estimate of the risk of hypertension and ESRD justifies culturing urine specimens from febrile infants as a strategy to prevent these complications. However, the quality of evidence about the future risks of ESRD and hypertension among infants with UTI later found to have VUR is tenuous at best. This is an area that needs additional investigation.

RECOMMENDATIONS

Who Should Be Evaluated for UTI?

Under the assumptions of the analysis, all febrile children between the ages of 2 months and 24 months with no obvious cause of infection should be evaluated for UTI, with the exception of circumcised males older than 12 months.

Minimal Test Characteristics of Diagnosis of UTI

To be as cost-effective as a culture of a urine specimen obtained by transurethral catheter or suprapubic tap, a test must have a sensitivity of at least 92% and a specificity of at least 99%. With the possible exception of a complete UA performed within 1 hour of urine collection by an on-site laboratory technician, no other test meets these criteria.

Performing a dipstick UA and obtaining a urine specimen by catheterization or tap for culture from patients with a positive LE or nitrite test result is nearly as effective and slightly less costly than culturing specimens from all febrile children.

Treatment of UTI

The data suggest that short-term treatment of UTI should not be for <7 days. The data do not support treatment for >14 days if an appropriate clinical response is observed. There are no data comparing intravenous with oral administration of medications.

Evaluation of the Urinary Tract

Available data support the imaging evaluation of the urinary tracts of all 2- to 24-month-olds with their first documented UTI. Imaging should include VCUG and renal ultrasonography. The method for documenting the UTI must yield a positive predictive value of at least 49% to justify the evaluation. Culture of a urine specimen obtained by bag does not meet this criterion unless the previous probability of a UTI is >22%.

The Management of Primary Vesicoureteral Reflux in Children

The following guideline for management of primary vesicoureteral reflux in children, developed by the American Urological Association Pediatric Vesicoureteral Reflux Clinical Guidelines Panel, has been endorsed by the American Academy of Pediatrics.

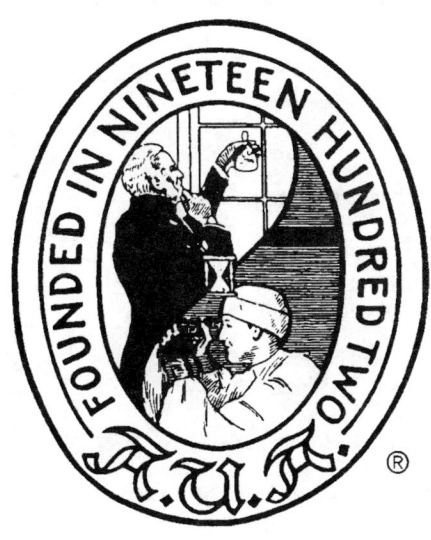

The American Urological Association
Pediatric Vesicoureteral Reflux
Clinical Guidelines Panel

Report on

The Management of Primary Vesicoureteral Reflux in Children

Clinical Practice Guidelines

Pediatric Vesicoureteral Reflux Clinical Guidelines Panel Members and Consultants

Members

Jack S. Elder, MD
(Panel Chairman)
Director of Pediatric Urology
Rainbow Babies/University Hospital
Professor of Urology and Pediatrics
Case Western Reserve University
    School of Medicine
Cleveland, Ohio

Craig Andrew Peters, MD
(Panel Facilitator)
Assistant Professor of Surgery
    (Urology)
Harvard University Medical School
Assistant in Surgery (Urology)
Children's Hospital
Boston, Massachusetts

Billy S. Arant, Jr., MD
Professor and Chairman
Department of Pediatrics
University of Tennessee College of
    Medicine—Chattanooga Unit
Medical Director
T.C. Thompson Children's Hospital
Chattanooga, Tennessee

David H. Ewalt, MD
Clinical Assistant Professor
Department of Urology
Children's Medical Center of Dallas
Dallas, Texas

Charles E. Hawtrey, MD
Professor of Pediatric Urology
Vice Chair, Department of Urology
University of Iowa
Iowa City, Iowa

Richard S. Hurwitz, MD
Head, Pediatric Urology
Kaiser Permanente Medical Center
Los Angeles, California

Thomas S. Parrott, MD
Clinical Associate Professor of
    Surgery (Urology)
Emory University School of
    Medicine
Atlanta, Georgia

Howard M. Snyder, III, MD
Associate Director
Division of Urology
Children's Hospital
Professor of Urology
University of Pennsylvania
    School of Medicine
Philadelphia, Pennsylvania

Robert A. Weiss, MD
Associate Professor, Pediatrics
Director, Pediatric Nephrology
New York Medical College
Valhalla, New York

Consultants

Steven H. Woolf, MD, MPH
Methodologist
Fairfax, Virginia

Vic Hasselblad, PhD
Statistician
Duke University
Durham, North Carolina

Gail J. Herzenberg, MPA
Project Director
Technical Resources International, Inc.
Rockville, Maryland

Michael D. Wong, MS
Information Systems Director
Technical Resources International, Inc.
Rockville, Maryland

Joan A. Saunders
Writer/Editor
Technical Resources International, Inc.
Rockville, Maryland

The Pediatric Vesicoureteral Reflux Clinical Guidelines Panel consists of board-certified urologists and nephrologists who are experts in vesicoureteral reflux in children. This *Report on the Management of Primary Vesicoureteral Reflux in Children* was extensively reviewed by over 50 urologists throughout the country in the summer of 1996. The Panel finalized its recommendations for the American Urological Association (AUA) Practice Parameters, Guidelines and Standards Committee, chaired by Joseph W. Segura, MD, in November 1996. The AUA Board of Directors approved these practice guidelines in November 1996.

The Summary Report also underwent independent scrutiny by the Editorial Board of the *Journal of Urology*, was accepted for publication in November 1996, and appeared in its May 1997 issue. *A Guide for Parents* and *Evidence Working Papers* have also been developed; both are available from the AUA.

The AUA expresses its gratitude for the dedication and leadership demonstrated by the members of the Pediatric Vesicoureteral Reflux Clinical Guidelines Panel and by the consultants affiliated with Technical Resources International, Inc., in producing this guideline.

ISBN 0-9649702-2-8

Introduction

Vesicoureteral reflux refers to the retrograde flow of urine from the bladder into the ureter and, usually, into the collecting system of the kidney. In most individuals, reflux results from a congenital anomaly of the ureterovesical junction, whereas in others it results from high-pressure voiding secondary to posterior urethral valves, neuropathic bladder or voiding dysfunction. Between 3–5 percent of girls and 1–2 percent of boys experience a urinary tract infection before puberty (Jodal and Winberg, 1987). Approximately 40 percent of children with a urinary tract infection have reflux (Bourchier, Abbott and Maling, 1984; Drachman, Valevici and Vardy, 1984). Urinary tract infection is the most common bacterial disease during the first 3 months of life (Krober, Bass, Powell, et al., 1985) and accounts for approximately 6 percent of febrile illnesses in infants (Hoberman, Chao, Keller, et al., 1993). Reflux is a predisposing factor for pyelonephritis, which can result in renal injury or scarring, also termed reflux nephropathy. The most serious late consequence of reflux nephropathy is renal insufficiency or end-stage renal disease. Between 3.1–25 percent of children and 10–15 percent of adults with end-stage renal disease have reflux nephropathy (Arant, 1991; Avner, Chavers, Sullivan, et al., 1995; Bailey, Maling and Swainson, 1993). In addition, reflux nephropathy may result in renin-mediated hypertension and cause morbidity in pregnancy (Martinell, Jodal and Lidin-Jason, 1990).

The primary goals in the management of vesicoureteral reflux in children are to prevent pyelonephritis, renal injury and other complications of reflux. Children with reflux may be managed either medically or surgically. The rationale for medical management is prevention of urinary tract infection with daily antimicrobial prophylaxis, regular timed voiding and, in some cases, anticholinergic medication. These children also undergo periodic screening of the urine for infection and radiologic reassessment of the urinary tract for reflux and renal injury. Many children show spontaneous reflux resolution while receiving medical management. Surgical management of reflux consists of repair of the ureterovesical junction abnormality.

Although vesicoureteral reflux is common, there is disagreement regarding the optimal management, even among specialists caring for these children (Elder, Snyder, Peters, et al., 1992; International Reflux Study Committee, 1981). Because of the lack of consensus regarding management of this common condition, the American Urological Association (AUA) convened a panel of experts to develop treatment guidelines for children with vesicoureteral reflux. The panel was charged with the task of producing practice recommendations based primarily on outcomes evidence from the scientific literature. This *Report on the Management of Primary Vesicoureteral Reflux in Children* is the result of the panel's efforts. The panel members represent various geographic areas, ages, professional activities (academic medical centers, private practice, health maintenance organizations) and expertise (pediatric urology, pediatric nephrology), allowing a broad perspective on the management of reflux.

The recommendations in this report are to assist physicians specifically in the treatment of vesicoureteral reflux in children diagnosed following a urinary tract infection. The recommendations apply to children aged 10 years and younger with unilateral or bilateral reflux with or without scarring. The report therefore deals only peripherally with the diagnostic methods of identifying vesicoureteral reflux, renal scarring and management of children with reflux identified incidentally or by screening of asymptomatic siblings. In addition, the report does not pertain to reflux associated with neuropathic bladder, posterior urethral valves, bladder exstrophy or fixed anatomic abnormalities, such as ectopic ureterocele and ectopic ureter.

Because treatment recommendations are made jointly with the parents of the child, *A Guide for Parents,* based on this report, is available to assist the physician in discussing treatment options with the parents. A summary of this report has been published in the *Journal of Urology*, May 1997.

Production and layout by

Joanna Taylor   Suzanne Boland Pope
Huey Chang   Lisa Emmons
Carlos Gonzalez   Tracy Kiely
Technical Resources International, Inc.   Betty Wagner
Rockville, Maryland   American Urological Association, Inc.
                                      Baltimore, Maryland

Copyright © 1997
American Urological Association, Inc.

Executive Summary:
Management of primary vesicoureteral reflux in children

Methodology

In developing recommendations for the management of primary vesicoureteral reflux in children, the AUA Pediatric Vesicoureteral Reflux Guidelines Panel extensively reviewed the available literature on the treatment of pediatric reflux from January 1965 through December 1994 and extracted all relevant data to estimate as accurately as possible desirable and undesirable outcomes of the alternative treatment modalities. The panel followed an explicit approach to the development of practice policies, supplemented by expert opinion. The panel synthesized the evidence using techniques described by Eddy, Hasselblad and Schachter (1992) and Cooper and Hedges (1994). The methodology for these analyses was described by Hasselblad (in press). For a full description of the methodology, see Chapter 2.

Background

Vesicoureteral reflux refers to the retrograde flow of urine from the bladder into the upper urinary tract. Reflux is a birth defect but also may be acquired. Vesicoureteral reflux predisposes an individual to renal infection (pyelonephritis) by facilitating the transport of bacteria from the bladder to the upper urinary tract. The immunologic and inflammatory reaction caused by a pyelonephritic infection may result in renal injury or scarring. Extensive renal scarring causes reduced renal function and may result in renal insufficiency, end-stage renal disease, renin-mediated hypertension, reduced somatic growth and morbidity during pregnancy.

The primary goals of treatment in children with reflux are to prevent renal injury and symptomatic pyelonephritis. Medical therapy is based on the principle that reflux often resolves with time. The basis for surgical therapy is that, in select situations, ongoing vesicoureteral reflux has caused or has a significant potential for causing renal injury

or other reflux-related complications and that elimination of the reflux condition will minimize their likelihood. Chapter 1 documents the various methods of diagnosis, treatment and surveillance and follow-up for children with primary vesicoureteral reflux.

Grading of reflux severity is important because more severe reflux is associated with higher rates of renal injury, and treatment success varies with reflux grade. The International Study Classification is the most common and is the grading system used in this report (International Reflux Study Committee, 1981).

Treatment alternatives and outcomes analysis

The panel considered 7 modalities as treatment alternatives, including:

- No treatment (intermittent antibiotic therapy for UTI);
- Bladder training (including timed voiding and other behavioral techniques);
- Antibiotic prophylaxis (continuous);
- Antibiotic prophylaxis and bladder training;
- Antibiotic prophylaxis, anticholinergics (for bladder instability), and bladder training;
- Open surgical repair; and
- Endoscopic repair.

Outcomes were identified as criteria by which effectiveness of treatment would be analyzed (see evidence matrix on page 21, Chapter 3), and the review of evidence was organized around this framework. The outcomes included intermediate outcomes (those not directly perceived by the patient or family but that are associated with or precede health outcomes), health outcomes (effects directly perceived in some way by patient or family), and harms of various forms of management. The following represents a brief summary of the statistical analysis that was conducted and that formed the basis of the treatment recommendations.

Intermediate outcomes

Reflux resolution—medical therapy (continuous antibiotic prophylaxis)

The database included 26 reports with data pertaining to reflux resolution after medical therapy, comprising 1,987 patients (1,410 girls and 304 boys—273 were not identified) and 2,902 ureters. The individual databases of Skoog, Belman and Majd (1987) and Arant (1992) and the data reported from the International Reflux Study, European Branch (Tamminen-Mobius, Brunier, Ebel, et al., 1992) were used to estimate the probability of reflux resolution with continuous antibiotic prophylaxis (see Figure 3 on page 24, Chapter 3). In general, a lower reflux grade correlated with a better chance of spontaneous resolution. Data for Grades I and II reflux showed no differences in regard to age at presentation or laterality (unilateral vs. bilateral). For Grade III, age and laterality were important prognostic factors, with increasing age at presentation and bilateral reflux decreasing the probability of resolution. Bilateral Grade IV reflux had a particularly low chance of spontaneous resolution. All of these estimates are subject to 2 restrictions: (1) estimates are only valid for up to 5 years after diagnosis; and (2) for Grade IV disease, estimates only apply to the time of diagnosis and are not age specific. No data were available for reflux resolution with intermittent antibiotic therapy.

In children with reflux and voiding dysfunction (frequency, urgency, urge incontinence, incomplete bladder emptying), available results from the series with control groups suggested that the reflux resolution rate increased with anticholinergic therapy and bladder training.

Reflux resolution—surgical therapy

In the articles reviewed by the panel, overall surgical success was reported in 959 of 1,008 patients (95.1 percent) and 7,731 of 8,061 ureters (95.9 percent). Surgical success was achieved in 108 of 109 ureters (99 percent) for Grade I, 874 of 882 (99.1 percent) for Grade II, 993 of 1,010 (98.3 percent) for Grade III, 386 of 392 (98.5 percent) for Grade IV and 155 of 192 (80.7 percent) for Grade V reflux.

For endoscopic therapy, most reports in the literature describe results of the use of polytetrafluoro-ethylene (Teflon™). Overall reflux was corrected in 77.1 percent of ureters after a single injection. Reflux was resolved after initial treatment in only 6 of 19 ureters (31.6 percent) with Grade V disease. Currently, no injectable substance has been approved for endoscopic antireflux surgery by the U.S. Food and Drug Administration.

Renal scarring

The panel felt that relevant data pertaining to renal scarring should be analyzed primarily from studies with a minimum of 5 years of follow-up. Four prospective trials comparing the outcomes of medical and surgical management included analysis of new renal scarring (Birmingham Reflux Study Group, 1987; Elo et al., 1983; Olbing et al., 1992; Weis et al., 1992). None of these trials showed a statistically significant difference in the rate of new renal scarring. In the European arm of the International Reflux Study, the rate of scarring was similar in patients receiving continuous antibiotic prophylaxis and those treated surgically (Olbing, Claesson, Ebel, et al., 1992). However, 80 percent of the new renal scars in the surgical group appeared by 10 months after randomization, whereas new renal scars appeared throughout the 5 years in the group managed medically (Tamminin-Mobius, Brunier, Ebel, et al., 1992). The Birmingham Reflux Study (1987) identified new scars after 5 years in only 6 percent and 5.2 percent of those treated medically and surgically, respectively, with no additional scars detected after 2 years of follow-up. In the prospective study by the Southwest Pediatric Nephrology Study Group of children younger than 5 years of age with Grades I, II or III reflux, normal kidneys at entry and with continuous antibiotic prophylaxis, 16 percent developed new scars (Arant, 1992). On the other hand, the International Reflux Study found new scars in 15.7 percent (medical) and 17.2 percent (surgical) of refluxing children in Europe and 21.5 percent (medical) and 31.4 percent (surgical) in North America (Olbing, Claesson, Ebel, et al., 1992; Weiss, Duckett and Spitzer, 1992). Few data were available to analyze the relationship between bacteriuria and new renal scarring in children with reflux.

Renal growth and function

On the basis of studies available to date, there is no evidence that renal growth is impaired in unscarred kidneys exposed to sterile reflux of any grade or that surgical correction of reflux facilitates growth of the kidney postoperatively. Surgical correction of reflux stabilizes the glomerular filtration rate but has not been shown to lead to long-term improvement.

Health outcomes

Urinary tract infection

The panel reviewed 41 articles that described the incidence of urinary tract infection in children with vesicoureteral reflux treated with antibiotic prophylaxis or reimplantation surgery. In children with Grades III to IV reflux, the incidence of pyelonephritis was approximately 2.5 times higher in patients treated with antibiotic prophylaxis than in those treated surgically. The incidence of cystitis in patients with vesicoureteral reflux was not significantly different in patients treated medically or surgically. In children treated medically, recurrent symptomatic urinary tract infections were more common in children with voiding dysfunction than in those with normal bladder function.

Hypertension

In the reports reviewed by the panel, no statistically significant difference was found in the risk of hypertension related to treatment modality. However, these studies indicated that renal scarring increases the relative risk of hypertension to 2.92 (95 percent confidence interval 1.2–7.1), compared to the risk without renal scarring.

Uremia

It was not possible to demonstrate that even optimal treatment of reflux and urinary tract infection can prevent progressive renal failure and ultimately uremia after severe bilateral reflux nephropathy has been diagnosed.

Somatic growth

No evidence substantiated an effect of reflux treatment on somatic growth.

Morbidity during pregnancy

The panel performed a limited search of pertinent literature pertaining to reflux, renal insufficiency and adverse outcomes of pregnancy. Although the available data suggest a greater risk of morbidity from pyelonephritis in women who have persistent reflux during pregnancy, the sample size is small and only limited conclusions can be based on this evidence. The panel reviewed 5 studies that demonstrated that women with renal insufficiency exhibit an increased incidence of toxemia, preterm delivery, fetal growth retardation, fetal loss and deteriorating renal function.

Harms of medical treatment

Adverse drug reactions

Potential adverse reactions to antimicrobial prophylaxis include minor effects, such as skin rash, nausea, vomiting, abdominal pain, a bad taste in the mouth, marrow suppression as well as more serious side effects. Few studies dealing with the medical management of reflux included information on any drug reaction.

Harms of surgery

Obstruction

A total of 33 studies provided rates of obstruction after ureteral reimplantation for reflux. The likelihood of obstruction in the 33 series ranged from 0 to 9.1 percent with a combined rate of 2 percent in studies published after 1986. The reoperation rate ranged from 0.3 to 9.1 percent with an overall prevalence of 2 percent. There was no difference among various surgical techniques.

A total of 15 series provided detailed information about postoperative ureteral obstruction following endoscopic treatment of reflux. The 15 series included refluxing ureters treated using polytetrafluoroethylene or collagen as the injected substance. Seven (0.40 percent) persistent obstructions were reported.

Contralateral reflux

The development of contralateral reflux after unilateral ureteral surgery has been reported in numerous series. Of 1,566 ureters considered at risk there was an overall incidence of 142 reported new cases (9.1 percent) of contralateral reflux. The surgical method of reimplantation did not influence the likelihood of new contralateral reflux. Contralateral reflux generally resolves with time and surgical intervention is not usually recommended for at least 1 year.

Recommendations

The panel generated its practice policy recommendations on the basis of evidence-based outcomes and panel opinion, reflecting its clinical experience in pediatric urology and pediatric nephrology. In this report, statements based on opinion are explicitly identified, and evidence-based recommendations are accompanied by appropriate references. Only a few recommendations could be derived purely from scientific evidence of a beneficial effect on health outcomes.

As a result, the recommendations were derived from a panel survey of preferred treatment options for 36 clinical categories of children with reflux. The treatment recommendations were classified as guidelines, preferred options and reasonable alternatives. Treatment options selected by 8 or 9 of the 9 panel members are classified as guidelines. Treatment options that received 5 to 7 votes are designated as preferred options, and treatment options that received 3 to 4 votes are designated as reasonable alternatives. Treatments that received no more than 2 votes are designated as having no support.

Assumptions

The recommendations listed on pages 585–587 are intended to assist physicians specifically in the treatment of vesicoureteral reflux in children diagnosed following a urinary tract infection. They apply only to children 10 years and younger with unilateral or bilateral reflux and with or without scarring. The recommendations assume that the patient has uncomplicated reflux (e.g., no voiding dysfunction, neuropathic bladder, posterior urethral valves, bladder exstrophy or fixed anatomical abnormalities).

Rationale for recommendations

Specific treatment recommendations for children with reflux with or without scarring are provided on pages 585–586. The panel's overall recommendations for all children follow. The panel's recommendations to offer continuous antibiotic prophylaxis as initial therapy are based on limited scientific evidence. Controlled studies comparing the efficacy of continuous antibiotic prophylaxis and intermittent therapy on health outcomes in children with reflux have not been performed. However, the opinion of the panel is that maintaining continuous urine sterility is beneficial in reducing the risk of renal scarring and this benefit outweighs the potential adverse effects of antibiotics.

Recommendations to proceed to surgery in children with reflux that has not resolved spontaneously are supported by limited scientific evidence: open antireflux surgery is 95–98 percent

effective in correcting reflux, and in children with Grades III–IV reflux the risk of clinical pyelonephritis is 2–2.5 times higher in children treated with continuous prophylaxis than in those treated surgically. Nevertheless, randomized controlled trials of such children have shown that most children treated medically do not develop a urinary tract infection while receiving prophylaxis.

Recommendations for more aggressive treatment of girls than boys (e.g., for persistent Grades III–IV reflux in school-aged children) are based on epidemiological evidence that girls have a higher risk of urinary tract infection than boys. Recommendations for more aggressive treatment of Grade V reflux (e.g., surgical repair as initial therapy) are based on panel opinion that such cases are unlikely to resolve spontaneously over time, surgery is effective in resolving severe reflux and these benefits outweigh the potential harms of surgery. More aggressive recommendations for children who have renal scarring at diagnosis are based on panel opinion that such patients have a higher risk of progressive scarring and decreased renal-functional reserve.

An important variable in the scope of treatment is the presence of voiding dysfunction, a common occurrence among children with reflux. Such children may require more aggressive treatment with anticholinergics and bladder training in addition to antibiotic prophylaxis. Surgical repair of reflux is slightly less successful in children with voiding dysfunction and, thus, a higher threshold is necessary before surgery is recommended in such patients. Consequently, children with reflux should be assessed for voiding dysfunction as part of the initial evaluation.

Literature limitations and research priorities

Limitations of the literature

The panel attempted to rely on published evidence whenever possible. Many studies that addressed a particular issue could not be used quantitatively in the various syntheses because of inconsistent reporting of data, limited follow-up, incomplete description of treatments or poorly defined patient populations. Analyses were also complicated by the existence of at least 5 methods

Treatment recommendations for children without scarring at diagnosis

Age at diagnosis: Infants (<1 year)

Initial treatment. Infants with Grades I–IV reflux should be treated initially with continuous antibiotic prophylaxis. In infants with Grade V reflux, continuous antibiotic prophylaxis is the preferred option for initial treatment.

Follow-up treatment. In infants who continue to demonstrate uncomplicated reflux, antibiotic prophylaxis should be continued. For patients with persistent Grades I–II reflux after this period of prophylaxis, there is no consensus regarding the role of continued antibiotic therapy, periodic cystography or surgery. Surgical repair is the preferred option, however, for patients with persistent unilateral Grades III–IV reflux. Patients with persistent bilateral Grades III–IV reflux or Grade V reflux should undergo surgical repair.

Age at diagnosis: Preschool children (ages 1–5 years)

Initial treatment. Preschool children with Grades I–II reflux or unilateral Grades III–IV reflux should be treated initially with continuous antibiotic prophylaxis. Continuous antibiotic prophylaxis is the preferred option in preschool children with bilateral Grades III–IV reflux. In patients with unilateral Grade V reflux, continuous antibiotic prophylaxis is the preferred option for initial treatment, although surgical repair is a reasonable alternative. In patients with bilateral Grade V reflux, surgical repair is the preferred option and continuous antibiotic prophylaxis is a reasonable alternative.

Follow-up treatment. In children who continue to demonstrate uncomplicated reflux, antibiotic prophylaxis should be continued. In children with persistent Grades I–II reflux, there is no consensus regarding the role of continued antibiotic therapy, periodic cystography or surgery. Surgery is the preferred option for children with persistent Grades III–IV reflux. Patients with persistent Grade V reflux should undergo surgical repair.

Age at diagnosis: School children (ages 6–10 years)

Initial treatment. School children with Grades I–II reflux should be treated initially with continuous antibiotic prophylaxis. Continuous antibiotic prophylaxis is the preferred option for initial treatment of patients with unilateral Grades III–IV reflux. In patients with bilateral Grades III–IV reflux, surgical repair is the preferred option, although continuous antibiotic prophylaxis is a reasonable alternative. Patients with Grade V reflux should undergo surgical repair.

Follow-up treatment. In children who continue to demonstrate uncomplicated reflux, antibiotic prophylaxis should be continued. In patients with persistent Grades I–II reflux after this period of prophylaxis, there is no consensus regarding the role of continued antibiotic prophylaxis, periodic cystography or surgery. Surgery is the preferred option for persistent reflux in children with Grades III–IV reflux.

Treatment recommendations for children with scarring at diagnosis

Age at diagnosis: Infants (<1 year)

Initial treatment. Infants with scarring at diagnosis and Grades I–IV reflux should be treated initially with continuous antibiotic prophylaxis. In infants with Grade V reflux and scarring, continuous antibiotic prophylaxis is the preferred option for initial treatment, and surgical repair is a reasonable alternative.

Follow-up treatment. In infants who continue to demonstrate uncomplicated reflux, antibiotic prophylaxis should be continued. In patients with persistent Grades I–II reflux after this period of prophylaxis, there is no consensus regarding the role of continued antibiotic prophylaxis, periodic cystography or surgery. In boys with persistent unilateral Grades III–IV reflux, surgical repair is the preferred option. Boys with persistent bilateral Grades III–IV reflux, girls with persistent Grades III–IV reflux, and boys and girls with persistent Grade V reflux should undergo surgical repair.

Age at diagnosis: Preschool children (ages 1–5 years)

Initial treatment. Preschool children with scarring at diagnosis and either Grades I–II reflux or unilateral Grades III–IV reflux should be treated initially with continuous antibiotic prophylaxis. Antibiotic therapy is the preferred option in children with bilateral Grades III–IV reflux and scarring, and surgical repair is a reasonable alternative. Surgery is the preferred option for patients with unilateral Grade V reflux. Patients with bilateral Grade V disease and scarring should undergo surgical repair as initial treatment.

Follow-up treatment. In children who continue to demonstrate uncomplicated reflux, antibiotic prophylaxis should be continued. In patients with persistent Grades I–II reflux after this period of prophylaxis, there is no consensus regarding the role of continued antibiotic prophylaxis, periodic cystography or surgery. Girls with persistent Grades III–IV reflux and boys with persistent bilateral Grades III–IV reflux should undergo surgical repair. Surgery is the preferred option for boys with persistent unilateral Grades III–IV reflux. For patients with persistent Grade V reflux who have not undergone surgery as initial treatment, surgical repair is the preferred option.

Age at diagnosis: School children (ages 6–10 years)

Initial treatment. School children with scarring at diagnosis and Grades I–II reflux should be treated initially with continuous antibiotic prophylaxis. In children with unilateral Grades III–IV reflux and scarring, antibiotic therapy is the preferred option. Patients with bilateral Grades III–IV reflux or Grade V reflux should undergo surgical repair as initial treatment.

Follow-up treatment. In children who continue to demonstrate uncomplicated reflux, antibiotic prophylaxis should be continued. In patients who have persistent Grades I–II reflux after this period of prophylaxis, there is no consensus regarding the role of continued antibiotic prophylaxis, periodic cystography or surgery. Patients with persistent unilateral Grades III–IV reflux who have not undergone surgery as initial treatment should undergo surgical repair.

Other recommendations for children with reflux

In children with vesicoureteral reflux, urethral dilation and internal urethrotomy are not beneficial. In addition, cystoscopic examination of the ureteral orifices does not appear to aid in predicting whether reflux will resolve. In children with symptoms of voiding dysfunction, urodynamic evaluation may be helpful, but evocative cystometry is unnecessary in children with reflux and a normal voiding pattern.

In children with reflux who are toilet trained, regular, volitional low-pressure voiding with complete bladder emptying should be encouraged. If it is suspected that the child is experiencing uninhibited bladder contractions, anticholinergic therapy may be beneficial.

The clinician should provide parents with information about the known benefits and harms of available options, including continuous antibiotic prophylaxis, surgery and intermittent antibiotic therapy. The clinician should indicate to what extent the estimates of benefits and harms are based on scientific evidence or on opinion and clinical experience. Given the general lack of direct evidence that any one treatment option is superior to another (especially when total benefits, harms, costs and inconvenience are considered), parent and patient preferences regarding treatment options should generally be honored.

In children for whom antireflux surgery is chosen, the panel does not recommend the endoscopic form of therapy because of the lack of proven long-term safety and efficacy of the materials used for injection and the lack of approval of such materials by the U.S. Food and Drug Administration.

Follow-up evaluation should be performed at least annually, at which time the patient's height and weight should be recorded and a urinalysis should be performed. If the child has renal scarring, the blood pressure should be measured. In deciding how often to obtain follow-up cystography in children managed medically, the clinician should take into consideration the likelihood of spontaneous resolution (see Figure 3 on page 24, Chapter 3), the risk of continued antibiotic prophylaxis and the risks of radiologic study. In general, cystography does not need to be performed more than once per year.

used for grading reflux, nonuniformity in characterizing reflux grade and patient population, and lack of a standard method for reporting outcomes. Only 3 prospective randomized controlled trials compared medical to surgical therapy—the Birmingham Reflux Study (1987), the International Reflux Study in Children (Olbing, Claesson, Ebel, et al., 1992; Weiss, Duckett and Spitzer, 1992), and a study from Erasmus University, Rotterdam, The Netherlands (Scholtmeijer, 1991). The literature on certain issues, such as complication rates of surgery and adverse drug reactions, was limited and in some cases so sparse that judgments were made on the basis of expert opinion.

Research priorities

The panel identified many research areas as needing further investigation. Presently, there is little information regarding health outcomes pertaining to reflux, and a significant priority should be to continue to acquire this information.

Basic research into the pathogenesis as well as the genetics of vesicoureteral reflux is needed. Further randomized controlled trials studying the role of medical and surgical therapy using dimercaptosuccinic acid scan for evaluation of renal scarring are indicated. Future studies should stratify results by patient gender, age and reflux grade, reporting reflux resolution both by rate of ureteral and patient resolution. Also worthwhile would be studies to confirm the panel's finding that resolution of Grade III reflux depends on patient age or laterality (unilateral vs. bilateral) and the finding

that resolution of Grades I and II reflux does not depend on age or laterality.

The extent to which reflux increases the risk of renal scarring associated with urinary tract infection and the mechanism of this effect deserves investigation. Comparison of the efficacy of intermittent and continuous antibiotic therapy would be beneficial. The role of voiding dysfunction in the pathogenesis of reflux and its risk on reflux complications, such as renal scarring and the complications of surgery, also deserve further investigation. Matched controlled studies of anticholinergic therapy and bladder training on reflux-related outcomes in children with voiding dysfunction are necessary.

Less traumatic methods of determining whether reflux is present should be developed as well as techniques of voiding cystourethrography that result in less radiation exposure. Analysis of the costs of reflux treatment and surveillance is important, particularly comparing those associated with medical and surgical therapy. The impact of screening at-risk populations and early medical or surgical intervention on reflux-related outcomes in such patients should be analyzed.

Development of minimally invasive techniques of antireflux surgery is indicated. Newer materials that can be used for endoscopic subureteral injection and that are safe in children should be studied.

The natural history of vesicoureteral reflux in adult women with persistent reflux deserves investigation, including an analysis of the morbidity of persistent reflux, and need for and efficacy of prophylaxis in pregnant and nonpregnant women.

SECTION 2

Policy Statements

• •

INTRODUCTION

This section of the *Pediatric Clinical Practice Guidelines & Policies: A Compendium of Evidence-based Research for Pediatric Practice* manual is composed of policy statements issued by the American Academy of Pediatrics (AAP) and is designed as a quick reference tool for AAP members, staff, and other interested parties. The collection of statements is arranged alphabetically, with abstracts where applicable. A Committee Index and Subject Index are also available. The enclosed CD-ROM contains the full text of all current policy statements (through December 2003). These materials should help answer questions that arise about the Academy's position on child health care issues. **However, it should be remembered that AAP policy statements do not indicate an exclusive course of treatment or serve as a standard of medical care. Variations, taking into account individual circumstances, may be appropriate.**

The policy statements have been written by AAP Committees, Task Forces, or Sections and approved by the AAP Board of Directors. Most of these statements have appeared previously in *Pediatrics, AAP News,* or *News & Comments* (the forerunner of *AAP News*).

This section does not contain all AAP policies. It does not include

- Press releases.
- Motions and resolutions that were approved by the Board of Directors. These can be found in the Board of Directors' minutes.
- Policies in manuals, pamphlets, booklets, or other AAP publications. These items can be ordered from the AAP Publications Catalog. A new catalog is updated biannually and sent to all AAP members; additional copies can be obtained by contacting the AAP.
- Testimony before Congress or government agencies.

Policy statements are reviewed every 3 years by the authoring body, at which time a recommendation is made that the policy be retired, revised, or reaffirmed without change. Until the Board of Directors approves a revision or reaffirmation, or retires a statement, the current policy remains in effect.

The AAP endorses and accepts as its policy the following statements that have been published by other organizations. Full text of these statements is available on the enclosed CD-ROM.

- Gifts to Physicians From Industry (American Medical Association), 8/01
- Pediatric Care in the Emergency Department, 11/03
- Principles and Guidelines for Early Hearing Detection and Intervention Programs (Year 2000 Position Statement) (Joint Committee on Infant Hearing), 10/00
- Targeted Tuberculin Testing and Treatment of Latent Tuberculosis Infection (American Thoracic Society and Centers for Disease Control and Prevention), 4/00 (*The Academy endorses and accepts as its policy the sections of this statement as it relates to infants and children.*)
- Type 2 Diabetes in Children and Adolescents (American Diabetes Association), 3/00

AMERICAN ACADEMY OF PEDIATRICS
Policy Statements
Current through December 2003
Full text of all titles listed below is available on the *Pediatric Clinical Practice Guidelines & Policies* CD-ROM included with this publication.

ACCESS TO PEDIATRIC EMERGENCY MEDICAL CARE
Committee on Pediatric Emergency Medicine
ABSTRACT. Hundreds of thousands of pediatric patients require some level of emergency care annually, and significant barriers limit access to appropriate services for large numbers of children. The American Academy of Pediatrics has a strong commitment to identify barriers to access to emergency care, work to surmount these obstacles, and encourage through education increased levels of emergency care available to all children. It is also crucial to involve and incorporate the child's medical home into emergency care, both during acute presentation when the medical home is identified and by assisting in locating a medical home for follow-up when none previously exists. (3/00)

ACETAMINOPHEN TOXICITY IN CHILDREN
Committee on Drugs
ABSTRACT. Acetaminophen is widely used in children, because its safety and efficacy are well established. Although the risk of developing toxic reactions to acetaminophen appears to be lower in children than in adults, such reactions occur in pediatric patients from intentional overdoses. Less frequently, acetaminophen toxicity is attributable to unintended inappropriate dosing or the failure to recognize children at increased risk in whom standard acetaminophen doses have been administered. Because the symptoms of acetaminophen intoxication are nonspecific, the diagnosis and treatment of acetaminophen intoxication are more likely to be delayed in unintentional cases of toxicity. This statement describes situations and conditions that may contribute to acetaminophen toxicity not associated with suicidal intentions. (10/01)

ADOLESCENT PREGNANCY—CURRENT TRENDS AND ISSUES: 1998
Committee on Adolescence
ABSTRACT. Although the prevention of unintended adolescent pregnancy is a primary goal of the American Academy of Pediatrics and society, many adolescents continue to become pregnant. Since the last statement on adolescent pregnancy was issued by the Academy in 1989, new observations have been recorded in the literature. The purpose of this new statement is to review current trends and issues on adolescent pregnancy to update practitioners on this topic. (2/99)

CLINICAL REPORT: ADOLESCENTS AND ANABOLIC STEROIDS: A SUBJECT REVIEW
Committee on Sports Medicine and Fitness
ABSTRACT. This revision of a previous statement by the American Academy of Pediatrics provides current information on anabolic steroid use by young athletes. It provides the information needed to enable pediatricians to discuss the benefits and risks of anabolic steroids in a well-informed, nonjudgmental fashion. (6/97, reaffirmed 5/00)

ADOLESCENTS AND HUMAN IMMUNODEFICIENCY VIRUS INFECTION: THE ROLE OF THE PEDIATRICIAN IN PREVENTION AND INTERVENTION
Committee on Pediatric AIDS and Committee on Adolescence
ABSTRACT. Half of all new human immunodeficiency virus (HIV) infections in the United States occur among young people between the ages of 13 and 24. Sexual transmission accounts for most cases of HIV during adolescence. Pediatricians can play an important role in educating adolescents about HIV prevention, transmission, and testing, with an emphasis on risk reduction, and in advocating for the special needs of adolescents for access to information about HIV. (1/01)

THE ADOLESCENT'S RIGHT TO CONFIDENTIAL CARE WHEN CONSIDERING ABORTION
Committee on Adolescence
ABSTRACT. In this statement, the American Academy of Pediatrics (AAP) reaffirms its position that the rights of adolescents to confidential care when considering abortion should be protected. The AAP supports the recommendations presented in the report on mandatory parental consent to abortion by the Council on Ethical and Judicial Affairs of the American Medical Association. Adolescents should be strongly encouraged to involve their parents and other trusted adults in decisions regarding pregnancy termination, and the majority of them voluntarily do so. Legislation mandating parental involvement does not achieve the intended benefit of promoting family communication, but it does increase the risk of harm to the adolescent by delaying access to appropriate medical care. The statement presents a summary of pertinent current information related to the benefits and risks of legislation requiring mandatory parental involvement in an adolescent's decision to obtain an abortion. The AAP acknowledges and respects the diversity of beliefs about abortion and affirms the value of voluntary parental involvement in decision making by adolescents. (5/96, reaffirmed 5/99)

ADVANCED PRACTICE IN NEONATAL NURSING
Committee on Fetus and Newborn
ABSTRACT. The advanced practice neonatal nurse's participation in newborn care continues to be accepted and supported by the American Academy of Pediatrics. Recognized categories of advanced practice neonatal nurse are the neonatal clinical nurse specialist and the neonatal nurse practitioner. Training and credentialing requirements have been updated recently and are endorsed in this revised statement. (6/03)

AGE LIMITS OF PEDIATRICS
Child and Adolescent Health Action Group (5/88, reaffirmed 9/92, 1/97, 3/02)

AGE FOR ROUTINE ADMINISTRATION OF THE SECOND DOSE OF MEASLES-MUMPS-RUBELLA VACCINE
Committee on Infectious Diseases
ABSTRACT. The purpose of this statement is to inform physicians of a modification in the recommendation of the appropriate age for routine administration of the second dose of measles-mumps-rubella (MMR) vaccine. The implementation of the two-dose measles vaccine schedule has improved the control of measles, but some outbreaks continue to occur in school children, although ≥95% of children in school have received one dose of vaccine. Because most measles vaccine failures are attributable to failure to respond to the first dose, that all children receive two doses of measles-containing vaccine is essential for the control of measles. Routine administration of the second dose of MMR vaccine at school entry (4 to 6 years of age) will help prevent school-based outbreaks. Physicians should continue to review the records of all children 11 to 12 years of age to be certain that they have received two doses of MMR vaccine after their first birthday. Documenting that all school children have received two doses of measles-containing vaccine by the year 2001 will help ensure the elimination of measles in the United States and contribute to the global effort to control and possibly eradicate measles. (1/98)

ALCOHOL USE AND ABUSE: A PEDIATRIC CONCERN
Committee on Substance Abuse
ABSTRACT. Alcohol use and abuse by children and adolescents continue to be a major problem. Pediatricians should interview their patients regularly about alcohol use within the family, by friends, and by themselves. A comprehensive substance abuse curriculum should be integrated into every pediatrician's training. Advertising of alcohol in the media, on the Internet, and during sporting events is a powerful force that must be addressed. Availability of alcohol to minors must be controlled, and interventions for the child and adolescent drinker and punitive action for the purveyor are encouraged. (7/01)

ALL-TERRAIN VEHICLE INJURY PREVENTION: TWO-, THREE-, AND FOUR-WHEELED UNLICENSED MOTOR VEHICLES
Committee on Injury and Poison Prevention
ABSTRACT. Since 1987, the American Academy of Pediatrics (AAP) has had a policy about the use of motorized cycles and all-terrain vehicles (ATVs) by children. The purpose of this policy statement is to update and strengthen previous policy. This statement describes the various kinds of motorized cycles and ATVs and outlines the epidemiologic characteristics of deaths and injuries related to their use by children in light of the 1987 consent decrees entered into by the US Consumer Product Safety Commission and the manufacturers of ATVs. Recommendations are made for public, patient, and parent education by pediatricians; equipment modifications; the use of safety equipment; and the development and improvement of safer off-road trails and responsive emergency medical systems. In addition, the AAP strengthens its recommendation for passage of legislation in all states prohibiting the use of 2- and 4-wheeled off-road vehicles by children younger than 16 years, as well as a ban on the sale of new and used 3-wheeled ATVs, with a recall of all used 3-wheeled ATVs. (6/00)

TECHNICAL REPORT: ALTERNATIVE DISPUTE RESOLUTION IN MEDICAL MALPRACTICE
John J. Fraser, Jr, MD, JD, and the Committee on Medical Liability
ABSTRACT. The purpose of this technical report is to provide pediatricians with an understanding of past crises within the professional liability insurance industry, the difficulties of the tort system, and alternative strategies for resolving malpractice disputes that have been applied to medical malpractice actions. Through this report, pediatricians will gain a technical understanding of common alternative dispute resolution (ADR) strategies. The report explains the distinctions between various ADR methods in terms of process and outcome, risks and benefits, appropriateness to the nature of the dispute, and long-term ramifications. By knowing these concepts, pediatricians faced with malpractice claims will be better-equipped to participate in the decision-making with legal counsel on whether to settle, litigate, or explore ADR options. (3/01)

CLINICAL REPORT: ALTERNATIVE ROUTES OF DRUG ADMINISTRATION—ADVANTAGES AND DISADVANTAGES (SUBJECT REVIEW)
Committee on Drugs
ABSTRACT. During the past 20 years, advances in drug formulations and innovative routes of administration have been made. Our understanding of drug transport across tissues has increased. These changes have often resulted in improved patient adherence to the therapeutic regimen and pharmacologic response. The administration of drugs by transdermal or transmucosal routes offers the advantage of being relatively painless. Also, the potential for greater flexibility in a variety of clinical situations exists, often precluding the need to establish intravenous access, which is a particular benefit for children.

This statement focuses on the advantages and disadvantages of alternative routes of drug administration. Issues of particular importance in the care of pediatric patients, especially factors that could lead to drug-related toxicity or adverse responses, are emphasized. (7/97, reaffirmed 10/00, 11/03)

ALUMINUM TOXICITY IN INFANTS AND CHILDREN
Committee on Nutrition (3/96, reaffirmed 4/00, 4/03)

AMBIENT AIR POLLUTION: RESPIRATORY HAZARDS TO CHILDREN
Committee on Environmental Health (6/93, reaffirmed 5/96)

APNEA, SUDDEN INFANT DEATH SYNDROME, AND HOME MONITORING
Committee on Fetus and Newborn
ABSTRACT. More than 25 years have elapsed since continuous cardiorespiratory monitoring at home was suggested to decrease the risk of sudden infant death syndrome (SIDS). In the ensuing interval, multiple studies have been unable to establish the alleged efficacy of its use. In this statement, the most recent research information concerning extreme limits for a prolonged course of apnea of prematurity is reviewed. Recommendations regarding the appropriate use of home cardiorespiratory monitoring after hospital discharge emphasize limiting use to specific clinical indications for a predetermined period, using only monitors equipped with an event recorder, and counseling parents that monitor use does not prevent sudden, unexpected death in all circumstances. The continued implementation of proven SIDS prevention measures is encouraged. (4/03)

APPROPRIATE BOUNDARIES IN THE PEDIATRICIAN-FAMILY-PATIENT RELATIONSHIP
Committee on Bioethics
ABSTRACT. All professionals are concerned about maintaining the appropriate limits in their relationships with those they serve. Romantic and sexual involvement between physicians and patients is unacceptable. Pediatricians also must strive to maintain appropriate professional boundaries in their relationships with the family members of their patients. Pediatricians should avoid behavior that patients and parents might misunderstand as having sexual or inappropriate social meaning. The acceptance of gifts or nonmonetary compensation for medical services has the potential to affect adversely the professional relationship. (8/99, reaffirmed 11/02)

ASSESSMENT OF MALTREATMENT OF CHILDREN WITH DISABILITIES
Committee on Child Abuse and Neglect and Committee on Children With Disabilities
ABSTRACT. Widespread efforts are continuously being made to increase awareness and provide education to pediatricians regarding risk factors of child abuse and neglect. The purpose of this statement is to ensure that children with disabilities are recognized as a population that is also at risk for maltreatment. The need for early recognition and intervention of child abuse and neglect in this population, as well as the ways that a medical home can facilitate the prevention and early detection of child maltreatment, should be acknowledged. (8/01)

THE ASSESSMENT AND MANAGEMENT OF ACUTE PAIN IN INFANTS, CHILDREN, AND ADOLESCENTS
American Academy of Pediatrics Committee on Psychosocial Aspects of Child and Family Health and the Task Force on Pain in Infants, Children, and Adolescents of the American Pain Society
ABSTRACT. Acute pain is one of the most common adverse stimuli experienced by children, occurring as a result of injury, illness, and necessary medical procedures. It is associated with increased anxiety, avoidance, somatic symptoms, and increased parent distress. Despite the magnitude of effects that acute pain can have on a child, it is often inadequately assessed and treated. Numerous myths, insufficient knowledge among caregivers, and inadequate application of knowledge contribute to the lack of effective management. The pediatric acute pain experience involves the interaction of physiologic, psychologic, behavioral, developmental, and situational factors. Pain is an inherently subjective multifactorial experience and should be assessed and treated as such. Pediatricians are responsible for eliminating or assuaging pain and suffering in children when possible. To accomplish this, pediatricians need to expand their knowledge, use appropriate assessment tools and techniques, anticipate painful experiences and intervene accordingly, use a multimodal approach to pain management, use a multidisciplinary approach when possible, involve families, and advocate for the use of effective pain management in children. (9/01)

ATHLETIC PARTICIPATION BY CHILDREN AND ADOLESCENTS WHO HAVE SYSTEMIC HYPERTENSION
Committee on Sports Medicine and Fitness
ABSTRACT. Children and adolescents who have systemic hypertension may be at risk for complications when exercise causes their blood pressures to rise even higher. The purpose of this statement is to make recommendations concerning the athletic participation of individuals with hypertension using the 26th Bethesda Conference on heart disease and athletic participation and of the Second Task Force on Blood Pressure Control in Children as a basis. (4/97, reaffirmed 5/00)

CLINICAL REPORT: ATLANTOAXIAL INSTABILITY IN DOWN SYNDROME: SUBJECT REVIEW
Committee on Sports Medicine and Fitness (7/95, reaffirmed 11/98, 5/00)

AUDITORY INTEGRATION TRAINING AND FACILITATED COMMUNICATION FOR AUTISM
Committee on Children With Disabilities
ABSTRACT. This statement reviews the basis for two new therapies for autism—auditory integration training and facilitative communication. Both therapies seek to improve communication skills. Currently available information does not support the claims of proponents that these treatments are efficacious. Their use does not appear warranted at this time, except within research protocols. (8/98, reaffirmed 5/02)

BICYCLE HELMETS
Committee on Injury and Poison Prevention
ABSTRACT. Bicycling remains one of the most popular recreational sports among children in America and is the leading cause of recreational sports injuries treated in emergency departments. An estimated 23 000 children younger than 21 years sustained head injuries (excluding the face) while bicycling in 1998. The bicycle helmet is a very effective device that can prevent the occurrence of up to 88% of serious brain injuries. Despite this, most children do not wear a helmet each time they ride a bicycle, and adolescents are particularly resistant to helmet use. Recently, a group of national experts and government agencies renewed the call for all bicyclists to wear helmets. This policy statement describes the role of the pediatrician in helping attain universal helmet use among children and teens for each bicycle ride. (10/01)

BREASTFEEDING AND THE USE OF HUMAN MILK
Provisional Section on Breastfeeding

ABSTRACT. This policy statement on breastfeeding replaces the previous policy statement of the American Academy of Pediatrics, reflecting the considerable advances that have occurred in recent years in the scientific knowledge of the benefits of breastfeeding, in the mechanisms underlying these benefits, and in the practice of breastfeeding. This document summarizes the benefits of breastfeeding to the infant, the mother, and the nation, and sets forth principles to guide the pediatrician and other health care providers in the initiation and maintenance of breastfeeding. The policy statement also delineates the various ways in which pediatricians can promote, protect, and support breastfeeding, not only in their individual practices but also in the hospital, medical school, community, and nation. (12/97)

CALCIUM REQUIREMENTS OF INFANTS, CHILDREN, AND ADOLESCENTS
Committee on Nutrition

ABSTRACT. This statement is intended to provide pediatric caregivers with advice about the nutritional needs of calcium of infants, children, and adolescents. It will review the physiology of calcium metabolism and provide a review of the data about the relationship between calcium intake and bone growth and metabolism. In particular, it will focus on the large number of recent studies that have identified a relationship between childhood calcium intake and bone mineralization and the potential relationship of these data to fractures in adolescents and the development of osteoporosis in adulthood. The specific needs of children and adolescents with eating disorders are not considered. (11/99)

CAMPHOR REVISITED: FOCUS ON TOXICITY
Committee on Drugs (7/94, reaffirmed 6/97, 5/00)

CARDIAC DYSRHYTHMIAS AND SPORTS
Committee on Sports Medicine and Fitness (5/95, reaffirmed 11/98, 5/00)

CARE OF ADOLESCENT PARENTS AND THEIR CHILDREN
Committee on Adolescence and Committee on Early Childhood, Adoption, and Dependent Care

ABSTRACT. Many children live with their adolescent parents, alone, or as part of an extended family. This statement updates a previous statement on adolescent parents and addresses specific medical and psychosocial risks specific to adolescent parents and their children. Challenges unique to the adolescent mother and her partner, as well as mitigating circumstances and protective factors that have been identified in the recent literature, are reviewed, along with suggestions for the pediatrician on models for intervention and care. (2/01)

CARE OF THE ADOLESCENT SEXUAL ASSAULT VICTIM
Committee on Adolescence

ABSTRACT. Sexual assault is a broad-based term that encompasses a wide range of sexual victimizations, including rape. Since the American Academy of Pediatrics published its last policy statement on this topic in 1994, additional information and data have emerged about sexual assault and rape in adolescents, the adolescent's perception of sexual assault, and the treatment and management of the adolescent who has been a victim of sexual assault. This new information mandates an updated knowledge base for pediatricians who care for adolescent patients. This statement provides that update, focusing on sexual assault and rape in the adolescent population. (6/01)

CARE OF CHILDREN IN THE EMERGENCY DEPARTMENT: GUIDELINES FOR PREPAREDNESS
American Academy of Pediatrics, Committee on Pediatric Emergency Medicine and American College of Emergency Physicians, Pediatric Committee

ABSTRACT. Children requiring emergency care have unique and special needs. This is especially so for those with serious and life-threatening emergencies. There are a variety of components of the emergency care system that provide emergency care to children that are not limited to children. With regard to hospitals, most children are brought to community hospital emergency departments (EDs) by virtue of their availability rather than to facilities designed and operated solely for children. Emergency medical services (EMS) agencies, similarly, provide the bulk of out-of-hospital emergency care to children. It is imperative that all hospital EDs and EMS agencies have the appropriate equipment, staff, and policies to provide high quality care for children. This statement provides guidelines for necessary resources to ensure that children receive quality emergency care and to facilitate, after stabilization, timely transfer to a facility with specialized pediatric services when appropriate. It is important to realize that some hospitals and local EMS systems will have difficulty in meeting these guidelines, and others will develop more comprehensive guidelines based on local resources. It is hoped, however, that hospital ED staff and administrators and local EMS systems administrators will seek to meet these guidelines to best ensure that their facilities or systems provide the resources necessary for the care of children. This statement has been reviewed by and is supported in concept by the Ambulatory Pediatric Association, American Association of Poison Control Centers, American College of Surgeons, American Hospital Association, American Medical Association, American Pediatric Surgical Association, American Trauma Society, Brain Injury Association Inc, Emergency Nurses Association, Joint Commission on Accreditation of Healthcare Organizations, National Association of Children's Hospitals and Related Institutions, National Association of EMS Physicians, National Association of EMTs, National Association of School Nurses, National Association of State EMS Directors, National Committee for Quality Assurance, and Society for Academic Emergency Medicine. (4/01)

CARE COORDINATION: INTEGRATING HEALTH AND RELATED SYSTEMS OF CARE FOR CHILDREN WITH SPECIAL HEALTH CARE NEEDS
Committee on Children With Disabilities
ABSTRACT. *Care coordination* is a process that links children with special health care needs and their families to services and resources in a coordinated effort to maximize the potential of the children and provide them with optimal health care. Care coordination often is complicated because there is no single entry point to multiple systems of care, and complex criteria determine the availability of funding and services among public and private payers. Economic and sociocultural barriers to coordination of care exist and affect families and health care professionals. In their important role of providing a medical home for all children, primary care pediatricians have a vital role in the process of care coordination, in concert with the family. (10/99)

CHANGING CONCEPTS OF SUDDEN INFANT DEATH SYNDROME: IMPLICATIONS FOR INFANT SLEEPING ENVIRONMENT AND SLEEP POSITION
Task Force on Infant Sleep Position and Sudden Infant Death Syndrome
ABSTRACT. The American Academy of Pediatrics has recommended since 1992 that infants be placed to sleep on their backs to reduce the risk of sudden infant death syndrome (SIDS). Since that time, the frequency of prone sleeping has decreased from >70% to ~20% of US infants, and the SIDS rate has decreased by >40%. However, SIDS remains the highest cause of infant death beyond the neonatal period, and there are still several potentially modifiable risk factors. Although some of these factors have been known for many years (eg, maternal smoking), the importance of other hazards, such as soft bedding and covered airways, has been demonstrated only recently. The present statement is intended to review the evidence about prone sleeping and other risk factors and to make recommendations about strategies that may be effective for further reducing the risk of SIDS. This statement is intended to consolidate and supplant previous statements made by this Task Force. (3/00)

CLINICAL REPORT: CHEMICAL-BIOLOGICAL TERRORISM AND ITS IMPACT ON CHILDREN: A SUBJECT REVIEW
Committee on Environmental Health and Committee on Infectious Diseases
ABSTRACT. There is an increasing threat that chemical and biological weapons will be used on a civilian population in an act of domestic terrorism. Casualties among adults and children could be significant in such an event. Federal, state, and local authorities have begun extensive planning to meet a chemical-biological incident by developing methods of rapid identification of potential agents and protocols for management of victims without injury to health care personnel. Because children would be disproportionately affected by a chemical or biological weapons release, pediatricians must assist in planning for a domestic chemical-biological incident. Government agencies should seek input from pediatricians and pediatric subspecialists to ensure that the situations created by multiple pediatric casualties after a chemical-biological incident are considered. This statement reviews key aspects of chemical-biological agents, the consequences of their use, the potential impact of a chemical-biological attack on children, and issues to consider in disaster planning and management for pediatric patients. (3/00)

CLINICAL REPORT: THE CHILD IN COURT: A SUBJECT REVIEW
Committee on Psychosocial Aspects of Child and Family Health
ABSTRACT. When children come to court as witnesses, or when their needs are decided in a courtroom, they face unique stressors from the legal proceeding and from the social predicament that resulted in court action. Effective pediatric support and intervention requires an understanding of the situations that bring children to court and the issues that will confront children and child advocates in different court settings. (11/99, reaffirmed 11/02)

CHILD LIFE SERVICES
Committee on Hospital Care
ABSTRACT. Child life programs have become the standard in large pediatric settings to address the psychosocial concerns that accompany hospitalization and other health care experiences. Child life programs facilitate coping and the adjustment of children and families in 3 primary service areas: 1) providing play experiences; 2) presenting developmentally appropriate information about events and procedures; and 3) establishing therapeutic relationships with children and parents to support family involvement in each child's care. Although other members of the health care team share these responsibilities for the psychosocial concerns of the child and the family, for the child life specialist, this is the primary role. The child life specialist focuses on the strengths and sense of well-being of children while promoting their optimal development and minimizing the adverse effects of children's experiences in a hospital setting. (11/00)

CHILDREN, ADOLESCENTS, AND ADVERTISING
Committee on Public Education (2/95)

CHILDREN, ADOLESCENTS, AND TELEVISION
Committee on Public Education
ABSTRACT. This statement describes the possible negative health effects of television viewing on children and adolescents, such as violent or aggressive behavior, substance use, sexual activity, obesity, poor body image, and decreased school performance. In addition to the television ratings system and the v-chip (electronic device to block programming), media education is an effective approach to mitigating these potential problems. The American Academy of Pediatrics offers a list of recommendations on this issue for pediatricians and for parents, the federal government, and the entertainment industry. (2/01)

CHILDREN IN PICKUP TRUCKS
Committee on Injury and Poison Prevention

ABSTRACT. Pickup trucks have become increasingly popular in the United States. A recent study found that in crashes involving fatalities, cargo area passengers were 3 times more likely to die than were occupants in the cab. Compared with restrained cab occupants, the risk of death for those in the cargo area was 8 times higher. Furthermore, the increased use of extended-cab pickup trucks and air bag-equipped front passenger compartments creates concerns about the safe transport of children. The most effective preventive strategies are the legislative prohibition of travel in the cargo area and requirements for age-appropriate restraint use and seat selection in the cab. Parents should select vehicles that are appropriate for the safe transportation needs of the family. Physicians have an important role in counseling families and advocating public policy measures to reduce the number of deaths and injuries to occupants of pickup trucks. (10/00)

CHOLESTEROL IN CHILDHOOD
Committee on Nutrition

ABSTRACT. This updated statement reviews the scientific justification for the recommendations of dietary changes in all healthy children (a population approach) and a strategy to identify and treat children who are at highest risk for the development of accelerated atherosclerosis in early adult life (an individualized approach). Although the precise fraction of risk for future coronary heart disease conveyed by elevated cholesterol levels in childhood is unknown, clear epidemiologic and experimental evidence indicates that the risk is significant. Diet changes that lower fat, saturated fat, and cholesterol intake in children and adolescents can be applied safely and acceptably, resulting in improved plasma lipid profiles that, if carried into adult life, have the potential to reduce atherosclerotic vascular disease. (1/98, reaffirmed 4/01)

CIRCUMCISION POLICY STATEMENT
Task Force on Circumcision

ABSTRACT. Existing scientific evidence demonstrates potential medical benefits of newborn male circumcision; however, these data are not sufficient to recommend routine neonatal circumcision. In circumstances in which there are potential benefits and risks, yet the procedure is not essential to the child's current well-being, parents should determine what is in the best interest of the child. To make an informed choice, parents of all male infants should be given accurate and unbiased information and be provided the opportunity to discuss this decision. If a decision for circumcision is made, procedural analgesia should be provided. (3/99)

CLIMATIC HEAT STRESS AND THE EXERCISING CHILD AND ADOLESCENT
Committee on Sports Medicine and Fitness

ABSTRACT. For morphologic and physiologic reasons, exercising children do not adapt as effectively as adults when exposed to a high climatic heat stress. This may affect their performance and well-being, as well as increase the risk for heat-related illness. This policy statement summarizes approaches for the prevention of the detrimental effects of children's activity in hot or humid climates, including the prevention of exercise-induced dehydration. (7/00)

CLIOQUINOL (IODOCHLORHYDROXYQUIN, VIOFORM) AND IODOQUINOL (DIIODOHYDROXYQUIN): BLINDNESS AND NEUROPATHY
Committee on Drugs (11/90, reaffirmed 2/94, 2/97, 2/00, 4/03)

COMBINATION VACCINES FOR CHILDHOOD IMMUNIZATION: RECOMMENDATIONS OF THE ADVISORY COMMITTEE ON IMMUNIZATION PRACTICES (ACIP), THE AMERICAN ACADEMY OF PEDIATRICS (AAP), AND THE AMERICAN ACADEMY OF FAMILY PHYSICIANS (AAFP)
Joint Statement

SUMMARY. An increasing number of new and improved vaccines to prevent childhood diseases are being introduced. Combination vaccines represent one solution to the problem of increased numbers of injections during single clinic visits. This statement provides general guidance on the use of combination vaccines and related issues and questions.

To minimize the number of injections children receive, parenteral combination vaccines should be used, if licensed and indicated for the patient's age, instead of their equivalent component vaccines. Hepatitis A, hepatitis B, and *Haemophilus influenzae* type b vaccines, in either monovalent or combination formulations from the same or different manufacturers, are interchangeable for sequential doses in the vaccination series. However, using acellular pertussis vaccine product(s) from the same manufacturer is preferable for at least the first three doses, until studies demonstrate the interchangeability of these vaccines. Immunization providers should stock sufficient types of combination and monovalent vaccines needed to vaccinate children against all diseases for which vaccines are recommended, but they need not stock all available types or brand-name products. When patients have already received the recommended vaccinations for some of the components in a combination vaccine, administering the extra antigen(s) in the combination is often permissible if doing so will reduce the number of injections required.

To overcome recording errors and ambiguities in the names of vaccine combinations, improved systems are needed to enhance the convenience and accuracy of transferring vaccine-identifying information into medical records and immunization registries. Further scientific and programmatic research is needed on specific questions related to the use of combination vaccines. (5/99, reaffirmed 3/02)

CONDOM USE BY ADOLESCENTS
Committee on Adolescence

ABSTRACT. The use of condoms as part of the prevention of unintended pregnancies and sexually transmitted diseases (STDs) in adolescents is evaluated in this policy statement. Sexual activity and pregnancies decreased slightly among adolescents in the 1990s, reversing trends that were present in the 1970s and 1980s, while condom use among adolescents increased significantly. These trends likely reflect initial success of primary and secondary prevention messages aimed at adolescents. Rates of acquisition of STDs and human immunodeficiency virus (HIV) among adolescents remain unacceptably high, highlighting the need for continued prevention efforts and reflecting the fact that improved condom use can decrease, but never eliminate, the risk of acquisition of STDs and HIV as well as unintended pregnancies. While many condom education and availability programs have been shown to have modest effects on condom use, there is no evidence that these programs contribute to increased sexual activity among adolescents. These trends highlight the progress that has been made and the large amount that still needs to be accomplished. (6/01)

CONFIDENTIALITY IN ADOLESCENT HEALTH CARE
Committee on Adolescence (4/89, reaffirmed 1/93, 11/97, 5/00)

TECHNICAL REPORT: CONGENITAL ADRENAL HYPERPLASIA
Section on Endocrinology and Committee on Genetics

ABSTRACT. The Section on Endocrinology and the Committee on Genetics of the American Academy of Pediatrics, in collaboration with experts from the field of pediatric endocrinology and genetics, developed this policy statement as a means of providing up-to-date information for the practicing pediatrician about current practice and controversial issues in congenital adrenal hyperplasia (CAH), including the current status of prenatal diagnosis and treatment, the benefits and problem areas of neonatal screening programs, and the management of children with nonclassic CAH. The reference list is designed to allow physicians who wish more information to research the topic more thoroughly. (12/00)

CONSENSUS REPORT FOR REGIONALIZATION OF SERVICES FOR CRITICALLY ILL OR INJURED CHILDREN
Committee on Pediatric Emergency Medicine and American College of Critical Care Medicine Society of Critical Care Medicine, Pediatric Section, Task Force on Regionalization of Pediatric Critical Care

ABSTRACT. The care of critically ill children has become more complex and demanding. This document establishes recommendations for developing regionalized integration of the care of these children into the emergency medical services system. These recommendations were developed by pediatricians with expertise in pediatric critical care, transport, and emergency medicine from the Committee on Pediatric Emergency Medicine, and the Pediatric Section of the Society of Critical Care Medicine Task Force on Regionalization of Pediatric Critical Care. The document was developed from existing guidelines from a number of professional organizations including the American Academy of Pediatrics and the Society of Critical Care Medicine, a thorough review of the literature, and expert consensus. (1/00)

A CONSENSUS STATEMENT ON HEALTH CARE TRANSITIONS FOR YOUNG ADULTS WITH SPECIAL HEALTH CARE NEEDS
American Academy of Pediatrics, American Academy of Family Physicians, and American College of Physicians-American Society of Internal Medicine

ABSTRACT. This policy statement represents a consensus on the critical first steps that the medical profession needs to take to realize the vision of a family-centered, continuous, comprehensive, coordinated, compassionate, and culturally competent health care system that is as developmentally appropriate as it is technically sophisticated. The goal of transition in health care for young adults with special health care needs is to maximize lifelong functioning and potential through the provision of high-quality, developmentally appropriate health care services that continue uninterrupted as the individual moves from adolescence to adulthood. This consensus document has now been approved as policy by the boards of the American Academy of Pediatrics, the American Academy of Family Physicians, and the American College of Physicians-American Society of Internal Medicine. (12/02)

CLINICAL REPORT: CONSENT BY PROXY FOR NONURGENT PEDIATRIC CARE
Jan Ellen Berger, MD, MJ and Committee on Medical Liability

ABSTRACT. Minor-aged patients are often brought to the pediatrician for nonurgent acute medical care or health supervision visits by someone other than their custodial parent or guardian. These surrogates can be members of the child's extended family, such as a grandparent or aunt. In cases of divorce and remarriage, a noncustodial parent or stepparent may accompany the patient. Sometimes, children are brought for care by adults living in the home who are not biologically or legally related to the child. In some instances, a child care professional (eg, au pair, nanny) brings the pediatric patient for medical care. This report identifies common situations in which pediatricians may encounter "consent by proxy" for nonurgent medical care for minors and explains the potential for liability exposure associated with these circumstances. The report suggests practical steps that balance the need to minimize the physician's liability exposure with the patient's access to health care. Key issues to be considered when creating or updating office policies for obtaining and documenting consent by proxy are offered. (11/03)

CONSENT FOR EMERGENCY MEDICAL SERVICES FOR CHILDREN AND ADOLESCENTS
Committee on Pediatric Emergency Medicine

ABSTRACT. Pediatric patients frequently seek medical treatment in the emergency department (ED) unaccompanied by a legal guardian. Current state and federal laws and medical ethics recommendations support the ED treatment of minors with an identified emergency medical condition, regardless of consent issues. Financial reimbursement should not limit the minor patient's access to emergency medical care or result in a breach of patient confidentiality. Every clinic, office practice, and ED should develop policies and guidelines regarding consent for the treatment of minors. The physician should document all discussions of consent and attempt to seek consent for treatment from the family or legal guardian and assent from the pediatric patient. Appropriate medical care for the pediatric patient with an urgent or emergent condition should never be withheld or delayed because of problems with obtaining consent. *This statement has been endorsed by the American College of Surgeons, the Society of Pediatric Nurses, the Society of Critical Care Medicine, the American College of Emergency Physicians, the Emergency Nurses Association, and the National Association of EMS Physicians.* (3/03)

THE CONTINUED IMPORTANCE OF SUPPLEMENTAL SECURITY INCOME (SSI) FOR CHILDREN AND ADOLESCENTS WITH DISABILITIES
Committee on Children With Disabilities

ABSTRACT. In 1996, as part of the Personal Responsibility and Work Opportunity Reconciliation (Welfare Reform) Act, Congress redefined the Supplemental Security Income (SSI) definition of disability for children and removed the individual functional assessment (IFA) step from the disability determination process. As a result, an estimated 100 000 SSI child beneficiaries have lost or will lose their SSI benefits. The publicity associated with this Congressionally mandated change might also have reduced the number of families applying for SSI benefits on behalf of their children because of a widely held belief that the eligibility criteria for disability benefits are now so restrictive that almost no children are determined to be eligible. The purpose of this statement is to provide updated information about the SSI Program's disability and financial eligibility criteria and disability determination process. This statement also discusses how pediatricians can help to ensure that all eligible children receive the SSI monies and associated benefits to which they are entitled. (4/01)

CONTRACEPTION AND ADOLESCENTS
Committee on Adolescence

ABSTRACT. The risks and negative consequences of adolescent sexual intercourse are of national concern, and promoting sexual abstinence is an important goal of the American Academy of Pediatrics. In previous publications, the American Academy of Pediatrics has addressed important issues of adolescent sexuality, pregnancy, sexually transmitted diseases, and contraception. The development of new contraceptive technologies mandates a revision of this policy statement, which provides the pediatrician with an updated review of adolescent sexuality and use of contraception by adolescents and presents current guidelines for counseling adolescents on sexual activity and contraceptive methods. (11/99)

CONTROVERSIES CONCERNING VITAMIN K AND THE NEWBORN
Committee on Fetus and Newborn

ABSTRACT. Prevention of early vitamin K deficiency bleeding (VKDB) of the newborn, with onset at birth to 2 weeks of age (formerly known as classic hemorrhagic disease of the newborn), by oral or parenteral administration of vitamin K is accepted practice. In contrast, late VKDB, with onset from 2 to 12 weeks of age, is most effectively prevented by parenteral administration of vitamin K. Earlier concern regarding a possible causal association between parenteral vitamin K and childhood cancer has not been substantiated. This revised statement presents updated recommendations for the use of vitamin K in the prevention of early and late VKDB. (7/03)

COPARENT OR SECOND-PARENT ADOPTION BY SAME-SEX PARENTS
Committee on Psychosocial Aspects of Child and Family Health

ABSTRACT. Children who are born to or adopted by 1 member of a same-sex couple deserve the security of 2 legally recognized parents. Therefore, the American Academy of Pediatrics supports legislative and legal efforts to provide the possibility of adoption of the child by the second parent or coparent in these families. (2/02)

TECHNICAL REPORT: COPARENT OR SECOND-PARENT ADOPTION BY SAME-SEX PARENTS

ABSTRACT. A growing body of scientific literature demonstrates that children who grow up with 1 or 2 gay and/or lesbian parents fare as well in emotional, cognitive, social, and sexual functioning as do children whose parents are heterosexual. Children's optimal development seems to be influenced more by the nature of the relationships and interactions within the family unit than by the particular structural form it takes. (2/02)

CLINICAL REPORT: CORD BLOOD BANKING FOR POTENTIAL FUTURE TRANSPLANTATION: SUBJECT REVIEW
Task Force on Cord Blood Banking

ABSTRACT. In recent years, umbilical cord blood, which contains a large number of hematopoietic stem cells, has been used successfully for allogeneic transplantation to treat a variety of pediatric genetic, hematologic, and oncologic disorders. It is a potential alternative when autologous or allogeneic transplantation with HLA-matched marrow is unavailable for children. This advance has resulted in the establishment of not-for-profit and for-profit cord blood banking programs for autologous and allogeneic transplantation. Many issues confront institutions that wish to establish such a program. Parents also seek information from their physicians about this new modality. This document is intended to provide information to guide physicians in responding to parents' questions about cord blood banking. The document also makes recommendations about appropriate ethical and operational standards, including informed consent policies, for the institutions that operate a program. (7/99)

CORPORAL PUNISHMENT IN SCHOOLS
Committee on School Health
ABSTRACT. The American Academy of Pediatrics recommends that corporal punishment in schools be abolished in all states by law and that alternative forms of student behavior management be used. (8/00, reaffirmed 6/03)

COUNSELING THE ADOLESCENT ABOUT PREGNANCY OPTIONS
Committee on Adolescence
ABSTRACT. When consulted by a pregnant adolescent, pediatricians should be able to make a timely diagnosis and to help the adolescent understand her options and act on her decision to continue or terminate her pregnancy. Pediatricians may not impose their values on the decision-making process and should be prepared to support the adolescent in her decision or refer her to a physician who can. (5/98, reaffirmed 1/01)

COUNSELING FAMILIES WHO CHOOSE COMPLEMENTARY AND ALTERNATIVE MEDICINE FOR THEIR CHILD WITH CHRONIC ILLNESS OR DISABILITY
Committee on Children With Disabilities
ABSTRACT. The use of complementary and alternative medicine (CAM) to treat chronic illness or disability is increasing in the United States. This is especially evident among children with autism and related disorders. It may be challenging to the practicing pediatrician to distinguish among accepted biomedical treatments, unproven therapies, and alternative therapies. Moreover, there are no published guidelines regarding the use of CAM in the care of children with chronic illness or disability. To best serve the interests of children, it is important to maintain a scientific perspective, to provide balanced advice about therapeutic options, to guard against bias, and to establish and maintain a trusting relationship with families. This statement provides information and guidance for pediatricians when counseling families about CAM. (3/01)

CULTURALLY EFFECTIVE PEDIATRIC CARE: EDUCATION AND TRAINING ISSUES
Committee on Pediatric Workforce
ABSTRACT. This policy statement defines culturally effective health care and describes its importance for pediatrics. The statement also defines cultural effectiveness, cultural sensitivity, and cultural competence and describes the importance of these concepts for training in medical school, residency, and continuing medical education. The statement is based on the premise that culturally effective health care is important and that the knowledge and skills necessary for providing culturally effective health care can be taught and acquired through 1) educational courses and other formats developed with the expressed purpose of addressing cultural competence and/or cultural sensitivity, and 2) educational components on cultural competence and/or cultural sensitivity that are incorporated into medical school, residency, and continuing medical education curricula. (1/99)

DEATH OF A CHILD IN THE EMERGENCY DEPARTMENT
Committee on Pediatric Emergency Medicine and the American College of Emergency Physicians (10/02)

DEVELOPMENTAL ISSUES FOR YOUNG CHILDREN IN FOSTER CARE
Committee on Early Childhood, Adoption, and Dependent Care
ABSTRACT. Greater numbers of young children with complicated, serious physical health, mental health, or developmental problems are entering foster care during the early years when brain growth is most active. Every effort should be made to make foster care a positive experience and a healing process for the child. Threats to a child's development from abuse and neglect should be understood by all participants in the child welfare system. Pediatricians have an important role in assessing the child's needs, providing comprehensive services, and advocating on the child's behalf.

The developmental issues important for young children in foster care are reviewed, including: 1) the implications and consequences of abuse, neglect, and placement in foster care on early brain development; 2) the importance and challenges of establishing a child's attachment to caregivers; 3) the importance of considering a child's changing sense of time in all aspects of the foster care experience; and 4) the child's response to stress. Additional topics addressed relate to parental roles and kinship care, parent-child contact, permanency decision-making, and the components of comprehensive assessment and treatment of a child's development and mental health needs. (11/00)

DEVELOPMENTAL SURVEILLANCE AND SCREENING OF INFANTS AND YOUNG CHILDREN
Committee on Children With Disabilities
ABSTRACT. Early identification of children with developmental delays is important in the primary care setting. The pediatrician is the best-informed professional with whom many families have contact during the first 5 years of a child's life. Parents look to the pediatrician to be the expert not only on childhood illnesses but also on development. Early intervention services for children from birth to 3 years of age and early childhood education services for children 3 to 5 years of age are widely available for children with developmental delays or disabilities in the United States. Developmental screening instruments have improved over the years, and instruments that are accurate and easy to use in an office setting are now available to the pediatrician. This statement provides recommendations for screening infants and young children and intervening with families to identify developmental delays and disabilities. (7/01)

DIAGNOSTIC IMAGING OF CHILD ABUSE
Section on Radiology
ABSTRACT. The role of imaging in cases of child abuse is to identify the extent of physical injury when abuse occurs, as well as to elucidate all imaging findings that point to alternative diagnoses. Diagnostic imaging of child abuse is based on both advances in imaging technology, as well as a better understanding of the subject based on scientific data obtained during the past 10 years. The initial recommendation was published in *Pediatrics* (1991;87:262–264). (6/00)

DISCLOSURE OF ILLNESS STATUS TO CHILDREN AND ADOLESCENTS WITH HIV INFECTION
Committee on Pediatric AIDS

ABSTRACT. Many children with human immunodeficiency virus (HIV) infection and acquired immunodeficiency syndrome are surviving to middle childhood and adolescence. Studies suggest that children who know their HIV status have higher self-esteem than children who are unaware of their status. Parents who have disclosed the status to their children experience less depression than those who do not. This statement addresses our current knowledge and recommendations for disclosure of HIV infection status to children and adolescents. (1/99, reaffirmed 2/02)

DISTINGUISHING SUDDEN INFANT DEATH SYNDROME FROM CHILD ABUSE FATALITIES
Committee on Child Abuse and Neglect

ABSTRACT. In most cases, when a healthy infant younger than 1 year dies suddenly and unexpectedly, the cause is sudden infant death syndrome (SIDS). SIDS is more common than infanticide. Parents of SIDS victims typically are anxious to provide unlimited information to professionals involved in death investigation or research. They also want and deserve to be approached in a nonaccusatory manner. This statement provides professionals with information and guidelines to avoid distressing or stigmatizing families of SIDS victims while allowing accumulation of appropriate evidence in potential cases of death by infanticide. (2/01)

ADDENDUM: DISTINGUISHING SUDDEN INFANT DEATH SYNDROME FROM CHILD ABUSE FATALITIES
Committee on Child Abuse and Neglect (9/01)

DO NOT RESUSCITATE ORDERS IN SCHOOLS
Committee on School Health and Committee on Bioethics

ABSTRACT. Increased medical knowledge and technology have led to the survival of many children who previously would have died of a variety of conditions. As these children with continuing life-threatening problems reach school age, families, professionals, and paraprofessionals have to deal with the challenges involved in their care. Some children may be at high risk of dying while in school. When families have chosen to limit resuscitative efforts, school officials should understand the medical, emotional, and legal issues involved. (4/00, reaffirmed 6/03)

DRUGS FOR PEDIATRIC EMERGENCIES
Committee on Drugs

ABSTRACT. This statement provides current recommendations about the use of emergency drugs for acute pediatric problems that require pharmacologic intervention. At each clinical setting, physicians and other providers should evaluate drug, equipment, and training needs. The information provided here is not all-inclusive and is not intended to be appropriate to every health care setting. When possible, dosage recommendations are consistent with those in stan-

dard references, such as the *Advanced Pediatric Life Support* (APLS) and *Pediatric Advanced Life Support* (PALS) textbooks. Additional guidance is available in the manual *Emergency Medical Services for Children: The Role of the Primary Care Provider,* published by the American Academy of Pediatrics, as well as in the PALS and APLS textbooks. (1/98)

ECHOCARDIOGRAPHY IN INFANTS AND CHILDREN
Section on Cardiology

ABSTRACT. It is the intent of this statement to inform pediatric providers on the appropriate use of echocardiography. Although on-site consultation may be impossible, methods should be established to ensure timely review of echocardiograms by a pediatric cardiologist. With advances in data transmission, echocardiography information can be exchanged, in some cases eliminating the need for a costly patient transfer. By cooperating through training, education, and referral, complete and cost-effective echocardiographic services can be provided to all children. (6/97, reaffirmed 3/03)

EDUCATION OF CHILDREN WITH HUMAN IMMUNODEFICIENCY VIRUS INFECTION
Committee on Pediatric AIDS

ABSTRACT. Treatment for human immunodeficiency virus (HIV) infection has enabled more children and youths to attend school and participate in school activities. Children and youths with HIV infection should receive the same education as those with other chronic illnesses. They may require special services, including home instruction, to provide continuity of education. Confidentiality about HIV infection status should be maintained with parental consent required for disclosure. Youths also should assent or consent as is appropriate for disclosure of their diagnosis. (6/00, reaffirmed 3/03)

EMERGENCY PREPAREDNESS FOR CHILDREN WITH SPECIAL HEALTH CARE NEEDS
Committee on Pediatric Emergency Medicine

ABSTRACT. Children with special health care needs are those who have, or are at risk for, chronic physical, developmental, behavioral, or emotional conditions and who also require health and related services of a type or amount not usually required by typically developing children. Formulation of an emergency care plan has been advocated by the Emergency Medical Services for Children (EMSC) program through its Children With Special Heath Care Needs Task Force. Essential components of a program of providing care plans include use of a standardized form, a method of identifying at-risk children, completion of a data set by the child's physicians and other health care professionals, education of families, other caregivers, and health care professionals in use of the emergency plan, regular updates of the information, 24-hour access to the information by authorized emergency health care professionals, and maintenance of patient confidentiality. (10/99, reaffirmed 8/02)

ENHANCING THE RACIAL AND ETHNIC DIVERSITY OF THE PEDIATRIC WORKFORCE
Committee on Pediatric Workforce

ABSTRACT. *Purpose.* This statement seeks to increase the awareness of the importance of diversity; to encourage the incorporation of principles of cultural competence into all aspects of pediatric education, training, and practice, as exemplified by practitioners, educators, and our national leadership; and finally to identify strategies for implementing this incorporation.

Key Concepts. The increasing cultural diversity of the population has significant implications for the pediatric workforce and for the provision of pediatric health services. Diversity within the pediatric workforce will enhance the potential for pediatricians to acquire the knowledge and practice skills needed to effectively address the health and wellness needs of children and families. Support from this diversity should be integrated into all aspects of education, including providing quality education for minority students and attracting and retaining minority faculty; and should be sought through collaboration locally, regionally, and nationally with organizations and community leaders.

Anticipated Outcomes. The Policy Statement recommendations will be used to inform educators, administrators, practitioners, and others in the development of curricula, programs, and initiatives to enhance the diversity of the pediatric workforce and increase the cultural competence of practitioners. (1/00)

ENVIRONMENTAL TOBACCO SMOKE: A HAZARD TO CHILDREN
Committee on Environmental Health

ABSTRACT. Results of epidemiologic studies provide strong evidence that exposure of children to environmental tobacco smoke is associated with increased rates of lower respiratory illness and increased rates of middle ear effusion, asthma, and sudden infant death syndrome. Exposure during childhood may also be associated with development of cancer during adulthood. This statement reviews the health effects of environmental tobacco smoke on children and offers pediatricians a strategy for promoting a smoke-free environment. (4/97, reaffirmed 10/00)

ETHICAL ISSUES WITH GENETIC TESTING IN PEDIATRICS
Committee on Bioethics

ABSTRACT. Advances in genetic research promise great strides in the diagnosis and treatment of many childhood diseases. However, emerging genetic technology often enables testing and screening before the development of definitive treatment or preventive measures. In these circumstances, careful consideration must be given to testing and screening of children to ensure that use of this technology promotes the best interest of the child. This statement reviews considerations for the use of genetic technology for newborn screening, carrier testing, and testing for susceptibility to late-onset conditions. Recommendations are made promoting informed participation by parents for newborn screening and limited use of carrier testing and testing for late-onset conditions in the pediatric population. Additional research and education in this developing area of medicine are encouraged. (6/01)

ETHICS AND THE CARE OF CRITICALLY ILL INFANTS AND CHILDREN
Committee on Bioethics

ABSTRACT. The ability to provide life support to ill children who, not long ago, would have died despite medicine's best efforts challenges pediatricians and families to address profound moral questions. Our society has been divided about extending the life of some patients, especially newborns and older infants with severe disabilities. The American Academy of Pediatrics (AAP) supports individualized decision making about life-sustaining medical treatment for all children, regardless of age. These decisions should be jointly made by physicians and parents, unless good reasons require invoking established child protective services to contravene parental authority. At this time, resource allocation (rationing) decisions about which children should receive intensive care resources should be made clear and explicit in public policy, rather than be made at the bedside. (7/96, reaffirmed 10/99, 6/03)

EVALUATION AND MEDICAL TREATMENT OF THE HIV-EXPOSED INFANT
Committee on Pediatric AIDS

ABSTRACT. As a result of the expanding human immunodeficiency virus (HIV) infection epidemic and recently published recommendations for routine HIV testing with consent for all pregnant women in the United States, pediatricians are becoming increasingly involved in providing care to infants born to HIV-infected women. This article provides guidelines about counseling the parent or care giver of the infant, use of antiretroviral therapy to reduce the risk of infection in the infant, medical treatment of the HIV-exposed infant, laboratory testing to determine the infection status of the infant, laboratory monitoring of hematologic and immunologic parameters, prophylaxis for *Pneumocystis carinii* pneumonia, and recommendations for immunizations and tuberculosis screening. (6/97)

EVALUATION OF THE NEWBORN WITH DEVELOPMENTAL ANOMALIES OF THE EXTERNAL GENITALIA
Committee on Genetics, Section on Endocrinology, and Section on Urology

ABSTRACT. The newborn with abnormal genital development presents a difficult diagnostic and treatment challenge for the primary care pediatrician. It is important that a definitive diagnosis be determined as quickly as possible so that an appropriate treatment plan can be established to minimize medical, psychological, and social complications. The purpose of this review is to identify which newborns among those with abnormal genital development need to be screened for intersexuality, to outline the investigations necessary, and to suggest indications for referral to a center with experience in the diagnosis and management of these disorders. An outline is also presented of the embryology of the external genitalia indicating where errors can arise to provide a framework for pediatricians to use when counseling families. Although the focus of this review is on newborns with what has been termed "ambiguous genitalia," it should be recognized that most genital abnormalities in newborns do not result in an ambiguous appearance. These anomalies include hypospadias, in which the genitalia are clearly malformed, although the sex is unquestionably male. (7/00)

EVALUATION AND PREPARATION OF PEDIATRIC PATIENTS UNDERGOING ANESTHESIA
Section on Anesthesiology and Pain Medicine (9/96)

EYE EXAMINATION IN INFANTS, CHILDREN, AND YOUNG ADULTS BY PEDIATRICIANS
Committee on Practice and Ambulatory Medicine, Section on Ophthalmology, American Association of Certified Orthoptists, American Association for Pediatric Ophthalmology and Strabismus and American Academy of Ophthalmology

ABSTRACT. Early detection and prompt treatment of ocular disorders in children is important to avoid lifelong visual impairment. Examination of the eyes should be performed beginning in the newborn period and at all well-child visits. Newborns should be examined for ocular structural abnormalities, such as cataract, corneal opacity, and ptosis, which are known to result in visual problems. Vision assessment beginning at birth has been endorsed by the American Academy of Pediatrics, the American Association for Pediatric Ophthalmology and Strabismus, and the American Academy of Ophthalmology. All children who are found to have an ocular abnormality or who fail vision assessment should be referred to a pediatric ophthalmologist or an eye care specialist appropriately trained to treat pediatric patients. (4/03)

CLINICAL REPORT: FACILITIES AND EQUIPMENT FOR THE CARE OF PEDIATRIC PATIENTS IN A COMMUNITY HOSPITAL
Ted D. Sigrest, MD, and the Committee on Hospital Care

ABSTRACT. Many children who require hospitalization are admitted to community hospitals that are more accessible for families and their primary care physicians but vary substantially in their pediatric resources. The intent of this clinical report is to provide basic guidelines for furnishing and equipping a pediatric area in a community hospital. (5/03)

FALLS FROM HEIGHTS: WINDOWS, ROOFS, AND BALCONIES
Committee on Injury and Poison Prevention

ABSTRACT. Falls of all kinds represent an important cause of child injury and death. In the United States, approximately 140 deaths from falls occur annually in children younger than 15 years. Three million children require emergency department care for fall-related injuries. This policy statement examines the epidemiology of falls from heights and recommends preventive strategies for pediatricians and other child health care professionals. Such strategies involve parent counseling, community programs, building code changes, legislation, and environmental modification, such as the installation of window guards and balcony railings. (5/01)

CLINICAL REPORT: FAMILIES AND ADOPTION: THE PEDIATRICIAN'S ROLE IN SUPPORTING COMMUNICATION
Deborah Borchers, MD, and Committee on Early Childhood, Adoption, and Dependent Care

ABSTRACT. Each year, more children join families through adoption. Pediatricians have an important role in assisting adoptive families in the various challenges they may face with respect to adoption. The acceptance of the differences between families formed through birth and those formed through adoption is essential in promoting positive emotional growth within the family. It is important for pediatricians to be informed about adoption and to share this knowledge with adoptive families. Parents need ongoing advice with respect to adoption issues and need to be supported in their communication with their adopted children. (12/03)

FAMILY-CENTERED CARE AND THE PEDIATRICIAN'S ROLE
Committee on Hospital Care

ABSTRACT. Drawing on several decades of work with families, pediatricians, other health care professionals, and policy makers, the American Academy of Pediatrics provides a definition of family-centered care. In pediatrics, family-centered care is based on the understanding that the family is the child's primary source of strength and support. Further, this approach to care recognizes that the perspectives and information provided by families, children, and young adults are important in clinical decision making. This policy statement outlines the core principles of family-centered care, summarizes the recent literature linking family-centered care to improved health outcomes, and lists various other benefits to be expected when engaging in family-centered pediatric practice. The statement concludes with specific recommendations for how pediatricians can integrate family-centered care in hospitals, clinics, and community settings as well as in more broad systems of care. (9/03)

FEMALE GENITAL MUTILATION
Committee on Bioethics

ABSTRACT. The traditional custom of ritual cutting and alteration of the genitalia of female infants, girls, and adolescents, referred to as female genital mutilation (FGM), persists primarily in Africa and among certain communities in the Middle East and Asia. Immigrants in the United States from areas where FGM is endemic may have daughters who have undergone a ritual genital procedure or may request that such a procedure be performed by a physician. The American Academy of Pediatrics (AAP) believes that pediatricians and pediatric surgical specialists should be aware that this practice has serious, life-threatening health risks for children and women. The AAP opposes all forms of FGM, counsels its members not to perform such ritual procedures, and encourages the development of community educational programs for immigrant populations. (7/98, reaffirmed 11/02)

FETAL ALCOHOL SYNDROME AND ALCOHOL-RELATED NEURODEVELOPMENTAL DISORDERS
Committee on Substance Abuse and Committee on Children With Disabilities

ABSTRACT. Prenatal exposure to alcohol is one of the leading preventable causes of birth defects, mental retardation, and neurodevelopmental disorders. In 1973, a cluster of birth defects resulting from prenatal alcohol exposure was recognized as a clinical entity called *fetal alcohol syndrome.* More recently, alcohol exposure in utero has been linked to a variety of other neurodevelopmental problems, and the terms *alcohol-related neurodevelopmental disorder* and *alcohol-related birth defects* have been proposed to identify infants so affected. This statement is an update of a previous statement by the American Academy of Pediatrics and reflects the current thinking about alcohol exposure in utero and the revised nosology. (8/00)

FETAL THERAPY—ETHICAL CONSIDERATIONS
Committee on Bioethics

ABSTRACT. Decisions to undertake fetal therapy involve a complex assessment of the best interests of the fetus and a pregnant woman's interest in her own health and freedom from unwanted invasion of her body. Pregnant women almost always accept a recommendation for fetal therapy that is approached collaboratively, especially if the therapy is of proven efficacy and has a low maternal risk. Fetal therapy of unproven efficacy should only be undertaken as part of an approved research protocol. In recommending fetal therapy of proven efficacy, physicians should respect maternal choice and assessment of risk. Under limited circumstances when fetal therapy would be effective in preventing irrevocable and substantial fetal harm with negligible risk to the health and well-being of the pregnant woman, should the pregnant woman be opposed to the intervention, physicians should engage in a process of communication and conflict resolution that may require consultation from an ethics committee and, in rare cases, require judicial review. A physician should never intervene without the woman's explicit consent before judicial review. (5/99, reaffirmed 11/02)

FIREARM-RELATED INJURIES AFFECTING THE PEDIATRIC POPULATION
Committee on Injury and Poison Prevention

ABSTRACT. This statement reaffirms the 1992 position of the American Academy of Pediatrics that the absence of guns from children's homes and communities is the most reliable and effective measure to prevent firearm-related injuries in children and adolescents. A number of specific measures are supported to reduce the destructive effects of guns in the lives of children and adolescents, including the regulation of the manufacture, sale, purchase, ownership, and use of firearms; a ban on handguns and semiautomatic assault weapons; and expanded regulations of handguns for civilian use. In addition, this statement reviews recent data, trends, prevention, and intervention strategies of the past 5 years. (4/00)

FIREWORKS-RELATED INJURIES TO CHILDREN
Committee on Injury and Poison Prevention

ABSTRACT. An estimated 8500 individuals, approximately 45% of them children younger than 15 years, were treated in US hospital emergency departments during 1999 for fireworks-related injuries. The hands (40%), eyes (20%), and head and face (20%) are the body areas most often involved. Approximately one third of eye injuries from fireworks result in permanent blindness. During 1999, 16 people died as a result of injuries associated with fireworks. Every type of legally available consumer (so-called "safe and sane") firework has been associated with serious injury or death. In 1997, 20 100 fires were caused by fireworks, resulting in $22.7 million in direct property damage. Fireworks typically cause more fires in the United States on the Fourth of July than all other causes of fire combined on that day. Pediatricians should educate parents, children, community leaders, and others about the dangers of fireworks. Fireworks for individual private use should be banned. Children and their families should be encouraged to enjoy fireworks at public fireworks displays conducted by professionals rather than purchase fireworks for home or private use. (7/01)

FOLIC ACID FOR THE PREVENTION OF NEURAL TUBE DEFECTS
Committee on Genetics

ABSTRACT. The American Academy of Pediatrics endorses the US Public Health Service (USPHS) recommendation that all women capable of becoming pregnant consume 400 µg of folic acid daily to prevent neural tube defects (NTDs). Studies have demonstrated that periconceptional folic acid supplementation can prevent 50% or more of NTDs such as spina bifida and anencephaly. For women who have previously had an NTD-affected pregnancy, the Centers for Disease Control and Prevention (CDC) recommends increasing the intake of folic acid to 4000 µg per day beginning at least 1 month before conception and continuing through the first trimester. Implementation of these recommendations is essential for the primary prevention of these serious and disabling birth defects. Because fewer than 1 in 3 women consume the amount of folic acid recommended by the USPHS, the Academy notes that the prevention of NTDs depends on an urgent and effective campaign to close this prevention gap. (8/99, reaffirmed 11/02)

FOLLOW-UP MANAGEMENT OF CHILDREN WITH TYMPANOSTOMY TUBES
Section on Otolaryngology and Bronchoesophagology

ABSTRACT. The follow-up care of children in whom tympanostomy tubes have been placed is shared by the pediatrician and the otolaryngologist. Guidelines are provided for routine follow-up evaluation, perioperative hearing assessment, and the identification of specific conditions and complications that warrant urgent otolaryngologic consultation. These guidelines have been developed by a consensus of expert opinions. (2/02)

FORGOING LIFE-SUSTAINING MEDICAL TREATMENT IN ABUSED CHILDREN
Committee on Child Abuse and Neglect and Committee on Bioethics

ABSTRACT. A decision to forgo life-sustaining medical treatment (LSMT) for a critically ill child injured as the result of abuse should be made using the same criteria as those used for any critically ill child. The parent or guardian of an abused child may have a conflict of interest when a decision to forgo LSMT risks changing the legal charge faced by a parent, guardian, relative, or acquaintance from assault to manslaughter or homicide. If a physician suspects that a parent or guardian is not acting in a child's best interest, further review and consultation should be sought in hopes of resolving the conflict. A guardian ad litem who will represent the child's interests regarding LSMT should be appointed in all cases in which a parent or guardian may have a conflict of interest. (11/00, reaffirmed 6/03)

GENERAL PRINCIPLES IN THE CARE OF CHILDREN AND ADOLESCENTS WITH GENETIC DISORDERS AND OTHER CHRONIC HEALTH CONDITIONS
Committee on Children With Disabilities

ABSTRACT. The intent of this statement is to describe the breadth of issues that have special pertinence to pediatricians who care for children and families affected by genetic disorders and other chronic health conditions. The Committee on Children With Disabilities believes that because these children are leading healthier and longer lives, pediatricians are the more highly qualified to serve them, by virtue of their training and experience, and to provide them a "medical home." This statement is designed to assist pediatricians in the treatment of these patients by describing their potential roles in relationship to their patients' changing needs, as they work with various members of the health care team and as they respond to the requirements of government agencies and various third-party payers. (4/97, reaffirmed 4/00)

GENERIC PRESCRIBING, GENERIC SUBSTITUTION, AND THERAPEUTIC SUBSTITUTION
Committee on Drugs (5/87, reaffirmed 6/93, 5/96, 6/99, 5/01)

GIFTS TO PHYSICIANS FROM INDUSTRY
American Medical Association (8/01)

GONORRHEA IN PREPUBERTAL CHILDREN
Committee on Child Abuse and Neglect

ABSTRACT. This statement updates a 1983 statement on this topic and reminds physicians that sexual abuse should be strongly considered when a gonorrheal infection is diagnosed in a child after the newborn period and before the onset of puberty. (1/98, reaffirmed 10/01)

GRADUATE MEDICAL EDUCATION AND PEDIATRIC WORKFORCE ISSUES AND PRINCIPLES
Task Force on Graduate Medical Education Reform (6/94)

GUIDANCE FOR EFFECTIVE DISCIPLINE
Committee on Psychosocial Aspects of Child and Family Health

ABSTRACT. When advising families about discipline strategies, pediatricians should use a comprehensive approach that includes consideration of the parent-child relationship, reinforcement of desired behaviors, and consequences for negative behaviors. Corporal punishment is of limited effectiveness and has potentially deleterious side effects. The American Academy of Pediatrics recommends that parents be encouraged and assisted in the development of methods other than spanking for managing undesired behavior. (4/98)

GUIDELINES FOR THE ADMINISTRATION OF MEDICATION IN SCHOOL
Committee on School Health

ABSTRACT. Many children who take medications require them during the school day. This policy statement is designed to guide prescribing physicians as well as school administrators and health staff on the administration of medications to children at school. The statement addresses over-the-counter products, herbal medications, experimental drugs that are administered as part of a clinical trial, emergency medications, and principles of student safety. (9/03)

GUIDELINES FOR DEVELOPING ADMISSION AND DISCHARGE POLICIES FOR THE PEDIATRIC INTENSIVE CARE UNIT
Committee on Hospital Care, Section on Critical Care, and the Society of Critical Care Medicine, Pediatric Section Admission Criteria Task Force

ABSTRACT. These guidelines were developed to provide a reference for preparing policies on admission to and discharge from pediatric intensive care units. They represent a consensus opinion of physicians, nurses, and allied health care professionals. By using this document as a framework for developing multidisciplinary admission and discharge policies, use of pediatric intensive care units can be optimized and patients can receive the level of care appropriate for their condition. (4/99)

GUIDELINES FOR EMERGENCY MEDICAL CARE IN SCHOOL
Committee on School Health

ABSTRACT. Minor and major illnesses and injuries can occur in children during the school day. This statement provides recommendations for emergency health care for children in school, including information about procedures, staff and their education, documentation, and parental notification. (2/01)

GUIDELINES FOR THE ETHICAL CONDUCT OF STUDIES TO EVALUATE DRUGS IN PEDIATRIC POPULATIONS
Committee on Drugs (2/95, reaffirmed 3/98, 5/01)

CLINICAL REPORT: GUIDELINES FOR THE EVALUATION OF SEXUAL ABUSE OF CHILDREN: SUBJECT REVIEW
Committee on Child Abuse and Neglect

ABSTRACT. This statement serves to update guidelines for the evaluation of child sexual abuse first published in 1991. The role of the physician is outlined with respect to obtaining a history, physical examination, and appropriate laboratory data and in determining the need to report sexual abuse. (1/99)

GUIDELINES FOR EXPERT WITNESS TESTIMONY IN MEDICAL MALPRACTICE LITIGATION
Committee on Medical Liability

ABSTRACT. The interests of the public and the medical profession are best served when scientifically sound and unbiased expert witness testimony is readily available to plaintiffs and defendants in medical negligence suits. As members of the physician community, as patient advocates, and as private citizens, pediatricians have ethical and professional obligations to assist in the administration of justice, particularly in matters concerning potential medical malpractice. The American Academy of Pediatrics believes that the adoption of the recommendations outlined in this statement will improve the quality of medical expert witness testimony in such proceedings and thereby increase the probability of achieving equitable outcomes. Strategies to enforce ethical guidelines should be monitored for efficacy before offering policy recommendations on disciplining physicians for providing biased, false, or unscientific medical expert witness testimony. (5/02)

GUIDELINES ON FORGOING LIFE-SUSTAINING MEDICAL TREATMENT
Committee on Bioethics (3/94, reaffirmed 11/97, 10/00)

GUIDELINES FOR HOME CARE OF INFANTS, CHILDREN, AND ADOLESCENTS WITH CHRONIC DISEASE
Committee on Children With Disabilities (7/95, reaffirmed 4/00)

GUIDELINES AND LEVELS OF CARE FOR PEDIATRIC INTENSIVE CARE UNITS
Committee on Hospital Care and Pediatric Section of the Society of Critical Care Medicine (7/93, reaffirmed 11/96)

GUIDELINES FOR MONITORING AND MANAGEMENT OF PEDIATRIC PATIENTS DURING AND AFTER SEDATION FOR DIAGNOSTIC AND THERAPEUTIC PROCEDURES
Committee on Drugs (6/92, reaffirmed 6/95, 6/98, 5/02)

GUIDELINES FOR MONITERING AND MANAGEMENT OF PEDIATRIC PATIENTS DURING AND AFTER SEDATION FOR DIAGNOSTIC AND THERAPEUTIC PROCEDURES: ADDENDUM
Committee on Drugs
ABSTRACT. The purpose of this addendum to the 1992 policy statement is to clarify some of the terms used in that document and to more thoroughly delineate the responsibilities of the practitioner when sedating children. (10/02)

GUIDELINES FOR OPHTHALMOLOGIC EXAMINATIONS IN CHILDREN WITH JUVENILE RHEUMATOID ARTHRITIS
Section on Ophthalmology and Section on Rheumatology (8/93, reaffirmed 8/99)

GUIDELINES FOR THE PEDIATRIC CANCER CENTER AND ROLE OF SUCH CENTERS IN DIAGNOSIS AND TREATMENT
Section on Hematology-Oncology
ABSTRACT. The intent of this statement is to delineate those personnel and facilities that are essential to provide state-of-the-art care for children and adolescents with cancer. This statement emphasizes the importance of a board-eligible or board-certified pediatric hematologist-oncologist and pediatric subspecialty consultants overseeing the care of all pediatric and adolescent cancer patients, and the need for facilities available only at a tertiary center as essential for the initial management and much of the follow-up for pediatric and adolescent cancer patients. In 1986, the Section on Oncology/Hematology of the American Academy of Pediatrics outlined the "Guidelines for the Pediatric Cancer Center and Role of Such Centers in Diagnosis and Treatment." Since that statement was published, significant changes in medical care reimbursement have prompted a review of the role of tertiary medical centers in the care of pediatric patients. The potential impact of these developments on the treatment of children with cancer led to a revision of the previous statement with the goal of delineating those elements that are necessary to ensure that current childhood cancer survival rates are not adversely impacted by requirements for care to be given at sites lacking essential personnel or equipment. (1/97)

GUIDELINES FOR PEDIATRIC CARDIOVASCULAR CENTERS
Section on Cardiology and Cardiac Surgery
ABSTRACT. Pediatric cardiovascular centers should aim to provide high-quality therapeutic outcomes for infants and children with congenital and acquired heart diseases. This policy statement describes critical elements and organizational features of centers in which high-quality outcomes have the greatest likelihood of occurring. Center elements include noninvasive diagnostic modalities, cardiac catheterization, cardiovascular surgery, and cardiovascular intensive care. These elements should be organizationally united in centers in which pediatric cardiac physician specialists and specialized pediatric staff work together to achieve and surpass existing quality-of-care benchmarks. (3/02)

GUIDELINES FOR PEDIATRIC EMERGENCY CARE FACILITIES
Committee on Pediatric Emergency Medicine (9/95, reaffirmed 10/98, 12/00)

GUIDELINES FOR THE PEDIATRIC PERIOPERATIVE ANESTHESIA ENVIRONMENT
Section on Anesthesiology and Pain Medicine
ABSTRACT. The American Academy of Pediatrics proposes the following guidelines for the pediatric perioperative anesthesia environment. Essential components are identified that make the perioperative environment satisfactory for the anesthesia care of infants and children. Such an environment promotes the safety and well-being of infants and children by reducing the risk for adverse events. (2/99, reaffirmed 10/02)

GUIDELINES FOR REFERRAL TO PEDIATRIC SURGICAL SPECIALISTS
Surgical Advisory Panel (7/02)

GUIDING PRINCIPLES, ATTRIBUTES, AND PROCESS TO REVIEW MEDICAL MANAGEMENT GUIDELINES
Task Force on Medical Management Guidelines
ABSTRACT. Few issues are more central to the ongoing debate about health care in the United States than concerns about cost and quality of medical care. The recent development and implementation of medical management guidelines that include recommendations for diagnostic and therapeutic interventions, hospital length of stay, intensity of service, home care, and access to specialists have often focused this debate on the potential trade-off between cost reductions and quality of care. The American Academy of Pediatrics recognizes that cost and quality are integrally related and that it is possible to reduce costs while maintaining and improving quality. The purpose of this statement is to help pediatricians and other health care providers interpret, evaluate, and improve medical management guidelines. (12/01)

GUIDING PRINCIPLES FOR MANAGED CARE ARRANGEMENTS FOR THE HEALTH CARE OF NEWBORNS, INFANTS, CHILDREN, ADOLESCENTS, AND YOUNG ADULTS
Committee on Child Health Financing
ABSTRACT. By including the precepts of primary care in the delivery of services, managed care can be a tool to increase access to a full range of health care clinicians and services. On the other hand, managed care can result in underutilization of appropriate services and reduced quality of care. Therefore, the American Academy of Pediatrics urges the use of the principles outlined in this statement in designing and implementing managed care for newborns, infants, children, adolescents, and young adults for several reasons. This policy statement replaces the 1995 policy statement, "Guiding Principles for Managed Care Arrangements for the Health Care of Infants, Children, Adolescents and Young Adults," and outlines the key principles of managed care for newborns, infants, children, adolescents, and young adults. (1/00)

THE HAZARDS OF CHILD LABOR
Committee on Environmental Health (2/95, reaffirmed 11/98)

CLINICAL REPORT: HEAD LICE
Committee on Infectious Diseases and Committee on School Health
ABSTRACT. Head lice infestation is associated with little morbidity but causes a high level of anxiety among parents of school-aged children. This statement attempts to clarify issues of diagnosis and treatment of head lice and makes recommendations for dealing with head lice in the school setting. (9/02)

HEALTH APPRAISAL GUIDELINES FOR DAY CAMPS AND RESIDENT CAMPS
Committee on School Health
ABSTRACT. The American Academy of Pediatrics recommends that specific guidelines be established for pre-camp health appraisals of young people in day and resident camps. Camp guidelines also should include reference to health maintenance, storage and administration of medication, and emergency medical services.

Although camps have diverse environments, there are general guidelines that apply to all situations, and specific recommendations are appropriate under special conditions. (3/00)

HEALTH CARE FOR CHILDREN AND ADOLESCENTS IN THE JUVENILE CORRECTIONAL CARE SYSTEM
Committee on Adolescence
ABSTRACT. Over the past decade, there has been a dramatic increase in the population of juvenile offenders in the United States. Juveniles detained or confined in correctional care facilities have been shown to have numerous health problems. Such conditions may have existed before incarceration; may be closely associated with legal problems; may have resulted from parental neglect, mental health disorders, or physical, drug, or sexual abuse; or may develop within the institutional environment. Delinquent youths are often disenfranchised from traditional health care services in the community. For these adolescents, health care provided through correctional services may be their major source of health services. Pediatricians and correctional health care systems have an opportunity and responsibility to help improve the health of this underserved and vulnerable group of adolescents. (4/01)

HEALTH CARE SUPERVISION FOR CHILDREN WITH WILLIAMS SYNDROME
Committee on Genetics
ABSTRACT. This set of guidelines is designed to assist the pediatrician to care for children with Williams syndrome diagnosed by clinical features and with regional chromosomal microdeletion confirmed by fluorescence in situ hybridization. (5/01)

HEALTH CARE OF YOUNG CHILDREN IN FOSTER CARE
Committee on Early Childhood, Adoption, and Dependent Care
ABSTRACT. Greater numbers of infants and young children with increasingly complicated and serious physical, mental health, and developmental problems are being placed in foster care. All children in foster care need to receive initial health screenings and comprehensive assessments of their medical, mental, dental health, and developmental status. Results of these assessments must be included in the court-approved social services plan and should be linked to the provision of individualized comprehensive care that is continuous and part of a medical home. Pediatricians have an important role in all aspects of the foster care system. (3/02)

HEALTH SUPERVISION FOR CHILDREN WITH ACHONDROPLASIA
Committee on Genetics (3/95, reaffirmed 10/98)

HEALTH SUPERVISION FOR CHILDREN WITH DOWN SYNDROME
Committee on Genetics
ABSTRACT. These guidelines are designed to assist the pediatrician in caring for the child in whom the diagnosis of Down syndrome has been confirmed by karyotype. Although the pediatrician's initial contact with the child is usually during infancy, occasionally the pregnant woman who has been given the prenatal diagnosis of Down syndrome will be referred for counseling. Therefore, these guidelines offer advice for this situation as well. (2/01)

HEALTH SUPERVISION FOR CHILDREN WITH FRAGILE X SYNDROME
Committee on Genetics (8/96, reaffirmed 10/99)

HEALTH SUPERVISION FOR CHILDREN WITH MARFAN SYNDROME
Committee on Genetics
ABSTRACT. This set of guidelines is designed to assist the pediatrician in caring for children with Marfan syndrome confirmed by clinical criteria. Although pediatricians usually first see children with Marfan syndrome during infancy, occasionally they will be called on to advise the pregnant woman who has been informed of the prenatal diagnosis of Marfan syndrome. Therefore, these guidelines offer advice for this situation as well. (11/96, reaffirmed 10/99, 10/02)

HEALTH SUPERVISION FOR CHILDREN WITH NEUROFIBROMATOSIS
Committee on Genetics (8/95, reaffirmed 10/98)

HEALTH SUPERVISION FOR CHILDREN WITH SICKLE CELL DISEASE
Section on Hematology/Oncology and Committee on Genetics
ABSTRACT. Sickle cell disease (SCD) is a group of complex genetic disorders with multisystem manifestations. This statement provides pediatricians in primary care and subspecialty practice with an overview of the genetics, diagnosis, clinical manifestations, and treatment of SCD. Specialized comprehensive medical care decreases morbidity and mortality during childhood. The provision of comprehensive care is a time-intensive endeavor that includes ongoing patient and family education, periodic comprehensive evaluations and other disease-specific health maintenance services, psychosocial care, and genetic counseling. Timely and appropriate treatment of acute illness is critical, because life-threatening complications develop rapidly. It is essential that every child with SCD receive comprehensive care that is coordinated through a medical home with appropriate expertise. (3/02)

CLINICAL REPORT: HEALTH SUPERVISION FOR CHILDREN WITH TURNER SYNDROME
Jaime L. Frías, MD, Marsha L. Davenport, MD, the
*   Committee on Genetics, and the Section on Endocrinology*
ABSTRACT. This report is designed to assist the pediatrician in caring for the child in whom the diagnosis of Turner syndrome has been confirmed by karyotyping. The report is meant to serve as a supplement to the American Academy of Pediatrics' "Recommendations for Preventive Pediatric Health Care" and emphasizes the importance of continuity of care and the need to avoid its fragmentation by ensuring a medical home for every girl with Turner syndrome. The pediatrician's first contact with a child with Turner syndrome may occur during infancy or childhood. This report also discusses interactions with expectant parents who have been given the prenatal diagnosis of Turner syndrome and have been referred for advice. (3/03)

CLINICAL REPORT: HEARING ASSESSMENT IN INFANTS AND CHILDREN: RECOMMENDATIONS BEYOND NEONATAL SCREENING
Michael Cunningham, MD and Edward O. Cox, MD the
*   Committee on Practice and Ambulatory Medicine and the*
*   Section on Otolaryngology and Bronchoesophagology*
ABSTRACT. Congenital or acquired hearing loss in infants and children has been linked with lifelong deficits in speech and language acquisition, poor academic performance, personal-social maladjustments, and emotional difficulties. Identification of hearing loss through neonatal hearing screening as well as objective hearing screening of all infants and children can prevent or reduce many of these adverse consequences. This report outlines the risk indicators for hearing loss, provides guidance for when and how to assess hearing loss, and addresses hearing referral resources for children of all ages. (2/03)

CLINICAL REPORT: HELPING CHILDREN AND FAMILIES DEAL WITH DIVORCE AND SEPARATION
Committee on Psychosocial Aspects of Child and Family Health
ABSTRACT. More than 1 million children each year experience their parents' divorce. For these children and their parents, this process can be emotionally traumatic from the beginning of parental disagreement and rancor, through the divorce, and often for many years thereafter. Pediatricians are encouraged to be aware of behavioral changes in their patients that might be signals of family dysfunction so they can help parents and children understand and deal more positively with the issue. Age-appropriate explanation and counseling is important so children realize that they are not the cause of, and cannot be the cure for, the divorce. Pediatricians can offer families guidance in dealing with their children through the troubled time as well as appropriate lists of reading material and, if indicated, can refer them to professionals with expertise in the emotional, social, and legal aspects of divorce and its aftermath. (11/02)

HEPATITIS C VIRUS INFECTION
Committee on Infectious Diseases
ABSTRACT. Hepatitis C virus (HCV) has become the most significant cause of chronic liver disease of infectious etiology in the United States. The recognition that HCV can be transmitted perinatally or through blood transfusions warrants particular attention by the pediatrician. The American Academy of Pediatrics recommends screening infants born to HCV-infected mothers and persons with risk factors for HCV infection such as injection drug use, transfusion of ≥1 U of blood or blood products before 1992, or hemodialysis should be screened for anti-HCV. Also, persons who received clotting factor concentrates before 1987, when effective inactivation procedures were introduced, also should be screened. Guidelines for counseling families of HCV-infected children are provided. (3/98)

HOME, HOSPITAL, AND OTHER NON–SCHOOL-BASED INSTRUCTION FOR CHILDREN AND ADOLESCENTS WHO ARE MEDICALLY UNABLE TO ATTEND SCHOOL
Committee on School Health
ABSTRACT. The American Academy of Pediatrics recommends that school-aged children and adolescents obtain their education in school in the least restrictive setting, that is, the setting most conducive to learning for the particular student. However, at times, acute illness or injury and chronic medical conditions preclude school attendance. This statement is meant to assist evaluation and planning for children to receive non–school-based instruction and to return to school at the earliest possible date. (11/00, reaffirmed 6/03)

HOMOSEXUALITY AND ADOLESCENCE
Committee on Adolescence (10/93, reaffirmed 11/96)

HORSEBACK RIDING AND HEAD INJURIES
Committee on Sports Medicine and Fitness (3/92, reaffirmed 5/98)

HOSPITAL DISCHARGE OF THE HIGH-RISK NEONATE—PROPOSED GUIDELINES
Committee on Fetus and Newborn

ABSTRACT. This policy statement is the first formal statement of the American Academy of Pediatrics on the issue of hospital discharge of the high-risk neonate. It has been developed, to the extent possible, on the basis of published, scientifically derived information. Four categories of high risk are identified: 1) the preterm infant, 2) the infant who requires technological support, 3) the infant primarily at risk because of family issues, and 4) the infant whose irreversible condition will result in an early death. The unique home care issues for each are reviewed within a common framework. Recommendations are given for four areas of readiness for hospital discharge: infant, home care planning, family and home environment, and the community and health care system. The need for individualized planning and physician judgment is emphasized. (8/98, reaffirmed 6/01)

THE HOSPITAL RECORD OF THE INJURED CHILD AND THE NEED FOR EXTERNAL CAUSE-OF-INJURY CODES
Committee on Injury and Poison Prevention

ABSTRACT. Proper record-keeping of emergency department visits and hospitalizations of injured children is vital for appropriate patient management. Determination and documentation of the circumstances surrounding the injury event are essential. This information not only is the basis for preventive counseling, but also provides clues about how similar injuries in other youth can be avoided. The hospital records have an important secondary purpose; namely, if sufficient information about the cause and mechanism of injury is documented, it can be subsequently coded, electronically compiled, and retrieved later to provide an epidemiologic profile of the injury, the first step in prevention at the population level. To be of greatest use, hospital records should indicate the "who, what, when, where, why, and how" of the injury occurrence and whether protective equipment (eg, a seat belt) was used. The pediatrician has two important roles in this area: to document fully the injury event and to advocate the use of standardized external cause-of-injury codes, which allow such data to be compiled and analyzed. (2/99, reaffirmed 5/02)

HOSPITAL STAY FOR HEALTHY TERM NEWBORNS
Committee on Fetus and Newborn (10/95, reaffirmed 10/98)

HOW PEDIATRICIANS CAN RESPOND TO THE PSYCHO-SOCIAL IMPLICATIONS OF DISASTERS
Committee on Psychosocial Aspects of Child and Family Health

ABSTRACT. Natural and human-caused disasters, violence with weapons, and terrorist acts have touched directly the lives of thousands of families with children in the United States. Media coverage of disasters has brought images of floods, hurricanes, and airplane crashes into the living rooms of most American families, with limited censorship for vulnerable young children. Therefore, children may be exposed to disastrous events in ways that previous generations never or rarely experienced. Pediatricians should serve as important resources to the community in preparing for disasters, as well as acting in its behalf during and after such events. (2/99)

HUMAN EMBRYO RESEARCH
Committee on Pediatric Research and Committee on Bioethics

ABSTRACT. In 1996, a ban on the use of US Department of Health and Human Services funds for research on the creation of human embryos and research that involved the injury or destruction of human embryos was signed into law. This ban was partially reversed in 2000 when the National Institutes of Health announced it would fund selective research on human pluripotent stem cells. Given the potential benefits to society, research using human embryos is an issue that deserves additional consideration. The American Academy of Pediatrics believes that, under certain conditions, research using human embryos and pluripotent stem cells is of sufficient scientific importance that the National Institutes of Health should fund it and that federal oversight is morally preferable to the currently unregulated private sector approach. (9/01)

HUMAN IMMUNODEFICIENCY VIRUS/ACQUIRED IMMUNODEFICIENCY SYNDROME EDUCATION IN SCHOOLS
Committee on Pediatric AIDS

ABSTRACT. The human immunodeficiency virus (HIV)/acquired immunodeficiency syndrome (AIDS) epidemic has grown during the past 15 years. Education remains a critical component of our efforts to prevent HIV infection/AIDS in school children and young adults. To accomplish this goal, school personnel should receive updated information about HIV infection/AIDS so that accurate teaching on this topic can be included in the K-12 health education curriculum. Informed pediatricians and nurses can serve as important resources for school health services and administration to provide current information for the curriculum. Each community should have a school health advisory committee that enlists community support and provides input to health education programs in schools. (5/98, reaffirmed 6/01)

HUMAN IMMUNODEFICIENCY VIRUS AND OTHER BLOOD-BORNE VIRAL PATHOGENS IN THE ATHLETIC SETTING
Committee on Sports Medicine and Fitness

ABSTRACT. Because athletes and the staff of athletic programs can be exposed to blood during athletic activity, they have a very small risk of becoming infected with human immunodeficiency virus, hepatitis B virus, or hepatitis C virus. This statement, which updates a previous position statement of the American Academy of Pediatrics, discusses sports participation for athletes infected with these pathogens and the precautions needed to reduce the risk of infection to others in the athletic setting. Each of the recommendations in this statement is dependent upon and intended to be considered with reference to the other recommendations in this statement and not in isolation. (12/99)

HUMAN IMMUNODEFICIENCY VIRUS SCREENING
Committee on Fetus and Newborn, Committee on Pediatric AIDS, and American College of Obstetricians and Gynecologists (7/99, reaffirmed 6/02)

TECHNICAL REPORT: HUMAN MILK, BREASTFEEDING, AND TRANSMISSION OF HUMAN IMMUNODEFICIENCY VIRUS TYPE 1 IN THE UNITED STATES

Jennifer S. Read, MD, MS, MPH, DTM&H, and the Committee on Pediatric AIDS

ABSTRACT. Transmission of human immunodeficiency virus type 1 (HIV-1) through breastfeeding has been conclusively demonstrated. The risk of such transmission has been quantified, the timing has been clarified, and certain risk factors for breastfeeding transmission have been identified. In areas where infant formula is accessible, affordable, safe, and sustainable, avoidance of breastfeeding has represented one of the main components of mother-to-child HIV-1 transmission prevention efforts for many years. In areas where affordable and safe alternatives to breastfeeding may not be available, interventions to prevent breastfeeding transmission are being investigated. Complete avoidance of breastfeeding by HIV-1-infected women has been recommended by the American Academy of Pediatrics and the Centers for Disease Control and Prevention and remains the only means by which prevention of breastfeeding transmission of HIV-1 can be absolutely ensured. This technical report summarizes the information available regarding breastfeeding transmission of HIV-1. (11/03)

HYPOALLERGENIC INFANT FORMULAS

Committee on Nutrition

ABSTRACT. The American Academy of Pediatrics is committed to breastfeeding as the ideal source of nutrition for infants. For those infants who are formula-fed, either as a supplement to breastfeeding or exclusively during their infancy, it is common practice for pediatricians to change the formula when symptoms of intolerance occur. Decisions about when the formula should be changed and which formula should be used vary significantly, however, among pediatric practitioners. This statement clarifies some of these issues as they relate to protein hypersensitivity (protein allergy), one of the causes of adverse reactions to feeding during infancy. (8/00)

IDENTIFICATION AND CARE OF HIV-EXPOSED AND HIV-INFECTED INFANTS, CHILDREN, AND ADOLESCENTS IN FOSTER CARE

Committee on Pediatric AIDS

ABSTRACT. As a consequence of the expanding human immunodeficiency virus (HIV) epidemic and major advances in medical management of HIV-exposed and HIV-infected persons, revised recommendations are provided for HIV testing of infants, children, and adolescents in foster care. Updated recommendations also are provided for the care of HIV-exposed and HIV-infected persons who are in foster care. (7/00, reaffirmed 3/03)

IDENTIFYING AND TREATING EATING DISORDERS

Committee on Adolescence

ABSTRACT. Pediatricians are called on to become involved in the identification and management of eating disorders in several settings and at several critical points in the illness. In the primary care pediatrician's practice, early detection, initial evaluation, and ongoing management can play a significant role in preventing the illness from progressing to a more severe or chronic state. In the subspecialty setting, management of medical complications, provision of nutritional rehabilitation, and coordination with the psychosocial and psychiatric aspects of care are often handled by pediatricians, especially those who have experience or expertise in the care of adolescents with eating disorders. In hospital and day program settings, pediatricians are involved in program development, determining appropriate admission and discharge criteria, and provision and coordination of care. Lastly, primary care pediatricians need to be involved at local, state, and national levels in preventive efforts and in providing advocacy for patients and families. The roles of pediatricians in the management of eating disorders in the pediatric practice, subspecialty, hospital, day program, and community settings are reviewed in this statement. (1/03)

IMMUNIZATION OF ADOLESCENTS: RECOMMENDATIONS OF THE ADVISORY COMMITTEE ON IMMUNIZATION PRACTICES, THE AMERICAN ACADEMY OF PEDIATRICS, THE AMERICAN ACADEMY OF FAMILY PHYSICIANS, AND THE AMERICAN MEDICAL ASSOCIATION

Committee on Infectious Diseases

ABSTRACT. This report, concerning the immunization of adolescents (ie, persons 11 to 21 years old, as defined by the American Medical Association [AMA] and the American Academy of Pediatrics [AAP]), is a supplement to previous publications (ie, MMWR. 1994;43 [No. RR-1]1-38; the AAP *1994 Red Book: Report of the Committee on Infectious Diseases; Summary of Policy Recommendations for Periodic Health Examination*, August 1996 from the American Academy of Family Physicians [AAFP]; and AMA *Guidelines for Adolescent Preventive Services [GAPS]: Recommendations and Rationale*). This report presents a new strategy to improve the delivery of vaccination services to adolescents and to integrate recommendations for vaccination with other preventive services provided to adolescents. This new strategy emphasizes vaccination of adolescents 11 to 12 years old by establishing a routine visit to their health-care providers. Specifically, the purposes of this visit are to a) vaccinate adolescents who have not been previously vaccinated with varicella virus vaccine, hepatitis B vaccine, or the second dose of the measles, mumps, and rubella (MMR) vaccine; b) provide a booster dose of tetanus and diphtheria toxoids; c) administer other vaccines that may be recommended for certain adolescents; and d) provide other recommended preventive services. The recommendations for vaccination of adolescents are based on new or current information for each vaccine. The most recent recommendations from the Advisory Committee on Immunization Practices (ACIP), AAP, AAFP, and AMA concerning specific vaccines and delivery of preventive services should be consulted for details. (3/97)

CLINICAL REPORT: IMMUNIZATION OF PRETERM AND LOW BIRTH WEIGHT INFANTS

Thomas N. Saari, MD the Committee on Infectious Diseases

ABSTRACT. Preterm (PT) infants are at increased risk of experiencing complications of vaccine-preventable diseases but are less likely to receive immunizations on time. Medically stable PT and low birth weight (LBW) infants should receive full doses of diphtheria, tetanus, acellular pertussis, Haemophilus influenzae type b, hepatitis B, poliovirus, and pneumococcal conjugate vaccines at a chronologic age consistent with the schedule recommended for full-term infants. Infants with birth weight less than 2000 g may require modification of the timing of hepatitis B immunoprophylaxis depending on maternal hepatitis B surface antigen status. All PT and LBW infants benefit from receiving influenza vaccine beginning at 6 months of age before the beginning of and during the influenza season. All vaccines routinely recommended during infancy are safe for use in PT and LBW infants. The occurrence of mild vaccine-attributable adverse events are similar in both full-term and PT vaccine recipients. Although the immunogenicity of some childhood vaccines may be decreased in the smallest PT infants, antibody concentrations achieved usually are protective. (7/03)

IMPACT OF MUSIC LYRICS AND MUSIC VIDEOS ON CHILDREN AND YOUTH

Committee on Public Education (12/96)

IMPLEMENTATION OF THE IMMUNIZATION POLICY

Committee on Practice and Ambulatory Medicine (8/95)

IMPLEMENTATION PRINCIPLES AND STRATEGIES FOR THE STATE CHILDREN'S HEALTH INSURANCE PROGRAM

Committee on Child Health Financing

ABSTRACT. This policy statement presents principles and implementation and evaluation strategies recommended for the State Children's Health Insurance Program (SCHIP). The statement summarizes the current status of SCHIP, the needs of uninsured children, and the potential benefits of SCHIP programs. Principles and recommended strategies include expanding eligibility, maximizing funding, providing comprehensive benefits, including pediatricians in program design and evaluation, providing adequate reimbursement and access to pediatricians, ensuring choices for families and pediatricians, and establishing simple administrative procedures. (5/01)

IMPROVING SUBSTANCE ABUSE PREVENTION, ASSESSMENT, AND TREATMENT FINANCING FOR CHILDREN AND ADOLESCENTS

Committee on Child Health Financing and Committee on Substance Abuse

ABSTRACT. The numbers of children, adolescents, and families affected by substance abuse have sharply increased since the early 1990s. The American Academy of Pediatrics recognizes the scope and urgency of this problem and has developed this policy statement for consideration by Congress, federal and state agencies, employers, national organizations, health care professionals, health insurers, managed care organizations, advocacy groups, and families. (10/01)

CLINICAL REPORT: "INACTIVE" INGREDIENTS IN PHARMACEUTICAL PRODUCTS: UPDATE (SUBJECT REVIEW)

Committee on Drugs

ABSTRACT. Because of an increasing number of reports of adverse reactions associated with pharmaceutical excipients, in 1985 the Committee on Drugs issued a position statement recommending that the Food and Drug Administration mandate labeling of over-the-counter and prescription formulations to include a qualitative list of inactive ingredients. However, labeling of inactive ingredients remains voluntary. Adverse reactions continue to be reported, although some are no longer considered clinically significant, and other new reactions have emerged. The original statement, therefore, has been updated and its information expanded. (1/97, reaffirmed 2/00)

THE INAPPROPRIATE USE OF SCHOOL "READINESS" TESTS

Committee on Early Childhood, Adoption, and Dependent Care and Committee on School Health (3/95, reaffirmed 4/98, 9/03)

INCREASING IMMUNIZATION COVERAGE

Committee on Community Health Services and Committee on Practice and Ambulatory Medicine

ABSTRACT. Despite many recent advances in vaccine delivery, the goal for universal immunization set in 1977 has not been reached. In 2001, only 77.2% of US toddlers 19 to 35 months of age had received their basic immunization series of 4 doses of diphtheria and tetanus toxoids and acellular pertussis (DTaP) vaccine, 3 doses of inactivated poliovirus vaccine, 1 dose of measles-mumps-rubella (MMR) vaccine, and 3 doses of Haemophilus influenzae type b (Hib) vaccine. Children who are members of a racial or ethnic minority, who are poor, or who live in inner-city or rural areas have lower immunization rates than do children in the general population. Additional challenges to vaccine delivery include the introduction of new childhood vaccines, ensuring a dependable supply of vaccines, bolstering public confidence in vaccine safety, and sufficient compensation for vaccine administration.

Recent research has demonstrated specific and practical changes physicians can make to improve their practices' effectiveness in immunizing children, including the following: 1) sending parent reminders for upcoming visits and recall notices; 2) using prompts during all office visits to remind parents and staff about immunizations needed at that visit; 3) repeatedly measuring practice-wide immunization rates over time as part of a quality improvement effort; and 4) having in place standing orders for registered nurses, physician assistants, and medical assistants to identify opportunities to administer vaccines. Pediatricians should work individually and collectively at local and national levels to ensure that all children receive all childhood immunizations on time. Pediatricians also can proactively communicate with parents to ensure they understand the overall safety and efficacy of vaccines. (10/03)

INDICATIONS FOR MANAGEMENT AND REFERRAL OF PATIENTS INVOLVED IN SUBSTANCE ABUSE

Committee on Substance Abuse

ABSTRACT. This statement addresses the challenge of evaluating and managing the various stages of substance use by children and adolescents in the context of pediatric practice. Approaches are suggested that would assist the pediatrician in differentiating highly prevalent experimental and occasional use from more severe use with adverse consequences that affect emotional, behavioral, educational, or physical health. Comorbid psychiatric conditions are common and should be evaluated and treated simultaneously by child and adolescent mental health specialists. Guidelines for referral based on severity of involvement using established patient treatment-matching criteria are outlined. Pediatricians need to become familiar with treatment professionals and facilities in their communities and to ensure that treatment for adolescent patients is appropriate based on their developmental, psychosocial, medical, and mental health needs. The family should be encouraged to participate actively in the treatment process. (7/00)

INFANT EXERCISE PROGRAMS

Committee on Sports Medicine and Fitness (11/88, reaffirmed 11/94, 5/98)

INFANT METHEMOGLOBINEMIA: THE ROLE OF DIETARY NITRATE

Committee on Nutrition (9/70, reaffirmed 4/94, 6/97, 4/00)

INFANTS WITH ANENCEPHALY AS ORGAN SOURCES: ETHICAL CONSIDERATIONS

Committee on Bioethics (6/92, reaffirmed 11/95, 11/98, 11/02)

INFECTION CONTROL IN PHYSICIANS' OFFICES

Committee on Infectious Diseases and Committee on Practice and Ambulatory Medicine

ABSTRACT. Infection control is an integral part of pediatric practice in outpatient settings as well as in hospitals. All employees should be educated regarding the routes of transmission and techniques used to prevent transmission of infectious agents. Policies for infection control and prevention should be written, readily available, updated annually, and enforced. The Centers for Disease Control and Prevention standard precautions for hospitalized patients with modifications from the American Academy of Pediatrics are appropriate for most patient encounters. As employers, pediatricians are required by the Occupational Safety and Health Administration (OSHA) to take precautions to protect staff likely to be exposed to blood or other potentially infectious materials while on the job. Key principles of infection control include the following: handwashing before and after every patient contact, separation of infected, contagious children from uninfected children, safe handling and disposal of needles and other sharp medical devices, appropriate use of personal protection equipment such as gloves, appropriate sterilization, disinfection and antisepsis, and judicious use of antibiotics. (6/00)

INFORMED CONSENT, PARENTAL PERMISSION, AND ASSENT IN PEDIATRIC PRACTICE

Committee on Bioethics (2/95, reaffirmed 11/98, 11/02)

INHALANT ABUSE

Committee on Native American Child Health and Committee on Substance Abuse (3/96, reaffirmed 5/99)

INITIAL MEDICAL EVALUATION OF AN ADOPTED CHILD

Committee on Early Childhood, Adoption, and Dependent Care (9/91)

THE INITIATION OR WITHDRAWAL OF TREATMENT FOR HIGH-RISK NEWBORNS

Committee on Fetus and Newborn (8/95, reaffirmed 10/98, 6/01)

INJURIES ASSOCIATED WITH INFANT WALKERS

Committee on Injury and Poison Prevention

ABSTRACT. In 1999, an estimated 8800 children younger than 15 months were treated in hospital emergency departments in the United States for injuries associated with infant walkers. Thirty-four infant walker-related deaths were reported from 1973 through 1998. The vast majority of injuries occur from falls down stairs, and head injuries are common. Walkers do not help a child learn to walk; indeed, they can delay normal motor and mental development. The use of warning labels, public education, adult supervision during walker use, and stair gates have all been demonstrated to be insufficient strategies to prevent injuries associated with infant walkers. To comply with the revised voluntary standard (ASTM F977-96), walkers manufactured after June 30, 1997, must be wider than a 36-in doorway or must have a braking mechanism designed to stop the walker if 1 or more wheels drop off the riding surface, such as at the top of a stairway. Because data indicate a considerable risk of major and minor injury and even death from the use of infant walkers, and because there is no clear benefit from their use, the American Academy of Pediatrics recommends a ban on the manufacture and sale of mobile infant walkers. If a parent insists on using a mobile infant walker, it is vital that they choose a walker that meets the performance standards of ASTM F977-96 to prevent falls down stairs. Stationary activity centers should be promoted as a safer alternative to mobile infant walkers. (9/01)

INJURIES RELATED TO "TOY" FIREARMS

Committee on Injury and Poison Prevention (3/87, reaffirmed 11/96)

CLINICAL REPORT: INJURIES IN YOUTH SOCCER: A SUBJECT REVIEW

Committee on Sports Medicine and Fitness

ABSTRACT. The current literature on injuries in youth soccer, known as football worldwide, has been reviewed to assess the frequency, type, and causes of injuries in this sport. The information in this review serves as a basis for encouraging safe participation in soccer for children and adolescents. (3/00)

IN-LINE SKATING INJURIES IN CHILDREN AND ADOLESCENTS

Committee on Injury and Poison Prevention and Committee on Sports Medicine and Fitness

ABSTRACT. In-line skating has become one of the fastest-growing recreational sports in the United States. Recent studies emphasize the value of protective gear in reducing the incidence of injuries. Recommendations are provided for parents and pediatricians, with special emphasis on the novice or inexperienced skater. (4/98, reaffirmed 1/02)

INSTITUTIONAL ETHICS COMMITTEES

Committee on Bioethics

ABSTRACT. In hospitals throughout the United States, institutional ethics committees (IECs) have become a standard vehicle for the education of health professionals about biomedical ethics, for the drafting and review of hospital policy, and for clinical ethics case consultation. In addition, there is increasing interest in a role for the IEC in organizational ethics. Recommendations are made about the membership and structure of an IEC, and guidelines are provided for those serving on an ethics committee. (1/01)

INSURANCE COVERAGE OF MENTAL HEALTH AND SUBSTANCE ABUSE SERVICES FOR CHILDREN AND ADOLESCENTS: A CONSENSUS STATEMENT

Joint Statement (10/00)

INTENSIVE TRAINING AND SPORTS SPECIALIZATION IN YOUNG ATHLETES

Committee on Sports Medicine and Fitness

ABSTRACT. Children involved in sports should be encouraged to participate in a variety of different activities and develop a wide range of skills. Young athletes who specialize in just one sport may be denied the benefits of varied activity while facing additional physical, physiologic, and psychologic demands from intense training and competition.

This statement reviews the potential risks of high-intensity training and sports specialization in young athletes. Pediatricians who recognize these risks can have a key role in monitoring the health of these young athletes and helping reduce risks associated with high-level sports participation. (7/00)

INVESTIGATION AND REVIEW OF UNEXPECTED INFANT AND CHILD DEATHS

Committee on Child Abuse and Neglect and Committee on Community Health Services

ABSTRACT. Although there is a continuing need for timely review of child deaths, no uniform system exists for investigation in the United States. Investigation of a death that is traumatic, unexpected, obscure, suspicious, or otherwise unexplained in a child younger than 18 years requires a scene investigation and an autopsy. Review of these deaths requires the participation of pediatricians and other professionals, usually as a child death review team. An appropriately constituted team should evaluate the death investigation process, review difficult cases, and compile child death statistics. (11/99, reaffirmed 10/02)

IRON FORTIFICATION OF INFANT FORMULAS

Committee on Nutrition

ABSTRACT. Despite the American Academy of Pediatrics' (AAP) strong endorsement for breastfeeding, most infants in the United States are fed some infant formula by the time they are 2 months old. The AAP Committee on Nutrition has strongly advocated iron fortification of infant formulas since 1969 as a way of reducing the prevalence of iron-deficiency anemia and its attendant sequelae during the first year. The 1976 statement titled "Iron Supplementation for Infants" delineated the rationale for iron supplementation, proposed daily dosages of iron, and summarized potential sources of iron in the infant diet. In 1989, the AAP Committee on Nutrition published a statement that addressed the issue of iron-fortified infant formulas and concluded that there was no convincing contraindication to iron-supplemented formulas and that continued use of "low-iron" formulas posed an unacceptable risk for iron deficiency during infancy. The current statement represents a scientific update and synthesis of the 1976 and 1989 statements with recommendations about the use of iron-fortified and low-iron formulas in term infants. (7/99, reaffirmed 11/02)

TECHNICAL REPORT: IRRADIATION OF FOOD

Katherine M. Shea, MD, MPH, and the Committee on Environmental Health

ABSTRACT. Recent well-publicized outbreaks of foodborne illness have heightened general interest in food safety. Food irradiation is a technology that has been approved for use in selected foods in the United States since 1963. Widespread use of irradiation remains controversial, however, because of public concern regarding the safety of the technology and the wholesomeness of irradiated foods. In this report, we describe the technology, review safety and wholesomeness issues, and give a historical perspective of the public controversy regarding food irradiation. (12/00)

CLINICAL REPORT: ISSUES IN THE APPLICATION OF THE RESOURCE-BASED RELATIVE VALUE SCALE SYSTEM TO PEDIATRICS: A SUBJECT REVIEW

Resource-Based Relative Value Scale Project Advisory Committee

ABSTRACT. In today's rapidly changing health care environment, it is crucial to understand the genesis and concepts of the Medicare Resource-based Relative Value Scale (RBRVS) physician fee schedule. Many third-party payers, including state Medicaid programs, Blue Cross-Blue Shield agencies, and managed care organizations are using variations of the Medicare RBRVS to determine physician reimbursement and capitation rates. Because the RBRVS fee schedule was originally created for Medicare only, pediatric-specific Current Procedural Terminology codes and pediatric practice expense issues were not included. The American Academy of Pediatrics agrees with the use of the Current Procedural Terminology codes and the RBRVS physician fee schedule and continues to work to rectify the inequities of the RBRVS system as they pertain to pediatrics. (10/98)

ISSUES RELATED TO HUMAN IMMUNODEFICIENCY VIRUS TRANSMISSION IN SCHOOLS, CHILD CARE, MEDICAL SETTINGS, THE HOME, AND COMMUNITY

Committee on Pediatric AIDS and Committee on Infectious Diseases

ABSTRACT. Current recommendations of the American Academy of Pediatrics (AAP) for infection control practices to prevent transmission of blood-borne pathogens, including human immunodeficiency virus (HIV) in hospitals, other medical settings, schools, and child care facilities, are reviewed and explained. Hand-washing is essential, whether or not gloves are used, and gloves should be used when contact with blood or blood-containing body fluids may occur. In hospitalized children, the 1996 recommendations of the Centers for Disease Control and Prevention (CDC) should be implemented as modified in the *1997 Red Book*. The generic principles of Standard Precautions in the CDC guidelines generally are applicable to children in all health care settings, schools, child care facilities, and the home. However, gloves are not required for routine changing of diapers or for wiping nasal secretions of children in most circumstances. This AAP recommendation differs from that in the CDC guidelines.

Current US Public Health Service guidelines for the management of potential occupational exposures of health care workers to HIV are summarized. As previously recommended by the AAP, HIV-infected children should be admitted without restriction to child care centers and schools and allowed to participate in all activities to the extent that their health and other recommendations for management of contagious diseases permit. Because it is not required that the school be notified of HIV infection, it may be helpful if the pediatrician notify the school that he or she is operating under a policy of nondisclosure of infection with blood-borne pathogens. Thus, it is possible that the pediatrician will not report the presence of such infections on the form. Because HIV infection occurs in persons throughout the United States, these recommendations for prevention of HIV transmission should be applied universally. (8/99, reaffirmed 2/02)

TECHNICAL REPORT: KNEE BRACE USE IN THE YOUNG ATHLETE

Committee on Sports Medicine and Fitness

ABSTRACT. This statement is a revision of a previous statement on prophylactic knee bracing and provides information for pediatricians regarding the use of various types of knee braces, indications for the use of knee braces, and the background knowledge necessary to prescribe the use of knee braces for children. (8/01)

LAWN MOWER-RELATED INJURIES TO CHILDREN

Committee on Injury and Poison Prevention

ABSTRACT. Lawn mower-related injuries to children are relatively common and can result in severe injury or death. Many amputations during childhood are caused by power mowers. Pediatricians have an important role as advocates and educators to promote the prevention of these injuries. (6/01)

TECHNICAL REPORT: LAWN MOWER-RELATED INJURIES TO CHILDREN

Gary A. Smith and the Committee on Injury and Poison Prevention

ABSTRACT. In the United States, approximately 9400 children younger than 18 years receive emergency treatment annually for lawn mower-related injuries. More than 7% of these children require hospitalization, and power mowers cause a large proportion of the amputations during childhood. Prevention of lawn mower-related injuries can be achieved by design changes of lawn mowers, guidelines for mower operation, and education of parents, child caregivers, and children. Pediatricians have an important role as advocates and educators to promote the prevention of these injuries. (6/01)

CLINICAL REPORT: LEARNING DISABILITIES, DYSLEXIA, AND VISION: A SUBJECT REVIEW

Committee on Children With Disabilities, American Academy of Pediatrics (AAP), American Academy of Ophthalmology (AAO), and American Association for Pediatric Ophthalmology and Strabismus (AAPOS)

ABSTRACT. Learning disabilities are common conditions in pediatric patients. The etiology of these difficulties is multifactorial, reflecting genetic influences and abnormalities of brain structure and function. Early recognition and referral to qualified educational professionals is critical for the best possible outcome. Visual problems are rarely responsible for learning difficulties. No scientific evidence exists for the efficacy of eye exercises ("vision therapy") or the use of special tinted lenses in the remediation of these complex pediatric developmental and neurologic conditions. (11/98, reaffirmed 5/02)

CLINICAL REPORT: MANAGED CARE AND CHILDREN WITH SPECIAL HEALTH CARE NEEDS: A SUBJECT REVIEW

Committee on Children With Disabilities

ABSTRACT. Barriers to access to health care frequently overshadow the opportunities for improvement through managed care, especially regarding children with special health care needs. This statement discusses such opportunities, identifies challenges, and proposes active roles for pediatricians, and families of patients to improve some aspects of managed care for children with special health care needs. (9/98)

MARIJUANA: A CONTINUING CONCERN FOR PEDIATRICIANS

Committee on Substance Abuse

ABSTRACT. Marijuana, the common name for products derived from the plant *Cannabis sativa*, is the most common illicit drug used by children and adolescents in the United States. Despite growing concerns by the medical profession about the physical and psychological effects of its active ingredient, Δ-9-tetrahydrocannabinol, survey data continue to show that increasing numbers of young people are using the drug as they become less concerned about its dangers. (10/99, reaffirmed 4/03)

MATERNAL PHENYLKETONURIA
Committee on Genetics
ABSTRACT. Elevated maternal phenylalanine levels during pregnancy are teratogenic and may result in growth retardation, significant psychomotor handicaps, and birth defects in the offspring of unmonitored and untreated pregnancies. Women of childbearing age with all forms of phenylketonuria, including mild variants such as hyperphenylalaninemia, should receive counseling concerning their risks for adverse fetal effects optimally before conceiving. The best outcomes occur when strict control of maternal phenylalanine levels is achieved before conception and continued throughout the pregnancy. (2/01)

MEASLES IMMUNIZATION IN HIV-INFECTED CHILDREN
Committee on Infectious Diseases and Committee on
  Pediatric AIDS
ABSTRACT. Children infected with human immunodeficiency virus (HIV) have had high rates of mortality attributable to measles, but until recently, measles vaccine was assumed to be safe for these children. A single fatal case of pneumonia attributable to vaccine type-measles virus has been documented in a young adult with acquired immunodeficiency syndrome. Because a protective immune response often does not develop in severely immunocompromised HIV-infected patients after immunization and some risk of severe complications exists, HIV-infected children, adolescents, and young adults who are severely immunocompromised (based on age-specific CD4 lymphocyte enumeration) attributable to HIV infection should not receive measles vaccine. All other HIV-infected children, adolescents, and young adults who are not severely immunocompromised should receive measles-mumps-rubella vaccine. (5/99, reaffirmed 10/01 COID)

MEDIA EDUCATION
Committee on Public Education
ABSTRACT. The American Academy of Pediatrics recognizes that exposure to mass media (ie, television, movies, video and computer games, the Internet, music lyrics and videos, newspapers, magazines, books, advertising, etc) presents both health risks and benefits for children and adolescents. Media education has the potential to reduce the harmful effects of media. By understanding and supporting media education, pediatricians can play an important role in reducing the risk of exposure to mass media for children and adolescents. (8/99)

MEDIA VIOLENCE
Committee on Public Education
ABSTRACT. The American Academy of Pediatrics recognizes exposure to violence in media, including television, movies, music, and video games, as a significant risk to the health of children and adolescents. Extensive research evidence indicates that media violence can contribute to aggressive behavior, desensitization to violence, nightmares, and fear of being harmed. Pediatricians should assess their patients' level of media exposure and intervene on media-related health risks. Pediatricians and other child health care providers can advocate for a safer media environment for children by encouraging media literacy, more thoughtful and proactive use of media by children and their parents, more responsible portrayal of violence by media producers, and more useful and effective media ratings. (11/01)

MEDICAID POLICY STATEMENT
Committee on Child Health Financing
ABSTRACT. This policy statement replaces the 1994 Medicaid Policy Statement. The new policy statement incorporates federal legislative changes and policy recommendations related to eligibility, outreach and enrollment, Medicaid managed care, covered benefits, access to pediatric care, and quality improvement plans. (8/99)

MEDICAL CONCERNS IN THE FEMALE ATHLETE
Committee on Sports Medicine and Fitness
ABSTRACT. Female children and adolescents who participate regularly in sports may develop certain medical conditions, including disordered eating, menstrual dysfunction, and decreased bone mineral density. The pediatrician can play an important role in monitoring the health of young female athletes. This revised policy statement provides updated and expanded information for pediatricians on these health concerns as well as recommendations for evaluation, treatment, and ongoing assessments of female athletes. (9/00)

MEDICAL CONDITIONS AFFECTING SPORTS PARTICIPATION
Committee on Sports Medicine and Fitness
ABSTRACT. Children and adolescents with medical conditions present special issues with respect to participation in athletic activities. The pediatrician can play an important role in determining whether a child with a health condition should participate in certain sports by assessing the child's health status, suggesting appropriate equipment or modifications of sports to decrease the risk of injury, and educating the athlete and parents on the risks of injury as they relate to the child's condition. This statement updates a previous policy statement and provides information for pediatricians on sports participation for children and adolescents with medical conditions. (5/01)

THE MEDICAL HOME
Medical Home Initiatives for Children With Special Needs
  Project Advisory Committee (7/02)

MEDICAL NECESSITY FOR THE HOSPITALIZATION OF THE ABUSED AND NEGLECTED CHILD
Committee on Hospital Care and Committee on
  Child Abuse and Neglect
ABSTRACT. The child suspected of being abused or neglected demands prompt evaluation in a protective environment where knowledgeable consultants are readily available. In communities without specialized centers for the care of abused children, the hospital inpatient unit becomes an appropriate setting for their initial management. Medical, psychosocial, and legal concerns may be assessed expeditiously while the child is housed in a safe haven awaiting final disposition by child protective services. The American Academy of Pediatrics recommends that hospitalization of abused and neglected children, when medically indicated or for their protection/diagnosis when there are no specialized facilities in the community for their care, should be viewed as medically necessary by both health professionals and third-party payors. (4/98, reaffirmed 5/01 COHC, reaffirmed 10/01 COCAN)

CLINICAL REPORT: MEDICAL STAFF APPOINTMENT AND DELINEATION OF PEDIATRIC PRIVILEGES IN HOSPITALS
Committee on Hospital Care

ABSTRACT. The review and verification of credentials and the granting of clinical privileges are required of every hospital to ensure that members of the medical staff are competent and qualified to provide specified levels of patient care. The credentialing process involves the following: 1) assessment of the professional and personal background of each practitioner seeking privileges; 2) assignment of privileges appropriate for the clinician's training and experience; 3) ongoing monitoring of the professional activities of each staff member; and 4) periodic reappointment to the medical staff on the basis of objectively measured performance. This statement examines the essential elements of a credentials review for initial and renewed medical staff appointments along with suggested criteria for the delineation of clinical privileges. Sample forms for the delineation of privileges can be found on the American Academy of Pediatrics Web site (http://www.aap.org/visit/cmte19.htm). Because of the differences in individual hospitals, no one method for credentialing is universally applicable. The medical staff of each hospital must, therefore, establish its own process based on the general principles reviewed in this statement. The issues of medical staff membership and credentialing have become very complex, and institutions and medical staffs are vulnerable to legal action. Consequently, it is advisable for hospitals and medical staffs to obtain expert legal advice when medical staff bylaws are constructed or revised. (8/02)

MENINGOCOCCAL DISEASE PREVENTION AND CONTROL STRATEGIES FOR PRACTICE-BASED PHYSICIANS (ADDENDUM: RECOMMENDATIONS FOR COLLEGE STUDENTS)
Committee on Infectious Diseases

ABSTRACT. The numbers of reported cases of meningococcal disease in 15- to 24-year-olds and outbreaks of meningococcal serogroup C disease, including outbreaks in schools and other institutions, have increased during the past decade. In response to outbreaks on college campuses, the American College Health Association has taken an increasingly proactive role in alerting college students and their parents to the risk of this disease and informing them about the availability of an effective vaccine. Recent epidemiologic studies have demonstrated an increased risk of disease in college students living in dormitories, particularly among freshmen, compared with similarly aged persons in the general population. At least 60% of these cases are potentially preventable by vaccination with the quadrivalent meningococcal A, C, Y, and W-135 polysaccharide vaccine. These findings support immunization of college students, particularly freshmen living in dormitories. Hence, college students and their parents should be informed by health care professionals at routine prematriculation visits and during college matriculation of the risk of meningococcal disease and potential benefits of immunization. Vaccine should be made available to those requesting immunization. College and university health services also should facilitate implementation of educational programs concerning meningococcal disease and availability of immunization services. (12/00, reaffirmed 10/01)

TECHNICAL REPORT: MERCURY IN THE ENVIRONMENT: IMPLICATIONS FOR PEDIATRICIANS
Lynn R. Goldman, MD, MPH; Michael W. Shannon, MD, MPH; and the Committee on Environmental Health

ABSTRACT. Mercury is a ubiquitous environmental toxin that causes a wide range of adverse health effects in humans. Three forms of mercury (elemental, inorganic, and organic) exist, and each has its own profile of toxicity. Exposure to mercury typically occurs by inhalation or ingestion. Readily absorbed after its inhalation, mercury can be an indoor air pollutant, for example, after spills of elemental mercury in the home; however, industry emissions with resulting ambient air pollution remain the most important source of inhaled mercury. Because fresh-water and ocean fish may contain large amounts of mercury, children and pregnant women can have significant exposure if they consume excessive amounts of fish. The developing fetus and young children are thought to be disproportionately affected by mercury exposure, because many aspects of development, particularly brain maturation, can be disturbed by the presence of mercury. Minimizing mercury exposure is, therefore, essential to optimal child health. This review provides pediatricians with current information on mercury, including environmental sources, toxicity, and treatment and prevention of mercury exposure. (7/01)

CLINICAL REPORT: MOLECULAR GENETIC TESTING IN PEDIATRIC PRACTICE: A SUBJECT REVIEW
Committee on Genetics

ABSTRACT. Although many types of diagnostic and carrier testing for genetic disorders have been available for decades, the use of molecular methods is a relatively recent phenomenon. Such testing has expanded the range of disorders that can be diagnosed and has enhanced the ability of clinicians to provide accurate prognostic information and institute appropriate health supervision measures. However, the proper application of these tests may be difficult because of their scientific complexity and the potential for negative, sometimes unexpected, consequences for many patients. The purposes of this subject review are to provide background information on molecular genetic tests, to describe specific testing modalities, and to discuss some of the benefits and risks specific to the pediatric population. It is likely that pediatricians will use these testing methods increasingly for their patients and will need to evaluate critically their diagnostic and prognostic implications. (12/00)

NEONATAL DRUG WITHDRAWAL
Committee on Drugs

ABSTRACT. Maternal drug use during pregnancy may result in neonatal withdrawal. This statement presents current information about the clinical presentation, differential diagnosis, therapeutic options, and outcome for the offspring associated with intrauterine drug exposure. (6/98, reaffirmed 5/01)

THE NEW MORBIDITY REVISITED: A RENEWED COMMITMENT TO THE PSYCHOSOCIAL ASPECTS OF PEDIATRIC CARE

Committee on Psychosocial Aspects of Child and Family Health
ABSTRACT. In 1993, the American Academy of Pediatrics adopted the policy statement "The Pediatrician and the 'New Morbidity.'" Since then, social difficulties, behavioral problems, and developmental difficulties have become a main part of the scope of pediatric practice, and recognition of the importance of these areas has increased. This statement reaffirms the Academy's commitment to prevention, early detection, and management of behavioral, developmental, and social problems as a focus in pediatric practice. (11/01)

NEWBORN SCREENING FOR CONGENITAL HYPOTHYROIDISM: RECOMMENDED GUIDELINES

Committee on Genetics and Section on Endocrinology (6/93, reaffirmed 10/96 COG)

NEWBORN SCREENING FACT SHEETS

Committee on Genetics (9/96, reaffirmed 10/99)

NOISE: A HAZARD FOR THE FETUS AND NEWBORN

Committee on Environmental Health
ABSTRACT. Noise is ubiquitous in our environment. High intensities of noise have been associated with numerous health effects in adults, including noise-induced hearing loss and high blood pressure. The intent of this statement is to provide pediatricians and others with information on the potential health effects of noise on the fetus and newborn. The information presented here supports a number of recommendations for both pediatric practice and government policy. (10/97, reaffirmed 10/00)

NONDISCRIMINATION IN PEDIATRIC HEALTH CARE

Committee on Pediatric Workforce
ABSTRACT. This policy statement reaffirms and consolidates the positions of the American Academy of Pediatrics relative to nondiscrimination in pediatric health care. It addresses pediatricians who provide health care and the infants, children, adolescents, and young adults who are entitled to optimal pediatric care. (11/01)

OFFICE-BASED COUNSELING FOR INJURY PREVENTION

Committee on Injury and Poison Prevention (10/94, reaffirmed 10/98)

ORAL AND DENTAL ASPECTS OF CHILD ABUSE AND NEGLECT

Joint Statement of the American Academy of Pediatrics Committee on Child Abuse and Neglect and the American Academy of Pediatric Dentistry Ad Hoc Work Group on Child Abuse and Neglect
ABSTRACT. In all states, physicians and dentists recognize their responsibility to report suspected cases of abuse and neglect. The purpose of this statement is to review the oral and dental aspects of physical and sexual abuse and dental neglect and the role of physicians and dentists in evaluating such conditions. This statement also addresses the oral manifestations of sexually transmitted diseases and bite marks, including the collection of evidence and laboratory documentation of these injuries. (8/99)

ORAL HEALTH RISK ASSESSMENT TIMING AND ESTABLISHMENT OF THE DENTAL HOME

Section on Pediatric Dentistry
ABSTRACT. Early childhood dental caries has been reported by the Centers for Disease Control and Prevention to be perhaps the most prevalent infectious disease of our nation's children. Early childhood dental caries occurs in all racial and socioeconomic groups; however, it tends to be more prevalent in low-income children, in whom it occurs in epidemic proportions. Dental caries results from an overgrowth of specific organisms that are a part of normally occurring human flora. Human dental flora is site specific, and an infant is not colonized until the eruption of the primary dentition at approximately 6 to 30 months of age. The most likely source of inoculation of an infant's dental flora is the mother or another intimate care provider, through shared utensils, etc. Decreasing the level of cariogenic organisms in the mother's dental flora at the time of colonization can significantly impact the child's predisposition to caries. To prevent caries in children, high-risk individuals must be identified at an early age (preferably high-risk mothers during prenatal care), and aggressive strategies should be adopted, including anticipatory guidance, behavior modifications (oral hygiene and feeding practices), and establishment of a dental home by 1 year of age for children deemed at risk. (5/03)

ORGANIZED SPORTS FOR CHILDREN AND PREADOLESCENTS

Committee on Sports Medicine and Fitness and Committee on School Health
ABSTRACT. Participation in organized sports provides an opportunity for young people to increase their physical activity and develop physical and social skills. However, when the demands and expectations of organized sports exceed the maturation and readiness of the participant, the positive aspects of participation can be negated. The nature of parental or adult involvement can also influence the degree to which participation in organized sports is a positive experience for preadolescents. This updates a previous policy statement on athletics for preadolescents and incorporates guidelines for sports participation for preschool children. Recommendations are offered on how pediatricians can help determine a child's readiness to participate, how risks can be minimized, and how child-oriented goals can be maximized. (6/01)

OUT-OF-SCHOOL SUSPENSION AND EXPULSION
Committee on School Health
ABSTRACT. Suspension and expulsion from school are used to punish students, alert parents, and protect other students and school staff. Unintended consequences of these practices require more attention from health care professionals. Suspension and expulsion may exacerbate academic deterioration, and when students are provided with no immediate educational alternative, student alienation, delinquency, crime, and substance abuse may ensue. Social, emotional, and mental health support for students at all times in all schools can decrease the need for expulsion and suspension and should be strongly advocated by the health care community. This policy statement, however, highlights aspects of expulsion and suspension that jeopardize children's health and safety. Recommendations are targeted at pediatricians, who can help schools address the root causes of behaviors that lead to suspension and expulsion and can advocate for alternative disciplinary policies. Pediatricians can also share responsibility with schools to provide students with health and social resources. (11/03)

PALLIATIVE CARE FOR CHILDREN
Committee on Bioethics and Committee on Hospital Care
ABSTRACT. This statement presents an integrated model for providing palliative care for children living with a life-threatening or terminal condition. Advice on the development of a palliative care plan and on working with parents and children is also provided. Barriers to the provision of effective pediatric palliative care and potential solutions are identified. The American Academy of Pediatrics recommends the development and broad availability of pediatric palliative care services based on child-specific guidelines and standards. Such services will require widely distributed and effective palliative care education of pediatric health care professionals. The Academy offers guidance on responding to requests for hastening death, but does not support the practice of physician-assisted suicide or euthanasia for children. (8/00, reaffirmed 6/03)

PARENTAL LEAVE FOR RESIDENTS AND PEDIATRIC TRAINING PROGRAMS
Committee on Early Childhood, Adoption, and Dependent Care and Section on Residents (11/95, reaffirmed 4/98 COECADC)

PARTICIPATION IN BOXING BY CHILDREN, ADOLESCENTS, AND YOUNG ADULTS
Committee on Sports Medicine and Fitness
ABSTRACT. Because boxing may result in serious brain and eye injuries, the American Academy of Pediatrics opposes this sport. This policy statement summarizes the reasons. (1/97, reaffirmed 5/00)

PEDIATRIC CARE IN THE EMERGENCY DEPARTMENT
Society for Academic Emergency Medicine
ABSTRACT. Physicians who have successfully completed an accredited Emergency Medicine residency and are certified in emergency medicine by the American Board of Emergency Medicine (ABEM) or the American Osteopathic Board of Emergency Medicine (AOBEM) ABEM/AOBEM or those who are certified in pediatric emergency medicine by ABEM or the American Board of Pediatrics (ABP) possess the knowledge and skills required to provide quality emergency medical care to childrenof all ages for a wide variety of illnesses, injuries or poisonings. To provide quality care, the emergency physician must have all necessary and age-appropriate medical equipment readily available. The emergency physician must also have access via consultation, admission, or transfer, to appropriate specialty and sub-specialty physicians, to who will provide any needed patient care after emergency department treatment. Physically separated care areas for children are not mandatory in order to provide high-quality care to patients of all ages. Although physically separate care areas for children are ideal, they are not mandatory to provide high-quality care. (11/03)

PEDIATRIC CARE RECOMMENDATIONS FOR FREESTANDING URGENT CARE FACILITIES
Committee on Pediatric Emergency Medicine
ABSTRACT. Freestanding urgent care centers are increasing as a source of after-hours pediatric care. These facilities may be used as an alternative to hospital emergency departments for the care and stabilization of serious and critically ill and injured children. The purpose of this policy statement is to provide recommendations for assuring appropriate stabilization in pediatric emergency situations and timely transfer to a hospital for definitive care when necessary. (5/99)

TECHNICAL REPORT: PEDIATRIC EXPOSURE AND POTENTIAL TOXICITY OF PHTHALATE PLASTICIZERS
Katherine M. Shea, MD, MPH and Committee on Environmental Health
ABSTRACT. Phthalates are plasticizers that are added to polyvinyl chloride (PVC) products to impart flexibility and durability. They are produced in high volume and generate extensive though poorly defined human exposures and unique childhood exposures. Phthalates are animal carcinogens and can cause fetal death, malformations, and reproductive toxicity in laboratory animals. Toxicity profiles and potency vary by specific phthalate. The extent of these toxicities and their applicability to humans remains incompletely characterized and controversial. Two phthalates, diethylhexyl phthalate (DEHP) and diisononyl phthalate (DINP), have received considerable attention recently because of specific concerns about pediatric exposures. Like all phthalates, DEHP and DINP are ubiquitous contaminants in food, indoor air, soils, and sediments. DEHP is used in toys and medical devices. DINP is a major plasticizer used in children's toys.

Scientific panels, advocacy groups, and industry groups have analyzed the literature on DEHP and DINP and have come to different conclusions about their safety. The controversy exists because risk to humans must be extrapolated from animal data that demonstrate differences in toxicity by species, route of exposure, and age at exposure and because of persistent uncertainties in human exposure data. This report addresses sensitive endpoints of reproductive and developmental toxicity and the unique aspects of pediatric exposures to phthalates that generate concern. DEHP and DINP are used as specific examples to illustrate the controversy. (6/03)

PEDIATRIC ORGAN DONATION AND TRANSPLANTATION
Committee on Hospital Care and Section on Surgery
ABSTRACT. Pediatric organ donation and organ transplantation can have a significant life-extending benefit to the young recipients of these organs and a high emotional impact on donor and recipient families. Pediatricians should become better acquainted with evolving national strategies involving organ procurement and organ transplantation to help acquaint families with the benefits of organ donation and to help shape public policies that will aid in efforts to provide a system of procurement, distribution, and finance that is fair and equitable to children and adults. Major issues of concern are availability and access; oversight and control; pediatric medical and surgical consultation throughout the organ donation and transplantation process; ethical, social, financial, and follow-up issues; insurance coverage issues; and public awareness of the need for organ donors of all ages. (5/02)

PEDIATRIC PHYSICIAN PROFILING
Committee on Practice and Ambulatory Medicine and Committee on Medical Liability
ABSTRACT. Employers, insurers, and other purchasers of health care services collect data to profile the practice habits of pediatricians and other physicians. This policy statement delineates a series of recommendations that should be adopted by health care purchasers to guide the development and implementation of physician profiling systems. (10/99)

PEDIATRIC PRIMARY HEALTH CARE
Committee on Pediatric Workforce (11/93, reaffirmed 6/01 AAP News)

PEDIATRIC WORKFORCE STATEMENT
Committee on Pediatric Workforce
ABSTRACT. This statement reviews current physician workforce projections, and identifies the factors that will have the most impact on future pediatric workforce projections. It discusses the key issues relating to the pediatric workforce: utilization of services, provision of care by both pediatricians and nonpediatricians, pediatric subspecialization, ethnic composition of the population and of the pediatric workforce, indebtedness, and geographic distribution. In a concluding series of recommendations, the statement addresses the steps that must be taken to ensure that all of America's infants, children, adolescents, and young adults have access to appropriate pediatric health care. (8/98)

THE PEDIATRICIAN AND CHILDHOOD BEREAVEMENT
Committee on Psychosocial Aspects of Child and Family Health
ABSTRACT. Pediatricians should understand and evaluate children's reactions to the death of a person important to them by using age-appropriate and culturally sensitive guidance while being alert for normal and complicated grief responses. Pediatricians also should advise and assist families in responding to the child's needs. Sharing, family support, and communication have been associated with positive long-term bereavement adjustment. (2/00)

PEDIATRICIANS' LIABILITY DURING DISASTERS
Committee on Pediatric Emergency Medicine and Committee on Medical Liability
ABSTRACT. This statement addresses the need for professional liability insurance coverage for pediatricians during disasters and suggests measures to ensure adequate coverage. (12/00)

THE PEDIATRICIAN'S ROLE IN ADVOCATING LIFE SUPPORT COURSES FOR PARENTS
Committee on Pediatric Emergency Medicine (7/94, reaffirmed 4/97)

THE PEDIATRICIAN'S ROLE IN COMMUNITY PEDIATRICS
Committee on Community Health Services
ABSTRACT. This policy statement offers pediatricians a concise definition of community pediatrics and provides a set of specific recommendations that underscore the critical nature of this important dimension of the profession. (6/99)

THE PEDIATRICIAN'S ROLE IN DEVELOPMENT AND IMPLEMENTATION OF AN INDIVIDUAL EDUCATION PLAN (IEP) AND/OR AN INDIVIDUAL FAMILY SERVICE PLAN (IFSP)
Committee on Children With Disabilities
ABSTRACT. The Individual Education Plan and Individual Family Service Plan are legally mandated documents developed by a multidisciplinary team assessment that specifies goals and services for each child eligible for special educational services or early intervention services. Pediatricians need to be knowledgeable of federal, state, and local requirements; establish linkages with early intervention, educational professionals, and parent support groups; and collaborate with the team working with individual children. (7/99, reaffirmed 11/02)

THE PEDIATRICIAN'S ROLE IN THE DIAGNOSIS AND MANAGEMENT OF AUTISTIC SPECTRUM DISORDER IN CHILDREN
Committee on Children With Disabilities
ABSTRACT. Primary care physicians have the opportunity, especially within the context of the medical home, to be the first point of contact when parents have concerns about their child's development or behavior. The goal of this policy statement is to help the pediatrician recognize the early symptoms of autism and participate in its diagnosis and management. This statement and the accompanying technical report will serve to familiarize the pediatrician with currently accepted criteria defining the spectrum of autism, strategies used in making a diagnosis, and conventional and alternative interventions. (5/01)

TECHNICAL REPORT: THE PEDIATRICIAN'S ROLE IN THE DIAGNOSIS AND MANAGEMENT OF AUTISTIC SPECTRUM DISORDER IN CHILDREN
Committee on Children With Disabilities
ABSTRACT. Primary care physicians have the opportunity, especially within the context of the medical home, to be the first point of contact when parents have concerns about their child's development or behavior. The goal of this policy statement is to help the pediatrician recognize the early symptoms of autism and participate in its diagnosis and management. This statement and the accompanying technical report will serve to familiarize the pediatrician with currently accepted criteria defining the spectrum of autism, strategies used in making a diagnosis, and conventional and alternative interventions. (5/01)

THE PEDIATRICIAN'S ROLE IN FAMILY SUPPORT PROGRAMS
Committee on Early Childhood, Adoption, and Dependent Care
ABSTRACT. Children's brain growth, general health, and development are directly influenced by emotional relationships during early childhood. Contemporary American life challenges families' abilities to promote successful developmental outcomes and emotional health for their children. Pediatricians are positioned to serve as family advisors and community partners in supporting the well-being of children and families. This statement recommends opportunities for pediatricians to develop their expertise in assessing the strengths and stresses in families, in counseling families about strategies and resources, and in collaborating with others in their communities to support family relationships. (1/01)

THE PEDIATRICIAN'S ROLE IN HELPING CHILDREN AND FAMILIES DEAL WITH SEPARATION AND DIVORCE
Committee on Psychosocial Aspects of Child and Family Health
(7/94)

THE PEDIATRICIAN'S ROLE IN THE PREVENTION OF MISSING CHILDREN
Committee on Early Childhood, Adoption, and Dependent Care
(1/92, reaffirmed 5/96)

CLINICAL REPORT: PERINATAL CARE AT THE THRESHOLD OF VIABILITY
Committee on Fetus and Newborn
ABSTRACT. In the United States, an increase in the number of births of extremely preterm infants and in their survival potential has occurred over the last decade. Determining the survival prognosis for the infant of a pregnancy with threatened preterm delivery between 22 and 25 completed weeks of gestation remains problematic. Many physicians and families encounter the difficulty of making decisions regarding the institution and continuation of life support for an infant born within this threshold period. This report addresses the process of counseling, assisting, and supporting families faced with the dilemma of an extremely preterm delivery. (11/02)

PERINATAL HUMAN IMMUNODEFICIENCY VIRUS TESTING
Committee on Pediatric AIDS (2/95, reaffirmed 10/96, 11/99)

TECHNICAL REPORT: PERINATAL HUMAN IMMUNODEFICIENCY VIRUS TESTING AND PREVENTION OF TRANSMISSION
Lynne M. Mofenson and the Committee on Pediatric AIDS
ABSTRACT. In 1994, the US Public Health Service published guidelines for the use of zidovudine to decrease the risk of perinatal transmission of human immunodeficiency virus (HIV). In 1995, the American Academy of Pediatrics and the US Public Health Service recommended documented, routine HIV education and testing with consent for all pregnant women in the United States. Widespread incorporation of these guidelines into clinical practice has resulted in a dramatic decrease in the rate of perinatal HIV transmission and has contributed to more than a 75% decrease in reported cases of pediatric acquired immunodeficiency syndrome (AIDS) since 1992. Substantial advances have been made in the treatment and monitoring of HIV infection; combination antiretroviral regimens that maximally suppress virus replication are now available. These regimens are recommended for pregnant and nonpregnant individuals who require treatment. Risk factors associated with perinatal HIV transmission are now better understood, and recent results from trials to decrease the rate of mother-to-child HIV transmission have contributed new strategies with established efficacy. However, perinatal HIV transmission still occurs; the Centers for Disease Control and Prevention estimates that 300 to 400 infected infants are born annually. Full implementation of recommendations for universal, routine prenatal HIV testing and evaluation of missed prevention opportunities will be critical to further decrease the incidence of pediatric HIV infection in the United States. This technical report summarizes recent advances in the prevention of perinatal transmission of HIV relevant to screening of pregnant women and their infants. (12/00, reaffirmed 3/03)

PERSONAL WATERCRAFT USE BY CHILDREN AND ADOLESCENTS
Committee on Injury and Poison Prevention
ABSTRACT. The use of personal watercraft (PWC) has increased dramatically during the past decade as have the speed and mobility of the watercraft. A similar dramatic increase in PWC-related injury and death has occurred simultaneously. No one younger than 16 years should operate a PWC. The operator and all passengers must wear US Coast Guard-approved personal flotation devices. Other safety recommendations are suggested for parents and pediatricians. (2/00)

PHYSICAL FITNESS AND ACTIVITY IN SCHOOLS
Committee on Sports Medicine and Fitness and Committee on School Health
ABSTRACT. Schools are in a uniquely favorable position to increase physical activity and fitness among their students. This policy statement reaffirms the American Academy of Pediatrics' support for the efforts of schools to include increased physical activity in the curriculum, suggests ways in which schools can meet their goals in physical fitness, and encourages pediatricians to offer their assistance. The recommendations in this statement are consistent with those published in 1997 by the Centers for Disease Control and Prevention. (5/00)

CLINICAL REPORT: PHYSICIANS' ROLES IN COORDINATING CARE OF HOSPITALIZED CHILDREN
Jack M. Percelay, MD, MPH, and the Committee on Hospital Care

ABSTRACT. The care of hospitalized children has become increasingly complex and intense and often involves multiple physicians beyond the traditional primary care attending physician. Pediatric and adult subspecialists and surgeons, teaching attending physicians, and hospitalists may all participate in the care of hospitalized children. This report summarizes the responsibilities of the primary care physician, attending physician, and other involved physicians to ensure that children receive appropriate, coordinated, and comprehensive inpatient care that is delivered within the context of their medical home and is appropriately continued on an outpatient basis. (3/03)

PLANNING FOR CHILDREN WHOSE PARENTS ARE DYING OF HIV/AIDS
Committee on Pediatric AIDS

ABSTRACT. Although the character of acquired immunodeficiency syndrome is changing into a chronic illness, it is estimated that by the end of this century, 80 000 children and adolescents in the United States will be orphaned by parental death caused by human immunodeficiency virus infection. Plans for these children need to be made to ensure not only a stable, consistent environment that provides love and nurturing, but also the medical and social interventions necessary to cope with the tragic loss. Pediatricians should become aware of local laws and community resources and initiate discussion early in the course of parental illness to facilitate planning for the future care and custody of the children. States need to adopt laws and regulations that provide flexible approaches to guardianship and placement of children orphaned by acquired immunodeficiency syndrome. (2/99, reaffirmed 2/02)

POISON TREATMENT IN THE HOME
Committee on Injury, Violence, and Poison Prevention

ABSTRACT. The ingestion of a potentially poisonous substance by a young child is a common event, with the American Association of Poison Control Centers reporting approximately 1.2 million such events in the United States in 2001. The American Academy of Pediatrics (AAP) has long concerned itself with this issue and has made poison prevention an integral component of its injury prevention initiatives. A key AAP recommendation has been to keep a 1-oz bottle of syrup of ipecac in the home to be used only on the advice of a physician or poison control center. Recently, there has been interest regarding activated charcoal in the home as a poison treatment strategy. After reviewing the evidence, the AAP believes that ipecac should no longer be used routinely as a home treatment strategy, that existing ipecac in the home should be disposed of safely, and that it is premature to recommend the administration of activated charcoal in the home. The first action for a caregiver of a child who may have ingested a toxic substance is to consult with the local poison control center. (11/03)

POLICY ON THE DEVELOPMENT OF IMMUNIZATION TRACKING SYSTEMS
Committee on Practice and Ambulatory Medicine (6/96)

CLINICAL REPORT: POSTEXPOSURE PROPHYLAXIS IN CHILDREN AND ADOLESCENTS FOR NONOCCUPATIONAL EXPOSURE TO HUMAN IMMUNODEFICIENCY VIRUS
Peter L. Havens, MD and Committee on Pediatric AIDS

ABSTRACT. Exposure to human immunodeficiency virus (HIV) can occur in a number of situations unique to, or more common among, children and adolescents. Guidelines for postexposure prophylaxis (PEP) for occupational and nonoccupational (eg, sexual, needle-sharing) exposures to HIV have been published by the US Public Health Service, but they do not directly address nonoccupational HIV exposures unique to children (such as accidental exposure to human milk from a woman infected with HIV or a puncture wound from a discarded needle on a playground), and they do not provide antiretroviral drug information relevant to PEP in children.

This clinical report reviews issues of potential exposure of children and adolescents to HIV and gives recommendations for PEP in those situations. The risk of HIV transmission from nonoccupational, nonperinatal exposure is generally low. Transmission risk is modified by factors related to the source and extent of exposure. Determination of the HIV infection status of the exposure source may not be possible, and data on transmission risk by exposure type may not exist. Except in the setting of perinatal transmission, no studies have demonstrated the safety and efficacy of postexposure use of antiretroviral drugs for the prevention of HIV transmission in nonoccupational settings. Antiretroviral therapy used for PEP is associated with significant toxicity. The decision to initiate prophylaxis needs to be made in consultation with the patient, the family, and a clinician with experience in treatment of persons with HIV infection. If instituted, therapy should be started as soon as possible after an exposure—no later than 72 hours—and continued for 28 days. Many clinicians would use 3 drugs for PEP regimens, although 2 drugs may be considered in certain circumstances. Instruction for avoiding secondary transmission should be given. Careful follow-up is needed for psychologic support, encouragement of medication adherence, toxicity monitoring, and serial HIV antibody testing. (6/03)

POSTNATAL CORTICOSTEROIDS TO TREAT OR PREVENT CHRONIC LUNG DISEASE IN PRETERM INFANTS
American Academy of Pediatrics Committee on Fetus and Newborn and Canadian Paediatric Society Fetus and Newborn Committee

ABSTRACT. This statement is intended for health care professionals caring for neonates and young infants. The objectives of this statement are to review the short- and long-term effects of systemic and inhaled postnatal corticosteroids for the prevention or treatment of evolving or established chronic lung disease and to make recommendations for the use of corticosteroids in infants with very low birth weight. The routine use of systemic dexamethasone for the prevention or treatment of chronic lung disease in infants with very low birth weight is not recommended. (2/02)

THE PRACTICAL SIGNIFICANCE OF LACTOSE INTOLERANCE IN CHILDREN
Committee on Nutrition (8/78, reaffirmed 12/93, 6/97, 4/00)

PRACTICAL SIGNIFICANCE OF LACTOSE INTOLERANCE IN CHILDREN: SUPPLEMENT
Committee on Nutrition (10/90, reaffirmed 12/93, 6/97, 4/00)

PRECAUTIONS CONCERNING THE USE OF THEOPHYLLINE
Committee on Drugs (4/92, reaffirmed 6/95, 6/98, 5/01)

TECHNICAL REPORT: PRECAUTIONS REGARDING THE USE OF AEROSOLIZED ANTIBIOTICS
Charles G. Prober, Philip D. Walson, Jim Jones, and the Committee on Infectious Diseases and Committee on Drugs

ABSTRACT. In 1998, the Food and Drug Administration (FDA) approved the licensure of tobramycin solution for inhalation (TOBI). Although a number of additional antibiotics, including other aminoglycosides, ß-lactams, antibiotics in the polymyxin class, and vancomycin, have been administered as aerosols for many years, none are approved by the FDA for administration by inhalation.

TOBI was approved by the FDA for the maintenance therapy of patients 6 years or older with cystic fibrosis (CF) who have between 25% and 75% of predicted forced expiratory volume in 1 second (FEV1), are colonized with *Pseudomonas aeruginosa*, and are able to comply with the prescribed medical regimen. TOBI was not approved for the therapy of acute pulmonary exacerbations in patients with CF nor was it approved for use in patients without CF. Currently, no other antibiotics are approved for administration by inhalation to patients with or without CF.

The purpose of this statement is to briefly summarize the data that supported approval for licensure of TOBI and to provide recommendations for its safe use. The pharmacokinetics of inhaled aminoglycosides and problems associated with aerosolized antibiotic treatment, including environmental contamination, selection of resistant microbes, and airway exposure to excipients in intravenous formulations, will be discussed. (12/00, reaffirmed 11/03)

PRECERTIFICATION PROCESS
Committee on Hospital Care
ABSTRACT. Precertification is a process still used by health insurance companies to control health care costs. Although we believe precertification is unnecessary and not cost-effective, in those instances where precertification is still being utilized, we suggest that the following procedures be adopted. This statement suggests guidelines that should help achieve this goal while allowing optimal access to care for children. (8/00)

PRENATAL GENETIC DIAGNOSIS FOR PEDIATRICIANS
Committee on Genetics (6/94, reaffirmed 10/97)

THE PRENATAL VISIT
Committee on Psychosocial Aspects of Child and Family Health
ABSTRACT. In their role as advocates for children and families, pediatricians are in an excellent position to support and guide parents during the prenatal period. Prenatal visits allow the pediatrician to gather basic information from parents, provide information and advice to them, and identify high-risk situations in which parents may need to be referred to appropriate resources for help. In addition, prenatal visits are the first step in establishing a relationship between the pediatrician and parents and help parents develop parenting skills. The prenatal visit may take several possible forms depending on the experience and preferences of the parents, competence and availability of the pediatrician, and provisions of the health care plan. (6/01)

PREVENTION OF AGRICULTURAL INJURIES AMONG CHILDREN AND ADOLESCENTS
Committee on Injury and Poison Prevention and Committee on Community Health Services
ABSTRACT. Although the annual number of farm deaths to children and adolescents has decreased since publication of the 1988 American Academy of Pediatrics statement, "Rural Injuries," the rate of nonfatal farm injuries has increased. Approximately 100 unintentional injury deaths occur annually to children and adolescents on US farms, and an additional 22 000 injuries to children younger than 20 years occur on farms. Relatively few adolescents are employed on farms compared with other types of industry, yet the proportion of fatalities in agriculture is higher than that for any other type of adolescent employment. The high mortality and severe morbidity associated with farm injuries require continuing and improved injury-control strategies. This statement provides recommendations for pediatricians regarding patient and community education as well as public advocacy related to agricultural injury prevention in childhood and adolescence. (10/01)

PREVENTION OF DROWNING IN INFANTS, CHILDREN, AND ADOLESCENTS
Committee on Injury, Violence, and Poison Prevention
ABSTRACT. Drowning is a leading cause of injury-related death in children. In 2000, more than 1400 US children younger than 20 years drowned. A number of strategies are available to prevent these tragedies. Pediatricians play an important role in prevention of drownings as educators and advocates. (8/03)

TECHNICAL REPORT: PREVENTION OF DROWNING IN INFANTS, CHILDREN, AND ADOLESCENTS
Ruth A. Brenner, MD, MPH and the Committee on Injury, Violence, and Poison Prevention
ABSTRACT. Drowning is a leading cause of injury-related death in children. In 2000, more than 1400 US children younger than 20 years drowned. Most (91%) of these deaths were unintentional and were not related to boating. For each drowning death, it is estimated that at least 1 to 4 children suffer a serious nonfatal submersion event, many of which leave children with permanent disabilities. Environmental strategies, such as installation of 4-sided fences around swimming pools, and behavioral strategies, such as increased supervision of children while around water, are needed to prevent these tragedies. (8/03)

PREVENTION OF HEPATITIS A INFECTIONS: GUIDELINES FOR USE OF HEPATITIS A VACCINE AND IMMUNE GLOBULIN

Committee on Infectious Diseases

ABSTRACT. The licensing of two inactivated hepatitis A vaccines for persons 2 years or older necessitates development of recommendations for pediatric use, as well as a review of the current indications for immune globulin (IG) in hepatitis A prophylaxis. Both vaccines are immunogenic and protective in children and adults. A single dose of vaccine induced antibody in 88% to 96% of subjects by 2 weeks and 97% to 100% by 1 month, and protected against subsequent hepatitis A virus (HAV) disease occurring 21 days after receipt of the dose in a community with endemic hepatitis A infection. However, completion of the full vaccine schedule is recommended to assure high antibody titers and likely long-term protection. The major pediatric indications for vaccine are: (1) travelers to areas with intermediate to high rates of endemic hepatitis A, (2) children living in defined and circumscribed communities with high endemic rates or periodic outbreaks of HAV infection, and (3) patients with chronic liver disease. Immune globulin is recommended for postexposure prophylaxis, as vaccine has not yet been demonstrated to be protective for this purpose. Except for travelers, recommendations for IG use are not changed from those in the current edition of the *Red Book*, and include contacts of cases in the home, child care centers, and other selected sites. (12/96, reaffirmed 2/00)

PREVENTION AND MANAGEMENT OF PAIN AND STRESS IN THE NEONATE

Committee on Fetus and Newborn, Committee on Drugs,
*   Section on Anesthesiology and Pain Medicine, Section*
*   on Surgery, and the Canadian Paediatric Society Fetus*
*   and Newborn Committee*

ABSTRACT. This statement is intended for health care professionals caring for neonates (preterm to 1 month of age). The objectives of this statement are to:
1. Increase awareness that neonates experience pain;
2. Provide a physiological basis for neonatal pain and stress assessment and management by health care professionals;
3. Make recommendations for reduced exposure of the neonate to noxious stimuli and to minimize associated adverse outcomes; and
4. Recommend effective and safe interventions that relieve pain and stress. (2/00, reaffirmed 4/03)

CLINICAL REPORT: PREVENTION AND MANAGEMENT OF POSITIONAL SKULL DEFORMITIES IN INFANTS

John Persing, MD, Hector James, MD, Jack Swanson, MD,
*   John Kattwinkel, MD, Committee on Practice and*
*   Ambulatory Medicine, Section on Plastic Surgery and*
*   Section on Neurological Surgery*

ABSTRACT. Cranial asymmetry may be present at birth or may develop during the first few months of life. Over the past several years, pediatricians have seen an increase in the number of children with cranial asymmetry, particularly unilateral flattening of the occiput. This increase likely is attributable to parents following the American Academy of Pediatrics "Back to Sleep" positioning recommendations aimed at decreasing the risk of sudden infant death syndrome. Although associated with some risk of deformational plagiocephaly, healthy young infants should be placed down for sleep on their backs. This practice has been associated with a dramatic decrease in the incidence of sudden infant death syndrome. Pediatricians need to be able to properly diagnose skull deformities, educate parents on methods to proactively decrease the likelihood of the development of occipital flattening, initiate appropriate management, and make referrals when necessary. This report provides guidelines for the prevention, diagnosis, and management of positional skull deformity in an otherwise normal infant without evidence of associated anomalies, syndromes, or spinal disease. (7/03)

PREVENTION OF MEDICATION ERRORS IN THE PEDIATRIC INPATIENT SETTING

Committee on Drugs and Committee on Hospital Care

ABSTRACT. Although medication errors in hospitals are common, medication errors that result in death or serious injury occur rarely. Even before the Institute of Medicine reported on medical errors in 1999, the American Academy of Pediatrics and its members had been committed to improving the health care system to provide the best and safest health care for infants, children, adolescents, and young adults. This commitment includes designing health care systems to prevent errors and emphasizing the pediatrician's role in this system. Human and device errors can lead to preventable morbidity and mortality. National and state legislative actions have heightened public awareness of these events. All involved persons, beginning with the physician and including every member of the health care team, must be better educated about and engaged in the several steps recommended to decrease these errors. The safe administration of medications to hospitalized infants and children requires additional specific safeguards that are above and beyond those for adult patients. Pediatricians should help hospitals develop effective programs for safely providing medications, reporting medication errors, and creating an environment of medication safety for all hospitalized pediatric patients. (8/03)

PREVENTION OF PEDIATRIC OVERWEIGHT AND OBESITY

Committee on Nutrition

ABSTRACT. The dramatic increase in the prevalence of childhood overweight and its resultant comorbidities are associated with significant health and financial burdens, warranting strong and comprehensive prevention efforts. This statement proposes strategies for early identification of excessive weight gain by using body mass index, for dietary and physical activity interventions during health supervision encounters, and for advocacy and research. (8/03)

TECHNICAL REPORT: PREVENTION OF PNEUMOCOCCAL INFECTIONS, INCLUDING THE USE OF PNEUMOCOCCAL CONJUGATE AND POLYSACCHARIDE VACCINES AND ANTIBIOTIC PROPHYLAXIS

Gary D. Overturf and the Committee on Infectious Diseases

ABSTRACT. Pneumococcal infections are the most common invasive bacterial infections in children in the United States. The incidence of invasive pneumococcal infections peaks in children younger than 2 years, reaching rates of 228/100 000 in children 6 to 12 months old. Children with functional or anatomic asplenia (including sickle cell disease [SCD]) and children with human immunodeficiency virus infection have pneumococcal infection rates 20- to 100-fold higher than those of healthy children during the first 5 years of life. Others at high risk of pneumococcal infections include children with congenital immunodeficiency; chronic cardiopulmonary disease; children receiving immunosuppressive chemotherapy; children with immunosuppressive neoplastic diseases; children with chronic renal insufficiency, including nephrotic syndrome; children with diabetes; and children with cerebrospinal fluid leaks. Children of Native American (American Indian and Alaska Native) or African American descent also have higher rates of invasive pneumococcal disease. Outbreaks of pneumococcal infection have occurred with increased frequency in children attending out-of-home care. Among these children, nasopharyngeal colonization rates of 60% have been observed, along with pneumococci resistant to multiple antibiotics. The administration of antibiotics to children involved in outbreaks of pneumococcal disease has had an inconsistent effect on nasopharyngeal carriage. In contrast, continuous penicillin prophylaxis in children younger than 5 years with SCD has been successful in reducing rates of pneumococcal disease by 84%.

Pneumococcal polysaccharide vaccines have been recommended since 1985 for children older than 2 years who are at high risk of invasive disease, but these vaccines were not recommended for younger children and infants because of poor antibody response before 2 years of age. In contrast, pneumococcal conjugate vaccines (Prevnar) induce proposed protective antibody responses (>.15 µg/mL) in >90% of infants after 3 doses given at 2, 4, and 6 months of age. After priming doses, significant booster responses (ie, immunologic memory) are apparent when additional doses are given at 12 to 15 months of age. In efficacy trials, infant immunization with Prevnar decreased invasive infections by >93% and consolidative pneumonia by 73%, and it was associated with a 7% decrease in otitis media and a 20% decrease in tympanostomy tube placement. Adverse events after the administration of Prevnar have been limited to areas of local swelling or erythema of 1 to 2 cm and some increase in the incidence of postimmunization fever when it is given with other childhood vaccines. Based on data in phase 3 efficacy and safety trials, the US Food and Drug Administration has provided an indication for the use of Prevnar in children younger than 24 months. (8/00)

CLINICAL REPORT: PREVENTION OF RICKETS AND VITAMIN D DEFICIENCY: NEW GUIDELINES FOR VITAMIN D INTAKE

Lawrence M. Gartner, MD, Frank R. Greer, MD and Section on Breastfeeding and Committee on Nutrition

ABSTRACT. Rickets in infants attributable to inadequate vitamin D intake and decreased exposure to sunlight continues to be reported in the United States. It is recommended that all infants, including those who are exclusively breastfed, have a minimum intake of 200 IU of vitamin D per day beginning during the first 2 months of life. In addition, it is recommended that an intake of 200 IU of vitamin D per day be continued throughout childhood and adolescence, because adequate sunlight exposure is not easily determined for a given individual. These new vitamin D intake guidelines for healthy infants and children are based on the recommendations of the National Academy of Sciences. (4/03)

PREVENTION OF SEXUAL HARASSMENT IN THE WORKPLACE AND EDUCATIONAL SETTINGS

Committee on Pediatric Workforce — Subcommittee on Women in Pediatrics

ABSTRACT. The American Academy of Pediatrics is committed to all its constituents supporting workplaces and educational settings free of sexual harassment. The purpose of this statement is to heighten awareness and sensitivity to this important issue, recognizing that institutions may have existing policies. (12/00)

CLINICAL REPORT: PREVENTION AND TREATMENT OF TYPE 2 DIABETES MELLITUS IN CHILDREN, WITH SPECIAL EMPHASIS ON AMERICAN INDIAN AND ALASKA NATIVE CHILDREN

Sheila Gahagan, MD and Janet Silverstein, MD the Committee on Native American Child Health and Section on Endocrinology

ABSTRACT. The emergence of type 2 diabetes mellitus in the American Indian/Alaska Native pediatric population presents a new challenge for pediatricians and other health care professionals. This chronic disease requires preventive efforts, early diagnosis, and collaborative care of the patient and family within the context of a medical home. (10/03)

CLINICAL REPORT: THE PREVENTION OF UNINTENTIONAL INJURY AMONG AMERICAN INDIAN AND ALASKA NATIVE CHILDREN: A SUBJECT REVIEW
Committee on Native American Child Health and Committee on Injury and Poison Prevention

ABSTRACT. Among ethnic groups in the United States, American Indian and Alaska Native (AI/AN) children experience the highest rates of injury mortality and morbidity. Injury mortality rates for AI/AN children have decreased during the past quarter century, but remain almost double the rate for all children in the United States. The Indian Health Service (IHS), the federal agency with the primary responsibility for the health care of AI/AN people, has sponsored an internationally recognized injury prevention program designed to reduce the risk of injury death by addressing community-specific risk factors. Model programs developed by the IHS and tribal governments have led to successful outcomes in motor vehicle occupant safety, drowning prevention, and fire safety. Injury prevention programs in tribal communities require special attention to the sovereignty of tribal governments and the unique cultural aspects of health care and communication. Pediatricians working with AI/AN children on reservations or in urban environments are strongly urged to collaborate with tribes and the IHS to create community-based coalitions and develop programs to address highly preventable injury-related mortality and morbidity. Strong advocacy also is needed to promote childhood injury prevention as an important priority for federal agencies and tribes. (12/99, reaffirmed 12/02 COIVPP, 5/03 CONACH)

PRINCIPLES OF CHILD HEALTH CARE FINANCING
Committee on Child Health Financing

ABSTRACT. Child health care financing must maximize access to quality, comprehensive pediatric and prenatal health care. This policy statement replaces the 1998 policy statement by the same title. Changes reflect recent state and federal legislation that affect child health care financing. The principles outlined in the statement will be used to evaluate the changing structure of child health care financing. (10/03)

YEAR 2000 POSITION STATEMENT: PRINCIPLES AND GUIDELINES FOR EARLY HEARING DETECTION AND INTERVENTION PROGRAMS
Joint Committee on Infant Hearing (10/00)

PRINCIPLES OF PATIENT SAFETY IN PEDIATRICS
National Initiative for Children's Health Care Quality Project Advisory Committee

ABSTRACT. The American Academy of Pediatrics and its members are committed to improving the health care system to provide the best and safest health care for infants, children, adolescents, and young adults. In response to a 1999 Institute of Medicine report on building a safer health system, a set of principles was established to guide the profession in designing a health care system that maximizes quality of care and minimizes medical errors through identification and resolution. This set of principles provides direction on setting up processes to identify and learn from errors, developing performance standards and expectations for safety, and promoting leadership and knowledge. (6/01)

PRIVACY PROTECTION OF HEALTH INFORMATION: PATIENT RIGHTS AND PEDIATRICIAN RESPONSIBILITIES
Pediatric Practice Action Group and Task Force on Medical Informatics

ABSTRACT. Pediatricians and pediatric medical and surgical subspecialists should know their legal responsibilities to protect the privacy of identifiable patient health information. Although paper and electronic medical records have the same privacy standards, health data that are stored or transmitted electronically are vulnerable to unique security breaches. This statement describes the privacy and confidentiality needs and rights of pediatric patients and suggests appropriate security strategies to deter unauthorized access and inappropriate use of patient data. Limitations to physician liability are discussed for transferred data. Any new standards for patient privacy and confidentiality must balance the health needs of the community and the rights of the patient without compromising the ability of pediatricians to provide quality care. (10/99)

PROFESSIONAL LIABILITY COVERAGE FOR RESIDENTS AND FELLOWS
Committee on Medical Liability

ABSTRACT. The American Academy of Pediatrics first developed a policy on professional liability coverage for pediatricians-in-training in 1989 and subsequently reaffirmed its basic position with slight modification in 1993. In this latest iteration of the statement, the original positions have been strengthened to address changes in the professional liability insurance industry, the structure and settings of residency training, and mandated reporting to health provider data banks. The new policy emphasizes the need to provide pediatricians in training with adequate professional liability insurance coverage and to educate residents and fellows on the importance of adequate and uninterrupted professional liability coverage—both during and after residency. (9/00)

PROMOTING EDUCATION, MENTORSHIP, AND SUPPORT FOR PEDIATRIC RESEARCH
Committee on Pediatric Research

ABSTRACT. Pediatricians have an important role to play in the advancement of child health research and should be encouraged and supported to pursue research activities. Education and training in child health research should be part of every level of pediatric training. Continuing education and access to research advisors should be available to practitioners and academic faculty. Recommendations to promote additional research education and support at all levels of pediatric training, from premedical to continuing medical education, as well as suggestions for means to increase support and mentorship for research activities, are outlined in this statement. (6/01)

PROMOTION OF HEALTHY WEIGHT-CONTROL PRACTICES IN YOUNG ATHLETES
Committee on Sports Medicine and Fitness (5/96, reaffirmed 10/99)

PROTECTIVE EYEWEAR FOR YOUNG ATHLETES
Committee on Sports Medicine and Fitness (8/96, reaffirmed 10/99)

PROVISION OF EDUCATIONALLY-RELATED SERVICES FOR CHILDREN AND ADOLESCENTS WITH CHRONIC DISEASES AND DISABLING CONDITIONS
Committee on Children With Disabilities

ABSTRACT. Children and adolescents with chronic diseases and disabling conditions often need related services. As medical home professionals, pediatricians can assist children, adolescents, and their families with the complex federal, state, and local laws, regulations, and systems associated with these services. Expanded roles for pediatricians in Individual Family Service Plan, Individualized Education Plan, and 504 Plan development and implementation are recommended.

The complex range of federal, state, and local laws, regulations, and systems for special education and related services for children and adolescents in public schools is beyond the scope of this statement. Readers are referred to the policy statement "The Pediatrician's Role in Development and Implementation of an Individual Education Plan (IEP) and/or an Individual Family Services Plan" by the American Academy of Pediatrics for additional background materials. (2/00)

TECHNICAL REPORT: THE PSYCHOLOGICAL MALTREATMENT OF CHILDREN
Committee on Child Abuse and Neglect

ABSTRACT. Psychological maltreatment is a common consequence of physical and sexual abuse but also may occur as a distinct entity. Until recently, there has been controversy regarding the definition and consequences of psychological maltreatment. Sufficient research and consensus now exist about the incidence, definition, risk factors, and consequences of psychological maltreatment to bring this form of child maltreatment to the attention of pediatricians. This technical report provides practicing pediatricians with definitions and risk factors for psychological maltreatment and details how pediatricians can prevent, recognize, and report psychological maltreatment. Contemporary references and resources are provided for pediatricians and parents. (4/02)

PSYCHOSOCIAL RISKS OF CHRONIC HEALTH CONDITIONS IN CHILDHOOD AND ADOLESCENCE
Committee on Children With Disabilities and Committee on Psychosocial Aspects of Child and Family Health (12/93, reaffirmed 10/96)

PUBLIC DISCLOSURE OF PRIVATE INFORMATION ABOUT VICTIMS OF ABUSE
Committee on Child Abuse and Neglect (2/91, reaffirmed 5/94, 9/00)

CLINICAL REPORT: RACE/ETHNICITY, GENDER, SOCIOECONOMIC STATUS—RESEARCH EXPLORING THEIR EFFECTS ON CHILD HEALTH: A SUBJECT REVIEW
Committee on Pediatric Research

ABSTRACT. Data on research participants and populations frequently include race, ethnicity, and gender as categorical variables, with the assumption that these variables exert their effects through innate or genetically determined biologic mechanisms. There is a growing body of research that suggests, however, that these variables have strong social dimensions that influence health. Socioeconomic status, a complicated construct in its own right, interacts with and confounds analyses of race/ethnicity and gender. The Academy recommends that research studies include race/ethnicity, gender, and socioeconomic status as explanatory variables only when data relevant to the underlying social mechanisms have been collected and included in the analyses. (6/00)

RADIATION DISASTERS AND CHILDREN
Committee on Environmental Health

ABSTRACT. The special medical needs of children make it essential that pediatricians be prepared for radiation disasters, including 1) the detonation of a nuclear weapon; 2) a nuclear power plant event that unleashes a radioactive cloud; and 3) the dispersal of radionuclides by conventional explosive or the crash of a transport vehicle. Any of these events could occur unintentionally or as an act of terrorism. Nuclear facilities (eg, power plants, fuel processing centers, and food irradiation facilities) are often located in highly populated areas, and as they age, the risk of mechanical failure increases. The short- and long-term consequences of a radiation disaster are significantly greater in children for several reasons. First, children have a disproportionately higher minute ventilation, leading to greater internal exposure to radioactive gases. Children have a significantly greater risk of developing cancer even when they are exposed to radiation in utero. Finally, children and the parents of young children are more likely than are adults to develop enduring psychologic injury after a radiation disaster. The pediatrician has a critical role in planning for radiation disasters. For example, potassium iodide is of proven value for thyroid protection but must be given before or soon after exposure to radioiodines, requiring its placement in homes, schools, and child care centers. Pediatricians should work with public health authorities to ensure that children receive full consideration in local planning for a radiation disaster. (6/03)

REAPPRAISAL OF LYTIC COCKTAIL/DEMEROL, PHENERGAN, AND THORAZINE (DPT) FOR THE SEDATION OF CHILDREN
Committee on Drugs (4/95, reaffirmed 3/98, 5/01)

RECOMMENDATIONS FOR THE PREVENTION OF PNEUMOCOCCAL INFECTIONS, INCLUDING THE USE OF PNEUMOCOCCAL CONJUGATE VACCINE (PREVNAR), PNEUMOCOCCAL POLYSACCHARIDE VACCINE, AND ANTIBIOTIC PROPHYLAXIS
Committee on Infectious Diseases

ABSTRACT. Heptavalent pneumococcal conjugate vaccine (PCV7) is recommended for universal use in children 23 months and younger, to be given concurrently with other recommended childhood vaccines at 2, 4, 6, and 12 to 15 months of age. For children 7 to 23 months old who have not received previous doses of PCV7, administration of a reduced number of doses is recommended. Two doses of PCV7 are recommended for children 24 to 59 months old at high risk of invasive pneumococcal infection—including children with functional, anatomic, or congenital asplenia; infection with human immunodeficiency virus; and other predisposing conditions—who have not been immunized previously with PCV7. Recommendations have been made for use of 23-valent pneumococcal polysaccharide (23PS) vaccine in high-risk children to expand serotype coverage. High-risk children should be given vaccines at the earliest possible opportunity. Use of antibiotic prophylaxis in children younger than 5 years with functional or anatomic asplenia, including children with sickle cell disease, continues to be recommended. Children who have not experienced invasive pneumococcal infection and have received recommended pneumococcal immunizations may discontinue prophylaxis after 5 years of age.

The safety and efficacy of PCV7 and 23PS in children 24 months or older at moderate or lower risk of invasive pneumococcal infection remain under investigation. Current US Food and Drug Administration indications are for administration of PCV7 only to children younger than 24 months. Data are insufficient to recommend routine administration of PCV7 for children at moderate risk of pneumococcal invasive infection, including all children 24 to 35 months old, children 36 to 59 months old who attend out-of-home care, and children 36 to 59 months old who are of Native American (American Indian and Alaska Native) or African American descent. However, all children 24 to 59 months old, regardless of whether they are at low or moderate risk, may benefit from the administration of pneumococcal immunizations. Therefore, a single dose of PCV7 or 23PS vaccine may be given to children 24 months or older. The 23PS is an acceptable alternative to PCV7, although an enhanced immune response and probable reduction of nasopharyngeal carriage favor the use of PCV7 whenever possible. (8/00)

RECOMMENDATIONS FOR PREVENTIVE PEDIATRIC HEALTH CARE
Committee on Practice and Ambulatory Medicine (3/00)

RECOMMENDATIONS FOR THE USE OF LIVE ATTENUATED VARICELLA VACCINE
Committee on Infectious Diseases (5/95, reaffirmed 6/98)

RECOMMENDED CHILDHOOD IMMUNIZATION SCHEDULE — UNITED STATES, 2003
Committee on Infectious Diseases (1/03)

RED REFLEX EXAMINATION IN INFANTS
Section on Ophthalmology

ABSTRACT. Red reflex examination is recommended for all infants. This statement describes the indications for and the technique to perform this examination, including indications for dilation of the pupils before examination and indications for referral to an ophthalmologist. (5/02)

REDUCING THE NUMBER OF DEATHS AND INJURIES FROM RESIDENTIAL FIRES
Committee on Injury and Poison Prevention

ABSTRACT. Smoke inhalation, severe burns, and death from residential fires are devastating events, most of which are preventable. In 1998, approximately 381 500 residential structure fires resulted in 3250 non-firefighter deaths, 17 175 injuries, and approximately $4.4 billion in property loss. This statement reviews important prevention messages and intervention strategies related to residential fires. It also includes recommendations for pediatricians regarding office anticipatory guidance, work in the community, and support of regulation and legislation that could result in a decrease in the number of fire-related injuries and deaths to children. (6/00)

REDUCING THE RISK OF HUMAN IMMUNODEFICIENCY VIRUS INFECTION ASSOCIATED WITH ILLICIT DRUG USE
Committee on Pediatric AIDS (12/94, reaffirmed 1/98)

REDUCTION OF THE INFLUENZA BURDEN IN CHILDREN
Committee on Infectious Diseases

ABSTRACT. Epidemiologic studies indicate that children with certain chronic conditions, such as asthma, and otherwise healthy children younger than 24 months are hospitalized for influenza and its complications at high rates similar to those experienced by the elderly. Currently, annual influenza immunization is recommended for all children 6 months and older with high-risk conditions. To protect these children more fully against the complications of influenza, increased efforts are needed to identify and recall high-risk children for annual influenza immunization. In addition, immunization of children 6 through 23 months of age and their household contacts and out-of-home caregivers is now encouraged to the extent feasible. The ultimate goal is a universal recommendation for influenza immunization. Issues that need to be addressed before institution of routine immunization of healthy young children include education of physicians and parents about the morbidity caused by influenza, adequate vaccine supply, and appropriate reimbursement of practitioners for influenza immunization. (12/02)

TECHNICAL REPORT: REDUCTION OF THE INFLUENZA BURDEN IN CHILDREN

ABSTRACT. Epidemiologic studies have shown that children of all ages with certain chronic conditions, such as asthma, and otherwise healthy children younger than 24 months (6 through 23 months) are hospitalized for influenza and its complications at high rates similar to those experienced by the elderly. Annual influenza immunization is already recommended for all children 6 months and older with high-risk conditions. By contrast, influenza immunization has not been recommended for healthy young children. To protect children against the complications of influenza, increased efforts are needed to identify and recall high-risk children. In addition, immunization of children between 6 through 23 months of age and their close contacts is now encouraged to the extent feasible. Children younger than 6 months may be protected by immunization of their household contacts and out-of-home caregivers. The ultimate goal is universal immunization of children 6 to 24 months of age. Issues that need to be addressed before institution of routine immunization of healthy young children include education of physicians and parents about the morbidity caused by influenza, adequate vaccine supply, and appropriate reimbursement of practitioners for influenza immunization. This report contains a summary of the influenza virus, protective immunity, disease burden in children, diagnosis, vaccines, and antiviral agents. (12/02)

REIMBURSEMENT FOR FOODS FOR SPECIAL DIETARY USE
Committee on Nutrition

ABSTRACT. Foods for special dietary use are recommended by physicians for chronic diseases or conditions of childhood, including inherited metabolic diseases. Although many states have created legislation requiring reimbursement for foods for special dietary use, legislation is now needed to mandate consistent coverage and reimbursement for foods for special dietary use and related support services with accepted medical benefit for children with designated medical conditions. (5/03)

RELIGIOUS OBJECTIONS TO MEDICAL CARE
Committee on Bioethics

ABSTRACT. Parents sometimes deny their children the benefits of medical care because of religious beliefs. In some jurisdictions, exemptions to child abuse and neglect laws restrict government action to protect children or seek legal redress when the alleged abuse or neglect has occurred in the name of religion. The American Academy of Pediatrics (AAP) believes that all children deserve effective medical treatment that is likely to prevent substantial harm or suffering or death. In addition, the AAP advocates that all legal interventions apply equally whenever children are endangered or harmed, without exemptions based on parental religious beliefs. To these ends, the AAP calls for the repeal of religious exemption laws and supports additional efforts to educate the public about the medical needs of children. (2/97, reaffirmed 10/00, 6/03)

RESIDENCY TRAINING AND CONTINUING MEDICAL EDUCATION IN SCHOOL HEALTH
Section on School Health (9/93)

RESTRAINT USE ON AIRCRAFT
Committee on Injury and Poison Prevention

ABSTRACT. Occupant protection policies for children younger than 2 years on aircraft are inconsistent with all other national policies on safe transportation. Children younger than 2 years are not required to be restrained or secured on aircraft during takeoff, landing, and conditions of turbulence. They are permitted to be held on the lap of an adult. Preventable injuries and deaths have occurred in children younger than 2 years who were unrestrained in aircraft during survivable crashes and conditions of turbulence. The American Academy of Pediatrics recommends a mandatory federal requirement for restraint use for children on aircraft. The Academy further recommends that parents ensure that a seat is available for all children during aircraft transport and follow current recommendations for restraint use for all children. Physicians play a significant role in counseling families, advocating for public policy mandates, and encouraging technologic research that will improve protection of children in aircraft. (11/01)

RETINOID THERAPY FOR SEVERE DERMATOLOGICAL DISORDERS
Committee on Drugs (7/92, reaffirmed 6/95, 6/98)

REVISED INDICATIONS FOR THE USE OF PALIVIZUMAB AND RESPIRATORY SYNCYTIAL VIRUS IMMUNE GLOBULIN INTRAVENOUS FOR THE PREVENTION OF RESPIRATORY SYNCYTIAL VIRUS INFECTIONS
Committee on Infectious Diseases and Committee on Fetus and Newborn

ABSTRACT. Palivizumab and Respiratory Syncytial Virus Immune Globulin Intravenous (RSV-IGIV) are licensed by the Food and Drug Administration for use in preventing severe lower respiratory tract infections caused by respiratory syncytial virus (RSV) in high-risk infants, children younger than 24 months with chronic lung disease (formerly called bronchopulmonary dysplasia), and certain preterm infants. This statement provides revised recommendations for administering RSV prophylaxis to infants and children with congenital heart disease, for identifying infants with a history of preterm birth and chronic lung disease who are most likely to benefit from immunoprophylaxis, and for reducing the risk of RSV exposure and infection in high-risk children. On the basis of results of a recently completed clinical trial, prophylaxis with palivizumab is appropriate for infants and young children with hemodynamically significant congenital heart disease. RSV-IGIV should not be used in children with hemodynamically significant heart disease. Palivizumab is preferred for most highrisk infants and children because of ease of intramuscular administration. Monthly administration of palivizumab during the RSV season results in a 45% to 55% decrease in the rate of hospitalization attributable to RSV. Because of the large number of infants born after 32 to 35 weeks' gestation and because of the high cost, immunoprophylaxis should be considered for this category of preterm infants only if 2 or more risk factors are present. High-risk infants should not attend child care during the RSV season when feasible, and exposure to tobacco smoke should be eliminated. (12/03)

TECHNICAL REPORT: REVISED INDICATIONS FOR THE USE OF PALIVIZUMAB AND RESPIRATORY SYNCYTIAL VIRUS IMMUNE GLOBULIN INTRAVENOUS FOR THE PREVENTION OF RESPIRATORY SYNCYTIAL VIRUS INFECTIONS

H. Cody Meissner, MD and Sarah S. Long, MD and the Committee on Infectious Diseases and Committee on Fetus and Newborn

ABSTRACT. Palivizumab and Respiratory Syncytial Virus Immune Globulin Intravenous (RSV-IGIV) are licensed by the Food and Drug Administration for use in preventing severe respiratory syncytial virus (RSV) infections in high-risk infants, children younger than 24 months with chronic lung disease (formerly called bronchopulmonary dysplasia), and certain preterm infants. This report summarizes the clinical trial information on which the guidance in the accompanying policy statement for administering RSV prophylaxis to certain children with a history of preterm birth, chronic lung disease, or congenital heart disease is based. On the basis of results of a recently completed clinical trial, palivizumab is appropriate for infants and young children with hemodynamically significant congenital heart disease. RSV-IGIV should not be used in children with hemodynamically significant heart disease. Palivizumab is preferred for most high-risk infants and children because of ease of intramuscular administration. Monthly administration of palivizumab during the RSV season results in a 45% to 55% decrease in the rate of hospitalization attributable to RSV. Because of the large number of infants born after 32 to 35 weeks' gestation and because of the high cost, immunoprophylaxis should be considered for this category of preterm infants only if 2 or more risk factors are present. (12/03)

RISK OF INJURY FROM BASEBALL AND SOFTBALL IN CHILDREN

Committee on Sports Medicine and Fitness

ABSTRACT. This statement updates the 1994 American Academy of Pediatrics policy statement on baseball and softball injuries in children. Current studies on acute, overuse, and catastrophic injuries are reviewed with emphasis on the causes and mechanisms of injury. This information serves as a basis for recommending safe training practices and the appropriate use of protective equipment. (4/01)

THE ROLE OF HOME-VISITATION PROGRAMS IN IMPROVING HEALTH OUTCOMES FOR CHILDREN AND FAMILIES

Council on Child and Adolescent Health

ABSTRACT. Traditional pediatric care is often based on the assumption that parents have the basic knowledge and resources to provide a nurturing, safe environment and to provide for the emotional, physical, developmental, and health care needs of their infants and young children. Unfortunately, many families have insufficient knowledge of parenting skills and an inadequate support system of friends, extended family, or professionals to help with these vital tasks. Home-visitation programs offer an effective mechanism to ensure ongoing parental education, social support, and linkage with public and private community services. This statement reviews the history and current research on home-visitation programs and provides recommendations about the pediatrician's role in supporting and using home visitation. (3/98, reaffirmed 5/01)

THE ROLE OF THE NURSE PRACTITIONER AND PHYSICIAN ASSISTANT IN THE CARE OF HOSPITALIZED CHILDREN

Committee on Hospital Care

ABSTRACT. The positions of nurse practitioner and physician assistant were created approximately 30 years ago. Since then, the role and responsibilities of these individuals have developed and grown and now may include involvement in the care of hospitalized patients. The intent of this statement is to suggest a manner in which nurse practitioners and physician's assistants may participate in and contribute to the care of the hospitalized child on the general inpatient unit, among other areas. (5/99, reaffirmed 11/01)

ROLE OF THE PEDIATRICIAN IN FAMILY-CENTERED EARLY INTERVENTION SERVICES

Committee on Children With Disabilities

ABSTRACT. There is growing evidence that early intervention services have had a positive influence on the developmental outcome of children with established disabilities or those considered "at risk" for disabilities and their families. Various federal and state statutes now mandate that community-based, coordinated, multidisciplinary, family-centered programs be established, which are accessible to serve children and families in need. The pediatrician, in close collaboration with the family and the early intervention team, plays a critical role in guiding the clinical and developmental aspects of the early intervention services provided. This role can be best served in the context of providing a medical home for children with special health care needs. The purpose of this statement is to assist the pediatrician in assuming a proactive role on the multidisciplinary team providing early intervention services. (5/01)

CLINICAL REPORT: THE ROLE OF THE PEDIATRICIAN IN IMPLEMENTING THE AMERICANS WITH DISABILITIES ACT: SUBJECT REVIEW

Committee on Children With Disabilities

ABSTRACT. In this statement, the American Academy of Pediatrics reaffirms the importance of the Americans With Disabilities Act (ADA), which guarantees people with disabilities certain rights to enable them to participate more fully in their communities. Pediatricians need to know about the ADA provisions to be able to educate and counsel their patients and patients' families appropriately. The ADA mandates changes to our environment, including reasonable accommodation to the needs of individuals with disabilities, which has application to schools, hospitals, physician offices, community businesses, and recreational programs. Pediatricians should be a resource to their community by providing information about the ADA and the special needs of their patients, assisting with devising reasonable accommodation, and counseling adolescents about their expanded opportunities under the ADA. (7/96, reaffirmed 10/00)

THE ROLE OF THE PEDIATRICIAN IN PRESCRIBING THERAPY SERVICES FOR CHILDREN WITH MOTOR DISABILITIES
Committee on Children With Disabilities

ABSTRACT. Pediatricians are often called upon to prescribe physical and occupational therapy service for children with motor disabilities. This statement defines the context in which rehabilitation therapies should be prescribed, emphasizing the identification and enhancement of the child's function and abilities. The statement encourages the pediatrician to work with teams including the parents, child, teachers, therapists, and other physicians. (8/96)

THE ROLE OF THE PEDIATRICIAN IN RECOGNIZING AND INTERVENING ON BEHALF OF ABUSED WOMEN
Committee on Child Abuse and Neglect

ABSTRACT. Pediatricians are in a position to recognize abused women in pediatric settings. Intervening on behalf of battered women is an active form of child abuse prevention. Knowledge of local resources and state laws for reporting abuse are emphasized. (6/98, reaffirmed 10/01)

THE ROLE OF THE PEDIATRICIAN IN RURAL EMSC
Committee on Pediatric Emergency Medicine

ABSTRACT. In rural America pediatricians can play a key role in the development, implementation, and ongoing supervision of emergency medical services for children (EMSC). Often the only pediatric resource for a large region, rural access pediatricians are more likely to treat pediatric emergencies in their own offices, and are a vital resource for rural physicians, or other rural health care professionals (physician assistants, nurse practitioners), and emergency medical technicians (EMTs) to improve system-wide EMSC by providing education about issues from prevention to rehabilitation, technical assistance in protocol writing, hospital care, and data accumulation, and as advocates for community and state legislation to support the goals of EMSC. (5/98, reaffirmed 6/00)

THE ROLE OF THE PEDIATRICIAN IN TRANSITIONING CHILDREN AND ADOLESCENTS WITH DEVELOPMENTAL DISABILITIES AND CHRONIC ILLNESSES FROM SCHOOL TO WORK OR COLLEGE
Committee on Children With Disabilities

ABSTRACT. The role of the pediatrician in transitioning children with disabilities and chronic illnesses from school to work or college is to provide anticipatory guidance and to promote self-advocacy and self-determination. Knowledge of the provisions of the key federal laws affecting vocational education is essential for the pediatrician's successful advocacy for patients. (10/00)

THE ROLE OF THE PEDIATRICIAN IN YOUTH VIOLENCE PREVENTION IN CLINICAL PRACTICE AND AT THE COMMUNITY LEVEL
Task Force on Violence

ABSTRACT. Violence and violent injuries are a serious threat to the health of children and youth in the United States. It is crucial that pediatricians define their role and develop the appropriate skills to address this threat effectively. From a clinical perspective, pediatricians should incorporate into their practices preventive education, screening for risk, and linkages to necessary intervention and follow-up services. As advocates, pediatricians should become involved at the local and national levels to address key risk factors and assure adequacy of preventive and treatment programs. There are also educational and research needs central to the development of effective clinical strategies. This policy statement defines the emerging role of pediatricians in youth violence prevention and management. It reflects the importance of this issue in the strategic agenda of the American Academy of Pediatrics for promoting optimal child health and development. (1/99, reaffirmed 5/02)

THE ROLE OF THE PRIMARY CARE PEDIATRICIAN IN THE MANAGEMENT OF HIGH-RISK NEWBORN INFANTS
Committee on Practice and Ambulatory Medicine and
*   Committee on Fetus and Newborn*

ABSTRACT. Quality care for high-risk newborns can best be provided by coordinating the efforts of the primary care pediatrician and the neonatologist. This ideally occurs in the newborn period, during the critical care and convalescing periods, and through the time of discharge. This statement offers guidelines for the primary care pediatrician involved in providing neonatal care, and discusses his/her individual and shared responsibilities, roles, and relationships with the neonatologist and the neonatal intensive care unit. (10/96)

THE ROLE OF THE SCHOOL NURSE IN PROVIDING SCHOOL HEALTH SERVICES
Committee on School Health

ABSTRACT. The school nurse has a crucial role in the provision of school health services. This statement describes the school nurse as a member of the school health services team and its relation to children with special health care needs. Recommendations for the professional preparation and education of school nurses also are provided. (11/01)

THE ROLE OF SCHOOLS IN COMBATTING SUBSTANCE ABUSE
Committee on Substance Abuse (5/95)

SAFE TRANSPORTATION OF NEWBORNS AT HOSPITAL DISCHARGE
Committee on Injury and Poison Prevention

ABSTRACT. All hospitals should set policies that require the discharge of every newborn in a car safety seat that is appropriate for the infant's maturity and medical condition. Discharge policies for newborns should include a parent education component, regular review of educational materials, and periodic in-service education for responsible staff. Appropriate child restraint systems should become a benefit of coverage by Medicaid, managed care organizations, and other third-party insurers. (10/99, reaffirmed 12/02)

SAFE TRANSPORTATION OF PREMATURE AND LOW BIRTH WEIGHT INFANTS
Committee on Injury and Poison Prevention and Committee on Fetus and Newborn

ABSTRACT. Special considerations are essential to ensure the safe transportation of premature and low birth weight infants. Both physical and physiologic issues must be considered in the proper positioning of these infants. This statement discusses current recommendations based on the latest research and provides guidelines for physicians who counsel parents of very small infants on the choice of the best car safety seats for their infants. (5/96, reaffirmed 4/99)

SAFEGUARDS NEEDED IN TRANSFER OF PATIENT DATA
Task Force on Medical Informatics, Section on Computers and Other Technologies, and Committee on Practice and Ambulatory Medicine

ABSTRACT. The intent of this statement is to provide practitioners with information to assist them in safeguarding the electronic storage and transmission of patient data. It lists safeguards that should be in place in pediatric practices that send facsimiles of patient data. Issues of protecting patient and provider confidentiality, maintaining the security of these data, and state and federal health data legislation are also addressed. (11/96, reaffirmed 2/01)

SAFETY IN YOUTH ICE HOCKEY: THE EFFECTS OF BODY CHECKING
Committee on Sports Medicine and Fitness

ABSTRACT. Ice hockey is a sport enjoyed by many young people. The occurrence of injury can offset what may otherwise be a positive experience. A high proportion of injuries in hockey appear to result from intentional body contact or the practice of checking. The American Academy of Pediatrics recommends limiting checking in hockey players 15 years of age and younger as a means to reduce injuries. Strategies such as the fair play concept can also help decrease injuries that result from penalties or unnecessary contact. (3/00)

SCHOOL BUS TRANSPORTATION OF CHILDREN WITH SPECIAL HEALTH CARE NEEDS
Committee on Injury and Poison Prevention (8/01)

SCHOOL HEALTH ASSESSMENTS
Committee on School Health

ABSTRACT. Comprehensive health assessments often are performed in school-based clinics or public health clinics by health professionals other than pediatricians. Pediatricians or other physicians skilled in child health care should participate in such evaluations. This statement provides guidance on the scope of in-school health assessments and the roles of the pediatrician, school nurse, school, and community. (4/00, reaffirmed 6/03)

SCHOOL HEALTH CENTERS AND OTHER INTEGRATED SCHOOL HEALTH SERVICES
Committee on School Health

ABSTRACT. This statement offers guidelines on the integration of expanded school health services, including school-based and school-linked health centers, into community-based health care systems. Expanded school health services should be integrated so that they enhance accessibility, provide high-quality health care, link children

to a medical home, are financially sustainable, and address both long- and short-term needs of children and adolescents. (1/01)

SCHOOL TRANSPORTATION SAFETY
Committee on School Health and Committee on Injury and Poison Prevention

ABSTRACT. The following policy statement is a revision of the American Academy of Pediatrics' 1985 statement entitled "School Bus Safety." It provides updated information regarding relevant federal regulations and outlines recommendations that can enhance community systems for addressing school bus safety education, awareness, and practices. Pediatricians can assist in this process by sharing these recommendations at both the community and state levels. (5/96, reaffirmed 4/99)

SCOPE OF HEALTH CARE BENEFITS FOR NEWBORNS, INFANTS, CHILDREN, ADOLESCENTS, AND YOUNG ADULTS THROUGH AGE 21 YEARS
Committee on Child Health Financing

ABSTRACT. The optimal health of children can best be achieved by providing access to comprehensive health care benefits. This policy statement replaces the 1993 statement, "Scope of Health Care Benefits for Infants, Children, and Adolescents Through Age 21 Years." Changes involve services and procedures specific to the delivery of comprehensive preventive, prenatal, postnatal, and mental health care. These services should be delivered by appropriately trained and board-eligible/certified pediatric providers, including primary care pediatricians, pediatric medical subspecialists, and pediatric surgical specialists. (12/97)

SCOPE OF PRACTICE ISSUES IN THE DELIVERY OF PEDIATRIC HEALTH CARE
Committee on Pediatric Workforce

ABSTRACT. In recent years, there has been an increase in the number of nonphysician pediatric clinicians and an expansion in their respective scopes of practice. This raises critical public policy and child health advocacy concerns. The American Academy of Pediatrics (AAP) believes that optimal pediatric health care depends on a team-based approach with coordination by a physician leader, preferably a pediatrician. The pediatrician is uniquely suited to manage, coordinate, and supervise the entire spectrum of pediatric care, from diagnosis through all stages of treatment, in all practice settings. The AAP recognizes the valuable contributions of nonphysician clinicians, including nurse practitioners and physician assistants, in delivering optimal pediatric care. The AAP also believes that nonphysician clinicians who provide health care services in underserved areas should be supported by consulting pediatricians and other physicians using technologies including telemedicine. Pediatricians should serve as advocates for optimal pediatric care in state legislatures, public policy forums, and the media and should pursue opportunities to resolve scope of practice conflicts outside state legislatures. The AAP affirms that as nonphysician clinicians seek to expand their scopes of practice as providers of pediatric care, standards of education, training, examination, regulation, and patient care are needed to ensure patient safety and quality health care for all infants, children, adolescents, and young adults. (2/03)

SCREENING FOR ELEVATED BLOOD LEAD LEVELS
Committee on Environmental Health

ABSTRACT. Although recent data continue to demonstrate a decline in the prevalence of elevated blood lead levels (BLLs) in children, lead remains a common, preventable, environmental health threat. Because recent epidemiologic data have shown that lead exposure is still common in certain communities in the United States, the Centers for Disease Control and Prevention recently issued new guidelines endorsing universal screening in areas with ≥27% of housing built before 1950 and in populations in which the percentage of 1- and 2-year-olds with elevated BLLs is ≥12%. For children living in other areas, the Centers for Disease Control and Prevention recommends targeted screening based on risk-assessment during specified pediatric visits. In this statement, the American Academy of Pediatrics supports these new guidelines and provides an update on screening for elevated BLLs. The American Academy of Pediatrics recommends that pediatricians continue to provide anticipatory guidance to parents in an effort to prevent lead exposure (primary prevention). Additionally, pediatricians should increase their efforts to screen children at risk for lead exposure to find those with elevated BLLs (secondary prevention). (6/98)

SCREENING EXAMINATION OF PREMATURE INFANTS FOR RETINOPATHY OF PREMATURITY
Section on Ophthalmology, American Association for Pediatric Ophthalmology and Strabismus, and American Academy of Ophthalmology

ABSTRACT. This statement revises a previous statement on screening of premature infants for retinopathy of prematurity originally published in 1997. (9/01)

SCREENING FOR RETINOPATHY IN THE PEDIATRIC PATIENT WITH TYPE 1 DIABETES MELLITUS
Section on Endocrinology and Section on Ophthalmology
(2/98)

SELECTING AND USING THE MOST APPROPRIATE CAR SAFETY SEATS FOR GROWING CHILDREN: GUIDELINES FOR COUNSELING PARENTS
Committee on Injury and Poison Prevention

ABSTRACT. Despite the existence of laws in all 50 states requiring the use of car safety seats or child restraint devices for young children, more children are still killed as passengers in car crashes than from any other type of injury. Pediatricians and other health care professionals need to provide up-to-date, appropriate information for parents regarding car safety seat choices and proper use. Although the American Academy of Pediatrics is not a testing or standard-setting organization, this policy statement discusses the Academy's current recommendations based on the peer-reviewed literature available at the time of publication and sets forth some of the factors that parents should consider before selecting and using a car safety seat. (3/02)

CLINICAL REPORT: SELECTING APPROPRIATE TOYS FOR YOUNG CHILDREN: THE PEDIATRICIAN'S ROLE
Danette Glassy, MD; Judith Romano, MD; and the Committee on Early Childhood, Adoption, and Dependent Care

ABSTRACT. Play is essential for learning in children. Toys are the tools of play. Which play materials are provided and how they are used are equally important. Adults caring for children can be reminded that toys facilitate but do not substitute for the most important aspect of nurture—warm, loving, dependable relationships. Toys should be safe, affordable, and developmentally appropriate. Children do not need expensive toys. Toys should be appealing to engage the child over a period of time. Information and resources are provided in this report so pediatricians can give parents advice about selecting toys. (4/03)

CLINICAL REPORT: SEVERE INVASIVE GROUP A STREPTOCOCCAL INFECTIONS: A SUBJECT REVIEW
Committee on Infectious Diseases

ABSTRACT. The course of severe invasive group A ß-hemolytic streptococcal (GABHS) infections is often precipitous, requiring prompt diagnosis and rapid initiation of appropriate therapy. Therefore, physicians must have a high index of suspicion of this disease, particularly in patients at increased risk (eg, those with varicella or diabetes mellitus). Although a relationship between the use of nonsteroidal antiinflammatory drugs and severe invasive GABHS infections has been suggested, at present data on which to base a clinical decision about the use or restriction of nonsteroidal antiinflammatory drugs in children with varicella are insufficient. When necrotizing fasciitis is suspected, prompt surgical drainage, debridement, fasciotomy, or amputation often is necessary. Many experts recommend intravenously administered penicillin G and clindamycin for the treatment of invasive GABHS infections on the basis of animal studies. Some evidence exists that intravenous immunoglobulin given in addition to appropriate antimicrobial and surgical therapy may be beneficial. Although chemoprophylaxis for household contacts of persons with invasive GABHS infections has been considered by some experts, the limited available data indicate that the risk of secondary cases is low (2.9 per 1000) and data about the effectiveness of any drug are insufficient to make recommendations. Because of the low risk of secondary cases of invasive GABHS infections in schools or child care facilities, chemoprophylaxis is not indicated in these settings. Routine immunization of all healthy children against varicella is recommended and is an effective means to decrease the risk of invasive GABHS infections. (1/98)

SEXUALITY, CONTRACEPTION, AND THE MEDIA
Committee on Public Education
ABSTRACT. Early sexual intercourse among American adolescents represents a major public health problem. Although early sexual activity may be caused by a variety of factors, the media are believed to play a significant role. In film, television, and music, sexual messages are becoming more explicit in dialogue, lyrics, and behavior. In addition, these messages contain unrealistic, inaccurate, and misleading information that young people accept as fact. Teens rank the media second only to school sex education programs as a leading source of information about sex. Recommendations are presented to help pediatricians address the effects of the media on sexual attitudes, beliefs, and behaviors of their patients. (1/01)

SEXUALITY EDUCATION FOR CHILDREN AND ADOLESCENTS
Committee on Psychosocial Aspects of Child and Family Health and Committee on Adolescence
ABSTRACT. Children and adolescents need accurate and comprehensive education about sexuality to practice healthy sexual behavior as adults. Early, exploitative, or risky sexual activity may lead to health and social problems, such as unintended pregnancy and sexually transmitted diseases, including human immunodeficiency virus infection and acquired immunodeficiency syndrome. This statement reviews the role of the pediatrician in providing sexuality education to children, adolescents, and their families. Pediatricians should integrate sexuality education into the confidential and longitudinal relationship they develop with children, adolescents, and families to complement the education children obtain at school and at home. Pediatricians must be aware of their own attitudes, beliefs, and values so their effectiveness in discussing sexuality in the clinical setting is not limited. (8/01)

SEXUALITY EDUCATION OF CHILDREN AND ADOLESCENTS WITH DEVELOPMENTAL DISABILITIES
Committee on Children With Disabilities (2/96, reaffirmed 4/00)

TECHNICAL REPORT: SHAKEN BABY SYNDROME: ROTATIONAL CRANIAL INJURIES
Committee on Child Abuse and Neglect
ABSTRACT. Shaken baby syndrome is a serious and clearly definable form of child abuse. It results from extreme rotational cranial acceleration induced by violent shaking or shaking/impact, which would be easily recognizable by others as dangerous. More resources should be devoted to prevention of this and other forms of child abuse. (7/01)

SKATEBOARD AND SCOOTER INJURIES
Committee on Injury, Violence, and Poison Prevention
ABSTRACT. Skateboard-related injuries account for an estimated 50 000 emergency department visits and 1500 hospitalizations among children and adolescents in the United States each year. Nonpowered scooter-related injuries accounted for an estimated 9400 emergency department visits between January and August 2000, and 90% of these patients were children younger than 15 years. Many such injuries can be avoided if children and youth do not ride in traffic, if proper protective gear is worn, and if, in the absence of close adult supervision, skateboards and scooters are not used by children younger than 10 and 8 years, respectively. (3/02)

SMALLPOX VACCINE
Committee on Infectious Diseases
ABSTRACT. After an extensive worldwide eradication program, the last nonlaboratory case of smallpox occurred in 1977 in Somalia. In 1972, routine smallpox immunization was discontinued in the United States, and since 1983, vaccine production has been halted. Stockpiled vaccine has been used only for laboratory researchers working on orthopoxviruses. In recent years, there has been concern that smallpox virus stocks may be in the hands of bioterrorists, and this concern has been heightened by the terrorist attack on the World Trade Center and the Pentagon on September 11, 2001. Because most of the population is considered to be nonimmune, there is debate as to whether smallpox immunization should be resumed. This statement reviews the current status of smallpox vaccine, the adverse effects that were associated with smallpox vaccine in the past, and the major proposals for vaccine use. The statement provides the rationale for a policy based on the so-called ring vaccination strategy recommended by the Centers for Disease Control and Prevention, in which cases of smallpox are rapidly identified, infected individuals are isolated, and contacts of the infected individuals as well as their contacts are immunized immediately. (10/02)

SNOWMOBILING HAZARDS
Committee on Injury and Poison Prevention
ABSTRACT. Snowmobiles continue to pose a significant risk to children younger than 15 years and adolescents and young adults 15 through 24 years of age. Head injuries remain the leading cause of mortality and serious morbidity, arising largely from snowmobilers colliding, falling, or overturning during operation. Children also were injured while being towed in a variety of conveyances by snowmobiles. No uniform code of state laws governs the use of snowmobiles by children and youth. Because evidence is lacking to support the effectiveness of operator safety certification and because many children and adolescents do not have the required strength and skills to operate a snowmobile safely, the recreational operation of snowmobiles by persons younger than 16 years is not recommended. Snowmobiles should not be used to tow persons on a tube, tire, sled, or saucer. Furthermore, a graduated licensing program is advised for snowmobilers 16 years and older. Both active and passive snowmobile injury prevention strategies are suggested, as well as recommendations for manufacturers to make safer equipment for snowmobilers of all ages. (11/00)

SOY PROTEIN-BASED FORMULAS: RECOMMENDATIONS FOR USE IN INFANT FEEDING
Committee on Nutrition

ABSTRACT. The American Academy of Pediatrics is committed to the use of maternal breast milk as the ideal source of nutrition for infant feeding. Even so, by 2 months of age, most infants in North America are formula-fed. Despite limited indications, the use of soy protein-based formula has nearly doubled during the past decade to achieve 25% of the market in the United States. Because an infant formula provides the largest, if not sole, source of nutrition for an extended interval, the nutritional adequacy of the formula must be confirmed and the indications for its use well understood. This statement updates the 1983 Committee on Nutrition review and contains some important recommendations on the appropriate use of soy protein-based formulas. (1/98, reaffirmed 4/01)

SPECIAL REQUIREMENTS FOR ELECTRONIC MEDICAL RECORD SYSTEMS IN PEDIATRICS
Task Force on Medical Informatics

ABSTRACT. Electronic medical record (EMR) systems, which are usually designed for adult care, must perform certain functions to be useful in pediatric care. This statement outlines these functions (eg, immunization tracking and pediatric dosing calculations) to assist vendors and standards organizations with software design for pediatric systems. The description of these functions should also provide pediatricians with a set of requirements or desirable features to use when evaluating EMR systems. Particular attention is paid to special aspects of pediatric clinical care and privacy issues unique to pediatrics. (8/01)

STERILIZATION OF MINORS WITH DEVELOPMENTAL DISABILITIES
Committee on Bioethics

ABSTRACT. Sterilization of persons with developmental disabilities has often been performed without appropriate regard for their decision-making capacities, abilities to care for children, feelings, or interests. In addition, sterilization sometimes has been performed with the mistaken belief that it will prevent expressions of sexuality, diminish the chances of sexual exploitation, or reduce the likelihood of acquiring sexually transmitted diseases. A decision to pursue sterilization of someone with developmental disabilities requires a careful assessment of the individual's capacity to make decisions, the consequences of reproduction for the person and any child that might be born, the alternative means available to address the consequences of sexual maturation, and the applicable local, state, and federal laws. Pediatricians can facilitate good decision-making by raising these issues at the onset of puberty. (8/99, reaffirmed 11/02)

STRENGTH TRAINING BY CHILDREN AND ADOLESCENTS
Committee on Sports Medicine and Fitness

ABSTRACT. Pediatricians are often asked to give advice on the safety and efficacy of strength training programs for children and adolescents. This review, a revision of a previous American Academy of Pediatrics policy statement, defines relevant terminology and provides current information on risks and benefits of strength training for children and adolescents. (6/01)

SUICIDE AND SUICIDE ATTEMPTS IN ADOLESCENTS
Committee on Adolescence

ABSTRACT. Suicide is the third leading cause of death for adolescents 15 to 19 years old. Pediatricians can help prevent adolescent suicide by knowing the symptoms of depression and other presuicidal behavior. This statement updates the previous statement by the American Academy of Pediatrics and assists the pediatrician in the identification and management of the adolescent at risk for suicide. The extent to which pediatricians provide appropriate care for suicidal adolescents depends on their knowledge, skill, comfort with the topic, and ready access to appropriate community resources. All teenagers with suicidal symptoms should know that their pleas for assistance are heard and that pediatricians are willing to serve as advocates to help resolve the crisis. (4/00)

SURFACTANT REPLACEMENT THERAPY FOR RESPIRATORY DISTRESS SYNDROME
Committee on Fetus and Newborn

ABSTRACT. Respiratory failure secondary to surfactant deficiency is a major cause of morbidity and mortality in low birth weight immature infants. Surfactant therapy substantially reduces mortality and respiratory morbidity for this population. The statement summarizes the indications for surfactant replacement therapy. Because respiratory insufficiency may be a component of multiorgan dysfunction in sick infants, surfactant should be administered only at institutions with qualified personnel and facilities for the comprehensive care of sick infants. (3/99)

SURVEILLANCE OF PEDIATRIC HIV INFECTION
Committee on Pediatric AIDS

ABSTRACT. Pediatric human immunodeficiency virus (HIV)/acquired immunodeficiency syndrome (AIDS) surveillance should expand to include perinatal HIV exposure and HIV infection as well as AIDS to delineate completely the extent and impact of HIV infection on children and families, accurately assess the resources necessary to provide services to this population, evaluate the efficacy of public health recommendations, and determine any potential long-term consequences of interventions to prevent perinatal transmission to children ultimately determined to be uninfected as well as for those who become infected. Ensuring the confidentiality of information collected in the process of surveillance is critical. In addition, expansion of surveillance must not compromise the established, ongoing surveillance system for pediatric AIDS. An expanded pediatric HIV surveillance program provides an important counterpart to existing American Academy of Pediatrics and American College of Obstetricians and Gynecologists recommendations for HIV counseling and testing in the prenatal setting. (2/98, reaffirmed 2/02)

SWIMMING PROGRAMS FOR INFANTS AND TODDLERS
Committee on Sports Medicine and Fitness and Committee on Injury and Poison Prevention

ABSTRACT. Infant and toddler aquatic programs provide an opportunity to introduce young children to the joy and risks of being in or around water. Generally, children are not developmentally ready for swimming lessons until after their fourth birthday. Aquatic programs for infants and toddlers have not been shown to decrease the risk of drowning, and parents should not feel secure that their child is safe in water or safe from drowning after participating in such programs. Young children should receive constant, close supervision by an adult while in and around water. (4/00)

TARGETED TUBERCULIN TESTING AND TREATMENT OF LATENT TUBERCULOSIS INFECTION
American Thoracic Society and Centers for Disease Control and Prevention (4/00) (The AAP endorses and accepts as its policy the sections of this statement as it relates to infants and children.)

THE TEENAGE DRIVER
Committee on Injury and Poison Prevention and Committee on Adolescence

ABSTRACT. Motor vehicle-related injuries continue to be of paramount importance to adolescents. This statement describes why teenagers are at particularly great risk, suggests topics suitable for office-based counseling, describes innovative programs, and proposes steps for prevention for pediatricians, legislators, educators, and other child advocates. (11/96, reaffirmed 11/99)

TESTING FOR DRUGS OF ABUSE IN CHILDREN AND ADOLESCENTS
Committee on Substance Abuse

ABSTRACT. The American Academy of Pediatrics (AAP) recognizes the abuse of psychoactive drugs as one of the greatest problems facing children and adolescents and condemns all such use. Diagnostic testing for drugs of abuse is frequently an integral part of the pediatrician's evaluation and management of those suspected of such use. "Voluntary screening" is the term applied to many mass non–suspicion-based screening programs, yet such programs may not be truly voluntary as there are often negative consequences for those who choose not to take part. Participation in such programs should not be a prerequisite to participation in school activities. Involuntary testing is not appropriate in adolescents with decisional capacity—even with parental consent—and should be performed only if there are strong medical or legal reasons to do so. The AAP reaffirms its position that the appropriate response to the suspicion of drug abuse in a young person is the referral to a qualified health care professional for comprehensive evaluation. (8/96, reaffirmed 5/99)

THERAPY FOR CHILDREN WITH INVASIVE PNEUMOCOCCAL INFECTIONS
Committee on Infectious Diseases

ABSTRACT. This statement provides guidelines for therapy of children with serious infections possibly caused by *Streptococcus pneumoniae*. Resistance of invasive pneumococcal strains to penicillin, cefotaxime, and ceftriaxone has increased over the past few years. Reports of failures of cefotaxime or ceftriaxone in the treatment of children with meningitis caused by resistant *S pneumoniae* necessitates a revision of Academy recommendations. For nonmeningeal infections, modifications of the initial therapy need to be considered only for patients who are critically ill and those who have a severe underlying or potentially immunocompromising condition or patients from whom a highly resistant strain is isolated. Because vancomycin is the only antibiotic to which all *S pneumoniae* strains are susceptible, its use should be restricted to minimize the emergence of vancomycin-resistant organisms. Patients with probable aseptic (viral) meningitis should not be treated with vancomycin. These recommendations are subject to change as new information becomes available. (2/97, reaffirmed 10/99)

TIMING OF ELECTIVE SURGERY ON THE GENITALIA OF MALE CHILDREN WITH PARTICULAR REFERENCE TO THE RISKS, BENEFITS, AND PSYCHOLOGICAL EFFECTS OF SURGERY AND ANESTHESIA
Section on Urology (4/96)

TOBACCO, ALCOHOL, AND OTHER DRUGS: THE ROLE OF THE PEDIATRICIAN IN PREVENTION AND MANAGEMENT OF SUBSTANCE ABUSE
Committee on Substance Abuse

ABSTRACT. During the past three decades, the responsibility of pediatricians to their patients and their patients' families regarding the prevention of substance abuse and the diagnosis and management of problems related to substance abuse has increased. The American Academy of Pediatrics (AAP) has highlighted the importance of such issues in a variety of ways, including its guidelines for preventive services. Nonetheless, many pediatricians remain reluctant to address this issue. The harmful consequences of tobacco, alcohol, and other drug use are a concern of medical professionals who care for infants, children, adolescents, and young adults. Thus, pediatricians should include discussion of substance abuse as a part of routine health care, starting with the prenatal visit and as a part of ongoing anticipatory guidance. Knowledge of the extent and nature of the consequences of tobacco, alcohol, and other drug use as well as the physical, psychological, and social consequences is important for pediatricians. Pediatricians should incorporate substance abuse prevention into daily practice, acquire the skills necessary to identify young people at risk for substance abuse, and provide or obtain assessment, intervention, and treatment as necessary. (1/98)

TOBACCO'S TOLL: IMPLICATIONS FOR THE PEDIATRICIAN
Committee on Substance Abuse

ABSTRACT. The disease of tobacco addiction, which is pervasive in the United States, begins in childhood and adolescence. Twenty-five percent of the population regularly uses tobacco, despite evidence that such use is the leading preventable cause of death in the United States. Tobacco use reportedly kills 2.5 times as many people each year as alcohol and drug abuse combined. According to 1998 data from the World Health Organization, there were 1.1 billion smokers worldwide and 10 000 tobacco-related deaths per day. Furthermore, in the United States, 43% of children aged 2 to 11 years are exposed to environmental tobacco smoke, which has been implicated in sudden infant death syndrome, low birth weight, asthma, middle ear disease, pneumonia, cough, and upper respiratory infection. Pediatricians play a crucial role in reducing both tobacco use (by children, adolescents, and their parents) and exposure to tobacco smoke and should rank this among their highest health prevention priorities. (4/01)

TOXIC EFFECTS OF INDOOR MOLDS
Committee on Environmental Health

ABSTRACT. This statement describes molds, their toxic properties, and their potential for causing toxic respiratory problems in infants. Guidelines for pediatricians are given to help reduce exposures to mold in homes of infants. This is a rapidly evolving area and more research is ongoing. (4/98, reaffirmed 4/02)

TRAMPOLINES AT HOME, SCHOOL, AND RECREATIONAL CENTERS
Committee on Injury and Poison Prevention and Committee on Sports Medicine and Fitness

ABSTRACT. The latest available data indicate that an estimated 83 400 trampoline-related injuries occurred in 1996 in the United States. This represents an annual rate 140% higher than was reported in 1990. Most injuries were sustained on home trampolines. In addition, 30% of trampoline-related injuries treated in an emergency department were fractures often resulting in hospitalization and surgery. These data support the American Academy of Pediatrics' reaffirmation of its recommendation that trampolines should never be used in the home environment, in routine physical education classes, or in outdoor playgrounds. Design and behavioral recommendations are made for the limited use of trampolines in supervised training programs. (5/99, reaffirmed 12/02)

THE TRANSFER OF DRUGS AND OTHER CHEMICALS INTO HUMAN MILK
Committee on Drugs

ABSTRACT. The American Academy of Pediatrics places emphasis on increasing breastfeeding in the United States. A common reason for the cessation of breastfeeding is the use of medication by the nursing mother and advice by her physician to stop nursing. Such advice may not be warranted. This statement is intended to supply the pediatrician, obstetrician, and family physician with data, if known, concerning the excretion of drugs into human milk. Most drugs likely to be prescribed to the nursing mother should have no effect on milk supply or on infant well-being. This information is important not only to protect nursing infants from untoward effects of maternal medication but also to allow effective pharmacologic treatment of breastfeeding mothers. Nicotine, psychotropic drugs, and silicone implants are 3 important topics reviewed in this statement. (9/01)

TECHNICAL REPORT: TRANSMISSIBLE SPONGIFORM ENCEPHALOPATHIES: A REVIEW FOR PEDIATRICIANS
Richard J. Whitley, MD, Noni MacDonald, MD, David M. Asher, MD, and Committee on Infectious Diseases

ABSTRACT. Transmissible spongiform encephalopathies (TSEs) are a family of rare, slowly progressive, and universally fatal neurodegenerative syndromes affecting animals and humans. Until recently, TSEs were of little interest to pediatricians. However, since the outbreak in adolescents and the association of TSEs with new-variant Creutzfeldt-Jakob disease (nvCJD), interest among pediatricians and the general public has increased. Even before bovine spongiform encephalopathy and nvCJD were linked, the recognition that iatrogenic Creutzfeldt-Jakob disease (CJD) had been acquired from administration of cadaveric human growth and gonadotropic hormones and from corneal and dura mater transplants prompted medical vigilance. Furthermore, recent concern about the potential for transmission of CJD by blood and blood products has raised awareness among public health and regulatory agencies, pediatricians, and the public, although no epidemiologic data support this concern. Because of worldwide concern (although no cases have been reported in North America), this review focuses on the potential impact of TSEs, particularly CJD and nvCJD, on the pediatric population. (11/00)

TRANSPORTING CHILDREN WITH SPECIAL HEALTH CARE NEEDS
Committee on Injury and Poison Prevention

ABSTRACT. Children with special health care needs should have access to proper resources for safe transportation. This statement reviews important considerations for transporting children with special health care needs and provides current guidelines for the protection of children with specific health care needs, including those with a tracheostomy, a spica cast, challenging behaviors, or muscle tone abnormalities as well as those transported in wheelchairs. (10/99, reaffirmed 12/02)

TREATMENT GUIDELINES FOR LEAD EXPOSURE IN CHILDREN
Committee on Drugs (7/95, reaffirmed 10/98, 11/01)

THE TREATMENT OF NEUROLOGICALLY IMPAIRED CHILDREN USING PATTERNING
Committee on Children With Disabilities

ABSTRACT. This statement reviews patterning as a treatment for children with neurologic impairments. This treatment is based on an outmoded and oversimplified theory of brain development. Current information does not support the claims of proponents that this treatment is efficacious, and its use continues to be unwarranted. (11/99, reaffirmed 11/02)

TRIATHLON PARTICIPATION BY CHILDREN AND ADOLESCENTS
Committee on Sports Medicine and Fitness
ABSTRACT. Triathlon is a sport combining swimming, cycling, and running in one continuous event. It is a relatively new sport for children and adolescents, and participation is growing rapidly. The purpose of this statement is to provide pediatricians and others with information on the participation in triathlons by young athletes. A list of triathlon events is given in the "Resources" section at the end of this statement. (9/96, reaffirmed 10/99)

TYPE 2 DIABETES IN CHILDREN AND ADOLESCENTS
American Diabetes Association (3/00)

ULTRAVIOLET LIGHT: A HAZARD TO CHILDREN
Committee on Environmental Health (8/99, reaffirmed 10/02)

UNIVERSAL ACCESS TO GOOD-QUALITY EDUCATION AND CARE OF CHILDREN FROM BIRTH TO 5 YEARS
Committee on Early Childhood, Adoption, and Dependent Care (3/96)

USE AND ABUSE OF THE APGAR SCORE
Committee on Fetus and Newborn, American Academy of Pediatrics; and Committee on Obstetric Practice, American College of Obstetricians and Gynecologists
ABSTRACT. This is a revised statement published jointly with the American College of Obstetricians and Gynecologists that emphasizes the appropriate use of the Apgar Score. The highlights of the statement include: (1) the Apgar Score is useful in assessing the condition of the infant at birth; (2) the Apgar score alone should not be used as evidence that neurologic damage was caused by hypoxia that results in neurologic injury or from inappropriate intrapartum treatment; and (3) an infant who has had "asphyxia" proximate to delivery that is severe enough to result in acute neurologic injury should demonstrate all of the following: (a) profound metabolic or mixed acidemia (pH <7.00) on an umbilical arterial blood sample, if obtained, (b) an Apgar score of 0 to 3 for longer than 5 minutes, (c) neurologic manifestation, eg, seizure, coma, or hypotonia, and (d) evidence of multiorgan dysfunction. (7/96, reaffirmed 10/97, 10/00)

THE USE OF CHAPERONES DURING THE PHYSICAL EXAMINATION OF THE PEDIATRIC PATIENT
Committee on Practice and Ambulatory Medicine (12/96, reaffirmed 11/99, 2/00)

USE OF CODEINE- AND DEXTROMETHORPHAN-CONTAINING COUGH REMEDIES IN CHILDREN
Committee on Drugs
ABSTRACT. Numerous prescription and nonprescription medications are currently available for suppression of cough, a common symptom in children. Because adverse effects and overdosage associated with the administration of cough and cold preparations in children have been reported, education of patients and parents about the lack of proven antitussive effects and the potential risks of these products is needed. (6/97, reaffirmed 5/00, 6/03)

USE OF INHALED NITRIC OXIDE
Committee on Fetus and Newborn
ABSTRACT. Approval of inhaled nitric oxide by the US Food and Drug Administration for hypoxic respiratory failure of the term and near-term newborn provides an important new therapy for this serious condition. This statement addresses the conditions under which inhaled nitric oxide should be administered to the neonate with hypoxic respiratory failure. (8/00, reaffirmed 4/03)

THE USE AND MISUSE OF FRUIT JUICE IN PEDIATRICS
Committee on Nutrition
ABSTRACT. Historically, fruit juice was recommended by pediatricians as a source of vitamin C and an extra source of water for healthy infants and young children as their diets expanded to include solid foods with higher renal solute. Fruit juice is marketed as a healthy, natural source of vitamins and, in some instances, calcium. Because juice tastes good, children readily accept it. Although juice consumption has some benefits, it also has potential detrimental effects. Pediatricians need to be knowledgeable about juice to inform parents and patients on its appropriate uses. (5/01)

USE OF PHOTOSCREENING FOR CHILDREN'S VISION SCREENING
Committee on Practice and Ambulatory Medicine and Section on Ophthalmology
ABSTRACT. This statement asserts that all children should be screened for risk factors associated with amblyopia. Guidelines are suggested for the use of photoscreening as a technique for the detection of amblyopia and strabismus in children of various age groups. The American Academy of Pediatrics favors additional research of the efficacy and cost-effectiveness of photoscreening as a vision screening tool. (3/02)

USE OF PSYCHOACTIVE MEDICATION DURING PREGNANCY AND POSSIBLE EFFECTS ON THE FETUS AND NEWBORN
Committee on Drugs
ABSTRACT. Psychoactive drugs are those psychotherapeutic drugs used to modify emotions and behavior in the treatment of psychiatric illnesses. This statement will limit its scope to drug selection guidelines for those psychoactive agents used during pregnancy for prevention or treatment of the following common psychiatric disorders: schizophrenia, major depression, bipolar disorder, panic disorder, and obsessive-compulsive disorder. The statement assumes that pharmacologic therapy is needed to manage the psychiatric disorder. This decision requires thoughtful psychiatric and obstetric advice. (4/00, reaffirmed 4/03)

USES OF DRUGS NOT DESCRIBED IN THE PACKAGE INSERT (OFF-LABEL USES)
Committee on Drugs

ABSTRACT. New regulatory initiatives have been designed to ensure that new drugs and biologicals include adequate pediatric labeling for the claimed indications at the time of, or soon after, approval. However, because such labeling may not immediately be available, off-label use (or use that is not included in the approved label) of therapeutic agents is likely to remain common in the practice of pediatrics. This policy statement was written to address questions practitioners have regarding off-label use. The purpose of off-label use is to benefit the individual patient. Practitioners may use their professional judgment to determine these uses. Practitioners should understand that the Food and Drug Administration does not regulate off-label use. (7/02)

VARICELLA VACCINE UPDATE
Committee on Infectious Diseases

ABSTRACT. Recommendations for routine varicella vaccination were published by the American Academy of Pediatrics in May 1995, but many eligible children remain unimmunized. This update provides additional information on the varicella disease burden before the availability of varicella vaccine, potential barriers to immunization, efforts to increase the level of coverage, new safety data, and new recommendations for use of the varicella vaccine after exposure and in children with human immunodeficiency virus infections. Pediatricians are strongly encouraged to support public health officials in the development and implementation of varicella immunization requirements for child care and school entry. (1/00)

WHEN INFLICTED SKIN INJURIES CONSTITUTE CHILD ABUSE
Committee on Child Abuse and Neglect

ABSTRACT. Child abuse should be considered as the most likely explanation for inflicted skin injuries if they are nonaccidental and there is any injury beyond temporary reddening of the skin. Minor forms of abuse may lead to severe abuse unless abusive skin injuries are identified and labeled as such and interventions are made. (9/02)

WIC PROGRAM
Provisional Section on Breastfeeding

ABSTRACT. This policy statement highlights the important collaboration between pediatricians and local Special Supplemental Nutrition Program for Women, Infants, and Children (WIC) programs to ensure that infants and children receive high-quality, cost-effective health care and nutrition services. Specific recommendations are provided for pediatricians and WIC personnel to help children and their families receive optimum services through a medical home. (11/01)

AMERICAN ACADEMY OF PEDIATRICS

Policy Statements
by Committee

(Current through December 2003)

Following is an alphabetical listing of the AAP Committees and the Policy Statements they authored. Full text of current statements can be found on the enclosed *Pediatric Clinical Practice Guidelines & Policies* CD-ROM. Policies that have been reaffirmed have reaffirmed dates listed following original date of issue.

COMMITTEE ON ADOLESCENCE

Adolescent Pregnancy—Current Trends and Issues: 1998, 2/99

Adolescents and Human Immunodeficiency Virus Infection: The Role of the Pediatrician in Prevention and Intervention (joint with Committee on Pediatric AIDS), 1/01

The Adolescent's Right to Confidential Care When Considering Abortion, 5/96, reaffirmed 5/99

Care of Adolescent Parents and Their Children (joint with Committee on Early Childhood, Adoption, and Dependent Care), 2/01

Care of the Adolescent Sexual Assault Victim, 6/01

Condom Use by Adolescents, 6/01

Confidentiality in Adolescent Health Care, 4/89, reaffirmed 1/93, 11/97, 5/00

Contraception and Adolescents, 11/99

Counseling the Adolescent About Pregnancy Options, 5/98, reaffirmed 1/01

Health Care for Children and Adolescents in the Juvenile Correctional Care System, 4/01

Homosexuality and Adolescence, 10/93, reaffirmed 11/96

Identifying and Treating Eating Disorders, 1/03

Sexuality Education for Children and Adolescents (joint with Committee on Psychosocial Aspects of Child and Family Health), 8/01

Suicide and Suicide Attempts in Adolescents, 4/00

The Teenage Driver (joint with Committee on Injury, Violence, and Poison Prevention), 11/96, reaffirmed 11/99

COMMITTEE ON BIOETHICS

Appropriate Boundaries in the Pediatrician-Family-Patient Relationship, 8/99, reaffirmed 11/02

Do Not Resuscitate Orders in Schools (joint with Committee on School Health), 4/00, reaffirmed 6/03

Ethical Issues With Genetic Testing in Pediatrics, 6/01

Ethics and the Care of Critically Ill Infants and Children, 7/96, reaffirmed 10/99, 6/03

Female Genital Mutilation, 7/98, reaffirmed 11/02

Fetal Therapy—Ethical Considerations, 5/99, reaffirmed 11/02

Forgoing Life-Sustaining Medical Treatment in Abused Children (joint with Committee on Child Abuse and Neglect), 11/00, reaffirmed 6/03

Guidelines on Forgoing Life-Sustaining Medical Treatment, 3/94, reaffirmed 11/97, 10/00

Human Embryo Research (joint with Committee on Pediatric Research), 9/01

Infants with Anencephaly as Organ Sources: Ethical Considerations, 6/92, reaffirmed 11/95, 11/98, 11/02

Informed Consent, Parental Permission, and Assent in Pediatric Practice, 2/95, reaffirmed 11/98, 11/02

Institutional Ethics Committees, 1/01

Palliative Care for Children (joint with Committee on Hospital Care), 8/00, reaffirmed 6/03

Religious Objections to Medical Care, 2/97, reaffirmed 10/00, 6/03

Sterilization of Minors With Developmental Disabilities, 8/99, reaffirmed 11/02

COMMITTEE ON CHILD ABUSE AND NEGLECT

Assessment of Maltreatment of Children With Disabilities (joint with Committee on Children With Disabilities), 8/01

Distinguishing Sudden Infant Death Syndrome From Child Abuse Fatalities, 2/01

Addendum: Distinguishing Sudden Infant Death Syndrome From Child Abuse Fatalities, 9/01

Forgoing Life-Sustaining Medical Treatment in Abused Children (joint with Committee on Bioethics), 11/00, reaffirmed 6/03

Gonorrhea in Prepubertal Children, 1/98, reaffirmed 10/01

Clinical Report: Guidelines for the Evaluation of Sexual Abuse of Children: Subject Review, 1/99

Investigation and Review of Unexpected Infant and Child Deaths (joint with Committee on Community Health Services), 11/99, reaffirmed 10/02

Medical Necessity for the Hospitalization of the Abused and Neglected Child (joint with Committee on Hospital Care), 4/98, reaffirmed 10/01

Oral and Dental Aspects of Child Abuse and Neglect (joint with American Academy of Pediatric Dentistry), 8/99

Technical Report: The Psychological Maltreatment of Children, 4/02, *Pediatrics electronic pages* (http://pediatrics.aappublications.org/cgi/content/full/109/4/e68)

Public Disclosure of Private Information About Victims of Abuse, 2/91, reaffirmed 5/94, 9/00

The Role of the Pediatrician in Recognizing and Intervening on Behalf of Abused Women, 6/98, reaffirmed 10/01

Technical Report: Shaken Baby Syndrome: Rotational Cranial Injuries, 7/01

When Inflicted Skin Injuries Constitute Child Abuse, 9/02

CHILD AND ADOLESCENT HEALTH ACTION GROUP (FORMERLY COUNCIL ON CHILD AND ADOLESCENT HEALTH)

Age Limits of Pediatrics, 5/88, reaffirmed 9/92, 1/97, 3/02

The Role of Home-Visitation Programs in Improving Health Outcomes for Children and Families, 3/98, reaffirmed 5/01

COMMITTEE ON CHILD HEALTH FINANCING

Guiding Principles for Managed Care Arrangements for the Health Care of Newborns, Infants, Children, Adolescents, and Young Adults, 1/00

Implementation Principles and Strategies for the State Children's Health Insurance Program, 5/01

Improving Substance Abuse Prevention, Assessment, and Treatment Financing for Children and Adolescents (joint with Committee on Substance Abuse), 10/01

Medicaid Policy Statement, 8/99

Principles of Child Health Care Financing, 10/03

Scope of Health Care Benefits for Newborns, Infants, Children, Adolescents, and Young Adults Through Age 21 Years, 12/97

COMMITTEE ON CHILDREN WITH DISABILITIES

Assessment of Maltreatment of Children With Disabilities (joint with Committee on Child Abuse and Neglect), 8/01

Auditory Integration Training and Facilitated Communication for Autism, 8/98, reaffirmed 5/02

Care Coordination: Integrating Health and Related Systems of Care for Children With Special Health Care Needs, 10/99

The Continued Importance of Supplemental Security Income (SSI) for Children and Adolescents With Disabilities, 4/01

Counseling Families Who Choose Complementary and Alternative Medicine for Their Child With Chronic Illness or Disability, 3/01

Developmental Surveillance and Screening of Infants and Young Children, 7/01

Fetal Alcohol Syndrome and Alcohol-Related Neurodevelopmental Disorders (joint with Committee on Substance Abuse), 8/00

General Principles in the Care of Children and Adolescents With Genetic Disorders and Other Chronic Health Conditions, 4/97, reaffirmed 4/00

Guidelines for Home Care of Infants, Children, and Adolescents With Chronic Disease, 7/95, reaffirmed 4/00

Clinical Report: Learning Disabilities, Dyslexia, and Vision: A Subject Review (joint with American Academy of Ophthalmology and American Association for Pediatric Ophthalmology and Strabismus), 11/98, reaffirmed 5/02

Clinical Report: Managed Care and Children With Special Health Care Needs: A Subject Review, 9/98

The Pediatrician's Role in Development and Implementation of an Individual Education Plan (IEP) and/or an Individual Family Service Plan (IFSP), 7/99, reaffirmed 11/02

The Pediatrician's Role in the Diagnosis and Management of Autistic Spectrum Disorder in Children, 5/01

Technical Report: The Pediatrician's Role in the Diagnosis and Management of Autistic Spectrum Disorder in Children, 5/01, *Pediatrics electronic pages* (http://pediatrics.aappublications.org/cgi/content/full/107/5/e85)

Provision of Educationally-Related Services for Children and Adolescents With Chronic Diseases and Disabling Conditions, 2/00

Psychosocial Risks of Chronic Health Conditions in Childhood and Adolescence (joint with Committee on Psychosocial Aspects of Child and Family Health), 12/93, reaffirmed 10/96

Role of the Pediatrician in Family-Centered Early Intervention Services, 5/01

Clinical Report: The Role of the Pediatrician in Implementing the Americans With Disabilities Act: Subject Review, 7/96, reaffirmed 10/00

The Role of the Pediatrician in Prescribing Therapy Services for Children With Motor Disabilities, 8/96

The Role of the Pediatrician in Transitioning Children and Adolescents With Developmental Disabilities and Chronic Illnesses From School to Work or College, 10/00

Sexuality Education of Children and Adolescents With Developmental Disabilities, 2/96, reaffirmed 4/00

The Treatment of Neurologically Impaired Children Using Patterning, 11/99, reaffirmed 11/02

STEERING COMMITTEE ON CLINICAL INFORMATION TECHNOLOGY (FORMERLY SECTION ON COMPUTERS AND OTHER TECHNOLOGIES AND TASK FORCE ON MEDICAL INFORMATICS)

Privacy Protection of Health Information: Patient Rights and Pediatrician Responsibilities (joint with Pediatric Practice Action Group), 10/99

Safeguards Needed in Transfer of Patient Data (joint with Committee on Practice and Ambulatory Medicine), 11/96, reaffirmed 2/01

Special Requirements for Electronic Medical Record Systems in Pediatrics, 8/01

COMMITTEE ON CODING AND NOMENCLATURE (FORMERLY COMMITTEE ON CODING AND REIMBURSEMENT)

Clinical Report: Issues in the Application of the Resource-Based Relative Value Scale System to Pediatrics: A Subject Review, 10/98

COMMITTEE ON COMMUNITY HEALTH SERVICES

Increasing Immunization Coverage (joint with Committee on Practice and Ambulatory Medicine), 10/03

Investigation and Review of Unexpected Infant and Child Deaths (joint with Committee on Child Abuse and Neglect), 11/99, reaffirmed 10/02

The Pediatrician's Role in Community Pediatrics, 6/99

Prevention of Agricultural Injuries Among Children and Adolescents (joint with Committee on Injury, Violence, and Poison Prevention), 10/01

COMMITTEE ON DRUGS

Acetaminophen Toxicity in Children, 10/01

Clinical Report: Alternative Routes of Drug Administration—Advantages and Disadvantages (Subject Review), 7/97, reaffirmed 10/00, 11/03

Camphor Revisited: Focus on Toxicity, 7/94, reaffirmed 6/97, 5/00

Clioquinol (Iodochlorhydroxyquin, Vioform) and Iodoquinol (Diiodohydroxyquin): Blindness and Neuropathy, 11/90, reaffirmed 2/94, 2/97, 2/00, 4/03

Drugs for Pediatric Emergencies, 1/98, *Pediatrics electronic pages* (http://pediatrics.aappublications.org/cgi/reprint/101/1/e13)

Generic Prescribing, Generic Substitution, and Therapeutic Substitution, 5/87, reaffirmed 6/93, 5/96, 6/99, 5/01

Guidelines for the Ethical Conduct of Studies to Evaluate Drugs in Pediatric Populations, 2/95, reaffirmed 3/98, 5/01

Guidelines for Monitoring and Management of Pediatric Patients During and After Sedation for Diagnostic and Therapeutic Procedures, 6/92, reaffirmed 6/95, 6/98, 5/02

Guidelines for Monitoring and Management of Pediatric Patients During and After Sedation for Diagnostic and Therapeutic Procedures: Addendum, 10/02

Clinical Report: "Inactive" Ingredients in Pharmaceutical Products: Update (Subject Review), 1/97, reaffirmed 2/00

Neonatal Drug Withdrawal, 6/98, reaffirmed 5/01

Precautions Concerning the Use of Theophylline, 4/92, reaffirmed 6/95, 6/98, 5/01

Technical Report: Precautions Regarding the Use of Aerosolized Antibiotics (joint with Committee on Infectious Diseases), 12/00, reaffirmed 11/03, *Pediatrics electronic pages* (http://pediatrics.aappublications.org/cgi/reprint/106/6/e89.pdf)

Prevention and Management of Pain and Stress in the Neonate (joint with Committee on Fetus and Newborn, Section on Anesthesiology and Pain Medicine, Section on Surgery, and Canadian Paediatric Society), 2/00, reaffirmed 4/03

Prevention of Medication Errors in the Pediatric Inpatient Setting (joint with Committee on Hospital Care), 8/03

Reappraisal of Lytic Cocktail/Demerol, Phenergan, and Thorazine (DPT) for the Sedation of Children, 4/95, reaffirmed 3/98, 5/01

Retinoid Therapy for Severe Dermatological Disorders, 7/92, reaffirmed 6/95, 6/98

The Transfer of Drugs and Other Chemicals Into Human Milk, 9/01

Treatment Guidelines for Lead Exposure in Children, 7/95, reaffirmed 10/98, 11/01

Use of Codeine- and Dextromethorphan-Containing Cough Remedies in Children, 6/97, reaffirmed 5/00, 6/03

Use of Psychoactive Medication During Pregnancy and Possible Effects on the Fetus and Newborn, 4/00, reaffirmed 4/03

Uses of Drugs Not Described in the Package Insert (Off-Label Uses), 7/02

COMMITTEE ON EARLY CHILDHOOD, ADOPTION, AND DEPENDENT CARE

Care of Adolescent Parents and Their Children (joint with Committee on Adolescence), 2/01

Developmental Issues for Young Children in Foster Care, 11/00

Clinical Report: Families and Adoption: The Pediatrician's Role in Supporting Communication, 12/03

Health Care of Young Children in Foster Care, 3/02

The Inappropriate Use of School "Readiness" Tests (joint with Committee on School Health), 3/95, reaffirmed 4/98, 9/03

Initial Medical Evaluation of an Adopted Child, 9/91

Parental Leave for Residents and Pediatric Training Programs (joint with Section on Residents), 11/95, reaffirmed 4/98

The Pediatrician's Role in Family Support Programs, 1/01

The Pediatrician's Role in the Prevention of Missing Children, 1/92, reaffirmed 5/96

Clinical Report: Selecting Appropriate Toys for Young Children: The Pediatrician's Role, 4/03

Universal Access to Good-quality Education and Care of Children From Birth to 5 Years, 3/96

COMMITTEE ON ENVIRONMENTAL HEALTH

Ambient Air Pollution: Respiratory Hazards to Children, 6/93, reaffirmed 5/96

Clinical Report: Chemical-Biological Terrorism and Its Impact on Children: A Subject Review (joint with Committee on Infectious Diseases), 3/00

Environmental Tobacco Smoke: A Hazard to Children, 4/97, reaffirmed 10/00

The Hazards of Child Labor, 2/95, reaffirmed 11/98

Technical Report: Irradiation of Food, 12/00

Technical Report: Mercury in the Environment: Implications for Pediatricians, 7/01

Noise: A Hazard for the Fetus and Newborn, 10/97, reaffirmed 10/00

Technical Report: Pediatric Exposure and Potential Toxicity of Phthalate Plasticizers, 6/03

Radiation Disasters and Children, 6/03

Screening for Elevated Blood Lead Levels, 6/98

Toxic Effects of Indoor Molds, 4/98, reaffirmed 4/02

Ultraviolet Light: A Hazard to Children, 8/99, reaffirmed 10/02

COMMITTEE ON FETUS AND NEWBORN

Advanced Practice in Neonatal Nursing, 6/03

Apnea, Sudden Infant Death Syndrome, and Home Monitoring, 4/03

Controversies Concerning Vitamin K and the Newborn, 7/03

Hospital Discharge of the High-Risk Neonate— Proposed Guidelines, 8/98, reaffirmed 6/01

Hospital Stay for Healthy Term Newborns, 10/95, reaffirmed 10/98

Human Immunodeficiency Virus Screening (joint with Committee on Pediatric AIDS and the American College of Obstetricians and Gynecologists), 7/99, reaffirmed 6/02

The Initiation or Withdrawal of Treatment for High-Risk Newborns, 8/95, reaffirmed 10/98, 6/01

Clinical Report: Perinatal Care at the Threshold of Viability, 11/02

Postnatal Corticosteroids to Treat or Prevent Chronic Lung Disease in Preterm Infants (joint with Canadian Paediatric Society), 2/02

Prevention and Management of Pain and Stress in the Neonate (joint with Committee on Drugs, Section on Anesthesiology and Pain Medicine, Section on Surgery, and Canadian Paediatric Society), 2/00, reaffirmed 4/03

Revised Indications for the Use of Palivizumab and Respiratory Syncytial Virus Immune Globulin Intravenous for the Prevention of Respiratory Syncytial Virus Infections (joint with Committee on Infectious Diseases), 12/03

Technical Report: Revised Indications for the Use of Palivizumab and Respiratory Syncytial Virus Immune Globulin Intravenous for the Prevention of Respiratory Syncytial Virus Infections (joint with Committee on Infectious Diseases), 12/03

The Role of the Primary Care Pediatrician in the Management of High-risk Newborn Infants (joint with Committee on Practice and Ambulatory Medicine), 10/96

Safe Transportation of Premature and Low Birth Weight Infants (joint with Committee on Injury, Violence, and Poison Prevention), 5/96, reaffirmed 4/99

Surfactant Replacement Therapy for Respiratory Distress Syndrome, 3/99

Use and Abuse of the Apgar Score (joint with American College of Obstetrics and Gynecologists), 7/96, reaffirmed 10/97, 10/00

Use of Inhaled Nitric Oxide, 8/00, reaffirmed 4/03

COMMITTEE ON GENETICS

Technical Report: Congenital Adrenal Hyperplasia (joint with Section on Endocrinology), 12/00

Evaluation of the Newborn With Developmental Anomalies of the External Genitalia (joint with Section on Endocrinology and Section on Urology), 7/00

Folic Acid for the Prevention of Neural Tube Defects, 8/99, reaffirmed 11/02

Health Care Supervision for Children With Williams Syndrome, 5/01

Health Supervision for Children With Achondroplasia, 3/95, reaffirmed 10/98

Health Supervision for Children With Down Syndrome, 2/01

Health Supervision for Children With Fragile X Syndrome, 8/96, reaffirmed 10/99

Health Supervision for Children With Marfan Syndrome, 11/96, reaffirmed 10/99, 10/02

Health Supervision for Children With Neurofibromatosis, 8/95, reaffirmed 10/98

Health Supervision for Children With Sickle Cell Disease (joint with Section on Hematology/Oncology), 3/02

Clinical Report: Health Supervision for Children With Turner Syndrome (joint with Section on Endocrinology), 3/03

Maternal Phenylketonuria, 2/01

Clinical Report: Molecular Genetic Testing in Pediatric Practice: A Subject Review, 12/00

Newborn Screening for Congenital Hypothyroidism: Recommended Guidelines (joint with Section on Endocrinology and American Thyroid Association Committee on Public Health), 6/93, reaffirmed 10/96

Newborn Screening Fact Sheets, 9/96, reaffirmed 10/99

Prenatal Genetic Diagnosis for Pediatricians, 6/94, reaffirmed 10/97

COMMITTEE ON HOSPITAL CARE

Child Life Services, 11/00

Clinical Report: Facilities and Equipment for the Care of Pediatric Patients in a Community Hospital, 5/03

Family-Centered Care and the Pediatrician's Role (joint with Institute for Family-Centered Care), 9/03

Guidelines for Developing Admission and Discharge Policies for the Pediatric Intensive Care Unit (joint with Section on Critical Care and Society of Critical Care Medicine), 4/99

Guidelines and Levels of Care for Pediatric Intensive Care Units (joint with Society of Critical Care Medicine), 7/93, reaffirmed 11/96

Medical Necessity for the Hospitalization of the Abused and Neglected Child (joint with Committee on Child Abuse and Neglect), 4/98, reaffirmed 5/01

Clinical Report: Medical Staff Appointment and Delineation of Pediatric Privileges in Hospitals, 8/02

Palliative Care for Children (joint with Committee on Bioethics), 8/00, reaffirmed 6/03

Pediatric Organ Donation and Transplantation (joint with Section on Surgery), 5/02

Clinical Report: Physicians' Roles in Coordinating Care of Hospitalized Children, 3/03

Precertification Process, 8/00

Prevention of Medication Errors in the Pediatric Inpatient Setting (joint with Committee on Drugs), 8/03

The Role of the Nurse Practitioner and Physician Assistant in the Care of Hospitalized Children, 5/99, reaffirmed 11/01

COMMITTEE ON INFECTIOUS DISEASES

Age for Routine Administration of the Second Dose of Measles-Mumps-Rubella Vaccine, 1/98

Clinical Report: Chemical-Biological Terrorism and Its Impact on Children: A Subject Review (joint with Committee on Environmental Health), 3/00

Combination Vaccines for Childhood Immunization: Recommendations of the Advisory Committee on Immunization Practices (ACIP), the American Academy of Pediatrics (AAP), and the American Academy of Family Physicians (AAFP), 5/99, reaffirmed 3/02

Clinical Report: Head Lice (joint with Committee on School Health), 9/02

Hepatitis C Virus Infection, 3/98

Immunization of Adolescents: Recommendations of the Advisory Committee on Immunization Practices, the American Academy of Pediatrics, the American Academy of Family Physicians, and the American Medical Association, 3/97

Clinical Report: Immunization of Preterm and Low Birth Weight Infants, 7/03

Infection Control in Physicians' Offices (joint with Committee on Practice and Ambulatory Medicine), 6/00

Issues Related to Human Immunodeficiency Virus Transmission in Schools, Child Care, Medical Settings, the Home, and Community (joint with Committee on Pediatric AIDS), 8/99, reaffirmed 2/02

Measles Immunization in HIV-Infected Children (joint with Committee on Pediatric AIDS), 5/99, reaffirmed 10/01

Meningococcal Disease Prevention and Control Strategies for Practice-Based Physicians (Addendum: Recommendations for College Students), 12/00, reaffirmed 10/01

Technical Report: Precautions Regarding the Use of Aerosolized Antibiotics (joint with Committee on Drugs), 12/00, reaffirmed 11/03, *Pediatrics electronic pages* (http://pediatrics.aappublications.org/cgi/reprint/106/6/e89.pdf)

Prevention of Hepatitis A Infections: Guidelines for Use of Hepatitis A Vaccine and Immune Globulin, 12/96, reaffirmed 2/00

Technical Report: Prevention of Pneumococcal Infections, Including the Use of Pneumococcal Conjugate and Polysaccharide Vaccines and Antibiotic Prophylaxis, 8/00

Recommendations for the Prevention of Pneumococcal Infections, Including the Use of Pneumococcal Conjugate Vaccine (Prevnar), Pneumococcal Polysaccharide Vaccine, and Antibiotic Prophylaxis, 8/00

Recommendations for the Use of Live Attenuated Varicella Vaccine, 5/95, reaffirmed 6/98

Recommended Childhood and Adolescent Immunization Schedule—United States, 2003, 1/03

Reduction of the Influenza Burden in Children, 12/02

Technical Report: Reduction of the Influenza Burden in Children, 12/02, *Pediatrics electronic pages* (http://pediatrics.aappublications.org/cgi/content/full/110/6/e80)

Revised Indications for the Use of Palivizumab and Respiratory Syncytial Virus Immune Globulin Intravenous for the Prevention of Respiratory Syncytial Virus Infections (joint with Committee on Fetus and Newborn), 12/03

Technical Report: Revised Indications for the Use of Palivizumab and Respiratory Syncytial Virus Immune Globulin Intravenous for the Prevention of Respiratory Syncytial Virus Infections (joint with Committee on Fetus and Newborn), 12/03

Clinical Report: Severe Invasive Group A Streptococcal Infections: A Subject Review, 1/98

Smallpox Vaccine, 10/02

Therapy for Children With Invasive Pneumococcal Infections, 2/97, reaffirmed 10/99

Technical Report: Transmissible Spongiform Encephalopathies: A Review for Pediatricians, 11/00

Varicella Vaccine Update, 1/00

COMMITTEE ON INJURY, VIOLENCE, AND POISON PREVENTION

All-Terrain Vehicle Injury Prevention: Two-, Three-, and Four-Wheeled Unlicensed Motor Vehicles, 6/00

Bicycle Helmets, 10/01

Children in Pickup Trucks, 10/00

Falls From Heights: Windows, Roofs, and Balconies, 5/01

Firearm-Related Injuries Affecting the Pediatric Population, 4/00

Fireworks-Related Injuries to Children, 7/01

The Hospital Record of the Injured Child and the Need for External Cause-of-Injury Codes, 2/99, reaffirmed 5/02

Injuries Associated With Infant Walkers, 9/01

Injuries Related to "Toy" Firearms, 3/87, reaffirmed 11/96

In-line Skating Injuries in Children and Adolescents (joint with Committee on Sports Medicine and Fitness), 4/98, reaffirmed 1/02

Lawn Mower-Related Injuries to Children, 6/01

Technical Report: Lawn Mower-Related Injuries to Children, 6/01, *Pediatrics electronic pages* (http://pediatrics.aappublications.org/cgi/content/full/107/6/e106)

Office-Based Counseling for Injury Prevention, 10/94, reaffirmed 10/98

Personal Watercraft Use by Children and Adolescents, 2/00

Poison Treatment in the Home, 11/03

Prevention of Agricultural Injuries Among Children and Adolescents (joint with Committee on Community Health Services), 10/01

Prevention of Drowning in Infants, Children, and Adolescents, 8/03

Technical Report: Prevention of Drowning in Infants, Children, and Adolescents, 8/03

Clinical Report: The Prevention of Unintentional Injury Among American Indian and Alaska Native Children: A Subject Review (joint with Committee on Native American Child Health), 12/99, reaffirmed 12/02

Reducing the Number of Deaths and Injuries From Residential Fires, 6/00

Restraint Use on Aircraft, 11/01

Safe Transportation of Newborns at Hospital Discharge, 10/99, reaffirmed 12/02

Safe Transportation of Premature and Low Birth Weight Infants (joint with Committee on Fetus and Newborn), 5/96, reaffirmed 4/99

School Bus Transportation of Children With Special Health Care Needs, 8/01

School Transportation Safety (joint with Committee on School Health), 5/96, reaffirmed 4/99

Selecting and Using the Most Appropriate Car Safety Seats for Growing Children: Guidelines for Counseling Parents, 3/02

Skateboard and Scooter Injuries, 3/02

Snowmobiling Hazards, 11/00

Swimming Programs for Infants and Toddlers (joint with Committee on Sports Medicine and Fitness), 4/00

The Teenage Driver (joint with Committee on Adolescence), 11/96, reaffirmed 11/99

Trampolines at Home, School, and Recreational Centers (joint with Committee on Sports Medicine and Fitness), 5/99, reaffirmed 12/02

Transporting Children With Special Heath Care Needs, 10/99, reaffirmed 12/02

COMMITTEE ON MEDICAL LIABILITY

Technical Report: Alternative Dispute Resolution in Medical Malpractice, 3/01

Clinical Report: Consent by Proxy for Nonurgent Pediatric Care, 11/03

Guidelines for Expert Witness Testimony in Medical Malpractice Litigation, 5/02

Pediatric Physician Profiling (joint with Committee on Practice and Ambulatory Medicine), 10/99

Pediatricians' Liability During Disasters (joint with Committee on Pediatric Emergency Medicine), 12/00

Professional Liability Coverage for Residents and Fellows, 9/00

COMMITTEE ON NATIVE AMERICAN CHILD HEALTH

Inhalant Abuse (joint with Committee on Substance Abuse), 3/96, reaffirmed 5/99

Clinical Report: Prevention and Treatment of Type 2 Diabetes Mellitus in Children, With Special Emphasis on American Indian and Alaska Native Children (joint with Section on Endocrinology), 10/03 (http://pediatrics.aappublications.org/cgi/reprint/112/4/e328)

Clinical Report: The Prevention of Unintentional Injury Among American Indian and Alaska Native Children: A Subject Review (joint with Committee on Injury, Violence, and Poison Prevention), 12/99, reaffirmed 5/03

COMMITTEE ON NUTRITION

Aluminum Toxicity in Infants and Children, 3/96, reaffirmed 4/00, 4/03

Calcium Requirements of Infants, Children, and Adolescents, 11/99

Cholesterol in Childhood, 1/98, reaffirmed 4/01

Hypoallergenic Infant Formulas, 8/00

Infant Methemoglobinemia: The Role of Dietary Nitrate, 9/70, reaffirmed 4/94, 6/97, 4/00

Iron Fortification of Infant Formulas, 7/99, reaffirmed 11/02

The Practical Significance of Lactose Intolerance in Children, 8/78, reaffirmed 12/93, 6/97, 4/00

Practical Significance of Lactose Intolerance in Children: Supplement, 10/90, reaffirmed 12/93, 6/97, 4/00

Prevention of Pediatric Overweight and Obesity, 8/03

Clinical Report: Prevention of Rickets and Vitamin D Deficiency: New Guidelines for Vitamin D Intake (joint with Section on Breastfeeding), 4/03

Reimbursement for Foods for Special Dietary Use, 5/03

Soy Protein-based Formulas: Recommendations for Use in Infant Feeding, 1/98, reaffirmed 4/01

The Use and Misuse of Fruit Juice in Pediatrics, 5/01

COMMITTEE ON PEDIATRIC AIDS

Adolescents and Human Immunodeficiency Virus Infection: The Role of the Pediatrician in Prevention and Intervention (joint with Committee on Adolescence), 1/01

Disclosure of Illness Status to Children and Adolescents With HIV Infection, 1/99, reaffirmed 2/02

Education of Children With Human Immunodeficiency Virus Infection, 6/00, reaffirmed 3/03

Evaluation and Medical Treatment of the HIV-Exposed Infant, 6/97

Human Immunodeficiency Virus/Acquired Immunodeficiency Syndrome Education in Schools, 5/98, reaffirmed 6/01

Human Immunodeficiency Virus Screening (joint with Committee on Fetus and Newborn and the American College of Obstetricians and Gynecologists), 7/99, reaffirmed 6/02

Technical Report: Human Milk, Breastfeeding, and Transmission of Human Immunodeficiency Virus Type 1 in the United States, 11/03

Identification and Care of HIV-Exposed and HIV-Infected Infants, Children, and Adolescents in Foster Care, 7/00, reaffirmed 3/03

Issues Related to Human Immunodeficiency Virus Transmission in Schools, Child Care, Medical Settings, the Home, and Community (joint with Committee on Infectious Diseases), 8/99, reaffirmed 2/02

Measles Immunization in HIV-Infected Children (joint with Committee on Infectious Diseases), 5/99

Perinatal Human Immunodeficiency Virus Testing, 2/95, reaffirmed 10/96, 11/99

Technical Report: Perinatal Human Immunodeficiency Virus Testing and Prevention of Transmission, 12/00, reaffirmed 3/03, *Pediatrics electronic pages* (http://pediatrics.aappublications.org/cgi/content/full/106/6/e88)

Planning for Children Whose Parents Are Dying of HIV/AIDS, 2/99, reaffirmed 2/02

Clinical Report: Postexposure Prophylaxis in Children and Adolescents for Nonoccupational Exposure to Human Immunodeficiency Virus, 6/03

Reducing the Risk of Human Immunodeficiency Virus Infection Associated With Illicit Drug Use, 12/94, reaffirmed 1/98

Surveillance of Pediatric HIV Infection, 2/98, reaffirmed 2/02

COMMITTEE ON PEDIATRIC EMERGENCY MEDICINE

Access to Pediatric Emergency Medical Care, 3/00

Care of Children in the Emergency Department: Guidelines for Preparedness (joint with American College of Emergency Physicians), 4/01

Consensus Report for Regionalization of Services for Critically Ill or Injured Children (joint with American College of Critical Care Medicine, Society of Critical Care Medicine), 1/00

Consent for Emergency Medical Services for Children and Adolescents, 3/03

Death of a Child in the Emergency Department: Joint Statement of the American Academy of Pediatrics and the American College of Emergency Physicians (joint with American College of Emergency Physicians), 10/02

Emergency Preparedness for Children With Special Health Care Needs, 10/99, reaffirmed 8/02, *Pediatrics electronic pages* (http://pediatrics.aappublications.org/cgi/content/full/104/4/e53)

Guidelines for Pediatric Emergency Care Facilities, 9/95, reaffirmed 10/98, 12/00

Pediatric Care Recommendations for Freestanding Urgent Care Facilities, 5/99

Pediatricians' Liability During Disasters (joint with Committee on Medical Liability), 12/00

The Pediatrician's Role in Advocating Life Support Courses for Parents, 7/94, reaffirmed 4/97

The Role of the Pediatrician in Rural EMSC, 5/98, reaffirmed 6/00

COMMITTEE ON PEDIATRIC RESEARCH

Human Embryo Research (joint with Committee on Bioethics), 9/01

Promoting Education, Mentorship, and Support for Pediatric Research, 6/01

Clinical Report: Race/Ethnicity, Gender, Socioeconomic Status—Research Exploring Their Effects on Child Health: A Subject Review, 6/00

COMMITTEE ON PEDIATRIC WORKFORCE

Culturally Effective Pediatric Care: Education and Training Issues, 1/99

Enhancing the Racial and Ethnic Diversity of the Pediatric Workforce, 1/00

Nondiscrimination in Pediatric Health Care, 11/01

Pediatric Primary Health Care, 11/93, reaffirmed 6/01

Pediatric Workforce Statement, 8/98

Prevention of Sexual Harassment in the Workplace and Educational Settings, 12/00

Scope of Practice Issues in the Delivery of Pediatric Health Care, 2/03

COMMITTEE ON PRACTICE AND AMBULATORY MEDICINE

Eye Examination in Infants, Children, and Young Adults by Pediatricians (joint with Section on Ophthalmology, American Association of Certified Orthoptists, American Association for Pediatric Ophthalmology and Strabismus, and American Academy of Ophthalmology), 4/03

Clinical Report: Hearing Assessment in Infants and Children: Recommendations Beyond Neonatal Screening (joint with Section on Otolaryngology and Bronchoesophagology), 2/03

Implementation of the Immunization Policy, 8/95

Increasing Immunization Coverage (joint with Committee on Community Health Services), 10/03

Infection Control in Physicians' Offices (joint with Committee on Infectious Diseases), 6/00

Pediatric Physician Profiling (joint with Committee on Medical Liability), 10/99

Policy on the Development of Immunization Tracking Systems, 6/96

Clinical Report: Prevention and Management of Positional Skull Deformities in Infants (joint with Section on Plastic Surgery and Section on Neurological Surgery), 7/03

Recommendations for Preventive Pediatric Health Care, 3/00

The Role of the Primary Care Pediatrician in the Management of High-risk Newborn Infants (joint with Committee on Fetus and Newborn), 10/96

Safeguards Needed in Transfer of Patient Data (joint with Steering Committee on Clinical Information Technology), 11/96, reaffirmed 2/01

The Use of Chaperones During the Physical Examination of the Pediatric Patient, 12/96, reaffirmed 11/99, 2/00

Use of Photoscreening for Children's Vision Screening (joint with Section on Ophthalmology), 3/02

COMMITTEE ON PSYCHOSOCIAL ASPECTS OF CHILD AND FAMILY HEALTH

The Assessment and Management of Acute Pain in Infants, Children, and Adolescents (joint with American Pain Society), 9/01

Clinical Report: The Child in Court: A Subject Review, 11/99, reaffirmed 11/02

Coparent or Second-Parent Adoption by Same-Sex Parents, 2/02

Technical Report: Coparent or Second-Parent Adoption by Same-Sex Parents, 2/02

Guidance for Effective Discipline, 4/98

Clinical Report: Helping Children and Families Deal With Divorce and Separation, 11/02

How Pediatricians Can Respond to the Psychosocial Implications of Disasters, 2/99

The New Morbidity Revisited: A Renewed Commitment to the Psychosocial Aspects of Pediatric Care, 11/01

The Pediatrician and Childhood Bereavement, 2/00

The Pediatrician's Role in Helping Children and Families Deal With Separation and Divorce, 7/94

The Prenatal Visit, 6/01

Psychosocial Risks of Chronic Health Conditions in Childhood and Adolescence (joint with Committee on Children With Disabilities), 12/93, reaffirmed 10/96

Sexuality Education for Children and Adolescents (joint with Committee on Adolescence), 8/01

COMMITTEE ON PUBLIC EDUCATION (FORMERLY COMMITTEE ON COMMUNICATIONS)

Children, Adolescents, and Advertising, 2/95

Children, Adolescents, and Television, 2/01

Impact of Music Lyrics and Music Videos on Children and Youth, 12/96

Media Education, 8/99

Media Violence, 11/01

Sexuality, Contraception, and the Media, 1/01

STEERING COMMITTEE ON QUALITY IMPROVEMENT AND MANAGEMENT

Clinical Practice Guideline: Diagnosis and Evaluation of the Child With Attention-Deficit/Hyperactivity Disorder, 5/00

Technical Report: Diagnosis of Attention-Deficit/Hyperactivity Disorder, 5/01

Clinical Practice Guideline: The Diagnosis, Treatment, and Evaluation of the Initial Urinary Tract Infection in Febrile Infants and Young Children, 4/99

Technical Report: Urinary Tract Infections in Febrile Infants and Young Children, 4/99, *Pediatrics electronic pages* (http://pediatrics.aappublications.org/cgi/reprint/103/4/e54)

Clinical Practice Guideline: Early Detection of Developmental Dysplasia of the Hip, 4/00

Technical Report: Developmental Dysplasia of the Hip, 4/00, *Pediatrics electronic pages* (http://pediatrics.aappublications.org/cgi/reprint/105/4/e57)

Clinical Practice Guideline: Long-term Treatment of the Child With Simple Febrile Seizures, 6/99

Technical Report: Treatment of the Child With Simple Febrile Seizures, 6/99, *Pediatrics electronic pages* (http://pediatrics.aappublications.org/cgi/reprint/103/6/e86)

Clinical Practice Guideline: The Management of Acute Gastroenteritis in Young Children, 3/96

Technical Report: Acute Gastroenteritis, 3/96

Clinical Practice Guideline: The Management of Minor Closed Head Injury in Children (joint with Commission on Clinical Policies and Research of the American Academy of Family Physicians), 12/99

Technical Report: Minor Head Injury in Children, 12/99, *Pediatrics electronic pages* (http://pediatrics.aappublications.org/cgi/reprint/104/6/e78)

Clinical Practice Guideline: Management of Sinusitis, 9/01

Technical Report: Evidence for the Diagnosis and Treatment of Acute Uncomplicated Sinusitis in Children: A Systematic Overview, 9/01, *Pediatrics electronic pages* (http://pediatrics.aappublications.org/cgi/reprint/108/3/e57)

Clinical Practice Guideline: The Neurodiagnostic Evaluation of the Child With a First Simple Febrile Seizure, 5/96

Technical Report: The Neurodiagnostic Evaluation of the Child With a First Simple Febrile Seizure, 5/96

Clinical Practice Guideline: Treatment of the School-Aged Child With Attention-Deficit/Hyperactivity Disorder, 10/01

COMMITTEE ON SCHOOL HEALTH

Corporal Punishment in Schools, 8/00, reaffirmed 6/03

Do Not Resuscitate Orders in Schools (joint with Committee on Bioethics), 4/00, reaffirmed 6/03

Guidelines for the Administration of Medication in School, 9/03

Guidelines for Emergency Medical Care in School, 2/01

Clinical Report: Head Lice (joint with Committee on Infectious Diseases), 9/02

Health Appraisal Guidelines for Day Camps and Resident Camps, 3/00

Home, Hospital, and Other Non–School-Based Instruction for Children and Adolescents Who Are Medically Unable to Attend School, 11/00, reaffirmed 6/03

The Inappropriate Use of School "Readiness" Tests (joint with Committee on Early Childhood, Adoption, and Dependent Care), 3/95, reaffirmed 4/98, 9/03

Organized Sports for Children and Preadolescents (joint with Committee on Sports Medicine and Fitness), 6/01

Out-of-School Suspension and Expulsion, 11/03

Physical Fitness and Activity in Schools (joint with Committee on Sports Medicine and Fitness), 5/00

The Role of the School Nurse in Providing School Health Services, 11/01

School Health Assessments, 4/00, reaffirmed 6/03

School Health Centers and Other Integrated School Health Services, 1/01

School Transportation Safety (joint with Committee on Injury, Violence, and Poison Prevention), 5/96, reaffirmed 4/99

COMMITTEE ON SPORTS MEDICINE AND FITNESS

Clinical Report: Adolescents and Anabolic Steroids: A Subject Review, 6/97, reaffirmed 5/00

Athletic Participation by Children and Adolescents Who Have Systemic Hypertension, 4/97, reaffirmed 5/00

Clinical Report: Atlantoaxial Instability in Down Syndrome: Subject Review, 7/95, reaffirmed 11/98, 5/00

Cardiac Dysrhythmias and Sports, 5/95, reaffirmed 11/98, 5/00

Climatic Heat Stress and the Exercising Child and Adolescent, 7/00

Horseback Riding and Head Injuries, 3/92, reaffirmed 5/98

Human Immunodeficiency Virus and Other Blood-borne Viral Pathogens in the Athletic Setting, 12/99

Infant Exercise Programs, 11/88, reaffirmed 11/94, 5/98

Clinical Report: Injuries in Youth Soccer: A Subject Review, 3/00

In-line Skating Injuries in Children and Adolescents (joint with Committee on Injury, Violence, and Poison Prevention), 4/98, reaffirmed 1/02

Intensive Training and Sports Specialization in Young Athletes, 7/00

Technical Report: Knee Brace Use in the Young Athlete, 8/01

Medical Concerns in the Female Athlete, 9/00

Medical Conditions Affecting Sports Participation, 5/01

Organized Sports for Children and Preadolescents (joint with Committee on School Health), 6/01

Participation in Boxing by Children, Adolescents, and Young Adults, 1/97, reaffirmed 5/00

Physical Fitness and Activity in Schools (joint with Committee on School Health), 5/00

Promotion of Healthy Weight-control Practices in Young Athletes, 5/96, reaffirmed 10/99

Protective Eyewear for Young Athletes (joint with American Academy of Ophthalmology), 8/96, reaffirmed 10/99

Risk of Injury From Baseball and Softball in Children, 4/01

Safety in Youth Ice Hockey: The Effects of Body Checking, 3/00

Strength Training by Children and Adolescents, 6/01

Swimming Programs for Infants and Toddlers (joint with Committee on Injury, Violence, and Poison Prevention), 4/00

Trampolines at Home, School, and Recreational Centers (joint with Committee on Injury, Violence, and Poison Prevention), 5/99, reaffirmed 12/02

Triathlon Participation by Children and Adolescents, 9/96, reaffirmed 10/99

COMMITTEE ON SUBSTANCE ABUSE

Alcohol Use and Abuse: A Pediatric Concern, 7/01

Fetal Alcohol Syndrome and Alcohol-Related Neurodevelopmental Disorders (joint with Committee on Children With Disabilities), 8/00

Improving Substance Abuse Prevention, Assessment, and Treatment Financing for Children and Adolescents (joint with Committee on Child Health Financing), 10/01

Indications for Management and Referral of Patients Involved in Substance Abuse, 7/00

Inhalant Abuse (joint with Committee on Native American Child Health), 3/96, reaffirmed 5/99

Marijuana: A Continuing Concern for Pediatricians, 10/99, reaffirmed 4/03

The Role of Schools in Combatting Substance Abuse, 5/95

Testing for Drugs of Abuse in Children and Adolescents, 8/96, reaffirmed 5/99

Tobacco, Alcohol, and Other Drugs: The Role of the Pediatrician in Prevention and Management of Substance Abuse, 1/98

Tobacco's Toll: Implications for the Pediatrician, 4/01

MEDICAL HOME INITIATIVES FOR CHILDREN WITH SPECIAL NEEDS PROJECT ADVISORY COMMITTEE

The Medical Home, 7/02

NATIONAL INITIATIVE FOR CHILDREN'S HEALTH CARE QUALITY PROJECT ADVISORY COMMITTEE

Principles of Patient Safety in Pediatrics, 6/01

PEDIATRIC PRACTICE ACTION GROUP

Privacy Protection of Health Information: Patient Rights and Pediatrician Responsibilities (joint with Steering Committee on Clinical Information Technology), 10/99

SECTION ON ANESTHESIOLOGY AND PAIN MEDICINE

Evaluation and Preparation of Pediatric Patients Undergoing Anesthesia, 9/96

Guidelines for the Pediatric Perioperative Anesthesia Environment, 2/99, reaffirmed 10/02

Prevention and Management of Pain and Stress in the Neonate (joint with Committee on Drugs, Committee on Fetus and Newborn, Section on Surgery, and Canadian Paediatric Society), 2/00, reaffirmed 4/03

SECTION ON BREASTFEEDING

Breastfeeding and the Use of Human Milk, 12/97

Clinical Report: Prevention of Rickets and Vitamin D Deficiency: New Guidelines for Vitamin D Intake (joint with Committee on Nutrition), 4/03

WIC Program, 11/01

SECTION ON CARDIOLOGY AND CARDIAC SURGERY

Echocardiography in Infants and Children, 6/97, reaffirmed 3/03

Guidelines for Pediatric Cardiovascular Centers, 3/02

SECTION ON CRITICAL CARE

Guidelines for Developing Admission and Discharge Policies for the Pediatric Intensive Care Unit (joint with Committee on Hospital Care and Society of Critical Care Medicine), 4/99

SECTION ON ENDOCRINOLOGY

Technical Report: Congenital Adrenal Hyperplasia (joint with Committee on Genetics), 12/00

Evaluation of the Newborn With Developmental Anomalies of the External Genitalia (joint with Committee on Genetics and Section on Urology), 7/00

Clinical Report: Health Supervision for Children With Turner Syndrome (joint with Committee on Genetics), 3/03

Newborn Screening for Congenital Hypothyroidism: Recommended Guidelines (joint with Committee on Genetics and American Thyroid Association Committee on Public Health), 6/93

Clinical Report: Prevention and Treatment of Type 2 Diabetes Mellitus in Children, With Special Emphasis on American Indian and Alaska Native Children (joint with Committee on Native American Child Health), 10/03 (http://pediatrics.aappublications.org/cgi/reprint/112/4/e328)

Screening for Retinopathy in the Pediatric Patient With Type 1 Diabetes Mellitus (joint with Section on Ophthalmology), 2/98

SECTION ON HEMATOLOGY/ONCOLOGY

Guidelines for the Pediatric Cancer Center and Role of Such Centers in Diagnosis and Treatment, 1/97

Health Supervision for Children With Sickle Cell Disease (joint with Committee on Genetics), 3/02

SECTION ON NEUROLOGICAL SURGERY

Clinical Report: Prevention and Management of Positional Skull Deformities in Infants (joint with Committee on Practice and Ambulatory Medicine and Section on Plastic Surgery), 7/03

SECTION ON OPHTHALMOLOGY

Eye Examination in Infants, Children, and Young Adults by Pediatricians (joint with Committee on Practice and Ambulatory Medicine, American Association of Certified Orthoptists, American Association for Pediatric Ophthalmology and Strabismus, and American Academy of Ophthalmology), 4/03

Guidelines for Ophthalmologic Examinations in Children With Juvenile Rheumatoid Arthritis (joint with Section on Rheumatology), 8/93, reaffirmed 8/99

Red Reflex Examination in Infants, 5/02

Screening Examination of Premature Infants for Retinopathy of Prematurity (joint with American Association for Pediatric Ophthalmology and Strabismus and American Academy of Ophthalmology), 9/01

Screening for Retinopathy in the Pediatric Patient With Type 1 Diabetes Mellitus (joint with Section on Endocrinology), 2/98

Use of Photoscreening for Children's Vision Screening (joint with Committee on Practice and Ambulatory Medicine), 3/02

SECTION ON OTOLARYNGOLOGY AND BRONCHOESOPHAGOLOGY

Follow-up Management of Children With Tympanostomy Tubes, 2/02

Clinical Report: Hearing Assessment in Infants and Children: Recommendations Beyond Neonatal

Screening (joint with Committee on Practice and Ambulatory Medicine), 2/03

SECTION ON PEDIATRIC DENTISTRY

Oral Health Risk Assessment Timing and Establishment of the Dental Home, 5/03

SECTION ON PEDIATRIC PULMONOLOGY

Clinical Practice Guideline: Diagnosis and Management of Childhood Obstructive Sleep Apnea Syndrome, 4/02

Technical Report: Diagnosis and Management of Childhood Obstructive Sleep Apnea Syndrome, 4/02, Pediatrics electronic pages (http://pediatrics.aappublications.org/cgi/reprint/109/4/e69)

SECTION ON PLASTIC SURGERY

Clinical Report: Prevention and Management of Positional Skull Deformities in Infants (joint with Committee on Practice and Ambulatory Medicine and Section on Neurological Surgery, 7/03

SECTION ON RADIOLOGY

Diagnostic Imaging of Child Abuse, 6/00

SECTION ON RESIDENTS

Parental Leave for Residents and Pediatric Training Programs (joint with Committee on Early Childhood, Adoption, and Dependent Care), 11/95

SECTION ON RHEUMATOLOGY

Guidelines for Ophthalmologic Examinations in Children With Juvenile Rheumatoid Arthritis (joint with Section on Ophthalmology), 8/93, reaffirmed 8/99

SECTION ON SCHOOL HEALTH

Residency Training and Continuing Medical Education in School Health, 9/93

SECTION ON SURGERY

Pediatric Organ Donation and Transplantation (joint with Committee on Hospital Care), 5/02

Prevention and Management of Pain and Stress in the Neonate (joint with Committee on Drugs, Committee on Fetus and Newborn, Section on Anesthesiology and Pain Medicine, and Canadian Paediatric Society), 2/00, reaffirmed 4/03

SECTION ON UROLOGY

Evaluation of the Newborn With Developmental Anomalies of the External Genitalia (joint with Committee on Genetics and Section on Endocrinology), 7/00

Timing of Elective Surgery on the Genitalia of Male Children With Particular Reference to the Risks, Benefits, and Psychological Effects of Surgery and Anesthesia, 4/96

SURGICAL ADVISORY PANEL

Guidelines for Referral to Pediatric Surgical Specialists, 7/02

TASK FORCE ON CIRCUMCISION

Circumcision Policy Statement, 3/99

TASK FORCE ON CORD BLOOD BANKING

Clinical Report: Cord Blood Banking for Potential Future Transplantation: Subject Review, 7/99

TASK FORCE ON GRADUATE MEDICAL EDUCATION REFORM

Graduate Medical Education and Pediatric Workforce Issues and Principles, 6/94

TASK FORCE ON INFANT SLEEP POSITION AND SUDDEN INFANT DEATH SYNDROME

Changing Concepts of Sudden Infant Death Syndrome: Implications for Infant Sleeping Environment and Sleep Position, 3/00

TASK FORCE ON MEDICAL MANAGEMENT GUIDELINES

Guiding Principles, Attributes, and Process to Review Medical Management Guidelines, 12/01

TASK FORCE ON VIOLENCE

The Role of the Pediatrician in Youth Violence Prevention in Clinical Practice and at the Community Level, 1/99, reaffirmed 5/02

JOINT STATEMENTS

Joint Statement of the American Academy of Pediatrics, the Advisory Committee on Immunization, and the American Academy of Family Physicians

Combination Vaccines for Childhood Immunization: Recommendations of the Advisory Committee on Immunization Practices (ACIP), the American Academy of Pediatrics (AAP), and the American Academy of Family Physicians (AAFP), 5/99, reaffirmed 3/02

Joint Statement of the American Academy of Pediatrics, the American Academy of Family Physicians, and the American College of Physicians-American Society of Internal Medicine

A Consensus Statement on Health Care Transitions for Young Adults With Special Health Care Needs, 12/02

Joint Statement of the American Academy of Pediatrics and the American Academy of Ophthalmology

Protective Eyewear for Young Athletes, 8/96, reaffirmed 10/99

Joint Statement of the American Academy of Pediatrics and the American Academy of Pediatric Dentistry

Oral and Dental Aspects of Child Abuse and Neglect, 8/99

Joint Statement of the American Academy of Pediatrics, the American Association of Certified Orthoptists, the American Association for Pediatric Ophthalmology and Strabismus, and the American Academy of Ophthalmology

Eye Examination in Infants, Children, and Young Adults by Pediatricians, 4/03

Joint Statements of the American Academy of Pediatrics, the American Association for Pediatric Ophthalmology and Strabismus, and the American Academy of Ophthalmology

Clinical Report: Learning Disabilities, Dyslexia, and Vision: A Subject Review, 11/98, reaffirmed 5/02

Screening Examination of Premature Infants for Retinopathy of Prematurity, 9/01

Joint Statement of the American Academy of Pediatrics and the American College of Critical Care Medicine, Society of Critical Care Medicine

Consensus Report for Regionalization of Services for Critically Ill or Injured Children, 1/00

Joint Statements of the American Academy of Pediatrics and the American College of Emergency Physicians

Care of Children in the Emergency Department: Guidelines for Preparedness, 4/01

Death of a Child in the Emergency Department: Joint Statement of the American Academy of Pediatrics and the American College of Emergency Physicians, 10/02

Joint Statements of the American Academy of Pediatrics and the American College of Obstetricians and Gynecologists

Human Immunodeficiency Virus Screening, 7/99, reaffirmed 6/02

Use and Abuse of the Apgar Score, 7/96, reaffirmed 10/97, 10/00

Joint Statement of the American Academy of Pediatrics and the American Pain Society

The Assessment and Management of Acute Pain in Infants, Children, and Adolescents, 9/01

Joint Statement of the American Academy of Pediatrics and the American Thyroid Association Committee on Public Health

Newborn Screening for Congenital Hypothyroidism: Recommended Guidelines, 6/93, reaffirmed 10/96

Joint Statements of the American Academy of Pediatrics and the Canadian Paediatric Society

Postnatal Corticosteroids to Treat or Prevent Chronic Lung Disease in Preterm Infants, 2/02

Prevention and Management of Pain and Stress in the Neonate, 2/00, reaffirmed 4/03

Joint Statement of the American Academy of Pediatrics and the Institute for Family-Centered Care

Family-Centered Care and the Pediatrician's Role, 9/03

Joint Statement of the American Academy of Pediatrics and Others

Insurance Coverage of Mental Health and Substance Abuse Services for Children and Adolescents: A Consensus Statement, 10/00

Joint Statement of the American Academy of Pediatrics and the Society of Critical Care Medicine

Guidelines for Developing Admission and Discharge Policies for the Pediatric Intensive Care Unit, 4/99

Guidelines and Levels of Care for Pediatric Intensive Care Units, 7/93, reaffirmed 11/96

ENDORSED CLINICAL PRACTICE GUIDELINES AND POLICY STATEMENTS
(The AAP endorses and accepts as its policy the following clinical practice guidelines and policy statements that have been published by other organizations.)

American Academy of Child and Adolescent Psychiatry and the Child Welfare League of America

Clinical Practice Guideline: Foster Care Mental Health Values

Clinical Practice Guideline: Mental Health and Substance Use Screening and Assessment of Children in Foster Care

American Academy of Neurology

Clinical Practice Guideline: Evaluating a First Nonfebrile Seizure in Children, 8/00

Clinical Practice Guideline: Neuroimaging of the Neonate, 6/02

Clinical Practice Guideline: Treatment of the Child with a First Unprovoked Seizure, 1/03

American College of Rheumatology

Clinical Practice Guideline: Guidelines for Referral of Children and Adolescents to Pediatric Rheumatologists, 6/02

American Diabetes Association

Type 2 Diabetes in Children and Adolescents, 3/00

American Medical Association

Gifts to Physicians From Industry, 8/01

American Orthopaedic Society for Sports Medicine

Clinical Practice Guideline: Concussion in Sports, 1999

American Thoracic Society and Centers for Disease Control and Prevention

(The AAP endorses and accepts as its policy the sections of this statement as they relate to infants and children.)

Targeted Tuberculin Testing and Treatment of Latent Tuberculosis Infection, 4/00

American Urological Association

Clinical Practice Guideline: Report on the Management of Primary Vesicoureteral Reflux in Children, 5/97

Centers for Disease Control and Prevention

Clinical Practice Guideline: Prevention of Perinatal Group B Streptococcal Disease, 8/02

Clinical Practice Guideline: Recommendations for Using Fluoride to Prevent and Control Dental Caries in the United States, 8/01

Centers for Disease Control and Prevention, Infectious Diseases Society of America, and the American Society of Blood and Marrow Transplantation

Clinical Practice Guideline: Guidelines for Preventing Opportunistic Infections Among Hematopoietic Stem Cell Transplant Recipients, 10/00

Family Violence Prevention Fund

Clinical Practice Guideline: Identifying and Responding to Domestic Violence: Consensus Recommendations for Child and Adolescent Health (endorsement will apply for 5 years unless sooner retired or revised by the FVPF), 9/02

Infectious Diseases Society of America

Clinical Practice Guideline: Practice Guidelines for the Treatment of Lyme Disease, 9/00

Inter-Association Task Force for Appropriate Care of the Spine-Injured Athlete

Clinical Practice Guideline: Prehospital Care of the Spine-Injured Athlete

Joint Committee on Infant Hearing

Year 2000 Position Statement: Principles and Guidelines for Early Hearing Detection and Intervention Programs, 10/00

National Asthma Education and Prevention Program

Clinical Practice Guideline: Guidelines for the Diagnosis and Management of Asthma, 2/98

National Athletic Trainers' Association

Clinical Practice Guideline: Lightning Safety for Athletics and Recreation, 12/00

National Diabetes Education Program

Clinical Practice Guideline: Helping the Student with Diabetes Succeed: A Guide for School Personnel, 6/03

North American Society for Pediatric Gastroenterology, Hepatology and Nutrition

Clinical Practice Guideline: Constipation in Infants and Children: Evaluation and Treatment, 3/00

Clinical Practice Guideline: Guidelines for Evaluation and Treatment of Gastroesophageal Reflux in Infants and Children

Clinical Practice Guideline: Helicobacter pylori Infection in Children: Recommendations for Diagnosis and Treatment, 11/00

Quality Standards Subcommittee of the American Academy of Neurology and the Child Neurology Society

Clinical Practice Guideline: Screening and Diagnosis of Autism, 8/00

Society for Academic Emergency Medicine

Pediatric Care in the Emergency Department, 11/03

Society of Critical Care Medicine, Infectious Disease Society of America, Society for Healthcare Epidemiology of America, Surgical Infection Society, American College of Chest Physicians, American Thoracic Society, American Society of Critical Care Anesthesiologists, Association for Professionals in Infection Control and Epidemiology, Infusion Nurses Society, Oncology Nursing Society, Society of Cardiovascular and Interventional Radiology, American Academy of Pediatrics, and the Healthcare Infection Control Practices Advisory Committee of the Centers for Disease Control and Prevention

Clinical Practice Guideline: Guidelines for the Prevention of Intravascular Catheter-Related Infections

US Department of Health and Human Services

Clinical Practice Guideline: Treating Tobacco Use and Dependence, 6/00

Subject Index

A

Abdominal pain
  recurrent, in asymptomatic children, 492
  unrelated to peptic ulcers, 491
Abdominal radiograph in diagnosing constipation, 117
Abortion, adolescent's right to confidential care when considering, 919
Abuse. *See* Assault; Child abuse; Sexual abuse; Substance abuse
Abused women, role of pediatrician in recognizing and intervening on behalf of, 263–264
Academic impairments in autism, 100
Acanthosis nigricans, 157
Access to pediatric emergency medical care, 919
Accidents. *See* Injuries
Acetabular dysplasias, 160, 313–314
Acetabulum, maldevelopments of, 308
Acetaminophen toxicity in children, 919
Achievement tests, effects of stimulant medication on, 85
Achondroplasia, health supervision for children with, 934
Acid suppressants for gastroesophageal reflux disease, 426, 433–435
Acquired immunodeficiency syndrome (AIDS). *See* Human immunodeficiency virus (HIV)
Active management of asthma, 11
Acute bacterial otitis media, 769
Acute bacterial sinusitis, 769, 770, 771, 773
Acute cervical fracture-dislocations, 858–859
Acute gastroenteritis, 399–419
  algorithms for, 411–412
  antidiarrheal compounds for, 406–408
  dehydration in, 404, 405–406
  electrolyte measurement in, 404
  intravenous therapy for, 405
  medications for, 406–407
  oral rehydration therapy in, 401–406
  rehydration and refeeding for, 402–404, 415
  research issues in, 408
  vomiting in, 404–405
Acute muscular spasm, 858
Acute otitis media, 770
Acute rheumatic fever, 713
Acute sinusitis, 783
Acyclovir, 516, 517–518
Adenoidectomy, 796, 811
Adenotonsillar hypertrophy, 796
Adenotonsillectomy, 799
Adenovirus, recommendations regarding, 523
Adjuvant therapies for sinusitis, 774–776
Admission policies for pediatric intensive care unit, 932
Adolescents
  advertising and, 923
  anabolic steroids and, 919
  assessment and management of acute pain in, 921
  asthma in, 22
  calcium requirements of, 922
  care of, as parents, 922
  chronic health conditions in, 932
  climatic heat stress and exercising in, 924
  condom use by, 925
  confidentiality in health care for, 925
  consent for medical services for, 926
  contraception and, 925, 926
  driving by, 962
  genetic disorders in, 932
  health care for, in juvenile correctional care system, 934
  health effects of intimate partner violence on, 239

homosexuality and, 935
human immunodeficiency virus infection in, 919
  in foster care, 937
    postexposure prophylaxis in, for nonoccupational exposure, 948
  immunization of, 937
  indicators of abuse in, 279
  instruction for, who are medically unable to attend schools, 935
  managed care for, 934
  personal watercraft use by, 947
  pregnancy of, 919
    counseling for, 927
    resources on, 288
  prevention of agricultural injuries among, 949
  psychosocial risks of chronic health conditions in, 953
  referral for intimate partner violence, 258
  referral to pediatric rheumatologists, 713–714
  right to confidential care when considering abortion, 919
  role of pediatricians in transitioning, with developmental disabilities and chronic illness, 957
  scope of health care benefits for, 958
  screening for intimate partner violence when patient is, 251–260
  as sexual assault victims, 922
  sexual education for, 960
  strength training by, 961
  substance abuse in
    prevention, assessment, and treatment financing in, 938
    testing for drugs in, 962
  suicide in, 961
  television and, 923
  triathlon participation by, 964
  type 2 diabetes in, 964
  as victims of violence, 256–257
Adoption
  coparent or second-parent, 926
  families and, 930
  initial medical evaluation of child in, 939
Adsorbents for acute gastroenteritis, 407
Adults. *See also* Young adults
  health effects of intimate partner violence on, 239
  indicators of abuse in, 279
Advanced practice in neonatal nursing, 920
Adverse Childhood Experiences (ACE) Study, 238–239
Advertising. *See also* Media
  children, adolescents, and, 923
Aerosolized antibiotics, precautions regarding use of, 949
Age, for routine administration of measles-mumps-rubella vaccine, 920
Age limits of pediatrics, 920
Ages and Stages Questionnaire in diagnosing autism, 98
Agricultural injuries, prevention of, among children and adolescents, 949
Agriculture, US Department of, 219
Aircraft, restraint use on, 955
Airflow obstruction, 15
Air pollution, ambient, 920
Airway inflammation in asthma, 11
Alaska Family Violence Prevention Project, 287
Alaska Native children, prevention of unintentional injury among, 952
Alcohol use, 920. *See also* Substance abuse
  fetal alcohol syndrome and, 930
  neurodevelopmental disorders related to, 930